Orthopaedic Surgery in Infancy and Childhood

Fifth Edition

Orthopaedic Surgery in Infancy and Childhood

Fifth Edition

Albert B. Ferguson, Jr., M.D.

Silver Professor of Orthopaedic Surgery and Chairman, Department of Orthopaedic Surgery, University of Pittsburgh

Chief of Orthopaedic Service, University of Pittsburgh Medical Center

Senior Staff—Children's Hospital, Presbyterian-University Hospital, Pittsburgh

Active Staff—Allegheny General Hospital, Pittsburgh

Chief Consultant—Veteran's Hospital (Oakland), Pittsburgh

Consultant—Mercy Hospital, St. Francis Hospital, St. Margaret's Hospital, Montefiore Hospital, Pittsburgh

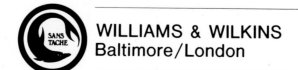

WILLIAMS & WILKINS
Baltimore/London

First Edition, 1957
Second Edition, 1963
Third Edition, 1968
Fourth Edition, 1975

Library of Congress Cataloging in Publication Data

Ferguson, Albert Barnett, 1919–
  Orthopaedic surgery in infancy and childhood.

  Includes bibliographical references and index.
  1. Pediatric orthopedia. I. Title.
[DNLM: 1. Orthopedics—In infancy and childhood.
WS270 F352o]
RD732.3.C48F47 1981   617′.3′0088054   80-23873
ISBN 0-683-03167-8

Composed and printed at the
Waverly Press, Inc.
Mt. Royal and Guilford Aves.
Baltimore, MD 21202, U.S.A.

PRECAUTION

I never dared to be radical when young

For fear it would make me conservative when old.

Robert Frost

Preface to the fifth edition

This volume has been in existence over twenty years. The emphasis on early surgery in children's deformities that started with the first volume has remained. As knowledge of the natural history of these deformities has been gained it is evident that they increase their morbidity with growth and, in many instances, make correction more difficult, amply justifying early surgery when indicated. Surgical skills and anesthesia safety have improved over the years as well. It would be rare now to see the extensive deformities in children that existed over twenty years ago.

The chapter on the foot has been completely rewritten by Pierce Scranton. Colin Moseley has brought his insight on unequal growth in children to the printed page. Carl Stanitski redid the Cerebral Palsy section to bring it up to date. David Bahnson and Carl Fackler have reviewed the philosophy in myelomeningocele and the accompanying problems brought on by growth. Additional information on Legg-Perthes disease has been added to the chapter on the hip. Illustrations have been added throughout. Many of the original operations that were first delineated in this volume have been further amplified.

More can be done for children with physical handicaps, with greater certainty and with their total welfare in mind. The volume owes a debt to the many orthopaedic surgeons who make the care of children their specialty and whose contributions we have tried to record.

The double-column format enables a more intensive use of each page, avoiding the necessity of having two volumes.

Although there are temptations to include childrens' fractures we have not done so in view of the excellent texts in this field. The temptation has occasionally been difficult to resist and post-traumatic situations have been included.

Albert B. Ferguson, Jr., M.D.

Preface to the fourth edition

There have been a number of objectives for this fourth edition. The illustrations, particularly those relating to surgical technique, have been increased in number, improved in quality, and made more informative. Information relating to any particular syndrome has been enlarged, with new information developed in greater depth and heavily referenced. Completeness has been a goal and all areas and types of disease and the relevant therapy increased in its coverage.

In addition, specific new material has been added, especially important here are "Developmental Anatomy" by John Ogden, specific scoliosis subjects by Charles Stone and William T. Green, Jr., the "Lower Extremity in Myelodysplasia" by Andrew Wissinger, "Hemophilia" by Ronald Hillegass, and "Amputations" by Mary Williams Clark.

Areas of recent interest and development such as congenital dislocation of the hip have been largely rewritten. New operations developed and followed by the author such as the treatment of plantar-flexed talus, dislocated hips and many others are included.

The fundamental approach to children's orthopaedics in a growing, maturing child is emphasized throughout.

The drawings, which are beautifully executed, are the work of Ron Filer, who very clearly grasps the principle being portrayed. Ann Eakins has taken great care with the photography, assuring that each illustration would clearly tell the message involved.

Mary Cosgrove has organized, typed and retyped and researched for material and is an indispensable part of the book's development.

With the help of many people this book is maturing into a valuable reference and text and is aimed to satisfy both the beginner and the highly trained orthopaedic surgeon. It is hoped that those who read it find it valuable.

A. B. F. Jr.

Preface to the first edition

This volume is the outgrowth of that period in life when the subject matter of orthopaedic surgery was laboriously amassed by running from text to text and article to article. Excellent though so many volumes are, none of them appeared to have gathered under one cover details regarding the many odd syndromes encountered in the practice of orthopaedic surgery dealing with infants and children. Pediatricians and residents have often indicated by their questions that they were undergoing a similar experience.

No syndrome, photograph or roentgenogram is presented which was not personally seen by the author. No feature of disease is reiterated which has not been a feature in our own experience.

Obviously no text arises without roots in the past, and the excellent volumes of Colonna, Howorth, Mercer, Platt, Wiles, Fairbank, Shands, Campbell, Luck, Smillie and DePalma have also served as references. This text does not include a consideration of fractures, for the subject is adequately covered in Walter Blount's recent book, *Fractures in Children.*

If clarity in visualizing these syndromes has been achieved, it is a reflection of the teaching of Joseph Barr, William T. Green and Albert B. Ferguson, Sr. They are not responsible for what others may deem as errors, however.

Certain areas in the book have been done by others. Frank Stelling has contributed his knowledge of reconstruction of the hand to the section on the upper extremity. Scoliosis is the work of William Donaldson of Pittsburgh. John Donaldson of Pittsburgh has added the chapter on the neck. Robert Klein encompasses rickets and scurvy from the metabolic point of view. Albert Ferguson, Sr., writes of defective formation of bone from cartilage. All these authors are deserving of my humble thanks in enabling a sound production of a book on orthopaedic surgery in the infant and childhood years.

The Children's Hospital of Pittsburgh is blessed with men of selfless spirit whose help has been invaluable. This is particularly true of Bertram Girdany, George Fetterman and Thomas Brower; although no one failed to respond when called upon. The pleasant and productive atmosphere of this hospital is a reflection of its guiding spirit and medical director, Edmund McCluskey.

The manuscript has been typed, retyped and retyped again by my secretary already overloaded with budgets, bills, and records. This type of dedication is typical of Mary Cosgrove.

My children and my wife, Louise, have taken night work, which deprived them of companionship, with good spirit. My wife's patient understanding is not found often in this world—without it such an arduous task could not be completed.

The drawings are the result of the talents of Margaret Croup except for those accompanying the section on the upper extremity. The photographs and roentgenogram reproductions were done by Albert Levine and James Stark. The patient cooperation exhibited by these worthy individuals has been a source of pleasure and has eased the task immeasurably.

The publishers and particularly Dick Hoover have been patient and have exhibited the skills of their profession with consummate ease.

Great care and effort have been used to duly credit thoughts, drawings and photographs whose origin might in any way be elsewhere. Should any omission have arisen, it is entirely inadvertent and not by conscious design.

The regional arrangement of the text will, we hope, make reference easy and invite a return visit.

A. B. F., Jr.

Contributors

DAVID H. BAHNSON, M.D.

Clinical Instructor in Orthopaedic Surgery, University of Pittsburgh School of Medicine. Staff of Children's Hospital and Presbyterian-University Hospital, University of Pittsburgh Medical Center. Co-Director, Myelomeningocele Orthopaedic Clinic.

MARY WILLIAMS CLARK, B.A., M.D.

Associate Clinical Professor of Orthopaedic Surgery, Louisiana State University. Assistant Clinical Professor of Orthopaedic Surgery, Tulane University School of Medicine. Director of Rehabilitation, Children's Hospital, New Orleans.

WILLIAM FIELDING DONALDSON, JR., B.A., M.D., F.A.C.S.

Clinical Professor of Orthopaedic Surgery, University of Pittsburgh. Senior Staff—Children's Hospital, Presbyterian-University Hospital, St. Francis Hospital, Shadyside Hospital, Pittsburgh. Attending Staff, Veteran's Hospital (Oakland), Pittsburgh. Consultant, St. Margaret's Hospital, Home for Crippled Children, Pittsburgh.

CARL D. FACKLER, M.D.

Associate Peachtree Orthopaedic Clinic, Atlanta, Georgia. Director, Myelodysplasia Clinic, Scottish Rite Hospital, Atlanta, Georgia.

WILLIAM THOMAS GREEN, JR., B.A., M.D., F.A.C.S.

Associate Professor, Orthopaedic Surgery, University of Pittsburgh. Senior Staff, Children's Hospital. Associate Staff, Presbyterian-University Hospital, Pittsburgh. Consultant, Veteran's Hospital (Oakland), John J. Kane Hospital, Pittsburgh.

RONALD CARL HILLEGASS, B.A., M.D.

Attending Staff, Roger Williams Hospital, Rhode Island Hospital, Providence, Rhode Island.

JAMES HENRY McMASTER, B.A., M.D.

Clinical Associate Professor of Orthopaedic Surgery, University of Pittsburgh. Senior Staff, Allegheny General Hospital, Pittsburgh. Associate Staff, Children's Hospital, Presbyterian-University Hospital, Pittsburgh. Consultant, Veteran's Hospital (Oakland).

COLIN F. MOSELEY, M.D., C.M., F.R.C.S.(C)

Orthopaedic Surgeon, Hospital for Sick Children, Toronto, Ontario, Canada. Lecturer, Faculty of Medicine, University of Toronto.

JOHN A. OGDEN, B.A., M.D.

Professor of Orthopaedic Surgery, Yale University Medical School. Director Orthopaedic Section, Human Growth and Development Unit, Yale University. Attending Staff, Yale-New Haven Hospital, Newington Children's Hospital, Connecticut. Consultant, Veteran's Hospital, West Haven, Connecticut.

PIERCE EDWARD SCRANTON, JR., B.A., M.D.

Clinical Instructor of Orthopaedic Surgery, University of Washington. Associate Staff, the Swedish Hospital, Providence Medical Center and Children's Orthopaedic Hospital and Medical Center, Seattle, Washington.

CARL LEON STANITSKI, B.S., M.D.

Clinical Assistant Professor of Orthopaedic Surgery, University of Pittsburgh. Associate Staff, Presbyterian-University Hospital, Children's Hospital and St. Margaret's Hospital, Pittsburgh. Orthopaedic Consultant, Cerebral Palsy Clinic, Children's Hospital.

FRANK H. STELLING, III, M.D., F.A.C.S.

Chief Surgeon, Shriners Hospital for Crippled Children, Greenville Unit, Greenville, South Carolina. Associate Clinical Professor of Orthopaedic Surgery, Medical University of South Carolina, Assistant Clinical Professor of Orthopaedic Surgery, Duke University School of Medicine. Chairman, Education, Orthopaedic Department, Greenville Hospital System.

CHARLES S. STONE, B.S., M.D

Clinical Assistant Professor of Orthopaedic Surgery, University of Pittsburgh. Associate Staff, Children's Hospital, Presbyterian-University Hospital, St. Francis Hospital. St. Margaret's Hospital, West Penn Hospital, Shadyside Hospital, Pittsburgh.

HAROLD EDWARD SWENSEN, B.S., M.D.

Clinical Associate Professor of Orthopaedic Surgery, University of Pittsburgh. Senior Staff, Children's Hospital, Presbyterian-University Hospital, West Penn Hospital, Pittsburgh. Consultant, Magee-Women's Hospital, Western Psychiatric Hospital, Pittsburgh.

Table of contents

Preface to the fifth edition vii
Preface to the fourth edition ix
Preface to the first edition xi
Contributors xiii

CHAPTER 1
Orthopaedic Treatment of Child-
hood Disability 1

Growth Affecting Skeleton 1
Skeletal Growth 1
Factors Affecting Growth 2
Prenatal 2
Postnatal 2
Relation of Growth to Orthopaedic
Conditions 3
Growth of Epiphysis 4
Development of Epiphysis and
Growth Plate—John Ogden, M.D. 4
Distinguishing Growth Lines from
Fracture Lines 17
X-ray Characteristics 17
Fracture Lines That Cannot Be
Seen 18
Multiple Trauma 19
Clinical Picture 19
Roentgen Picture 19
Treatment 20
Motor Development 21
Secondary Effects of Immobiliza-
tion 22
Joint Stability Maintained by Atmos-
pheric Pressure 22
Fluid Behavior 23
Childhood Amputees 27
Juvenile Amputations and Congenital
Limb Deficiencies—Mary Williams
Clark, M.D. 27
Acquired Amputations 28
Surgical Principles 28
Surgical Techniques 29
Comprehensive Care Principles .. 29
Rigid Dressing 29
Exercise Program and Stump Care 29
Skin Care 30
Psychologic Support 30
Prosthetic Fitting 31
Timing 31
Prosthetic Prescription 31
Training 38
Lower Extremity 38
Upper Extremity 39
Long Term Follow-Up 40
Congenital Limb Deficiencies 41
Classification 41
Treatment Principles 41
Surgical "Conversion" 42
Specific Congenital Anomalies ... 42

Proximal Femoral Focal Deficiency 42
Fibular Meromelia 43
Tibial Meromelia 43
Elective Revision 46
Developmental Anatomy—John Og-
den, M.D. 47
Upper Extremity 47
Shoulder 47
Elbow 47
Wrist 47
Hand 47
Vertebral Column 50
Lower Extremity 50
Hip 51
Congenital Hip Dislocation 58
Knee 61
Ankle 62
Foot 62
Clubfoot 63
How to Read an Orthopaedic X-ray
Film, Self-Teaching 66
Introduction 66
Program 66

CHAPTER 2
Unequal Growth in Children—Colin
F. Moseley, M.D. 81

The Source of Longitudinal Growth . 81
The Control of Longitudinal Growth . 82
Genetic Control 82
Vascular Control 82
Mechanical Control 82
Hormonal Control 82
Pattern of Normal Growth 82
Causes of Discrepancy 83
Effects of Leg Length Discrepancy . 84
Clinical Assessment 86
Radiologic Assessment 88
Methods of Prediction 90
"Rule-of-Thumb" Method 90
Growth Remaining Method 91
Straight Line Graph Method 92
Clinical Considerations 93
Anticipated Discrepancy 94
Location of Discrepancy 95
Cause 95
Paralysis 97
Age 98
Sex 98
Unpredictability 98
Angular Deformity 98
Scoliosis 98
Anticipated Height 98
Patient Preparation 98
Associated Surgery 98
Nonsurgical Treatment 98
Surgical Treatment 98

Shortening Procedures 99
Epiphyseodesis 99
Epiphyseal Plate Stapling 99
Surgical Shortening 100
Tibial Shortening 100
Femoral Shortening 100
Lengthening Procedures 101
Growth Stimulation 101
Surgical Lengthening 101
Femoral Lengthening 102
Tibial Lengthening 104
Complications of Lengthening ... 106
Innominate Osteotomy 108
Partial Closure of the Growth Plate . 108

CHAPTER 3
Epiphyseal, Metaphyseal, and Diaphyseal Affections 115

Epiphyseal Affections 115
Dysplasia Epiphysialis Hemimelica 115
Clinical Picture 115
Pathology 116
Treatment 117
Epiphyseal Chondroblastoma ... 117
Clinical Picture 117
Pathology 118
Roentgen Picture 118
Treatment 118
Chondrodystrophia Calcificans
Congenita (Stippled Epiphyses,
Fairbank's Disease) 118
Roentgen Features 118
Prognosis 119
Spondyloepiphyseal Dysplasia
(Pseudoachondroplasia) 119
Clinical Picture 119
Roentgen Picture 119
Treatment 120
Ellis-van Creveld Syndrome 122
Treatment 123
Pleonosteosis 123
Clinical Picture 123
Treatment 123
Diastrophic Dwarfism 123
Clinical Picture 124
Roentgen Features 124
Treatment 124
Metaphyseal Affections 124
Morquio's Syndrome 124
Etiology 126
Clinical Picture 126
Roentgen Findings 126
Differential Diagnosis 127
Treatment 127
Familial Metaphyseal Dysplasia ... 128
Solitary Bone Cyst 129
Etiology 130
Clinical Picture 130
Roentgen Findings 131
Pathology 131

Treatment 131
Aneurysmal Bone Cyst 134
Etiology 134
Clinical Picture 134
Roentgen Picture 134
Pathology 135
Treatment 135
Tibia Vara 136
Clinical Picture 136
Roentgen Findings 137
Prognosis 137
Treatment 137
Surgical Treatment 138
Osteopoikilosis (Osteopathia Con-
densus Disseminata) 139
Diaphyseal Affections 140
Marfan's Syndrome (Arachnodac-
tyly) 140
Etiology 141
Clinical Picture 144
Roentgen Picture 145
Treatment 145
Progressive Diaphyseal Dysplasia 146
Etiology 147
Clinical Picture 147
Roentgen Features 147
Pathology 148
Treatment 148
Infantile Cortical Hyperostosis ... 148
Clinical Picture 149
Roentgen Picture 149
Pathology 151
Treatment 151
Osteoid Osteoma 151
Clinical Picture 152
Roentgen Examination 153
Pathology 153
Etiology 153
Treatment 154
Pseudarthroses in Childhood 154
Treatment 155

CHAPTER 4
Foot Disorders—Pierce E. Scranton,
Jr., M.D. 161

Principles in the Examination of the
Foot 161
Physiologic Toe-in Gait 162
Clinical Picture 163
Roentgen Appearance 163
Treatment 163
Operative Treatment 164
Pes Valgus 165
Flat Feet in Childhood 167
Pediatric Flexible Pes Valgus (Plan-
tar-flexed Talus) 167
Roentgen Appearance 168
Physical Examination 170
Treatment 171
Disabling Flat Feet 174

Kidner Operation 177
Modified Giannestras Procedure . 177
Hoke Operation 177
Giannestras Procedure 180
Congenital Vertical Talus 180
Clinical Picture 181
Roentgen Appearance 181
Treatment 182
Coleman Approach 182
Naviculectomy 184
Tarsal Coalitions (Peroneal Spastic
Flat Foot) 185
Treatment 187
Neurogenic Flat Feet 191
Congenital Clubfeet (Talipes Equi-
novarus) 192
Etiology 192
Clinical Picture 195
Treatment 196
Serial Casting Technique 196
Denis-Browne Splints 197
Resistant Clubfeet 197
Surgical Anatomy of Clubfoot ... 201
Posteromedial Release 201
Follow-up Therapy 206
Severe or Recurrent Clubfeet 206
Astragalectomy 208
Recurring Clubfeet below Age 5 . 208
Anterior Tibial Transplant 208
Posterior Tibial Transplant 208
Rocker-bottom Foot 209
Uncorrected Clubfeet after Age 5 . 210
Triple Arthrodesis 211
Overcorrected Clubfoot 212
Metatarsus Varus 213
Clinical Picture 214
Treatment 214
Mobile Foot 214
Fixed Foot 218
Operative Treatment 218
Combination of Positional Metatarsus
Varus of One Foot and Calcaneal Val-
gus of the Other 221
Metatarsus Atavicus (Morton's Foot) 222
Metatarsus Primus Varus (Bunions) . 222
Clinical Appearance 222
Roentgen Appearance 223
Treatment 223
Silver Procedure 224
Akins Procedure 225
Mitchell or Wilson Procedure 225
Proximal Osteotomy or Lapidus
Procedure 227
Cavus Feet 229
Etiology 229
Clinical Appearance 229
Diagnosis 231
Treatment 232
Vascular Disorders (Osteochon-
droses) 234

Köhler's Disease 234
Etiology 234
Clinical Picture 234
Roentgen Findings 235
Treatment 235
Freiberg's Disease 235
Clinical Picture 236
Roentgen Findings 236
Treatment 236
Painful Heels in Children 236
Operative Treatment 237
Stress Fractures 238
Achilles Tendonitis 239
Congenital Anomalies 239
Overlapping Fifth Toes 241
Supernumerary Digits 242
Multiple Tarsal Anomalies 242

CHAPTER 5
The Knee 249

Positional Deformities 249
Apparent Bowlegs 249
Uterine Packing Syndrome 249
Clinical Findings 249
Roentgen Appearance 249
Treatment 250
Developmental Genu Valgum 250
Treatment 251
Osteochondritis Dissecans 252
Pathology 252
Etiology 253
Clinical Picture 253
Roentgen Findings 254
Treatment 254
Discoid Meniscus 256
Normal Development 256
Etiology 256
Clinical Picture 257
Treatment 257
Osgood-Schlatter Disease 258
Etiology 258
Clinical Picture 258
Roentgen Findings 259
Treatment 259
Popliteal Cysts 260
Clinical Picture 260
Roentgen Findings 260
Treatment 261
Monarticular Arthritis 261
Etiology 262
Clinical Picture 262
Laboratory Findings 263
Treatment 263
Foreign Body Knee 263
Septic Arthritis of Knee 265
Etiology 265
Clinical Picture 265
Joint Fluid Findings 265
Treatment 265

Tuberculosis of Knee 266
  Etiology 266
  Pathology 266
  Clinical Picture 267
  Roentgen Findings 267
  Treatment 267
Congenital Dislocation of the Knee   269
  Clinical Picture 269
  Treatment 270
Genu Valgum 271
  Treatment 271
  Surgical Correction 272
Recurrent Dislocation of Patella   272
  Etiology 273
  Mechanism 274
  Clinical Picture 274
  Roentgen Findings 275
  Treatment 275
  Elevation of the Tibial Tubercle   278
  Larson-Johansson Disease (Osteo-
  chondritis of Patella) 280
  Roentgen Findings 281
  Treatment 281
Osteochondroma of Distal Femoral
Epiphysis 281
  Treatment 281

CHAPTER 6
The Hip 285

Congenital Hip Disease 285
  Etiology 289
  Mechanics of Iliopsoas 291
  Acetabular Index 293
  C-E Angle 298
  Anteversion 298
  Relation of Hip to Spine 299
Dysplastic Hip 301
  Roentgen Signs 301
  Treatment 301
Subluxated Hip 302
  Treatment 303
Pathology and Recognition of Con-
genital Dislocation of Hip 304
  Clinical Picture 306
  Signs Due to Weakness of Hip
  Abductors 308
  Differential Diagnosis 309
Treatment of Congenital Dislocation
of Hip under Age 2 311
  Median Adductor Approach 312
  Evaluation of Reduction 316
  Closed Reduction 321
Treatment of Dislocated Hip at Age
2–4 322
  Iliofemoral Incision 323
  Anteversion Osteotomy 324
  Treatment of Primary Anterior Con-
  genital Dislocation 324
  Salter's Osteotomy 325

Treatment of Dislocated Hip after Age
4 328
  Osteotomy of Acetabulum 328
  Acetabuloplasty 330
  Operation 330
  Other Procedures 332
  Criteria of Reduction 334
Neurogenic Dislocation of Hip 335
  Treatment 338
Developmental Coxa Vara 340
  Roentgen Findings 342
  Clinical Picture 343
  Course 343
  Pathology 343
  Treatment 344
  Early Cases 344
  Late Cases 344
Slipped Capital Femoral Epiphysis   346
  Etiology 347
  Pathology 348
  Clinical Picture 348
  Roentgen Signs 348
  Treatment 348
  Southwick Biplane Osteotomy   351
  Wedge   Osteotomy   and   Klein
  Procedure 352
  Postoperative Treatment 354
  Cartilage Necrosis 357
Synovitis of Hip 357
  Etiology 358
  Clinical Features 358
  Roentgen Findings 358
  Differential Diagnosis 359
  Treatment 360
Legg-Perthes Disease 360
  Significance 360
  Past Contributions 361
  One Vascular Insult or Multiple Vas-
  cular Insults 366
  Pathology 366
  First Stage 366
  Second Stage 366
  Third Stage 367
  Pathologic Specimens from Pa-
  tients with Legg-Perthes Disease   367
  Blood Supply to the Central Seg-
  ment of the Femoral Head 369
  Stress within the Femoral Head   371
  Surgical Treatment of Aseptic Ne-
  crosis in Child and Adult 371
  Conservative Treatment 374
  First Goal 374
  Development of Osteoarthritis   377
  Summary 391
Epiphyseal Dysplasia 393
  Multiple   Epiphyseal   Dysplasia
  Congenita 393
  Clinical Picture 393
  Roentgen Findings 393
  Treatment 394

CHAPTER 7
Congenital Orthopaedic Conditions 395

Hemihypertrophy 395
  Treatment 395
  Local Giantism 395
  Other Causes of Limb Enlarge-
  ment 396
  Arteriovenous Fistula 396
  Hemangiomas 396
  Lymphatic Aberrations 396
  Lymphangiosarcoma 396
  Neurofibroma 396
Ehlers-Danlos Syndrome 397
  Clinical Picture 397
  Treatment 397
Proximal Femoral Focal Deficiency
(Congenital Short Femur) 397
  Clinical Picture 398
  Classification 398
  Treatment 400
Congenital Absence of Fibula (Par-
axial Hemimelia (Fibula)) 403
  Clinical Picture 403
  Pathology 404
  Treatment 404
Absent Tibia (Paraxial Hemimelia
(Tibia)) 405
  Treatment 405
Congenital Amputations and Con-
stricting Bands 407
  Treatment 407
Cleidocranial Dysostosis 408
  Clinical Picture 408
  Treatment 408
Congenital Posterior Angulation of Ti-
bia with Talipes Calcaneus 408
  Treatment 409
Radioulnar Synostosis 410
  Treatment 410
Milroy's Disease 411
  Clinical Picture 412
  Treatment 412
Congenital Dislocation of Radial
Head 412
  Clinical Picture 412
  Treatment 412
Ulnar-deficient Extremity 416
Nail-Patella Syndrome (Osteo-ony-
chodystrophy) 417

CHAPTER 8
Defective Formation of Bone 419

Chondrodystrophies 419
  Chondrodystrophia Fetalis (Achon-
  droplastic Dwarfism) 419
  Local Chondrodystrophies 419
Chondrodysplasias 421
  Peripheral Conversion Defects . . 424
  Single Peripheral Metaphyseal

Chondrodysplasia 424
Multiple Peripheral Metaphyseal
Chondrodysplasia (Diaphyseal
Aclasia) 425
Unilateral Multiple Peripheral and
Central Metaphyseal Chondrodys-
plasia (Ollier's Disease) 426
Peripheral Epiphyseal Chondro-
dysplasia 427
Submarginal Conversion Defects . 429
Benign Nonosteogenic Fibroma . . 430
Melorrheostosis 430
Multiple Enchondromas 433
Central Conversion Defects 434
Gargoylism 438
Achondrogenesis—John Ogden,
M.D. 439
Humerus Varus—John Ogden, M.D. 441

CHAPTER 9
**Metabolic and Generalized Ortho-
paedic Conditions** 443

Hystiocytosis X 443
  Clinical Features 443
  Roentgen Features 443
  Histologic Features 443
Gaucher's Disease 444
  Treatment 444
Mucopolysaccharidoses 445
  MPS Type I (Hurler's Syndrome) . 445
  Roentgen Findings 446
  Laboratory Findings 446
  MPS Type II (Hunter's Syndrome) 446
  MPS Type III (Sanfilippo's Syn-
  drome) 447
  MPS Type IV (Morquio's Syn-
  drome) 447
  MPS Type V (Scheie's Syndrome) 447
  MPS Type VI (Maroteau-Lamy Syn-
  drome; Polydystrophic Dwarfism) 447
Eosinophilic Granuloma 448
  Pathology 448
  Roentgen Findings 448
  Clinical Picture 448
  Differential Diagnosis 449
  Treatment 450
Resistant Rickets and Other Disor-
ders of Calcium and Phosphate Me-
tabolism—Robert Klein, M.D. 450
  Some Metabolic Changes in
  Rickets 451
  Action of Vitamin D and Parathyroid
  Hormone 451
  Action of Vitamin D in Refractory
  Rickets 452
  Renal Phosphate-losing Rickets . 453
  Renal Phosphate-retaining Rickets 453
  Hypercalcemia 454
  Refractory Rickets 454

Scurvy—Robert Klein, M.D. 456
Hemophilia—Ronald Hillegass, M.D. 458
  History and Incidence 458
  Etiology 459
  Clinical Picture 459
  Diagnosis 460
  Pathology 460
  Treatment 461
  Specific Problems 464
  Acute Hemarthrosis 464
  Muscle and Soft-tissue Bleeding . 466
  Chronic Synovitis and Arthritis . . . 467
  Preventive Treatment 467
Rheumatoid Arthritis in Children . . . 470
  Age and Sex Incidence 471
  Mode of Onset 471
  Systemic Manifestations 471
  Rheumatoid Arthritis without Meta-
  bolic Involvement 472
  Clinical Picture 472
  Treatment 474
  Correction of Deformity 474
  Bivalved Cast Routine 475
  Synovectomy in Childhood—Rheu-
  matoid 475
  Regimen of Therapy 476
  Comparison of Therapy 477
Generalized Affections 478
  Fibrous Dysplasia 478
  Clinical Picture 478
  Roentgen Findings 480
  Pathology 482
  Treatment 482
  Osteopetrosis 483
Osteogenesis Imperfecta 487
  Bauze's Classification 487
  Mild 487
  Severe 488
  Clinical Picture 488
  Pathology 489
  Roentgen Findings 489
  Healing of Fracture 489
  Treatment 489
Osteopathia Striata 491
Maffucci's Syndrome (Multiple Carti-
lage Tumors Associated with Heman-
giomas of the Extremity 493
  X-ray Examination 493
  Pathology 495
  Treatment 495

CHAPTER 10
Affections of Muscle 497

Pseudohypertrophic Muscular Dys-
trophy 497
  Etiology 497
  Clinical Picture 497
  Serum Enzymes in Muscular
  Dystrophy 499

Pathology 499
Differential Diagnosis 500
Treatment 500
Dermatomyositis 502
  Etiology 502
  Clinical Picture 502
  Pathology 502
  Treatment 502
Arthrogryposis Multiplex Congenita 503
  Etiology 503
  Clinical Picture 503
  Roentgen Picture 503
  Pathology 503
  Treatment 504
Myositis Ossificans (Circumscripta) . 506
  Clinical Picture 507
  Pathology 508
  Treatment 508
Persistent Adducted Femurs (Posi-
tional) 508
  Physical Examination 509
  Treatment 509

CHAPTER 11
Benign and Malignant Tumors of
Bone 511

Benign Tumors in Childhood 511
  Osteogenic Fibroma and Osteoid
  Osteoma 511
  Roentgen Findings 513
  Pathology 513
  Treatment 513
  Nonosteogenic Fibroma (Benign
  Cortical Defect) 514
  Pathology 515
  Treatment 515
  Osteochondroma 515
  Experimental Osteochondroma . . 516
  Clinical Picture 517
  Treatment 521
  Simple Bone Cyst 522
  Treatment 523
  Aneurysmal Bone Cyst 523
  Roentgen Appearance 524
  Pathology 524
  Treatment 524
  Chondromyxoid Fibroma 525
  Roentgen Appearance 525
  Pathology 525
  Treatment 526
  Desmoplastic Fibroma 526
  Roentgen Appearance 527
  Pathology 527
  Treatment 527
  Chondroblastoma 528
  Roentgen Appearance 528
  Pathology 529
  Treatment 529
  Eosinophilic Granuloma 529

Treatment 531
Giant Cell Tumor 531
Roentgen Appearance 531
Pathology 532
Treatment 532
Congenital Generalized Fibroma-
tosis 533
Malignant Tumors—James H. Mc-
Master, M.D. 534
Osteogenic Sarcoma 534
Symptoms 535
Physical Examination 535
Laboratory Data 536
Pathology 536
Classification 536
Treatment 539
Ewing's Sarcoma 541
Original Description 541
Clinical Picture 541
Symptoms 541
Signs 541
X-ray Examination 542
Laboratory Data 542
Pathology 542
Differential Diagnosis 543
Treatment 543
Course 543
Neuroblastoma 544
Treatment 545
Reticulum Cell Sarcoma 547

CHAPTER 12
The Neck and Shoulder 549

Congenital Deformities 549
Spina Bifida 549
Etiology 549
Clinical Picture 549
Treatment 549
Klippel-Feil Syndrome 549
Etiology 549
Clinical Picture 549
Treatment 549
Sprengel's Deformity 550
Etiology 551
Clinical Picture 551
Treatment 551
Green Procedure 552
Discussion 555
Absence of Muscles or Muscle
Groups 559
Familial Nuchal Rigidity 559
Etiology 559
Clinical Picture 559
Treatment 559
Acquired Deformities 560
Deformity Due to Position in Utero   560
Etiology 560
Clinical Picture 560
Treatment 560

Muscular Torticollis 561
Embryology of Sternocleidomas-
toid Muscle 561
Etiology 562
Pathology 563
Clinical Picture 563
Treatment 564
Rotary Subluxations 564
Clinical Picture 565
Pathology 565
Treatment 565

CHAPTER 13
Infections of the Bones and Joints.   567

Septic Arthritis—Harold Swensen,
M.D. 567
Etiology 567
Clinical Picture 567
Pathology 568
X-ray Appearance 568
Diagnosis 569
Treatment 570
Gonococcal Arthritis 580
Tuberculosis of Hip 581
Clinical Picture 581
Pathology 582
Roentgen Picture 582
Treatment 582
Retroperitoneal Abscess 585
Pyogenic Infection of Hip 585
Clinical Picture 586
Roentgen Picture 586
Treatment 587
Reconstruction of Old Septic Hip .   589
Osteomyelitis 589
Etiology 590
Clinical Picture 591
Advent of Antibiotics 592
Pathology 593
Roentgen Picture 594
Treatment 597
Inflammation of Intervertebral Disc
Space in Children 601
Laboratory Findings 601
Roentgen Findings 603
Treatment 603
Course 603

CHAPTER 14
Neurogenic Affections 607

Poliomyelitis 607
History 607
Diagnosis 608
Acute Stage 608
Onset 608
Clinical Picture 609
Differential Diagnosis 609
Treatment 609

Convalescent Stage **610**
Pathology **610**
Treatment **611**
Chronic or Residual Poliomyelitis . **613**
Clinical Description **613**
Bracing **614**
Lower Extremities **614**
Knee **614**
Hip **614**
Trunk **615**
Neck **615**
Upper Extremity **615**
Progressive Resistance Exercise . **616**
Stretching Exercises **616**
Functional Training **616**
Reconstruction of Paralytic Patient **617**
Unstable Foot **617**
Knee **620**
Hip **620**
Shoulder **621**
Elbow **621**
Progressive Muscular Atrophy of
the Peroneal Type (Peroneal Atro-
phy, Charcot-Marie-Tooth Disease)
Pierce E. Scranton, Jr., M.D. **623**
Clinical Picture **623**
Inheritance **625**
Neurophysiology **625**
Treatment **625**
Paraplegia in Childhood **627**
Lordosis **627**
Pelvic Obliquity **627**
Collapsing Spine **627**
Kyphosis **627**
Treatment **627**
Neurofibromatosis **629**
Clinical Picture **629**
Recognition **629**
Skeletal Lesions **629**
Scoliosis **631**
Nonunion **631**
Orbital Defects **631**
Overgrowth **631**
Sarcoma **631**
Radial Nerve Paralysis Associated
with Fractures of Humerus **632**
Congenital Indifference to Pain . . . **632**

CHAPTER 15
Myelomeningocele—David H. Bahnson, M.D. **635**

Terminology **635**
Embryology **636**
Natural History and Ethical Con-
siderations **638**
Treatment **639**
General Principles **639**
Orthopaedic Management **640**
Specific Treatment Considerations . **641**

Thoracic Level **642**
Spine **642**
Hips **642**
Knee **643**
Feet **645**
Upper Lumbar Level **645**
Spine **646**
Hips **647**
Knee **647**
Feet **647**
Lower Lumbar Level **648**
Spine **648**
Hips **648**
Knee **649**
Feet **650**
Sacral Level **650**
Spine **650**
Hips **651**
Knee **651**
Feet **651**
Fractures **651**
Spinal Deformities in Myelodyspla-
sia—Carl D. Fackler, M.D. **655**
Natural History and Classification. **657**
Clinical Management **657**
Observation **657**
Bracing **657**
Surgical Management **658**
Lumbar Kyphosis **660**
Scoliosis with Lordosis **660**
Scoliosis with Thoracic Kyphosis . **660**
Increased Lumbar Lordosis **660**
Spinal Deformity with Diastema-
tomyelia **663**

CHAPTER 16
Cerebral Palsy—Carl L. Stanitski,
M.D. **665**

Definition **665**
Prevalence **666**
Classification **666**
Assessment **669**
Prognosis **674**
Goals **678**
Management **679**
Surgical Treatment **681**
Hips **682**
Knee **687**
Foot and Ankle **688**
Spine **693**
Upper Extremity **700**

CHAPTER 17
The Upper Extremity—Frank Stelling, M.D. **709**

Congenital Anomalies **709**
Radial Meromelia (Hemimelia),
Complete or Incomplete **709**

Associated Anomalies 711
Muscular Defects 711
Vascular Defects 712
Treatment 712
Conservative Treatment 712
Surgical Treatment 712
Congenital Flexion and Adduction
Deformity of Thumb (Pollex Varus,
Thumb-clutched Hand, Congenital
Clasped Hand) 715
Treatment 715
Stenosing Tenovaginitis of
Thumb—"Trigger Thumb" 716
Pathology 716
Clinical Picture 716
Treatment 717
Syndactylism 717
Treatment 717
Polydactylism 726
Treatment 726
Cleft Hand 728
Treatment 730
Megalodactylism 730
Treatment 730
Annular Grooves and Congenital
Amputations 730
Treatment 732
Brachydactylism 733
Treatment 733
Agenesis and Incomplete Devel-
opment 733
Treatment 735
Absence of Thumb 737
Symphalangism 745
Triphalangeal Thumb 745
Cerebral Palsy 745
Splinting and Physical Therapy .. 746
Surgical Treatment 747
Poliomyelitis 756
Arthrodeses 757
Tendon Transplantation 757
Opposition 758
Rerouting of Extensor Pollicis
Longus 759
Reinforcement of Pulley for Oppo-
nens Transfers 759
Finger Flexion 760
Restoration of Finger Function by
Tenodesis 763
Rheumatoid Arthritis 764
Treatment 765
Trauma 769
Volkmann's Ischemic Contracture 769
Etiology 769
Pathology 770
Clinical Picture 771
Treatment 773
Early Phase 773
Late Phase 774
Reconstruction 775

Wringer Arm 777
Pathogenesis and Pathology 777
Clinical Examination 778
Treatment 778
Lacerations of Hand and Fingers . 779
Burns 788
Treatment 789
Early 789
Late 792
Brachial Palsy—Birth Type 795
Etiology 799
Pathology 801
Clinical Picture 801
Early 801
Late 802
Treatment 802

CHAPTER 18
The Spine 805

Posture in Early Adolescents 805
Treatment 805
Back Pain in Children—Differential
Diagnosis 805
Congenital Kyphosis 807
Etiology 807
Clinical Picture 808
Morquio's Syndrome 808
Hurler's Syndrome 808
Kyphosis Associated with Single
Areas of Bony Anomaly 808
Treatment 809
Vertebral Plana (Calvé's Disease) .. 809
Clinical Picture 809
X-ray Picture 809
Treatment 810
Spondylolisthesis 810
Etiology 810
Clinical Picture 810
Roentgen Findings 812
Treatment 813
Tuberculosis of Spine 814
Etiology 815
Pathology 815
Clinical Picture 816
Laboratory Findings 816
Roentgen Findings 817
Treatment 817
Paraplegia 819
Preadolescent and Adolescent
Kyphosis 821
Etiology 821
Normal Spine Development 822
Clinical Picture 823
Roentgen Picture 823
Treatment 823
"Cast Syndrome" 824
Congenital Spinal Deformities—
Charles S. Stone, M.D. 825
Embryology 825

Classification 827
Congenital Scoliosis 827
Natural History 828
Treatment Plan 829
Milwaukee Brace 831
Surgical Treatment 831
Posterior in Situ Fusion 831
Cast Correction and Posterior
Fusion 831
Halo-Femoral Traction and Poste-
rior Fusion 832
Spinal Osteotomy 832
Congenital Kyphosis 834
Classification and Natural History 834
Diagnosis and Preoperative Evalu-
ation 835
Early Posterior Fusion 836
Later Fusion in Moderate Deform-
ity 837
Severe Kyphotic Deformity without
Paraplegia 837
Paraplegia 837
Anterior Decompression and Strut
Graft Arthrodesis 837
Myelomeningocele Spinal Deform-
ity 839
Pelvic Obliquity 840
Lumbar Kyphosis 841
Kyphectomy 841

Congenital Scoliosis 842
Developmental Lordoscoliosis ... 843
Treatment 843
Nonoperative Treatment of Kypho-
scoliosis—William T. Green, Jr.,
M.D. 849
Milwaukee Brace 850
Scoliosis—William F. Donaldson, Jr.,
M.D. 855
Functional Scoliosis 858
Structural Scoliosis 859
Idiopathic Scoliosis 862
History 869
Physical Findings 869
X-ray Findings 870
Adolescent Idiopathic Scoliosis .. 873
Postpoliomyelitis Scoliosis 907
Congenital Scoliosis 913
von Recklinghausen's Neurofibro-
matosis 915
Postempyema and Post-thoraco-
plasty Scolioses 916
Muscular Dystrophy 916
Postirradiation Scoliosis 917
Summary 918
Postlumboperitoneal Shunt Lor-
dosis 920
Index 927

CHAPTER 1

Orthopaedic Treatment of Childhood Disability

The child is a growing, maturing individual, a fact that must be kept in mind in the treatment phases of orthopaedic disability.

Braces must be used to enlarge, not limit, a child's horizon. All aspects of the child's development must be given attention at a time when the tendency is to rivet the attention on the single aspect of a deformity or loss of function under treatment. If treatment is always thought of in terms of total function of the child, these things can be brought into proper perspective. Surgical decisions are accurately made when the contribution of the surgical procedure to the total function of the child is ascertained. Decisions for long term hospitalization or physiotherapy must be made only after being weighed against the removal of the child from an area where emotional and intellectual development can be served. The rapid improvement in function occasionally possible with surgery is a point in its favor if it returns the child to a growth environment with greater opportunity to take part in it.

Many procedures fail because of a poor concept of what is necessary to make them work and increase the child's function. The procedure includes the postoperative period and the type of cast, traction, or physical therapy, the return home with adequate instruction for the parents and child, and the follow-up in the years following so that maximum function is achieved.

Factors which tend to make a deformity recur, such as growth, must be considered in on-going care. Unbalanced muscle pull and diseased tissue must be corrected or the limb braced until they can be corrected. The natural vigor of the child's tissues aids in regeneration of tissues if protection of the area is continued sufficiently long. During this period the hobbling effect of the treatment must be minimized so that the child can still take part in learning activities of all types.

GROWTH AFFECTING SKELETON

Many orthopaedic diseases may represent the development of a congenital abnormality. The variation usually appears in the specific age group in which the particular portion of the skeleton normally is differentiated. Growth may affect the degree of development of an abnormality such as scoliosis. The effect of growth on the development of deformity in the presence of unbalanced musculature of the limb is a very important underlying consideration in orthopaedics. The growing child with one muscle group dominating another, as in poliomyelitis, must be braced; but the unbraced adult with the same clinical picture does not necessarily develop a deformity.

Some understanding of human skeletal growth and its effects is essential to an understanding of orthopaedic disease.

Skeletal Growth

In order to appreciate growth at a given age, two types of studies may be done. Cross sectional studies, to be significant, require a large number of children, but they are more commonly carried out than longitudinal studies because of the time involved in studying one child throughout his growth period. From cross sectional studies, the mean measurement of any particular skeletal attribute is obtained. From longitudinal studies, the rate of change can be determined. Longitudinal studies are quite readily available to the orthopaedist because he usually follows up a patient throughout the growth period when a particular abnormality is present.

There is an exponential fall in the rate of mean gain in standing height for the human being except for two periods. The first delay

1

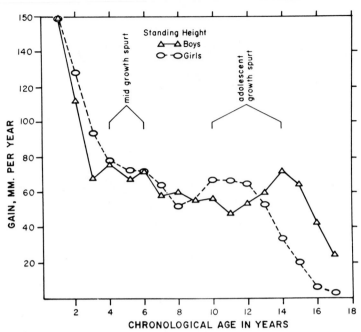

Figure 1.1. Note the declination in height per year as growth progresses. The two periods during which this rate of decline levels off are known as the midgrowth spurt and the adolescent growth spurt. (Reproduced with permission of J. B. Lippincott Co., from R. Duthie: The significance of growth in orthopaedic surgery, *Clinical Orthopaedics*, *14:* 7, 1959. Prepared from data that originally appeared in K. Simmons: *The British Foundation Study of Child Growth and Development, II. Physical Growth and Development*, Monograph, Society for Research in Child Development, Vol. 9, No. 1, Serial 37, 1944.)

in this fall is noted between 5½ and 7 years and is called the midgrowth spurt. The second delay is the adolescent growth spurt between 13 and 15 years (Fig. 1.1).

The growth rates in boys and girls are essentially the same except for the following variations. Boys may be slightly longer at birth, and they may grow slightly faster in the first year. Girls begin their adolescent growth spurt 2 years earlier than boys (at 11 instead of 13 years). During this spurt, they grow faster and larger than boys, but, slowing quickly, they are finally smaller than boys in all dimensions except pelvic width. The boys, commencing their adolescent growth spurt 2 years later, go on to grow for a longer period and to larger dimensions.

Because their growth period is longer, the boys have longer legs. Hormonal influences give the boys wider shoulders and the girls a wider pelvis. In boys there is also a relative increase in the amount of growth of the trunk

(sitting height) to that of the legs (Fig. 1.2). The tremendous variation in this pattern in any one individual, racial group, or body type is readily evident.

Factors Affecting Growth

PRENATAL

The influence of inherited factors is accepted. Such orthopaedic conditions as achondroplasia, spina bifida, dislocation of the hip, and osteogenesis imperfecta in genetic studies have been shown to result from a single gene mutation. The state of health of the mother also obviously affects the developing fetal skeleton.

POSTNATAL

Environmental and sociologic factors may influence the onset of puberty. Genetic fac-

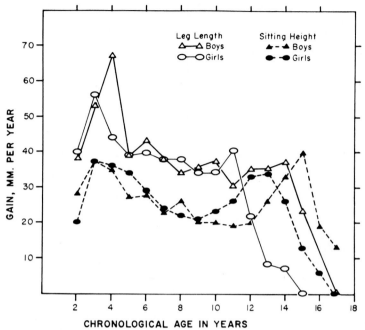

Figure 1.2. Gain in millimeters per year in sitting height and leg length is contrasted in boys and girls. The later increase in leg length and sitting height of boys is evident. (Reproduced with permission of J. B. Lippincott Co., from R. Duthie: The significance of growth in orthopaedic surgery, *Clinical Orthopaedics*, 14: 7, 1959. Prepared from data that originally appeared in K. Simmons: *The British Foundation Study of Child Growth and Development, II. Physical Growth and Development*, Monograph, Society for Research in Child Development, Vol. 9, No. 1, Serial 37, 1944.)

tors are also still of importance. The state of health of the individual can result in skeletal dwarfism. Dietary factors are important.

Relation of Growth to Orthopaedic Conditions

The so-called osteochondritides are distinguished by their preference for a specific age group and often for a specific sex. If all cases were considered to occur at a physiologic rather than a chronologic age, their relationship to a specific age might be still more remarkable. Girls, because of their earlier skeletal maturation, would be expected to experience an earlier onset of these diseases, and, in osteochondritis involving the spine and Osgood-Schlatter disease, they do in fact (Fig. 1.3).

Tumors such as osteogenic sarcoma, neuroblastoma, and Ewing's chondrosarcoma and giant cell sarcoma are distinguished by their occurrence in specific age groups.

Scoliosis is a noteworthy anomaly in terms of relating growth to skeletal disease. That the curve in idiopathic scoliosis ceases to progress when spine growth is complete is documented (Fig. 1.4). Paralytic curvatures that have been doing well often develop into severe deformity during the adolescent growth spurt.

Temporary deformities that normally occur during development, such as genu valgus, which appears between the ages of 2 and 4 years and gradually improves thereafter, internal tibial torsion, and anteversion of the hip, are evidence of the influence of growth on the skeleton. The examples are many, for the influence of growth can be seen in most skeletal changes—normal and abnormal—of childhood.

Osteochondritis of:	Usual Age at Diagnosis	Range of Age Incidence	Sex Incidence	Year of Appearance of Epiphysis MALE	FEMALE
Upper Femoral Epiphysis (Legg-Calve-Perthes' Disease)	5 - 9	3½ - 15	M > F	1	½
Tuberosity of Tibia (Osgood-Schlatter's Disease)	12 - 15	10 - 23	M > F	11	11
Navicular Bone (Kohler's Disease)	3 - 8	2½ - 10	M > F	2 - 4	2 - 4
Calcanean Tubercles (Haglund's Disease)	8½ - 15	8 - 22	M > F	10	8
Head of Second Metatarsal Bone (Freiberg's Disease)	10 - 18	10 - 45	F > M	3	2
Upper and Lower Epiphyses of Vertebrae (Scheuermann's Disease)	10 - 21	•	M > F	10	10

Figure 1.3. Relationship of some orthopaedic conditions in childhood to specific age groups. Growth and its effects may be a prime underlying factor in delineating these age groups. (Reproduced with permission of J. B. Lippincott Co., from R. Duthie: The significance of growth in orthopaedic surgery, *Clinical Orthopaedics, 14:* 7, 1959.)

References

1. Crompton, C. W.: Physiological age, a fundamental principle, *Child Dev., 15:* 1, 1944.
2. Duthie, R. B.: The significance of growth in orthopedic surgery, *Clin. Orthop., 14:* 7, 1959.
3. Price, C. H. S.: Osteogenic sarcoma; an analysis of the sex and age incidence, *Br. J. Cancer, 9:* 558, 1955.
4. Simmons, K., and Todd, T. W.: Growth of well children: analysis of stature and weight, 3 months to 13 years, *Growth, 2:* 93, 1938.

GROWTH OF EPIPHYSIS

There is a startling ability of the epiphysis to recover from injury. This is substantiated by animal experiments. On the other hand, trauma (the effects of which are virtually undiscernible on the roentgenogram) may result in real growth inhibition and subsequent deformity in the human (Fig. 1.5).

Selye[4] removed the entire epiphysis in rats and found that a complete new functional epiphysis developed in 12- to 15-day-old rats. This potential was confined to very young animals and did not occur in mature rats. Ford and Key[1] found that drilling the central portion of the epiphyseal plate produced no deformity in rabbits, whereas peripheral damage caused extensive changes. Langenskiold and Edgren[3] produced small central areas of destruction with x-ray and found that there was ingrowth of cartilage cells from the surrounding undamaged areas and no

deformity resulted with growth. Friedenberg[2] found after partial resection of the epiphysis in rabbits that the shortening and deformity that occurred were related to the remaining length of the undamaged epiphyseal line and the extent of reactive bone bridging the epiphyseal line. There was no evidence of cartilage regeneration. Normal growth in the remnants of the epiphyseal line occurred in some specimens where there was obvious bridging.

References

1. Ford, L. T., and Key, J. A.: A study of experimental trauma to the distal femoral epiphysis in rabbits, *J. Bone Joint Surg., 38A:* 84, 1956.
2. Friedenberg, L. A.: Reaction to partial surgical resection of the epiphysis, *J. Bone Joint Surg., 39A:* 332, 1957.
3. Langenskiold, A., and Edgren, W.: Imitation of chondrodysplasia by localized roentgen ray; an experimental study of bone growth, *Acta Chir. Scand., 99:* 352, 1949.
4. Selye, H.: On the mechanism controlling growth in long bones, *J. Anat., 68:* 289, 1934.

DEVELOPMENT OF EPIPHYSIS AND GROWTH PLATE

An understanding of the dynamic development of the growth plate is implicit to comprehension of the multiple problems of

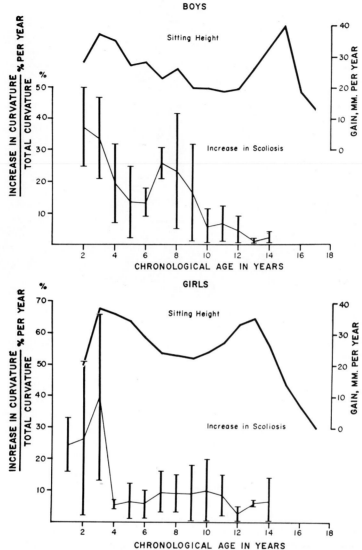

Figure 1.4. Relation of increase in curvature in children with infantile scoliosis to the gain in millimeters per year in sitting height.

pediatric orthopaedics. This structure is responsible for the enlargement of immature bone, by elaboration of both cellular constituents and intercellular matrices. The most important aspect of the growth plates is that they provide for a controlled rapid expansion of preformed cartilage models.

A discrete structure that can be classified as a growth plate appears relatively late in the development of long bones, and even later in the development of epiphyses, apophyses, and the small bones of the wrist and ankle. Initially the axial skeleton and shortly thereafter the limb buds from mes-

enchymal condensations that begin conversion to cartilage by the fifth to sixth weeks. These small cartilagenous anlagen then enlarge by interstitial and appositional expansion of cells throughout their length, particularly at the ends. The cartilage cells in the center of the anlage then begin to hypertrophy (Fig. 1.6a). A periosteal cuff forms around the center of the anlage by the end of the sixth week. The hypertrophic central cartilage continues to mature and calcify and subsequently begins ossification concomitant with the penetration of the irruption artery. The central shaft converts to bone and leaves

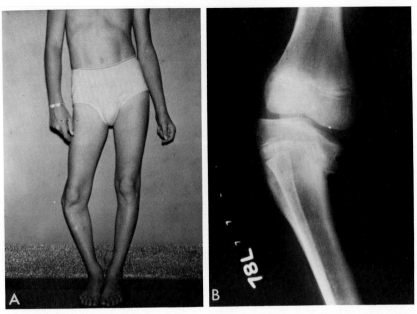

Figure 1.5. (*A*) This 14-year-old boy has shortening and angulation of the tibia secondary to epiphyseal injury. (*B*) The growth arrest occurred medially at the proximal tibial epiphysis. The continued growth of a major portion of the lateral segment produced the severe deformity.

cartilage at each end. This junction between bone and cartilage is initially not a discrete structure (Fig. 1.6 *b*). By the third month these junctional cartilage cells have assumed a.typical columniated appearance (Fig. 1.6 *c*). From this point of differential development, further specialization of the growth plate is contingent upon the type of bone and varies considerably.

There are two basic types of growth plate, discoid and spherical. Most primary growth plates of the long bones are discoid—a relatively planar area of rapidly differentiating and maturing cartilage between the epiphysis and metaphysis. These contribute to longitudinal as well as circumferential increase in bone size. These discoid growth plates are also found between apophyses and shafts. There are several anatomic variations. In shorter, tubular bones, such as the metacarpals, metatarsals, and phalanges, two discoid growth plates are initially present, but, with further skeletal growth and maturation, only one end of the bone forms a true epiphysis. The growth plate at the opposite end becomes juxtaposed to the developing articular cartilage and more closely resembles a spherical, rather than discoid, growth plate (Fig. 1.7). The growth plate of the calcaneal

apophysis, although discoid, curves around the posteroinferior body of the calcaneus. A spherical growth plate is found in the small bones of the wrist and ankle, as well as in early development of the secondary ossification centers of the epiphyses and apophyses. The growth plate surrounds an evolving ossific nucleus that is analogous to the metaphysis. In the small bones of the wrist and ankle, as well as the apophyses, this spherical growth plate gradually assumes the contour of the bone. In the epiphyses the spherical growth plate and ossification centers enlarge and lead to juxtaposition of the spherical secondary center growth plate and discoid primary growth plate (Fig. 1.8), temporarily creating a bipolar growth zone between the epiphyseal ossification center and the metaphysis. The spherical secondary center growth plate is eventually replaced by a subchondral bone plate where it is apposed to the primary discoid growth plate. However, the spherical growth plate does remain along the epiphyseal borders and under the articular surface to allow expansion of the epiphysis commensurate with diametric growth of the shaft. The vertebral body initially has a spherical growth plate (Fig. 1.9), which disappears by gradual expansion of

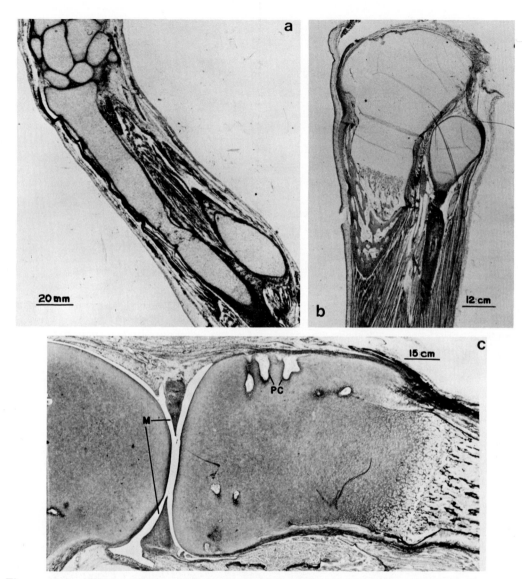

Figure 1.6. Stages in the early development of the growth plate. Readings refer to crown-rump length of the embryo or fetus. At 20 mm (a), a midshaft periosteal cuff is beginning to form. No growth plate is present. At 12 cm (b), the primary ossification center has extended along the shaft. There is a distinct margin between cartilage and bone. But the characteristic columniation is not yet present. By 15 cm (c), about 4½ months, the growth plate has assumed its characteristic appearance. Also, the chondroepiphysis is now beginning to develop a circulatory (cartilage canal) system.

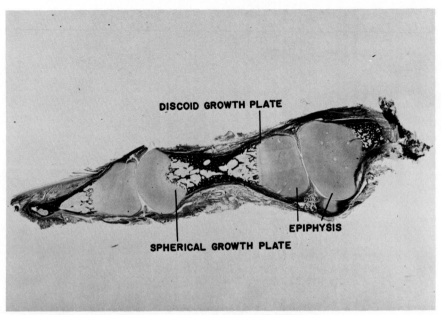

Figure 1.7. First phalanx of the foot in a full term fetus. Note the contour differences between the proximal (discoid) growth plate and the distal (spherical) growth plate. Also note that the ends of the phalanges and metatarsal that will form true epiphyses have a cartilage canal system, whereas the distal end of the proximal phalanx, which does not form bony epiphysis, has no cartilage canal system.

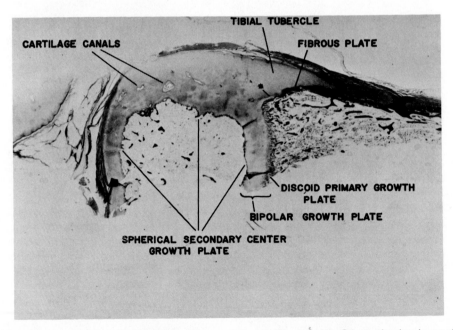

Figure 1.8. Proximal, anterior tibia from a 15-month-old girl. Of particular importance is that the growth plate stops at the beginning of the tibial tubercle (*) and does not extend down the posterior aspect of the tubercle, as is usually described. Instead, this area is comprised of fibrous tissue.

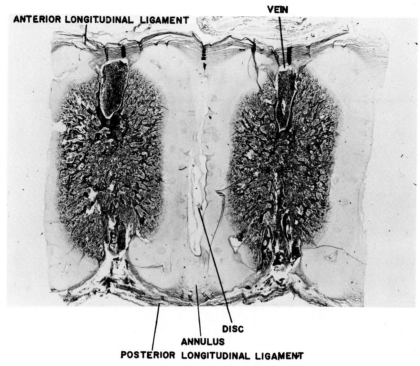

Figure 1.9. Lumbar vertebrae from a 2-month-old neonate. Both the anterior and posterior longitudinal ligaments are well developed. The disc (nucleus pulposus) occupies a much larger area than in the adult.

the ossification center and becomes two parallel discoid growth plates on the upper and lower surfaces of the vertebral body. However, no true vertebral epiphyses develop (in essence, the intervertebral disc occupies the analogous anatomic position of the epiphysis). The bipolar growth plate of the triradiate (acetabular) cartilage develops by the juxtaposition of spherical growth plates of the various pelvic ossification centers.

The growth plate has a characteristic and virtually unchanging architectural pattern from early fetal life to skeletal maturation. The structure can be arbitrarily broken down into different zones using either histologic or functional criteria—the zone of growth, the zone of cartilage maturation, and the zone of transformation (Fig. 1.10).

The zone of growth is concerned with longitudinal and diametric expansion of the bone. It is the only area where cell addition and multiplication occurs (the other regions are concerned with matrix elaboration and transformation to bone). The resting cells are intimately associated with the blood vessels

that cover the zone of growth (E-vessels). These vessels may be instrumental in providing undifferentiated cells that will become the resting chondrocytes. Additional resting cells are also elaborated peripherally through the perichondrial ring (zone of Ranvier). The next stage in the zone of growth is cell division. This occurs in transverse and longitudinal directions and leads to the formation of the cell columns characteristic of the growth plate. These cell columns constitute about one-half of the overall height of the growth plate. The randomly dispersed collagen of the resting/dividing regions becomes longitudinally oriented along these cell columns.

The next area is the zone of cartilage transformation. In this zone the intercellular matrix undergoes the significant biochemical changes necessary for eventual ossification. The matrix becomes metachromatic and calcifies. The chondrocytes become hypertrophic, a reflection of their increased metabolic activity. The fate of these chondrocytes at the end of the zone of cartilage transformation is controversial—some believe that

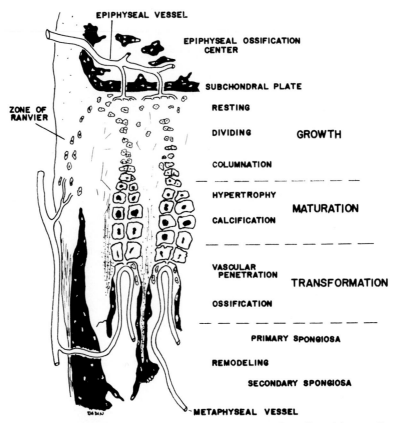

Figure 1.10. Schematic depiction of the architecture of a discoid growth plate. The spherical growth plate is similar, but there is no subchondral plate and the cell columns are quite short.

the cells degenerate, whereas others believe the cells modulate to become osteoblasts. It is quite likely that both processes occur.

The last zone is that of cartilage transformation. The cartilage matrix is replaced by bone. Most characteristic of the region is vascular invasion (M-vessels). Electron microscopy has confirmed that these capillary loops are a closed circulation. They undoubtedly are a source of cells necessary to the formation of bone. Osteoblasts elaborate osteoid on the preformed calcified cartilage, transforming it to bone. This bone surrounding cartilage is the primary spongiosa. By remodeling, this bone is replaced by a more mature secondary spongiosa. In the neonatal skeleton this zone of very active bone formation and remodeling is the weakest structurally, and fractures during birth or infancy occur in this region of the metaphysis, rather than through the growth plate itself, as in the classical Salter I or II injury of the older child.

The growth plate derives blood supply from three major regions, the epiphyseal circulation (E-vessels), the metaphyseal circulation (M-vessels), and the perichondrial circulation.

The epiphyseal circulation varies considerably, depending upon whether the epiphysis is principally cartilage or bone. The vessels enter in regions characteristic for each epiphysis, usually in the regions of capsular and perichondrial attachment. In the apophyses there is extensive vascular penetration along the tendinous insertions.

Vessels enter the chondroepiphyses in cartilage canals (Fig. 1.11). These canals course throughout the cartilage, supplying discrete regions, with minimum anastomosis between major canal systems. These canal systems send branches down to the resting cell region of the growth plate. Occasionally these vessels communicate across the growth plate, anastomosing with the metaphyseal circulation (Fig. 1.12). The vessels that cross the growth plate tend to be found in the larger epiphyses (proximal and distal femur, proximal humerus) for several months, but they become less frequent as the secondary ossification center forms and enlarges. By the time the subchondral plate is formed, no vessels cross the growth plate.

The cartilage canals have several important characteristics. First, and most important, they supply discrete regions within the epiphysis, with virtually no anastomosis between canalicular systems of adjacent regions. Second, the canals enter the epiphysis at fairly regular intervals along the growth plate periphery, but much more irregularly in other regions of the epiphysis. Third, the canals probably serve as a source of chondroblasts for interstitial enlargement of the epiphysis. Fourth, the canals are surrounded by a more dense area of cartilage and intercellular matrix that probably renders an internal support system to the chondroepiphysis and protects the canals from collapse during load-bearing stress (Fig. 1.13). And fifth, the canals

play an integral role in the development of the secondary ossification center (Fig. 1.14).

Once the ossification center begins to form and enlarge, the epiphyseal circulatory pattern changes. Several cartilage canal systems send vessels into the ossification center, creating significant anastomoses between canal systems that previously were virtually endarterial. Enlargement of the ossification center leads to the formation of a subchondral bone plate adjacent to the growth plate. Small branches cross this bone plate and form vascular expansions that supply regions containing several cell columns (Fig. 1.15). The proximity of vessels and resting cells suggests that the resting cells may originate from vascular endothelium or perivascular tissue. These arborizing vessels never penetrate between cell columns. There do not appear to be any anastomoses between these perforating arteries after they cross the subchondral plate. However, before crossing the bony plate there are extensive anastomoses.

If a portion of the epiphyseal circulation is compromised, the zones of growth and transformation associated with the affected vessels cannot undergo appropriate cell division and maturation. The unaffected surrounding growth plate continues to grow longitudinally, resulting in the affected portion being "pulled" toward the metaphysis (Fig. 1.17). The rate of growth of the cells adjacent to the infarcted area would be more compromised (by tethering effect) than the rate of growth of cells much further away. If the involved area is peripherally situated, this results in tilting of the epiphysis relative to the metaphysis. If the circulatory compromise occurs while the epiphysis is still primarily cartilaginous, the infarcted area may continue to grow, but at a significantly decreased rate compared to adjacent growth plate. But in the older child with an ossification center, the damaged segment of the growth plate may be "pulled" far enough into the metaphysis to allow a bony bridge to replace the damaged cartilage, connecting the metaphysis and epiphyseal ossification center. If a large enough segment of the growth plate is replaced by a bone bridge, an epiphyseodesis may result. If the subchondral plate is damaged during the injury to the epiphyseal circulation, significant epiphyseodesis invariably results.

The metaphyseal circulation is derived primarily from the nutrient artery. However,

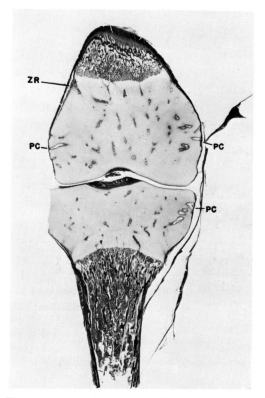

Figure 1.11. Sagittal section of the knee of a 7-month-old fetus showing the extensive cartilage canal system. (*RZ*, zone of Ranvier; *PC*, perichondrium.)

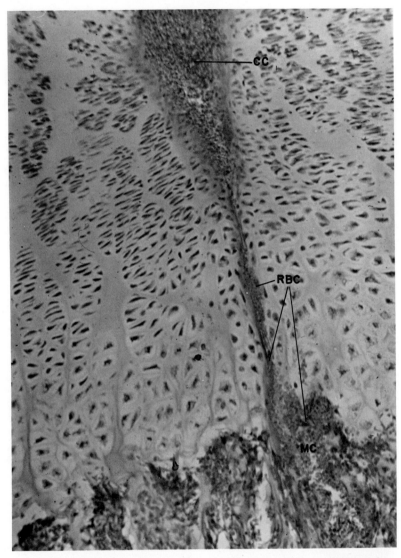

Figure 1.12.   A blood vessel crossing the growth plate of the proximal femur in a full term fetus. (*CC*, cartilage (epiphyseal) canal; *RBC*, red blood cells in the communicating canal; *MC*, metaphyseal circulation.)

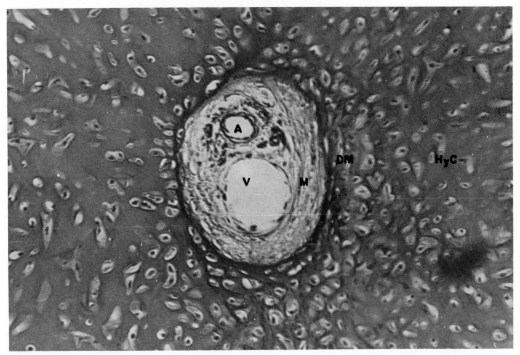

Figure 1.13. Representative cartilage canal in a 2-month-old neonate, showing the artery (*A*), vein (*V*), undifferentiated mesenchymal tissue (*M*), the densely stained matrix surrounding the canal (*DM*), and the differentiating and maturing hyaline cartilage (*HyC*).

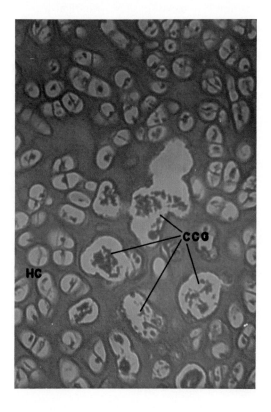

Figure 1.14. Cartilage canal glomerular ending (*CCG*) in the middle of a group of hypertrophic hyaline cartilage cells (*HC*), from the early ossification center of the proximal humerus of a 2-month-old neonate.

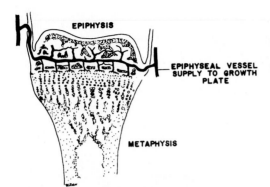

Figure 1.15. Epiphyseal circulation, with vessels penetrating the subchondral bone plate to supply the growth plate.

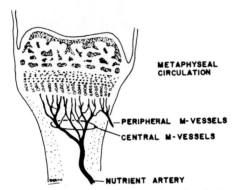

Figure 1.16. Metaphyseal circulation, with contributions from the perichondral and nutrient circulations.

small branches from the perichondrial circulation also enter the periphery of the metaphysis (Fig. 1.16). The terminal portions of both arterial systems form a series of parallel loops that penetrate between the trabeculae of the primary spongiosa to reach the end of the hypertrophic region. These vessels do not form an open communication with the "empty" lacunae. The venule sides of the loops terminate as large sinusoids. These capillary loops and venous sinusoids are not associated with any reticuloendothelial system, which, along with the rheologic changes in this type of network, may explain the predisposition to infection localization adjacent to the growth plate.

Interruption of the metaphyseal circulation has no effect on chondrogenesis and maturation of the growth plate, but transformation to bone is blocked. This causes significant widening of the affected portion as more

cartilage is added in the resting/maturation regions, while no cartilage is replaced by bone in the transformation region (Fig. 1.17). When the metaphyseal circulation is reestablished (which occurs quickly, since the metaphyseal circulation has significant anastomoses near the terminal loops), the broad, already calcified region is rapidly penetrated and ossified, returning the growth plate to normal width.

The perichondral circulation, besides providing branches to the metaphyseal circulation peripherally, also supplies the peripheral regions of the growth plate in a region called the zone of Ranvier. This region is necessary to the appositional enlargement of the growth plate. Compromise of the vessels probably causes decreased diametric expansion of the growth plate.

Characteristically, growth of long bones is considered a *longitudinal* phenomenon. However, the growth plates may expand in two other significant ways. The discoid growth plate must also grow in a diametric, or latitudinal direction. This occurs by cell division and matrix expansion within the plate (interstitial expansion) or by cell addition at the peripheral zone of Ranvier (appositional expansion). The spherical growth plate expands primarily by rapid interstitial expansion, with radially directed "longitudinal" growth that corresponds to the longitudinal metaphyseal erosion of the discoid growth plate (Fig. 1.18). Such interstitial expansion of the epiphyseal growth plate occurs throughout the existence of the ossification

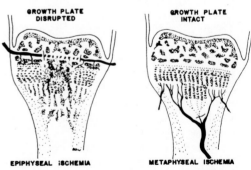

Figure 1.17. Disruption of the epiphyseal circulation usually leads to damage to the structural integrity of the growth plate, whereas metaphyseal ischemia results in widening of the growth plate but leaves the basic structure intact.

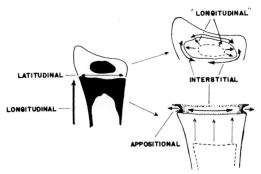

Figure 1.18. Types of growth in the discoid and spherical growth plates.

center, even after it has assumed the general contour of the epiphysis. Interstitial growth in the discoid growth plate is probably directly related to the epiphyseal ossification center. When there is a chondroepiphysis, or even when a small epiphyseal ossification center is present, the pliable hyaline epiphyseal cartilage continuous with the growth plate probably does not present a mechanical barrier to interstitial expansion. But with increasing development of the epiphyseal ossification center, a discrete subchondral bone plate forms, to which the underlying portions of the discoid growth plate become "attached." Further interstitial, latitudinal expansion of the discoid growth plate is precluded in the areas under this subchondral plate (Fig. 1.19). When the secondary ossification center approximates the diametric size of the juxtaposed metaphysis, latitudinal expansion of the discoid growth plate is possible only at the periphery (appositional growth).

Two regions of the developing skeleton show growth variations that can be explained by the presence or absence of this mechanical limitation to interstitial expansion. The distal humerus of the neonate has a capitulum and trochlea of approximately equal cross sectional areas. The ossification center of the capitulum develops during the third to fifth months, and thus presents an early limitation to interstitial expansion of that portion of the distal humeral growth plate associated with the capitulum. In contrast, the ossification center of the trochlea does not appear until 7 to 8 years of age, allowing both interstitial as well as appositional expansion of the distal humeral growth plate associated with the trochlea. The mature trochlea is considerably

larger than the mature capitulum. Eventually these two ossification centers coalesce and permit continued expansion of the distal humerus in fully integrated fashion. The proximal femur similarly shows the appearance of two separate ossification centers (capital femur and greater trochanter) at different times. However, the central region, which will eventually become the intertrochanteric groove, never has a limiting bony plate and continues interstitial expansion, contributing to the length of the femoral neck (Fig. 1.20).

In the epiphysis, the articular cartilage and nonarticular contours do not present as rigid a limiting structure to interstitial expansion of the spherical growth plate of the epiphyseal ossification center.

The effects of force on growth cartilage and epiphyseal cartilage are incompletely understood. Physiologic stress seems necessary for continued, orderly development of both discoid and spherical growth plates. These stresses may result from compression or tension forces. All growth plates must be able to respond initially to both compression and tension-induced stress. However, as each growth plate develops, it may become primarily responsive to either compression (epiphyseal growth plates) or tension (apophyseal growth plates). Because a growth plate, such as the proximal femur, may develop into one section that responds to tension (under the greater trochanter), it is reasonable to assume that there is a biologic range of compression-tension response for each growth plate. Within this physiologic range, increasing tension or compression probably accelerates growth, whereas decreasing tension or compression decelerates growth. Beyond the physiologic limits of compression,

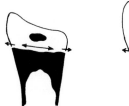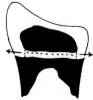

Figure 1.19. Maturation of the ossification center precludes further interstitial enlargement of the growth plate and limits latitudinal expansion to appositional growth.

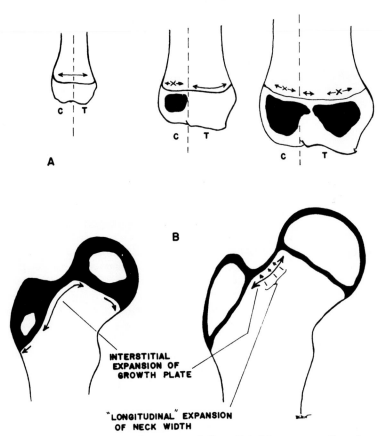

Figure 1.20. (A) Sequential development of the distal humerus. Development of the ossification center of the capitulum (C) first limits interstitial expansion on the lateral half of the distal humeral growth plate. Eventual development of the trochlear (T) ossification center then limits interstitial enlargement of the medial half of the distal humeral growth plate. These two ossification centers then fuse, completely stopping interstitial expansion. (B) Sequential development of the proximal femur. Unlike the distal humerus, the two initially separate ossification centers do not fuse, allowing continued interstitial expansion to form the length of the femoral neck. In addition, this portion of the growth plate also grows "longitudinally," contributing to overall neck diameter. Disruption of this region can lead to shortening and narrowing of the femoral neck.

growth may be significantly decreased. The response (i.e., rate of growth) is probably greater to compression than tension (e.g., the differential rates of growth of the capital femoral and greater trochanteric sections of the proximal femoral growth plate).

The discoid growth plate is never completely planar, but rather is variably convoluted, because each growth plate tends to align its various regions to be perpendicular to the absorbed forces in each region. This minimizes shear stresses within the discoid growth plate. Similarly, the spherical growth plates of the epiphyses, carpus, and tarsus

respond to compression and tension forces *within* the chondroepiphysis and from characteristic shapes that best respond to the stress patterns (e.g., the nonspherical shape of the early proximal tibial ossification center).

When the hyaline cartilage of the chondroepiphysis first forms, there is no significant difference histochemically between the cartilage at the joint surface and the cartilage within the epiphysis. But during the last month of intrauterine development and particularly during the first year of life, significant changes occur such that the articular cartilage becomes histochemically different from the underlying hyaline cartilage. Further, this articular cartilage will not calcify or ossify. If a piece of articular cartilage is embedded in the hyaline cartilage, the epiphyseal ossification center will develop all around it, but the cartilage will remain unchanged. As skeletal maturity is reached, a tidemark develops that delineates articular cartilage from underlying mature epiphyseal cartilage and subchondral bone.

BY JOHN OGDEN, M.D.

DISTINGUISHING GROWTH LINES FROM FRACTURE LINES*

Distinguishing the growth line from the fracture line can be a very troublesome medicolegal problem. A knowledge of their characteristics and features in their occurrence is at times helpful.

This is illustrated in spondylolisthesis, where the defect in the neural arch may be pointed out after trauma as due to the injury. The clue to the correct diagnosis is furnished by the sacrum. Ordinarily its superior border is the same width as the inferior border of the fifth lumbar vertebra. With forward slip of the vertebra, however, the sacrum builds up an anterior prominence resulting in the widening of its superior border, which would not be present if the injury were a fracture.

X-ray Characteristics

A fracture line varies in width and has sharp angles and edges. A growth line is the same width all the way across with rounded edges (Fig. 1.22).

The suture lines of a skull are growth lines. Here the line has maintained its width throughout or, if narrowing, does so in a symmetrical artistic manner, one edge of the line undulating with the other. Inspection reveals apparently sharp angles to actually be rounded or blunted.

The problem of distinguishing growth lines from fracture lines is not always easy. The pull off fracture at the base of the fifth metatarsal is a good example. The shell of bone forming a separate growth center in this area can easily be mistaken for fracture unless the fundamental characteristics of the fracture line are borne in mind (Fig. 1.21).

The accessory growth center at the medial or lateral malleolus about the ankle joint is similarly difficult and leads us to several additional characteristics that may be helpful. Soft-tissue swelling in the area of injury helps lead the eye to the injured area but may be stimulated by ankle sprain. More important

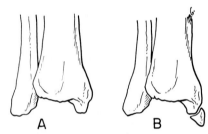

Figure 1.21. An accessory center of ossification, when it is combined with the parent bone, forms a bone that is larger than the normal size of the particular bone. Diagram of the normal (A) is compared with an accessory ossification center (B) at the medial malleolus; the combined size of the ossification center and the medial malleolus is larger than normal.

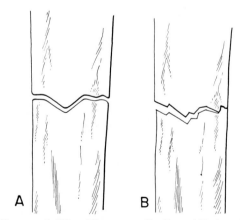

Figure 1.22. The growth line (A) is of equal width throughout and has rounded points rather than sharp angles. The fracture line (B) is of uneven width and has sharp angles.

---

* This section, "Distinguishing Growth Lines from Fracture Lines," is reprinted from A. B. Ferguson, Jr.: Growth lines versus fracture lines, *Journal of the Medical Association of Georgia, 46:* 55, 1957.

is the fact that the accessory center in combination with the parent bony area is always larger than the expected size of the part with a single growth center. In cases in which for one reason or another the growth line is difficult to see, this point may assume great importance.

Some areas where separate growth centers occur normally include the lower pole of the patella, where the characteristic growth line can be seen separating the apophysis from the parent bone (Fig. 1.23).

Fracture Lines That Cannot Be Seen

Where the fracture line is invisible to ordinary roentgen technique, other signs must be relied upon.

The epiphyseal line fracture when little or no displacement of the epiphysis has occurred is one of these. It must be recognized that the epiphyseal line fracture occurs on the metaphyseal side of the line and always takes with it a triangle of metaphyseal bone, however small.

Where the epiphyseal line appears intact, a search for this triangle of metaphyseal bone will frequently lead to the diagnosis, which otherwise might be missed. Where epiphyseal displacement is marked, there is no diagnostic problem—in these cases the triangular area of metaphyseal bone can be seen. Common areas for this type of fracture are the distal radius and the lateral condyle of the humerus. In either case the soft-tissue swelling and slight elevation of the metaphyseal cortex may be the only leads.

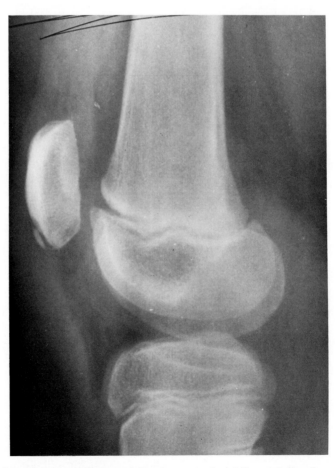

Figure 1.23. Apophysis ossifiying at the lower pole of the patella. A growth line, not a fracture line, divides it from the parent bone. Note the rounded edges and constant width of the line.

In infants, in whom the growth center for the epiphysis has not yet been seen, the diagnostic problem becomes even more difficult. Epiphyseal line fractures at this time of life are frequently called dislocations if seen early before a calcifying callus is seen, or bone tumors when seen late with a massive and apparently wild growth of bone engulfing the metaphyseal area.

The reason for the appearance of dislocation is obvious. The metaphysis and diaphysis of the involved bone no longer have the expected anatomic relationship to the joint. The epiphysis, however, remains in the joint, the fracture allowing the remainder of the bone to displace away from it. The small triangle of metaphyseal bone will be present, however, still attached to the epiphysis. Knowledge of the weakness of this area as compared to the possibility of dislocation helps and will prevent useless manipulation to reduce the joint. Such fractures surround themselves with such exuberant callus that rapid remodeling in the presence of good general limb alignment tends to obliterate all evidence of the fracture. The displacement into varus or valgus at either side of the knee joint may be troublesome, however, and require several years to recover normal alignment.

The two most common areas in which this injury is mistaken for dislocation are the elbow and hip.

MULTIPLE TRAUMA

The chief complaint when infants and children subject to multiple trauma are seen is unexplained inability to use a limb. Some patients, however, arrive with multiple contusions and occasionally with obvious severe injuries and poor systemic conditions verging on shock. Investigation of the circumstances of an obvious severe injury leads, in the usual course of events, to an uncovering of the family situation that is responsible for the injury.

Diagnosis of the more isolated, but recurring, disability requires more subtlety. These children come to orthopaedic attention as diagnostic problems from the roentgenographic point of view. Confusion with metabolic bone disease may arise.

Clinical Picture

In addition to soft-tissue contusions, swelling at the distal end of one or more of the long bones is often seen. On examination, the general health is usually found to be good, although malnutrition of the infant or child may be present. The initial history of the injury is vague, because the person bringing the child attempts to conceal the true nature of events from the examiner.

Roentgen Picture

The usual injury is an epiphyseal fracture without marked displacement. Such fractures are recognized by the triangular area of metaphysis that is fractured off in the process of even a minimal displacement (Figs. 1.24–1.26). They take place on the metaphyseal side of the epiphyseal line but are always accompanied by the metaphyseal fragment as well. Suspicion of the diagnosis is aroused by evidences of other trauma. These may consist of fractures of a minimal nature so far as displacement is concerned and in various

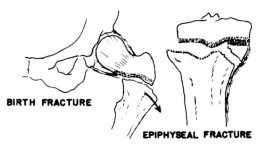

BIRTH FRACTURE

EPIPHYSEAL FRACTURE

Figure 1.24 (*Left*).   The typical birth fracture at the ends of long bones is an epiphyseal fracture. When the epiphysis has not ossified, the fracture may be mistaken for dislocation due to displacement of the shaft in relation to the joint. In the diagram, the femoral head is stippled to indicate its location, but all that is seen by roentgenogram is the small triangle of metaphysis carried with it. Epiphyseal fracture is much more likely than dislocation secondary to birth trauma.

Figure 1.25 (*Right*).   Epiphyseal fracture is recognized by the small triangular fragment of the metaphysis that is carried with the epiphysis even when displacement is minimal.

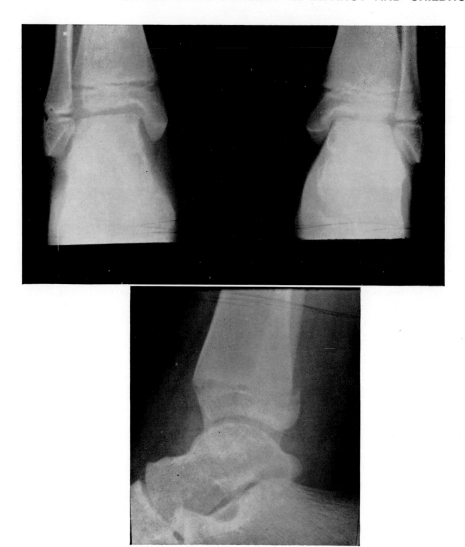

Figure 1.26. Anteroposterior view (*top*) of the distal tibial epiphyseal line bilaterally is not very remarkable. The lateral view (*bottom*) shows the slight displacement of the epiphysis and the small triangle of metaphysis carried with it posteriorly.

stages of healing. Rib fractures or old healed malunions may be noted. Confusion sometimes arises because of thickening of the diaphysis caused by repeated subperiosteal hemorrhages. These result in bizarre-appearing bones without evidence of normal remodeling (Fig. 1.27).

Treatment

The individual fractures are usually without marked displacement and require the usual plaster immobilization. Of far more importance is the attempt to save these children from further injury. A close interrogation of the person bringing the child to medical attention in most cases brings to light the reason for the child's dilemma.

Possible causes include psychiatric disturbance in the mother or father, alcoholism in the family, or brutality from other children. The physician who makes the diagnosis is responsible for following through with a social investigation of the family background and for procuring the help of whatever agencies may be available to seek a solution to the situation.

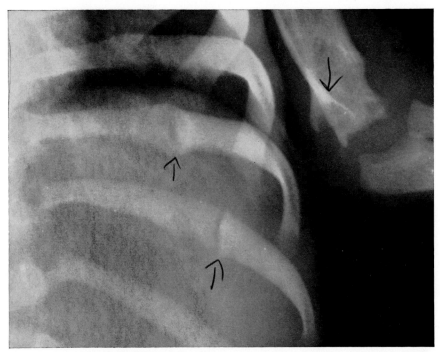

Figure 1.27. In a child with multiple trauma, fractures in various stages of healing can be seen. Here, the two rib fractures, one almost healed, are evident, and ossification at the distal end of the humerus due to old epiphyseal fracture is seen. Note also the widening of the medullary canal of the distal humerus due to repeated subperiosteal hemorrhages and the remodeling that is not quite sufficient to withstand repeated episodes of trauma.

References

1. Caffey, J.: Multiple fractures in long bones of infants suffering from chronic subdural hematoma, *Am. J. Roentgenol.*, *56:* 163, 1946.
2. Friedman, M. S.: Traumatic periotitis in infants and children, *J.A.M.A., 166:* 1840, 1958.
3. Miller, D. S.: Fractures among children. I. Parental assault as causative agent, *Minn. Med., 42:* 1209, 1959.
4. Silverman, F. N.: Roentgen manifestations of unrecognized skeletal trauma in infants, *Am. J. Roentgenol., 69:* 413, 1953.

MOTOR DEVELOPMENT

Some standard pattern of motor development must be borne in mind by the physician examining children. It is well to remember, for instance, that to prefer to use one upper extremity rather than the other before the age of 1 year is abnormal. Before the age of 18 months, such a preference raises the suspicion of the examiner and suggests the possibility of underlying neural damage, such as might exist with hemiplegia in cerebral palsy.

A normal sequence of motor events is roughly as follows (Fig. 1.28). In the first 2 weeks, the infant exhibits mass activity of the limbs, and the eyes focus on light and on the face of the observer. Crying occurs with discomfort. At 1 month, the chin and chest are up and the eyes follow a moving object. At 3 or 4 months, the infant laughs and brings the hand to the mouth. The feet push, and the reach for a rattle occurs. In the 6- to 8-month range, the infant learns to sit alone, to transfer a toy from one hand to the other, and to pull the hair of an observer. By 8 or 9 months, the youngster stands with support. By 11 or 12 months, he can pull himself up to stand; and at 12 or 14 months he can walk, repeat words, recognize sounds, and name a few objects. Running starts at 16–18 months. By 24 months, the child climbs on furniture and jumps off, obeys simple commands, and

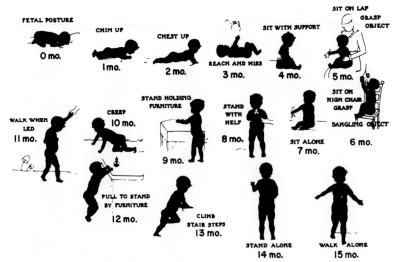

Figure 1.28. A general guide to the development of motor skills in a child. There is wide normal variation.

investigates objects of interest. He opens cupboards and drawers and begins to use simple sentences.

All such indications of timing are rough approximations and guides, not absolute rules.

Secondary Effects of Immobilization

Immobilization removes a child from an opportunity for learning experience. In addition, immobilization results in an adjustment of the muscles of the limb or trunk to a new fixed position.

This adjustment is termed "myostatic" contracture. It may be defined as the adaptation of an innervated muscle to a new functional length. Such a process cannot occur in a flail muscle without tone. It cannot occur in joint capsule or synovia that is in a normal state, except over a very prolonged period of time when the collagen fibers could become reoriented to new stresses. The principal cause for joint stiffness when a plaster cast is removed is the development of a myostatic contracture in the muscles.

There are no joint adhesions in the normal joint, although they may exist in the inflamed or diseased joint. Trauma and the development of edema inflammation and fibrin deposits in tendon sheaths, torn muscle bellies, and around joint capsules may aid this process.

The treatment of myostatic contracture is active exercise controlled by the patient. Passive stretching may tear tissues and compound the process. The treatment of limited motion at the elbow resulting in flexion contracture, for instance, is active flexion and extension of the elbow—not carrying a pail of water. This latter type of passive stretching results in a painful, still further limited elbow with muscle spasm.

Immobilization atrophy is not a loss of water in the muscle, but a total loss of muscle tissue, the relative percentage of water remaining the same.

Immobilization of the total patient results in a negative nitrogen balance, with loss of protein and mineral from the skeleton. Where the process is rapid, there may be secondary complications in areas such as the genitourinary tract.

JOINT STABILITY MAINTAINED BY ATMOSPHERIC PRESSURE**

There are a number of factors involved in the support of a human joint: ligaments, the

---

** This section, "Joint Stability Maintained by Atmospheric Pressure," is reprinted in part from K. Semlak and A. B. Ferguson, Jr.: Joint stability maintained by atmospheric pressure; an experimental study, *Clinical Orthopaedics, 68:* 294, 1970.

architectural shape of the joint, muscle pull, and atmospheric pressure. How great is the role of atmospheric pressure? We carried out a number of experiments in an attempt to accurately calculate this force in its role of aiding joint stability.

Human metacarpophalangeal joints and knees were subject to distraction to the point at which vaporization occurred in the joint and the effect of atmospheric pressure was neutralized. Determination of the force necessary to do this combined with the surface area of the joint made it possible to calculate the force of atmospheric pressure supporting the joint. It was shown that this force in an intact congruous joint is much larger than that necessary to stretch the joint ligaments.

Fluid Behavior

The syringe experimental model offers an opportunity to test the behavior of various types of fluids in both atmospheric pressure and partial vaccum without the complicating factors present in the joint. Synovial fluid has some of the physical properties of an aqueous solution, such as surface tension. To show that the plunger in the syringe is not held by surface tension alone, the following experiment was performed. The distraction force necessary to pull the plunger from the syringe creating a vapor phase was determined at atmospheric pressure for water, glycerin, liquid petrolatum, isopropyl alcohol, normal saline solution, and synovial fluid obtained from human knees where the effusion was due either to traumatic causes or degenerative arthritis. The same experiment was carried out in a vacuum jar, and the level of vaccum required to permit the plunger to fall from the syringe was determined for the above fluids. A fixed weight of 143 g/cm^2 was attached to the plunger. The results, shown in Table 1.1, indicate that, in its ability to initiate vaporization, synovial fluid most closely resembles pure water. Synovial fluid as an aqueous dialysate of plasma contains 2.5 g of plasma protein per 100 ml (about one-third as much as plasma), of which 60–75% is albumin, and about 0.36 g of hyaluronate per 100 ml. The forces needed to cause formation of a gas bubble inside the syringe when synovial fluid is used lie between the amount needed for an aqueous solution and that needed for an organic solution.

Table 1.1
Pressure effects on fluids

Substance	Pressure of distraction force at 20 C and 750 mm Hg	Vacuum required to cause distraction at weight of 143 g/cm^2 and 20 C*
	g/cm^2	mm Hg
H$_2$O	984	100
Glycerin	1010.5	92
Liquid petrolatum	948	103
Isopropyl alcohol	940	118
Normal saline solution (0.9%)	1010	102
Synovial fluid	965	96‡
	955	92‡

* All vacuum measurements are the averages from 3 experiments.

† Obtained from degenerative arthritis.

‡ Obtained from traumatic effusion.

Organic fluids with a lower heat of vaporization would be expected to distract with lower forces than required by water. However, the increased viscosity of these organic fluids and their decreased heat conductivity do affect the kinetics and reduce the rate of nucleation and growth of a gas bubble, thus leading to an expectation that the forces required would be quite similar to an aqueous solution.

It is apparent that atmospheric pressure forms an almost solid bar to distraction of the joint until it is overcome. Either considerable laxity of the walls or incongruity of the joint so that a seal cannot be obtained, the rapid appearance of increasing volumes of fluid, or communication with the atmosphere negates this affect. The failure of a vapor phase to appear in the synovial fluid marks this situation, and progressive distraction resisted solely by the soft tissues occurs (Figs. 1.29 and 1.30).

The amount of nitrogen, oxygen, and carbon dioxide dissolved in synovial fluid was calculated as 3.80 ml/100 ml from the partial pressures determined on 5 fluid samples. The small amounts of synovial fluid present in normal joints would not be sufficient to produce a gas bubble of 1–2 ml seen in these experiments. The vapor phase produced in

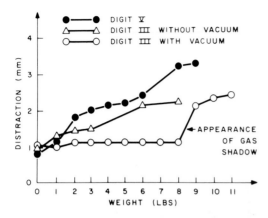

Figure 1.29. Distraction curve of the third and fifth metacarpophalangeal joints. Note the continuous distraction of the fifth metacarpophalangeal joint. The third metacarpophalangeal joint shows negligible distraction until the appearance of a vapor phase. Insertion of a needle into the metacarpophalangeal joint of the third finger gives a distraction curve illustrated by the *triangle*. With a vapor phase constantly in the joint, the soft tissues are the only resisting force to distraction.

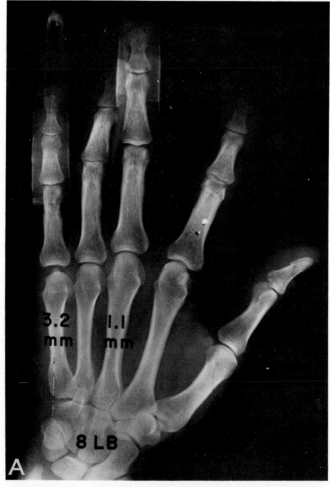

Figure 1.30. (*A*) The third and fifth metacarpophalangeal joints are under an 8-lb distraction force and the fifth distracts to 3.2 mm; the third is unaffected. (*B*) Increasing the force to 11 lb on the third metacarpophalangeal joint causes distraction to 2.8 mm with the formation of a gas bubble in the joint. (*C*) Inserting an open needle to the atmosphere and to the joint negates the effect.

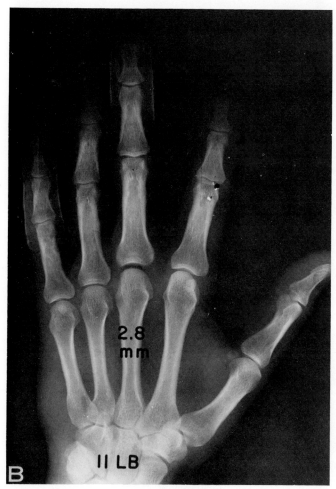

Figure 1.30B

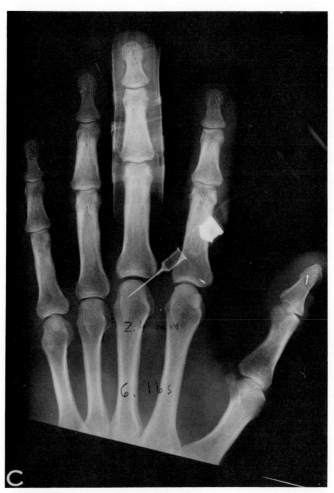

Figure 1.30 C

the joint by distraction disappeared quickly. Contrast air injected into a joint for arthrography usually remained for several days.

The initial nucleation apparently comes from gas in solution in synovial fluid. It must be augmented by the vapor phase of the fluid, however, to produce a bubble of the size seen.

Both the knee and metacarpophalangeal joint experiments detailed here reveal that if the joint is not effectively sealed against atmospheric pressure either by damage to its intact structure or by excess joint fluid, the distracting force is immediately thrown on the ligaments. The difference in the force necessary to distract the joint between a knee with an effusion and one without points out the considerable role that atmospheric pressure may play. In the experiment, a 5-kg force was all that was necessary to stretch the ligaments of a knee with a surface area of 50 cm^2 when it contained an effusion. This contrasts with a calculated value of a 60-kg force necessary to distract the intact joint.

Thus, a patient with a joint effusion has a greater risk of stretching his knee ligaments than a patient with a normal joint who has atmospheric pressure as a real force aiding stability. This may explain the development of ligamentous laxity in a joint with a chronic effusion.

Excess fluid or a readily available reservoir of fluid will negate the effect of atmospheric pressure by supplying additional fluid to eliminate the pressure on it and prevent vaporization. The vaporization is taken as a mark of the reality of force being exerted on the fluid rather than in itself a form of resistance. Women retaining fluid thus have available a reservoir to negate this effect. The effect is more evident in very congruous joints than in those with eccentric anatomic formation.

These experiments suggest that atmospheric pressure is an important force aiding joint stability and protecting ligaments from being overstretched.

References

1. Evans, W. A., Jr.: The roentgenological demonstration of the true articular space, *Am. J. Roentgenol.*, *43*: 860, 1940.
2. Fick, R.: *Anatomie and Mechanid der Gelenke.* Jena: G. Fischer, 1911.
3. Fuiks, D. M., and Grayson, C. H.: Vacuum pneumoarthrography and spontaneous occurrence of the gas in the joint spaces, *J. Bone Joint Surg.*, *32A;* 933, 1950.
4. Gerschow, C. I.: Internal derangement of the knee joint; the diagnostic scope of soft tissue roentgenogram examination and the vacuum technique demonstration of the meniscus, *Am. J. Roentgenol.*, *54:* 338, 1945.

CHILDHOOD AMPUTEES

In discussing childhood amputees, one includes not only those children with traumatic loss of a limb or a segment of it, but those with congenital conditions that either primarily or secondarily require a prosthetic appliance and training for maximal function. There has been a great increase in the amount of function that can be achieved for children with an amputation through improved equipment, increased knowledge, and better training.

The child is a unit in a family situation, and the orthopaedist must recognize that rehabilitation can be achieved for the child only if the family supports and desires it. Unless the family wants prosthetic restoration of a limb and increased function for the child, the program will fail. So much depends on guidance by the family that if it is lacking the child will not use the prosthetic device and will fail to develop skill in its use. The family must be educated along with the child.

The amputee clinic for the child includes among its personnel the orthopaedic surgeon, the physical therapist, the occupational therapist, the prosthetist, and the medical social worker. Following up treated patients and finding untreated ones depends on the skill of the social worker, without whose work the program will fall short of its objectives.

Children grow as adults do not, and the level of proficiency achieved varies among the different age groups. In setting goals the physical therapist, occupational therapist, and surgeon must bear in mind the child's age, future problems, and development.

JUVENILE AMPUTATIONS AND CONGENITAL LIMB DEFICIENCIES

Juvenile amputees include children with congenital limb deficiencies and those with acquired amputations for trauma, tumor, or other disease. They need long term care and concern, and their problems fall properly in the orthopaedic field. Fortunately, knowledge, equipment, and techniques are constantly improving and provide increasingly better function for these patients. All orthopaedists should be familiar with current principles of good treatment and stay aware of the new developments in this changing area.

How many juvenile amputees are there in the United States? We have some statistics available from the 31 participating clinics in the National Research Council's Cooperative Child Amputee Research Program. During 1972 the clinics saw 644 new patients, an average of 20 per year for each clinic.[12] Of these, 66% had congenital problems. Several years ago two large clinics saw congenital problems reflect increased local care of children with uncomplicated acquired amputations outside of regional clinics; this means that the absolute number of new amputees per year is probably even greater than that shown by clinic statistics.

Acquired Amputations

About 35–45% of all juvenile amputations are acquired.[5] Trauma causes approximately 70% of these, and power tools (including farm machines), vehicular accidents, and gunshots or explosions are almost equally responsible.

The most common nontraumatic cause of amputation in children is tumor; the most common childhood malignant tumor of the extremities is osteogenic sarcoma. Vascular and neurogenic disease or malformation are the most common other diseases that can require amputation. About 70% of all acquired amputations are of the lower extremity, and most of these are below the knee.

SURGICAL PRINCIPLES

The severity and extent of trauma usually dictate the amputation level that it causes, but there are some general principles that can apply to both traumatic and surgical amputations in children.

A. Save all length possible, whether lower or upper extremity. The greater the length, the greater the proprioception and the longer the lever arm for control of the prosthesis.

Use skin grafts if necessary to preserve length. Today's prosthetic fabrication techniques for plastic total contact sockets allow comfortable weight bearing with some relief of grafted skin and few breakdown problems.

Open amputations for markedly contaminated wounds or very short stumps are feasible to preserve length and prevent infection. Skin traction and frequent dressing changes in the first postoperative week provide a good granulating surface suitable for grafting.

B. Save epiphysis whenever possible, for two reasons: to preserve length (and assure adequate length after growth) and to prevent the complication of bony overgrowth, which is very common after section of a long bone in children. The contributions of the various epiphyses to growth are shown in Tables 1.2 and 1.3.

C. If section of a long bone is necessary, avoid stripping periosteum of the portion of the bone which will remain; to do so will allow the raised periosteal remnants to produce irregular new bone growth, which will be painful under a prosthesis, and may cause a ring sequestrum if circumferential.

D. It is better not to use techniques of myodesis which require drilling near the bone end; the drilled holes may increase the tendency to bony overgrowth.

E. Handle nerves with care and do the least possible amount of trauma to them. Pull

Table 1.2
Epiphyseal growth contributions

Epiphysis	Contribution	
	Proximal	Distal
	%	%
Humerus	80	20
Radius	20	80
Ulna	25	75
Femur	30	70
Fibula	60	40
Tibia	55	45

Table 1.3
Contribution to total lower extremity growth by individual epiphyses

Epiphysis	Contribution
	%
Proximal femur	10
Distal femur	40
Proximal tibia	30
Distal tibia	20

them gently distally and cut sharply with one stroke of a fresh scalpel blade, allowing them to retract from the scar area. Attempts to reduce neuroma formation by injection, ligation, or banding have all proved to increase scarring and are no longer believed to be good practice. Vessels on larger nerves, such as the sciatic and the tibial, may be dissected free and clamped or ligated separately.

F. Remember that rigid dressing immediately postoperatively, according to the principles detailed by Burgess et al.,[8, 9] can markedly decrease edema formation and speed healing. This dressing is as appropriate in children as in adults. (See further discussion below.)

SURGICAL TECHNIQUES

The details of the operative procedures are covered well in *Campbell's Operative Orthopaedics*[11] and the July 1972 issue of *Orthopaedic Clinics of North America.*[25] These are as applicable to children as adults, bearing in mind the principles outlined above.

COMPREHENSIVE CARE PRINCIPLES

A. Rigid Dressing. Casting in the operating room immediately after amputation (with sterile lambswool distally, then elastic plaster over a spandex stump sock, padded with felt or foam to relieve bony prominences, reinforced with standard plaster, and suspended from a waist or shoulder belt) will prevent the development of edema and has proved far superior to "conventional" elastic wrapping for below-knee stumps.[22] It is also applicable to upper extremity amputations. The techniques are more complicated and the results less easy to achieve with above-knee stumps or proximal disarticulations.

A pylon attachment for standing may be added immediately or deferred for 1 or 2 weeks and applied after a cast change reveals the wound to be healing well. A report on the use of semi-rigid unna paste dressings has been published,[20] but we have no long term experience with it. It appears promising for such difficult to cast areas as above-elbow and above-knee stumps.

B. Exercise Program and Stump Care. No matter what stump dressing and weight-bearing routine is followed, an exercise program taught and encouraged daily by a physical therapist is essential. The program should be taught preoperatively if possible so that postoperatively it is familiar and will be easier in spite of discomfort. It should include active strengthening exercises to the unaffected extremities and active range of motion exercises to the stump, followed by strengthening as healing allows. Walking should begin in parallel bars and progress to crutches, whether or not partial weight bearing in a pylon cast is allowed.

Flexion contractures occur easily at the hip, shoulder, and knee and interfere with the fitting and use of a prosthesis. Once present they are difficult to get rid of; it is far better to prevent them instead. Postoperative elevation of the bed in Trendelenberg position is better than using pillows to decrease edema. Pillows under below-knee stumps can allow the knee to flex and should be discouraged. Wheelchairs for below-knee amputees should have an extension board under the affected limb to keep the knee straight. All lower extremity amputees should spend several half-hours each day lying prone to prevent hip flexion contractures. Active range of motion exercises for the involved shoulder should be begun early for the upper extremity amputee. External rotation and abduction of the stump should be discouraged in above-knee amputees.

Stump wrapping with elastic bandages is an important part of an amputee's self-care and must be taught to the child or his parents. Even those patients dressed initially with a rigid cast must begin stump wrapping when the cast is discontinued. Wrapping is an art which must be practiced so that the compression is always greatest distally and gradually decreases proximally with no proximal constriction. This means that below-knee stump wrapping must be carried above the knee, because suspension of a wrap that ends below the knee depends on tightness proximally, producing constriction. An above-knee stump wrapping must be carried around the waist in a spica for the same reasons. Few individuals can wrap a stump well, but those involved with amputee care should learn. A new stump must always be wrapped when the prosthesis is not on, and rewrapped when the bandages slide or curl at the edges (several times a day, at least). After 6 months to 1 year, the stump will no longer swell when out of the prosthesis, and wrapping may be discontinued.

C. Skin Care. The skin on the stump needs to be kept clean and dry. Sometimes patients and family have a disturbing tendency to treat the wrapped limb as something apart from the patient, to be surprised that it needs to be washed, and to be shocked that they will be expected to wrap it themselves. Occasionally nurses also suffer the same misconceptions, but on a well organized orthopaedic floor with good communication among doctors, nurses, and patients this should not remain a problem for long.

Both stump and prosthetic socket should be washed daily with soap and water and dried thoroughly. Dry skin is the best defense against bacterial invasion. Skin softeners are not necessary and may predispose to maceration and superficial infection. Occasionally an area of skin subject to pressure is slow to develop the thickened keratin layer it needs, and some patients have found that patting the area with wet tea bags and allowing it to dry is helpful. It may be the tannic acid in the tea that produces the desired effects; it is, at least, not harmful.

Specific Skin Problems. (1) *Reactive hyperemia.* Reddening of the skin, particularly in the areas of pressure, subsides with time as the skin adapts; both the keratin layer and the living skin layers increase in thickness. (2) *Stump edema syndrome.* Later development of reactive hyperemia (beyond the initial prosthetic training period) may progress to a serous ooze with some capillary rupture. Treatment: stop wearing prosthesis, wrap with elastic bandages, and elevate. (3) *Contact dermatitis.* This may be a primary irritation or an allergy. The first is due to a substance which is itself an irritant (soap, turpentine). Some patients use such substances in an effort to toughen the skin or clean it. Allergic reactions are due to a substance to which the patient has been exposed and become allergic. Common allergens for amputees are nickel, chrome, polyester resins, lacquer, dyes, and antioxidants used in foam rubber. In all these cases the dermatitis is limited to the area of contact, which helps in the identification of the offending agent. (4) *Epidermoid cysts.* Usually occurring at or near the brim of the socket, they appear at points of rolling friction, pushing keratin fragments into the dermis; they rarely occur if the prosthesis is well fitted and well aligned. Treatment: stop wearing the prosthesis, incise and drain or excise the cyst, realign and fit the prosthesis. (5) *Pyogenic infections.* (a) Folliculitis: superficial; usually occurs early with wearing of a new prosthesis. Treatment: an antibiotic ointment or lotion. (b) Furuncles: treat as elsewhere with incision and drainage. (c) Hidradenitis: infection in the apocrine sweat glands, in the axilla and groin; these glands empty into the hair follicles, secrete slowly and with thick secretion; infections of them are deep seated and difficult to treat, sometimes requiring wide excision and skin grafting. (6) *Fungal infections.* These infections usually occur in the groin and more often in fat people, whose skin is less dry than that of thin people. As amputees have loss of heat-radiating surface, they begin to sweat at lower temperatures, and wet intertriginous areas predispose to these infections. They are characteristically patches of red scaly dermatitis which enlarge and clear in the center. Treatment: Griseofulvin orally. *Candida albicans* infection typically produces red, moist, oozing skin, with small pimples at the periphery with candida yeast spores present in the pus. This occurs frequently in diabetics and obese patients. Treatment: topical Nystatin. (7) *Tumors.* Warts, keratoses, etc., under a prosthesis can produce painful pressure points and should be removed if they do. All suspicious nodules should, of course, be biopsied.

Teaching the parents the details of stump care and exercise programs and allowing them to help the therapist before discharge of the patient will help ensure success of the program at home.

D. Psychologic Support. Children having to undergo amputation have a great deal of adjustment to make before they can come eventually to acceptance. Most go though a denial-anger—depression-bargaining-acceptance cycle similar to that described in dying or grieving people,[19] although the phases or the cycle are not always equally evident or in the same order. Some patients have to accept both the fact of an amputation and that of having a malignancy and an uncertain future. They need help with this; someone must be able to listen, to offer answers to the many questions, and to understand when the anger comes out in words and actions. Fear is worse when it is of things unknown, and knowing in advance some details of the dressing, the exercising, and the fitting of the prosthesis can help a patient make the fear manageable. Experienced nurses can be very helpful in this area; we have at times been lucky enough to have available a nurse clinical specialist who has more time available than the floor nurses or the doctors and who spends it with these patients and their families, to the benefit of all. The details of management can be frightening to the patient if given too soon or at a time when he is worrying about something else, and all of those who care (in all senses) for these patients must be alert for the signs that show when they need to talk and about what. Reviewing current material on dying and grief reactions[19] is worthwhile.

PROSTHETIC FITTING

A. Timing. If long term follow-up is not to be done by the primary surgeon, early consultation with an appropriate physician is necessary. If immediate postoperative ambulation with the cast-pylon technique is planned, the prosthetist or a physician experienced with the technique should be present at the time of the amputation to apply the cast.

If there is any doubt about the potential healing of the stump (e.g., if the amputation was done for ischemia), it may be best to delay weight bearing.[22] A rigid dressing is still useful, and the wound may be checked at 1 week or 10 days. If the wound is healing well, a second cast can be applied with a weight-bearing pylon attached, or a mold for an intermediate prosthesis may be taken by the prosthetist. The intermediate ("temporary") limb has a plastic total-contact socket with a modular adjustable pylon attached; it may be covered with cosmetic foam. It can usually be made in less than 1 week, and in the interim the stump may be recast (and will remain the same size) or elastic wrapping may be begun (with the advantage of continued stump shrinkage and usually perfect fit with a stump sock).

The permanent prosthesis can be made when the stump is no longer shrinking noticeably and there are no areas of palpable edema. The further, slower shrinkage of the stump which occurs over 6–8 months can be accommodated for by adding 3- or 5-ply wool stump socks as necessary. A child requires a new prosthesis because of growth or

wear every 18 months on the average, but in the first year after amputation the time may be closer to every 6 or 8 months. Upper extremity prostheses need replacement less frequently because length requirements are less precise than for lower extremities.

Some physicians delay prosthetic fitting of patients with malignant tumors for an arbitrary number of months after amputation or omit it altogether if a metastasis is present. Statistics show that patients with metastases use a prosthesis for an average of 1 year, and many longer.[5] Now that fitting and fabrication techniques take only 1 or 2 weeks and inpatient gait training another week, denying a prosthesis and the independence it allows to any patient seems totally unjustified.

B. Prosthetic Prescription. Prescription is legally and traditionally the sole responsibility of the physician, but the advice of experienced prosthetists and therapists can be invaluable. Each case of acquired amputation is individual and has its own particular considerations. Current laminated sockets, fabricated over a mold of the stump, allow total contact, which distributes pressure evenly. These are more comfortable and more efficient than the previously used open-ended sockets. Following is a list of the most frequently used prostheses for each level of amputation and some of the options follows.

Lower Extremity
1. Hemipelvectomy: Plastic total-contact socket with Canadian hip joint, single-axis knee, and SACH (solid-ankle-cushion-heel) foot.
2. Hip disarticulation (Fig. 1.31): Same as above.
3. Above-knee (Fig. 1.32): Quadrilateral total-contact socket; may be suction; may be used with hip joint and pelvic belt or a Silesian belt. May use single-axis, constant-friction knee joint or hydraulic knee unit; SACH foot.
4. Through-knee: Knee disarticulartion-type plastic total-contact socket, with entrance panel for molded suspension, or the new silastic air-pocket "diaphragm" suspension: SACH foot.
5. Below-knee (Fig. 1.33): Patellar-tendon bearing (PTB) total-contact socket with either cuff or wedge suspension; SACH foot. Occasionally knee joint side hinges and thigh lacer may be necessary, but the

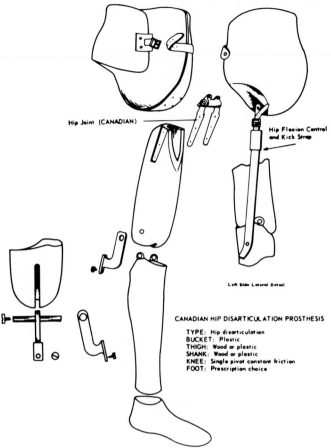

Figure 1.31. Hip disarticulation prosthesis, Canadian type.

Hip Joint (CANADIAN)

Hip Flexion Control
and Kick Strap

Left Side Lateral Detail

CANADIAN HIP DISARTICULATION PROSTHESIS

TYPE: Hip disarticulation
BUCKET: Plastic
THIGH: Wood or plastic
SHANK: Wood or plastic
KNEE: Single pivot constant friction
FOOT: Prescription choice

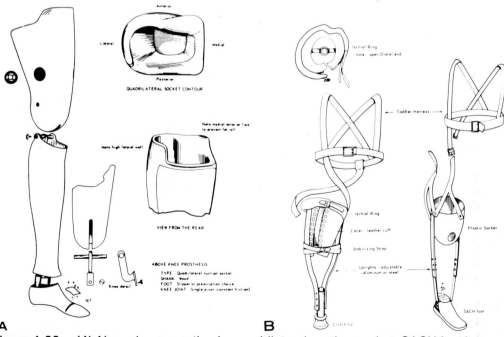

Anterior

Lateral — Medial

Posterior

QUADRILATERAL SOCKET CONTOUR

Note medial anterior lips
to prevent fat roll

Note high lateral wall

VIEW FROM THE REAR

ABOVE KNEE PROSTHESIS

TYPE: Quadrilateral suction socket
SHANK: Wood
FOOT: Slipper or prescription choice
KNEE JOINT: Single pivot (constant friction)

Knee detail

Ischial Ring
note open Distal end

Toddler Harness

Ischial Ring

Lacer: leather cuff

Stabilizing Strap

Uprights adjustable
(aluminum or steel)

Plastic Socket

SACH foot

Crutch tip

A   B

Figure 1.32. (A) Above-knee prosthesis, quadrilateral suction socket; SACH foot is now preferred. (B) The toddler's harness for the early walker.

32

thigh lacer has the disadvantage of usually producing quadriceps atrophy.

6. Symes (Fig. 1.34) socket with front, side, or back entrance panel: Of the new and promising (and more cosmetic) silastic air panel suspension.

7. Partial foot: Shoe fillers, some attached to molded heel and ankle sockets.

Upper Extremity

1. Shoulder disarticulation and forequarter amputation: Molded shoulder cap and extension over opposite shoulder; or a chest-strap harness; shoulder hinge with motion in two planes to allow for dressing, abducting over chair arm, etc.; mechanical or motorized aids can improve operation of elbow flexion or elbow lock. (Terminal devices will be discussed separately below.)

2. Above-elbow (Fig. 1.35): Total-contact plastic socket with figure-of-eight harness, positive locking elbow (with 11 locking positions and turntable to allow internal and external rotation—without the humeral condyles, shoulder rotation cannot be transferred to the prosthesis).

3. Elbow disarticulation: Same as for above-elbow, but the currently available outside locking hinges have only 7 locking positions available, as opposed to the 11 of the more bulky "inside" positive locking elbows, and are not as durable.

4. Below-elbow (Fig. 1.46): Total-contact double-wall plastic socket, with figure-8 or single loop (figure-9) harness, triceps cuff, single pivot hinges, and constant-friction wrist unit. Polycentric hinges allow more antecubital space; multiple-action or step-up hinges allow more flexion for a very short stump, when used with a split socket. It is more common to use a preflexed socket to achieve full flexion with a very short stump. A triceps *pad* (smaller than cuff) and flexible hinges allow pronation and supination if the stump is long enough; 50% of available rotation of a forearm stump is lost in the harnessing, therefore only long below-elbow stumps will have enough useful rotation to take advantage of flexible hinges.

5. "Muenster" below-elbow socket: A molded supracondylar fit with olecranon-notch molding (Fig. 1.37); for very short below-elbow stumps; eliminates separate

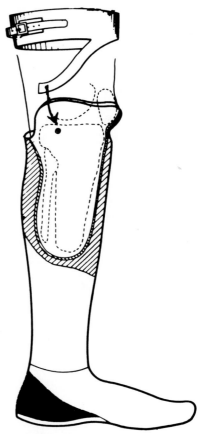

Figure 1.33. Below-knee prosthesis, patellar tendon-bearing type (PTB), with cuff suspension and SACH foot.

suspension and only harnessing necessary if for cable control of the terminal device. Does limit flexion to about 90°.

6. Wrist disarticulartion: Fitted as for a long below-elbow stump; an oval constant-friction wrist is available that can be laminated into the socket more easily and takes slightly less room than the standard below-elbow constant-friction wrist unit.

7. Partial hand: There are no really useful partial hand prostheses at present; surgical reconstruction of pinch and grasp is necessary.

8. Harnessing: As described above, a cable is anchored to the harness and the prosthesis so that the body motions of shoulder flexion and scapular abduction (when necessary) will exert tension on the cable and open the terminal device; the first part of these motions will cause a second cable to flex the elbow and lock it for an above-

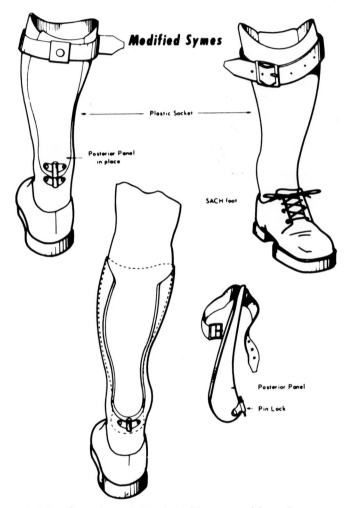

Figure 1.34. Syme's prosthesis, with removable entrance panel.

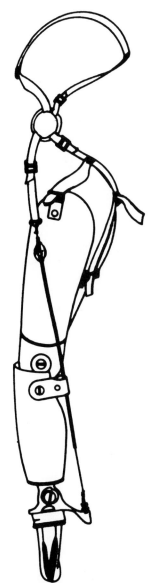

Figure 1.35. Above-elbow prosthesis, with figure-8 harness, standard positive locking elbow, and hook terminal device.

elbow amputee. Voluntary-opening terminal devices close by rubber bands about the bases of the fingers of the device, exerting about 1 lb of pressure per rubber band.

9. Other wrist units. *Flexion*: Necessary only with bilateral upper extremity amputations to bring one terminal device close to the body. *Quick-change*: Useful for those who wear both a hook terminal device and a cosmetic hand; allows easy one-handed change.

10. Terminal devices: All available for children are voluntary-opening devices. Voluntary-closing devices are available for adolescents and adults and are useful for those activities requiring more precise regulation of pinch force.

11. Standard adult terminal devices, suitable for adolescents:

   Dorrance 5: Stainless steel; weight, 7 oz.

   Dorrance 5X (Fig. 1.38): Same, with Neoprene lining of fingers for better prehension.

   Dorrance 5XA: Same as 5X in aluminum; weight, 3 oz.

   Dorrance 7 (Fig. 1.39): "Farmer's hook" stainless steel; weight, 8 oz. Adapted for nail, knife, and tool holding.

12. Smaller devices, suitable for children:

   Dorrance 8: Weight is 5¾ oz, otherwise equivalent to Dorrance 5.

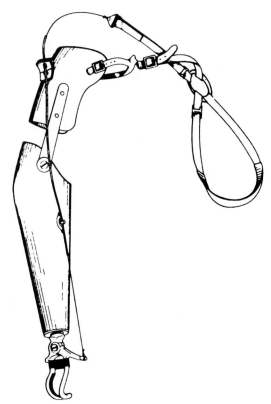

Figure 1.36. Below-elbow prosthesis standard, with triceps cuff, single-pivot hinges, and hook terminal device.

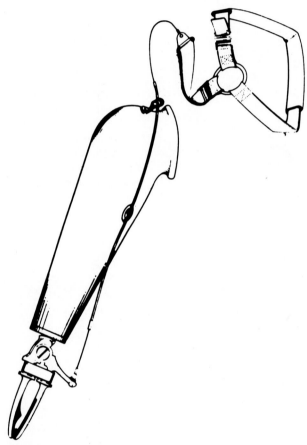

Figure 1.37. Below-elbow prosthesis, Muenster type, with figure-9 harness for cable control of terminal device.

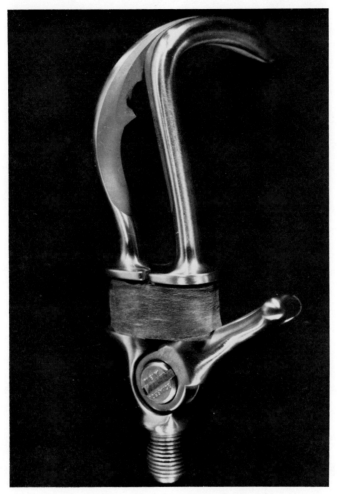

Figure 1.38. Dorrance 5X terminal device.

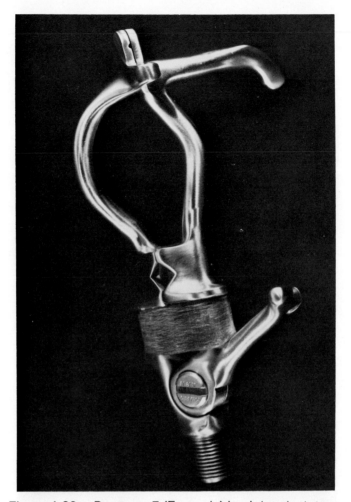

Figure 1.39. Dorrance 7 (Farmer's) hook terminal device.

Dorrance 8X: Weight is 5¾ oz, equivalent to Dorrance 5X.

Dorrance 88X: Aluminum; weight 2⅓ oz, equivalent to 5XA: 4⅜ inches long; suitable for ages 10–14 years.

Dorrance 99X (Fig. 1.40): Aluminum; weight, 2 oz, 3⅜ inches long; suitable for ages 3–6 years.

Dorrance 10P: Plastisol-covered fingers; 3½ inches long; weight, 3 oz; for 3–6 years.

Dorrance 12P: Plastisol-covered fingers; 2¾ inches long; weight, 2 oz; steel; for 1–4 years.

Plastic mitt: 2¼ inches long; weight 2 oz; useful for 6 months to 1 year.

Myoelectric prostheses are now in the experimental stages, and will probably become the most useful prostheses in the near future when they are perfected. They operate by utilizing action potentials of the remaining muscles of the stump to activate a controller switch which allows a battery to supply power to the prosthesis.

TRAINING

A. Lower Extremity. Gait training should be begun by an experienced physical therapist on a daily schedule. Inpatient training for several days is best because the patient's early efforts can be supervised and awkward body movements changed before they become bad habits. The limb should be delivered to the training facility after final fitting for check out by the physician or therapist according to a protocol. If training is to be outpatient, the limb should not go home with the patient until both he and his parents are familiar with the correct gait pattern.

Ambulation begins in parallel bars and progresses usually to crutches, then to one or two canes, and then to independence. Training should include steps (with and without railings), ramps, rough ground, and falling and getting up again while wearing the prosthesis.

It is helpful to keep in mind the normal progression of gait in childhood, from toddling at about 1 year to an adult heel-toe pattern at about age 5 years. The gait sought with an artificial limb should be kept appropriate to the child's age. Children can usually

be taught to use crutches at about age 3; younger children can toddle independently, in a sling walker or around furniture.

B. Upper Extremity. This training should also be done daily, by an experienced physical therapist or occupational therapist; it can be accomplished within about a week for a unilateral amputee old enough to cooperate well. Training periods for children are limited by their attention span, which has been estimated at *1 min* for each year of age. At the present time initial training with a hook type of terminal device is highly recommended and is actually a rule in some clinics, even for patients who are sure (or whose parents are sure) they will only accept a cosmetic hand. Functional hand prostheses are currently far

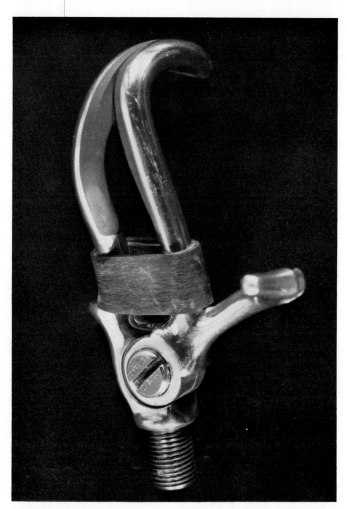

Figure 1.40. Dorrance 99X terminal device. Note scale compared to Figure 1.38; wrist-connect threaded units are the same size.

from satisfactory—their action is less precise, and they are far less durable. Even appearance-conscious adolescents usually use a hook at school and work and a hand only for social events, if at all (Fig. 1.41).

Training is mainly work on the body control motions necessary to activate the terminal device (below-elbow) and the elbow flexion and lock (above-elbow). Patients with shoulder disarticulations or forequarter amputations need work on breathing exercises as well to increase chest expansion and decrease the energy expenditure necessary for operation of the limb.

Both child and parents should learn how to watch for impending skin and fit problems. Some children show a distressing tendency to gain weight rapidly after amputation; the parents must understand that rapid changes in weight will affect prosthetic fit and attention to careful diet may be necessary.

LONG TERM FOLLOW-UP

Children with amputations should be followed every 3 or 4 months at a minimum until growth is complete. The average time between new prostheses is 18 months but during growth spurts may be much less. Limb lengthening without fabrication of a whole new prosthesis is necessary an average of every 6 months.

Overgrowth is a common complication after transverse section of a growing long bone, occurring in 16% of Dr. Aitken's cases.[1] It is appositional new bone laid down distally, and epiphyseodesis will not prevent or halt it. The only treatment is stump revision when the prosthesis is no longer comfortable, and this may have to be repeated several times. Although overgrowth is not epiphyseal, once skeletal maturity is reached, overgrowth stops. It occurs most frequently in humerus, fibula, and tibia, in that order.

Follow-up is best done in a children's amputee clinic, staffed by a physician (orthopaedist, physiatrist, or pediatrician), certified prosthetist(s), physical therapists, occupational therapists, and social worker; frequently the staff includes a nurse-specialist and a psychologist or psychiatrist.[20] The presence of all these people together allows easy exchange of information and evaluation of the patient from the various points of view.

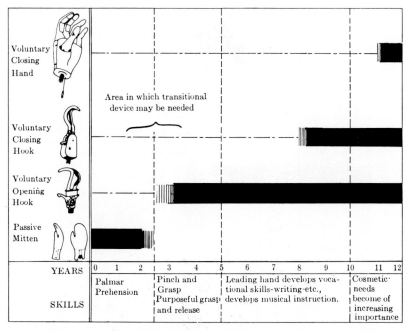

Figure 1.41. This chart, showing the development of prehension by age, helps in the fitting of terminal devices for upper extremity prostheses. (From G. T. Aiken and C. F. Frantz: Management of the child amputee, Instructional Course Lecturer; American Academy of Orthopaedic Surgeons, 1960.)

Another advantage is the chance children and parents have to see and know others with similar problems.

Congenital Limb Deficiencies

About 60% of all juvenile amputees are the result of congenital limb deficiencies; about 70% of these are upper extremity problems. About one-third of congenital limb-deficient patients have more than one limb involved, and 10% are quadrimembral (Fig. 1.42).[5]

The term "congenital amputee" is an inaccurate but shorter way to speak of children with congenital limb anomalies. True congenital amputations, usually due to a constricting band with a developed but gangrenous or separated limb present, are very rare. However, failure of the limbs to develop occurs in many various ways, most of which can be best treated prosthetically and managed as amputees whether or not they have in fact had an amputation.

CLASSIFICATION

The variety of forms of developmental limb anomalies makes classification necessary for better communication. There have been in the past many classification systems in use simultaneously and without international agreement. In 1975, a 17-member international committee presented its recommendations for a new international terminology,[15,16,18] which has been included by the World Health Organization in its revision of standard nomenclature.

In this system, deficiencies are classified as *transverse* or *longitudinal.* The transverse deficiencies are those in which *all* elements distal to a particular level are missing; they are labeled T- (with L or R added to designate left or right limb) and the level at which the limb terminates is named. For example, "T-L, Fo, upper ⅓" indicates a left short-below-elbow-equivalent stump.

The longitudinal deficiencies are all those other than transverse and are labeled L/, with L or R added. All *missing* skeletal elements are named, using two-letter abbreviations, with "total" or "partial" added as necessary. The term "ray" may be used to refer to metacarpal or metatarsal and all of its corresponding phalanges. Thus, a left radial "club-

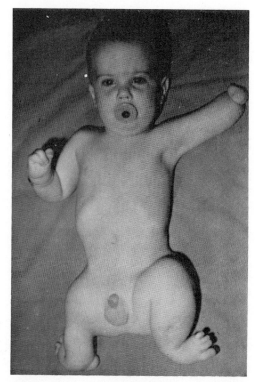

Figure 1.42. Many problems for rehabilitation exist for a child with multiple anomalies of the upper and lower extremities.

hand" with two missing radial digits is "L/L Ra total, Ca [carpal] partial, Rays 1,2."

As it will take several years for this nomenclature to become widely used, and we are following patients whose deficiencies have been classified with the older systems, a review of Burtch's revision[10] of Frantz and O'Rahilly's classification[13] will be useful. In clinical practice, the terms amelia, phonomelia, and PFFD (proximal femoral focal deficiency) will probably continue to be used. However, a good understanding and consistent use of the new nomenclature in charting are a necessity for accurate record keeping, documentation of incidence, and better care of patients.

TREATMENT PRINCIPLES

Aitken and Lambert[5] emphasized that the major problems which may be presented by upper extremity anomalies are (1) loss of prehension, (2) lack of promimal power and stability, (3) difficulty with hand placement due to limitation of proximal joint motion, (4) malrotation, and (5) severe length inequalities. Problems of lower extremity anomalies are (1) severe length inequalities, (2) instability impairing weight bearing, and (3) malalignment.

These problems will be present in varying degrees in individual cases but must be evaluated and accommodated for in some way. Current plastic fabricating techniques allow the fitting of nonstandard prostheses; these are most successful when the *most distal stable* joint in the limb is identified and everything distal to it is treated as stump for purposes of fitting. This identification of the joint with the most useful range of motion and adequate motor power allows prescription as for an amputation above or below the knee or elbow; the anomalous limb becomes an amputation homologue.

Timing of prosthetic fitting should be based on consideration of normal developmental patterns. As far as possible a child should progress through his motor and social skills at appropriate ages, and, if he needs a prosthesis to do so, that is the best indication for fitting.

At 6 months of age, the average child begins to creep and sit; he also begins to use palmar grasp for objects. At 8 or 9 months he is pulling up to stand, and is using a "3-jaw-chuck" finger grasp. At 1 year he can stand unsupported and has mastered release of objects held in his hand. Exploring his world by crawling, standing, and reaching is necessary for his mental and social development. A child with a severe leg length inequality needs a prosthesis when he begins to stand. If he has a lower extremity amelia severe enough to impair his sitting balance, he needs to be fitted with a plastic "bucket" to sit in, at 6 months or younger. Early fitting of upper extremity prostheses, even with nongrasping "mitten" hands, allows normal crawling patterns, and normal two-handed examination of objects at arm's length. Also, the earlier that children are fitted the sooner they become accustomed to the harnessing, and the artificial limb becomes incorporated in their own body image.

Development of motor power and coordination allows modification of the initial prosthesis at an appropriate time, such as a cable-activated terminal device at 12–18 months. An elbow lock control cannot usually be operated before about 3 years of age, and before that time a constant-friction passive joint is used. At 2–3 years of age an above-knee prosthesis can be articulated at the knee; normally knee flexion patterns are not present in a child's gait before this age. Timing of these steps must depend on evaluation of the individual child and his progress in development, as most children are not "average."

SURGICAL "CONVERSION"

Amputation of part of an anomalous limb may be thought of as "surgical conversion" to a more standard amputation stump. In lower extremity anomalies, it may be necessary to allow proper weight-bearing function of the limb and a better gait. In upper extremities, it is almost never indicated because all portions of the limb may be useful to the child for tactile sensation and examination of objects without a prosthesis, *and* almost any movable part, however small, can be utilized to push a switch, pull a lock, etc., to conserve energy in the use of a prosthesis. For these reasons primary surgical conversion is not recommended in the upper extremity. In large clinics approximately 50% of anomalous lower extremities require surgical conversion, but in most cases this is not done until after fitting around the original has proved inadequate. There are probably only three congenital lower extremity problems whose usual life history is well enough known to make primary surgical conversion an accepted method of treatment. These are proximal femoral focal deficiency, fibular meromelia, and tibial meromelia; they will be discussed in greater detail below.

SPECIFIC CONGENITAL ANOMALIES

A. Proximal Femoral Focal Deficiency (PFFD). In the past 15 years much work has been done to differentially diagnose and classify this problem, which is not uncommon. It may be difficult to distinguish at birth from infantile or congenital coxa vera, or "congenital short femur" of another etiology. In 1967, Aitken[4] presented a classification which allows consideration of the natural history of each type and treatments appropriate for each.

The classification is based on radiologic

findings. Clinically the patients all present with a shortened, flexed, and externally rotated thigh; in some instances the shortening is such that the foot on the affected side is at the level of the opposite knee.

In Classes A and B, both an adequate acetabulum and a femoral head are present, with a short femoral segment. Initially there is no connection between the femoral shaft and head, but at maturity in Class A there is bony connection, usually with subtrochanteric varus and occasionally with a pseudarthrosis. In Class B there is never any bony connection between head and shaft, and probably no cartilaginous connection.

In Classes C and D, there is no femoral head, and the acetabulum is severely dysplastic or absent. In Class C, an ossified tuft is present at the proximal end of the short femoral shaft; in Class D this is absent.

These classes (and some of the conditions with which PFFD may be confused clinically) may not be clear radiologically until age 6 months or 1 year.

Treatment usually involves a combination of surgery and prosthetic treatment. Initially a platform brace may be fitted to equalize leg lengths, but this is usually an awkward and ugly appliance; a nonstandard prosthesis fitted over the foot with the foot in equinus may be better. A modified Syme's amputation (ankle disarticulation with Syme's flap) simplifies future fitting and eliminates the unsightly anterior bulge of a prosthesis fitted over the foot.

Arthrodesis of the knee can stabilize the lever arm of the limb and considerably reduce the limp. King has shown that this can be done as early as 3–4 years of age; if done carefully and stabilized with a Küntscher rod, the epiphyses remain open and continue to contribute to needed length.[4,14]

Stabilization or reconstruction about the hip can only be useful in Classes A and B and is not uniformly successful. Attempts at hip fusion have not been successful.

Rotation osteotomies of the tibia through 180°, to allow the foot to be fitted as a below-knee stump, have been found by Van Nes[28] to yield good results. Their disadvantages and a high incidence of derotation with growth and the need to use a platform brace to preserve the foot until the patient is large enough to have the operation.

In cases of bilateral PFFD consideration should be given to preserving the feet (without rotation) so that around the house the patient may ambulate without prostheses. Knee arthrodesis in these cases is also believed to interfere with independent (nonprosthetic) ambulation.

B. Fibular Meromelia. This deficiency is one of the most frequent congenital limb deformities and often occurs with other anomalies (for instance, it is seen in more than 50% of all patients with PF). The major problem it presents is leg length discrepancy, which is progressive. Kruger[3] found that this discrepancy was, unfortunately, greater in those patients who retained a normal foot (intercalary deficiency) and less in those with terminal deficiencies and only a partial foot remaining. Many of these patients have associated shortening of the ipsilateral femur; the tibia is also frequently bowed anteriorly at the junction of the middle and distal thirds; both of these problems increase the leg length discrepancy.

Modified Syme amputation (as described above, or fusing the os calcis and attached heel pad to the distal tibia) offers many advantages to these patients, e.g., the avoidance of multiple osteotomies, lengthening procedures, and procedures to stabilize the ankle, and the better cosmesis of a prosthesis compared to a plateform brace (Fig. 1.43).

Keeping the heel pad correctly located after a Syme's amputation is a difficult problem in a growing child. The use of a Steinman pin through the pad into the tibia and a well molded cast for 6 weeks postoperatively is helpful.

C. Tibial Meromelia. This deficiency is less common; it may be partial or complete and may be associated with distal reduplication (the only reduction deformity documented to do this). It is also known to occur in siblings and in more than one generation of the same family, often with a familial incidence of clawhand deformities as well.

The fibular head lies more proximal than normally and is lateral and posterior at the knee. Clinically the patients present with a flexed knee and varus foot; the foot may be complete (intercalary deficit) or incomplete, and associated tarsal anomalies are common.

As leg length discrepancy in the unilateral cases precludes normal use of the foot, it cannot usually be preserved. Achievement of a useful knee, to be fitted with a below-knee prosthesis, can sometimes be accomplished by centralization of the proximal fibula. Myers[23] in 1905 published one of the first reports of this operation, with a 5-year follow-up, but it was Brown[6,7] who reintroduced it. Brown and Pohnert emphasized in their follow-up review[7] attachment of the patellar ligament to the fibula, hamstring releases if necessary, and obtaining and maintaining full extension. The biggest postoperative difficulty is flexion deformity, and secondary release or other procedures may be necessary and are worthwhile. The earlier this procedure is performed, of course, the better adaptation of proximal fibular cartilage to form a joint with the femur will occur; Brown recommended operating as early as possible; the patient will have a limb suitable for a below-

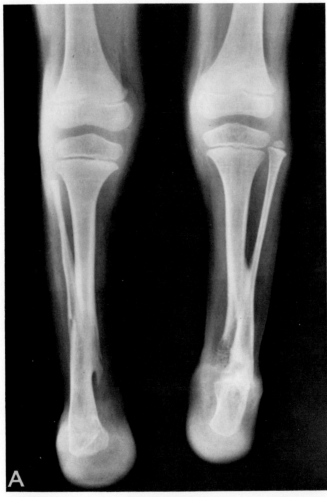

Figure 1.43. A useful termination for the amputation stump in childhood is the heel pad still attached to the os calcis. (*A*) Anteroposterior view shows os calcis firmly united to the hypertrophied distal end of the fibula, which had previously been united to the remnant of the proximal tibia. (*B*) Lateral view shows firm adherence of the heel pad to the os calcis. This prevents many of the complications of amputation in childhood. The heel pad stays in place, and the bone does not grow through the skin. (*C*) To get the heel pad (still attached to the os calcis) into the weight-bearing end of the amputation stump, a portion of the os calcis remains, as outlined by the lines drawn from *A* to *B*. The os calcis segment is then tilted up against the denuded distal tibial epiphysis and held there by an intramedullary pin until healed.

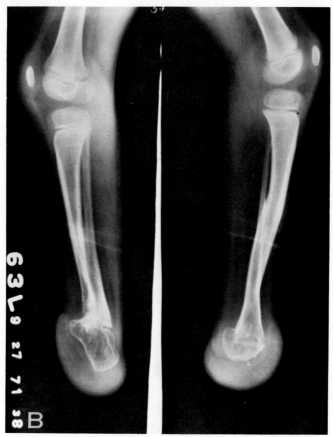

Figure 1.43*B*

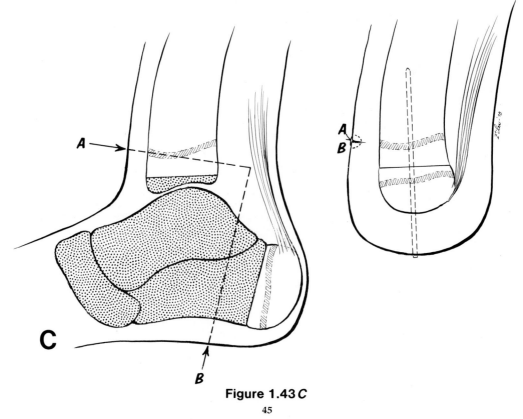

Figure 1.43*C*

knee prosthesis. Knee joints and a thigh lacer must be used because of persistent mediolateral instability. Strengthening exercises for the quadriceps and hamstrings are important postoperatively.

If a portion of the tibia is present proximally, the fibula can be transferred centrally into it; this has to be done after a portion of the tibial remnant has ossified, to allow bone-to-bone apposition.

Bilateral cases may cause consideration of ways to preserve the feet, but instability at the ankle is usually extreme, and short stature is marked. These patients are best treated by ankle disarticulation and Brown procedure, or by knee disarticulation if these fail.

BY MARY WILLIAMS CLARK, M.D.

Elective Revision

Elective revisions of the stump have one fundamental etiology peculiar to children. This is bone overgrowth, which results in stretching of the soft tissues over the stump end, ulceration, trophic changes, and a non-functional situation. Painful and functionally limiting neuromas occur in children as they do in adults.

The fibula is a particularly troublesome bone with respect to overgrowth and its secondary sequelae, perhaps because of its narrow cross sectional diameter and poor adherence to the skin over it. Overgrowth does not necessarily follow the growth potential of the proximal epiphysis.

Bursae are a complication particularly in childhood. It is not unusual to find them in anyone who plays basketball or football, not in a wheelchair, but as one of the active participants. This kind of activity, seldom practiced by the adult, tears at the stump and its tissue, which is not intended for weight bearing. Bursae thus formed usually require surgical excision, but the stump does not necessarily need to be shortened.

References

1. Aitken, G. T.: Amputation as a treatment for certain lower extremity congenital abnormalities, *J. Bone Joint Surg.*, *41A*: 1267, 1959.
2. Aitken, G. T. (ed.): *The Child with an Acquired Amputation*, Washington, D.C.: National Academy of Sciences, 1972.
3. Aitken, G. T. (ed.): *Selected Lower Limb Anomalies*, Washington, D.C.: National Academy of Sciences, 1971.
4. Aitken, G. T. (ed.): *P.F.F.D.: Congenital Anomalies*, Washington, D.C.: National Academy of Sciences, 1969.
5. Aitken, G. T., and Lambert, C.: The Management of the Juvenile Amputee, Manual and Lectures for Prosthetics 631, Prosthetic-Orthotic Center, Northwestern University Medical School, 1972.
6. Brown, F. W.: Construction of a knee joint in congenital total absence of the tibia; a preliminary report, *J. Bone Joint Surg.*, *47A*: 695, 1965.
7. Brown, F. W., and Pohnert, W. H.: Construction of a knee joint in meromelia tibia; a 15-year follow-up study, *J. Bone Joint Surg.*, *54A*: 1333, 1972.
8. Burgess, E. M., and Romano, R. L.: Immediate post-surgical prosthetic fitting, *Bull. Prosthetic Res.*, *10*(4), 1965.
9. Burgess, E. M., Romano, R. L., and Zettl, J. H.: Management of Lower Extremity Amputees, TR 10-5, Veteran's Administration, Washington, D.C., 1969.
10. Burtch, R. L.: Nomenclature for congenital skeletal limb deficiencies; a revision, *Artif. Limbs*, *10*: 24, 1966.
11. Crenshaw, A. H. (ed.): *Campbell's Operative Orthopedics*, St. Louis: C.V. Mosby Co., 1971.
12. Fishman, S.: Report of NYU Studies, 1972 Clinic Chiefs Meeting, Atlanta, 1972.
13. Frantz, C. H., and O'Rahilly, R.: Congenital skeletal limb deficiencies, *J. Bone Joint Surg.*, *43A*: 1202, 1961.
14. *Inter-Clinic Information Bulletin*, New York University Postgraduate Medical School, New York; monthly publication.
15. Kay, H. W.: A proposed international terminology for the classification of congenital limb deficiencies. *Inter-Clinic Information Bulletin*, *13*(9), April, 1974.
16. Kay, H. W.: Clinical applications of the new international terminology for the classification of congenital limb deficiencies. *Inter-Clinic Information Bulletin*, *14*(3), March, 1975.
17. Kay, H. W., and Dolan, C. M. E.: Some guidelines for operation of child amputee clinics, *Inter-Clinic Information Bulletin*, *7*(9), 1968.
18. Kay, H. W., et al.: The proposed international terminology for the classification of congenital limb deficiencies. *Dev. Med. Child Neurol.*, *17*(3), suppl. 34, 1975.
19. Kübler-Ross, E.: *On Death and Dying*, New York: Macmillan, 1969.
20. LaForest, N. T., and Regon, L. W.: The physical therapy program after an immediate semirigid dressing and temporary below-knee prosthesis, *Phys. Ther.*, *53*: 497, 1973.
21. Levit, F.: Dermatological Considerations, Lecture for Prosthetics 622, Prosthetic-Orthotic Center, Northwestern University Medical School, 1971.
22. Mooney, V.: Comparison of post-operative stump management, *J. Bone Joint Surg.*, *53A*: 241, 1971.
23. Myers, T. H.: *Am. J. Orthop. Surg.*, *3*: 72, 1905.
24. Myers, T. H.: Further report on a case of congenital absence of the tibia, *Am. J. Orthop. Surg.*, *8*: 398, 1910.
25. *Orthopedic Clinics of North America*, *3*(2), July 1972; Amputation Surgery and Prosthetics.

26. Schoenberg, B., Carr, A. C., Peretz, D., and Kutscher, A. H.: *Loss and Grief: Psychological Management in Medical Practice*, New York: Columbia University Press, 1970.
27. Swinyard, C. (ed.): *Limb Development and Deformity*, Springfield, Ill.: Charles C Thomas, 1969.
28. Van Nes, C. P.: Rotation-plasty for congenital defects of the femur, *J. Bone Joint. Surg.*, 32B: 12, 1950.

DEVELOPMENTAL ANATOMY

The gross anatomy of the infant or child exhibits marked differences from the adult. This is most manifest in the musculoskeletal system. Inasmuch as a complete survey of anatomic changes from birth to physeal closure is not feasible, salient areas will be emphasized.

Upper Extremity

The upper limbs are relatively long compared to the rest of the body. Their overall length averages 16.5 cm, which is about the same as the lower limb. Structurally and functionally the upper limb is better developed than the lower limb.

SHOULDER

The clavicle is the first bone to form a primary ossification center, about the sixth week of development. It forms an epiphysis and discoid growth plate at the proximal end (sternoclavicular joint), while the distal (acromioclavicular) end has a subarticular spherical growth plate analogous to that in the phalanges (Fig. 1.7). The scapula forms a large, flat ossification center with two significant discoid growth plates, one along the medial edge and one adjacent to the glenoid. Like the acetabulum, the glenoid is entirely composed of hyaline cartilage at birth, with some fibrocartilage along the rim. The proximal humerus develops an ossification center just before or after birth. Figure 1.44 *A* shows the proximal humerus of a neonate. The ossification center is just beginning to form. By 15 months (Fig. 1.44 *B*) the first epiphyseal ossification center has appeared and the second one has started in the region of the greater tuberosity. The proximal humeral growth plate contributes 40% of the length of the upper extremity and 80% of the length of the humerus.

ELBOW

Development of the distal humerus has been alluded to in a previous section. No ossification centers are present at birth, but during the first year the ossification center appears in the capitellar portion of the distal humeral epiphysis. The ossification center of the trochlear portion of the epiphysis does not appear until approximately 7 years. The distal humerus contributes 10% of the length of the upper extremity and 20% of the length of the humerus. The proximal radius has no ossification center until 3 years of age, whereas the proximal ulnar ossification center appears at 7–8 years. The proximal ulna shows considerable variation in the structure of the growth plate (Fig. 1.45). The most proximal portion is a normally structured plate, engaged in longitudinal growth. But the segment under the elbow joint has narrower, shorter cell columns (a reflection of the lessening role in longitudinal development of this area of the proximal ulna). The proximal radial and ulnar growth plates contribute 11% of the overall length of the upper extremity and, respectively, 25% and 20% of radial and ulnar length. Only 21% of overall arm length occurs at the elbow.

WRIST

The distal radius and ulna are relatively underdeveloped (Fig. 1.46). The radial growth plate is slightly more proximal than the ulnar growth plate. Both epiphyses are of similar volume, a relationship that will change very rapidly over the next 2–3 years. The distal radial and ulnar growth plates contribute 39% of overall length of the upper extremity and, respectively, 75% and 80% of radial and ulnar length. The carpal bones do not begin to ossify until the end of the first year of life. The pisiform does not develop until just before puberty.

HAND

The newborn hand is functionally very mature, being capable of relatively strong grasp. The length is about one-quarter that of the upper extremity (about 4–5 cm). The

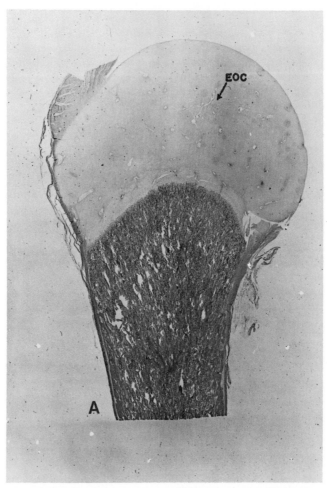

Figure 1.44. (*A*) Neonatal humerus. The epiphysis is entirely cartilaginous. The epiphyseal ossification center (*EOC*) is just beginning to form. This area is shown in more detail in Figure 1.8. (*B*) Proximal humerus from a 15-month-old infant, showing two well developed ossification centers. The *arrow* indicates a blood vessel connecting the two centers. Cartilage transformation is occurring around this vessel.

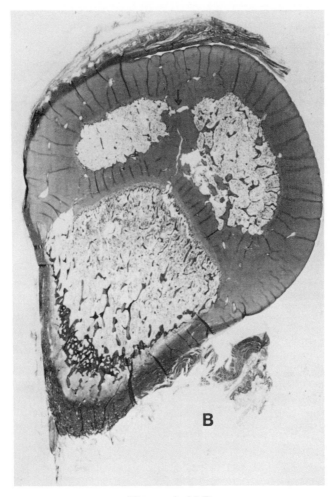

Figure 1.44 B

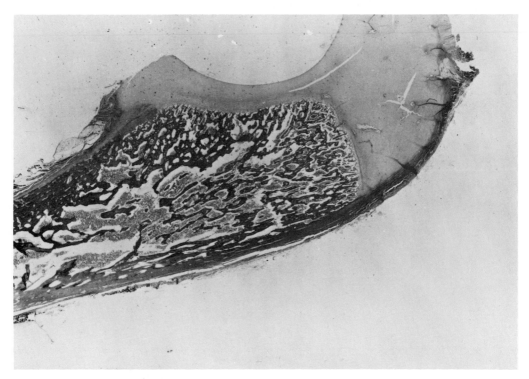

Figure 1.45. Olecranon from a 2-month-old infant. The portion of the growth plate oriented perpendicular to the longitudinal axis has a normal architecture, whereas that part under the joint has much shorter cell columns and is primarily undergoing interstitial rather than longitudinal growth.

phalanges develop similarly to the toe phalanx shown previously (Fig. 1.7), i.e., a discoid growth plate and epiphysis at one end and a slowly diminishing chondroepiphysis and spherical growth plate at the other end.

VERTEBRAL COLUMN

The average neonatal vertebral column is 19–20 cm from C1 to L5, with the thoracic spine comprising 50% of the length and the cervical and lumbar regions 25% each. With development, the thoracic portion remains about the same, but the cervical decreases and the lumbar increases. There are *no* fixed curves at birth, unless a structural abnormality is present. The spine is so flexible that the dissected column can be bent into a semicircle. After birth the thoracic spine rapidly develops and stabilizes a fixed curve. The cervical curve develops a few weeks later as the infant begins to lift his head. The lumbar curve does not develop until the child begins to stand and walk. At birth each vertebra

(except C1 and C2) has three separate ossification centers (one in the body and two in the posterior elements). The atlas (C1) has only two ossification centers (both in the posterior elements), whereas the axis (C2) has four centers (two posterior, one in the body, and one in the odontoid process). Most of the vertebra is comprised of hyaline cartilage. The nucleus pulposus is relatively large in the neonate, with a much smaller anulus (Fig. 1.9).

Lower Extremity

Relative to the upper limbs the legs are poorly developed at birth, both structurally and functionally. They are proportionately much smaller than the upper limbs, when considering final adult size. Intrauterine positioning is much more manifest, causing significant flexion and abduction at the hip, flexion at the knees, and supination at the foot. There is moderate resistance to manip-

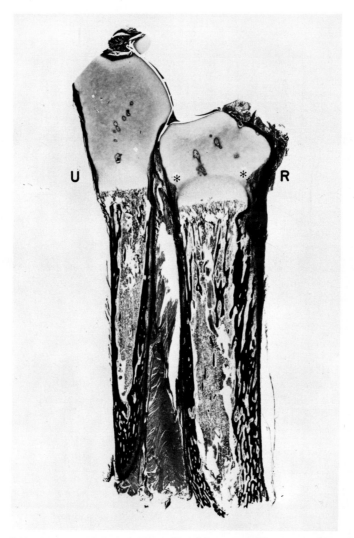

Figure 1.46. Distal radius (*R*) and ulna (*U*) of a neonate. The growth plate of the ulna is more distal than the radius. The radius has a more significant zone of Ranvier (*).

ulative correction of these positional "contractures."

HIP

The neonatal femur is a straight bone that averages 8.5 cm in length. The femoral head is approximately 1 cm in diameter. A femoral neck is virtually nonexistent. The head is incompletely covered by the acetabulum. The ligamentum capitum femoris is relatively long. The musculature is better developed medially than laterally. Because hip disorders are a major problem in infants, the detailed anatomy will be discussed.

The femoral nerve, artery, and vein are relatively large structures that occupy the middle one-third of the proximal lower leg (Fig. 1.47). The adductor muscle group is much better developed than the abductor group. The iliopsoas is separated from the overlying nerve and blood vessels by a fascial sleeve that creates a tunnel from the inguinal ligament to the lesser trochanter (Fig. 1.48). The role of the iliopsoas functionally varies, depending upon the position of the femur relative to the pelvis. When the hip is neutral, the iliopsoas crosses only a small portion of the medial femoral head and acetabular rim. With flexion the iliopsoas relaxes signifi-

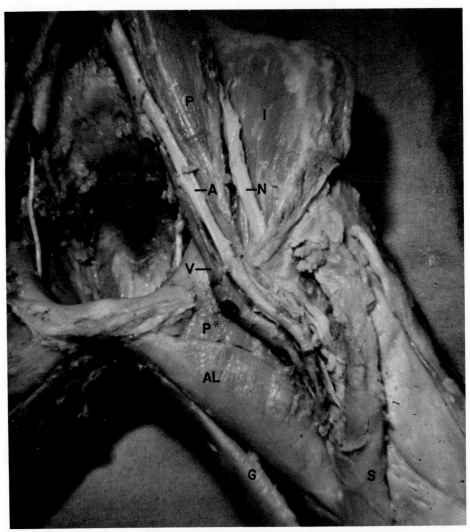

Figure 1.47. Superficial anatomy of the infant thigh. (*P*, psoas; *I*, iliacus; *A*, femoral artery; *N*, femoral nerve; *V*, femoral vein; *P**, pectineus; *AL*, adductor longus; *G*, gracilis; *S*, sartorius.)

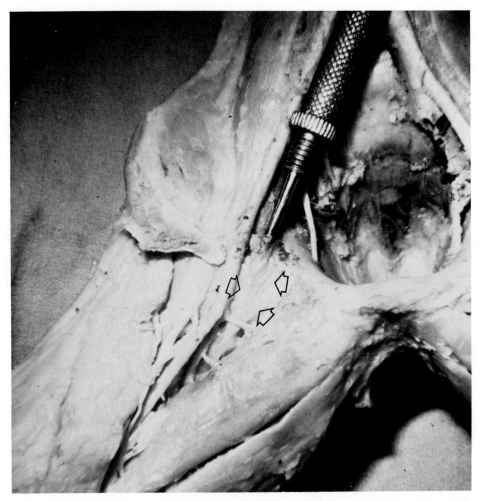

Figure 1.48. Fascial tunnel separating the iliopsoas from the overlying neurovascular structures.

cantly. But with increasing abduction, the iliopsoas translocates laterally to cover more of the femoral head and cross the acetabulum rim more laterally and superiorly (Fig. 1.49). As the iliopsoas shifts laterally, its function changes to a significant hip abductor.

The hip capsule is attached to the proximal femur along the groove between femoral head and greater trochanter (intraepiphyseal groove). In the neonate the medial most attachment of the capsule to the proximal femur is adjacent to the growth plate. Therefore, most of the proximal femoral growth plate at this stage is extra-articular. With subsequent development the growth plate eventually becomes an intra-articular structure. The capsular attachments on the acetabular side are several millimeters beyond the labrum and not directly at the edge of the labrum (Fig. 1.50). The labrum is then an intra-articular, rather than periarticular structure.

The acetabulum is composed of two significantly different types of cartilage during early development (Fig. 1.51). The most peripheral portion of the labrum is composed of fibrocartilage, whereas the bulk of the labrum and acetabulum is composed of hyaline cartilage. The limbus forms from hypertrophy of the fibrocartilaginous portion of the acetabulum. The labrum, especially the fibrocartilaginous portion, can be easily deformed by manual pressure (Fig. 1.52).

The proximal femur of the neonate has a single epiphysis and a single growth plate (Fig. 1.51). This is transversely oriented, just above the lesser trochanter. However, as the infant grows, differential growth rates cause

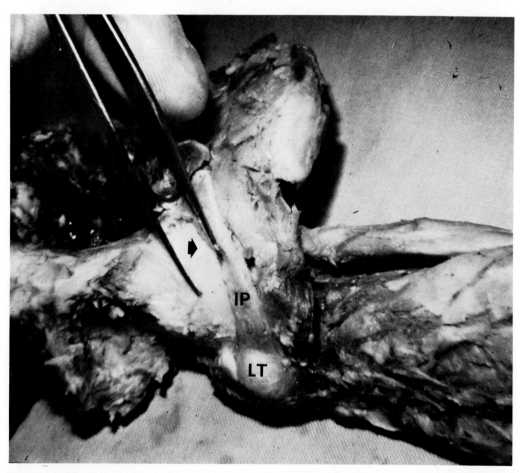

Figure 1.49. Lateral translocation of the iliopsoas (*IP*) when the hip is flexed and abducted. (*LT*, lesser trochanter.)

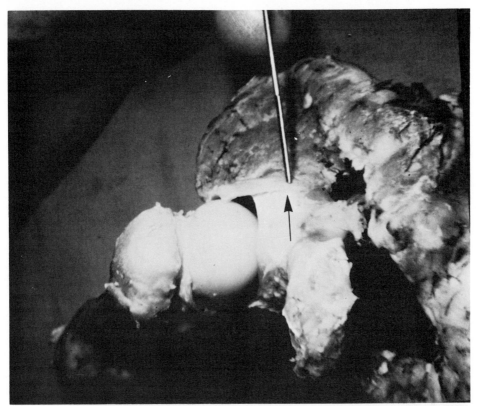

Figure 1.50. Attachment of hip joint capsule several millimeters beyond the acetabular rim, leaving a potential space between the rim and capsule. This area fills with dye in an arthrogram, visualizing the "rose thorn."

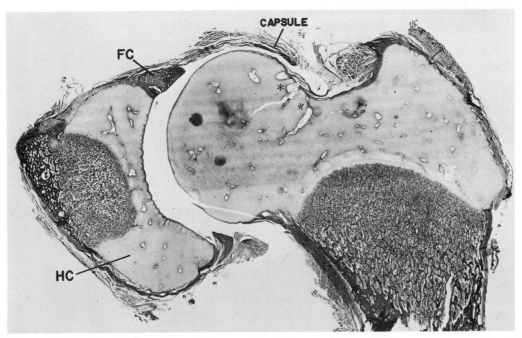

Figure 1.51. Sagittal section of the proximal femur and acetabulum of a 2-month-old infant. Note the extensive cartilage canal system, with major penetrating canals (*) from the interepiphyseal groove. (*FC*, fibrocartilaginous acetabular rim; *HC*, hyaline cartilage of the acetabulum.) The articular cartilage of the acetabulum is histochemically different (darker staining).

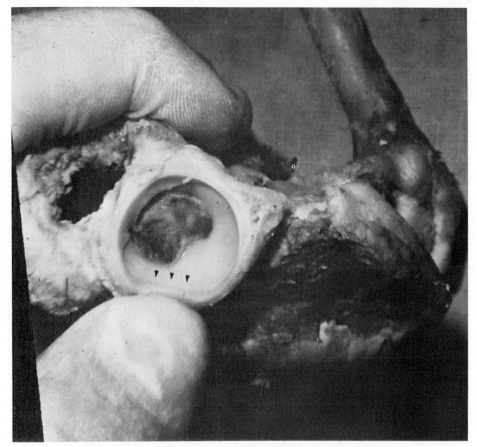

Figure 1.52. Deformity of the posterior acetabular rim.

the central portion of the epiphysis to grow faster both longitudinally as well as interstitially, such that the growth plate becomes "pyramidal." The proximal femoral growth plate contributes 15% of the overall leg length and 30% of femoral length.

The blood supply of the proximal femur stems primarily from the deep (profunda) femoral artery, which gives off two significant branches—the lateral and medial circumflex arteries. The lateral circumflex artery divides into ascending, transverse, and descending branches. The transverse branch goes between the rectus femoris and iliopsoas to reach the anterolateral proximal femur (Fig. 1.53). Several branches ramify over the greater trochanter, and a small branch courses in the intraepiphyseal groove to anastomose with the terminal portion of the medial circumflex artery. The medial circumflex artery goes between the iliopsoas and adductor muscles to reach the medial side of

the proximal femur just above the lesser trochanter (Fig. 1.54). Small branches enter the epiphysis just above the growth plate. The medial circumflex artery then continues around to the posterior surface to reach the intraepiphyseal groove. The artery courses along this groove onto the anterior portion to anastomose with the lateral circumflex termination. The major penetrating arteries to the epiphysis and growth plate arise from the medial circumflex artery posteriorly in the intraepiphyseal groove. This artery in the intraepiphyseal groove is subject to compression during positioning.

Positioning significantly affects the relationship between the intraepiphyseal groove and its contained arteries and the acetabulum, and thereby affects the circulation to the proximal femur. When hips are put through various ranges of motion or held in the commonly used treatment positions, the superior and posterior acetabulum fits tightly into the

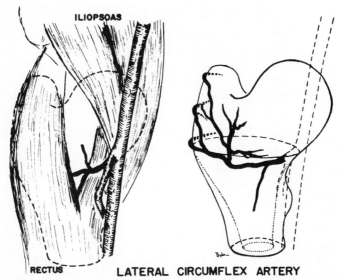

Figure 1.53. Lateral circumflex arterial circulation. The artery stems from the profound femoris and crosses the iliopsoas and then goes between the two heads of the rectus femoris to reach the anterior proximal femur, where distribution is primarily to the trochanteric region.

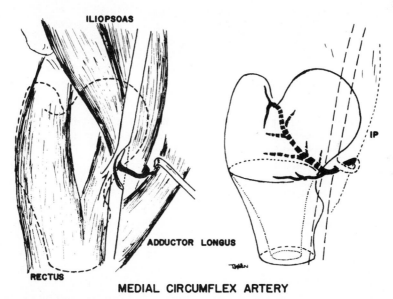

Figure 1.54. Medial circumflex arterial circulation. The artery usually stems from the profunda femoris. It crosses the iliopsoas and then wraps around the iliopsoas tendon to reach the medial portion of the proximal femur. It then courses along the posterior intraepiphyseal groove, providing the major blood supply to the chondroepiphysis and central and medial portions of the growth plate.

intraepiphyseal groove, interlocking similar to pieces of a jigsaw puzzle (Fig. 1.55). Not much pressure is necessary to firmly wedge the labrum into the groove, especially with increasing abduction, compromising the space available in the groove for the blood vessels that supply the femoral head. In the Lorenz and "frog-leg" positions, the labrum

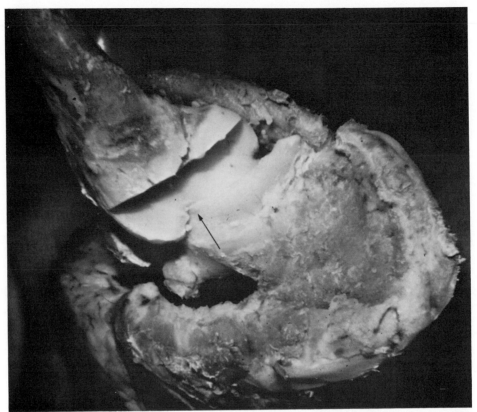

Figure 1.55. Abduction and flexion cause impingement between the rim of the acetabulum and the intraepiphyseal groove.

and groove are maximally compressed together. In less extreme treatment positions, such as the "human position" of Salter, compression in the intraepiphyseal groove is minimized. Thus, one of the major effects of treatment in positions emphasizing marked abduction is to variably occlude the blood supply as it courses along the posterior intraepiphyseal groove.

Circulatory compromise may also occur as the medial circumflex artery courses between the iliopsoas and adductor group. By abducting the hip the medial circumflex artery may be stretched and partially occluded as it courses over the iliopsoas tendon (Fig. 1.56). Internal rotation increases the degree of stretching. There may also be arterial compression deeper, between the iliopsoas tendon and the pectineus/adductor muscles. One of the beneficial effects of adductor tenotomy may be to lessen such arterial compression.

Congenital Hip Dislocation. The pathologic anatomy of congenital hip dislocation will be discussed in detail in the section dealing with hip disease. However, some normal anatomy is pertinent to discuss here. The ligamentum capitum femoris is relatively long. If the capsule is transected, the femoral head can be dislocated over the lateral rim, but it cannot be dislocated into the usual superoposterior position due to limitation imposed by the ligamentum capitum femoris (Fig. 1.57). The intact capsule and its intrinsic supporting ligaments further limit lateral motion of the femoral head.

The adductor/pectineus muscle group is much better developed than the abductors (gluteus medius, minimus) and external rotators, which tends to direct the femoral head into a more uncovered position. The iliopsoas is significantly displaced when the hip is dislocated (Fig. 1.58). The iliopsoas crosses the evacuated acetabulum, creating the char-

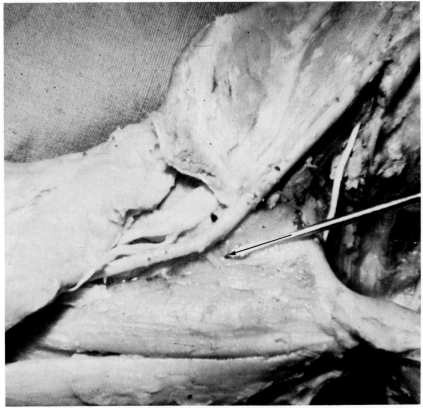

Figure 1.56. Abduction and flexion stretch the medial circumflex, as it is fixed where it courses between the iliopsoas and the adductor longus.

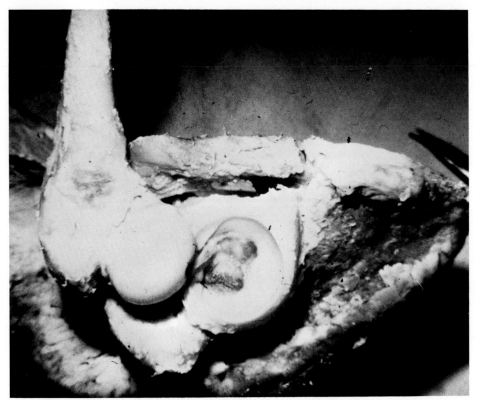

Figure 1.57. With the ligamentum capitum femoris intact, the femoral head can be displaced only to the acetabular rim.

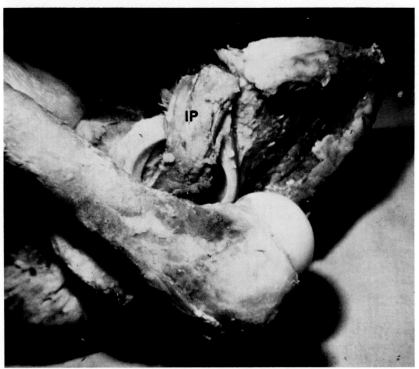

Figure 1.58. When the hip is completely dislocated, the iliopsoas (*IP*) crosses the vacated acetabulum, compressing the capsule into the joint and causing the "hourglass" constriction.

acteristic hourglass capsular contraction. The iliopsoas also pulls the dislocated head back against the labrum, deforming it initially, and even invaginating the fibrocartilaginous portion. This inverted fibrocartilaginous rim may hypertrophy to create the pathologic limbus.

KNEE

The distal femoral chondroepiphysis characteristically has a secondary ossification center at birth (Fig. 1.59). The distal femoral growth plate makes the most significant contribution to overall leg length (40%), as well as femoral length (70%). The proximal tibia may have a secondary ossification center at birth. This rapidly expands because of growth and forces across the knee during the first year of life (Fig. 1.60). The proximal tibia contributes 27% of overall leg length and 55% of tibial length. Thus the knee growth plates contribute 67% of the entire leg length, a significant difference compared to the elbow contribution to arm length. The tibial tubercle does not develop an ossification center until relatively late (8–10 years). This may

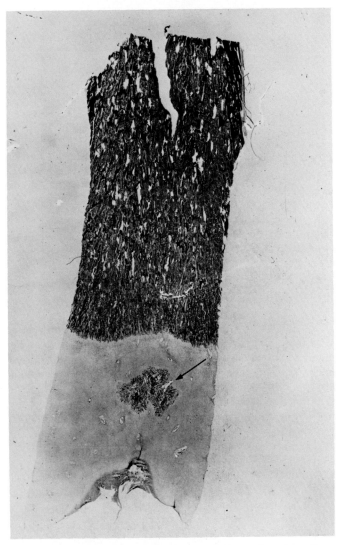

Figure 1.59. Distal femoral epiphysis of a newborn, showing the well developed ossification center that is present at birth. The *arrow* indicates a cartilage canal artery entering the vascular system of the ossification center.

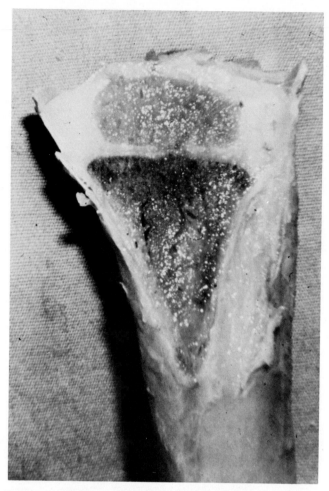

Figure 1.60. Proximal tibial epiphysis of a 15-month-old infant, showing the well developed ossification center.

arise as a separate ossification center or may extend from the main proximal tibial ossification center. It is classically taught that the growth plate of the proximal tibia turns to extend downward under the tibial tubercle. This does *not* occur. The cellular growth plate is replaced by a fibrous plate between the tibial tubercle cartilage and proximal tibial metaphysis (Fig. 1.61). This fibrous plate is more susceptible to shear stress than the cellular growth plate, and this may explain how the tibial tubercle pulls away in a disease such as Osgood-Schlatter's.

ANKLE

The distal tibia and fibula are entirely cartilagenous at birth, while the talus and cal-

caneus have already commenced ossification. Significant blood vessels enter the lateral side of the tibial epiphysis (Fig. 1.62). This blood supply may be injured in a fracture of Tillaux. The distal tibia (and fibula) contribute 18% of overall leg length and 45% of tibial length.

FOOT

By the end of the second fetal month the developing foot is formed but markedly supinated. Not until the seventh fetal month does the process of gradual pronation commence, although at birth and for the first few weeks of life many children may still have some supination. Pronation occurs because of structural changes in the shape of the talus

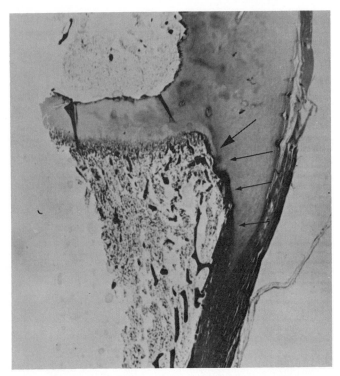

Figure 1.61. Section of the tibial tubercle showing the end of the cellular growth plate (*large arrow*) and the fibrous "growth" plate under the tibial tubercle.

and calcaneus and by the rapid growth of the medial side of the foot. At birth the foot is capable of considerable dorsiflexion because of the shape of the articular surface of the body of the talus. In contrast, plantar flexion may be limited, partially because of shortness of the foot extensor tendons. The feet are relatively long and narrow compared to the rest of the lower extremity, with an average length of 6.5 cm (the hip to heel length averages 16–18 cm). The foot appears to have no arches because of a thick, fibrous, plantar fat pad. The longitudinal arch of the neonate is actually relatively higher than during later development. Failure of the transition from a supinated to a pronated foot, along with intrauterine positioning, probably play a major role in the evolution of the clubfoot.

Clubfoot. The clubfoot that proves resistant to treatment or recurs after nonoperative treatment usually has significant chronic alterations in the anatomy of the ankle, subtalar, and midtarsal articulations. There are major soft-tissue contractures. The head and neck of the talus become structurally deformed, even while the body of the talus

retains a relatively normal relationship with the mortise.

The most important "joint" is a multiple articulation that includes the talonavicular joint and the anterior and middle talocalcaneal joints. These articulations have a common synovial cavity that is separate from the posterior subtalar articulation. The anterior calcaneus and navicular are maintained as a structural unit by strong ligaments, the most important of which is the inferior calcaneonavicular, or spring ligament. This "joint" can be considered a ball-and-socket joint, with the head of the talus (ball) articulating in the calcaneonavicular complex (socket).

Normal plantar flexion of the foot includes supination of the forefoot and calcaneovarus. The calcaneovarus occurs by a pivotal motion focused at the middle of the calcaneus: the anterior portion moves downward and medial, while the posterior portion moves upward and lateral. Concomitantly, the navicular, which must move integrally with the anterior calcaneus, also moves medially, but it rotates instead of going downward. This exposes a greater portion of the talar head laterally, because the talus is normally unable to significantly abduct and adduct within the ankle mortise.

In the resistant or recurrent clubfoot, pathologic contractures of the soft tissue prevent the reduction of the calcaneonavicular complex on the head of the talus. These posterior, medial, and subtalar soft-tissue contractures are more significant than the structural deformity of the talus. Figures 1.63 A and 1.63 B show gross and schematic depictions of these contractures. The posterior contractures involve the posterior cap-

sules of the ankle and subtalar joints, the heel cord, and the posterior tibiofibular and calcaneofibular ligaments. These latter contractures also lead to a more posterior displacement of the fibula. The medial contractures include the deltoid and spring ligaments; the talonavicular joint capsule; the posterior tibial, flexor digitorum longus, and flexor hallucis longus tendons; and the anterior tibial and extensor hallucis longus tendons. Subtalar contractures involve the anterior subtalar interosseous ligament and the bifurcated (Y) ligament.

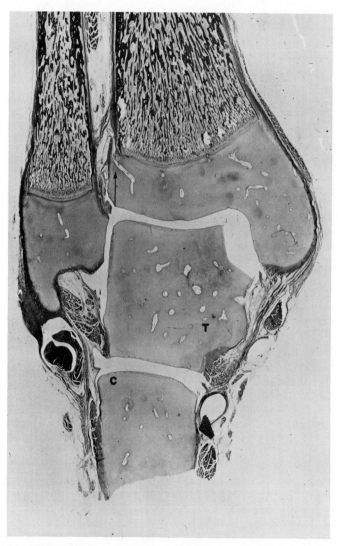

Figure 1.62. Distal tibia, fibula, calcaneus (*C*), and talus (*T*) of a 2-month-old infant. This sagittal section is posterior to the ossified portions of the talus and calcaneus. The *arrow* indicates a major vessel entering the lateral side of the tibial epiphysis.

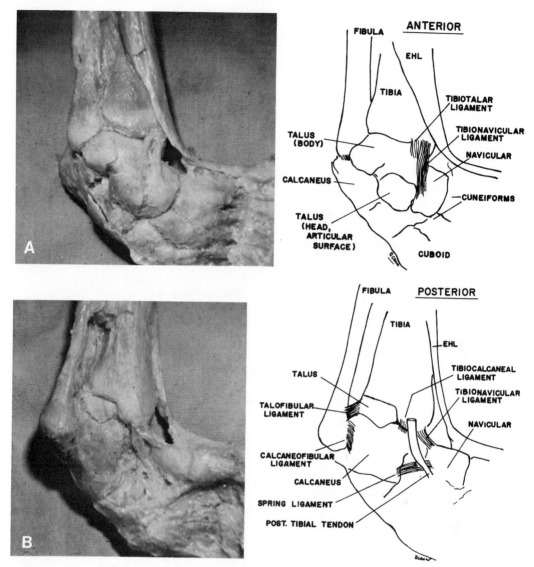

Figure 1.63. (A) Gross and schematic anatomy of a resistant clubfoot (A) Anterior view. (B) Posterior view.

Because the talus has no musculotendinous connections, its position and shape are mediated by surrounding structures. As the talus is forced into equinus, the posterior calcaneus is displaced upward and lateral. This is due to contractures of the posterior capsule, the heel cord, and the calcaneofibular ligament. Because the calcaneus pivots centrally, the anterior segment is displaced downward, medially, and under the head of the talus. In this position contractures of the deltoid and spring ligaments and posterior tibial tendon worsen and accentuate the deformity and undoubtedly play a role in the deformation of the more cartilaginous head and neck of the talus. The navicular is displaced medial to the head of the talus and may even articulate with the medial malleolus. The severity of the contractures juxtaposes the navicular bone, the sustentaculum tali, and the medial malleolus. The pathologically contracted ligaments form a dense medial mass that obscures the joint lines and neck of the talus anteriorly and posteriorly.

BY JOHN OGDEN, M.D.

HOW TO READ AN ORTHOPAEDIC X-RAY FILM, SELF-TEACHING

INTRODUCTION

This is a program on the fundamentals of x-ray diagnosis of bone and joint lesions. It is arranged as a branching program. It begins with a single major concept or idea. You read this. You are then asked a question and given a number of possible answers from which you select one you think is correct. Only one answer is actually correct. The others are selected because they are typical or plausible mistakes.

The answers are numbered, and they have been scrambled in the remainder of this portion of the text. Turn to the numbered answers that you selected.

If you are correct, you will be given additional new material followed by an option for an additional question, and thus will advance through the material.

If you are incorrect, you will be given a short explanation of why and asked to return to the original numbered segment from which you started. You may then select another answer.

Remember, this material is not arranged in consecutive order and you must progress by numbered segments, choosing your next reading on the basis of the options offered you at the end of each portion of new material.

PROGRAM

1

The important attribute that anyone reading orthopaedic x-ray films must have is that of making an observation of the individual roentgen features present on the film. These changes in various combinations lead one to surmise the pathologic process that is taking place. Ultimately, with logical reasoning and the addition of other facts about the patient, such as age and sex, the observer is led to the diagnosis.

All of this depends on the observation of individual roentgen features. It must be looked at in detail rather than in a total impression. A beginning is made when one can distinguish fluid and muscle density from fat density, bone density, and metallic density.

On an x-ray film there are a number of densities apparent. Air or gas is least dense. Fat, as exemplified in subcutaneous tissue, is next in density. The third density is that of water, which is exemplified by muscle density in the soft tissues. Bone is obviously more dense than any of these. If one contrasted bone and metal on the x-ray film, he would expect metal to be most dense.

Water density is:

Less dense than fat	32
Less dense than muscle	13
More dense than bone	39
More dense than fat	17

2

YOUR ANSWER: Bone density is the density of medullary contents of the bone.

You are incorrect. Bone density is principally formed by the extremely dense cortex.

Return to number 33 and try again.

3

YOUR ANSWER: A swelling is most likely to be associated with a tumor.

You are incorrect. A swelling is caused by inflammatory edema. This could occur with a tumor but is not likely. Most likely is the x-ray definition of a mass caused by growth of the tumor. It has well defined edges as it displaces normal tissue.

Return to number 6 and try again.

4

YOUR ANSWER: The metaphysis is more likely to be the seat of disease than other areas of the bone because embolic phenomena lodge in the metaphysis due to the formation of endarterial loops in this area.

You are correct. Infection, tumor, and metabolic products all tend to lodge in the metaphysis, carried there by the general circulation.

Blood-borne bacteria lodging in the metaphysis would produce an inflammation. This would first be evident on the x-ray film as a soft-tissue swelling. Nine to 11 days later one might have sufficient destruction of the cortex to distinguish the lesion in the bone.

The swelling associated with osteomyelitis would involve the deep soft tissues next to the bone. Deep soft-tissue swelling can be distinguished from superficial soft-tissue swelling involving the subcutaneous tissues. Superficial soft-tissue swelling is associated with cellulitis rather than osteomyelitis.

An osteomyelitis first is evident on the x-ray film as:

An area of bone destruction in the metaphysis	5
An area of superficial swelling centered about the metaphysis	52
An area of deep soft-tissue swelling centered about the metaphysis	61
An area of bone destruction in the diaphysis	25

5

YOUR ANSWER: An osteomyelitis first is evident on the x-ray film as an area of bone destruction in the metaphysis.

You are incorrect. The change of bone destruction is a late change only visible when enough of the cortex has been destroyed. The first change is a deep soft-tissue swelling centered about the metaphysis.

Return to number 4 and try again.

6

YOUR ANSWER: A swelling obscures the fat lines running through the muscle density areas because swellings have density comparable to muscle.

You are correct. Swellings have water density comparable to muscle density and, therefore, eliminate contrast areas within the muscle shadow. In the illustration for frame 6 there is a swelling about the distal femoral metaphysis. It is partly obscured by the wrapping holding the infant to the x-ray cassette,

but note that its exact limits are hard to determine.

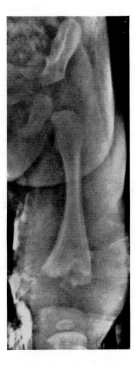

A swelling enlarges an area of water density. A mass also enlarges an area of water density. A mass has a clear-cut and distinct edge, in contrast to a swelling which has indistinct edges gradually fading into the shadow created by other soft tissues. A mass would be most likely to be associated with a tumor or an infection? If you answered tumor, you were correct.

Between these two which would be most likely to be associated with swelling?

Tumor	3
Infection	56

7

YOUR ANSWER: Tumor bone tends to a pattern which is around rather than in the tumor.

You are incorrect. Tumor bone is formed by the tumor and is the distinguishing feature of osteogenic sarcoma. Bone formed around the tumor is a reaction of the host and formed by normal tissues.

Return to number 59 and try again.

8

YOUR ANSWER: *B* is more dense than *D*.

You are incorrect. *B* is the subcutaneous tissue or fat. It is not as dense as bone.

Return to number 17 and try again.

9

YOUR ANSWER: A bone cyst could be larger than evident on the x-ray film.

You are correct. What is seen is those areas where the cortex has been thinned. Actual cystic involvement could extend beyond this point, involving or replacing the medullary contents as in *A* or *B* in figure for frame 9.

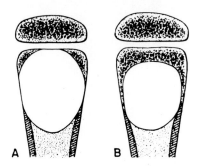

Ordinarily lines of contrasting density are seen running through the area occupied by muscle. These are created by fat lying in tissue planes. A swelling has vague outlines fading into the water density but obscures these fat lines, rendering the shadow relatively homogeneous. These lines are obscured because a swelling has water density.

A swelling obscures the fat lines running through the muscle density areas because:

Swellings have fat density.　　　　41
Swellings have air density.　　　　51
Swellings have density comparable to　6
　muscle.

10

YOUR ANSWER: A tumor that is designated an osteogenic sarcoma always arises from marrow elements.

You are incorrect. Arising from marrow elements is not a characteristic of osteogenic sarcoma.

Return to number 36 and try again.

11

YOUR ANSWER: Total destruction of the bone area occupied is characteristic of metastases from breast carcinoma.

You are incorrect. The roentgen appearance of breast carcinoma may be one of varying degrees of sclerosis giving rise to alternate areas of density as the host tissues are excited to lay down bone.

Return to number 53 and try again.

12

YOUR ANSWER: The number of visible vessel lines would be expected to increase with a swelling.

This is true. Vascular dilation is associated with inflammation. An inflammation causes a swelling. One can see evidence of this increased vascularity in the subcutaneous tissue where the vessel lines of water density contrast with the fat density of subcutaneous tissue.

An area of active destruction in the metaphysis of a long bone associated with soft-tissue swelling would presumably be an infection. An area of active desturction in a bone associated with a mass would presumably be a malignant tumor.

Active destruction is associated with either osteomyelitis or a malignant process.

Osteomyelitis can be distinguished from destruction of bone due to malignancy by:

The nature of destructive line　　　24
The decision as to whether a mass or　59
　a swelling accompanies the destruction
The area of bone involved　　　　35

13

YOUR ANSWER: Water density is less dense than muscle.

You are incorrect. Water density and muscle density are synonymous so far as x-ray interpretation is concerned.

Return to number 1 and try again.

14

YOUR ANSWER: The metaphysis is more likely to be the seat of disease than other areas of the bone because it is the most active portion of the bone from the standpoint of metabolism.

You are incorrect. It is true that metabolism is most active in the metaphysis. Bone as an organ mirrors body states in this area, but disease phenomena are transmitted to this area from the rest of the body and the nature of the metaphyseal circulation becomes extremely important.

Return to number 42 and try again.

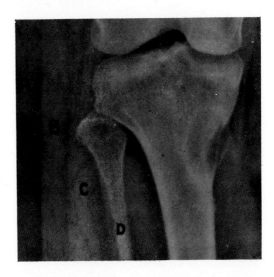

The illustration is the roentgen picture of an extremity. The various densities are tagged with letters. Select the proper answer below.

B is more dense than D.	8
B is less dense than A.	21
B is less dense than C.	33

15

YOUR ANSWER: Numbers 1 and 3 are true; number 2 is false.

You are incorrect. Metastases from the thyroid are totally lytic, and prostatic metastases can be both sclerotic and lytic. However, leukemia with its cellular infiltrates tends to run between bone trabeculae, giving rise to a lagging type of destruction by roentgenogram.

Return to number 28 and try again.

16

YOUR ANSWER: The diagnosis would be fracture line if soft-tissue swelling were present.

You are incorrect. Soft-tissue swelling does not differentiate a growth line from a fracture line, because this finding could accompany either.

Return to number 46 and try again.

17

YOUR ANSWER: Water density is more dense than fat.

This is correct. Fat does not contain water, and its structure is such that it is not as dense on the roentgen film as water density, as exemplified by muscle shadows on the x-ray film.

18

YOUR ANSWER: The diagnosis would be fracture line if the radiolucent line was of uneven width with sharp angles and irregular edges.

You are correct. The growth line, by contrast, has even width and rounded edges.

A fracture line is associated with soft-tissue swelling. Would you expect this to be deep soft-tissue swelling or superficial soft-tissue swelling? If you said deep soft-tissue swelling, you were correct, because the onset of the swelling, at least, is due to the developing hematoma about the fracture. Where the injury has been crushing in nature, the superficial tissues may be swollen as well.

A fracture line is most likely associated with:

Deep soft-tissue swelling	20
No soft-tissue swelling	63
Superficial soft-tissue welling	54

19

YOUR ANSWER: Bone density is principally formed by the cortex.

You are correct. A lesion in the bone, if it involved the medullary contents only and not the cortex, might not be visible on the roentgen film.

A, B, and C in the figure illustrate varying degrees of involvement of the cortex in fibrous dysplasia. If the medullary lesion was similar in density to the medullary contents and did not involve cortex, it would not be evident on the roentgen film.

A lesion of bone is going to be most evident on the x-ray film if it affects the medullary contents of the bone or the cortex? If you answered cortex, this is true. Here we have a very dense substance by x-ray. It can overlay a considerable medullary lesion and make it impossible to be seen. To be seen by roentgenogram, a lesion must create a contrast.

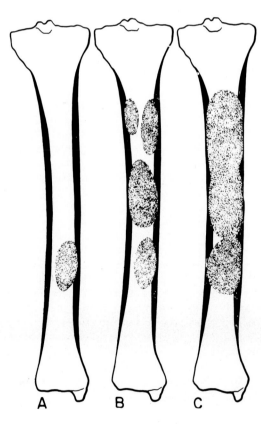

A   B   C

A bone cyst could be:

Larger than evident on the x-ray film	9
Smaller than evident on the x-ray film	48

20

YOUR ANSWER: A fracture line is most likely associated with deep soft-tissue swelling.

You are correct. The developing hematoma associated with a fracture soon makes deep soft-tissue swelling evident.

A vertebral fracture produces a typical deformity. Soft-tissue swelling cannot be ascertained through the overlying structures. The deformity due to trauma occurs by fracturing the superior cortex. This produces an angulation of the anterior margin as the anterior cortex is broken and decreases the height of the vertebra anteriorly.

The deformity of a vertebra due to osteoporosis is quite different. Here the intervertebral disc, being of fluid nature and relatively incompressible, maintains its height. The vertebra loses height more anteriorly than posteriorly, but without pushing out the superior, anterior angle of the vertebra. Both superior and inferior cortices are depressed in rounded fashion by pressure from the intervertebral disc, giving rise to a biconcave vertebra.

In the drawings for frame 20, select the vertebral outline which is due to fracture.

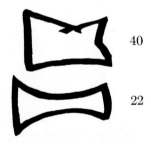

40

22

21

YOUR ANSWER: *B* is less dense than *A*.

A is the background density of the film itself. *B* is subcutaneous tissue of fat density recording a shadow against the background density and consequently more dense.

Return to number 17 and try again.

22

YOUR ANSWER: The vertebral outline in the figure for frame 20 is due to fracture. You are correct.

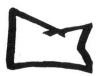

The compression and fracture of the superior cortex breaks out an anterior beak superiorly as the anterior cortex also fractures. This is a typical vertebral fracture outline.

The density of a bone is a reflection of its metabolic equilibrium with the body. This equilibrium cannot be maintained if the blood supply to a bone or a portion of it is cut off. The bone about this area remains responsive to changes in this equilibrium, but the dead bone remains at a static density. Thus, disuse that accompanies the pain associated with this lesion leaves the dead portion at its original density as the bone about it loses density.

The roentgen appearance of avascular bone is such that it is more dense than the surrounding bone.

To recognize the avascular state of a segment of a bone by roentgenogram:

More calcium salt must go into the avascular segment.	23
The original density of the bone segment must change.	57
A contrasting change in density is necessary in the bone about it.	47

23

YOUR ANSWER: To recognize the avascular state of a segment of bone by roentgenogram, more calcium salt must go into the avascular segment.

You are incorrect. Because there is no longer a vascular penetration of this segment, it is impossible for additional metabolic products to be deposited.

The density of this segment remains the same. The bone about it becomes less dense, increasing the contrast between the two.

Please return to number 22 and try again.

24

YOUR ANSWER: Osteomyelitis can be distinguished from destruction of bone due to malignancy by the nature of the destructive line.

You are incorrect. In both cases active destruction of bone is present. This is distinguished by a minutely spiculated rather than a smooth edge.

Return to number 12 and try again.

25

YOUR ANSWER: An osteomyelitis first is evident on the x-ray film as an area of bone destruction in the diaphysis.

You are incorrect. Osteomyelitis is blood borne to the metaphysis, not the diaphysis, and the metaphysis is the characteristic location for it. The diaphysis is a relatively inactive portion of the bone principally used for support.

Return to number 4 and try again.

26

YOUR ANSWER: Numbers 1, 2, and 3 are true.

You are correct. Metastases from the thyroid are totally lytic, whereas prostatic metastases vary with lytic and sclerotic areas. The cellular infiltrates of leukemia tend to give the appearance of lagging destruction.

When a bone has an accessory bone next to it separated by a growth line, the combined mass of the two is greater than you would expect the bony structure to occupy normally (*B*).

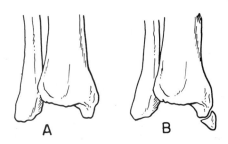

Where a fragment of bone has been fractured away from its parent bone, you would expect the combined mass of the two to be equal to the expected mass of the bone normally.

One would also expect to see the bed from which the fragment had been torn.

An accessory bone is separated from the parent bone by a radiolucent line.

It is helpful in determining whether a fracture exists to note:

Whether the mass of the parent bone   46
and the bone fragment is greater
or equal to the area normally
occupied by the undivided bone

Whether the parent bone and the   60
bone fragment have a mass less
than the area normally occupied
by the undivided bone

27

YOUR ANSWER: Avascular segments of bone may arise in various ways. The entrance of new blood vessels into the avascular segment is visible roentgenographically as areas of lesser density.

You are correct. The areas of lesser density occur about the newly vascular areas as old bone is resorbed.

There is another important distinction that can be made roentgenographically as an aid in diagnosis. This is the distinction between ossification and calcification.

Ossification has bone structure, and individual bone stria can be seen. Calcification is homogenous and structureless. When examined pathologically, it is also amorphous.

Amorphous calcification occurs as a deposit in degenerative areas in bursae, tendons, and in metabolic disease. Ossification may occur as a repair process or as a reaction to tumor or infection.

If an adventitious area of calcific density has definite structure visible in the roentgenogram, it could be termed:

Ossification   55

Calcification   37

28

YOUR ANSWER: Total destruction of the bone area occupied is characteristic of metastases from lung and thyroid carcinoma.

You are correct. Lung and thyroid carcinoma metastases, when present in bone, totally destroy all bone visible in the roentgenogram within the area occupied by the tumor. Little reaction is excited in the host bone, and, consequently, bony reaction about the tumor is not prominent.

Metastases such as those from breast and prostate exhibit lytic areas of increased density as well. Here new bone is laid down around the exciting lesion.

1. A metastases from the thyroid would tend to give a totally lytic area in bone.

2. A leukemic lesion would tend to give lagging destruction.

3. A prostatic metastasis might look both more dense and less dense than the surrounding bone.

In the three statements above:

Numbers 1 and 2 are true; number 3   49
is false.

Numbers 1 and 3 are true; number 2   15
is false.

Numbers 1, 2, and 3 are true.   26

29

YOUR ANSWER: The number of visible vessel lines would be decreased with a swelling.

You are incorrect. Vessel lines are normally not remarkable on the x-ray film. It is true that the swelling in its central portion obscures vessel lines by rendering the whole area of water dense and homogeneous. At the periphery, however, in areas of lesser density, the vessel lines caused by vascular dilation become well marked in the presence of inflammation.

Return to number 56 and try again.

30

YOUR ANSWER: Tumor bone tends to a pattern determined by the stress on the bone.

You are incorrect. Because the bone is destroyed, the normal engineering stresses are no longer present and the pattern of the bone that is formed is grossly irregular.

Return to number 59 and try again.

31

YOUR ANSWER: Avascular segments of bone may arise in various ways. The entrance of new blood vessels into the avascular segment is visible roentgenographically as increasing density of bone about the avascular segment.

You are incorrect. Increasing density of the uninvolved bone may indicate greater use of the extremity, but it does not necessarily foretell the entrance of new blood vessels into the avascular segment.

Return to number 47 and try again.

32

YOUR ANSWER: Water density is less dense than fat.

You are incorrect. Fat contains no water and its roentgenographic density is less than water, as exemplified by the muscle shadows on the x-ray film.

Return to number 1 and try again.

33

YOUR ANSWER: *B* is less dense than *C.*

You are correct. Subcutaneous tissue is less dense than muscle or water density.

If you contrasted gas or air and fat or subcutaneous tissue, fat or subcutaneous tissue would be most dense. If you contrasted water density and fat density, water density would be most dense. Bone has a very dense cortex, but one would expect the interior contents of the bone to have water density if they could be x-rayed isolated from the cortex.

Bone density is the density of the medullary contents of the bone.	2
Bone density is principally formed by the cortex.	19
The interior contens of the bone would be less dense than fat density.	45

34

YOUR ANSWER: A tumor tracks irregularly along the easiest anatomic route.

You are incorrect. An infection tracts irregularly, but a tumor grows concentrically. An infection is associated with poorly defined deep soft-tissue swelling, a tumor with a mass with clean-cut edges.

Return to number 61 and try again.

35

YOUR ANSWER: Osteomyelitis can be distinguished from destruction of bone due to malignancy by the area of bone involved.

You are incorrect. It is true that blood-borne osteomyelitis is typically a metaphy-seal disease. However a malignant tumor could be a metaphyseal lesion as well.

Return to number 12 and try again.

36

YOUR ANSWER: A tumor expands in concentric fashion into a rounded mass.

You are correct. A tumor will grow in all directions until it meets an anatomic obstacle. This gives rise to a rounded mass with clean-cut edges.

A bone tumor with well defined mass producing tumor bone.

A bone tumor producing tumor bone is an osteogenic sarcoma. This tumor destroys bone in the area it occupies. Some malignant bone lesions, particularly those arising from cells in the medullary canal, tend to infiltrate through and around bone trabeculae, displacing normal marrow elements. This gives rise to a type of destruction designated as "lagging" destruction. It is found in lesions such as Ewing's tumor.

A tumor that is designated an osteogenic sarcoma:

Infiltrates through the bone marrow giving rise to lagging destruction	62
Always arises from marrow elements	10
Always produces tumor bone	53

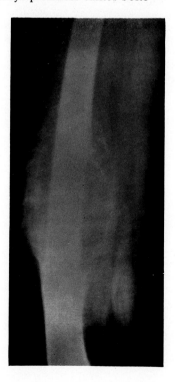

37

YOUR ANSWER: An adventitious area of calcific density having definite structure visible in the roentgenogram is termed calcification.

You are incorrect. Definite structure is not a characteristic of calcification. Calcification represents a toothpaste-like deposit occurring particularly in tendons and bursae about joints. It does not have bone formation within it. The ability to distinguish it from ossification is a great aid in differential diagnosis by roentgenogram.

Please return to number 27 and try again.

38

YOUR ANSWER: Avascular segments of bone may arise in various ways. The entrance of new blood vessels into the avascular segment is visible roentgenographically as areas of greater density.

You are incorrect. The new blood vessels remove the avascular bone (dense segments still apparent have not yet been invaded). New bone formation will be of normal bone density.

Return to number 47 and try again.

39

YOUR ANSWER: Water is more dense than bone.

You are incorrect. Bone contains water and, in addition, mineral. It is consequently more dense than water or muscle density on the x-ray film.

Return to number 1 and try again.

40

YOUR ANSWER:

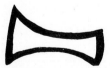

You are incorrect. The rounded compression of both superior and inferior cortices results in a biconcave vertebra. This is due to compressible bone in the presence of fluid-incompressible disc material. Such a compression is secondary to osteoporosis. A fracture principally affects the superior cortex, producing anterior breaking, and the anterior cortex breaks as well.

Return to number 20 and try again.

41

YOUR ANSWER: A swelling obscures fat lines running through the muscle density area because swellings have fat density.

You are incorrect. Fat density would obviously not obscure an area of fat density.

Return to number 9 and try again.

42

YOUR ANSWER: Tumor bone tends to a pattern which is grossly irregular within the tumor.

You are correct. Tumor bone is within the area occupied by the tumor. Because the bone has been destroyed in this area, the normal engineering stresses are no longer present and the pattern is grossly irregular.

X-ray features such as a mass or a swelling or benign or active destruction can now be distinguished. We are aware of the fact that a lesion in bone may not be readily distinguished unless it involves the cortex. A simple cyst involving the metaphysis is shown in the figure for frame 42.

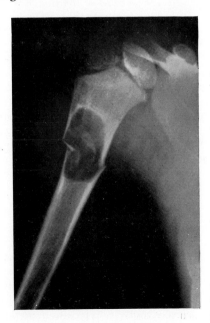

Of diagnostic importance also is the location of the lesion. The metaphysis is the portion of the bone converted from the cartilage of the epiphyseal line until it becomes remodeled into diaphysis. The diaphysis serves a supporting function, lying between the metaphysis at either end. The metaphysis is an area of active blood supply, endarterial loops, and formation of blood elements. As an active metabolic area it is more likely to be the seat of embolic disease, such as blood-borne infection. The epiphyseal area caps the metaphysis and supports the articular cartilage. It is less likely to be the seat of embolic disease than the metaphysis because its blood supply is frequently limited by the extension of the joint cavity about it. A giant cell tumor tends to arise in the epiphysis; a simple bone cyst, because it arises in the bone laid down from the epiphyseal line, is in the metaphysis.

The metaphysis is more likely to be the seat of disease than other areas of the bone because:

It is the most active portion of the bone from the standpoint of metabolism.	15
It lies midway between the diaphysis and the epiphysis.	43
Embolic phenomena lodge in the metaphysis due to the formation of endarterial loops in this area.	4

43

YOUR ANSWER: The metaphysis is more likely to be the seat of disease than other areas of the bone because it lies midway between the diaphysis and the epiphysis.

You are incorrect. The mere fact of location is not important. Each of these areas of the bone has its own specific function, and, of all the area, the metaphysis is the most active and has a peculiar endarterial loop formation which is typical of it.

Return to number 42 and try again.

44

YOUR ANSWER: Total destruction of the bone area occupied is characteristic of metastases from prostatic carcinoma.

You are incorrect. Prostatic carcinoma may have both lytic and sclerotic areas of bone involvement as the host tissues are excited to varying degrees of reactive bone formation.

Return to number 53 and try again.

45

YOUR ANSWER: The interior contents of the bone would be less dense than fat density.

You are incorrect. The isolated medullary contents of the bone would have water density of greater density than fat alone.

Return to number 33 and try again.

46

YOUR ANSWER: It is helpful in determining whether a fracture exists to note whether the mass of the parent bone and bone fragment is greater or equal to the area normally occupied by the individual bone.

You are correct. If the combined mass is greater than the expected size of an individual bone, this tends to indicate that this is an accessory bone and the line is a growth line.

In the figure A represents a growth line and B a fracture line.

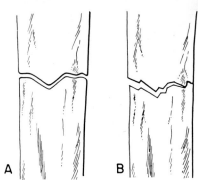

A fracture line has sharp angles, irregular edges, and uneven width.

A growth line separating an accessory bone from its parent has even width throughout. Its edges are rounded.

With trauma to the area, soft-tissue swelling could be present in either event.

The diagnosis would be fracture line if:

Soft-tissue swelling were present	16
The radiolucent line was of even width throughout with rounded edges	58
The radiolucent line was of uneven width with sharp angles and irregular edges	18

47

YOUR ANSWER: To recognize the avascular state of a segment of bone by roentgenogram, a contrasting change in density is necessary in the bone about it.

You are correct. The avascular segment is no longer in contact with the metabolic equilibrium of the body; consequently, it remains at its original density. This will only be apparent if the bone about it loses density. Note the density of the femoral epiphysis on the reader's *right* compared to the femoral neck in the figure.

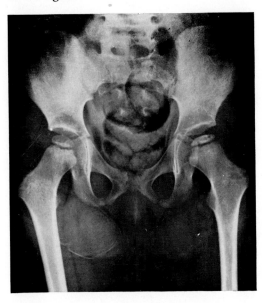

Areas of lesser density appearing in the previously dense avascular femoral epiphysis.

Bone that exhibits greater than normal density may arise typically at the femoral epiphysis, which has a perilous blood supply. As bone is revascularized, areas of lesser density appear due to the invasion of new blood vessels. The extension of infection in bone may isolate segments of it from its blood supply. These fragments are called sequestra. Trauma may divide the blood supply in bones such as the carpal scaphoid. If new blood vessels then invade the avascular bone, one would expect it to become less dense.

Avascular segments of bone may arise in various ways. The entrance of new blood vessels into the avascular segment is visible roentgenographically as:

Areas of greater density	38
Increasing density of bone about the avascular segment	38
Areas of lesser density	27

48

YOUR ANSWER: A bone cyst could be smaller than evident on the x-ray film.

You are incorrect. This could not be true because the area seen is the area where the cortex has actually been made thin by the pathologic lesion. Consequently, at least the area seen to be involved on the x-ray film must be involved.

Return to number 19 and try again.

49

YOUR ANSWER: Numbers 1 and 2 are true; number 3 is false.

You are incorrect. Metastases from the thyroid tend to be totally lytic, and leukemia tends to infiltrate rather than grow across an area, giving rise to lagging destruction. However, prostatic metastases do tend to be both lytic and sclerotic.

Return to number 28 and try again.

50

YOUR ANSWER: A tumor cannot be differentiated from an infection.

You are incorrect. Both the irregular tracking nature of the bone destruction by an infection and the poorly defined inflammatory swelling in the deep tissues which accompany it distinguish infection from tumor.

Return to number 61 and try again.

51

YOUR ANSWER: A swelling obscures fat lines running through the muscle density area because swellings have air density.

You are incorrect. Air, being less dense than fat, would not obscure it.

Return to number 9 and try again.

52

YOUR ANSWER: An osteomyelitis first is evident on the x-ray film as an area of superficial swelling centered about the metaphysis.

You are incorrect. Superficial soft-tissue swelling is associated with cellulitis. An osteomyelitis involving the bone involves the deep soft tissue of muscle density. It is centered at the metaphysis.

Return to number 4 and try again.

53

YOUR ANSWER: A tumor that is designated an osteogenic sarcoma always produces tumor bone.

You are correct. Tumor bone is bone actually produced by the tumor cells. It is not bone produced by the host tending to wall off the tumor such as the periosteal cuff at either side. Tumor bone is irregular and lacks alignment along stress patterns.

By contrast with lesions that exhibit lagging destruction, in which the advancing destructive edge is poorly visualized, some types of bone metastases totally destroy the bone within the area they occupy. Tumor bone is not formed. Metastases from the lung, thyroid, and kidney have this characteristic, for example. Would you expect leukemia to have this total type of destruction or an infiltrative (lagging) type of destruction?

Other metastases exhibit not only active destruction but tend to excite the host tissues to lay down bone in reaction to it, thereby tending to wall it off.

Total destruction of bone area occupied is characteristic of:

Metastases from breast carcinoma	11
Metastases from prostatic carcinoma	44
Metastases from lung and thyroid carcinoma	28

54

YOUR ANSWER: A fracture line is most likely associated with superifical soft-tissue swelling.

You are incorrect. The fracture occurs beneath the deep soft tissues and swelling would appear there first. The superficial tissues may be injured and subsequently swell due to the same trauma.

Return to number 18 and try again.

55

YOUR ANSWER: An adventitious area of calcific density having definite structure visible in the roentgenogram is termed ossification.

The presence of definite bone stria in this area of calcific density is a guideline to ossification. Your ability to distinguish structure as compared to amorphorus calcific density is a useful tool in differential diagnosis of bone and joint disease by roentgenogram.

56

YOUR ANSWER: A swelling would be likely to be associated with an infection.

You are correct. A swelling is caused by inflammatory edema rather than growth. Consequently its edges fade gradually into the other soft-tissue densities. The inflammation involves all tissues in the area, which is reflected by their conversion to water density. The *arrow* in the figure for frame 56 indicates a deep soft-tissue swelling about the metaphysis consistent with early osteomyelitis.

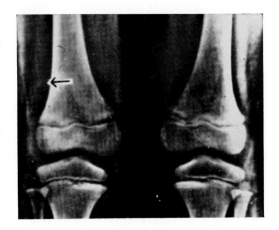

Because a lesion in bone is frequently hidden until it involves the cortex, it may involve a considerable portion of the bone in which it is not seen. A bone is like a metal pipe: unless the wall of the tube is thinned, the x-ray film will not record what is inside. Consequently, the soft-tissue shadows may be a very important guide to a lesion in the skeleton.

A swelling, because it is associated with inflammation, often creates a reaction in tissue about it. The vessel lines running through the fat show a greater contrast with the subcutaneous tissue than is normal.

The number of visible vessel lines would be expected to be:

Increased	12
Decreased	29

57

YOUR ANSWER: To recognize the avascular state of a segment of bone by roentgenogram, the original density of the bone segment must change.

You are incorrect. The original density of the bone segment cannot change because it is avascular. Contrast is created only by changing the density of the bone still alive.

Please return to number 22 and try again.

58

YOUR ANSWER: The diagnosis would be fracture line if the radiolucent line was of even width throughout with rounded edges.

You are incorrect. These features distinguish a growth line. A fracture line has sharp angles, irregular edges, and uneven width.

Return to number 46 and try again.

59

YOUR ANSWER: Osteomyelitis can be distinguished from destruction of bone due to malignancy by the decision as to whether a mass or a swelling accompanies the destruction.

You are correct. Active destruction is present in both conditions. A swelling with poorly defined edges is typical of the inflammation about an infection. A mass with globular shape and clearly defined edges is typical of a tumor.

Active destruction of bone is distinguished by a fine, spiculated irregular edge. Destruction associated with a benign lesion has a relatively smooth edge. There often tends to be some condensation of bone density about it.

Active destruction is associated with malignant tumor or infection.

An osteogenic sarcoma would have a junction with bone about it which is a fine spiculated irregular edge. An osteogenic sarcoma is also distinguished by the fact that it produces tumor bone. Tumor bone consists of gross bone stria which are laid down in an irregular pattern and do not conform to the stress patterns usually visible in the arrangement of bone trabeculae.

Tumor bone tends to a pattern:

Which is around rather than in the tumor	7
Which is grossly irregular within the tumor	42
Determined by the stress on the bone	30

60

YOUR ANSWER: It is helpful in determining whether a fracture exists to note whether the parent bone and the bone fragment have a mass less than the area normally occupied by the undivided bone.

You are incorrect. In determining whether this is a fracture fragment or an accessory bone, the only important consideration relates to the fact that an accessory bone, if combined with the parent bone, would be of greater than normal size.

Return to number 26 and try again.

61

YOUR ANSWER: An osteomyelitis first is evident on the x-ray film as an area of deep soft-tissue swelling centered about the metaphysis.

You are correct. The metaphysis is the area of localization for blood-borne bacteria. It is not necessary to wait for the development of bone destruction to make the diagnosis of osteomyelitis. This change occurs so late that considerable damage may already have been done.

Osteomyelitis is associated with active destruction and a deep soft-tissue swelling. It also behaves in a characteristic manner in bone as compared with tumor. An infection tends to track irregularly as if it had pseudopods reaching out to find the easiest way out of the bone. A tumor, on the other hand, tends to expand concentrically until it reaches an anatomic obstacle. It then tends to a globular form. A tumor also tends to be associated with a soft tissue mass rather than a swelling.

A tumor:

Expands in concentric fashion into a rounded mass	36

Tracks irregularly along the easiest   34
    anatomic route

Cannot be differentiated from an   50
    infection by roentgenogram

Tumors that destroy in this manner, infiltrating through the bone, tend to arise from marrow cells.

Return to number 36 and try again.

62

YOUR ANSWER: A tumor that is designated an osteogenic sarcoma infiltrates through the bone marrow, giving rise to lagging destruction.

You are incorrect. Lagging destruction is typical of tumors such as Ewing's sarcoma.

63

YOUR ANSWER: A fracture line is most likely associated with no soft-tissue swelling.

You are incorrect. The nature of the pathology of a fracture with developing hematoma makes this statement impossible.

Return to number 18 and try again.

CHAPTER 2

Unequal Growth in Children

COLIN F. MOSELEY, M.D.

Disturbed growth and leg length discrepancy have been common problems for the orthopaedic surgeon for many years because there are so many conditions that can affect the dynamics of the growth plate. However, the changing pattern of disease over the past two decades and additions to our armamentarium for evaluation and treatment have produced a significant evolution in the way in which these problems are approached. Prior to the introduction of effective immunization, poliomyelitis contributed about one-third of all cases of leg length discrepancy and, although there were exceptions, the magnitude of these discrepancies tended to be small and amenable to relatively uncomplicated methods of correction. With the disappearance of that disease, discrepancies of congenital origin have increased their relative incidence, and these are frequently discrepancies of greater magnitude that are associated with other anomalies and are more difficult to treat. Improvements in methods of evaluation and prediction have made the timing of epiphyseodesis more reliable and have facilitated the determination of the future course of discrepancies. The surgical technique and the device for lengthening the long bones have been refined, and it has been demonstrated that lengthening can be performed to a greater degree and with fewer complications than had previously been the case. Finally, it is now clear that partial closure of the growth plate does not always lead to progressive deformity because, in some cases, the area of partial closure can be excised, allowing normal growth to continue. This evolution in the character of unequal growth in children makes it all the more important for the orthopaedic surgeon who deals with these problems to remain conversant with concepts of growth and, in particular, asymmetrical growth and its correction.

THE SOURCE OF LONGITUDINAL GROWTH

Bones, like trees, do not grow by expanding their substance (interstitial growth) but by adding on to their surfaces (appositional growth). Longitudinal growth of the long bones occurs mainly in the growth plates with a small contribution from epiphyseal enlargement. The growth plate demonstrates a series of histologic changes from the epiphyseal to the metaphyseal side that reflect the transition that each cell passes through over a period of approximately 24 hours. The growth plate has been well described elsewhere,[15] but it is useful in this context to appreciate the mechanism by which the plate actually grows. All growth occurs in that very narrow zone between the tops of the cell columns and the last intact transverse septum, a transition that takes each cell approximately 24 hours to pass through. The onset of calcification marks the cessation of growth and the transformation to bone. There are several direct contributions to longitudinal growth:

1. Multiplication of Cells. The cells in the columns are replaced every 24 hours, and the plate advances by the length of a column each day.

2. Hypertrophy of Cells. As the cells pass from the tips of the columns into the zone of cell hypertrophy, their transverse diameters increase by 50% and their longitudinal dimensions by 300%. This one mechanism produces about 20 μ of growth per cell.

3. Cartilage Synthesis. The cells in the columns increase their volumes of endoplasmic reticulum by at least 10 times as they hypertrophy, indicating that they are very active metabolically and are adding to the quantity of material in the plate.

THE CONTROL OF LONGITUDINAL GROWTH

The factors that control rate of growth are not clearly understood, but certain influences are evident.

Genetic Control. In spite of variations in other factors, the various growth plates grow at rates that bear constant relationships to one another. For example, in the normal child the proximal femoral growth plate grows approximately half as fast as the distal plate, not only during the years of slow growth but during the growth spurt as well. If the growth of a plate is impaired by an abnormal genetic compliment (for example in hemihypertrophy or the congenital short femur) or damaged by past disease or radiation, its rate of growth nevertheless maintains a constant, although slowed, relationship to the growth of other plates.[43,50] There is also a relatively consistent relationship between longitudinal growth and skeletal age such that, for children of the same genetic stock, skeletal age provides a fairly accurate index of the proportion of adult leg length achieved.[5]

Vascular Control. It is widely held that increased vascularity in the region of a growth plate increases the rate of growth of that plate. This effect is poorly understood, however, and is not consistent, inasmuch as there are cases in which hemangiomatous involvement occurs in the short limb. Nevertheless, hypervascularity is thought to be the basis of the lengthening that accompanies fracture healing[2,8] and osteomyelitis and that sometimes follows periosteal stripping[26] and arteriovenous fistual formation.[57] The vascular supply to the cells at the tips of the cell columns is derived from epiphyseal arteries, and any interruption to the vascular supply of the epiphysis, such as occurs in Legg-Perthes disease, will affect the growth of the epiphyseal plate.

Mechanical Control. It seems that mechanical factors can both accelerate and decelerate growth. Stapling of the plate slows and stops growth, whereas, on the other hand, the shortening of legs paralyzed by poliomyelitis is thought to be due to a reduction in the forces applied by the musculature of the limb but may also be due to changes in vascularity. Damage to a part of the plate by trauma or infection can slow growth in that portion only, leading to progressive angular deformity.

Hormonal Control. Hormonal, nutritional, and metabolic factors are responsible for the relatively consistent changes in growth rate that occur throughout life and that are the basis of growth charts.[5] They affect the limbs symmetrically, however, and are not responsible for discrepancies in length.

PATTERN OF NORMAL GROWTH

Growth can be examined from many different aspects, depending on the interest of the examiner. In the present context, however, growth will be thought of as the relationship between leg length and skeletal age, a relationship that has been well documented by Anderson et al.[6] One must always remember that growth in length of the legs correlates better with skeletal age than with chronologic age and that, in examining patterns of growth, the chronologic age can be virtually ignored. The "tall" teenager, for example, may be tall only with respect to chronologic age and not skeletal age, and he may, in fact, be a "short" child with advanced maturity.

The results of the study of Anderson et al.[6] can be depicted graphically (Fig. 2.1). These growth curves, showing the pattern of growth in boys, illustrate that the curves of both the tibia and femur have the same shape, indicating that they grow proportionately throughout life. The curves for girls are roughly the same shape with the difference that their growth stops at about skeletal age 15, whereas boys stop at about 17. Two important features appear in the growth curve. The first is that growth is faster at birth than it ever will be again, both in absolute and relative terms. The second is that there is no inflection point in the graph; there is no point at which the growth rate increases. At first glance this would seem to show that there is no growth spurt, but in fact it shows that the growth spurt occurs only with respect to chronologic age and not with respect to skeletal age. This is because the skeletal age undergoes rapid change concurrently with increasing leg length and the rate with respect to skeletal age, therefore, does not change significantly. The growth spurt might be more precisely thought of as a maturation spurt. It must be remembered that this graph refers to growth in normal plates of Cauca-

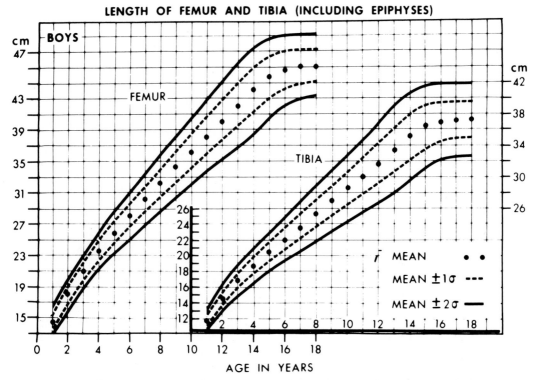

LENGTH OF FEMUR AND TIBIA (INCLUDING EPIPHYSES)

Figure 2.1. Growth curves of the femur and tibia in boys with respect to skeletal age. Both curves have the same shape indicating that they grow proportionately, and there is no upward inflection point that would suggest a growth spurt. (Redrawn from M. Anderson, W. T. Green, and M. B. Messner: Growth and predictions of growth in the lower extremities, *Journal of Bone and Joint Surgery*, 45A: 1, 1963.)

sian children, and extrapolation beyond this group must be made with care.

Using Harris lines and other markers, it has been possible to determine the contributions made by the individual epiphyseal plates to the growth of the whole bone and to that of the entire leg (Fig. 2.2). The largest contributions to growth are made by the plates about the knee, and it follows that the largest discrepancies result from interference with the growth of those plates.

CAUSES OF DISCREPANCY

A comprehensive list of causes of leg length discrepancy is shown in Table 2.1. Listing the etiologies is less useful than understanding pathogensis, but certain general comments are in order here.

Discrepancies of congenital origin are frequently associated with other abnormalities that may play a more important role in the treatment plan. The treatment of the discrep-

ancy associated with fibular hemimelia, for example, frequently involves prosthetic fitting after amputation of what would be a useless and problematic foot. Similarly, treatment of proximal focal femoral deficiency often involves attention to the stability of the hip and the production of an efficient lever arm for prosthetic use, the discrepancy itself being a problem of secondary importance.

Trauma may produce leg length discrepancy by several means. Stimulation of growth of neighboring epiphyseal plates frequently occurs after fractures of long bones in young children, and this is likely due to hyperemia induced by the healing process that occurs during the first year or so of healing.[2] Unfortunately, this phenomenon occurs somewhat unpredictably and, therefore, cannot usually be used to the patient's advantage, especially because fractures sometimes result in premature closure of the adjacent growth plate. Malunions also may produce discrepancies in length, through overriding, overdistraction, or angulation. The most frequent concern in fractures in children is that of damage

CONTRIBUTION TO INDIVIDUAL BONE   **CONTRIBUTION TO ENTIRE LEG**

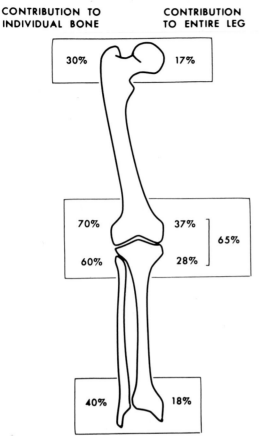

Figure 2.2. The contributions made by the individual growth plates of the limb are constant regardless of the absolute rate of growth. These figures neglect the minor contributions made by the epiphyses themselves.

to the growth plate that inhibits or arrests growth, resulting in either asymmetrical growth with angulation or discrepancy in length or both. The classification of epiphyseal plate injuries proposed by Salter and Harris (Fig. 2.3 *A-E*) provides a sound system of terminology and gives an idea of the relative risk of growth impairment after these injuries.[52] The portion of these fractures that occurs transversely through the plate tends to occur at about the junction of the zone of cell hypertophy and the metaphysis. Therefore, types one and two are unlikely to cause growth disturbance because those fractures do not violate the zone of cell columns and, therefore, do not injure the germinal cells. Types three and four, on the other hand, do traverse this zone and are more likely to

injure those cells and disturb growth. The chance of growth disturbance can be minimized in these types by anatomic reduction that prevents formation of a bony bridge. The prognosis is always in doubt, however, because any of these types may be accompanied by a type V crushing injury that is not evident radiologically.

Discrepancies resulting from generalized skeletal diseases, such as rickets, pose a different sort of problem. Because the course of the disease is variable and unpredictable, so is the rate of growth; therefore, it is impossible for the surgeon to make valid predictions about future growth. Epiphyseodesis becomes a less dependable means of correction, and treatment may best be delayed until growth has ceased. Except for this group of conditions, however, longitudinal growth follows fairly predictable patterns and, of particular importance, the relative rate of growth of the short leg and the growth inhibition remain constant after the primary disease process or healing process is past, regardless of the cause.[44]

EFFECTS OF LEG LENGTH DISCREPANCY

There are several compensatory mechanisms that the patient with a leg length discrepancy makes use of when he stands or walks. Young children with minor discrepancies tend to stand and walk on the toes of the short leg and have little or no limp. The older child and the adolescent, in the absence of an equinus contracture, tend to flex the knee on the long side in order to bear weight on both heels. A functional pelvic tilt is often present as is a slightly lurching gait as the child tends to vault over the long leg. With larger discrepancies, more than one of these mechanisms may be present. Patients with pelvic tilt must develop a functional lumbar scoliosis convex to the short side to balance the spine, and this scoliosis almost always disappears when the patient is sitting or when the discrepancy is obliterated by a heel lift or by placing blocks under the heel of the short leg. A short leg limp is usually detectable with discrepancies greater than 1 cm and begins to become disfiguring or diabling at about 2 cm.

In the short term, leg length discrepancies can cause both discomfort and increased energy requirements. The pelvic tilt causes increased pressure of the iliotibial tract on the greater trochanter and can result in greater trochanteric bursitis. It is possible that tendinitis of the muscles about the hip can result from the disordered mechanics, but such symptoms are rare in children. An increase in the energy requirement of gait is caused by an increase in the vertical travel of the pelvis and center of gravity of the body because this travel must be effected by muscular action. The asymmetry of the legs affects the energy requirement of standing as well, and electromyographic studies have shown that a completely relaxed stance is impossible with even small discrepancies.[55]

Although the compensatory mechanisms and short term effects are immediately apparent, it is the long term effects that are of greater significance and that prompt the orthopaedic surgeon to correct the disability even if it is not presently disabling. Disorders

Table 2.1
Causes of leg length discrepancies during the age of bone growth*

	By growth retardation	By growth stimulation
I. Congenital	Congenital hemiatrophy with skeletal anomalies (fibular aplasia, femoral aplasia, coxa vara etc.), dyschondroplasia (Ollier's disease), dysplasia epiphysealis punctata, multiple exostoses, CDH; clubfoot	Partial giantism with vascular abnormalities (Klippel-Trenaunay, Parkes-Weber) Hemarthrosis due to hemophilia
II. Infection	Epiphyseal plate destruction due to osteomyelitis (femur, tibia), tuberculosis (hip, knee joint, foot), septic arthritis	Diaphyseal osteomyelitis of femur or tibia, Brodie's abscess Metaphyseal tuberculosis of femur or tibia (tumor albus) Septic arthritis Syphilis of femur or tibia Elephantiasis a a result of soft-tissue infections Thrombosis of femoral or iliac veins
III. Paralysis	Poliomyelitis, other paralysis (spastic)	
IV. Tumors	Osteochondroma (solitary exostosis) Giant cell tumors Osteitis fibrosa cystica generalisata Neurofibromatosis (Recklinghausen)	Hemangioma, lymphangioma Giant cell tumors Osteitis fibrosa cystica generalisata Neurofibromatosis Recklinghausen Fibrous dysplasia (Jaffe-Lichtenstein)
V. Trauma	Damage of the epiphyseal plate (dislocation, operation, etc.) Diaphyseal fractures with marked overriding of fragments Severe burns	Dia- and metaphyseal fractures of femur or tibia (Osteosynthesis!) Diaphyseal operations (stripping of periosteum, bone graft removal osteotomy etc.)
VI. Mechanical	Immobilization of long duration by weight-relieving braces	Traumatic arteriovenous aneurysms
VII. Others	Legg-Calvé-Perthes' disease Slipped upper femoral epiphysis Damage to femoral or tibial epiphyseal plates due to radiation therapy	

* Reproduced with permission from W. Taillard and E. Morscher: *Beinlangenunterschiede*, Basel: Karger, 1965.

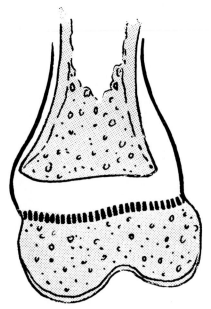

Figure 2.3. (*A*) Salter-Harris type one epiphyseal injury. Because the fracture does not cross the zone of proliferating cells, growth disturbance is very uncommon unless there is an associated type V crushing injury. (Reproduced with permission form R. B. Salter and W. R. Harris: Injuries involving the epiphyseal plate, *Journal of Bone and Joint Surgery, 45A:* 587, 1963.)

little time standing still on both legs, yet cases of structural scoliosis definitely exist, as do cases in which what seems to be a compensatory functional scoliosis cannot be completely corrected by equalizing leg lengths.[53] The fact that up to one-third of curves are not compensatory at all but are to the opposite side supports the hypothesis that they are caused not only by the static influence of standing posture but also by the dynamic forces of movement and gait.[53,55]

Although it is easy to rationalize a relationship between degenerative disc disease with low back pain and leg length discrepancy, attempts to demonstrate it on a statistical basis have been contradictory,[26,34,51] and such a relationship has not yet been proven to exist.

CLINICAL ASSESSMENT

There are certain conditions that can masquerade as leg length discrepancy such that certain patients with that presenting com-

of the hip and low back are of principle concern in spite of the fact that conclusive evidence for cause-effect relationships is lacking in most cases.

Pauwels has described the pattern of pressure distribution between the femoral head and acetabulum on the long side where the center-edge (CE) angle is decreased.[45] He has calculated that increased pressures are present and that the pressure gradient is higher at the acetabular lip, producing higher shear stresses on the articular cartilage at that point. It seems reasonable to suspect that the long term effect of these mechanical changes would be early degenerative arthritis of the hip, but in fact such an effect has not been clearly proved. Despite the lack of proof, however, the high proportion of so-called idiopathic arthritis encourages one to believe that such a relationship exists.

The effects on the spine are also debatable. It is maintained by some that structural scoliosis cannot result because children spend so

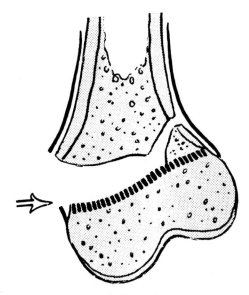

Figure 2.3. (*B*) Salter-Harris type two injury. Like the type one injury, the fracture does not cross the growth area and growth disturbance is uncommon. (Reproduced with permission from R. B. Salter and W. R. Harris: Injuries involving the epiphyseal plate, *Journal of Bone and Joint Surgery, 45A:* 587, 1963.)

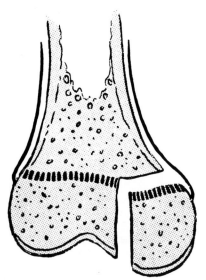

Figure 2.3. (*C*) Salter-Harris type three injury. In this case the fracture line crosses both the growing cells and the articular surface and, therefore, must be repositioned precisely. Growth disturbance is more common than with types one and two. (Reproduced with permission from R. B. Salter and W. R. Harris: Injuries involving the epiphyseal plate, *Journal of Bone and Joint Surgery, 45A:* 587, 1963.)

plaint have no discrepancy whatever. Cerebral palsy, flexion contractures of the hip and knee, equinus and other deformities of the foot, angular deformities of the limbs, scoliosis, and fixed pelvic obliquity must all be taken into account in the clinical assessment.

Although clinical measurement is not as accurate as radiologic measurement, it is an essential part of the assessment because it guards against technical errors and more easily takes into account differences in the sizes of the feet or of the halves of the pelvis. There are three basic ways of assessing leg length clinically. The first, the apparent length, is measured from the umbilicus to the medial malleolus and is affected by position and by contractures. It is somewhat less useful than the second parameter, the true length, which is measured from the anterior superior iliac spine to the tip of the medial malleolus, taking a reading at the level of the knee joint as well, if necessary. These measurements correspond well to the lengths of the long bones but do not take into account differences below the ankle or above the hip that may be functionally important. The third method involves placing blocks under the heel on the short side to bring the iliac crests level and the lumbar spine straight and ver-

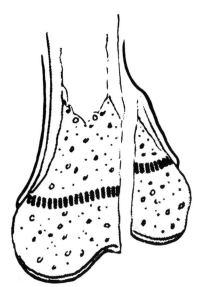
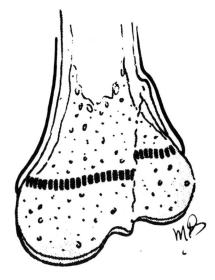

Figure 2.3. (*D*) Salter-Harris type four injury. This injury crosses the growth area of the epiphyseal plate as well as the articular surface and must be anatomically reduced. The diagram on the right shows that a metaphyseal-epiphyseal bony bridge will form if the fracture is allowed to heal in a displaced position. (Reproduced with permission from R. B. Salter and W. R. Harris: Injuries involving the epiphyseal plate, *Journal of Bone and Joint Surgery, 45A:* 587, 1963.)

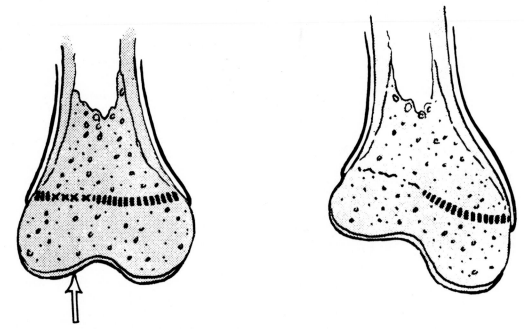

Figure 2.3 (*E*) Salter-Harris type V injury. In this type the cells of the growth plate are injured by crushing, and the injury is not radiologically detectable until growth disturbance appears. This type of injury may be a component of any of the other types. (Reproduced with permission from R. B. Salter and W. R. Harris: Injuries involving the epiphyseal plate, *Journal of Bone and Joint Surgery*, *45A:* 587, 1963.)

tical. This method takes into account such things as the hypoplastic foot and the pelvis that has undergone an innominate osteotomy. Any difference between the height of the blocks and the discrepancy measured by other means must be fully explained before proceeding with treatment.

Some importance is sometimes placed on certain other clinical findings in anticipating future growth, including the appearance of secondary sexual characteristics, age at menarche, heights of parents and siblings, and present growth rate. These criteria are of limited usefulness, however, because none has been documented as precisely as the relationship between leg length and skeletal age itself and none can be used to predict future growth as accurately as the growth remaining method or the straight line graph.

RADIOLOGIC ASSESSMENT

The lengths of the legs can be measured extremely accurately radiologically, and several methods exist to do so. The most accurate method is the scanogram, which is a modification described by Bell and Thompson of a technique previously described by Green et al.[28] It involves the placement of a radiopaque scale beneath the patient and separate exposures of the hips, knees, and ankles so that the central x-ray beam passes through the reference point and perpendicular to the film. This eliminates magnification due to divergence of the beam, and true measurements can be made directly from the image of the scale (Fig. 2.4). The joints of the two limbs can be exposed together if the discrepancy is small so that three exposures suffice, but with larger discrepancies the fact that the joints lie at very different levels necessitates separate exposures of the six joints.

Because children under the age of 6 cannot lie still long enough for the multiple exposures of the scanogram, they are better suited to the teleoroentgenogram, which is a single exposure of the entire lengths of the limbs on a 34-inch film with a long tube-to-film distance (usually 72 inches). This technique introduces magnification but has the advantage of demonstrating angular deformities; therefore, it is sometimes useful in older patients as well (Fig. 2.5).

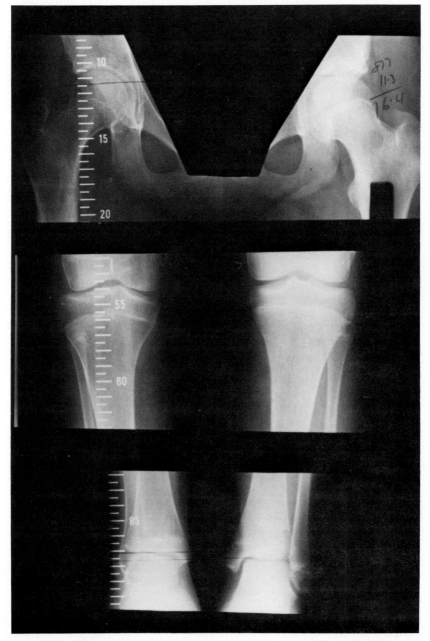

Figure 2.4. Scanogram. In this case the discrepancy was mild so that three exposures, including both sides at a time, were sufficient.

A useful adjunct to these techniques is an anteroposterior film of the pelvis and hips with the patient standing with both heels on the floor and the legs straight. If this position is impossible, then the heel can be blocked up to the appropriate height as determined clinically. The difference in elevation of the femoral heads and iliac crests on the film, taking into account the height of the blocks, gives a precise evaluation of the true discrepancy, including the effects of the feet and pelvis. Any discrepancy between this measurement and other clinical and radiologic measurement must be explained.

Inasmuch as growth, in the present context, is the relationship of leg length to skeletal age, the measurement of leg length should be accompanied on each occasion by an assess-

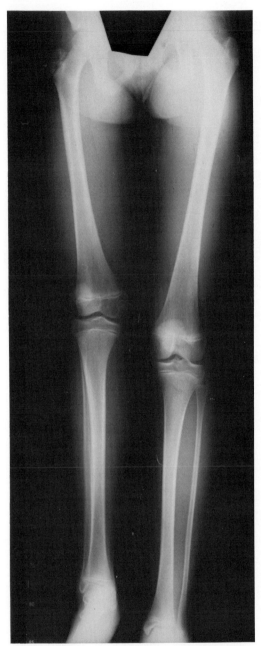

Figure 2.5. Teleoroentgenogram. Although this technique involves a magnification factor of uncertain magnitude, it is useful in cases with angular deformity.

much as a year apart, but it is with respect to these standards that the growth curves were originally developed and they remain our best source. Additional difficulty is encountered with those patients in whom the order of appearance and rates of development of the ossification centers do not follow the pattern described in that atlas. A more recent method attempts to resolve that difficulty by assigning numerical scores to each of 20 landmarks about the hand and wrist and combining those scores to obtain the skeletal age.[56] This method must be used with caution, however, because it does not correspond exactly to the other and has not yet been correlated with leg lengths.

Because there is some observer variation in the assessment of skeletal age and also some variation in the choice of landmarks for measuring leg length, it is important for the surgeon to review all films personally before taking an irrevocable surgical step. To describe the patient's pattern of growth, it is useful to have assessments at least annually during the growing years and more frequently when the time for surgical correction is drawing near. Although not so important for very young children, it is essential to obtain simultaneous skeletal age films whenever leg length is assessed after the age of 8 or so.

METHODS OF PREDICTION

Inasmuch as equality of leg length at maturity is the goal, prediction of future growth and discrepancy at maturity is of the essence and must be based on accurate and valid data. Three methods of prediction are in current use and will be described here in order of increasing complexity and accuracy. Much of the discussion to follow concerning assessment and treatment assumes the short leg to be the abnormal one. This is not always true, however, and certain comments must be qualified accordingly.

"Rule of Thumb" Method

This method was originally described by White and Stubbins[64] and has been recently reiterated by Menelaus.[40] It makes use of the following criteria: (1) the distal femoral epiphyseal plate grows ⅜ inch per year, and the proximal tibial ¼ inch per year; and (2) girls

ment of skeletal age. This is customarily done by comparing an x-ray film of the patient's left hand and wrist with the standards for boys and girls published in atlas form by Greulich and Pyle.[29] A certain inherent error is unavoidable because the standards are as

stop growing at 14 and boys at 16 years of skeletal age. The surgeon planning an epiphyseodesis can predict the amount of shortening that will result by multiplying the rate of growth by the number of years of growth remaining. Although this is a useful rule of thumb and enables one to know when the time to consider epiphyseodesis is approaching, it is only a rough approximation because growth does not occur at a constant rate in the last few years and does not stop abruptly. When making a decision regarding surgery, it should only be used in conjunction with a more accurate method.

Growth Remaining Method

The growth data gathered by Anderson et al. have been further refined and represented in a graph (Fig. 2.6) that illustrates the re-

maining growth potential of the individual growth plates about the knee for girls and boys with respect to skeletal age.[6] It enables the surgeon to predict the amount of shortening that will result from an epiphyseodesis on a more accurate basis than the previous method. Both, however, suffer from several sources of error: (1) they are based on a single estimate of skeletal age and are subject to the inherent error of that technique; (2) they do not take into account the growth percentile of the child and, therefore, will not recognize that a child who is tall for his skeletal age will undergo slightly more shortening than expected after epiphyseodesis; (3) the final result of an epiphyseodesis depends not only on the shortening of the long leg but also on the ability of the short leg to catch up. This method does not take the ability to catch up into consideration, and thus its accuracy is impaired in cases where there is a significant degree of growth inhibition and a relatively

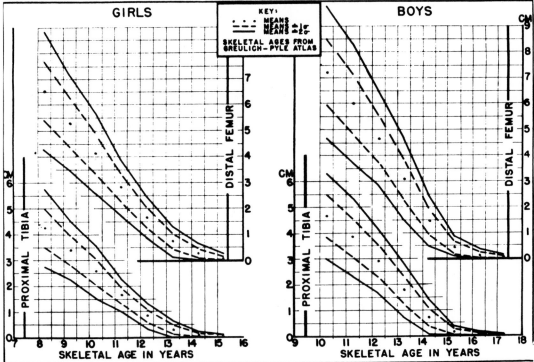

Figure 2.6. The growth remaining graph. This graph is an alternative way of depicting the data represented by Figure 2.1. It is the keystone of the growth remaining method for scheduling epiphyseodesis. (Reproduced with permission from M. Anderson, W. T. Green, and M. B. Messner: Growth and predictions of growth in the lower extremities, *Journal of Bone and Joint Surgery, 45A: 1, 1963.*)

long period of growth remaining. Nevertheless, it is a widely and successfully used clinical tool and is sufficiently accurate for the majority of clinical situations.

Straight Line Graph Method

This method differs from the other two in that it predicts the absolute leg lengths and the discrepancy at maturity as well as the anticipated correction. It utilizes data from several visits to establish the pattern of past growth and thereby to predict future growth. It makes use of a special graph (Fig. 2.7) and a unique method of plotting leg length and skeletal age data that makes it possible to maintain a written record of growth that can be interpreted quickly, accurately, and without mathematical calculations. It can be used

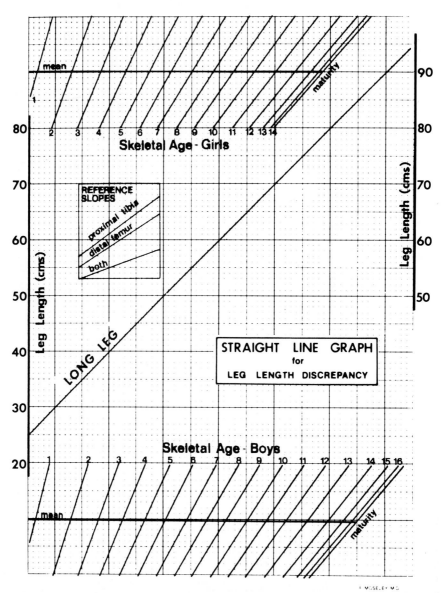

Figure 2.7. The straight line graph for leg length discrepancy. When used according to the steps outlined in the following figures, this method allows depiction of the pattern of past growth, the prediction of future growth, and the prediction of the effects of the various operative procedures available to correct discrepancies. (Reproduced with permission from C. F. Moseley: A straight line graph for leg length discrepancies, *Journal of Bone and Joint Surgery*, 59A: 174, 1977.)

THE DEPICTION OF ONE ASSESSMENT

At each visit to the hospital obtain these three values:

1. The length of the long leg measured by orthoroentgenogram from the most superior part of the femoral head to the middle of the articular surface of the tibia at the ankle,
2. The length of the short leg, and
3. The radiologic estimate of skeletal age.

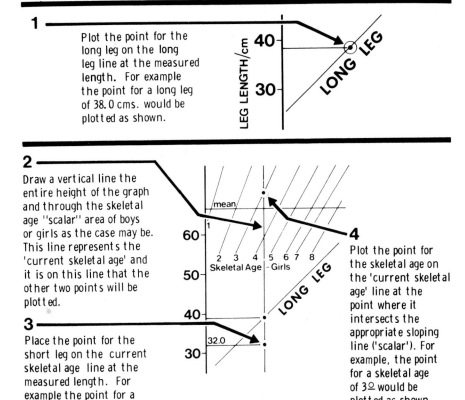

1

Plot the point for the long leg on the long leg line at the measured length. For example the point for a long leg of 38.0 cms. would be plotted as shown.

2

Draw a vertical line the entire height of the graph and through the skeletal age "scalar" area of boys or girls as the case may be. This line represents the 'current skeletal age' and it is on this line that the other two points will be plotted.

3

Place the point for the short leg on the current skeletal age line at the measured length. For example the point for a short leg at 32.0 cm. would be plotted as shown.

4

Plot the point for the skeletal age on the 'current skeletal age' line at the point where it intersects the appropriate sloping line ('scalar'). For example, the point for a skeletal age of 3♀ would be plotted as shown.

Figure 2.8. (A) The straight line graph method. These steps show the method of plotting the three data points obtained at a single visit.

to determine either the correct time for epiphyseodesis or the correct amount to lengthen the short leg because in some cases overcorrection will be necessary because of increasing discrepancy. The child's growth percentile and the growth inhibition in the short leg are automatically taken into account and, because several estimations of skeletal age are used, errors in single estimations tend to be "averaged out." Step-by-step instructions for its use are shown in Figure 2.8 A–E, and the reader is referred to the original descriptions for further discussion.[43,44] This method is used to its best advantage if simultaneous skeletal age and leg length x-rays are done at each visit and if the child is followed for at least 1 year to be certain of his pattern of growth.

CLINICAL CONSIDERATIONS

The anticipated discrepancy at maturity is the overriding criterion in formulating a treatment plan but certain other clinical factors demand considerations.

B THE DEPICTION OF PAST GROWTH

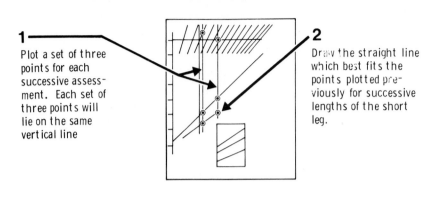

1 Plot a set of three points for each successive assessment. Each set of three points will lie on the same vertical line

2 Draw the straight line which best fits the points plotted previously for successive lengths of the short leg.

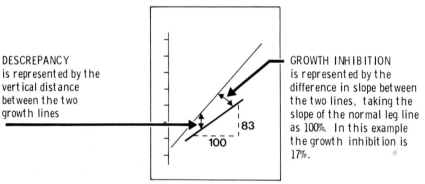

DESCREPANCY is represented by the vertical distance between the two growth lines

GROWTH INHIBITION is represented by the difference in slope between the two lines, taking the slope of the normal leg line as 100%. In this example the growth inhibition is 17%.

Figure 2.8. (*B*) By plotting points for successive visits, the pattern of past growth can be depicted and analyzed.

Anticipated Discrepancy. Because prediction of the discrepancy at maturity is so important, it must be done using a reliable method and must be based on reliable data. With respect to this criterion, there are certain cut-off points that aid the surgeon in formulating a treatment plan. These cut-off points are flexible and must be adapted to the needs of the individual patient.

Discrepancies of less than 2 cm do not require treatment, but patients with a noticeable limp will occasionally appreciate a heel lift. Discrepancies between 2 and 6 cm usually deserve treatment, either with a heel lift or with a surgical procedure. An epiphyseodesis is the best approach during the growing years because it is virtually free from complications and entails little disability.

Shortening procedures are less prone to complications than lengthenings and are, therefore, preferable in adult patients.

One is usually unwilling to introduce shortening of more than 6 cm into a limb, because of both the disproportionate appearance and the possibility that full muscle strength will not be regained. Therefore, correction of more than 6 cm usually requires a lengthening procedure. Correction of more than 8 cm requires a combination of procedures because that is the practical limit of a single lengthening procedure. Discrepancies that are anticipated to exceed 15 cm are usually considered to be beyond correction, although Wagner has reported one case with a total of 22 cm of length gained after three lengthenings.[60]

In patients too old for correction by epiphyseodesis, surgical lengthenings are appropriate for lesser discrepancies than otherwise and may be considered for corrections of 4 cm or more.

Location of Discrepancy. In general, one strives not only to equalize leg lengths but also to make the knees level. It is preferable to lengthen the short bone of the short leg, and it is also preferable, when performing a shortening or epiphyseodesis, to do it in the bone that is more shortened on the other side. This factor is not strong enough in itself to justify shortening two bones when correction can be achieved by shortening one.

Cause. Discrepancies of congenital origin may be so severe that equalization is not a reasonable goal. If the final discrepancy is anticipated to be greater than 15 cm amputation of the foot and fitting of a prosthesis is likely to be the best approach. Amstutz's finding that the limbs maintain their relative

Ⓒ THE PREDICTION OF FUTURE GROWTH

1* Extend to the right the growth line of the short leg.

2* Draw the horizontal straight line which best fits the points plotted previously in the skeletal age area.

GROWTH PERCENTILE— is represented by the position of that horizontal line and indicates whether the child is 'taller' or 'shorter' that the mean.

SKELETAL AGE SCALE— is represented by the intersections of this horizontal line with the scalars in the skeletal age area.

The <u>Maturity Point</u> is the intersection of the <u>line</u> with the maturity scalar.

3* Through the maturity point draw a vertical line, the <u>Maturity Line</u>. This line represents maturity and the cessation of growth. Its intersections with the growth lines of the two legs represents their anticipated lengths at maturity.

Maturity point.
Anticipated discrepancy at maturity.

* In keeping a child's graph up to date it is recommended that these lines be drawn in pencil. The addition of further data makes this method more accurate and may require slight changes in the positions of these lines.

Figure 2.8. (*C*) The straight line graph method. Using points already plotted, the graph can be used to predict the extent of future growth and the magnitude of the eventual discrepancy at maturity.

THE EFFECT OF SURGERY

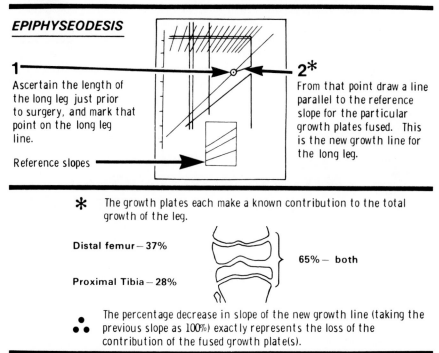

EPIPHYSEODESIS

1 Ascertain the length of the long leg just prior to surgery, and mark that point on the long leg line.

Reference slopes

2* From that point draw a line parallel to the reference slope for the particular growth plates fused. This is the new growth line for the long leg.

* The growth plates each make a known contribution to the total growth of the leg.

Distal femur — 37%

Proximal Tibia — 28%

65% — both

∙∙ The percentage decrease in slope of the new growth line (taking the previous slope as 100%) exactly represents the loss of the contribution of the fused growth plate(s).

LENGTHENING

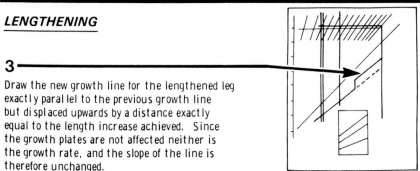

3 Draw the new growth line for the lengthened leg exactly parallel to the previous growth line but displaced upwards by a distance exactly equal to the length increase achieved. Since the growth plates are not affected neither is the growth rate, and the slope of the line is therefore unchanged.

Figure 2.8. (*D*) The straight line graph method. The immediate and ultimate affects of epiphyseodesis and leg length discrepancy can be predicted.

lengths during growth aids in predicting the ultimate discrepancy.[4] The congenital short femur may be associated with absence of the tibia or fibula or with an abnormal foot or hip, necessitating other surgical procedures that must be included in the treatment plan. The congenital short femur frequently has a hypoplastic lateral condyle that can predispose to posterior subluxation of the lateral tibial plateau during the lengthening process and lengthening of the biceps tendon and

release of the iliotibial band should be considered as prophylactic measures.

Certain bone abnormalities that produce growth disturbance may also affect the bone in such a way that the preferred form of treatment cannot be undertaken. For example, in Ollier's disease it may be impossible to lengthen the bone because there may be no solid bone in which to place the pins. Previous osteomyelitis may also preclude lengthening because of the danger of repeated infection. Diseases that follow unpredictable courses may make it impossible to predict future growth, and in those cases correction of the discrepancy is best left until maturity.

Posttraumatic discrepancies follow predictable patterns. The overgrowth that follows fractures of long bones occurs only during the healing period, tapering off at about 6 months and stopping at about 1 year when the growth rate of the bone returns to normal. If growth of a plate is completely arrested by

trauma, then the effect will be virtually identical to an epiphyseodesis and the final result can be predicted using the straight line graph. Later epiphyseodesis of the same plate in the contralateral limb will only serve to perpetuate the present discrepancy and will not correct it. The prognosis in epiphyseal plate injuries must always be guarded until it is certain that a type V injury has not occurred.

Paralysis. If significant weakness exists in the short leg, then perfect equalization may not be the best goal. The patient with a drop

 # THE TIMING OF SURGERY

EPIPHYSEODESIS

1 Project the growth line of the short leg to intersect the maturity line, taking into account the effect of a lengthening procedure if necessary.

2 From the intersection with the maturity line draw a line whose slope is equal to the reference slope for the proposed surgery.

3 The point at which this line meets the growth line of the long leg indicates the point at which the surgery should be done. Note that this point is defined, not in terms of the calendar, but in terms of the length of the long leg

LENGTHENING
Since lengthening procedures do not affect the rate of growth, the timing of this procedure is not critical and will be governed by clinical considerations.

 # POST-SURGICAL FOLLOW-UP

1 Data is plotted exactly as before except that the first point plotted is that for the length of the short leg which is placed on the growth line established for the short leg pre-operatively.

2 Draw the vertical straight line through that point representing the current skeletal age and place the points for the long leg and the skeletal age on it.

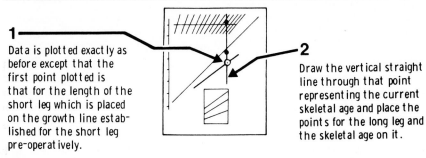

Figure 2.8. (*E*) The straight line graph method indicates a correct time to perform epiphyseodesis and can be used to continue follow-up postoperatively (*F*).

foot or with weakness of the hip or knee flexors may be better off with some residual discrepancy to facilitate the foot in clearing the floor during swing phase.

Age. Because lengthening procedures require the understanding and cooperation of the patient in maintaining knee motion and in protected weight bearing, they are best not done before the age of 10 and are best done during the growing years because of the decline in osteogenesis that occurs thereafter. Inasmuch as the possible amount of lengthening is related to the original length of the bone, more length can be added to the longer bones of older children.

Sex. Cosmesis is usually more important to girls than to boys, but the surgeon must avoid compromising the functional result for cosmetic reasons. Cosmesis is becoming less important to girls as cultural attitudes change and pants and long skirts become more fashionable. Boys usually consider it more important to be tall, and they may be less willing than girls to accept shortening procedures.

Unpredictability. In the case of diseases of changing severity and variable effects, such as the metabolic bone diseases, the inability to predict the ultimate discrepancy with accuracy usually necessitates waiting until maturity before undertaking correction.

Angular Deformity. Angular deformity should be corrected before undertaking correction of length because straightening the limb can increase its true length and angular deformity also predisposes to complications during the lengthening process.

Scoliosis. The presence of scoliosis or fixed oblique lumbar take-off must be carefully assessed before equalizing leg lengths because the spine may become unbalanced, leaving the patient with a worse problem than the original one. The patient must be able to compensate through the spine for the leveling of the pelvis; this can be assessed preoperatively by blocking up the heel on the short side.

Anticipated Height. Short children may prefer lengthening to shortening because the latter reduces standing height by exactly half the amount of the shortening.

Patient Preparation. It is important for the patient to have realistic expectations and to realize that the correction of leg length inequality will be only that. It will not restore normal girth, nor will it restore normal gait to a patient whose limp is due partly to muscle weakness or spasticity. Patients about to undergo lengthening must understand the demands to be made upon them with respect to the maintainance of knee motion and prolonged protected weight bearing and must be well motivated to cooperate.

Associated Surgery. Other surgery may have to be included in the treatment plan. It may be required for an associated defect, as in fibular hemimelia; for the cause of the discrepancy, as in malunion with both shortening and angulation; or may result from the correction itself, as in the relative heel cord tightness that occurs with tibial lengthening.

NONSURGICAL TREATMENT

Small discrepancies can be treated with a heel lift and larger ones with more complex shoe modifications, but this approach becomes decreasingly satisfactory with increasing discrepancies because it is only effective when the modified shoe is worn and involves a lifetime of inconvenience and expense. The height of the heel lift should be chosen to bring the leg lengths within 2 cm of being equal, and a sole lift of half the height of the heel lift is optional. The weight of the shoe and ankle instability set a practical limit of about 6 cm on the height of the lift. Very large discrepancies are best treated with a prosthesis with the foot either in equinus or amputated. This subject is covered more fully elsewhere in this text.

SURGICAL TREATMENT

Surgical procedures designed to correct leg length discrepancies involve either shortening the long leg or lengthening the short leg. The shortening procedures will be covered first in this section. The indication for all such procedures is the presence of the discrepancy itself, and the magnitude of the anticipated discrepancy at maturity guides the surgeon, by way of the guidelines discussed in the previous section, toward an appropriate plan of treatment. Given this indication, the case must meet every pertinent prerequisite; these will be presented for each procedure.

Shortening Procedures

Shortening can be achieved either by slowing down the growth rate of the long leg or by resecting a portion of one of its bones. In either case the disadvantage exists that it is the normal leg that is undergoing the procedure and the result will be two abnormally short legs. These procedures compensate for the problem but do not correct it. They have the advantage, however, of lower complication rates than the lengthening procedures.

Epiphyseodesis. Because of its technical simplicity and virtual freedom from complications, epiphyseodesis is the treatment of choice for all cases that meet its prerequisites. It has disadvantages because it is performed on the long leg and thereby produces two abnormally short legs, reduces height, and leaves the patient slightly disproportionate, but these are usually minor considerations. The first description of a technique for permanent arrest of growth of an epiphyseal plate was by Phemister in 1933, and several variations have more recently been described.[27,47,64] In principle, epiphyseodesis involves removal of a block of bone that crosses the plate and its later replacement in an altered orientation to promote formation of a bony bridge. The principle behind this procedure is to slow down the growth of the long leg, allowing the short leg to catch up.

There are two prerequisites for this procedure. The first is a discrepancy of 2–6 cm; less than that does not warrant surgical correction, and more tends to result in persistent muscle weakness, excessive decrease in height, and disproportion and is usually better treated by lengthening. The second prerequisite is an accurate prediction of the future discrepancy and the effect of the surgical procedure showing that the desired correction will be obtained. This prediction must be based on valid and accurately collected data and can be determined using one of the methods described above.

Epiphyseodesis may be performed on the distal femoral plate, the proximal tibial plate, or both, depending on the rate of correction desired. These procedures slow down the rate of growth of the leg by 37%, 28%, and 65%,

respectively. The chosen plate is approached through longitudinal incisions over its medial and lateral aspects. In the case of the distal femur, the quadriceps muscle can be retracted anteriorly to expose periosteum. The level of the plate can be determined by passing a needle through periosteum but I prefer to incise it longitudinally and to locate the plate by stripping periosteum from bone from the metaphysis toward the epiphysis. It strips easily from bone but is firmly adherent to the perichondral ring at the level of the plate. Flaps of periosteum are raised to allow the removal of a rectangular window of bone approximately 2 cm 1½ cm and ½ cm thick that crosses the plate with about two-thirds of its area on the metaphyseal side. The plate is then clearly visible in the base of the window and is curetted using a curette slightly wider than the plate, keeping it in view in the depth of the defect so formed. Partial curettage of the plate is then carried out leaving enough intact so that postoperative protective immobilization is not necessary and knee stiffness is thereby avoided. The window is then rotated 180 degrees and replaced so that the plate is bridged by solid bone. It is impacted into place and the periosteum closed over it. The same procedure can be used for the medial aspect of the proximal tibial plate, but on the lateral aspect the fibula must be dealt with. It is approached from the anterolateral aspect, taking care to avoid the peroneal nerve, and the plate is completely obliterated with a rongeur or a curette. The lateral aspect of the tibial plate can then be approached anterior to it. The variations on this technique differ only in the shape of the cortical block and its orientation when replaced. They offer no distinct advantage, and the choice is one of individual preference.

Complications are rare and result from errors in prediction of the extent of correction or errors in technique. Errors in prediction should occur only rarely because it is possible to predict the extent of correction to within 1 cm in 95% of children who have had accurate data collected for a period of at least 1 year preoperatively.[44] Partial or complete failure of the plate to close can occur only with gross errors in technique. Knee stiffness can result from postoperative immobilization.

Epiphyseal Plate Stapling. This procedure was devised by Bount in 1949 at a time when the prediction of future growth and the effect of epiphyseodesis could not be predicted with the accuracy and confidence of today.[11] It is based on the hypothesis that epiphyseal plate growth can be arrested temporarily by placing staples across it and that growth will later resume when the staples are removed. If that were the case, the surgeon could apply the staples early and remove them at precisely the moment of perfect correction. Unfortunately, premature plate closure sometimes occurs and growth does not consistently resume. Therefore, stapling must be considered an alternate means of permanent epiphyseal plate arrest. Its indication and prerequisites are virtually the same as those for epiphyseodesis and must be assessed in comparison with that procedure.

Epiphyseal plate stapling is technically more exacting than epiphyseodesis and is prone to complications in that errors in placement of the staples can lead to asymmetrical or incomplete growth arrest or penetration of a time into the articular cartilage or joint space of the knee. These potential problems and the likelihood of a second procedure to remove troublesome staples tip the balance strongly in favor of epiphyseodesis.

Surgical Shortening. Shortening procedures are performed only after the cessation of growth when it is too late to consider epiphyseodesis. They have the advantage that the final discrepancy requiring correction is known so that exactly the desired amount of correction can be achieved without having to make predictions. These are, however, more extensive surgical procedures, are more prone to complications than epiphyseodesis, and should probably be restricted to discrepancies of greater than 2.5 cm.

Tibial Shortening. The indications for tibial and femoral shortening are different because tibial shortening is a two bone procedure, involves greater postoperative disability, is more prone to complications, and cannot safely achieve as much shortening. The indication is a discrepancy in the range of 2.5 to 3 cm; less than that does not warrant extensive surgery, and more than that is likely to leave permanent muscle weakness with impaired control of the ankle and foot. The prerequisites include the following. The patient must be too old to be corrected by epiphyseodesis. There can be no compromise of the vascularity or health of the bone or

soft tissues of the calf. Cosmesis and the levels of the knees must be very important to the patient because, if that were not the case, the preferred technique of femoral shortening would be utilized.

The details of the procedure will not be described here, but in principle the operation is usually done in the proximal third of the bone to avoid the tendency for nonunion that exists in the distal third. The usual technique involves a step cut with screw fixation, however a transverse osteotomy with plate fixation could be used to obviate postoperative immobilization.[10,41] The resected portion should be used as a bone graft, and, if screw fixation has been chosen, protection in plaster will be necessary.

Tibial shortenings may go on to nonunion, may develop compartment syndromes, may have persistent weakness if excessive shortening is attempted, and may have problems with stiffness after immobilization. The very narrow indication and possible complications make this an infrequently used procedure.

Femoral Shortening. Femoral shortening has several advantages over tibial shortening. Methods of internal fixation are secure enough to allow the patient to be weight bearing without external immobilization shortly after the procedure; the thigh is not prone to compartment syndromes; much greater correction can be achieved without persistent muscle weakness; the femur is not so prone to nonunion; only one bone need be dealt with, and the procedures are technically less demanding.

The indication is desired correction of 2.5–6 cm because less than that does not warrant major surgery, and more than that may result in permanent muscle weakness. The prerequisites are a mature patient and suitable bone stock to accept internal fixation.

The literature is replete with methods for accomplishing femoral shortening, most of historic interest only. With advances in the biomechanics of internal fixation, the surgeon should not be satisfied with a technique that keeps the patient immobilized or disabled for a long postoperative convalescence because both midshaft osteotomy with intramedullary rod fixation and subtrochanteric osteotomy with blade-plate fixation will allow the patient to be up and weight bearing a few days after surgery.[9,41] In the former technique, the femur is approached laterally along the intermuscular septum and is exposed subperiosteally. The osteotomy should be done where the medullary canal is narrowest, and a step cut may be used to control rotation. If a step cut is used, reaming should be done to within ½ mm of the rod size and should be done before the osteotomy is fashioned to avoid splitting the bone because the corners of the step cut act as stress risers. Reaming must be done to a slightly greater extent than one would do for a fracture because removal of the segment will reduce the length of contact between rod and cortex. Winquist et al. have reported a closed technique for femoral shortening and intramedullary fixation, but it requires special equipment and expertise and is not for general use.[65] If the osteotomy is performed at the subtrochanteric or intertrochanteric level, special attention must be given to avoiding rotational deformity because the shapes of the cut bone ends do not match after removal of the segment. A strong unit, such as the Richards screw or ASIF blade-plate, should be used to allow early weight bearing.

The complications include those that accompany all major surgery, but infection and mechanical breakdown of the fixation system are the major concerns.

Lengthening Procedures

Lengthening can theoretically be accomplished either by stimulation of growth of the short leg or by surgical lengthening of one or both of the bones in that leg. These procedures have the advantage of being performed on the abnormal leg so that the result is two legs of normal length, thereby correcting the discrepancy rather than just compensating for it. Also, complications, if they occur, will involve an already abnormal limb.

Growth Stimulation. Stimulation of growth in the short limb is a very appealing approach to leg length discrepancies because it strikes at the heart of the defect. Many methods have been attempted over the years to accomplish this, attesting to the fact that none of them produces reliable and satisfactory results. The procedures described to stimulate growth fall into several categories based on the mechanism involved: (1) periosteal elevation[36,66]; (2) metaphyseal implan-

tation of foreign material[31,46]; (3) arteriovenous fistula formation[35,58]; (4) sympathectomy[32]; (5) repeated osteotomy[23]; (6) obliteration of nutrient foramen[16]; (7) electrical stimulation.

The first six of these methods derived from observation of situations in which stimulation of growth occurs when it is not the primary goal, and their rationalizations are clear. The seventh method is mentioned, not because it has been shown to be effective, but for the sake of completeness, because electrical current stimulates connective tissue cells in other circumstances and investigation into its effects on the longitudinal growth of bones is currently under way. These techniques have proven disappointing, inasmuch as lengthening is minimal, inconsistent, and unpredictable. Several such procedures may have to be undertaken in one child to effect sufficient lengthening; hence they have been largely abandoned and will not be described here.

Surgical Lengthening. Surgical lengthening was performed first by Codivilla in 1905,[18] and the history of this approach has been a waxing and waning of enthusiasm linked to changes in technique and expected improvements in the rate of complications. The improvement in the complication rate resulting from each new variation in technique has never been as great as anticipated. Even tody, after significant advances in fixation and technique, surgeons are still well advised to use this approach only if epiphyseodesis and shortening are inappropriate.

The literature is replete with procedures for leg lengthening, but only the author's preferred technique (based on that of Wagner) will be described in detail here. The reader is referred to the following authors for their original descriptions and recommendations: Abbott and Crego,[1] Anderson,[7] Bost,[12] Bost and Larson,[13] Cauchoix and Morel,[17] Codivilla,[18] Coleman and Noonan,[20] Compere,[22] Eyring,[24] Gross,[30] Herron et al.[33] Magnusson,[39] Millis and Hall,[42] Putti,[48] Wagner,[59,61,62] and Westin.[63] The procedures described differ mainly with respect to three parameters; the site of the lengthening (tibia, femur, pelvis, diaphysis, physis), the rate of elongation (immediate, slow), and the method of fixation.

Historically, the method that has been used with the greatest satisfaction over the longest period of time has been that of Anderson, who developed a stable fixation device and achieved lengthening slowly over a period of weeks. Those concepts of site and rate of elongation and of fixation have undergone only minor modifications since. Wagner has developed a protocol with significant advantages over that of Anderson, but the changes have been in technique and technology and not in principle. The major practical difference has been with respect to lengthening of the femur, which was fraught with complications using the Anderson device partly because the method of fixation was cumbersome. With the Wagner technique, this problem has been largely overcome and femoral lengthening can be utilized with less risk. Lengthening through the pelvis by an innominate osteotomy can achieve compensation and has specific indications. One other variation exists concerning the site of elongation, and that is the choice between diaphyseal or physeal lengthening. In actuality, at the present time this is a purely academic issue because physeal distraction has been done only experimentally and then with an unacceptably high complication rate.[25,54]

The reports concerning instantaneous lengthening show that it is possible to achieve up to 4.5 mm of length by this means, but they also report high complication rates even in cases of shortening due to overriding of fractures where one might expect fewer complications.[17,33] This approach is certainly less attractive than either epiphyseodesis or shortening, and is an advantage only in that definitive fixation can be applied immediately.

With respect to internal fixation, both the Anderson and the Wagner devices offer stable fixation and reliable means for gradual elongation. The Wagner device, however, is more flexible in that it provides for adjustments in two planes, can be applied easily to the femur, and is sufficiently light and compact to allow ambulation with partial weight bearing. It is worth noting at this point that the smaller Wagner device intended for the forearm bones or for the lower extremity in small children is not at all adjustable except for the lengthening itself. The external fixators customarily used for fractures are much less satisfactory because they do not provide a convenient means for gradual elongation. In general, plates have been used for final internal fixation when necessary, and special plates are available that are solid in the middle over the lengthening gap.

Femoral Lengthening. The prerequisites for this procedure are normal femoral bone and surrounding soft tissues, a discrepancy that will be greater than 4 cm, is either too great or too late to be corrected by epiphyseodesis, is not suitable for shortening, and is either mainly in the femur or will not result in unsightly disproportion if corrected through the femur. Also, significant angular deformities should have been corrected, and the hip and knee joints should be stable. Special attention should be paid to the knee of the congenitally short femur that is apt to have a hypoplastic lateral femoral condyle and lax ligaments predisposing it to subluxation during lengthening.

The technique which I prefer is identical to that of Wagner except in the method of the osteotomy. The orthopaedic surgeon is well advised to become fully conversant with the technique, the possible difficulties, and the ways to handle them before undertaking this procedure. The protocol involves five stages and three operations: osteotomy and application of the lengthening device, gradual lengthening, removal of the device and internal fixation with or without bone grafting, consolidation in the lengthening gap, and, lastly, removal of the plate (Fig. 2.9).

The first phase takes place in the operating room with the patient in the lateral position and under general anesthesia. An image intensifier should be available. Four Shanz screws are passed through stab wounds in the skin into the femur, two proximally and two distally. They should be in the coronal plane, should be perpendicular to the long axis of the bone, should engage both cortices, and should be placed with the bevel of the tip vertical for best transfer of the distraction force. The order of placement of the screws is not critical, but I place the proximal screw first at the level of the lesser trochanter. I next place the most distal screw about 3 cm proximal to the distal femoral growth plate because it is desirable to have the screws as far apart as possible and the cortex thins out excessively more distal than that. Great care must be taken to ensure that this screw is also in the coronal plane because the lengthening device does not permit adjustment to compensate for rotational malalignment. It is useful to have an unscrubbed

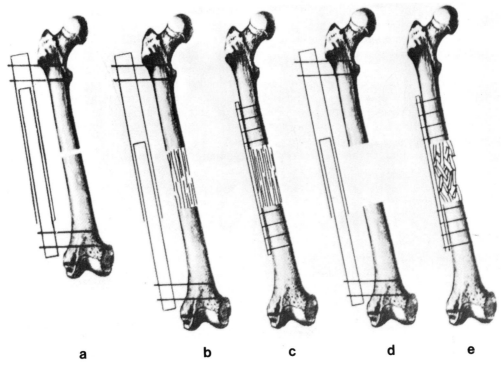

a b c d e

Figure 2.9. Diagrammatic representation of the steps in femoral lengthening. (*a*) Application of the device and osteotomy. (*b* and *c*) If abundant callus is present in the lengthening gap at the conclusion of distraction, then plating can be carried out without grafting. (*d* and *e*) If insufficient callus is present in the lengthening gap, then autogenous bone graft is carried out at the time of plating.

assistant stand in line with the pins to direct the surgeon while he places the screws. The other two screws are then placed using those holes in the special guide that result in the screws of each pair being relatively farther apart. The distraction device is then adjusted so that its scale reads zero, is applied to the pins to ensure an appropriate fit, and is then removed. An osteoclasis is then performed through percutaneous drill holes, and the bone fragments are angulated in all directions to ensure that the periosteum is completely severed. The device is then reapplied and tightened on the pins using the image intensifier to ensure correct alignment. Because there is a tendency for the bone to develop varus during elongation, it is advisable to introduce slight valgus of 5 to 10 degrees at the time of initial application. Elongation of 1 cm is carried out immediately, and the stab wounds through which the pins pass are elongated about 1 cm toward the nearest end of the bone to allow the pins room to travel during elongation and to prevent pressure on

the skin that would cause pain and could lead to necrosis and infection. The knee is then fully flexed to produce tracts for the pins during postoperative knee movement.

This first phase differs appreciably if the shortening of the femur is of congenital origin, because in these cases it is essential to perform a formal lengthening of the iliotibial band. This is done through a longitudinal incision on the lateral aspect of the thigh by incising the deep fascia longitudinally along the anterior and posterior margins of the band. The band itself is then transected by an oblique incision that extends the entire length of the exposure, and the deep fascia is cut circumferentially as far anteriorly and posteriorly as can be reached. In these cases the femur is approached along the intermuscular septum, a formal osteotomy is done, and the periosteum is cut at the same level. Cutting the periosteum does not seem to inhibit osteogenesis and may prevent pain due to stretching. Because of the high incidence of posterior subluxation of the tibia in our own series, I lengthen the hamstring tendons at this time, but as yet there is insufficient evidence to recommend this routinely.

During the second phase, that of gradual elongation, the patient is allowed to ambulate on crutches with touch weight bearing but should remain in hospital under supervision. The device is lengthened 1.5 mm per day by turning the knob through one full turn, and most children can be permitted to carry this out themselves as long as the reading on the scale of the device is monitored daily. The pin sites are cleansed daily and dressed with antibiotic ointment. The patient's blood pressure, ranges of knee flexion and extension, and the scale of the device are read daily and recorded on a chart kept by the bed. The skin incisions should be elongated using local infiltration analgesia when the pins approach their ends, and this is usually required about once a week. The femur is x-rayed weekly and if angulation of greater than 15 degrees is found then it must be corrected under general anesthesia, because a greater degree of angulation is difficult to correct at the time of later plating. The patient's primary daily goal should be to achieve at least 60 degrees of knee flexion and to avoid a knee flexion contracture of more than 20 degrees. Using gravity by sitting over the edge of the bed or by lying prone helps to achieve these goals, and moving through that range several times each day suffices. Very close attention is paid to the range of knee motion and, if the range does not reach those limits, then the elongation is interrupted until the range improves. It is usually this criterion that heralds the end of the elongation phase (Fig. 2.10A).

When the desired amount of length has been achieved, taking into account any future increase of the discrepancy, or when the clinical situation demands it, elongation is halted and a decision must be made as to the third phase. One must decide whether or not to apply internal fixation and, if fixation is chosen, whether or not to bone graft. My own choice has always been to plate the bone, use a bone graft, and remove the device except in cases of pin tract infection where the hazard of deep infection prevents it. The plate is placed on the posterior surface of the femur and is curved slightly to match the anterior bow of the bone to reduce the risk of breakage (Fig. 2.10B). Wagner suggested that, on occasion, especially with young children, the device can be left in place and the bone allowed to heal without further surgical intervention. He also suggested that if the tissue in the lengthening gap is relatively solid and forming bone well then a bone graft is unnecessary; but if this phase is entered into immediately after elongation ceases the tissue in the elongation gap never meets those criteria, and I have used a bone graft from the iliac crest in every case. If plating is decided against, the device is left in place until the bone is solid enough to permit its removal, and Wagner suggested that osteogenesis can be encouraged by using the distraction device to exert compression on the tissue in the lengthening gap. The decision regarding removal of the device must be made on the basis of the radiologic appearance of the bone in the gap, but reliable criteria regarding bone strength are lacking, and fracture through the gap is a hazard.

The patient spends the fourth phase as an outpatient, partial weight bearing on crutches, and is taught with a bathroom scale to exert 30 lb of foot pressure on the floor. The limb is assessed at intervals, and the patient can be expected to regain almost full knee flexion in about 1 year. When the bone has healed and has remodeled to form a solid circumferential cortex, consideration can be given to removing the plate, and that constitutes the fifth phase (Fig. 2.10 C).

Tibial Lengthening. The prerequisites for tibial lengthening are virtually the same as for femoral lengthening with the obvious difference that they apply to the calf rather than to the thigh. The principles of lengthening the tibia are very similar to those stated above, with certain specific exceptions (Fig. 2.11).

Because the leg is a two bone segment and the stability of the ankle must be maintained, holding screws are used above and below the osteotomy site to maintain the relationship between the fibula and tibia. They should not be lagged, but should be tapped in both bones and must maintain the normal separation between them. The fibula is osteotomized transversely through the same lateral incision, and, although the tibia can also be osteotomized through this incision by exposing it across the interosseous membrane, it is easier and safer to do it through a separate medial incision, particularly if a power saw is used. The device itself is placed in a similar

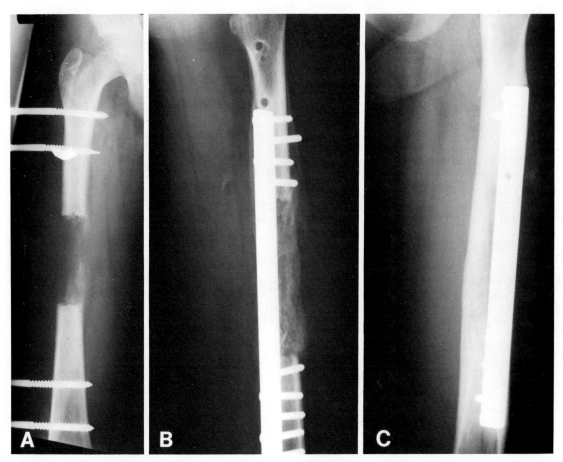

Figure 2.10. Femoral lengthening. (*A*) At the conclusion of distraction, flimsy callus is present in the lengthening gap. (*B*) The lengthened bone is fixed internally by means of a plate and bone graft is added. (*C*) Six months later, osteogenesis is proceding satisfactorily and remodeling is producing a tubular bone. (Reproduced with permission from H. Wagner: Surgical lengthening or shortening of femur and tibia; technique and indications, *Progress in Orthopaedic Surgery*, *1:* 71, 1977.)

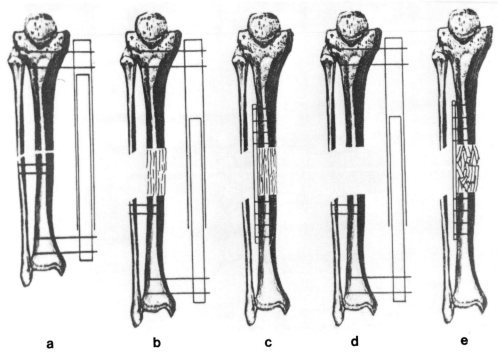

a   b   c   d   e

Figure 2.11.   Tibial lengthening. (*a*) Application of the device, osteotomy and insertion of fibulotibial screws. (*b* and *c*) Internal fixation of a lengthened bone with profuse callus in the lengthening gap. (*d* and *e*) When insufficient callus is present in the lengthening gap, autogenous bone is added at the time of plating.

fashion except that it is placed medially. A formal lengthening of the heel cord is usually required and can be done either before or during the elongation phase (Fig. 2.12 *A* and *B*).

Complications of Lengthening. Complications of lengthening are frequent, and neither the surgeon nor the patient should have unreasonable expectations in that regard. It is important to be aware of them, to avoid them if possible, and to treat them appropriately when they occur. Complications can be general or can be localized to adjacent joints, soft tissues, or to the lengthened bone itself.

General Complications. It is common for hypertension to develop during the lengthening process, and the systolic pressure may be elevated by 20 mm Hg or so. This generally appears early and regresses soon after the lengthening stops. Psychologic problems have also been reported, including emotional lability, anorexia, and weight loss, but they are seldom of serious magnitude.[19]

Joint Complications. Femoral lengthening can cause problems with both the hip and the knee. If instability of either joint is present it

should be corrected before the lengthening is undertaken. Congenital short femurs are often associated with ligamentous laxity of the knee, and a hypoplastic lateral femoral condyle and posterior subluxation of the tibia occurred in 7 of 9 patients in our series. If knee extension is encouraged in the presence of subluxation, then hinging can occur with damage to the joint surface. Serious consideration should be given to routinely lengthening the hamstrings, particularly biceps, because the subluxations are partially rotatory with the lateral side moving first. Because subluxation is accompanied by a loss of knee extension, careful monitoring of knee extension will alert one to its occurrence. A significant permanent loss of extension has occurred in as many as one-third of patients in some reports.[3] Deformity at the ankle occurs in about 80% of tibial lengthenings, with equinus and valgus being the most common.[49] Valgus occurs at the subtalar joint, not at the ankle, and is caused by tension in the heel cord and in the peroneal tendons. It is not the result of migration of the distal fibular fragment and occurs even when nor-

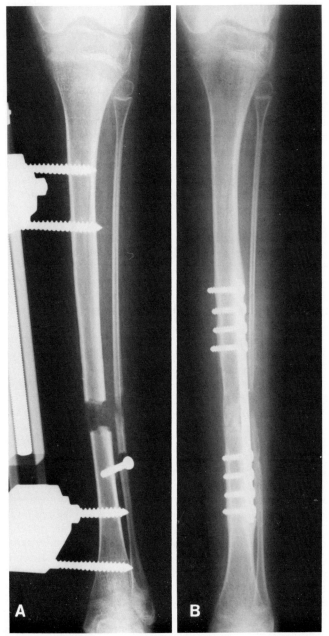

Figure 2.12. Tibial lengthening. (*A*) During the period of distraction. (*B*) After plating and bone grafting. (Reproduced with permission from H. Wagner: Surgical lengthening or shortening of femur and tibia; technique and indications, *Progress in Orthopaedic Surgery, 1:* 71, 1977.)

mal configuration of the ankle is maintained. Early, and perhaps routine, lengthening of the heel cord and peroneal tendons is recommended to avoid it.

Soft-tissue Complications. Serious discharge occurs around the pins in almost all patients, and daily care of the pin sites is essential to prevent this from becoming a more serious soft-tissue infection. Infection in the lengthening gap, particularly if the bone has been plated, is a serious and difficult problem, and plating should be deferred or rejected if anything more than the most innocent pin tract drainage exists. Vascular compromise may occur, especially with tibial lengthening, and it has been suggested that the claw toes and cavus feet that sometimes follow this procedure may, in fact, be caused by occult vascular insufficiency.[21] Certain authors perform routine fasciotomy to avoid this complication. Motor and sensory symptoms occur in about one-third of patients. The sensory symptoms are generally transient, but permanent weakness has been reported in about 10% of cases.[49] This is likely the result of permanent changes within the muscle, perhaps on the basis of vascular compromise.

Complications in the Lengthening Gap. These problems are, with the exception of infection, mechanical in nature. Fracture may occur early or late, whether or not the bone has been plated. Plates should not be removed early, but substitution of a less rigid plate may be advisable if remodeling and consolidation are not proceding satisfactorily in order to stimulate osteogenesis by allowing the bone to bear a greater proportion of the load. Angulation should not be a long term problem, because angulation of more than 15 degrees can be corrected during the lengthening period, and lesser angulation can be corrected at the time of plating.

Innominate Osteotomy. In certain instances it is appropriate to correct leg length discrepancy through the pelvis using an innominate osteotomy as described by Salter, but with a rectangular rather than a triangular graft.[42] Up to 2.5 cm can be gained in this way. This approach has advantages over lengthening long bones in that the hip of the short leg maintains coverage, the healing and rehabilitation period is short, and the complication rate is less. The indications are very narrow, however, because it is unusual to undertake lengthening procedures for discrepancies of such small magnitude. Nevertheless, for the patient who requires lengthening rather than shortening and who will be adequately corrected by a gain of 2.5 cm, this may be the procedure of choice.

PARTIAL CLOSURE OF THE GROWTH PLATE

Many of the same processes that disturb the growth plate causing leg length discrep-

ancies occasionally involve only a part of the plate, producing a local arrest and bony bridge. The remainder of the plate may continue to grow more or less normally but be tethered by the bony bridge. If the bridge is peripheral, then angular deformity results; if central, the plate can become tented, resulting in deformation of the adjacent joint.

Langenskjold[37,38] and Bright[14] have shown that the bony bridge can be resected surgically and that normal or improved growth will resume in an encouragingly high proportion of cases. It is small, peripheral bridges that give the best results after resection, but this approach is indicated in most cases because, even if unsuccessful, the patient's condition is not worsened and more traditional methods can still be used.

It is important before undertaking resection to establish the size and location of the plate exactly in order to plan the approach and to assess the likelihood of success. Regular and oblique x-rays, tomograms, and computerized tomography are all useful in that regard. Resection may be attempted even for large bridges.

Peripheral bridges may be approached directly and should be completely removed with a curette until normal plate can be seen throughout the margin of the surgical defect. The defect should then be filled with fat (Langenskjold) or silastic (Bright), because both of these substances seem to inhibit osteogenesis and reformation of the bony bridge. Fat is conveniently available in the subcutaneous tissues and avoids the introduction of foreign material. Bridges that are close to the periphery can still be approached in this way if only a minimal part of normal growth plate need be sacrificed (Fig. 2.13).

Central bridges are more challenging to excise because they must be approached through the metaphysis and accurate localization is essential. This is best done by introducing a guide wire through metaphyseal cortex and into the bridge under x-ray control. Its position is confirmed in two views, and then the surgical approach can be carried out along it. A complete ring of intact growth plate around the depths of the surgical defect confirms adequate excision.

If successful, the plate will resume more or less normal growth, and the surgical defect in the bone will be left behind as the plate grows away from it. If the first attempt is unsuccessful, then a second attempt is some-

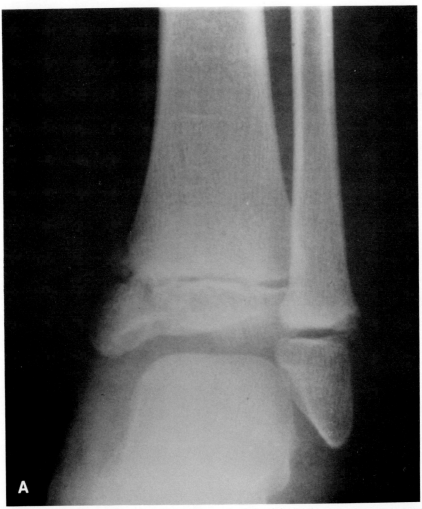

Figure 2.13. Partial closure of the epiphyseal plate due to trauma. (*A*) The initial x-ray shows a minimally displaced type three fracture of the medial malleolus and a type two fracture of the distal fibula with a very small metaphyseal flake. Immobilization in the form of a long leg cast was applied without reduction. (*B*) Further displacement occurred during the healing process and after removal of the plaster, deformation of the articular surface secondary to a partial growth arrest from a bony bridge in the medial aspect of the plate was evident. (*C* and *D*) The bony bridge was excised through a medial approach through the plate. Six months later no further deformation of the articular surface had occurred and the epiphyseal plate seemed to be growing away from the surgical defect and leaving it behind in the metaphysis.

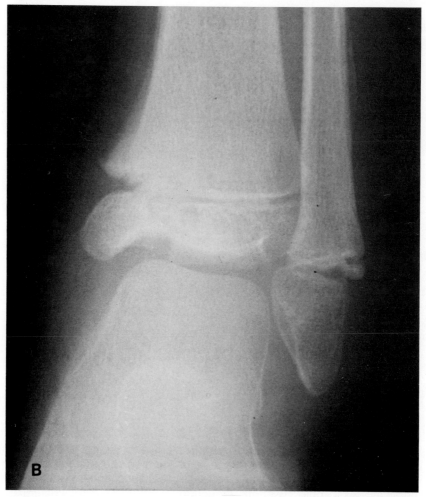

Figure 2.13 *B.*

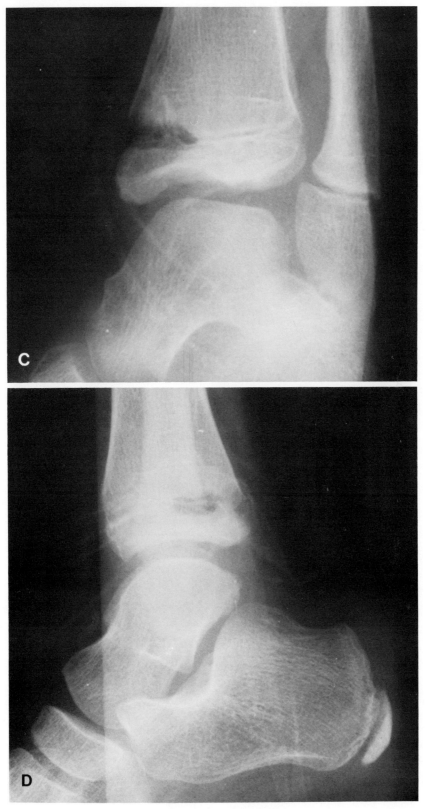

Figure 2.13 *C* and *D*.

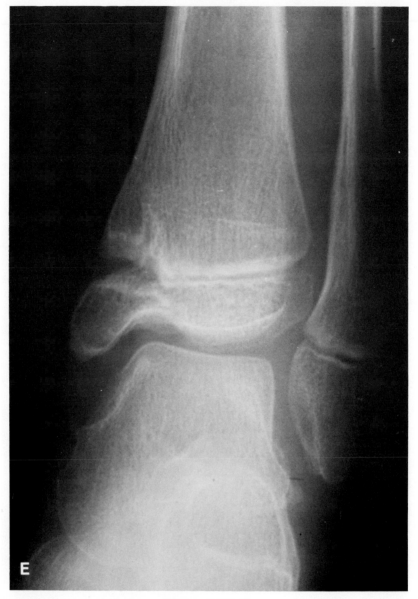

Figure 2.13 *E.*

times indicated because there is little to be lost.

If resection of the bony bridge proves unsuccessful and must be abandoned, then more traditional methods must be used. If there is only slowing rather than complete arrest of growth in the plate and the contour of the adjacent joint is preserved, then repeated osteotomies may adequately correct angulation while preserving growth potential.

If there is no growth potential worth preserving, then it is best to complete the arrest by epiphyseodesis, thereby obviating recurring angular deformities and osteotomies to correct them, and to resign the patient to later procedures for equalization of length.

References

1. Abbott, L. C., and Crego, C. H.: Operative lengthening of the femur, *South. Med. J.,* *21:* 823, 1928.

2. Aitken, A. P., Blackett, C. W., and Ciacotti, J. J.: Overgrowth of the femoral shaft following fractures in childhood, *J. Bone Joint Surg.*, 21: 334, 1939.

3. Allan, P. G.: Bone lengthening, *J. Bone Joint Surg.*, 30B: 490, 1948.

4. Amstutz, H. C.: Natural history and treatment of congenital abscence of the fibula, *J. Bone Joint Surg.*, 54A: 349, 1972.

5. Anderson, M., and Green, W. T.: Lengths of the femur and tibia; norms derived from orthoroentgenograms of children from five years of age until epiphyseal closure, *Am. J. Dis. Child.*, 75: 279, 1948.

6. Anderson, M., Green, W. T., and Messner, M. B.: Growth and predictions of growth in the lower extremities. *J. Bone Joint Surg.*, 45A: 1, 1963.

7. Anderson, W. V.: Leg lengthening, *J. Bone Joint Surg.*, 34B: 150, 1952.

8. Bisgard, J. D.: Longitudinal overgrowth of long bones with special reference to fractures, *Surg. Gynecol. Obstet.*, 62: 823, 1936.

9. Blount, W. P.: Blade-plate internal fixation for high femoral osteotomies, *J. Bone Joint Surg.*, 25: 319, 1943.

10. Blount, W. P.: *Fractures in Children*, Baltimore: Williams & Wilkins, 1954.

11. Blount, W. P., and Clark, G. R.: Control of bone growth by epiphyseal stapling; preliminary report, *J. Bone Joint Surg.*, 31A: 464, 1949.

12. Bost, F. C.: Operative lengthening of the bones of the lower extremity. American Academy of Orthopaedic Surgeons, Instructional Course Lecture, 1, 1944.

13. Bost, F. C., and Larson, L. J.: Experiences with lengthening of the femur over an intrameduallary rod, *J. Bone Joint Surg.*, 38A: 567, 1956.

14. Bright, R. W.: Operative correction of partial epiphyseal plate closure by osseous-bridge resection and silicone-rubber implant, *J. Bone Joint Surg.*, 56A: 665, 1974.

15. Brighton, C. T.: Structure and function of the growth plate, *Clin. Orthop.*, 136: 22, 1978.

16. Brookes, M.: Femoral growth after occlusion of the principal nutrient canal in day-old rabbits, *J. Bone Joint Surg.*, 39B: 563, 1957.

17. Cauchoix, J., and Morel, G.: One stage femoral lengthening, *Clin. Orthop.*, 136: 66, 1978.

18. Codivilla, A.: On the means of lengthening in the lower limbs, the muscles and tissues which are shortened through deformity, *Am. J. Orthop. Surg.*, 2: 353, 1905.

19. Coleman, S. S.: Current concepts of tibial lengthening, *Orthop. Clin. North Am.*, 3: 201, 1972.

20. Coleman, S. S., and Noonan, T. D.: Anderson's method of tibial lengthening by percutaneous osteotomy and gradual distraction; experiences with 31 cases, *J. Bone Joint Surg.*, 49A: 263, 1967.

21. Coleman, S. S., and Stevens, P. M.: Tibial lengthening, *Clin. Orthop.* 136: 92, 1978.

22. Compere, E. L.: Indications for and against the leg lengthening operation, *J. Bone Joint Surg.*, 18: 692, 1936.

23. Compere, E. L., and Adams, C. O.: Studies of the longitudinal growth of long bones: the influence of trauma to the diaphysis, *J. Bone Joint Surg.*, 19: 922, 1937.

24. Eyring, E. J.: Staged femoral lengthening, *Clin. Orthop.*, 136: 83, 1978.

25. Fishbane, M. D., and Riley, L. M.: Continuous transphyseal traction: experimental observations, *Clin. Orthop.*, 136: 120, 1978.

26. Gernet, W.: Die Verkurzungsosteotomie an den unteren extremitaten, *Mang. Dis.*, 1966.

27. Green, W. T., and Anderson, M. A.: Experiences with epiphyseal arrest in correcting discrepancies in length of the lower extremities in infantile paralysis, *J. Bone Joint Surg.*, 29: 659, 1947.

28. Green, W. T., Wyatt, G. M., and Anderson, M.: Orthoroentgenography as a method of measuring the bones of the lower extremity, *J. Bone Joint Surg.*, 28: 60, 1946.

29. Greulich, W. W., and Pyle, S. I.: *Radiographic Atlas of the Skeletal Development of the Hand and Wrist*, Stanford, Calif.: Stanford University Press, 1950.

30. Gross, R. H.: An evaluation of tibial lengthening procedures, *J. Bone Joint Surg.*, 53A: 693, 1971.

31. Haas, S. L.: Stimulation of bone growth, *Am. J. Surg.*, 95: 125, 1958.

32. Harris, R. I., and McDonald, J. L.: The effect of lumbar sympathectomy upon the growth of legs paralysed by anterior poliomyelitis, *J. Bone Joint Surg.*, 18: 35, 1936.

33. Herron, L. D., Amstutz, H. C., and Sakai, D. N.: One staged femoral lengthening in the adult, *Clin. Orthop.*, 136: 74, 1978.

34. Hult, L.: The munkfors investigation: a study of the frequency and causes of the stiff neck-brachialgia and lumbago-sciatica syndromes as well as observations on certain signs and symptoms from the dorsal spine and the joints of the extremities in industrial and forest workers, *Acta Orthop. Scand. Suppl.*, 16: 1, 1954.

35. James, J. M., and Jennings, W. K.: Effect of induced arteriovenous fistula on leg length; ten year observations, *Proc. Mayo Clinic*, 36: 1, 1961.

36. Khoury, S. C., Silberman, F. S., and Cabrine, R. L.: Stimulation of the longitudinal growth of long bones by periosteal stripping, *J. Bone Joint Surg.*, 45A: 1679, 1963.

37. Langenskjold, A.: An operation for partial closure of an epiphyseal plate in children, and its experimental basis, *J. Bone Joint Surg.*, 57B: 325, 1975.

38. Langenskjold, A., and Osterman, K.: Surgical treatment of partial closure of the epiphyseal plate, *Reconstr. Surg. Traumatal.*, 17: 48, 1979.

39. Magnusson, P. B.: Lengthening of shortened bones of the leg by operation, *Surg. Gynecol. Obstet.*, 17: 63, 1913.

40. Menelaus, M. B.: Correction of leg length discrepancy by epiphyseal arrest, *J. Bone Joint Surg.*, 48B: 336, 1966.

41. Merle D'Aubigne, R., and Dubousset, J.: Surgical correction of large leg length discrepancies in the lower extremities of children and adults, *J. Bone Joint Surg.*, 53A: 411, 1971.

42. Millis, M. B., and Hall, J. E.: Transiliac lengthening of the lower extremity; a modified innominate osteotomy for the treatment of postural imbalance, *J. Bone Joint Surg.*, 61A: 1182, 1979.

43. Moseley, C. F.: A straight line graph for leg length discrepancies, *J. Bone Joint Surg.*, 59A: 174, 1977.

44. Moseley, C. F.: A straight line graph for leg length discrepancies, *Clin. Orthop.*, 136: 33, 1978.

45. Pauwels, F.: Des affections de la hanche d'origine mecanique et de leur traitement par l'osteotomie d'adduction, *Rev. Chir. Orthop.*, 37: 22, 1951.

46. Pease, C. N.: Local stimulation of growth of long

bones; a preliminary report, *J. Bone Joint Surg., 34A:* 1, 1952.

47. Phemister, D. B.: Operative arrestment of longitudinal growth of bones in the treatment of deformities, *J. Bone Joint Surg., 15:* 1, 1933.

48. Putti, V.: Operative lengthening of the femur, *Surg. Gynecol. Obstet., 58:* 318, 1934.

49. Rangaswami, S.: Limb lengthening operations. Thesis, University of Liverpool, 1979.

50. Ring, P. A.: Congenital short femur; simple femoral hypoplasia. *J. Bone Joint Surg., 41B:* 73, 1959.

51. Rush, W. A., and Steiner, H. A.: Study of lower extremity length, inequality, *Am. J. Roentgenol., 56:* 616, 1946.

52. Salter, R. B., and Harris, W. R.: Injuries involving the epiphyseal plate, *J. Bone Joint Surg., 45A:* 587, 1963.

53. Scheller, M. L.: Uber den einflub der beinverkurzung auf die wirbelsaule. *Mang. Dis. Koln,* 1964.

54. Sledge, C. B., and Noble, J.: Experimental limb lengthening by epiphyseal distraction, *Clin. Orthop., 136:* 111, 1978.

55. Taillard, W., and Morscher, E.: *Beinlangenunterschiede,* Basel: Karger, 1965.

56. Tanner, J. M., Whitehouse, R. M., Marshall, W. A., Healy, M. J. R., and Goldstein, H.: *Assessment of Skeletal Maturity and Prediction of Adult Height (TW 2 Method),* London: Academic Press, 1975.

57. Vanderhoeft, P. J., Kelly, P. J., Janes, J. M., and Peterson, L. F. A.: Growth and structure of bone distal to an arteriovenous fistula: quantitative analysis of the tetracycline induced transverse growth patterns, *J. Bone Joint Surg., 45B:* 582, 1963.

58. Vesely, D. C., and Mears, T. M.: Surgically induced arteriovenous fistula; its effect upon inequality of leg length, *South. Med. J., 57:* 129, 1964.

59. Wagner, H.: Operative beinverlangerung, *Chirurg, 42:* 260, 1971.

60. Wagner, H.: Technik und indikation der operativen verkurzung und verlangerung von ober - und untershenkel, *Orthopade, 1:* 59, 1972.

61. Wagner, H.: Surgical lengthening or shortening of femur and tibia; technique and indications, *Prog. Orthop. Surg., 1:* 71, 1977.

62. Wagner, H.: Operative lengthening of the femur, *Clin. Orthop., 136:* 125, 1978.

63. Westin, G. W.: Femoral lengthening using a periosteal sleeve; report of 26 cases, *J. Bone Joint Surg., 49A:* 83, 1967.

64. White, J. W., and Stubbins, S. G., Jr.: Growth arrest for equalizing leg lengths, *J. A. M. A., 126:* 1146, 1944.

65. Winquist, R. A., Hansen, S. T., and Pearson, R. E.: Closed intrameduallary shortening of the femur, *Clin. Orthop., 136:* 54, 1978.

66. Yabsley, R. H., and Harris, W. R.: The effect of shaft fractures and periosteal stripping on the vascular supply to epiphyseal plates, *J. Bone Joint Surg., 47A:* 551, 1965.

CHAPTER 3

Epiphyseal, Metaphyseal, and Diaphyseal Affections

EPIPHYSEAL AFFECTIONS

Dysplasia Epiphysialis Hemimelica

This entity was described in 1950 by Trevor,[3] who named it "tarsoepiphyseal aclasis." It is not limited to the tarsus, nor is the tarsus constantly involved. It is an epiphyseal disease that, in a sense, represents an osteochondroma of the epiphysis. Involvement of the astragalus is striking, and the tarsal bones represent the most common site (Figs. 3.1 and 3.2).

CLINICAL PICTURE

In reported cases, this disease is most common in the male. It is usually recognized in childhood.

A swelling at either the medial or the lateral side of the ankle or knee is the most common presenting complaint. Such a swelling is bony and hard, and, because of the abnormal growth of the epiphysis on one side, deformity of the part distal to it, as, for instance, genu valgus or varus, may be apparent. There may be limitation of motion of the affected joint, and symptoms of internal derangement of the joint may arise as the growth progresses. Ligaments and tendons have to slide over these prominences and may lock on one side.

The medial side of the epiphysis is the usual site of involvement. The distal femoral epiphysis and the talus are most commonly subject to this abnormal growth. Progression is most severe in the early years of life, but it may continue through the growth period. It tends to cease as the epiphyseal lines close.

The x-ray appearance is that of an abnormal mass and an eccentric epiphyseal enlargement. There appear to be multiple centers of ossification irregularly and disorderly distributed in the involved area of the epiphysis. Diagnosis by the roentgenogram requires primarily knowledge of this condition, because epiphyseal diseases are few and none have the eccentric disorderly appearance of bone-forming elements and distortion of epiphyseal shape present here.

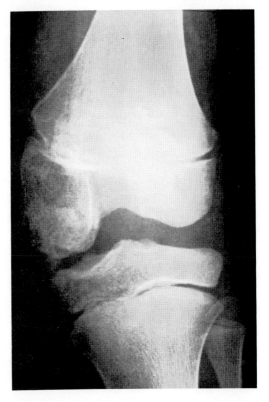

Figure 3.1. Epiphyseal osteochondroma of the medial condyle of the femur. Such a lesion belongs to the condition known as dysplasia epiphysialis hemimelica. It produces marked deformity and may be surgically remodeled to the expected anatomic shape of the bone. To permit the lesion to produce secondary deformity increases the disaster stemming from overgrowth of the lesion.

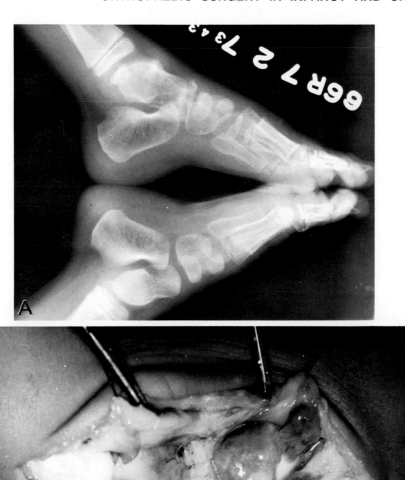

Figure 3.2. (*A*) Epiphyseal osteochondroma involving the talus and navicular with irregular ossific masses. The normal foot is shown beneath for contrast. (*B*) Exposure of cartilage-capped enlargement coming from both talus and navicular and in line with the medial ray of the foot, consistent with dysplasia epiphysialis hemimelica described by Trevor.

PATHOLOGY

The mass, when visualized at operation, has a smooth, glistening, bluish cartilage surface. Its irregularly convoluted surface joins the area of normal epiphyseal cartilage in a manner that permits no clear-cut distinction. It becomes a matter of judgment as to where the epiphysis ends. Examined by microscope, the cartilage is more hyperplastic than normal, and active enchondral ossification is taking place at multiple centers within it. The appearance is very similar to that of an osteochondroma. All the elements taken by themselves are parts of normal growth; only the pattern and the organization have become disorderly.

TREATMENT

It is noteworthy that experience generally indicates that these epiphyses can be attacked surgically to remove the excess mass and to shape the epiphysis into something regarded as normal for a given location and a given child. There has been no particular tendency for the growth to recur, and functional improvement has been good. It is not a question of removing the lesion entirely but of reshaping the epiphysis into a functioning part. Judgment has to be used in preserving other elements of the joint.

References

1. Donaldson, J. S., Sankey, H. H., Girdany, B. R., and Donaldson, W. F.: Osteochondroma of the distal femoral epiphysis, *J. Pediatr., 43:* 212, 1953.
2. Fairbank, T. J.: Dysplasia epiphysialis hemimelica, *J. Bone Joint Surg., 38B:* 237, 1956.
3. Trevor, D.: Tarso epiphyseal aclasis: a congenital error of epiphyseal development, *J. Bone Joint Surg., 32B:* 204, 1950.

Epiphyseal Chondroblastoma

This lesion seems to be a distinct entity that occurs in the epiphyses of adolescents. It arises from proliferation of the chondroblast and produces foci of chondroid matrix. For a long time after Codman[1] in 1931 described 9 cases that occurred in the proximal end of the humerus, it was known as Codman's tumor (Fig. 3.3). One suspects that this tumor is not yet completely understood. It has certain similarities to giant cell tumor in that it occurs in the epiphysis, but it differs in that it begins to develop (before the epiphyseal line closes) from the chondroblast. Giant cell tumor occurs only after the epiphysis is ossified.

Ewing[2] first noted this tumor in 1928, and he considered it a variant of the giant cell tumor. Jaffe and Lichtenstein[3] in 1942 described the lesion in further detail and renamed it a benign chondroblastoma of bone.

It is a rare tumor arising principally at the ends of long bones.

CLINICAL PICTURE

The lesion produces pain. The child is usually adolescent, the tumor rarely having been noted before the age of 10. In the series of Kunkel et al.,[4] one patient was age 8. Tumors noted just after the epiphyseal lines have closed, when the patient is in the early 20s, are suspected of having originated just prior to closure of the epiphyseal line, when the chondroblast was still active. The usual

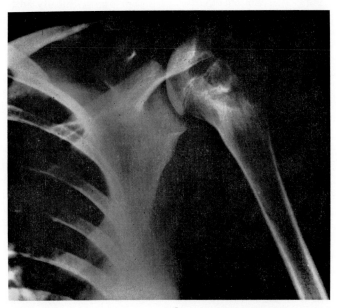

Figure 3.3. Epiphyseal chondroblastoma (so-called Codman's tumor). The tumor involves the proximal humeral epiphysis and extends into the metaphysis.

duration of symptoms before the patient is seen is 1–2 years. Limitation of motion of the adjacent joint and occasionally swelling may be seen. A mass may be palpated if the tumor has been present for considerable time.

PATHOLOGY

The gross appearance is not very helpful, the principle feature being the epiphyseal location. With increasing duration, the lesion may extend into the metaphysis and break through the cortex, but it is usually overlain by subperiosteal bone if it does so. It may erode the articular surface. The material feels gritty when it is cut. Microscopically, the diagnosis depends on recognition of the chondroblast as the basic proliferating cell. This cell is larger than normal and has a well defined cytoplasmic membrane. Areas filled with sheets of these cells are found to be quite uniform in nature. The cellular areas lie in a matrix of hyalin, of myxoid material, and of collagenized connective tissue. Deposits of amorphous calcium lie in this matrix. Giant cells are present. Mitotic figures are rare.

ROENTGEN PICTURE

Location in an epiphysis is characteristic. The calcium in the matrix of the tumor may give it a hazy appearance, or definite foci of increased density may be seen within the radiolucent area occupied by the lesion. The lesion may be very small, occupying but a small portion of the epiphysis, or it may occupy most of the epiphysis and extend into the metaphysis. When it does so, subperiosteal new bone may wall off the lesion. The edge of the lesion in contact with bone is rather well defined and may be walled off sclerotically.

TREATMENT

The features of this tumor are quite characteristic, and the course is benign. Biopsy, however, is indicated. Surgical excision seems to be a satisfactory means of ablating the lesion. It may be necessary to fill the resulting defect with bone grafts. Recurrences are rare and respond to second excisions. It is generally thought that radiation therapy should be avoided.

References

1. Codman, E. A.: Epiphyseal chondromatous giant cell tumors of the upper end of the humerous, *Surg. Gynecol. Obstet.*, 52: 543, 1931.
2. Ewing, J.: The classification and treatment of bone sarcoma, 365–376, *Report of the International Conference on Cancer*; Bristol: John Wright & Sons, 1928.
3. Jaffe, H. L., and Lichtenstein, L.: Benign chondroblastoma of bone; reinterpretation of the so-called calcifying or chondromatous giant cell tumor, *Am. J. Pathol.*, 18: 969, 1942.
4. Kunkel, M. G., Dahlin, D. C., and Young, H. H.: Benign chondroblastoma, *J. Bone Joint Surg.*, 38A: 817, 1956.
5. Valls, J., O'Holeghi, C. E., and Schajowicz, F.: Epiphyseal chondroblastoma of bone, *J. Bone Joint Surg.*, 33A: 997, 1951.

Chondrodystrophia Calcificans Congenita (Stippled Epiphyses, Fairbank's Disease)

This condition cannot be recognized from the roentgen film alone. It is associated with flexion contractures and congenital cataracts.

Several types of roentgen findings may be confused with the more serious classic form of the disease. A child with clinically normal extremities may be noted to have multiple ossification centers, for the epiphyses of coalescence may be seen. The epiphyseal centers appear none the worse for this method of ossification as growth progresses, and the child goes on to normal growth and development both clinically and roentgenographically as the centers fully coalesce.

Very rarely, areas of calcification in the articular cartilage are seen in infancy. These areas are amorphous. The child goes on to normal development. There is no apparent relation to calcinosis and no detectable disturbance of calcium metabolism.

The irregular ossification of the epiphyses that is clinically serious is associated with flexion contractures of the knees, hips, elbows, wrists, and fingers (Fig. 3.4). The involved limb is short and readily detectable when unilateral congenital cataracts are noted. The skull is normal. The child is hypotonic and remains in the lower growth percentiles.

ROENTGEN FEATURES

The epiphyses of the distal femur and proximal tibia are most commonly involved.

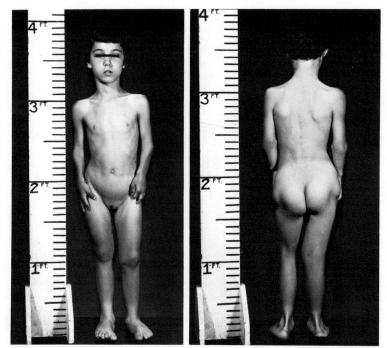

Figure 3.4. Shortening of the long bones, flaring of the epiphyseal metaphyseal area, and irregular shape of the small bones of the hands and feet are all features of chondrodystrophic bone formation with multiple joint involvement due to deformity.

Multiple ossification centers give a stippled appearance. The upper extremity often shows changes around the elbow joint. The ossification centers may be distributed like a necklace of pearls through the epiphysis. Irregular outlines of the bones of the tarsus may be visible. Where growth is affected, the bones are short and thick.

PROGNOSIS

A number of these infants seem to have little resistance to infection and die before 1 year of age.

Little is known of the underlying abnormality. The cartilage of the epiphysis may contain fibrous areas in which normal cartilage structure is lost and degenerative changes occur. There is extreme vascular invasion of the cartilage. Occasional areas of mucoid degeneration may calcify.

Spondyloepiphyseal Dysplasia (Pseudoachondroplasia)

There is shortening of the long bones in this disease. It becomes evident after the second year of extrauterine growth, but is usually not apparent before this age group. It is transmitted as a Mendelian dominant (Fig. 3.5).

CLINICAL PICTURE

The child is short or dwarfed when seen at age 4 and over, but is not apparently dwarfed at birth. The skull is not involved and the facies consequently normal. Painful hips and a gluteus medius limp are the clinical features that bring the patient to medical attention. The disease is compatible with a normal life expectancy.

ROENTGEN PICTURE

The long bones show many features of chondrodystrophy. Such bone as is formed has normal texture and microscopically is undistinguishable from normal bone. The bones are short and broad and tend to be widened in the metaphyseal area to accommodate the irregular epiphyses.

The gross irregularity in shape of the formed epiphyses is the distinguishing characteristic. Particularly evident are the hips

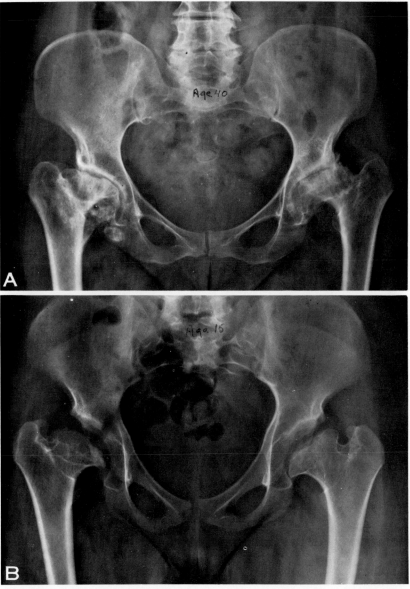

Figure 3.5. Spondyloepiphyseal dysplasia in (*A*) mother age 40, (*B*) daughter age 15, and (*C*) son age 14. The gross irregularity of the proximal femoral epiphyses can be expected to lead to the arthritis present at age 40. (*D*) The spine shows progressive diminution of height of the proximal lumbar vertebra and irregular notching of the anterior angles of the vertebral bodies.

with irregularity so gross that it leads to secondary arthritic changes. The knees may also be affected.

The vertebrae are similarly involved with diminished height and irregular shape and widening. There is hypoplasia of the upper lumbar vertebrae and deficient ossification at the anterior angle of the vertebrae.

The pelvis is normal except for the hip joints and tends to be broad.

TREATMENT

Unfortunately the gross joint irregularities are already the seat of extensive pathology when seen. There is no known prevention

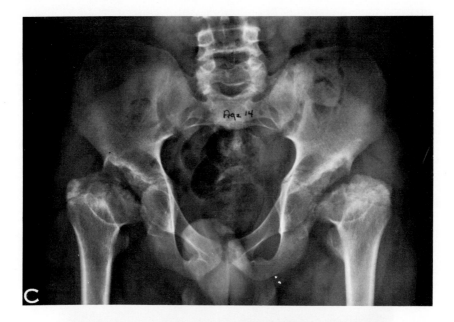

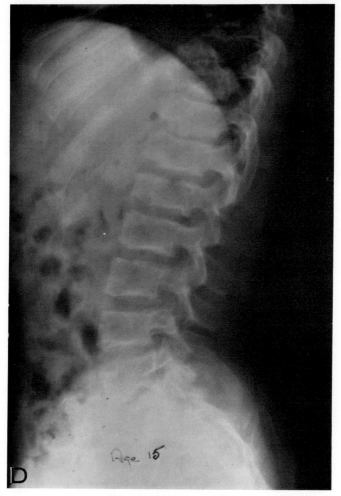

Figure 3.5 (*C* and *D*)

for the specific abnormality in growth of the epiphyses and vertebrae.

The joints can be aided by orthopaedic measures appropriate to the individual case and respond to these measures including replacement in a normal way.

Ellis-van Creveld Syndrome

For those who like to consider generalized disturbance of bone formation from cartilage which has a particular distribution as a syndrome, this entity appears fairly clear cut (Fig. 3.6).

The youngster shows a shortening of the extremities that is most pronounced distally. The teeth and nails are underdeveloped (ec-todermal dysplasia). There is bilateral poly-dactyly with fused or duplicated metacarpals. Delayed maturation of the primary ossification center of the phalanges, deformity of the proximal end of the tibial epiphysis, and possible association with congenital heart disease complete the picture.

The child looks somewhat like an achondroplastic dwarf, although his deformity is not so severe. The skull is normal, and there is no nasal deformity. The trunk is normal in length for the child's age, but the limb are disproportionately short. The polydactyly is evident, and other minor anomalies or variations may be associated with this malformation. The dentition is retarded. Intelligence is normal; at least, retarded intelligence is not part of the syndrome.

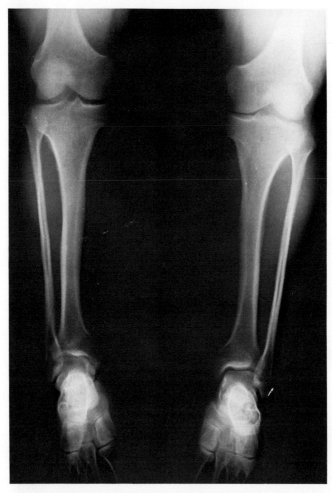

Figure 3.6.   Shortening and irregular shape of the distal long bones, a feature of Ellis-van Creveld syndrome and diastrophic dwarfism.

The acetabuli may be slightly hypoplastic. The shortening of the long bones, which is most marked in the lower leg and the lower arm, is evident. The anomalies of the meta-carpals are varieties of duplication or fusion and polydactylism. The depression of the lateral proximal tibial epiphysis has appeared in cases reviewed by the author to be due to an epiphyseal osteochondroma of the lateral condyle of the femur.

Osteochondromas and other forms of chondrodysplasia arising from the metaphy-seal side of the epiphyseal line are not pres-ent.

TREATMENT

Recognition of the youngster as having a form of achondroplastic dwarfism with other anomalies is the first step. Explanation to the parents and care of the psychologic hazards of this situation for both the parents and the child are important. The youngster should be followed to full maturity to obtain maximal function.

Pleonosteosis

This is a rare congenital and hereditary syndrome which principally involves the skeletal system. André Leri,[1] who de-scribed the anomaly in 1921, used the prefix "pleon" to signify the superabundance of the changes.

There is enlargement of the epiphyses and precocious and excessive ossification of bones arising from cartilage, which give rise to limitation of the joints of the body. Wat-son-Jones[3] noted an increase in the collage-nous tissue of major ligaments and the pres-ence of fibrocartilage and mucinous material. There was a marked absence of elastic fibers.

CLINICAL PICTURE

The hands are short and spadelike, the stature is short, and mongoloid facies may be present. The digits have flexion contractures; the thumb is broad, and the first metacarpal is in a valgus position. There may be such skin changes as accentuated skin creases, thickened hollow palms, and a condition re-sembling scleroderma on the hands and fore-arms. The knees may be in valgus and may have a hyperextension deformity.

The disease is apparent early in life and becomes more obvious with growth. The pathogenesis of the syndrome is not known. The hereditary transmission seems to occur by means of a dominant autosomal gene.

TREATMENT

The individual deformity has to be evalu-ated along orthopaedic lines as at the knees and in the hands. In general no treatment is indicated except in cases in which a noticea-ble deformity can be improved in appearance and function.

References

1. Leri, A.: Une maladie congenitale et hereditaire de l'ossification: la pleonosteosis familiale, *Bull. Mém. Soc. Méd. Hôp. Paris, 75:* 1228, 1921.
2. Rukavina, J. S., Falls, H. F., Holt, J. F., and Block, W. D.: Leri's pleonosteosis, *J. Bone Joint Surg., 41A:* 397, 1959.
3. Watson-Jones, R.: Leri's pleonosteosis, carpal tunnel compression of the median nerve and Morton's metatarsalgia, *J. Bone Joint Surg., 3B:* 560, 1949.

Diastrophic Dwarfism

It is possible to separate out from the entities of Morquio's chondrodystrophy, achondroplasia, multiple epiphyseal dyspla-sia, and arthrogryposis an entity which re-sults in considerable deformity and dwarfism below 5 feet in height.

A typical diastrophic dwarf would present as an infant with finger deformities, short finger and broad palm, hypermobile thumb, bilateral clubfeet, and dysplastic or dislocated hip. In addition, there would be thickened and protruding external ears (Figs. 3.7 and 3.8).

The condition affects both sexes equally and is quite rare. It is transmitted by a single autosomal gene and has a distribution in the offspring of a particular union typical of this type of transmission. This separates it from achondroplastic dwarfism, which is a mutant condition from normal parents, or arthrogry-posis, which is not transmitted by hereditary patterns.

The condition was described by Jackson[1] in 1951, Lamy and Marateaux[2] in 1960, and in a clear-cut description by Stover et al. in 1963.[3]

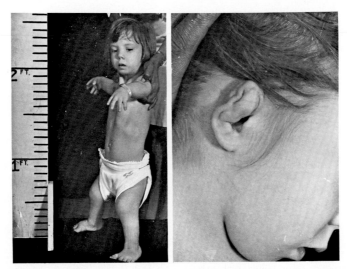

Figure 3.7 (*Left*). Diastrophic dwarfism with short extremities and enlargements around epiphyseal areas.

Figure 3.8 (*Right*). Deformed ear in diastrophic dwarfism.

CLINICAL PICTURE

The interphalangeal joints of the fingers may be fixed in a hyperextension contracture and they are short. The thumb, by contrast, is held away from the palms but has loose capsular structure and is hypermobile. The ears are thickened, protruding, and irregular shaped. Cleft palate has been reported as an occasional associated anomaly. The clubfeet and limited abduction at the hips with trochanters above Nélaton's line are evident in most, but not all, cases.

ROENTGEN FEATURES

The femurs reveal delay in appearance of the epiphyses. Where the distal bony epiphysis does appear, it tends to be medially displaced, and, as development of both the femoral and tibial epiphyses progresses, they are flattened with flaring metaphyses and somewhat irregular in outline. At the hips there may be a coxa vara rather than dislocated epiphysis made difficult to recognize by the late development of the bony center. Occasionally both ulna and fibula are short with bowing of the radius and flaring of the distal metaphysis. The first metacarpal is typically rudimentary and very short. The phalanges ossify in an irregular manner (Figs. 3.9–3.11).

A structural scoliosis appears early and progresses in severity toward adulthood.

TREATMENT

All adults reported have been well under 5 feet, varying from 3 feet to 4 feet, 6 inches. There is some muscle involvement, as shown by abnormal electromyographic motion units and occasional denervation fibrillations. An elevated serum glutamic oxaloacetic transaminase has been reported.

All of this is to emphasize that the equinovarus feet are difficult to correct, with muscle imbalance frequently an accompaniment that must result in early tendon transplant. The hips are difficult to correct due to the epiphyseal deformity. The treatment follows the standard attacks on the various deformities with psychiatric support for both parent and child afflicted with dwarfism.

References

1. Jackson, W. P. M.: Irregular familial chondroosseous defect, *J. Bone Joint Surg.*, *33B:* 420, 1951.
2. Lamy, M., and Marateaux, P.: L'anisme diastrophique, *Presse méd.*, *68: 1977*, 1960.
3. Stover, C., Hayes, J. Y., and Holt, J. F.: Diastrophic dwarfism, *Am. J. Roentgenol.*, *89:* 914, 1963.

METAPHYSEAL AFFECTIONS

Morquio's Syndrome

The entity called Morquio's syndrome was first described by Morquio[3] in 1929 as a "form of familial osseous dystrophy." Chon-

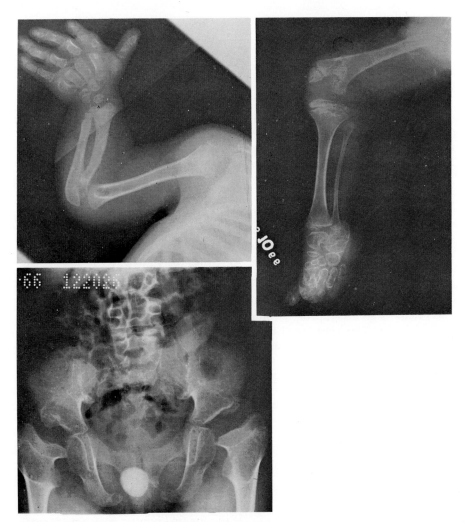

Figure 3.9 (*Top, left*). In the upper extremity the roentgenogram reveals the thumb held away from the palm, the short broad metacarpals and phalanges, and the bowed radius with flaring metaphysis, a picture that is consistent with diastrophic dwarfism.

Figure 3.10 (*Bottom*). The hip joints exhibit gross malformation with widening of the proximal femoral metaphysis and lateral displacement of the femoral shaft. The acetabulum mirrors the incongruity of the proximal femur. The ossification center for the proximal femoral epiphysis is delayed in its appearance.

Figure 3.11 (*Right*). The distal femoral epiphysis has a displacement of its ossification center. The shortened tibia and flared metaphysis are also evident.

drodystrophy is characterized by an altered rate in the formation of bone from cartilage.

The characteristics of this disease include dwarflike stature, a marked kyphos usually centering at the dorsolumbar junction, and involvement of the hips and other major joints in the changes of chondrodystrophy. These are noted clinically as enlargements and deformity. The bones of the skull and face are not involved, and the intelligence is normal.

In infancy there is little to raise the suspicion of Morquio's syndrome. The short trunk relative to the extremities gradually becomes evident with growth. There is often ligamentous laxity and lack of coordination, resulting in a delayed walking age. Corneal opacities and dental abnormalities develop with maturity.

The disease has been recorded slightly more frequently in male patients, but both sexes are affected. According to Fairbanks, more than one member of a family is involved in about one-third of the cases.

ETIOLOGY

There is apparently an autosomal recessive mode of inheritance. Keratosulfate is found in the urine in childhood, gradually ceasing past puberty. The nature of the disturbances producing widespread disturbances of bone structure and shape, ligamentous laxity, and corneal opacities is still unknown.

CLINICAL PICTURE

The presence of Morquio's syndrome is ordinarily not recognized until after the child begins to walk. The disease is symptomless until the patient is older and secondary changes have developed in joints. The standing posture is characteristic. The spine is in flexion, and there is an accentuated kyphos at the midspine area. The knees tend to be flexed and the feet pronated. Valgus at the knee is quite common. As the age of the patient progresses, these deformities tend to become more severe. The gait tends to be a bilateral Trendelenburg type that results in waddling owing to the varus deformity at the hips.

The head may appear enlarged in relation to the short trunk and extremities, but usually it is normal in size and shape for the chronologic age. The kyphos and round back result in a lordotic curve through the lumbar area; the curve is usually quite short and accentuated. The shortening of the spine is out of proportion to that of the extremities. The hands may reach the knee level. There is limited extension of the spine, and in older patients there may be some lateral elevation resulting in mild scoliosis.

In achondroplastic dwarfs the proximal portion of the extremities may be excessively short, but this is not true in chondrodystrophy. In the lower extremities in particular, the ends of the bones in the epiphyseal and metaphyseal areas may be enlarged. Such enlargements are more readily noted at the knee than elsewhere.

Motion at the hip hoint, which is usually involved in the disease, is often limited, and flexion contractures of mild degree are frequently present. There may be an inability to extend the knee completely. However, cases of excessive ligamentous laxity about the joints have been described. Enlargement of the interphalangeal joints is not common, but it may occur. The hand is broad and has broad and blunt fingers.

Narrowing of the chest anteriorly and protrusion of the sternum is common. The chin may be prominent, and a short, flat nose is characteristic. The corneal opacities seen by slit lamp examination appear early. The shoulders and elbows may be limited in terms of full extension (elbow) or abduction (shoulder).

Keratosulfate is found in the urine. Life expectancy is limited with cardiopulmonary involvement resulting in demise prior to age 40.

ROENTGEN FINDINGS

Although the rate of formation of bone from cartilage may be altered, there is no area of persistent failure of ossification as there is in chondrodysplasia. Delayed growth of cartilage and failure of remodeling produces short, broad bones.

In the vertebrae, the transverse and anteroposterior diameters are increased. The upper and lower surfaces are irregular and poorly defined. The anterior border may be much smaller than the posterior, so that the vertebra may be wedge shaped (Fig. 3.12). The wedging may appear to be more at the expense of either the upper or lower half rather than symmetric, however.

At an area of kyphosis, one vertebra, usually the first lumbar, may appear smaller and more irregularly wedged than the others, and it may be displaced posteriorly. The epiphyseal lines of the long bones are widened, deepened, and irregular. The metaphyseal areas are broad and out of proportion to the diaphyses. Not all epiphyses are necessarily involved.

The ribs are more horizontal than usual and may present an expansion at either end. The hips are involved, the changes becoming more evident with increasing age (Fig. 3.13). The femoral heads show marked epiphyseal irregularity and flattening. The femoral necks are shortened and broad, and they tend toward a varus deformity. According to Fairbanks, these changes are markedly progressive; the child may appear normal early in life only to develop changes later. Other joints may or may not be involved.

The metacarpals and phalanges are short and expanded at their extremities. Ossifica-

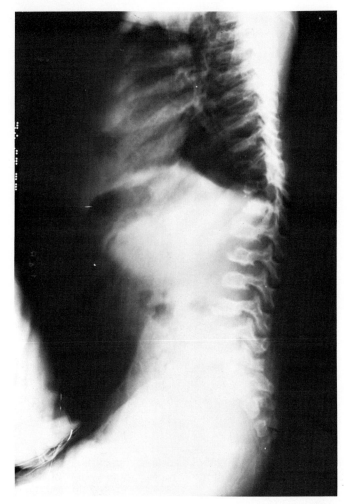

Figure 3.12.   The spine in Morquio's syndrome with abnormal shape, flattening, and increased anteroposterior diameter of the vertebrae.

tion in the bones of the hand may be delayed and may be irregular in outline when it does appear.

DIFFERENTIAL DIAGNOSIS

Achondroplasia is differentiated clinically and roentgenographically. The spine is of normal height; the prominent buttocks and lumbar lordosis with a round back or kyphos are characteristic. The shortening of the limbs occurs principally in the proximal segments. Joint degenerative changes are not seen, and genu valgum is not a feature. The bone is affected by failure to form in some areas rather than by slowness and irregularity of the rate of formation.

In "dysostosis multiplex" or gargoylism the patient is mentally deficient, the facial features coarsened and heavy, the liver and spleen enlarged, and the cornea cloudy.

Tuberculosis and other causes of dorsal vertebral collapses and subsequent kyphos are readily distinguished clinically. It should be remembered that chondrodystrophy of Morquio's type is a generalized disease and that roentgenograms reveal the generalized involvement.

TREATMENT

There may be frequent respiratory tract infections requiring treatment. Hernias, loss of hearing, visual problems, and ear infec-

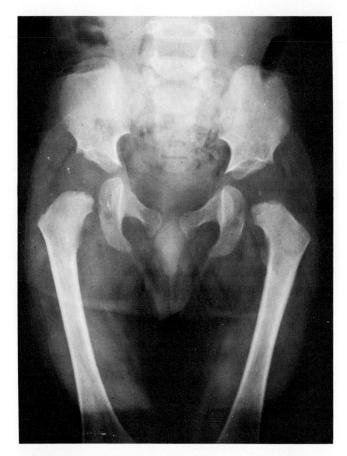

Figure 3.13.   Involvement of epiphyseal and articular cartilage at the hip in Morquio's syndrome. The tendency toward a flat acetabular roof is apparent.

tions all complicate the disease. The teeth may be of poor quality and require attention.

The use of the Milwaukee brace may be necessary to stabilize progressive kyphosis. The prominent genu valgum may complicate the walking disability to the point of requiring elective correction. The ligamentous laxity at the knee makes correction difficult and soft-tissue reefing and subsequent bracing is often required.

References

1. Gordenich, I. F., and Lenzi, L. Morquio-Ullrich disease; new mucopolysaccharidosis, *J. Bone Joint Surg., 46A:* 743, 1964.
2. Langer, L. O., Jr., and Carey, L. S.: The roentgenographic features of the k.s. mucopolysaccharidosis of Morquio, *Am. J. Roentgenol., 97:* 1, 1966.
3. Morquio, L.: Sur une forme de dystrophie osseuse familiale, *Bul. Soc. Pediatr. Paris, 27:* 145, 1929.
4. Schenk, F. A., and Haggerty, J.: Morquio's disease;

radiologic and morphologic study. *Pediatrics, 34:* 839, 1964.

Familial Metaphyseal Dysplasia

A rare bone disease, familial metaphyseal dysplasia was described in 1931 by Edwin Pyle.[2] Its outstanding feature is a failure to remodel of bone laid down by growth from the epiphyseal line. The cases previously described in the literature have had a familial incidence. The distribution is symmetric, and the metaphyseal areas of long bones are involved. The wide, flask-shaped metaphyses may result in confusion with Gaucher's disease. Phalanges, metacarpals, and metatarsals may also be involved.

By roentgen examination, the lack of involvement of bone originating from fetal or membranous material is striking; therefore, the pictures show beautifully the relative percentages of growth from either end of a long bone (Figs. 3.14 and 3.15). The area laid down by any one epiphyseal line has not been subject to remodeling. With the increased width there is a lack of normal development of bone cortex. The vertebrae may have an increased anteroposterior diameter. The pubis and ischii may be markedly widened. Skull changes, particularly a decrease in the transverse diameter at the base, may be noted.

The clinical picture is not striking. The osseous lesions ordinarily are found incidentally on a routine x-ray examination. Valgus at the knee has resulted in discovery of the anomaly is some children. Osteotomy may

be necessary if the deformity justifies it. Treatment is ordinarily not otherwise indicated.

References

1. Feld, H., Switzer, R. A., Dexter, M. W., and Langer, E. M.: Familial metaphyseal dysplasia, *Radiology*, 65: 206, 1955.
2. Pyle, E.: Case of unusual bone development, *J. Bone Joint Surg.*, 13: 874, 1931.

Solitary Bone Cyst

A solitary bone cyst is usually brought to the attention of the orthopaedic surgeon by pathologic fracture. Rarely, it may be incidentally found on roentgen examination. Although found in the adult, this lesion is pe-

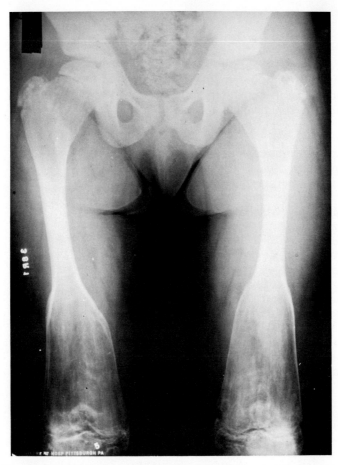

Figure 3.14. Familial metaphyseal dysplasia with failure of bone laid down by the epiphyses to remodel. This disease indicates nicely the amount of growth from one epiphysis as compared to another.

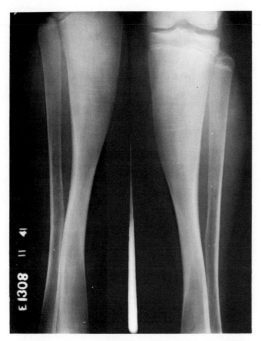

Figure. 3.15. Note small area of original fetal bone compared with unremodeled areas above and below in both tibia and fibula (familial metaphyseal dysplasia).

culiarly a disease of children and young adults. It has been termed osteitis fibrosa, but it is not associated with the generalized skeletal changes found in hyperparathyroidism, which is followed by polycystic lesions in the bones and bone atrophy.

Silver[5] reviewed the so-called "benign cyst of the bones" in 1912. In 97 cases, only 18 patients were past the age of 20 years. The usual age group in which bone cysts are discovered is that from 6 to 15 years. In addition to the long bones, the calcaneus is sometimes affected. The vast majority of cysts occur in the humerus or femur, however. There is a tendency for the lesion to predominate in males.

ETIOLOGY

The underlying prime factor that causes the area immediately adjacent to an epiphyseal line to become productive of cyst tissue rather than of bone is unknown. Trauma and hemorrhage have been suggested, but there are two opposing theories of the mechanism. The first assumes that the epiphyseal line in difficulty gives rise not to normal bone but to cyst tissue. This process may already have eased when the patient is first seen, and an area of normal bone may be visualized distal to the epiphyseal line. The walls of the cyst are never wider than the width of the epiphyseal line in solitary bone cyst.

The second theory notes that the mechanism of production may be an exaggeration of the resorptive phase, during which calcified cartilage is replaced by bone. This phase, which is characterized by a proliferation of vessels and giant cells, according to Geschickter and Copeland,[4] may produce a loss of structure when it is exaggerated and may thus result in the cyst.

The location is conspicuously that of areas of high rates of growth and extensive remodeling. What part trauma plays in the picture is still unknown.

CLINICAL PICTURE

Pain, swelling, and mild deformity may be complaints that caused the patient to seek medical attention. The pain is quite low grade except in instances of acute fracture, and, as a result, it may have existed for considerable time before the patient is seen. There may have been no preceding symptoms. When the cyst occurs in areas such as the femoral neck, hemorrhage into the joint may initially result in confusion with entities that may cause pain and spasm at the hips.

The site of these complaints is characteristic (Fig. 3.16). The most common area involved is the proximal femur. It is usually apparent on viewing the x-ray film that either the trochanteric epiphysis or the capital femoral epiphyseal line is more closely related to the cyst. The second most common site is the proximal tibia. Other long bone sites may occasionally be involved. The older the patient and the longer the duration of symptoms, the further removed from the epiphyseal line the cyst may reasonably be found.

So-called acute bone cysts may have a duration of but a few months and are regarded by Geschickter and Copeland as giant cell variants that may be related to giant cell tumor. These cysts have not progressed down the shaft with growth but are situated close to the epiphyseal line. Garceau and Gregory,[3] in tabulating the incidence of healing of the cyst in those cases with fracture, found that it was 15% both in their own cases and in those in the literature (Fig. 3.17).

ROENTGEN FINDINGS

This lesion is not actually expansile, although superficially it may appear so. There is an area of loss of normal bone structure which is contained within thinned cortex. The actual width of the cyst is never greater than the width of the epiphyseal line. The cyst area has not been subject to remodeling, but this process has taken place distal to it. When the cyst is removed from the epiphyseal line, it is seen that remodeling has also taken place proximal to it. The remodeling of the normal bone results in the expanded appearance of the cyst by contrast. When the width of the lesion is greater than that of the epiphyseal line from which it may have arisen, serious doubt of the diagnosis of solitary bone cyst should arise. Lesions such as syphilitic gumma and giant cell tumor should be considered.

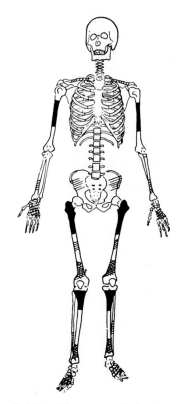

Figure 3.16. Diagram of distribution of solitary bone cyst. Solid black areas are most frequently affected. (From C. T. Geschichter and M. M. Copeland: *Tumors of Bone*, J. B. Lippincott, Philadelphia, 1949.)

The juncture of the cyst with the normal cortex is a symmetric one; that is, the normal cortex thins on both its exterior and its interior surfaces to the width of the cortex overlying the lesion.

PATHOLOGY

The cyst wall on examination at operation may be greatly thinned and may fracture on slight pressure. There may be little or no lining, but some areas of fibrous tissue are usually found (Fig. 3.18). The cyst contents usually consist of fluid either yellow or reddened by recent hemorrhage. Except in the region of recent fracture, there is no indication that new bone formation is going on exteriorly.

In the areas of fibrous tissue lining the wall there is no evidence of fibrous tissue proliferation, but there are occasionally osteoblasts and new bone. The more central fibrous tissue, if present, is quite loose and myxomatous.

Evidence of old hemorrhages is sometimes noted. In the areas of fresh hemorrhage a giant cell reaction may be present. Bone formation from cartilage is not seen; and when there is osteoblastic activity, it takes place in fibrous tissue.

The so-called giant cell variant of the solitary bone cyst may tend more to be subcortical and most frequently is found in the region of the greater trochanter of the femur. The tissue is featured by numerous giant cell areas close to the epiphyseal line in a stroma of considerable intercellular tissue and fibroblasts.

TREATMENT

The solitary bone cyst lends itself well to carefully performed surgery. A belief has arisen that fracture heals cysts of this type, but this belief is not borne out by experience. When the cyst is small, i.e., when its long axis is ½ inch or less, the healing reaction about a fracture line extending approximately ¼ inch on either side of it may indeed ablate the cyst or render it of little consequence. In larger cysts, such a reaction is not expected.

If the cyst has suffered a recent fracture, its healing reaction may be utilized by surgery performed during the phase of callus proliferation. Not all cysts must have surgery, however.

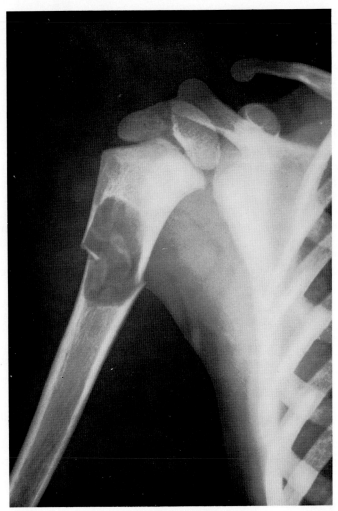

Figure 3.17.   Fracture in solitary bone cyst. The fracture will not result in healing of the cyst.

The optimal time for operation in a case of cyst which has rendered the bone mechanically inadequate arises when a centimeter or more of normal bone has been laid down between the epiphyseal line and the cyst itself. Attempts to ablate the cyst when there is no evidence that normal bone is being developed from the epiphyseal line may be followed by recurrence. Garceau and Gregory have emphasized the high recurrence rate in patients operated on below the age of 10.

The operation has two aims: (1) to remove the contents of the cyst and (2) to stimulate a repair reaction which will cause bone to be laid down in the cyst area. At surgery, the area involved is usually wider than the expected width of bone subject to remodeling

and has a bluish cast. Normal-bleeding bone should be visualized at both proximal and distal ends of the cyst cavity after curettement. There is occasionally a small quantity of fibrous tissue that can be obtained by curetting. It is helpful to displace the wall segment removed in order to visualize the cyst to the far side so that it abuts against the remaining wall, thereby obliterating the cyst cavity. Bone grafts are used to fill the cavity remaining (Fig. 3.19).

Bone grafts are inserted so that contact with the parent bone is made at both ends of the cyst. If chips are used, large cystic spaces that the bone would have difficulty in bridging are avoided, and the cavity is not packed so tightly that development of the repair reaction is impeded. Autogenous bone is preferable but may be impractical in the presence of large cystic areas. Where bone bank bone is used, match stick grafts derived from ribs are inserted into the cyst cavity so that they run longitudinally and have good contact in normal cancellous bone areas.

Carefully performed operative procedures in a patient in whom the cyst area is removed from the epiphyseal line by normal cancellous bone 1 cm or more in depth, and in the older child, may be expected to yield good results.

References

1. Alldrédge, R. H.: Localized fibrocystic disease of bone: results of treatment in 152 cases, *J. Bone Joint Surg., 24:* 795, 1942.

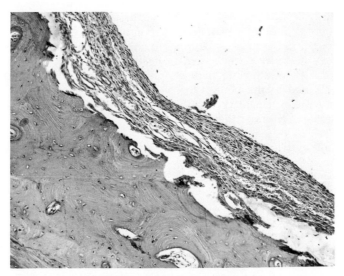

Figure 3.18. Fibrous lining membrane from wall of simple bone cyst.

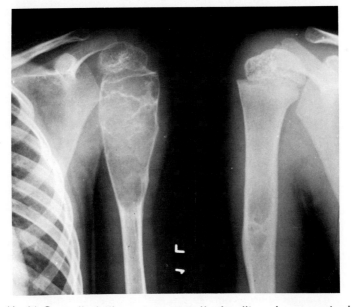

Figure 3.19. (*Left*) So called "immature state" of solitary bone cyst with epiphyseal lines still directly adjacent to the cyst. (*Right*) Postoperative view after bone grafting. (Courtesy of Elmer King, M.D.)

2. Elinslic, R. C.: Fibrocystic diseases of the bone, *Br. J. Surg.*, *2:* 17, 1914.
3. Garceau, G. J., and Gregory, C. F.: Solitary unicameral bone cyst, *J. Bone Joint Surg.*, *36A:* 267, 1954.
4. Geschickter, C. T., and Copeland, M. M.: *Tumors of Bone*, Ed. 3; Philadelphia: J. B. Lippincott, 1949.
5. Silver, D.: The so-called benign cyst of the bones, *Am. J. Orthop. Surg.*, *9:* 563, 1912.
6. Stewart, M. J., and Hamel, H. A.: Solitary bone cyst, *South. Med. J.*, *43:* 927, 1950.

Aneurysmal Bone Cyst

This lesion of bone once was classified within a group of conditions known as "atypical giant cell tumor." Jaffe and Lichtenstein[3] in 1942 reclassified it as an individual entity. It seems to be confined to the young, the youngest reported patient being 2 years and 3 months and the majority under the age of 30 years.

Aneurysmal bone cyst is a benign lesion occurring in the metaphyses of long bones and occasionally in the spine and flat bones (Fig. 3.20). It produces local pain and symptoms secondary to its pressure on adjacent structures. It destroys bone and thus gives rise to the characteristic described as a "blow out."

ETIOLOGY

The cause is unknown. Aberrant vessel formation has been suggested by Donaldson.[2] Jaffe and Lichtenstein[3] suggested that the lesion is engrafted onto some preexisting lesion in bone, such as a nonossifying fibroma or fibrous dysplasia. Trauma seems to draw attention to the lesion but is not a primary cause.

There are characteristics in the pathology which have led some observers to the belief that the lesion is essentially a hemangioma in bone. In one of Donaldson's cases reported in 1962, roentgenograms of the involved bone had been made in connection with a femoral fracture. A metaphysis that appeared normal upon roentgen examination was shown distal to the fracture at that time; 1½ years after healing of the fracture, the area involved was the site of an aneurysmal bone cyst.

CLINICAL PICTURE

The patient is usually under 30 years of age. Pain at the site of involvement is the most frequent presenting complaint. In patients with spine lesions, paraplegia as well as back pain may be the presenting complaint. The involved area may have collapsed with trauma or manipulation.

Swelling and tenderness are present over the involved area. There is an equal incidence in males and females.

ROENTGEN PICTURE

In the long bones, the aneurysmal bone cyst is located in the metaphysis. It is ovoid

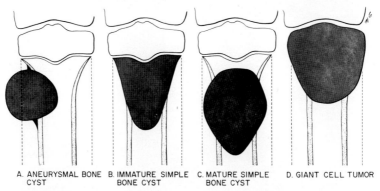

A. ANEURYSMAL BONE CYST   B. IMMATURE SIMPLE BONE CYST   C. MATURE SIMPLE BONE CYST   D. GIANT CELL TUMOR

Figure 3.20. *Dotted line* represents the width of the adjacent epiphyseal plate and its metaphysis. The *shaded areas* represent the typical sites of involvement in a long bone with various types of cystlike lesions of bone. The aneurysmal bone cyst is frequently eccentric. The immature bone cyst is metaphyseal; it abuts directly on the epiphyseal line and usually extends entirely across the metaphysis. The mature simple cyst is not remodeled, as the normal bone around it is, and the result is an apparent expansion of the lesion as the epiphysis starts laying down normal bone. The giant cell tumor involves the epiphyseal area in an older age group after the epiphyseal line has closed. (From W. A. Donaldson: *Journal of Bone and Joint Surgery, 44A:* 25, 1962).

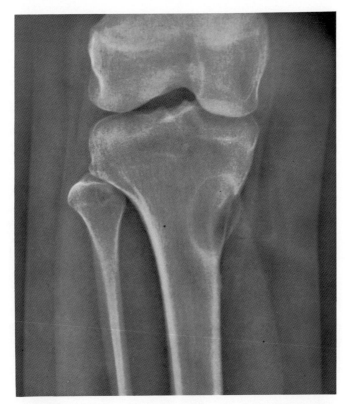

Figure 3.21. Aneurysmal bone cyst in a 19-year-old girl. The eccentric position of the lesion is well demonstrated. The cortex has been destroyed, and the lesion is covered by a thin shell of new bone.

in shape and usually eccentrically located (Fig. 3.21). The cortex overlying it has been destroyed, and the lesion is not bounded by a thin shell of new bone. The edge is benign in character rather than actively destructive. In the spine, it is usually found in the posterior elements, such as the spinous processes and lunimae, rather than in the body of the vertebra, although it may advance into the posterior portion of the vertebra. The lesion may produce a mass that balloons out from its original site.

PATHOLOGY

Although the metaphyses of long bones and spine are the most frequent site, it has been found in the calcaneous, clavicle, scapula, ilium, occiput metacarpals, and metatarsals. When exposed surgically, the lesion is covered by a thin layer of subperiosteal bone. Beneath this lies a bloody, red tissue which is soft. Occasionally, the area may be filled with fluid, but there is a well marked lining. Microscopically, the lesion contains numerous blood-filled spaces contained by fibrous tissue septa with osteoid. There are giant cells of the foreign body type that vary greatly in density from area to area. In the septa, in addition to active fibroblasts and osteoid, some areas of immature bone may be seen.

TREATMENT

Aneurysmal bone cyst is a benign lesion apparently capable of increasing to great size if untreated. Its secondary effects, such as paraplegia, are most serious.

The lesion responds to curettement, which is apparently, however, not always sufficient. In one of the author's cases, a previous procedure consisting of curettement and replacement with bone chips had failed to cure the conditions. In this case, the area was resected en bloc and cure resulted. In contrast to simple bone cysts, these cysts seem to respond beneficially to x-ray therapy in doses varying between 600 and 2,000 R.

The surgical approach, especially in children, seems preferable, however, because growth areas may be affected. Roentgen therapy may be necessary in surgically inaccessible areas.

References

1. Coley, B. L., and Miller, L. B.: Atypical giant cell tumor, *Am. J. Roentgenol.*, *47:* 541, 1942.
2. Donaldson, W. F.: Aneurysmal bone cyst, *J. Bone Joint Surg.*, *44A:* 25, 1962.
3. Jaffe, H. L., and Lichtenstein, L.: Solitary unicameral bone cyst with emphasis on the roentgen picture, pathologic appearance, and pathogenesis, *Arch. Surg.*, *44:* 1004, 1942.
4. Lichtenstein, L.: Aneurysmal bone cyst: a pathological entity commonly mistaken for giant cell tumor and occasionally for hemangioma and osteogenic sarcoma, *Cancer*, *3:* 279, 1950.

Tibia Vara

Three forms of tibia vara are encountered in childhood. By far the commonest of these is tibia vara or bowlegs associated with growth stress. Such a condition is commonly seen in orthopaedic and pediatric practice. This form of tibia vara is associated with internal tibial torsion and is of mild degree. It is present at birth—apparently a remnant of intrauterine position—and persists with sleeping on the stomach.

Deformity due to asymmetric growth of the proximal tibial epiphyseal line with apparent osteochondritis (or Blount's disease) is occasionally seen and must be particularly considered in unilateral tibia vara. Varus deformity of the tibia due to various forms of rickets and other growth disturbances of the epiphyseal line, such as chondrodystrophy, is not quite rare. When tibia vara is associated with generalized disease, such as osteogenesis imperfecta, it is usually an incidental part of a generalized deformity.

CLINICAL PICTURE

Complaint of the deformity is not ordinarily made until the child begins to walk and the rolling gait, the wide-spaced knees, and the secondary pronation of the foot become evident (Figs. 3.22 and 3.23). Infants are seen

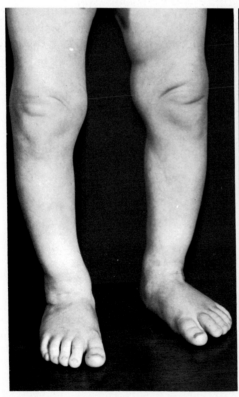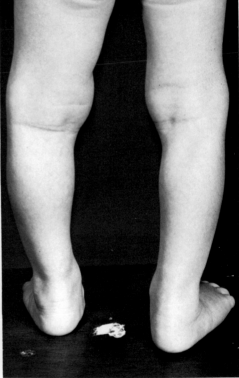

Figure 3.22   (*Left*). Patient with tibia vara. Note the change of angle in the proximal tibial area and secondary pronation of feet.
Figure 3.23   (*Right*). Posterior view.

usually because the associated internal tibial torsion has resulted in turning inward of the foot to a sufficient degree to alarm the parents.

Infants with tibia vara due to growth stress are most often quite stocky and unusually active. Those with Blount's disease do not exhibit evidence of generalized disease. However, in instances of rachitic and other growth disturbances of the epiphyseal line, there is usually a generalized diminished rate of growth as well.

ROENTGEN FINDINGS

The findings on the x-ray film are most helpful in differentiating among the various causes of tibia vara.

Growth Stress. Here the angulation takes place in the proximal tibia (Fig. 3.24). The epiphyseal line is normal. There is a characteristic increase in width of the medial cortex that is most prominent at the junction of the proximal and middle thirds. The plane of knee ankle joint faces slightly medialward instead of lying parallel to that of the knee. The deformity is equal in both legs.

Blount's Disease. The height of the proximal tibial epiphysis is diminished on its medial aspect, and the epiphyseal line is narrowed and irregular on this side. The metaphysis immediately below this area is irregularly ossified, and there is breaking medially. The diminished growth in this area causes angulation to take place proximally. The deformity is often unilateral.

Rickets. The irregularity and widening of the epiphyseal line are evident at once. The fraying of the metaphysis, its cuplike deformity, and generalized osteoporosis are later changes. The angulation of the tibia, in contradistinction to that due to growth stress, takes place at the junction of the mid and distal thirds, and there is maximal thickening of the medial cortex in this area. A similar angulation of the distal femur helps to contribute to the deformity.

PROGNOSIS

Growth Stress. The deformity has a tendency to improve with weight bearing and growth (Fig. 3.25). Eventually, at approximately age 3–4 years, it actually tends to pass over to genu valgum.

Blount's Disease. The condition tends to subside spontaneously after a 3- to 4-year

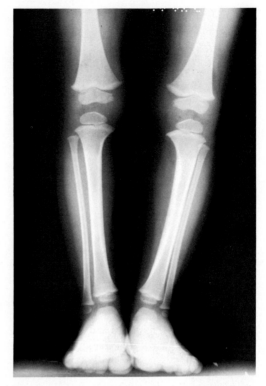

Figure 3.24. Weight-bearing roentgenogram in tibia vara due to growth stress. Note the medial facing of the distal tibial surface and secondary pronation of feet.

period, and there is reconstitution of the epiphyseal line and filling in of the irregularly calcified medial metaphysis (Fig. 3.26).

Rickets. The response to antirachitic therapy is dependent on the type of rickets involved and is discussed elsewhere.

TREATMENT

Tibia vara results in medial facing of the ankle joint and secondary pronation of the foot to get it flat on the floor. To avoid this foot position, the foot must be supported by a longitudinal arch pad. A ⅛-inch inner heel wedge is added to support the pad and to stimulate medial growth. After adequate alignment of the foot with the leg, the child is followed, as growth itself tends to straighten the leg if the deformity is due to growth stress. Osteotomy of the tibia is not necessary.

In Blount's disease the foot is similarly supported. The activity of the disease is followed by roentgenogram. When the disease is quiescent and growth restored to normal,

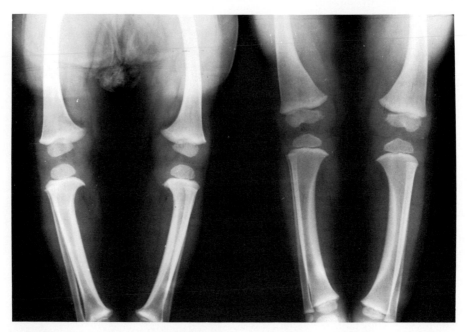

Figure 3.25.   Prominent breaking of medial metaphysis of both femora and tibiae. (*Left*) The tendency toward irregular ossification at the proximal tibia is no longer present. (*Right*) One year later the deformity still appears severe, but one may expect these legs to straighten through growth with appropriate foot support.

surgical correction by osteotomy may be considered if the deformity is of sufficient degree. Braces which are built with partial correction of the malalignment are sometimes used in an endeavor to prevent the development of severe deformity.

The rachitic bowleg with deformity in the distal third of the tibia does not have the tendency toward spontaneous correction that exists in angulation of the upper third. It is obviously poor judgment to attempt correction in the presence of active disease; but once the disease is controlled, osteotomy may be considered. This may involve correction of the femur as well, in order to get knee and ankle aligned in the same plane.

In Blount's disease the diminished growth of the medial epiphysis is apparent as it loses height. The metaphysis appears pinched and beaked medially. The metaphysis bone in this area is often laid down irregularly. Chung, Mitchell, and Gregg, at Children's Hospital in Philadelphia, have devised a measurement of the deformity. A line is drawn parallel to the inferior surface of the proximal tibial epiphysis. From the center of this line

a second line is projected to the medial beak. Deformity that is well established erects an angle of 30 degrees or more and indicates the need for surgical correction.

SURGICAL TREATMENT

Once the diagnosis is definitely established, early surgery is indicated. This is necessitated by the progressive nature of the disease, the favorable response in the growth center by at least partial elimination of weight-bearing compressive forces, and the difficulty in achieving a cosmetic correction at one level once the tibia vara becomes severe.

Chung initiated a manual osteoclasis in the proximal metaphysis as a means of avoiding complications such as compartment syndromes that have attended surgery in the proximal tibia in children.

A proximal Steinman pin is inserted in the proximal tibial metaphysis as close to the epiphyseal line as can be done without injury to the epiphyseal line. A second pin is placed approximately 1 inch distal to the first pin.

Through a stab wound, numerous drill holes are made transversly outlining the osteoclasis line. Not only is the varus corrected, but some external rotation of the distal fragment can be achieved as well when necessary to avoid hyperextension at the osteoclasis site. A second drilling in the distal fibula allows osteoclasis of this bone as well, assuring correction of the deformity. A plaster cast (long leg) is necessary for 6 weeks.

Early correction of tibia vara due to Blount's disease is indicated. There is no correction necessary in growth stress tibia vara.

Osteopoikilosis (Osteopathia Condensus Disseminata)

This condition is characterized by dense calcific densities irregularly spotted about the ends of the long bone of the extremities. They are found in the small bones of the hands and feet as well (Figs. 3.27 and 3.28).

The appearance was described by Stredi in 1905. It is of importance only to avoid confusion with clinical entities of more serious import. The opacities are of gross size, giving a bizarre appearance of the roentgenogram of the skeleton, but not affecting the external

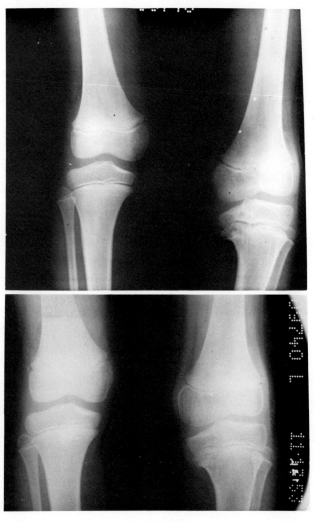

Figure 3.26. Blount's disease. (*Top*) Irregular ossification and diminished height of metaphysis and epiphysis medially on right. (*Bottom*) Healing in previously affected area.

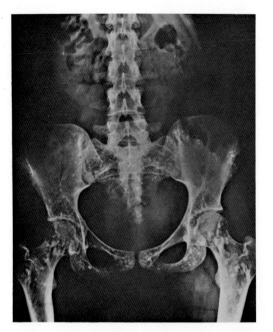

Figure 3.27. Dense sclerotic areas articulating with the normal bone stria are observed tending to a metaphyseal location in the proximal femur (osteopoikilosis).

form or function of the skeleton. It is a familial condition and may be accompanied by hereditary multiple exostoses. The opacities articulate with the normal trabeculae about them but are flat expanses of unvarying density. The nodules tend to be spherical and occasionally elongated. Microscopic examination reveals that they are composed of dense lamellated bone, similar to cortical bone.

Reference

1. Hinson, A.: Familial osteopoikilosis, *Am. J. Surg.*, 45: 566, 1939.

DIAPHYSEAL AFFECTIONS

Marfan's Syndrome (Arachnodactyly)

Marfan's syndrome, also known as arachnodactyly, is a relatively rare familial disorder of unknown etiology in which there are widespread abnormalities of the skeletal, cardiovascular, and ocular systems. In 1896, Marfan[9] made the first report of the syndrome which now bears his name and de-

scribed the long extremities and long, spidery fingers, the hallmark of the skeletal abnormalities (Figs. 3.29 and 3.30). In 1902, Achard coined the name arachnodactyly to describe the spider-like fingers seen in the classical case of Marfan's syndrome, and this term and the eponym have been used interchangeably to describe the syndrome ever since. Since then, it has been estimated that between 350 and 400 cases have been reported in the literature, including detailed pathologic studies of more than 70 cases.

McKusick[10] suggested the term "Marfan syndrome" for this generalized disease involving mesodermal tissue and producing an undefined defect. Although the disease is known as arachnodactyly in orthopaedic circles because the skeletal abnormalities it causes often bring the patient to medical

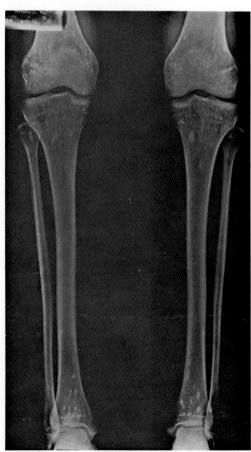

Figure 3.28. In the tibia the tendency of the opacities to occupy a metaphyseal location in osteopoikilosis is evident.

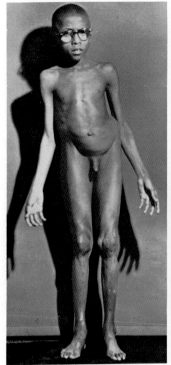 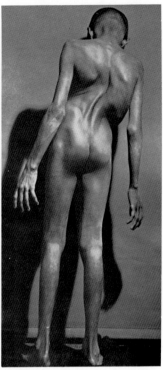

Figure 3.29 (*Left*) and **Figure 3.30** (*Right*). Diagnosis: arachnodactyly. Note long extremities and digits, scoliosis, and eye defect.

attention, Marfan's syndrome is probably a better term since not all patients exhibit skeletal manifestations. "Arachnodactyly" refers to the long "spider-like" fingers. Marfan suggested "dolichostenomelia," which emphasized long extremities.

Marfan's syndrome is characterized by excessive length of the long bones, loose joints and ligaments, ectopia lentis, dilation of the aorta, and defects such as inguinal hernia (Figs. 3.31 and 3.32).

The disease affects approximately 1.5 per 100,000 population. According to McKusick, at least 85% of the cases actually can be shown to have been inherited as autosomal dominants when appropriate genetic studies are conducted, with the remaining 15% being spontaneous mutations. It has also been shown the incidence is the same in both sexes and in both whites and Negroes.

ETIOLOGY

That the disease is transmitted as a dominant trait was brought to medical attention by Weve[17] of Utrecht in 1931, who designated the disease "dystrophia—mesodermalis congenita—typus Marfans."

In 1958, Tijo and Puck first reported variability in size of human satellited chromosomes. At first no significance was ascribed to the variation in satellite size, but in 1960 Tijo, Puck, and Robinson[16] described the results of chromosome studies in 2 patients with Marfan's syndrome and noted that 1 of the patients possessed a tremendously enlarged satellite on one member of pair 21 while the other patient had a similarly greatly enlarged satellite on one member of pair 13. Handmaker[5] presented evidence in 1963 that there was no correlation between enlarged satellites and Marfan's syndrome. He found that in chromosome studies of 8 patients with Marfan's syndrome, none of them possessed a chromosome satellite enlarged any greater than those observed in any of their unaffected relatives.

In an experiment performed in 1961, Procop[12] reported an increase in urinary bound hydroxyproline excretion in patients with Marfan's syndrome. His values demonstrated that, whereas normal subjects ex-

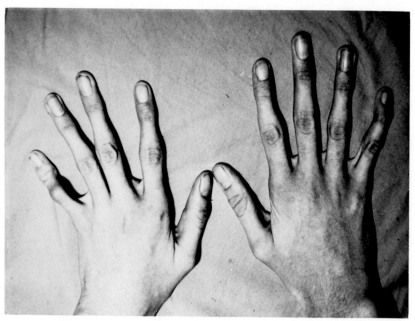

Figure 3.31. Elongated metacarpals and phalanges result in long, graceful hands in Marfan's syndrome.

creted less than 34 mg of hydroxyproline per day, those with Marfan's syndrome excreted between 38 and 90 mg per day. Jones et al.[6, 7] confirmed this in 1964 when they compared urinary hydroxyproline excretion in Marfan's syndrome with age-matched controls. They found that preadolescent and adult patients with Marfan's syndrome consistently excreted greater amounts of hydroxyproline than did the controls. The vast majority of the urinary hydroxyproline in both of these studies was excreted bound to peptides and the amount of free hydroxyproline was consistently insignificant. Stetten[15] found that exogenous ^{15}N-labeled hydroxyproline was not incorporated into collagen but rather remains as free hydroxyproline and is excreted as such in the urine. From this it was inferred that, without significant hydroxyproline in the exogenous form, most of the hydroxyproline in the body and in the urine must be derived from the breakdown of collagen. Therefore, Procop suggested that the increased hydroxyproline excretion in the urine of subjects with Marfan's syndrome must indicate a more rapid than normal rate of collagen breakdown in this condition.

An association between the abnormalities produced in experimental animals fed *Lathyrus odoratus* (sweet pea) seeds and the ab-

normalities of Marfan's syndrome has also been postulated. Ponseti and Shepard found that white rats fed a diet containing 50% *Lathyrus odoratus* seeds all developed kyphoscoliosis—apparently the result of osteoporosis and collapse of several vertebrae. Aneurysms of the thoracic aorta in 6 of 16 rats were also found, and histopathologic studies on these demonstrated marked medial necrosis. They concluded that the sweet pea seeds contained a toxic factor which had its primary effect on the development of mesodermal structures. In 1954 these same investigators[11] found that rats fed *Lathyrus odoratus* developed epiphyseal plates containing a cartilage matrix that appeared to lose cohesion, and the same diets produced loosening and detachments of the tendinous and ligamentous insertions with such defects as recurrent shoulder dislocations.

Subsequently, the toxic agent of the sweet pea seed has been identified as being β-amino-propionitrile (BAPN). Rats fed BAPN have been found to have an increased amount of soluble collagen that could be extracted in neutral salts and also a comparable increase in urinary hydroxyproline peptides. Jasin and Ziff concluded that the increased amounts of bound hydroxyproline in the urine represented an increase in this soluble collagen fraction. In 1963, Gross[4] found that guinea pigs fed 0.5–1.0 mg of BAPN/kg/day showed an increase in the amount of collagen that was extractable in neutral salts and that this soluble collagen would not reprecipitate with prolonged incubation as would normal soluble collagen. He proposed that previously formed intramolecular bonds and intermolecular bonds in the normal collagen molecule had been disrupted by the BAPN.

Macek et al.[8] stated in 1967 that the fibroblasts form a basic molecule of the tropocollagen which consists of three polypeptide chains. In the youngest developmental forms the individual chains are not cross linked so that this form of collagen, which is called α-collagen, is very labile and degradates easily. During fibrillogenesis, the three fundamental chains of tropocollagen are cross linked together to a higher degree, and further tropocollagen units aggregate. This is how β-collagen, and, from this, gradually insoluble collagen forms are formed.

In summary, these studies have shown that there is an increase in urinary hydroxyproline excretion in Marfan's syndrome, and this is thought to represent collagen breakdown, that lathyrism results in many Marfan-like abnormalities, and the lathyrism produces an increased urinary hydroxyproline excretion due to a block in collagen cross linking.

The problem that arises with any hypothesis as to the basic defect in Marfan's syndrome is that it must explain the wide variety of clinical manifestations involving the skeletal, cardiovascular, and ocular systems.

Pathologic studies have shown that aortic aneurysms in patients with Marfan's disease show a form of medial necrosis in which there is marked disarrangement of the normal orientation of the elastic lamellae with whorls of elastic fibers, increased vascularization, and large areas of cystic degeneration. However, if it is remembered that there is a large component of collagen in the wall of the aorta, an explanation of the histologic findings might go as follows: the collagen may actually act to hold the elastic fibers in their normal lamellar orientation and thus a defective collagenous element may result in disorganization of the elastic fibers in the wall of the aorta. The increased vascularity observed may result from dilation of the vasa vasorum. Ectopia lentis and myopia could also readily be explained by a possible defect in collagen, because both of these (i.e., the suspensory ligament of the lens and the sclera of the eye) are largely collagenous structures.

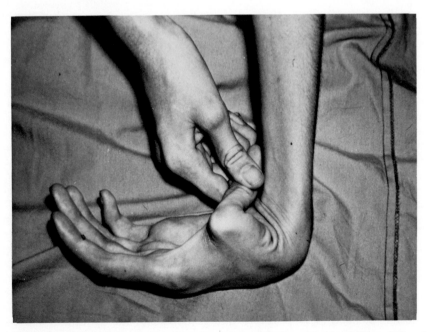

Figure 3.32. Excess laxity of the ligaments permits excess mobility of the joints in arachnodactyly.

CLINICAL PICTURE

The dislocated lens that accompanies the development of pigeon chest deformity or scoliosis may bring the patient to medical attention. Later in life, back pain, joint pain, and effusion may occur. Cardiac symptoms may occur at an early age, but usually begin in the late teenage group. Once left-sided failure has occurred, the prognosis, as in syphilitic aortitis, is very grave, the patient seldom living more than 2 years.

The orthopaedist is often consulted because of deformity, which may consist of pronated feet, scoliosis, or round back deformity. Some patients have subluxated elbows. The patient is usually thin and notes generalized weakness. There is no evidence that the muscles are involved, however, and there is a normal creative coefficient.

The edge of the dislocated lens may be visualized on dilating the pupil. Retinal detachment is not uncommon. The sclerae may be blue, and the patient may be myopic.

An increase in pubis-sole height over that of pubis to vertex is a common abnormality, although the total height is not necessarily increased. Some patients are unusually tall.

Some diagnostic ratios have been given. A hand-to-height ratio greater than 11% or a foot-to-height ratio greater than 15% are thought to be diagnostic. A middle finger that is one and a half times greater than the metacarpal is easily ascertained. Elasticity of the tissues is often noted by a high-riding patella due to stretching out of the patellar tendon.

In 1960, Sinclair, Kitchin, and Turner[14] suggested a new measurement which they found useful in making the diagnosis of arachnodactyly. They averaged the ratios of the length to the width of the second through fifth metacarpals and found that 80% of normal subjects had values between 7.0 and 8.0, with the other 20% having values below 7. In patients with Marfan's syndrome, they found that over 90% had values between 8½ and 10. Another useful measure for the diagnosis of Marfan's syndrome is the ratio of the distance from the vertex to the pubis and the distance from the pubis to the sole. In normal whites this ratio varies with a mean of 1.08 to 0.94 between the ages of 4 and 14, respectively; in Marfan's syndrome the ratio is much lower,

with an average of approximately 0.85 at 14 years of age. The reason for the reduction in this ratio in Marfan's syndrome is not difficult to appreciate when one considers the fact that not only are the extremities longer but also the frequently found kyphoscoliosis reduces the numerator of the ratio.

Kyphoscoliosis is not ordinarily noted before 10 years of age, but may become quite severe as growth progresses. The pigeon breast deformity is often present anteriorly. Most of the spine deformity is in the thoracic spine.

The aortic dilation begins at the aortic ring and involves the ascending aorta; the patient may develop a dissecting aneurysm.

The two most outstanding features of the cardiovascular system in Marfan's syndrome are: (1) dilation of the aortic ring with resultant aortic insufficiency and (2) dissecting aneurysm of the ascending aorta. However, the many other cardiovascular complications associated with Marfan's syndrome include abdominal aortic aneurysms, mitral regurgitation secondary to redundant chordae tendinae, atrial septal defects, tetralogy of Fallot, coarctation of the aorta, and even one reported case of patent ductus arteriosus.

The joints hyperextend, and the limbs are flail-like.

The ocular manifestations of Marfan's syndrome are numerous, but the most important include: (1) ectopia lentis—usually bilateral—in which the suspensory ligaments of the lens are relaxed or fragmented with the lower ligaments most frequently being the most defective so that the lens is displaced upward; (2) myopia—secondary to the excessive length of the eyeball, which is again thought to be due to a defect in the connective tissue elements of the sclera; (3) spontaneous retinal detachment; (4) coloboma of the iris or lens; and (5) associated blue sclera.

Other manifestations of the disease include: (1) congenital cystic lung disease, which may result in spontaneous pneumothorax; (2) small skin papules that occur most often over the neck and are composed of what histologically looks like whorls of elastic fibers in continuity with the dermis (these occur rarely in Marfan's syndrome, but, when they do, they are also virtually pathognomonic of the syndrome and have been given the name Meischer's elastoma); and (3) striae of the skin over the pectoral region are also frequent.

Mental retardation is not a conspicuous component of the syndrome.

ROENTGEN PICTURE

The excessive length of the bone compared to its width is apparent (Figs. 3.33 and 3.34). The long bones tend to be especially long distally. The increased length of the finger as compared to the metacarpal is apparent on a film of the hand. Skeletal maturation is normal.

TREATMENT

The various systems that can be involved in this disease demand highly specialized care in each area. Both cardiac and ocular systems must be thoroughly evaluated initially to determine the need for referral.

The orthopaedic complaints can be individually dealt with, although the total condition affecting the patient still remains unsolvable in terms of remedy for the fundamental metabolic defect.

Generalized weakness demands a resistive exercise program. The training effect from these exercises in these patients is less than normal, but sufficient help is apparent to the patient that a carefully graded program is indicated.

Because the scoliosis can be expected to be progressive, early bracing (Milwaukee-Blount brace) is indicated with regular visits

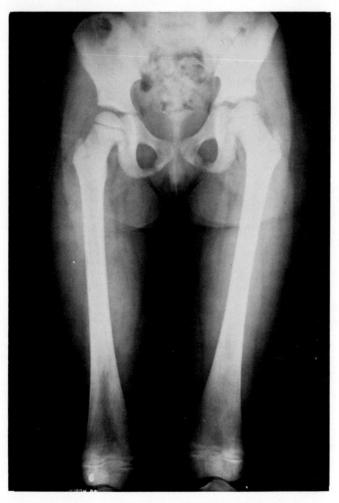

Figure 3.33. Femora in arachnodactyly.

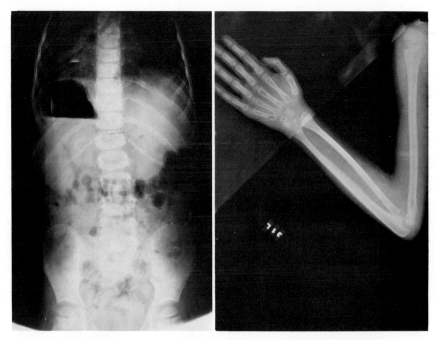

Figure 3.34. Roentgenogram of a patient with arachnodactyly. There is unusual length of long bones and phalanges and a mild scoliosis.

for evaluation of progression and consideration of fusion when indicated.

The long feet may lead to symptoms, with arch supports an early necessity. Eventually, triple arthrodesis may be indicated.

References

1. Aegerter E., and Kirkpatrick, J. A.: *Orthopedic Diseases*, p. 123; Philadelphia: W. B. Saunders, 1958.
2. Bacchus, H.: A quantitative abnormality in serum mucoproteins in the Marfan syndrome, *Am. J. Med.*, 25: 744, 1958.
3. Goodman, R. M.: Thoughts on various genetic disorders of connective tissue, *Med. Times*, 94: 1361, 1966.
4. Gross, J.: An intermolecular defect of collagen in experimental lathyrism, *Biochim. Biophys. Acta*, 71: 250, 1963.
5. Handmaker, S. D.: The satellited chromosomes of man with reference to the Marfan's syndrome, *Am. J. Hum. Genet.*, 15: 11, 1963.
6. Jones, C. R., et al.: Urinary hydroxyproline excretion in normal children and adolescents, *Proc. Soc. Exp. Biol. Med.*, 115: 85, 1964.
7. Jones, C. R., et al: Urinary hydroxyproline excretion in Marfan's syndrome as compared with age matched controls, *Proc. Soc. Exp. Biol. Med.*, 116: 931, 1964.
8. Macek, J., Hurych, J., Chvapil, M., and Kadecova, V.: Study on fibroblasts in Marfan's syndrome, *Hum. Genet.*, 3: 87, 1967.
9. Marfan, A. B.: Une corde déformation congenitale des quatre membres plus prononcée aux extrémités characterisée par l'allongement des os avec un certain degré d'amincissement, *Bull. Mém. Soc. Méd. Hôp. Paris*, 13: 220, 1896.
10. McKusick, V. A.: *Heritable Disorders of Connective Tissues*, Ed. 2; St. Louis: C. V. Mosby, 1960.
11. Ponseti, I. V., and Shepard, R. S.: Lesions of the skeletal and of other mesodermal tissues in rats fed sweet pea seeds, *J. Bone Joint Surg.*, 36A: 1031, 1954.
12. Procop, D. J.: Significance of urinary hydroxyproline in man, *J. Clin. Invest.*, 40: 843, 1961.
13. Sinclair, R. J. G.: The Marfan syndrome, *Bull. Rheum Dis.*, 8: 153, 1958.
14. Sinclair, R. J., Kitchin, A. H., and Turner, R. W.: The Marfan syndrome, *Q. J. Med.*, 29: 19, 1960.
15. Stetten, M. R.: Dietary N^{15}-hydroxyproline, *J. Biol. Chem.*, 181: 31, 1949.
16. Tijo, J. H., Puck, T. T., and Robinson, A.: The human satellited chromosomes in normal patients and in two patients with Marfan's syndrome, *Proc. Natl. Acad. Sci.*, 46: 532, 1960.
17. Weve, H.: Neben Arachnodaktylie, *Arch. Angenh.*, 104: 1, 1931.

Progressive Diaphyseal Dysplasia

A rare disease, progressive diaphyseal dysplasia is characterized by muscular wasting, progressive laying down of subperiosteal new bone in the diaphyseal areas of long bones, and mild neuromuscular disturbances. The syndrome has also been termed Englemann's disease.

ETIOLOGY

The cause is unknown. Some observers have likened the anomaly to muscular dystrophy because of the progressive muscular weakness and familial incidence. Instances of the disease have been found in relatives of the patient who were unaware of any disorder.

CLINICAL PICTURE

Males seem to be more commonly affected. The disease is usually discovered in the 4- to 10-year age group. Easy fatigue or a gait abnormality usually bring the patient for examination. The latter may consist of waddling, difficulty in going up or down stairs, or limp. The patients are frequently underweight and show general growth disturbance. Pain is not a feature.

The legs are thinned, the reflexes may be hyperactive, and there may be swelling and prominence of the diaphyseal areas of long bones. Tenderness is not prominent. The complete blood count, serum, calcium, phosphorous, and alkaline phosphatase have not been noted to be remarkable.

ROENTGEN FEATURES

Neuhauser et al.[1] emphasized the symmetric skeletal distribution of the diaphyses of the long bones and the thickening of the cortex from both the periosteal and the endosteal sides (Figs. 3.35–3.37). The epiphyses and metaphyses are normal, and there is an abrupt termination of the lesion in extremities that are relatively long for the individual.

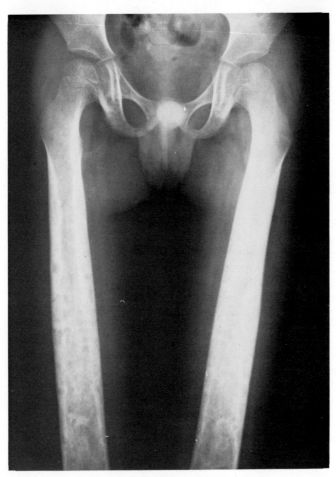

Figure 3.35. Progressive diaphyseal dysplasia. The diaphysis is widened and the cortex is widened from both periosteal and endosteal sides.

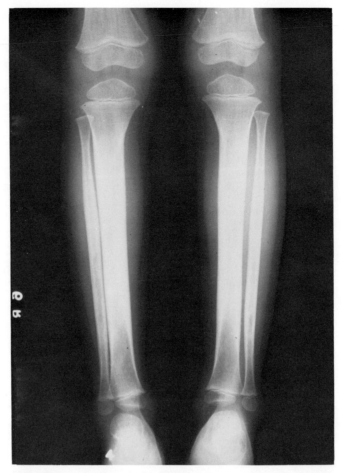

Figure 3.36. Involvement of diaphysis of the tibiae and fibulae in progressive diaphyseal dysplasia. Note the symmetry of involvement.

PATHOLOGY

Thickening of the periosteum accompanied by alteration of the cortex by bone resorption and accretion results in a change to bone of the cancellous type. The marrow frequently is fibrous and has mononuclear and hematopoietic foci. There is no evidence of the effect of an inflammatory agent. Cartilage formation at the epiphyseal line and conversion to bone in the metaphysis are apparently normal.

TREATMENT

Some individuals noted to have the disease are able to live full lives without disabling muscular weakness. Some follow a progressive, downhill course. Muscle exercises, including resistive ones to strengthen available musculature, have been of some value. No medication has been proved to alter the course of the disease.

References

1. Neuhauser, E. B. D., Schwachman, H., Wittenborg, M., and Cohen, J.: Progressive diaphyseal dysplasia, *Radiology, 51:* 11, 1948.
2. Riley, C. M., and Schwachman, H.: Unusual osseous disease with neurologic changes, *Am. J. Dis. Child., 66:* 150, 1943.

Infantile Cortical Hyperostosis

This is an infantile disease in which the diaphysis of long bones, the mandible, and the scapula are characteristically involved by the deposition of subperiosteal new bone. It was first reported in the German literature by

Roske in 1930, but was brought to American attention principally by Caffey (1939), whose name is sometimes given to this disease. The mandibular swelling, a principal sign, has led to an erroneous diagnosis of osteomyelitis in many cases (Fig.s 3.38 and 3.39). The disease occurs in the first 6 months of life and is more common in the male.

CLINICAL PICTURE

Swelling about the jaw without heat or redness leads to a suspicion of the diagnosis. Swelling over the scapula is also especially characteristic, but not as frequent. The infant is usually irritable and may have a low grade fever which runs a chronic course. Leukocytosis usually accompanies the fever.

The swelling is often tender and asymmetric. The tibia, humerus, and clavicle are often involved in conjunction with the mandible and scapula (Fig. 3.40). The small bones of the hands and feet, along with the vertebrae, are exempt.

ROENTGEN PICTURE

Subperiosteal swelling occurs along the diaphysis, usually starting centrally and then spreading throughout the length. It may appear more marked on one side than on the other. The edges of this new subperiosteal bone are smooth; it is laid upon the cortex in layers and separated from it by a thin dark line. In later stages, the subperiosteal new bone and the old cortex are not well delineated from each other (Fig. 3.41) the area of new bone tending to become confluent. The new bone laid down in the scapular region is more masslike and is sometimes confused

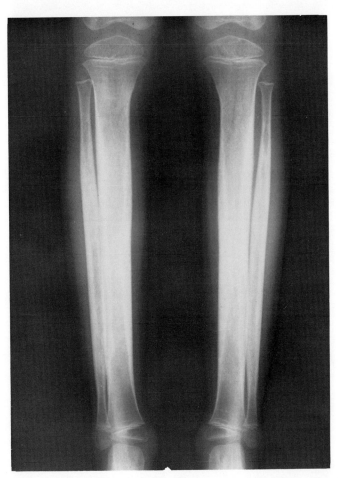

Figure 3.37. Same case as in Figure 3.36. Three years later the cortex is beginning to have a mottled appearance.

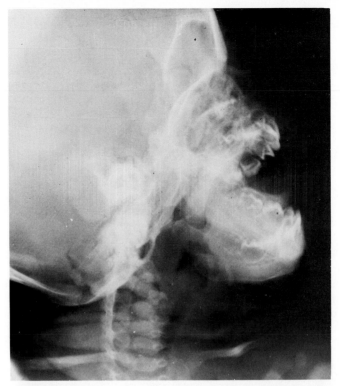

Figure 3.38. Involvement of mandible in infantile cortical hyperostosis, lateral view.

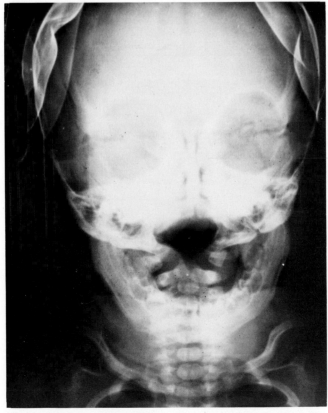

Figure 3.39. Anterior view of patient seen in Figure 3.38. Clinically, swelling due to this bony reaction may be mistaken for osteomyelitis.

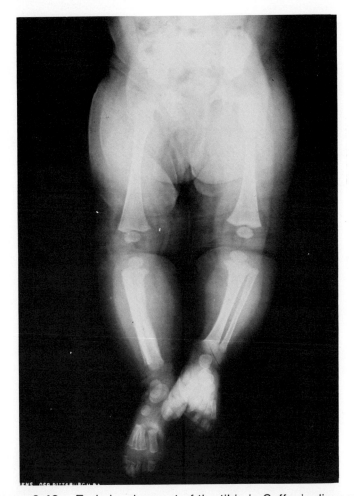

Figure 3.40. Early involvement of the tibia in Caffey's disease.

with tumor. The lesion may be differentiated from osteomyelitis by the fact that the accompanying deep soft-tissue swelling is diaphyseal rather than metaphyseal.

PATHOLOGY

Biopsies have revealed the areas of subperiosteal bone formation but have not shown signs of active inflammation. The marrow is often vascular and exhibits fibrosis and activity of cells in the form of osteoclasts. Cultures of these lesions have been sterile.

TREATMENT

The disease is self-limited; it runs for 10 or 11 months at the longest. It is not affected by antibiotics. The swelling subsides, and the bones appear normal eventually by roentgenogram. The disease is more widespread than osteomyelitis and does not exhibit bone destruction. Scurvy is inappropriate to the age group in which this disease arises. When the bone heals, it does so by widening the medullary cavity so that the cortex lies in the area of bony thickening (Fig. 3.42). As the bone increases in width and length, the developing bone catches up with the increased width created by the disease, so that with sufficient growth the bone is reconstructed.

Reference

1. Caffey, J., and Silverman, W. A.: Infantile cortical hyperostoses, *Am. J. Roentgenol.*, *54:* 1, 1945.

Osteoid Osteoma

Recognition of the osteoid osteoma lesion followed the publication in 1935 of a paper

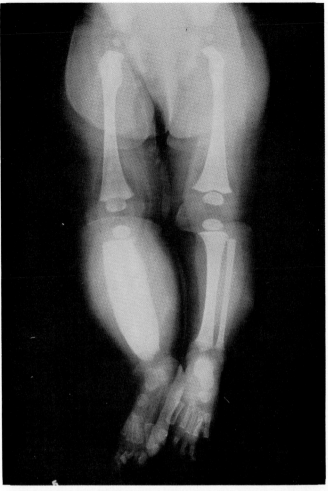

Figure 3.41. Severe involvement with obliteration of bony architecture by bony reaction in Caffey's disease.

by Jaffe[1] which revealed its clinical and pathologic characteristics. It is seen as a cause of chronic bone pain in children, adolescents, and young adults. The nature of the lesion is still in doubt. Opinion supports a benign neoplasm, chronic infection, and unusual bone repair. Due to its unusual pathology and difficulty in classification, it has occupied the attention of many writers. Notable reviews were published by Jaffe[2] in 1945 and by Sherman[3] in 1947.

CLINICAL PICTURE

The entity is more common in males, and the majority of cases occur in the age group between 6 and 12 years. It is rare in Negroes. The two most common areas of involvement are the tibia and the femoral neck. Involve-

ment of a vertebra is not unusual. Other bones may be involved.

The usual patient is seen because of pain that began insidiously but has lasted for many months. The pain is accentuated at night, is localized, and may be relieved by aspirin. It characteristically has gradually increased in severity until medical advice is sought.

If the osteoma is in the lower extremity, examination frequently reveals an antalgic limp. There is usually quite severe atrophy of the soft tissues. A location close to a joint may cause limitation of motion. Superficial locations cause muscle spasm, limitation of motion, and tenderness on palpation of the spine of the involved vertebra. There is no fever and no abnormality of routine blood studies.

ROENTGEN EXAMINATION

The characteristic picture is that of a radiolucent nidus surrounded by sclerosis (Fig. 3.43). There may be a central calcified area within the nidus. Demonstration of the radiolucent center may be quite difficult in the presence of excessive sclerosis. With a cortical location, the periosteum is often raised, and there may be considerable thickening of the bone. Lesions in an early stage of development and causing minimal bony reaction may easily be missed.

PATHOLOGY

There is a vascular fibrous tissue stroma which may be quite cellular. Occasional giant cells may be found. Most characteristic is an irregular deposition of osteoid tissue throughout the nidus (Fig. 3.44). Some of the osteoid trabeculae may become bone. Surrounding the nidus are areas of hypertrophic

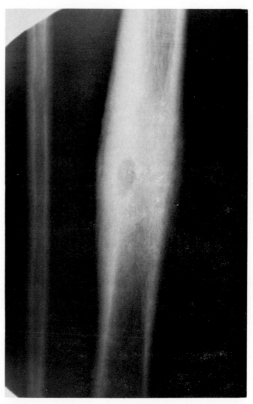

Figure 3.43. Subperiosteal and endosteal ossification in diaphysis of tibia in osteoid osteoma. The area of the nidus is well delineated.

bone, often with intervening fibrous tissue rather than marrow between the layers. There is no evidence of acute or chronic inflammation.

ETIOLOGY

Aside from occasional cultured organisms from the group that commonly are thought of as contaminants, there is no evidence that osteoid osteoma is an infection. There is no clinical response to infection and no pathologic evidence of it. Jaffe supported the theory that these are benign neoplasms, but there is no evidence that this "tumor" grows. The nidus is always small.

The lesion may represent repair after trauma which for some reason cannot be carried to its full conclusion. This inhibition excites the outpouring of further bony calcification to wall off the defect. The repair under difficulty may be caused by a vascular lesion.

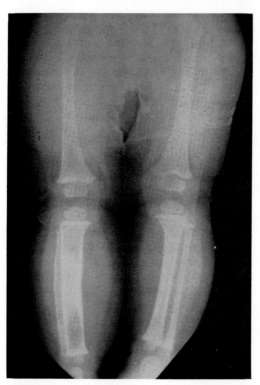

Figure 3.42. Healing in which the widened shape is maintained and results in a widened medullary cavity. Eventually growth in length and width at the metaphysis will obliterate this evidence of disease. This represents the expected result after Caffey's disease.

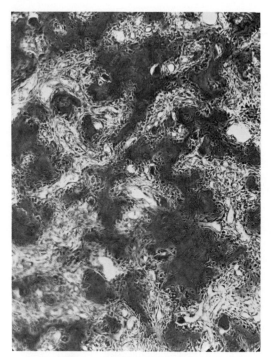

Figure 3.44. Osteoid formation from osteoid osteoma.

TREATMENT

The course of mature osteoid osteoma seems to be chronic persistence of the lesion. Some authors have reported cases in which after a period of years the nidus and pain cleared, although bony sclerosis was still evident.

The response to surgical removal of the nidus is dramatic and satisfactory. It is appropriate to ensure removal of the essential part of the lesion—the nidus. This is done by inserting drills above and below the area presumed to contain the lesion. An x-ray is then taken in the operating room. When the nidus is demonstrated to lie between the drills, it is removed en bloc.

References

1. Jaffe, H. L.: Osteoid osteoma; a benign osteoblastic tumor composed of osteoid and atypical bone, *Arch. Surg., 31:* 709, 1935.
2. Jaffe, H. L.: Osteoid-osteoma of bone, *Radiology, 45:* 319, 1945.
3. Sherman, M. S.: Osteoid-osteoma (review of the literature and report of 30 cases), *J. Bone Joint Surg., 29:* 918, 1947.
4. Wallace, G. T.: Some surgical aspects of osteoid-osteoma, *J. Bone Joint Surg., 29:* 777, 1947.

Pseudarthroses in Childhood

Pseudarthroses in childhood have various backgrounds. The congenital type is rare by comparison with other anomalies. They are noted at birth or shortly thereafter and are most frequent in the mid or distal third of the tibia or fibula (Fig. 3.45). They have also been found in the femur, clavicle, humerus, ulna, and first rib.

Strangely, some pseudarthroses appear to develop with gradual narrowing of the bone. The medullary cavity becomes sclerosed, and a fracture, either spontaneous or induced, occurs. The end result of both types appears the same. The area of the pseudarthrosis consists of the meeting place of two narrowed bony structures, both of which have lost their medullary cavity. Green and Rudo[4] reported the finding of neurofibroma at the site of the pseudarthrosis, and others have confirmed their finding. However, in some cases little is noted other than a binding structure of dense connective tissue about the pseudarthrosis (Fig. 3.46).

The area of pseudarthrosis is sometimes bound by a bulbous mass consisting of irregularly distributed cartilage and fibrous tissue. When this is the case, there is no marked narrowing of the bone, but there may be adjacent cystic changes in the bone.

Boyd and Sage[2] reported 15 cases of congenital pseudarthrosis of the tibia and noted that 2 presented the microscopic picture of fibrous dysplasia in the tissue between the bone ends. Moore[6] noted that, of 178 cases reported from the Shrine Hospitals of North America, 17 were recorded as revealing neurofibromatosis at the site of the pseudarthrosis. Aegerter[1] has suggested that neurofibromatosis, fibrous dysplasia, and congenital pseudarthrosis are in some way related. Fibrous dysplasia here may represent an inability to produce normal bone in one or more areas and a metaplasia into primitive bone. The hamartomatous proliferation of fibrous tissue may lead to a mistaken diagnosis of neurofibroma. Aegerter believed that the fibroblastic masses seen in all three conditions have a common cause, namely, an alteration of the nerve pathways to the areas in which they occur. The alteration may be a neurofibromatous mass or masses in the nerves supplying the area, but the definitive presence of neurofibroma in the bone has not yet been adequately delineated.

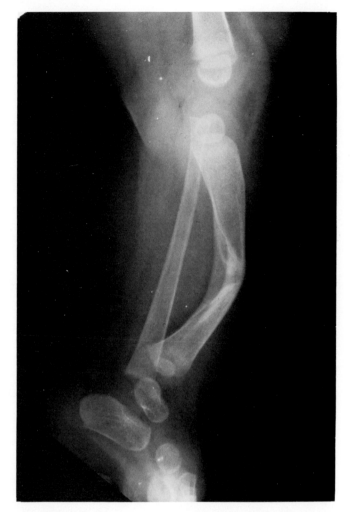

Figure 3.45.   Congenital anterior angulation of the tibia possibly preliminary to pseudarthrosis.

The author has seen tibiae that appeared normal by roentgenogram, go on, after a simple childhood fracture, to develop this lesion. In some, the development of cystlike lesions seems clearly to be a part of the disease; such lesions either inhibit union or threaten union after it is obtained. In these cases, the microscopic picture most closely resembles that of fibrous dysplasia. On the other hand, fractures in children with previously diagnosed fibrous dysplasia have gone on to heal without difficulty.

TREATMENT

If operation is delayed, considerable overlapping often occurs. In some cases, the bone at the pseudarthrosis narrows, and considerable atrophy of the distal fragment makes reconstruction still more difficult (Fig. 3.47). The author believes, as Boyd does, that operation should be performed as soon as the general condition of the patient is at the optimum. The parents should clearly understand that operative procedures may have to be repeated, and, if union is obtained and cystic changes or narrowing of the bone begin to threaten that union, regrafting should not be delayed (Fig. 3.48).

The history of treatment includes many well thought out and noble attempts to secure union, but many of these attempts have been quite discouraging.

J. R. Moore[7] has described a procedure in which each of the united fragments of the

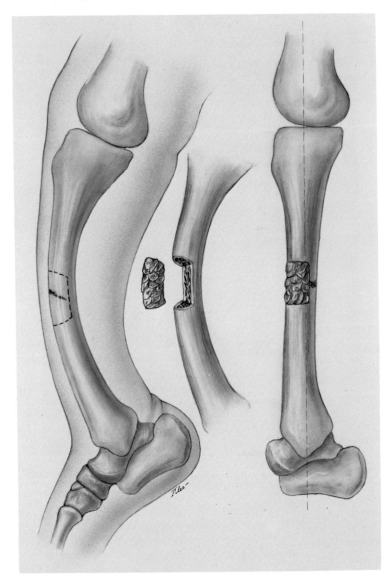

Figure 3.46.   Diagram of delayed osteotomy used in correcting angulation when bone healing is suspect. (*Left and center*) initial operation dividing one-half of the involved bone and leaving mass of bone chips. (*Right*) Second operation dividing the second half of the bone when callus has formed at the first area.

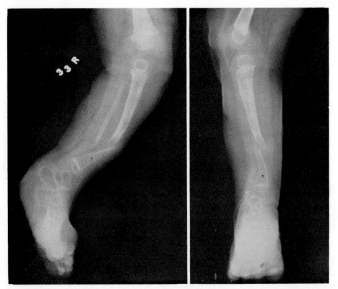

Figure 3.47. Pseudarthrosis of tibia and fibula with narrowing of bone progressively toward the involved area.

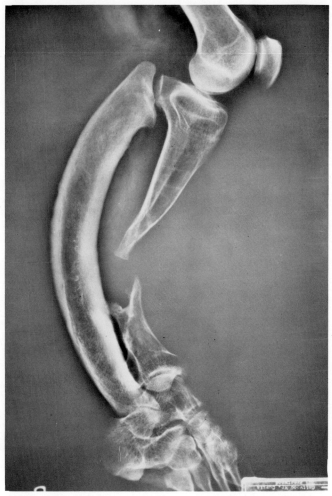

Figure 3.48. Hypertrophy of the fibula in old unresolved congenital nonunion of the tibia.

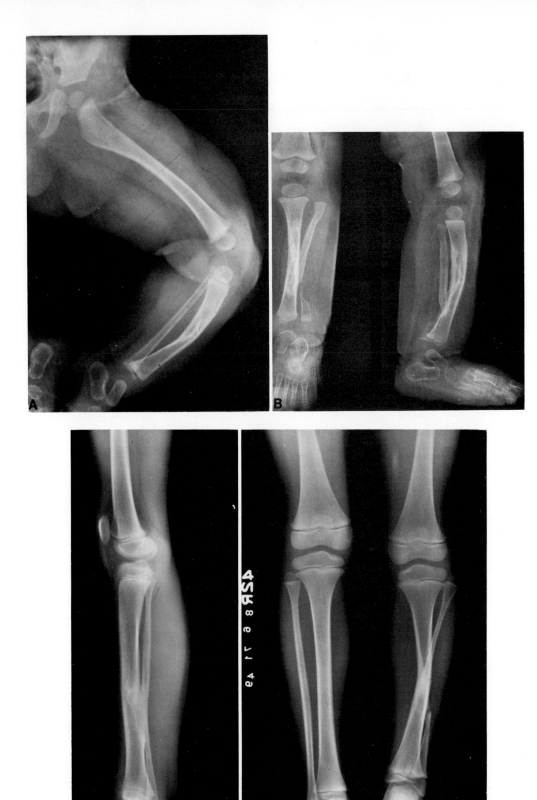

Figure 3.49. (*A*) Anterior angulation of the tibia with beginning narrowing of the medullary canal. (*B*) Implantation of fibula into distal portion of bowed tibia. (*C*) Straightening of the tibia 4 years later. (*D*) Remaining lateral bow of the tibia with nonunion of the fibula.

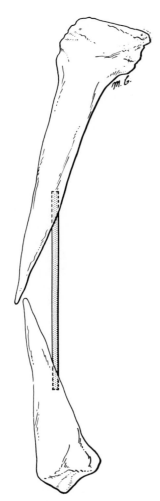

pass graft technique in which a tibial cortical and cancellous graft from the opposite leg is inserted into the proximal and distal tibial fragments (Fig. 3.50). The graft is posterior and does not directly attack the pseudarthrosis. It is so placed that the stress of use is transmitted through it and causes hypertrophy.

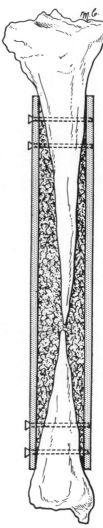

Figure 3.50. Diagram of by-pass cortical graft of McFarland. Bone chips may also be used to fill in the interval between the graft and the parent bone.

tibia is held by two transfixing pins and placed in an Abbott leg-lengthening apparatus (Fig. 3.49). An os novum type of graft is raised on the opposite tibia and, along with a smaller fibular graft, is used 18 days later to bridge the defect. The pertinent points in technique, as detailed by Moore, are that (1) the bone grafts must overlap the fragments by 2 inches or more, (2) fixation with four pins is essential, (3) the graft is held in position until a well defined medullary cavity has appeared, and (4) the graft should not be delayed more than 18 days.

MacFarland[5] has used two procedures. One is a double onlay graft that was later described again by Boyd. The second is a by-

Figure 3.51. Double onlay grafts for pseudarthrosis with double fixation of both proximal and distal end bone chips filling in the area of bone narrowing. (Modified from H. B. Boyd: Congenital pseudarthrosis, *Journal of Bone and Joint Surgery*, 30A: 274, 1948, and J. R. Moore: Autogenous bone graft in the delayed treatment of congenital pseudarthrosis, *Journal of Bone and Joint Surgery*, 31A: 23, 1949.)

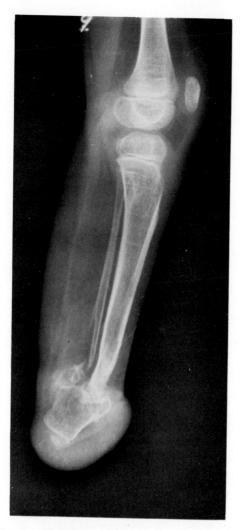

Figure 3.52. Amputation occasionally may be necessary for failure to achieve union of congenital tibial lesion. Use of the heel as above achieves good end bearing stump without problem of the bone growing through the soft tissues.

MacFarland has favored the by-pass technique rather than the double onlay graft (Fig. 3.51), as he believes the former is more certain to produce a good result.

Charnley[3] has successfully used intramedullary fixation, including tibia and os calis, along with grafting but without lengthening.

Whatever method is used, the chances of success are slim unless the greatest care is taken to ensure that no fundamental principle in the treatment of nonunion is neglected (Fig. 3.52). Such principles include elimination of infection, adequate fixation, good soft-tissue coverage; wide bone contact, good general health of the patient, and placement so that the graft will be functional. Once union is secured, regrafting should not be delayed if the bone shows a tendency to narrow in any portion. Gradually increased and protected weight bearing helps to develop the bone.

References

1. Aegerter, E. E.: The possible relationship of neurofibromatosis, congenital pseudarthrosis, and fibrous dysplasia, *J. Bone Joint Surg.*, *32A*: 618, 1950.
2. Boyd, H. B., and Sage, F. P.: Congenital pseudarthrosis of the tibia, *J. Bone Joint Surg.*, *40A*: 1245, 1958.
3. Charnley, J.: Congenital pseudarthrosis of the tibia treated by the intramedullary nail, *J. Bone Joint Surg.*, *38A*: 283, 1956.
4. Green, W. T., and Rudo, W.: Pseudarthrosis and neurofibromatosis, *Arch. Surg.*, *46*: 639, 1940.
5. MacFarland, B.: Pseudarthrosis of the tibia in childhood, *J. Bone Joint Surg.*, *33B*: 36, 1951.
6. Moore, B. H.: Peripheral nerve changes associated with congenital deformities, *J. Bone Joint Surg.*, *26*: 282, 1944.
7. Moore, J. R.: Delayed autogenous bone graft in treatment of congenital pseudarthrosis, *J. Bone Joint Surg.*, *31A*: 23, 1949.

CHAPTER 4

Foot Disorders

PIERCE E. SCRANTON, JR. M.D.

The human foot is an appendage uniquely evolved, assisting man in the assumption of an erect posture and gait. It is a specialized structure of 26 bones, the articulations of which serve as levers and "torque-converters," allowing efficient gait. In the course of assuming an erect, ambulating posture, the foot has come to serve a variety of functions.

The first and foremost function is that of proprioception. Nowhere is this better illustrated than in blind children (Fig. 4.1). The foot provides important proprioceptive input, such as body position, motion, and the nature of surface terrain. The elimination of this proprioceptive function in the diabetic, myelomeningocoel or neuropathic foot will result in an alteration of the entire body habitus.

A second function of the foot is that of providing balance and support. The foot serves as a passive platform, an interface between the limbs and ground. Thus, in walking, the inertia and momentum of the upper limbs and body provide the motive force, with the foot serving as a passive balance platform during each stance phase of the gait cycle.

Next, the foot can serve to assist in either acceleration or deceleration of the gait cadence. Acceleration is most commonly seen in the running individual, where the contraction of the long flexors of the foot and gastroc soleus muscle groups serve to provide propulsive push-off. Similarly, the controlled lengthening of these flexors can serve to decelerate the forward acceleration of the tibia on the talus during the latter half of stance phase. Thus, it is possible to descend a hill in a controlled fashion or, when running, to change direction rapidly or even stop.

The final function of the foot is that of providing shock absorption. With each step, there is an impact force as the body's center of gravity shifts toward the supporting foot. In running gait, where the individual is airborne during swing phase, each foot is subjected to the impact force of the entire body's

weight times the acceleration of gravity. This has been calculated as a force of approximately 2.5 times the body weight. Through a controlled lengthening of the flexors of the foot and knee flexion, this sudden impact force can be absorbed.

In managing pediatric disorders of the foot, it is helpful to keep in mind these five functions. In addition to a thorough knowledge of the foot's anatomic relationships, it is vital to have an understanding of the functional requirements of the patient to be treated. The birth history, chronology of the foot disorder, and the treatment expectations of the child, the child's parents, and the physician must all be carefully delineated.

PRINCIPLES IN THE EXAMINATION OF THE FOOT

Foot disorders may be primary to the foot itself, or they may be secondary to disorders delineated in the family history, birth history, or the examination of the back, hips, or tibia. For this reason, it is helpful to develop a systematized method of evaluation. In the initial examination, the child's parents should be questioned closely regarding family history and the patient's birth history. Disorders such as Charcot-Marie-Tooth disease, bunions, the "delta deformity" in toes, etc. may all have a positive family history. The birth and gestational history are equally important in evaluating infants and children with pes planus, clubfeet, gait disturbances, etc. It is particularly important to determine whether the gestation was complicated or uncomplicated, term or premature, and whether the delivery presentation was vertex or breach or whether cesarean section was necessary. Did the infant do well immediately and come home from the hospital with the mother, or was it necessary to observe or treat the infant further in the hospital?

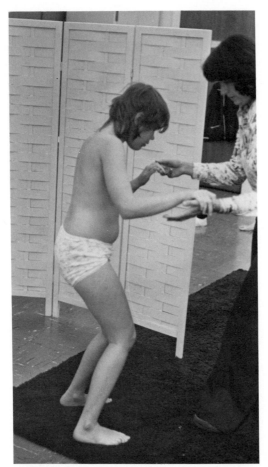

Figure 4.1. The broad-based, flexed stance of blind children. Proprioception by the foot assists in balance and orientation.

ciated with being examined by a doctor. Although most younger children are quite sensitive about their physical appearance, it is nevertheless imperative to watch them walking and occasionally running, without skirts or pants, observing the leg or foot. Appropriate examination gowns and some degree of privacy should, therefore, be available. Another point is that of allaying the fears in toddler patients who are afraid of strangers and most particularly of doctors, whom they associate with getting shots or stitches. It is thus prudent to allow toddlers to remain in the arms of the parent as much as possible. The child can sit in the parent's lap, be dressed and undressed by the parent, and, if it is necessary to observe walking or running, the parent can hold the child's hand, improving cooperation and easing groundless fears.

Any good foot examination begins at the back and works downward. Posterior skin markers such as a hairy patch, dimple, or hemangioma may be important findings with regard to the etiology of a foot disorder. The hips should be carefully examined, evaluating alignment, muscular strength, and range of motion. Infants presenting with a foot disorder should always be evaluated carefully to rule out hip dysplasia. The alignment of the patella, lower legs, malleoli, and knee and ankle motion should all be observed. If indicated, the subtalar motion may be checked by plantar flexing the ankle and exerting a varus-valgus stress across the heel. Dorsiflexing and supinating the foot will "lock" the subtalar joint, prohibiting this motion.

Once the history and actual physical examination are complete, the child should be observed walking and then running in a hallway of suitable length. It is particularly important to include running in the analysis to observe for signs of ataxia, spasticity, or posturing that might not otherwise be noted. Further laboratory and roentgenographic studies may then be ordered, as indicated. In the author's opinion, however, a careful history and physical examination in the fashion described will yield more useful information about a patient than any other study.

Finally, from a historic standpoint, the child's progression through developmental motor milestones is important. A chart giving the average age at achievement is shown in Chapter 1. However, the importance of allowing for a broad variation in what is considered normal cannot be overemphasized. For example, it is not uncommon for a child not to stand or walk until 16 or 18 months. Some children will not talk until 3 or 4 years of age. What is most important is to regard the child's motor milestones, birth history, and family history each in the light of the others. Only after putting together the entire picture, along with the physical examination, can any significance be attached to any one item.

In evaluating the child who has a potential foot disorder, there are several techniques that will help to smooth out anxieties asso-

PHYSIOLOGIC TOE-IN GAIT

Children are frequently seen who have been brought in by parents or relatives with the complaint that the child's feet "turn in." Frequently they have been previously evaluated by several other physicians. During the initial history and evaluation, a grandmother or in-law may become quite dominant, and in such families it may be more difficult to manage the interfamily friction than the child's in-toeing.

Most in-toeing is seen in toddlers under the age of 2. The birth history may not be of assistance, even if abnormalities were present, because these children have generally progressed through their motor milestones without difficulty, achieving early independent walking between 8 and 12 months. The parents will usually relate that the in-toeing seems to be more pronounced and tripping more frequent when the child is tired.

Clinical Picture

Because this discussion is concerned with physiologic in-toeing, etiologies discussed elsewhere, such as congenital clubfeet, spastic cerebral palsy, and other neuromuscular disorders, will not be included. The child with physiologic in-toeing has a normal back, and the foot examination will also be normal, with the exception of mild compensatory pronation. On stress, the foot will passively abduct well past neutral, and, if the child is cooperative, active abduction will also achieve adequate external rotation. Because the feet and back are normal, the in-toeing must arise somewhere between the hips and ankles.

Internal tibial torsion is believed to represent one potential physiologic component of the toe-in gait. The etiology is unclear but may involve an intrauterine positional phenomenon. In the in-toeing child with normal hips, there will frequently appear to be an internal twisting of the distal malleoli relative to the axis of motion of the leg, as measured from the estimated center of the patella and anterior tibial tubercle (Fig. 4.2 *A* and *B*). This alignment may frequently be seen in association with physiologic bowing of the tibia (see Chapter 9).

Anteversion at the hips is a second cause for symmetrical physiologic in-toeing. On observing the child walk, it will be apparent that the entire leg turns in, as well as the foot. The limb may appear to be well aligned, without evidence of genu varum or physiologic bowing. In contrast to those children with internal tibial torsion, children with anteversion of the hips may have considerable external tibial torsion (Fig. 4.3*B*). In general, on physical examination, the hips readily rotate internally past 90 degrees or more. However, the most important finding is that there is a significant increase in internal rotation relative to external rotation (at least 20 degrees greater). Lastly, children with anteverted hips frequently sit on the floor with the knees flexed and the heels under the buttocks (Fig. 4.3*A*).

Roentgen Appearance

There are no bony deformities present in internal torsion. Comparing internal and external rotation anteroposterior roentgenograms, it will be noted that on internal rotation the fibula is not brought into normal lateral relief, but still overlaps and is posterior to the tibia, relative to the normal adult leg. In the hip, the femoral head has a normal height in relation to the trochanter. In the anteroposterior view, it may seem as though the femoral neck angle is increased, but a second view with full external rotation of the hips will confirm that the femoral neck angle is normal in the range of 135 degrees.

Treatment

There is no place for bracing, twister cables, corrective shoes, or operative intervention in the child with physiologic in-toeing who is under 5 years of age. As the foot is normal, corrective shoes with reverse lasts, arches, wedges, or twister heels are definitely contraindicated. The most difficult part of the treatment will be that of assuring the parents that the in-toeing will correct with growth alone.

In the child with persistent anteversion of the hips, the characteristic internally rotated sitting posture must be prohibited. From a practical point of view, the only way to accomplish this is to insist that the child "sit like an Indian" with the hips externally rotated, or to provide the child with a small chair, making it impossible to tuck the heels under the buttocks. This becomes the child's television-viewing chair and play chair. It will

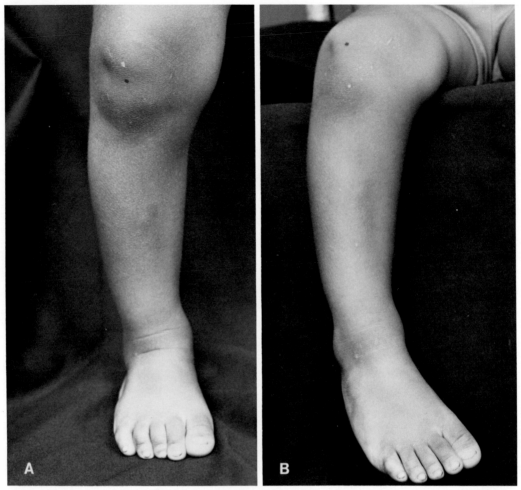

Figure 4.2. (A) The child with internal torsion of the tibia has secondary pronation of the foot. This pushes the fibula posteriorly but does not fill out the medial calf so that leg appears bowed. (B) In internal tibial torsion the axis of the malleoli appear "internally twisted" relative to the axis of the leg itself. The dot at the knee marks the center of the patella. The appearance is created by the fibula gliding forward at the distal tibial-fibula joint.

take up to 5 years of growth to achieve correction.

Operative Treatment

At some time after age 5 or 6, a child with severe, persistent in-toeing may require surgery. Usually these children have a family history of parents or relatives who also had severe, persistent in-toeing. The physical and roentgenographic evaluation must be carefully performed to ensure that there is no occult neuromuscular deficit present. In ad-

dition, the site of abnormal version must be localized. The activity level of the child must be assessed, and the degree to which the in-toeing interferes in keeping up with peers.

When in-toeing is persistent and severe, a derotational osteotomy at the level of the proximal tibia, distal femur, or proximal femur may be performed (Fig. 4.4). Because of the potential for problems with the peroneal nerve and/or compartment syndromes, we prefer not to derotate at the proximal tibia. On the fracture table, the proximal femurs may be operated upon through small lateral incisions. Threaded Steinman pins are inserted in parallel fashion, the osteotomy performed between the pins, and the appropriate, symmetrical correction "dialed" by rotating the legs outward. The incisions should be small and closed cosmetically. The pins are incorporated into the spica cast. If proximal femoral, derotational osteotomies are performed, the child should be maintained in the spica cast for 8–12 weeks, depending upon the child's age and healing. Proximal tibial or distal femoral derotational osteotomies may be ambulated much sooner in protective casts after pin removal.

PES VALGUS

Flat feet in children pose a significant diagnostic challenge. To begin with, although the entire foot may appear "flat," the deformity may be due to a variety of bony or soft-tissue disorders found separately or in combination in the hindfoot, midfoot, forefoot, or upper limb. The age of presentation and the multitude of entirely separate etiologies have resulted in a great deal of confusion in both diagnosis and management. For example, in outlining principles in the conservative management of flat feet, various authors have termed this condition: relaxed flat foot, pes planus, flat foot, pes planovalgus, pronated foot, etc. It has thus been difficult to determine exactly what condition was being treated and, if there were discrepancies in results, why.

The recent classification proposed by Bleck seems to bring order to this confusion (Fig. 4.5). Undoubtedly, as time passes, there will be exceptions and additions to this proposed

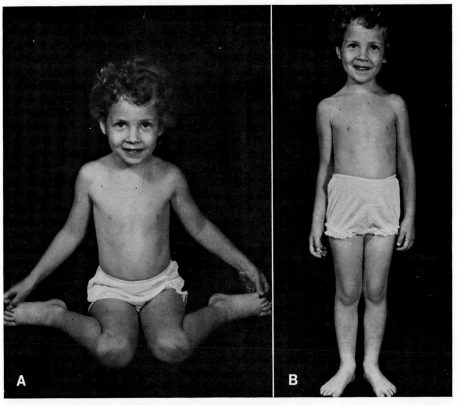

Figure 4.3. (*A*) The sitting posture that allows persistent anteversion and subsequent in-toeing gait in the older child. A youngster with this sitting posture characteristically has relaxed ligaments allowing this posture. (*B*) On standing, the child who has been subject to the anteverted sitting posture stands with external torsion of the tibia, a secondary effect of the posture. To bring the foot forward in line with a forward progression, the knee must turn in.

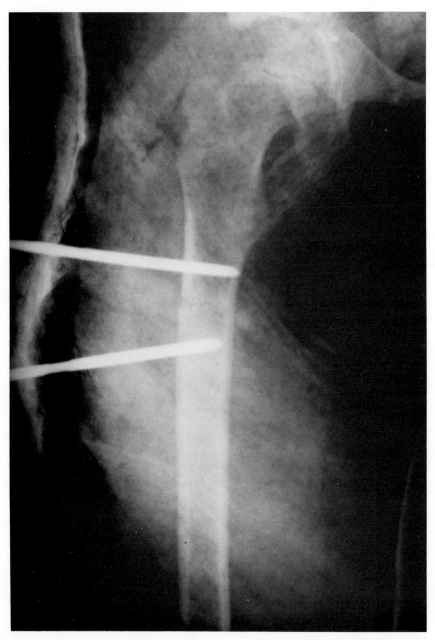

Figure 4.4. A proximal femoral derotational osteotomy, held with threaded Steinman pins incorporated in a spica cast.

I. Static
  A. Plantar flexed talus, rigid (congenital vertical talus)
  B. Plantar flexed talus, flexible (probably the "hypermobile flat foot")
  C. Z-foot with metatarsus varus ("skewfoot" — McCormick and Blount)
  D. Calcaneal equinus (dorsiflexion angle < 10°)
  E. Medial deviation of the talar neck (probably the medial deviation of the talonavicular joint — Giannestras)

II. Arthritic
  A. Tarsal coalitions (peroneal spastic flat foot)

III. Paralytic
  A. Flaccid — lower motor neuron
  B. Spastic — upper motor neuron

Figure 4.5. The classification for pes valgus. (Reproduced with permission from *Clinical Orthopaedics and Related Research, 122:* 89, 1977.)

system. However, experience would seem to dictate that the vast majority of all pediatric flat feet will find a category within this classification.

Flat Feet in Childhood

True structural malalignment leading to pes valgus in childhood is often difficult to discern (Fig. 4.6). Most children in the "toddler" age group do appear to have flat feet but in fact have an "arch" obscured by fat. As walking progresses and skeletal growth continues, this fat disappears. Children with the appearance of a flat foot may also have secondary pronation of the foot in response either to physiologic bowing of the limb or internal tibial torsion. As growth and straightening ensue, the feet come closer together during gait, and with supination an arch appears.

Another reason for the foot to appear flat when in fact there is no structural abnormality is found in blind children (Fig. 4.7). Although the foot seems quite pronated, this is in response to the broad-based, flexed knees and hips gait of the blind. In this population, cerebral palsy, ligamentous laxity, and structural abnormalities should be ruled out. However, once the pathologic etiologies have been eliminated, this pronated foot should not be treated with arch supports or corrective devices, because this pronation is a helpful adaptation of the blind, assisting in proprioception and ambulation.

Pediatric Flexible Pes Valgus (Plantar-flexed Talus)

Pediatric pes valgus (flexible flat feet) is commonly missed in a child's early years, primarily because our culture tends to cover the feet with shoes and socks. Once the child has passed the toddler stage and there is evidence of persistent flattening of the foot with complaints of fatigue after playing, it is apparent that further evaluation is necessary. As this type of foot has not been grossly flat from birth, chances are that it represents the flexible flat foot with plantar-flexed talus as classified by Bleck. Frequently there will be other signs of this laxity, as evidenced by hyperextension at the elbow, hyperabduction of the thumb, and excessive symmetrical laxity in the knees.

The symptoms that may be associated with weak feet are often not recognized. The child who seems lazy, dislikes long walks, and comes indoors while the rest of his age group is still out playing may be suffering from foot strain. When actual pain is complained of, it is frequently located not in the foot but in the calf. This leg discomfort has two characteristics: it is intermittent, and it tends to occur at the end of the day.

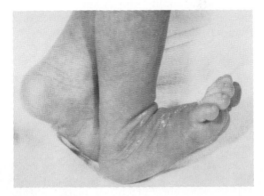

Figure 4.6. Calcaneovalgus feet in infancy with excessive dorsiflexion and tight anterior tibial tendon. This foot is "positional," and serial stretching or casting will assist correction.

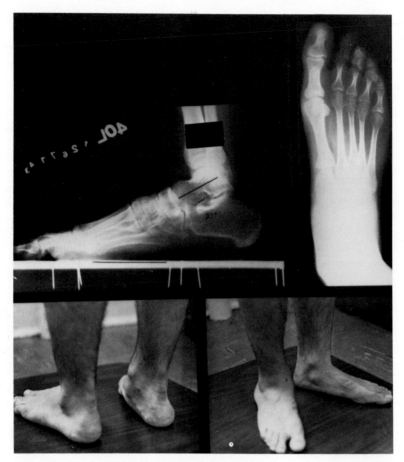

Figure 4.7. The forefoot pronation in the congenitally blind is a functional adaptation to the broad-based, flexed stance. There are no structural abnormalities and nonoperative or operative correction should not be attempted.

On first standing, the infant's feet are almost invariably pronated, spread apart in a wide-based stance for balance, gripping for support. Standing barefoot in this position stretches out the ligaments of the medial side of the foot. Gradually, as the feet come closer together, they supinate. The infantile fat is redistributed as the child's activity increases. As a preventive measure, a child should be in firm shoes with a heel as soon as he gains upright posture. The child whose foot is not responding to increased activity is ordinarily not recognized until the age of 2 or later.

Why is it a good practice to place a toddler in high-top shoes? There is really one reason—in order to keep them on. The infant's heel is rounded and not developed posteriorly. High shoes are not worn to support the ankle, which is a tight nortise. The stiff counter of the heel holds the os calcis upright and thereby aligns the subtalar joint where inversion and eversion take place. It follows that the time when oxfords can be worn is shown by the ability of the child to keep these low shoes on without walking out of them. This can be determined by trial and error at the shoe store.

Roentgen Appearance

As is true for almost all foot x-rays, standing views are mandatory. For flexible pes valgus, plantar-flexed talus, standing anteroposterior and lateral roentgenograms will confirm the diagnosis (Fig. 4.8). The anteroposterior view will delineate the axis of talus and calcaneus. These axes should normally not diverge more than approximately 18 degrees.

The lateral view reveals the axis of the talus, which bisects that of the calcaneus. This should measure approximately 26.5 ± 5 degrees in normal feet. In the flexible plantar-flexed talus foot, this angle is increased (Fig. 4.9). That this deformity is due to ligamentous laxity is easily shown by re-x-raying with a corrective arch support or medial insert. The lateral talocalcaneal angle will significantly diminish.

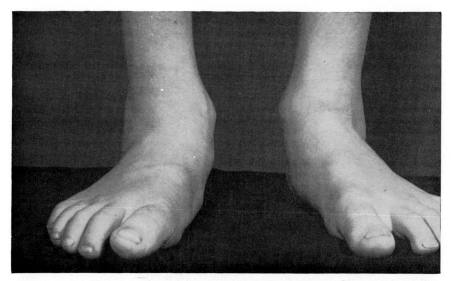

Figure 4.8. The hypermobile flat foot with short short Achilles tendon results in severe pronation.

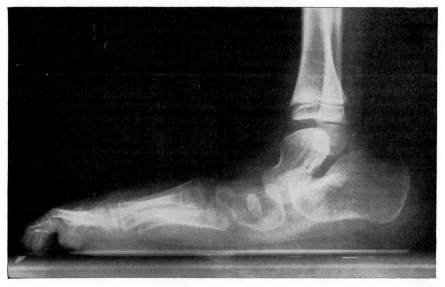

Figure 4.9. A lateral standing roentgenogram of the weight-bearing foot, showing the plantar-flexed talus, depressed navicular, loss of the medial arch, and subluxation of the talar head over the anterior portion of the os calcis. Note, however, the navicular is still in normal relation to the talar head, in contradistinction to congenital vertical talus when this joint is dislocated.

Physical Examination

The examiner finds not a structural flat foot, but a foot functioning in a position that throws strain on its ligaments and muscles and does not use its bony support. The degree of arch medially and longitudinally is noted in recumbency. Most feet are well arched in this position, but some feet are architecturally flat, even when not weight bearing. The tightness of the heel cord is noted by dorsiflexing the foot in inversion while the knee is straight. A foot normally should be able to dorsiflex at least 10 degrees above the right ankle when examined in this way (Fig. 4.10).

When the child is standing, the position of the os calcis in relation to the weight-bearing line out from the tibia is the degree of pronation of the foot. It is best noted from the posterior view with the foot at eye level. As the talus is plantar flexed, the medial side of the foot comes into prominence (Fig. 4.11). Pressure on the medial side of the foot reveals whether or not the talus can be passively corrected into an upright position. The contrast between the weight-bearing and the non-weight-bearing position is important from the standpoint of strain.

The alignment of the leg affects the foot. Tibia vara with a medial facing of the ankle mortise means that the foot must pronate to

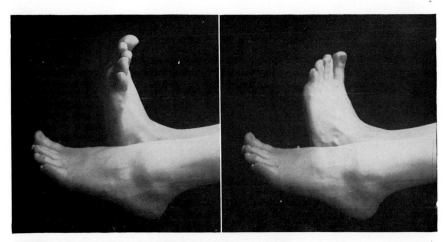

Figure 4.10.   The foot everted (*left*) dorsiflexes further than the foot inverted (*right*).

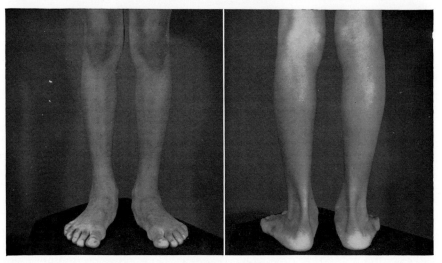

Figure 4.11.   Pronated feet with prominence of the talonavicular area medially and a valgus position of the os calcis in the posterior view.

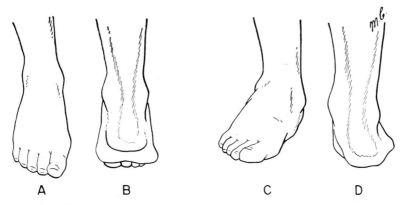

Figure 4.12. The foot with ligamentous laxity is normally constituted without weight bearing (*A* and *B*). With weight bearing the foot pronates and the os calcis goes into a valgus position (*C* and *D*).

bring its weight-bearing surface onto the ground. Internal torsion of the tibia may be confused with the tibia vara deformity or may be part of it. Internal torsion is noted by placing the knee facing directly to the examiner and dorsiflexing the foot in line with the ankle joint. It should be in the same plane as the knee. Deviation of the ankle joint medially in relation to the plane of the knee joint may be due to internal torsion. A facing outward or laterally of the coronal plane of the ankle joint in relation to the knee is external torsion.

Valgus at the knee may also develop in children with pronated feet. This is particularly true in youngsters with chubby thighs, whose legs are widely separated on weight bearing. This genu valgum is probably the product of the same relaxed ligamentous structure that allows the foot to pronate (Figs. 4.12–4.15).

Treatment

Children with ligamentous laxity who have flexible pes valgus, plantar-flexed talus, require corrective orthotics or shoe inserts for a period of at least 3 years. The prime goal in treatment is the restoration of the arch. As this is easily done merely with pressure applied at the medial talonavicular region, the single most important corrective device is thus some sort of medial arch support.

Arch supports have evolved on a regional basis, but each variation still basically provides medial support. Thus, depending on the regional availability of these devices, one

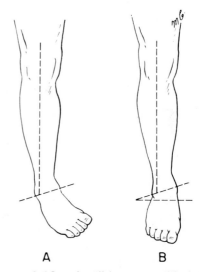

Figure 4.13. In tibia vara with internal torsion there is a medial facing of the distal tibial surface at the ankle joint, resulting in the necessity for the foot to pronate to bear weight on its medial side.

might prescribe a "navicular-cookie," a Helfet corrective heel seat, a UCBL insert (University of California Biomechanics Laboratory), a medial arch support with Thomas heel, or a Whitman steel arch support. It is important that this support be constructed correctly and that it be comfortable to the child. Recurrent blisters and pain with walking will mean that the corrective device will simply not be used. To prepare the parents for coping with problems in the initial adjustment to the arch support, they should be advised that it will take at least 2 weeks for the child to become accustomed to the insert.

With an appropriate heel cup, a medial arch pad or support helps to prevent rotation of the foot within the shoe. This increases the effectiveness of a medial heel wedge, which is designed to tilt the hindfoot into inversion (Figs. 4.16–4.20). The usual well tolerated medial heel wedge height is 1/8 inch. If the hindfoot is controlled, the forefoot will follow. Medial arch supports that are carried too far forward result in difficulty in fitting the foot over them into the shoe.

The subastragalar area is the point at which support is needed most. The usual height for a medial arch support in childhood is 3/8 inch. A medial prolongation of the heel may be used in addition to the wedge. This so-called "Thomas" heel is a part of shoes that are sold as "orthopaedic shoes."

Straight-last shoes (plumb-line) disguise in-toeing by the child and can be used when the forefoot tends to turn medialward or to adduct in relation to the hindfoot.

Exercises for the feet of an inverting or supinating type have been of little help in the treatment of flat or pronated feet in childhood. However, there is one exception to this: the case of a tight heel cord. Because the foot can dorsiflex further in inversion, the youngster is forced into a weak mechanical position in order to get his heel on the ground in the presence of tight heel cords. No progress in the direction of improvement of the feet can be expected while the heel cord remains tight. The mother can stretch this tendon when the child is small by inverting and dorsiflexing the foot while the knee is extended. When the child is older, he or she can be taught heel cord stretching exercises as illustrated in Figure 4.21. Such exercises need not be done to the point of boredom, but they should be done regularly and thoroughly at least once each day. It usually takes 3–4 months to notice improvement.

Correction of foot and gait problems do not take place instantaneously when corrective measures are applied, but only with further development and growth of the foot.

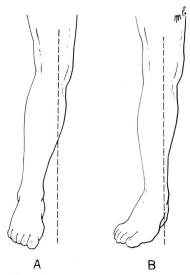

Figure 4.14. The weight-bearing line is brought medialward by valgus at the knee as in (*A*). External torsion of the tibia rotates the foot outward and away from the weight-bearing line (*B*).

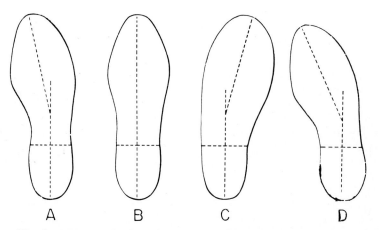

Figure 4.15. Varying types of shoe lasts controlling the relationship of hindfoot to forefoot: (*A*) regular; (*B*) Straight; (*C*) forefoot abduction; (*D*) forefoot adduction.

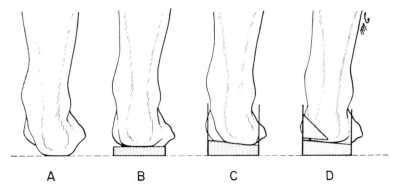

A   B   C   D

Figure 4.16.   The effect of various measures on the position of the os calcis is shown. In (*B*) a normal heel alone improves the position, but this effect is increased further by a medial wedge combined with a longitudinal arch. A medial wedge alone is not sufficient to keep the heel from the valgus (*C*), but when it is combined with a pad, the full effect of both is felt (*D*).

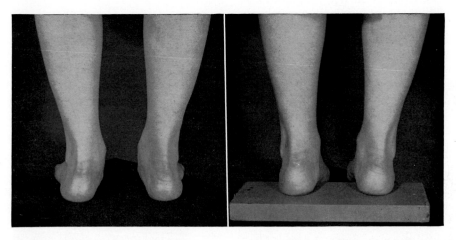

Figure 4.17.   The effect of a heel alone on foot position. Valgus of the os calcis is largely corrected.

Stiff plates of steel or plastic tend to make the foot rigid and to wed the child permanently to their use. Flexible but firm supports seem preferable. Pasted-in longitudinal arch supports such as are commonly seen commercially are inadequate as a general rule, because a fully adequate support necessarily gives the child some slight difficulty in getting his foot into the shoe.

This problem is avoided by not building the pad too far forward. Its most important function in the simple pronated foot of childhood is to control the hindfoot; the forefoot must necessarily fall in line. A longitudinal arch pad ends behind the first metatarsal head and extends posteriorward to the end of the arch and inward (lateralward) from there

to tilt the os calcis into an upright position by its support.

After 2–3 years of wearing the insert, the talocalcaneal diversion in the anteroposterior roentgenogram and the plantar-flexed talus seen in the lateral generally correct. To ensure that the insert device is providing correction, it is a good practice to take a lateral standing roentgenogram with the child wearing the corrective shoes. After the initial years with the corrective insert, the patient may require the use of inexpensive, removable arch supports that can be moved from shoe to shoe. This is optional and dependent upon the degree of correction achieved and the extent to which the patient may or may not have symptoms.

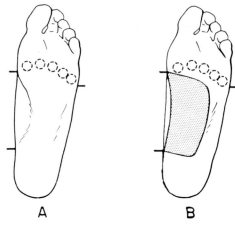

Figure 4.18. In tracing a foot for medial arch support, the area just proximal to the first and fifth metatarsal head is marked, as well as the posterior termination of the medial arch. Keeping the anterior end of the pad behind these prominences is important for comfort and for fitting the pad into the shoe. The pad is brought well toward the middle of the foot posteriorly to support the subtalar area.

attempts to provide support. The inactivity engendered by these painful, fatigued feet discourages parents and affects the child's personality and development. In our experience, these patients generally present after age 10, at a time when their peers are beginning to play vigorously and explore athletic potential. Prominent among these children is

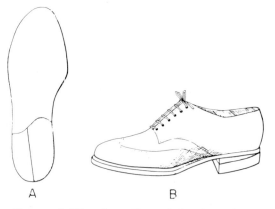

Figure 4.20. Location of the inner heel wedge to aid in inverting the os calcis.

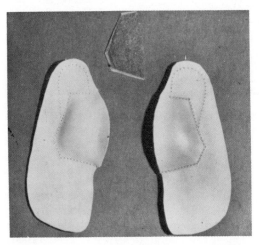

Figure 4.19. Leather arch supports with felt insert. The extra felt is inserted when the first becomes compressed.

DISABLING FLAT FEET

There are children who have a complete collapse of the arch, resulting in severe disability (Fig. 4.22). This collapse will be persistent despite prolonged and well executed

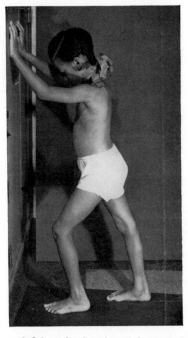

Figure 4.21. In heel cord stretching in the older child, the heel of the posterior limb is kept on the ground. The elbows flex as the child gently dorsiflexes the ankle, stretching the cord.

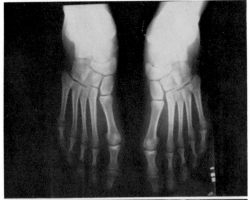

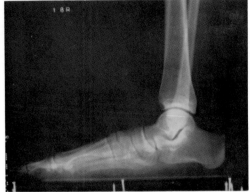

Figure 4.22. Roentgenogram of disabling feet. The overlap of the talus on calcaneus indicates the degree of hindfoot valgus.

a long and frustrating history of repeated, failed attempts with corrective orthotics.

Two types of deformities are commonly found in early adolescence: a calcaneus in equinus and valgus (Bleck's classification D) and the talonavicular or naviculocuneiform sag described by Giannestras (Bleck's classification E).

The first disorder represents a flat foot in which the primary deformity is found in hindfoot valgus and equinus (Fig. 4.22). The posterior portion of the arch is lost through an equinus calcaneus, while pronation occurs because of a valgus relationship between the talus and calcaneus. There may be a slight degree of associated talonavicular sag, but clinically and roentgenographically the deformity is predominant at the hindfoot. Therefore, treatment considerations must be directed posteriorly.

Two procedures have been described for this type of foot. Giannestras advocated cor-

rection of the hindfoot deformity through a Grice-type, extra-articular, subtalar arthrodesis that forced the calcaneus out of valgus (Fig. 4.23). The number of patients requiring this procedure has not been large, and there has been a high incidence of degenerative talonavicular beaking. It is this author's opinion that the creation of a subtalar "tarsal coalition" in an otherwise neurologically normal child should not be performed.

The operative procedure of choice would seem to be the Chambers procedure. Miller reported a long term follow-up of the Chambers procedure in 81 feet. The results were good or excellent in 95%. The procedure involves a soft-tissue release of the talonavicular joint, the posterior capsule, and a tendo achillis lengthening. This is coupled with an elevation of the anterolateral facet of the calcaneus, just behind the calcaneocuboid joint (in effect, an anterior, reverse Dwyer)

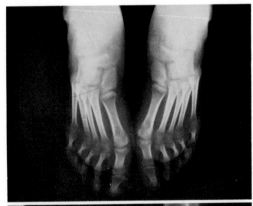

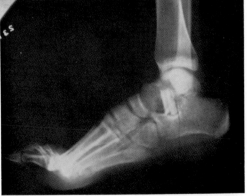

Figure 4.23. The foot shown in Figure 4.22 was treated by a Grice, subtalar, extra-articular arthrodesis. The os calcis has been brought under the talus, evident in both the anteroposterior and lateral views.

(Fig. 4.24). A long leg cast is applied for 4 weeks, followed by a short leg walking cast for 8 weeks. Care is taken to mold a supportive arch into the cast.

The majority of adolescents presenting with symptomatic static pes valgus are found under Bleck's classification E, or Giannestras' talonavicular and/or naviculocuneiform sag. Here the hindfoot relationships are usually relatively normal. The forefoot, however, is pronated due to collapse of the main arch. These individuals characteristically complain a great deal of fatigue and aching in the calf and arch after prolonged activity, due to tibialis posterior strain. Often there will be an accessory navicular in association with this deformity, a clue that there may be an aberrant insertion of the posterior tibialis tendon.

The muscular support is quite important to maintenance of the arch. Even though it has been argued quite vehemently that the alignment of the bones and ligamentous structures are the sole sources of arch maintenance, the role of the anterior and posterior tibialis muscles in relation to the arch have now become more clearly defined. The arch

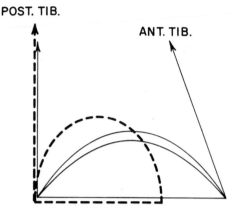

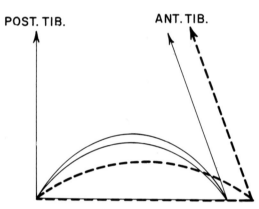

Figure 4.25. A diagrammatic representation of the effects of overpull on the arch of either the anterior or posterior tibialis muscles. A tight posterior tibialis increases the arch (to a certain extent the peroneus longus assists in this) and a tight anterior tibialis will flatten the arch.

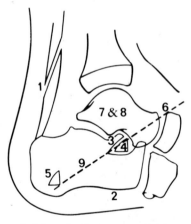

Figure 4.24. A diagrammatic representation of the Chambers procedure. The operative procedure consists of (1) a tendo achillis lengthening; (3) a bone flap is raised against the shoulder of the talus; (4) the bone graft itself in place; (5) the donor area for the graft; (6) reduction of the talonavicular joint; (7 and 8) reduction of equinus and the body of the talus. The *dotted line* is the path of the incision. (Reproduced with permission from *Clinical Orthopaedics and Related Research, 122:* 97, 1977.)

should be regarded as a bow (Fig. 4.25). A tightening of the posterior tibialis supports or enhances the strength of the arch. Overpull of the anterior tibialis will act to flatten the arch. This principle was shown in Giannestras' illustration of the unilateral increased arch in a young girl several years after an unrecognized laceration of the anterior tibialis tendon. The action of this tendon to distally flatten the arch prompted Giannestras to incorporate a release of this tendon in the operative treatment of pes valgus, attaching it to reinforce the posterior tibialis.

The importance of the posterior tibialis in assisting in arch support was illustrated by

Smith and associates, who reported on 10 patients with severe, unilateral pes valgus resulting from unrecognized posterior tibialis laceration. From these observations on the changes in arch structure after interruption of muscle function, it would seem that, although bony alignment and ligamentous structures are probably primary in arch preservation, the muscular contribution must not be ignored.

A variety of operative procedures are available to correct the pes valgus of talonavicular sag. The Kidner, Hoke, Giannestras, and modified Giannestras procedures will each provide a satisfactory correction. The Kidner and modified Giannestras procedures involve soft-tissue surgery only and are reserved for the child under 13 years of age for whom naviculocuneiform arthrodesis would be contraindicated. The Hoke and Giannestras procedures include naviculocuneiform arthrodesis and should be performed only after age 13. An adducted cavus foot can result from premature medial tarsal epiphyseal closure.

Kidner Operation

We have employed this procedure primarily upon younger patients with moderately symptomatic flat feet who also have an accessory navicular. A nonoperative trial of well fitted arch supports must be attempted in these patients for at least 3 months. Upon failure of such a trial, the Kidner procedure should be employed (Fig. 4.26).

The Kidner operation excises the accessory navicular or medial tuberosity of the navicular and transposes the posterior tibial tendon into a groove on the inferior surface of this bone. In this operation, a curvilinear incision over the medial aspect of the foot and outlining the navicular area is made. As the flap is retracted, the insertion of the posterior tibial tendon is seen. This is carefully outlined in order to save a flap of soft tissue both inferiorly and superiorly over the navicular. The accessory navicular is completely delineated and then excised. Bone wax may be packed into the attachment to the navicular to prevent the occurrence of an exostosis. The inferior flap is dissected underneath the navicular, and the undersurface of the navicular is exposed. A groove of varying depth will be found here. The tendon of the posterior tibial muscle is now dissected from its

navicular attachment, care being taken to keep it intact and continuous and its distal portion radiating under the cuneiform. It is then brought under the navicular to act in slinglike support. A stay suture is needed to ensure that the tendon is held in place. The previously devised flaps are now sewn over the exposed surface of the navicular. This is a relatively simple procedure with an evident purpose—to reconstitute the medial arch.

Modified Giannestras Procedure

This procedure was developed by the author as an abbreviated form of that described by Nicholas Giannestras in 1973 and again in 1976. It is indicated for the child with persistent severe naviculocuneiform sag, aged 8–12. The procedure described here involves a modification of the Giannestras incision that will result in improved venous drainage. Also, the wedge naviculocuneiform fusion is eliminated, which is otherwise contraindicated in this age group.

The incision is S-shaped, beginning over the anterior tibialis, ending plantarly at the distal insertion of the posterior tibialis (Fig. 4.27a). The anterior tibialis is released. The medial capsule overlying the naviculocuneiform joint is turned back in a flaplike fashion, retaining the proximal attachment (Fig. 4.27b). The posterior tibialis is moved inferiorly as in the Kidner procedure and then tightened by advancing it upon itself approximately 0.5 cm with nonabsorbable suture. The anterior tibialis is sutured into the posterior tibialis. The foot is then held with the naviculojoint in the corrected position and the medial capsular flap sewn beneath the anterior tibialis, advancing it distally (Fig. 4.27d). The child is then maintained in a cast, non-weight bearing for 4 weeks, followed by a short leg walking cast for 8 weeks. Again, the arch support is molded into each cast. After the casts are removed, a steel-shanked oxford with arch supports is worn.

Hoke Operation

The Hoke procedure is primarily for the "in-between" foot that does have some calcaneal equinus in addition to prominent talonavicular sag. It should only be performed in the skeletally mature foot, as arthrodesis

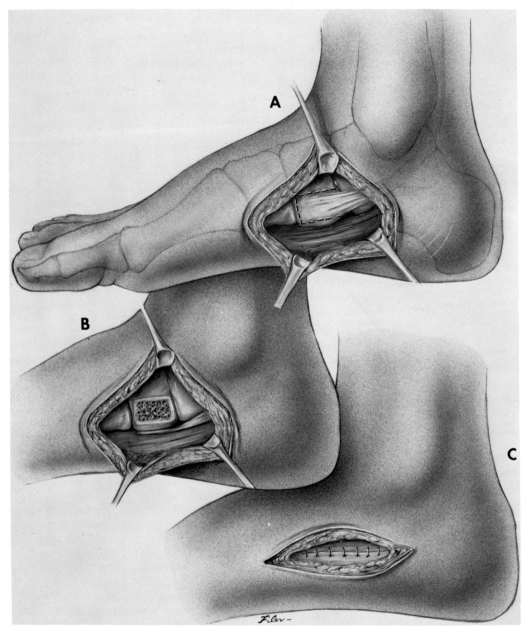

Figure 4.26. The Kidner operation for symptomatic flat feet. (*A*) Posterior tibial insertion on the navicular tuberosity is visualized. The area to be removed with a thin shell of bone is outlined by the *dotted line*. (*B*) The bare surface of the navicular is visualized above the inferior surface of the navicular where a subcortical flap has been raised. The posterior tibial insertion is placed beneath this flap. (*C*) The soft tissues are repaired, holding the posterior tibial insertion in place. A cast is then applied.

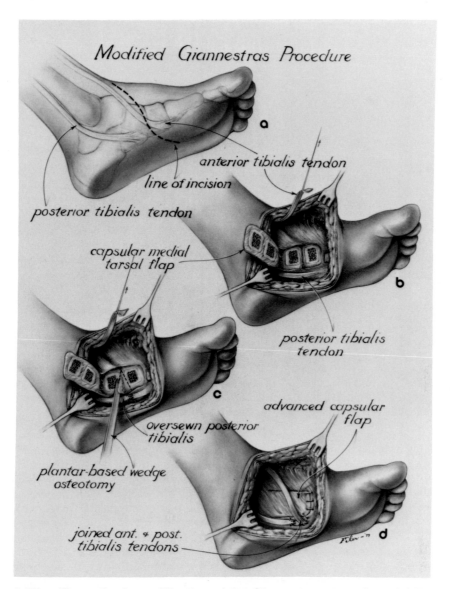

Figure 4.27. The author's modification of the Giannestras procedure. (*a*) The altered skin incision will protect venous drainage and not risk damage to superficial sensory nerves. (*b*) The insertion of the anterior tibial is freed, and a subperiosteal flap of medial capsule overlying the naviculocuneiform joint is removed. (*c*) The posterior tibialis is moved laterally and plantarly, oversewing it upon itself. If the child has a skeletally mature foot, the plantar-based wedge osteotomy may be performed and held in approximation with a catgut suture. (*d*) The anterior tibialis is joined to the posterior tibialis, and the capsular flap is advanced distally.

across the naviculocuneiform joint in a growing foot will produce the forefoot cavus adductus deformity.

The Hoke operation involves lengthening the tendo achillis as the first step. The naviculocuneiform joint is then exposed. The ar-

ticular cartilage is removed from the articular surface of both navicular and the cuneiforms both first and second (Fig. 4.28).

The foot and the distal end of the first metatarsal are then forced into equinus. In this position, a rectangular block is removed

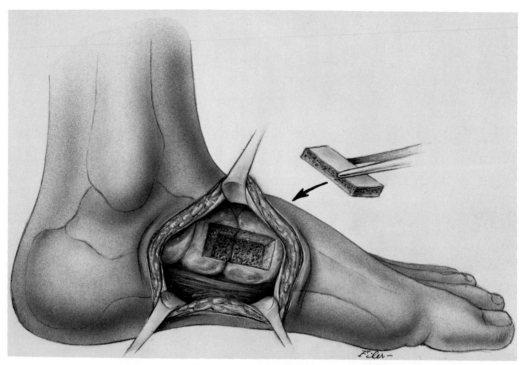

Figure 4.28. In the Hoke operation, a bone graft, in the form of a rectangle taken from the tibial cortex, is placed into a cancellous bone slot made to involve navicular and cuneiform bone. The medial arch is reconstituted before the cuts are made.

from both the navicular and cuneiform. Careful carpentry is involved, because an accurately sized bone is needed. This is taken from the tibial cortex and fitted as an inlay graft across the joint and into the rectangle formed in both the navicular and cuneiform. The cast to immobilize the patient postoperatively starts as a plaster slipper holding the foot in equinus and the heel in varus. The foot is then brought up to neutral, and a long leg cast incorporates the slipper.

The cast is held for 6 weeks followed by crutch walking for 3–4 months with a medial support shoe and longitudinal arch pad and partial weight bearing. When the fusion appears fully formed and swelling of the operative site gone, the crutches are discarded, but the shoes are used for the next several years.

Giannestras Procedure

This procedure is thoroughly outlined in Giannestras' text, *Foot Disorders*. It has yielded gratifying results in our hands, and

has been reported as yielding an 87% excellent to good result in 146 feet.

The procedure itself is as outlined in the "modified" section, with the only addition being that of the plantar-based wedge naviculocuneiform osteotomy (Fig. 4.27c). This is held together by a large catgut stay suture and not by a medial staple, which would later cause painful bursitis with shoe wear.

The patient should remain non-weight bearing for an initial 6 weeks, followed by a walking cast for 6 weeks. After cast removal, the child should go immediately into rigid shanked oxfords with arch supports. It may require up to 6 months before ambulation is normal after any of these described procedures.

CONGENITAL VERTICAL TALUS

Infants and children presenting with a congenital vertical talus (plantar-flexed talus, rigid in Bleck's classification) are relatively uncommon. In a 15-year period, only 12 such

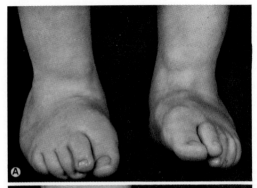

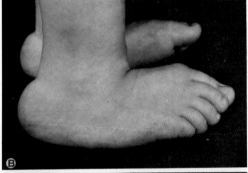

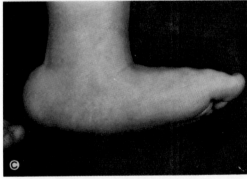

Figure 4.29. (A) Anterior view of foot with superior dislocation of the forefoot carried into supination in a child with congenital vertical talus. (B) Lateral view of foot, making the dislocation superiorly more evident with resultant loss of the lateral arch of the foot. (C) Medial view of foot with prominence in the center of the medial arch produced by the head of the astragalus.

patients were seen on the Orthopaedic Service at Children's Hospital in Pittsburgh, Pennsylvania. The etiology of this deformity is probably multifactorial. It is most commonly seen in association with arthrogryposis multiple congenital or spastic cerebral palsy. It may also be seen as an isolated, congenital, idiopathic deformity, or its clini-

cal appearance may be inadvertently created by incorrect casting techniques in the treatment of a clubfoot (the so-called "rocker-bottomed foot").

Clinical Picture

The superficial appearance of the congenital vertical talus foot is that of plantar convexity, with calcaneal equinovalgus (Fig. 4.29). The forefoot appears abducted, the head of the talus is prominent medially, and the valgus hindfoot has a tight heel cord. The important feature that differentiates this foot from the plantar-flexed talus (flexible) or calcaneal equinovalgus foot is that this deformity is rigid and cannot be reduced.

When the infant starts to walk, the gait is not normal, for the persistent midfoot dislocation deprives the child of a normal push-off (Fig. 4.30). This is in spite of the fact that the talus itself will exhibit normal range of motion in dorsiflexion-plantar flexion.

Roentgen Appearance

The most helpful views in evaluating this deformity are dorsiflexion and plantar flexion

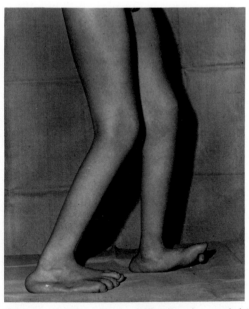

Figure 4.30. The difficulty in weight bearing with congenital vertical talus uncorrected is painfully apparent in this older child. Such feet are extremely disabling.

laterals. The equinus position of the hindfoot will persist despite forced dorsiflexion. With plantar flexion, in the flexible foot, the navicular will maintain its alignment with the head of the talus. However, the navicular will remain dislocated dorsally in the congenital vertical talus foot. In the neonate, the navicular has not ossified, and discerning this relationship will be quite difficult (Figs. 4.31–4.33). Because the cuboid ossifies earlier, it is frequently helpful to use this bone as a marker to estimate where the navicular is. If, on plantar flexion, the ossific center of the cuboid is above the axis of the talus, it can be predicted that there is dorsal navicular dislocation.

Treatment

The true congenital vertical talus foot cannot be successfully managed by manipulative reduction. To begin with, most of these feet occur in the arthrogrypotic or cerebral palsy patient. Thus, the combination of dorsal navicular dislocation and hindfoot equinovalgus, coupled with aberrant neuromuscular function, doom serial casting to failure. In the neonate, serial casting is initially valuable as a means of stretching the soft tissues, making later surgery easier. Further, it will buy time, providing some correction as the child grows

to a size where surgery is feasible. In these infants, after 8–12 weeks of serial casting, a Denis-Browne bar may be used in an effort to hold the improved position and still allow further growth. By age 6 months, most infants may be large enough to perform technically precise surgery.

The goal of operative treatment is to restore the talotarsal alignment and correct hindfoot equinovalgus. Two schools of thought prevail regarding the operative management. Coleman and associates reported a two-stage approach, designed to correct both the hind- and midfoot deformities, restoring and preserving bony architecture. Eyre-Brook, Stone, Robbins, and Clark all reported excellent correction by naviculectomy and/or posterior release.

COLEMAN APPROACH

As the surgery is quite extensive, it is necessary to perform the correction in two stages. The first stage consists of a dorsolateral approach to the midfoot. A Batchelor-type subtalar, extra-articular arthrodesis is performed, wedging the fibular strut graft in to correct the valgus deformity of the calcaneus. Through the anterior aspect of this incision, all extensor tendons and the anterior tibialis are identified and lengthened in a Z-fashion. The dorsal capsule overlying the

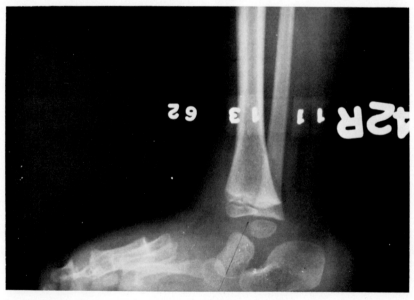

Figure 4.31. Congenital vertical talus. A lateral roentgenogram reveals the forefoot dislocated superiorly in relation to the plantar-flexed talus.

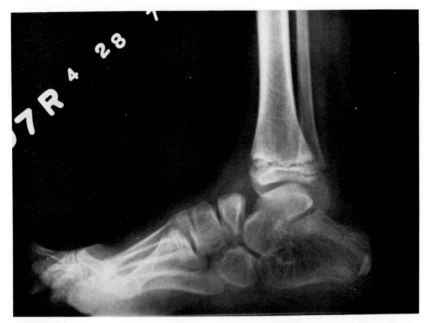

Figure 4.32. A 9-year follow up of patient seen in Figure 4.31 reveals that the navicular had not been retained in an anatomic relationship to the talar head, and the consequent deformity of the tarsal bone is obvious.

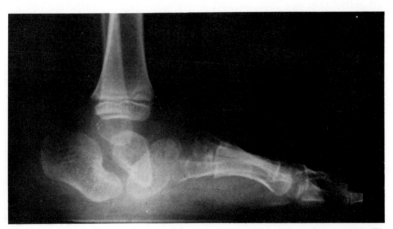

Figure 4.33. The vertical talus deformity uncorrected in the older child. The navicular and the entire forefoot are dislocated in relation to the hindfoot. The os calcis, the talus, and the cuboid form a triumvirate, creating a weight-bearing prominence that is extremely difficult to walk upon.

dislocated navicular is incised, and the talo-navicular joint is reduced. This reduction is maintained with K-wire fixation. At no time during this initial procedure is the foot dor-siflexed, and after wound closure the foot is placed in a long leg cast in equinus for 8 weeks.

The second stage of the procedure consists of a posterior lengthening and medial repair. The posterior ankle joint and subtalar joints are released, and the tendo achillis is lengthened. The posterior tibialis is translo-cated plantarly and advanced, similar to the Kidner procedure. Again, a long leg cast is applied, with attention placed now on molding an arch into the cast and holding the foot at neutral. After cast removal, the child should wear an oxford with arch support, with or without braces, depending upon the child's neurologic status.

The disadvantage of this procedure is that it is quite extensive surgery, performed over two stages. The child will be immobilized in a long leg cast for at least 3 months, confined to home or hospital. Further, the subtalar arthrodesis predisposes the child to later, painful degenerative talonavicular changes that may ultimately require a triple arthrodesis.

The advantages of this procedure are equally important. To begin with, it offers a means of reconstruction, preserving and restoring the bony architecture. In the child over the age of 24 months, a naviculectomy may not be appropriate due to the inadequate remodeling potential at the newly formed talocuneiform joint. Thus, the Coleman procedure will serve as a salvage for the late-presenting congenital vertical talus patient. Further, it provides excellent correction, forestalling or eliminating the necessity for a later triple arthrodesis. As most of these children present with arthrogryposis or spastic cerebral palsy, their functional demands upon the foot will not be so great as to predispose to painful, degenerative talonavicular changes. Therefore, this procedure should be remembered as one approach to the operative reduction of the congenital vertical talus.

NAVICULECTOMY

Excision of the navicular should be considered in the child under 24 months of age with congenital vertical talus. The rationale behind the procedure may be based upon Dilwyn Evans' concept of visualizing the foot as having a medial column and a lateral column. In the congenital vertical talus foot, the medial column is too long, with resultant dorsal dislocation of the navicular (Fig. 4.34). Rather than performing a radical lateral release, in an effort to lengthen and to equalize the lateral column, a simple naviculectomy provides the correction. Further, when done at a younger age, remodeling at the talocuneiform joint will result in an excellent articulation without the production of degenerative arthritis (Figs. 4.35 and 4.36 A and B).

The naviculectomy and posterior release may be performed in one procedure through a medial incision, extending from the plantar aspect of the first cuneiform to the posterior margin of the Achilles tendon. The navicular itself is removed by sharp, subperiosteal dissection. The anterior tibialis tendon is dissected from the navicular, and it is determined whether sutures are necessary to attach it more firmly to the first cuneiform. The posterior tibialis is advanced distally, oversewing it upon its cuneiform attachments. A posterior capsular release of the ankle and subtalar joints is performed, in combination with a tendo achillis lengthening.

An additional lateral incision may or may not be necessary to assist in levering up the talar head. This lateral incision is made over the sinus tarsi and brought up on the dorsum sufficiently to expose the head of the talus. A joker or small periosteal elevator is inserted beneath the talar neck to prevent it from sinking into equinus at the time the foot is held in reduction and transfixed with a K-wire.

With the hindfoot held in neutral and the forefoot aligned with the corrected talus, a K-

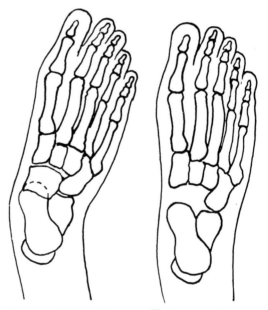

Figure 4.34. Diagrammatic dorsal views of the foot with a congenital vertical talus. Shortening the medial column by naviculectomy balances the columns. (Reproduced with permission from *Journal of Bone and Joint Surgery, 59A:* 822, 1977).

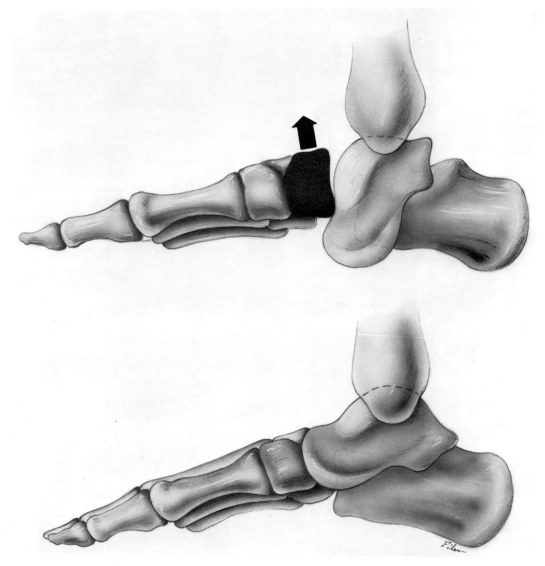

Figure 4.35. A diagrammatic lateral view illustrating the dorsal abutment of the navicular. A simple naviculectomy, rather than a radical two-stage procedure, results in correction.

wire is used to transfix the first metatarsal, cuneiform, and talus to hold this corrected position. A long leg cast is applied with a well molded arch. This is changed at 6 weeks, at which time the wire is removed. The second cast is maintained for 6 weeks, after which time the child is placed in high-top straight-last shoes with a medial arch, Thomas heel, and 1/8-inch medial wedge. A single lateral upright brace with a medial T-strap may be necessary for at least 1 year, and arch supports will probably be necessary for several years. The talus and cuneiform adapt with secondary growth into a well formed joint and normal-appearing foot (Fig. 4.36). Because of this remodeling, it is often not apparent that the navicular is missing in later roentgenograms.

TARSAL COALITIONS (PERONEAL SPASTIC FLAT FOOT)

Occasionally children will present, generally between the ages of 8 and 12, with the

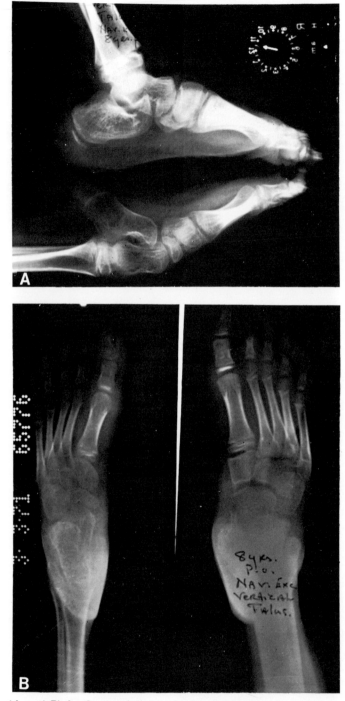

Figure 4.36. (*A* and *B*) An 8-year follow-up of a child's foot in which the navicular was excised in infancy to allow reduction of the forefoot in relation to the hindfoot. The subsequent remodeling of the tarsal bones is evident with maintenance of the medial arch of the foot.

recent onset of painful flat feet. This pain is dissimilar to the vague midfoot aching and calf pain commonly seen in static flat feet. The pain localizes to the lateral aspect of the hind- and midfoot, "deep inside." Because the patient resists attempts to invert the foot and the peroneal tendons appear to tighten during such inversion attempts, this condition has been referred to as a "peroneal spastic flat foot." Occasionally the extensor tendons may join the resisted inversion.

There are many underlying etiologies to the so-called peroneal spastic flat foot. Inflammatory lesions to the subtalar joint, such as tuberculus, infectious, and rheumatoid arthritis, all may present with pain and peroneal tendon spasm. Osteoid osteoma has been associated with peroneal spasm, as has posttraumatic subtalar irritation. Depending upon the site of irritation, the foot sometimes may be held in supination and inversion.

It is important to rule out congenital bony anomalies, such as tarsal coalitions. Talocalcaneal, talonavicular, calcaneonavicular, and calcaneocuboid coalitions all may produce midtarsal and subtalar strain with resultant peroneal spasm. Therefore, although there is apparent rigidity due to peroneal spasm, the lack of motion is in fact due to congenital fusion between one or more of these tarsal bones.

In a report by Harris and Beath, the most significant and frequent anomaly was a talocalcaneal bridge, rather than a calcaneonavicular bar. Such a bridge is apparently a variation similar to that which produces the os sustentaculum and may actually represent fusion of the accessory bone at either end. A similar bone, calcaneus secondarius, is the basis of the calcaneonavicular bar. Embryologic failure of segmentation is believed to represent a possible etiology.

The bridge may be bony, cartilaginous, or fibrous. The limitation of subtalar joint motion causes a characteristic talonavicular impingement. This will later cause the characteristic dorsal lipping of the talus. A Harris view, or 45 degree posteranterior view, of the os calcis is necessary to demonstrate the subtalar joint and its pathology (Fig. 4.37 A–C). However, 30 degree and 60 degree views may also be necessary. If the coalition is more anterior, at the sustentaculum tali, tomograms may be necessary.

The age at presentation is variable, depending upon the location of the coalition and whether there is a mature synfibrosis, synchondrosis, or synostosis. Talonavicular coalitions will ossify at 3–5 years of age, calcaneonavicular at 8–12, and talocalcaneal at 12–16. If the bridge is incomplete and some motion persists, the coalition may be discovered only by accident when a foot x-ray is taken for other reasons.

Treatment

Peroneal spastic flat feet must be thoroughly investigated to determine the etiology. Standard arteroposterior, lateral, oblique, and Harris view roentgenograms should delineate a coalition. If none is discovered, a work-up for infections or rheumatoid arthritis should be started, in addition to hindfoot tomograms to rule out an occult, anterior talocalcaneal coalition. For arthritic conditions, rest and anti-inflammatory agents are helpful. A bivalved cast with daily exercise periods will alleviate symptoms.

Should a talonavicular, talocalcaneal or calcaneocuboid coalition be discovered, nonoperative treatment should be attempted for as long as possible. Intermittent treatment with a short leg walking cast and analgesics is helpful. A special shoe with a SACH heel and rocker bottom sole, with or without a double upright short leg brace, may be of assistance. The alternative to this is surgery, a triple arthrodesis, because of the location of these particular coalitions. Therefore, an adequate trial of nonoperative therapy must be attempted.

The calcaneonavicular coalition is unique, compared with the other types, in that early recognition and excision will result in a complete relief of symptoms. Synfibroses retain suitable motion such that they are generally asymptomatic, and, therefore, no surgery is indicated. However, large synchondroses or synostoses will restrict subtalar motion, causing painful spasm. If these are excised before secondary degenerative talonavicular beaking occurs, complete and permanent relief will be obtained. Figure 4.38 A and B is an illustration of such a calcaneonavicular bar without degenerative beaking. Complete excision, such as illustrated in Figure 4.39, is

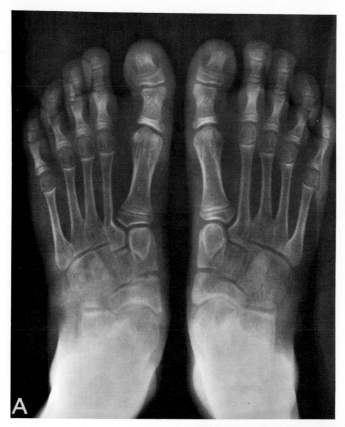

Figure 4.37. The calcaneal-talar bar is easy to miss by roentgenogram. In (*A*) the production of the forefoot due to peroneal spasm is evident. In (*B*) no definite bar is shown connecting os calcis and the navicular (oblique view). In (*C*) the union of the medial side of the subtalar joint is shown with the talus and os calcis joined (45 degree posteroanterior view of the os calcis).

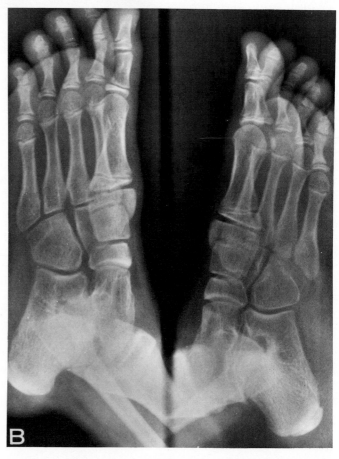

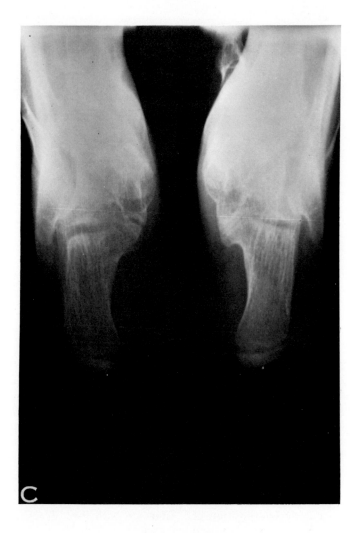

Fig. 4.37 (C)

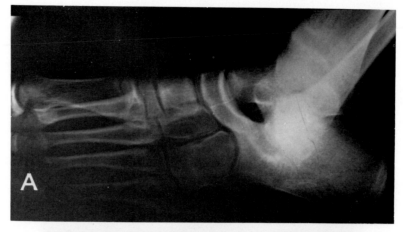

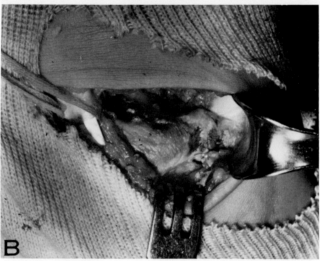

Figure 4.38. (*A*) In this oblique roentgenogram of the foot, the calcaneonavicular bar is clearly shown. A union such as this may be fibrous, cartilaginous, or osseous. In the young child, resection frequently yields normal foot function, but, in the older child, a triple arthrodesis is necessary to cure the condition. (*B*) At operation the bar is visualized adjacent to the retractor. The peroneal tendons are retracted by tape, and the skin inferiorly by a rake.

necessary or there will be a recurrence. Cowell has advocated a muscle interposition of the extensor digitorum brevis into the excised coalition space in an effort to prevent synostosis recurrence. In our experience, if the excision is adequate and bone wax is used on the excised calcaneal and navicular margins, there will not be recurrence. Early motion and weight bearing, as tolerated, in a compression dressing will assist in the prevention of recurrence. If the child is maintained in a cast, the immobilization will only enhance bone formation.

Occasionally a patient will present at a later age with the calcaneonavicular bar in combination with degenerative talonavicular beaking (Fig. 4.40). It is tempting to consider excision and avoid a triple arthrodesis. However, because of the degenerative changes, the total increase in joint motion will exacerbate foot pain and ultimately lead to the triple arthrodesis. Therefore, upon recognition of degenerative changes, a triple arthrodesis is the procedure of choice.

In performing the triple arthrodesis, the bar must be excised or it will maintain the pes valgus deformity. Furthermore, as these are painful flat feet, the arthrodesis should be performed in such a way that the arch is restored. The technique of inlay grafting described by Williams and Menelaus will provide a satisfactory arthrodesis in addition to correction of the deformity. If necessary, a small medial incision over the talonavicular joint will enhance visualization and ensure adequate apposition of these bones, which might otherwise be difficult.

NEUROGENIC FLAT FEET

Although pes valgus may occur because of a variety of neurologic disorders (myelomeningocoel, athetoid, spastic, or flaccid cerebral palsy), we are primarily concerned here with

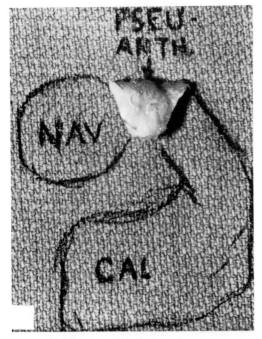

Figure 4.39. The resection of a calcaneonavicular bar must be complete. This diagrammatic illustration of the calcaneus and navicular has the resected bar specimen in place. Even though this specimen is fairly large, it has been incorrectly removed in a wedgelike fashion, a common tendency in this resection. The excision should be square so that the deeper portion is not closely approximated.

the hindfoot equinovalgus produced by the spastic gastroc-soleus muscle groups. As this deformity is not the result of static ligamentous inadequacy but rather the product of neuromuscular imbalance, treatment is necessarily different.

Initially, children with progressive, spastic pes valgus may be treated by bracing and corrective shoes. A steel-shanked oxford with medial arch support, 1/8-inch medial wedge, and a single upright short leg brace with medial T-strap may provide all the stabilization that is necessary. If the degree of spasticity is severe, there will be a history of tendo achillis lengthenings and hamstring releases or transfers. Tight hamstrings in combination with tight heel cords will accentuate the pes valgus.

Once bracing and/or upper leg muscular releases and/or transfers have not resulted in an arrest of progressive spastic pes valgus, surgery is indicated. The Grice procedure, or extra-articular subtalar arthrodesis, is the operation of choice for those children between the ages of 6–12 (Fig. 4.41). At 13 years of age or older, a triple arthrodesis by inlay graft technique may be necessary.

The Grice procedure has been established as quite effective in controlling progressive, spastic pes valgus. It is not without its pitfalls, however, and is a technically demanding procedure. In the younger child, if a large tibial bone block for graft is removed, tibial overgrowth will be stimulated, relative to the fibula. This relative shortening will create a valgus deformity at the ankle, thus compounding the original problem. To avoid the problems of tibial overgrowth, Batchelor devised the fibular strut graft as an alternative source of bone graft. However, if the graft is removed from the distal two-thirds of the fibula, the incidence of fibular pseudarthrosis is very high, again creating valgus instability at the ankle. Therefore, in younger children, the fibular strut graft should come from the upper fibula. The tibial strut graft can be taken from children over the age of 10 without fear of stimulating tibial overgrowth.

There is the legitimate concern that this subtalar arthrodesis can create the identical problems of the tarsal coalition, resulting in later painful degenerative talonavicular beaking. However, in this patient population, the incidence of later degenerative changes is surprisingly small. Undoubtedly, this is due

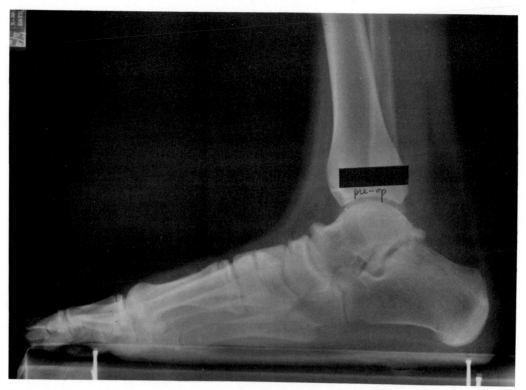

Figure 4.40. The standing lateral roentgenogram of a 14-year-old male with an occult, anterior, talocalcaneal coalition. Degenerative talonavicular beaking has already occurred, and this painful foot must be treated by triple arthrodesis.

to the limited functional requirements placed upon the feet by this patient population.

CONGENITAL CLUBFEET (TALIPES EQUINOVARUS)

Congenital clubfoot is one of the oldest known and treated deformities of mankind. Since the days of Hippocrates, various methods of manipulation, strapping, and binding have been used in its correction. The condition occurs once in every 1,000 births and is approximately twice as common in males as in females. The characteristic deformity has three elements: forefoot adduction, inversion, and equinus of the foot (Fig. 4.42). Such a foot has been termed talipes equinovarus. Although some reports have indicated an equal distribution between unilateral and bilateral types, most authorities say that the unilateral type is slightly more common.

Etiology

Duraswaimi produced this deformity in chick embryos after treating the developing embryo by injecting insulin into its milieu in the egg. Beckham and associates produced stiff, deformed feet in chicks by paralyzing chick embryos for an 8-day period. It was hypothesized that the lack of normal tendon movement contributed to the stiff, deformed development of the foot. This work correlated nicely with the studies of Isaacs and associates, whose histologic, histochemical, and electron microscopic studies suggested a neuromuscular deficit as a strong possibility in the production of this deformity.

Bechtol and Mossman, in dissecting two fetal specimens, found evidence favoring abnormality of muscle growth resulting in failure of the muscles to keep pace with skeletal development. However, they believed that the relative shortening of the muscle fibers was due to degeneration. Flinchum, in study-

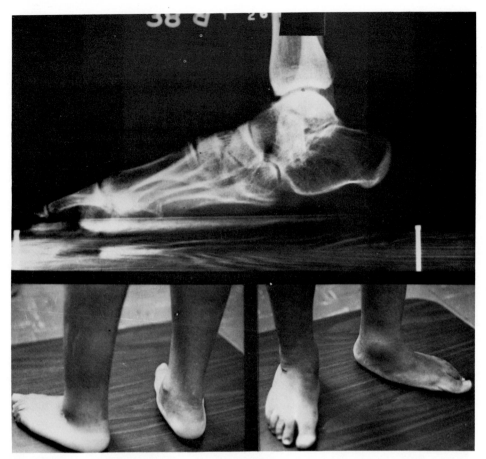

Figure 4.41. The standing lateral roentgenogram and photographs of a child with severe spastic cerebral palsy and calcaneoequinovalgus. This foot was treated 5 years earlier by a Grice, extra-articular, subtalar arthrodesis. The fitting of braces was made easier. Note the absence of degenerative talonavicular beaking.

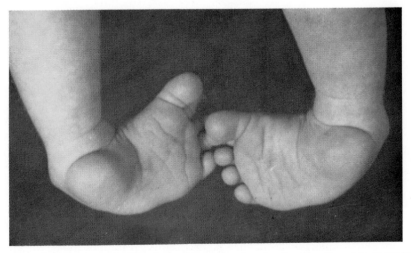

Figure 4.42. Clubfeet, posterior view. Revealing forefoot adduction, hindfoot inversion, and equinus.

ing a 6½-month, premature infant, found the peroneal muscles on the involved side to be about one-half the size of those on the normal side. This suggested an imbalance between medial and lateral musculature. Stewart, in his dissection of clubfeet, found abnormal insertions of the anterior tibial tendon apparently playing a part in producing adduction and supination of the forefoot. Other authors have emphasized abnormalities of the ligaments (Brockman) and of nerves (Moore), and the older German authors discussed bony anomaly. These studies would seem to at least narrow down the etiology to faulty and incomplete development involving the neuromuscular structures that control the position of the foot.

The production of a neuromuscular deficit is multifactorial, however, and this has led to a certain degree of confusion both in speculating upon the etiology and in evaluating treatment. Severe clubfeet are seen in asso-

ciation with arthrogryposis multiplex congenita, myelomeningocoel, cerebral palsy, familial traits, and as a spontaneous occurrence with no prior family history. Stewart notes a familial and racial predilection in his study of Hawaiian Island inhabitants. Then there are those so-called "positional clubfeet," which are easily treated and represent only a uterine packing phenomenon rather than a true clubfoot.

It is evident that at least some clubfeet have an intrinsic deformity of the astragalus. This has been shown by Sherman, among others, in postmortem dissection. The body of the astragalus is in its normal position in the ankle mortise. From this point, the head and neck of the astragalus are deviated medialward. Cartilage covers the head of the astragalus, but when the forefoot is brought into a corrected position, the navicular is actually further medial than this cartilage-covered area (Figs. 4.43 and 4.44). This bony deform-

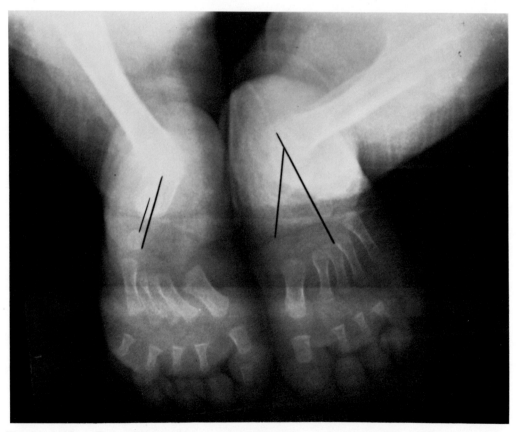

Figure 4.43. The anteroposterior roentgenogram of a normal foot (*left*) and clubfoot (*right*). The forefoot adduction and supination is obvious, and the "stacking" of the calcaneus beneath the talus (as compared to the normal divergence on the left) reveals the degree of hindfoot involvement.

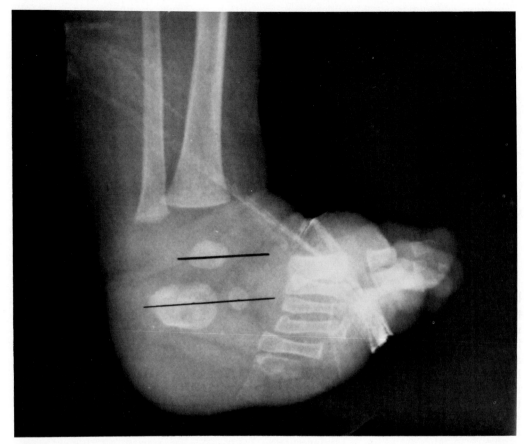

Figure 4.44. The lateral roentgenogram of a congenital clubfoot. The axes of the talus and calcaneus are parallel. In forced dorsiflexion they should be convergent and the hindfoot should follow the forefoot.

ity helps to account for the peculiar flat-topped outline of the astragalus in a lateral x-ray of the foot, because most of the astragalus is oblique rather than lateral to the x-ray when the film is taken. The external torsion of the lower limb may frequently be associated with clubfoot, still further accentuating this position by holding the body of the astragalus in the opposite direction to the deformed position of the head and neck.

Clinical Picture

The orthopaedist hopes to see a patient with a foot in equinovarus immediately after birth. The immediate problem is to differentiate the positional foot from the fixed "clubfoot." The clubfoot cannot be passively corrected. Stimulation of the peroneal muscles by stroking the lateral side of the foot reveals a deficiency in their action and an inability to evert the foot. Should the foot be mobile, the expectation is that it can be readily and easily corrected. True clubfoot deformities are fixed. The foot has fixed forefoot adduction, fixed inversion particularly noted in the hindfoot, and equinus of the hindfoot carrying the forefoot with it.

The calf size should be compared. Smallness of the involved calf may be noted at birth before treatment is begun. It tends particularly to be associated with the more rigid types of clubfoot, such as those seen in arthrogryposis.

The degree of internal or external torsion of the tibia should be noted. We have seen clubfeet in which there was a surprising degree of external rotation of the malleoli. This should be differentiated from the external rotational deformity or "horizontal breach talus" deformity that may occur from chronic, inappropriate casting techniques.

In other instances, we have noted a marked degree of bilateral internal torsion, even when only one foot had a clubfoot deformity. It is particularly helpful to note this before treatment, because an excellent foot correction may be achieved only to have distraught parents seek help elsewhere when their child's physiologic toe-in gait becomes manifest.

In these children, the hips must be carefully checked for associated dysplasia or frank dislocation. This is certainly associated with arthrogryposis, but it may occur in isolated instances where there is otherwise no evidence of arthrogryposis. The opposite foot may not have a true clubfoot, but rather a less severe deformity such as metatarsus adductus.

Treatment

Forcible methods of manipulation have been found in the past to be associated with the development of rigid, insufficiently corrected feet. Such manipulation was particularly done by means of the Thomas wrench—a tool found in the hospital instrument cupboard, but now seldom used. Kite has been responsible for an emphasis on gentle correction and an insistence on fully correcting one portion of the deformity before continuing treatment to other portions. If fundamental casting principles are followed, most clubfeet can be corrected into pliable, fully useful feet. Severe clubfeet with atrophied calves will prove very resistant and require other means.

Plaster casts in various forms, constructed either in sections or as a complete unit, are used by some orthopaedists. Some prefer Denis-Browne splints for continued control after casting. Whatever method is used, the results should be carefully assessed, both clinically and by roentgenogram, to ensure that full correction of all elements is obtained.

Serial Casting Technique

In Kite's method, the most important part of casting is the initial manipulation. This consists of traction on the forefoot followed by gentle lateral abduction (Fig. 4.45A). This traction distracts the medially displaced navicular, allowing it to swing laterally around the head of the talus. Attempts to correct forefoot adduction by merely forcibly ab-

ducting the foot or by wedging the cast should be condemned. This type of manipulation will result in impingement of the navicular on the talar head (Fig. 4.46) with the production of either navicular deformity or the external rotational deformity described by Miller.

The infant's foot may be painted with tincture of benzoin before applying cotton webril. This will diminish the likelihood that the cast will be kicked off by the child. We prefer to use 1/2-inch cotton webril, obtained by cutting a 1-inch roll in half with a cast knife or scalpel blade. Using this 1/2-inch roll will eliminate a great deal of overlapped, loose webril, which can create problems in such a small foot.

After application of the benzoin, gentle manipulation, and wrapping with webril, the initial half of the Kite slipper is applied, using 1-inch LPL-Gypsona. Several wraps around the distal forefoot are taken, followed by looping three gypsona folds back and forth underneath the midfoot and also looping three folds around the hindfoot (Fig. 4.45 B). These folds are wrapped in with the remaining gypsona, taking care not to impinge upon the anterior ankle. The hardening slipper may then be molded, correcting hindfoot varus, forefoot adduction, and molding in a small arch (Fig. 4.45 C). During this initial slipper molding, at no time is equinus corrected. The remaining portion of the cast is then applied (short leg or long leg). If adequate correction of hindfoot varus is being achieved, with each serial cast the ankle may be dorsiflexed by gentle pressure beneath the arch (Fig. 4.45 D). Attempts at dorsiflexion by elevating the forefoot should be discouraged, as this will tend to produce the so-called rocker-bottomed foot (Fig. 4.47 A and B).

If the foot can be corrected by serial casting, the usual time for correction started at birth is 6–8 weeks. The foot should be held in an overcorrected position for several weeks to ensure the maintenance of correction. The foot brought merely to neutral will revert to its former position. The corrected foot must have motions corresponding to those of the "normal" foot. The correction should be confirmed by x-ray. Both os calcis and astragalus should be out of equinus, and on forced dorsiflexion they should follow the foot. The long axis of the astragalus should run down the long axis of the first metatarsal. The supination of both hindfoot and forefoot should be fully corrected so that, on the anteroposterior x-ray, the shadows of the astragalus and os calcis do not overlie each other: the os calcis should have been brought out laterally from beneath the astragalus. A lateral of the foot should show an angle of at least 15 degrees convergence of the talus and calcaneus.

To assist in maintaining a satisfactory correction, the infant may be placed in a Denis-Browne bar for up to 3 months. This will help to avoid the supination-adduction forces that occur when the infant sleeps prone, on the stomach.

Denis-Browne Splints

This form of treatment is not commonly performed, nor is it as efficient as casts in the correction of equinus. Bell and Grice have described in detail the method of strapping the foot to the splint. Minute attention to method is necessary to avoid loosening of the foot from the plate and skin decubitii. Tincture of benzoin is applied to the foot.

The forefoot is first held to the plate by a circular strap. Bringing the plate to the foot is more effective than trying to hold the foot in a corrected position while applying adhesive.

Two straps then crisscross over the dorsum and attach to the rear flange of the plate to keep the foot from slipping forward, the dorsum being protected by a felt pad. One of these straps comes up under the cuboid area of the foot. The foot is held firmly against the plate as adhesive running down the back of the calf is split just above the heel, carried forward, and attached to the plate. Further straps are added to hold the hindfoot to the lateral flange. There should be no play between the plate and foot when the application is finished, and the color of the toes should be normal.

The other foot is also strapped. When the plate is attached to a connecting bar in varying degrees of external rotation, the forefoot adduction and the inversion are corrected. In later stages, the cross bar can be bent in a V to achieve still further correction.

The feet are suspended by a cord to the bar so that the baby can kick freely and procure dynamic correction. When the process is correctly done, a very pliable, well corrected foot can be obtained.

RESISTANT CLUBFEET

Clubfeet in arthrogryposis multiplex congenita, myelomeningocoel, and cerebral palsy will resist correction attempts by serial casting. In addition, there are those feet in otherwise normal infants that will also resist manipulation and serial casting. Operative treatment should never be attempted until an adequate trial of casting has been tried and the foot is large enough so that technically precise surgery can be performed without difficulty.

What constitutes an adequate trial of serial casting is a point of debate, still to be resolved. In the American Academy of Orthopaedic Surgeons' Instructional Lectures, Kite stated that there was not an infant's foot that could not be corrected by serial casting. Wood Lovell conceded that some feet would require surgery, but approximately 2 years of serial casting should be attempted. Turco believed that if serial casting by an experienced orthopaedist over 3 months had not yielded correction, operative release was indicated. However, he believed technically precise surgery could not be done until at least 1 year of age. After 3 months' casting, therefore, the infant's feet were held in a Denis-Browne bar until surgery at 1 year of age.

Bleck reported upon the operative treatment of 33 resistant clubfeet in which it was clearly indicated from an early point in treatment that correction was not progressing. In these feet, the common finding was that of a hypoplastic, medially deviated talar neck. It was apparent that the earlier the patient received surgery, the less stiffness and the better the correction. Late surgical treatment after prolonged casting resulted in permanent bony deformity, occasionally requiring a lateral approach in the method of Dilwyn Evans.

If it is true that a significant percentage of resistant congenital clubfeet have evidence of neuromuscular abnormalities and talar structural deformity, it would seem to make sense that early correction would be beneficial both from the standpoint of corrective remodeling and in reducing unnecessary immobilization.

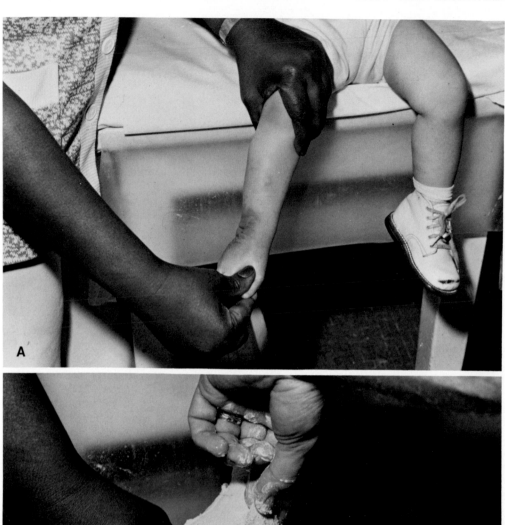

Figure 4.45. (*A*) To begin serial casting, the infant's anterior tibia is grasped for countertraction, while the forefoot is distracted and then brought into abduction. Note the redundant skin folds laterally, characteristic of the clubfoot. (*B*) After applying tincture of benzoin and 1/2-inch webril, the "slipper" is applied. Three folds of plaster around the forefoot and hindfoot serve to "cradle" the corrected forefoot. These folds are then "tied in" with the remaining plaster, taking care to avoid the anterior ankle. (*C*) The

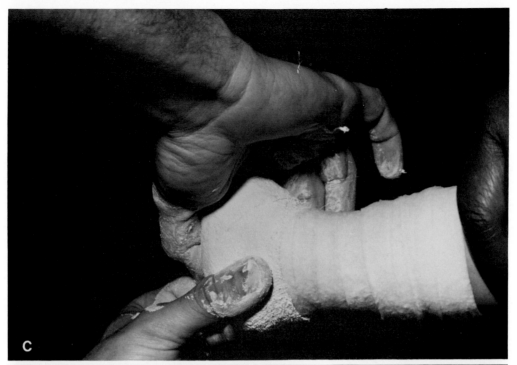

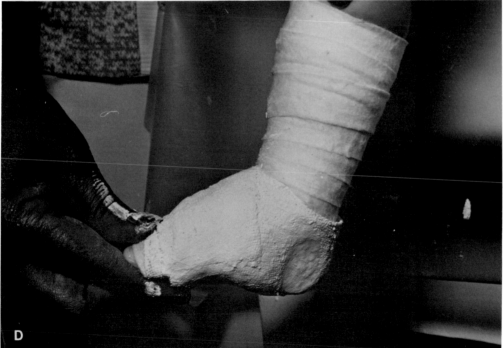

Fig. 4.45 (C and D)

forefoot and hindfoot may be manipulated simultaneously. For the patient's right foot, the surgeon's left thumb corrects hindfoot varus while the left index finger serves as a lateral "post" to push against. The surgeon's right thumb and web space assist in molding an arch as well as correcting forefoot adduction. The right index finger assists the left in providing the lateral "post." (*D*) The "slipper" has now been completed. If the hindfoot has been resistant to correction of varus deformity, the forefoot is left in equinus. If the correction of hindfoot varus is complete, the equinus may be serially corrected both by pulling down on the hindfoot and pushing up at the level of the arch. The remainder of the cast is applied (long leg cast if the infant is small, short leg cast for a larger child).

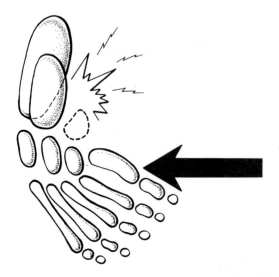

Figure 4.46. A diagrammatic representation of the effect of wedging a cast in the attempts at serial correction. If traction is not applied when correcting forefoot adduction, the unossified, medially subluxed navicular will abut against the talus. Either permanent talonavicular deformity will be created or the hindfoot as well will be levered against the fibula, creating external rotation deformity at the ankle.

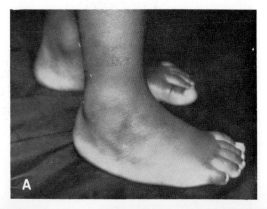

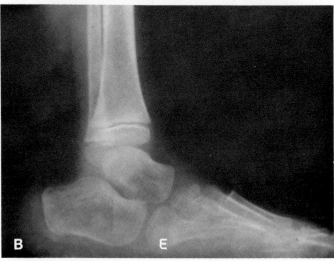

Figure 4.47. (*A*) The "rocker-bottom" foot will be produced if the forefoot is brought out of equinus before the hindfoot varus is corrected. The clinical appearance is that of reversal of the lateral arch and cuboid prominence. (*B*) Uncorrected equinus with break at midfoot and relative dorsiflexion of the forefoot in "rocker-bottom" foot.

For this reason, we attempt careful serial casting in all clubfeet for a period of 12 weeks. If there is marked resistance to correction or if, despite apparent correction, it is obvious roentgenographically that hindfoot correction has not been achieved, then surgery is contemplated.

It is our belief that the child's foot should be corrected by the time the child is ready to walk. We can see no advantage to obstinate, prolonged casting, which will only produce a stiff foot and delay the child's advancement through the normal development of motor milestones. Thus, after 12 weeks of careful serial casting, if there is evidence of failure, the infant is maintained in a Denis-Browne bar to hold what correction has been achieved. The bar is utilized for a 3-month period while the child is continuing to grow. The parents are advised regarding the ipsilateral atrophied calf, the smaller foot, the resistance to correction, and the likelihood that, even after excellent correction has been achieved, the child's foot and calf will remain smaller and not be as effective as the normal side. At 6 months of age a tourniquet will easily fit on an infant's leg and, in our opinion, surgery can be precisely performed without fear of inadequate release or overcorrection.

Surgical Anatomy of Clubfoot

Turco described the talocalcaneonavicular joint well as a ball-and-socket joint separate from the posterior subtalar joint. The socket is formed by the navicular anteriorly, dorsomedially by the talonavicular joint capsule, deltoid ligament, and posterior tibial tendon. The lateral support is the bifurcated (Y) ligament, and inferiorly the head of the talus is supported by the middle and anterior subtalar articular surfaces of the calcaneus and spring ligament. The surgical correction must be concentrated here and at the hindfoot. The cup formed by these structures moves around the ball (head of the talus) and expands and contracts through the fibroelastic ligaments. The clubfoot has been described as a subluxation of the talocalcaneonavicular joint.

When the talus is in fixed equinus, the posterior tuberosity of the os calcis is displaced laterally and superiorly in relation to it. The structures now fixing the position are the posterior talocalcaneal capsule, heel cord,

and the calcaneofibular ligament. Anteriorly the deltoid and spring ligaments, the posterior tibial tendon, and the subtalar interosseous ligament resist correction.

In resistant clubfeet, the stressed dorsiflexed lateral x-ray reveals a failure of the calcaneus to dorsiflex. If full dorsiflexion of the os calcis can be achieved at operation and held for at least 4 months, Turco has noted an absence of recurrent deformity.

Posteromedial Release

In the medial release procedure described by Turco, sharp dissection is used through a long medial incision beginning at the base of the first metatarsal and running posteriorly to the tendo achillis (Fig. 4.48 A).

The posterior tibial tendon is identified, and both its sheath and that of the flexor digitorum longus tendon are divided around and above the medial malleolus. The neurovascular bundle is mobilized and retracted gently with an umbilical tape. When retracted, the flexor hallucis longus tendon is freed from its sheath (Fig. 4.48 B).

The master knot of Henry is a fibrocartilaginous structure attached to the undersurface of the navicular and enveloping the flexor digitorum longus and flexor hallucis longus tendons as they cross over one another. This structure is excised (Fig. 4.48 C).

Once these structures have been mobilized, a posterior, medial, and subtalar release is made. The tendo achillis is lengthened by a Z-plasty, detaching the medial half from the os calcis (Fig. 4.48 D).

Anterior retraction of the neurovascular bundle and flexor hallucis longus tendon brings the posterior aspect of the ankle into view. A posterior capsulotomy of the ankle joint is then done. The posterior capsule of the posterior component of the subtalar joint is divided along with the calcaneofibular ligament. This is seen deep in the wound and is important to reach. Retracting the neurovascular bundle posteriorly, the posterior insertion of the superficial deltoid ligament of the calcaneus is divided (Fig. 4.48 E).

Medially, the posterior tibial tendon is cut approximately 1 cm above the medial malleolus and allowed to retract (Fig. 4.48 F). The distal portion is followed down to its insertion at the talonavicular joint. The deltoid ligament on navicular and talonavicular cap-

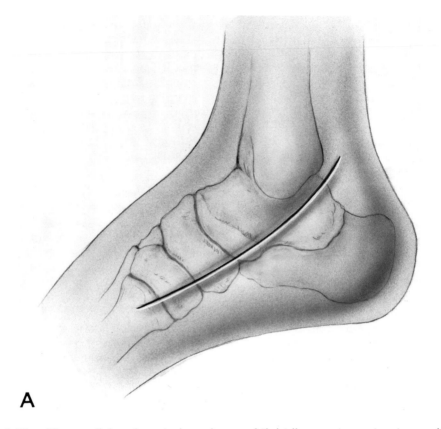

A

Figure 4.48. The medial and posterior release of tight ligamentous structures should not be postponed when the foot is evidently resistant to cast treatment. If this is done, immobilization atrophy becomes excessive, the cartilage of the small bones of the foot is deformed, and motion of the joint becomes limited. (These drawings have had a liberal inspiration from both Turco and Bost in their articles on medial release, but have been modified according to our concepts as well.) (*A*) The incision extends posteriorly beyond the peroneal tendons and forward sufficiently to visualize the naviculocuneiform joint. (*B*) The neurovascular bundle can be isolated and drawn to either side to avoid damage to it during the course of the procedure. (*C*) The posterior tibial tendon and the flexor digitorum longus are identified, and the sheaths of both divided are posteriorly around the medial malleolus. The "master knot of Henry" is a fibrocartilaginous structure attached to the undersurface of the navicular and enclosing the flexor hallucis longus and flexor digitorum longus as they cross over one another. This structure is excised. (*D*) The Achilles tendon is lengthened by a Z-plasty. The neurovascular bundle and flexor hallucis longus are retracted anteriorly to bring the posterior ankle and subtalar joint into view. (*E*) Once visualized, the capsulotomy of the talotibial and subtalar joint is performed. The calcaneofibular ligament can be divided deep in the wound, as well as the talofibular ligament. (*F*) The posterior tibial tendon is cut just above the medial malleolus and allowed to retract. (*G*) The ligaments medially are then divided including those shown plus the spring ligament and the attachment of the posterior tibial tendon inferior to the navicular after it is no longer needed to pull the point toward the surgeon. When the heel is everted, the deltoid ligament can be cut to completely release the os calcis anteriorly and posteriorly. (*H*) When the heel deformity is completely corrected, the navicular is then correctly reduced onto the head of the talus and held with a Kirschner wire. This can project through the cast and be removed 3 weeks postoperatively.

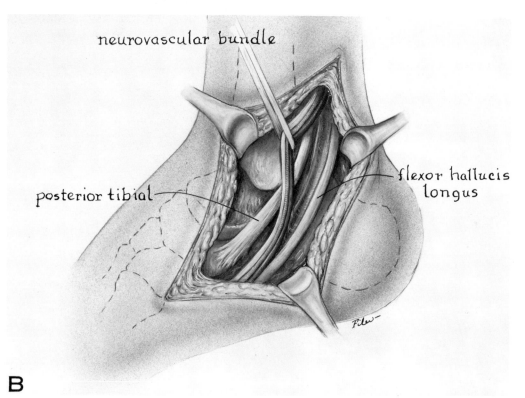

neurovascular bundle

posterior tibial

flexor hallucis longus

B

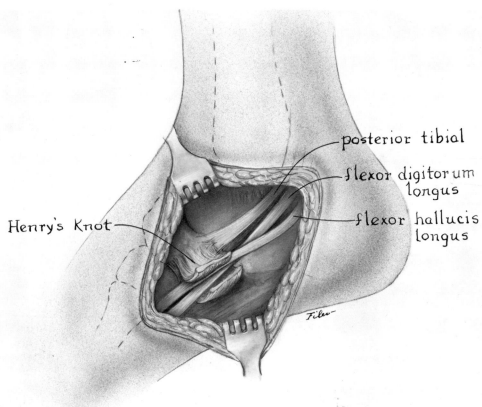

posterior tibial

flexor digitorum longus

flexor hallucis longus

Henry's Knot

C

Fig. 4.48 (*B* and *C*)

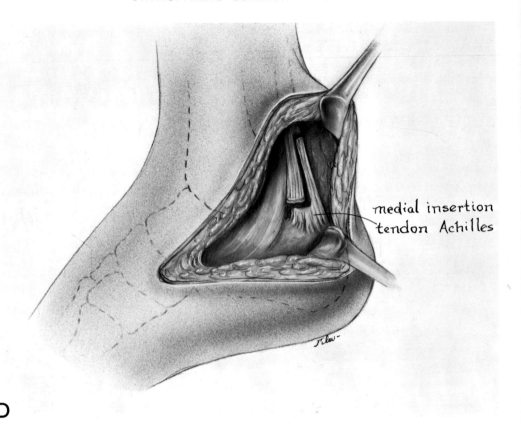

D

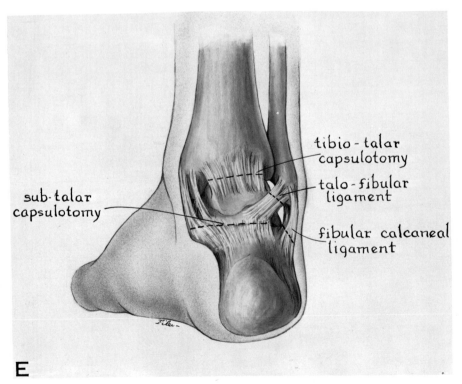

E

Fig. 4.48 (*D* and *E*)

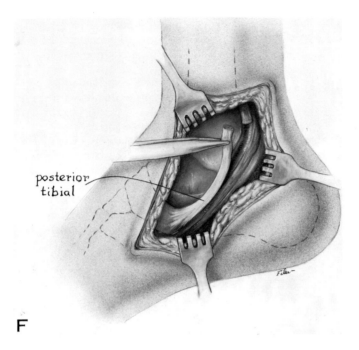

F

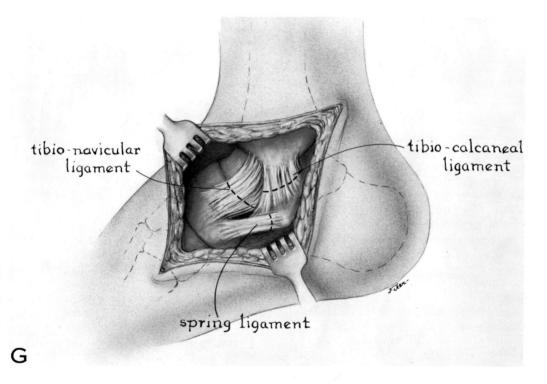

G

Fig. 4.48 (*F* and *G*)

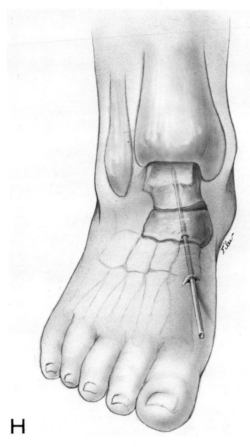

H

Fig. 4.48 (H)

A Kirschner wire inserted on the dorsum of the foot transfixes the talonavicular joint once it is correctly reduced—avoiding over-correction (Fig. 4.48 *H*). The foot is dorsiflexed to a right angle, and the tendo achillis is approximated with sutures. The Kirschner wire is left in place for 6 weeks.

Turco recommends cast changes at 3 and 6 weeks and, after 4 months of immobilization, a Denis-Browne bar with everted feet for sleeping for 1 year. The child should remain in high-top straight-last shoes with a medial arch for at least 1 year of ambulation.

A wire through the superior posterior portion of the calcaneus may be used to control the position of the calcaneus as the plaster is applied; it is incorporated in the plaster. The wire is removed at 3 weeks, the plaster at 6 weeks.

Follow-up Therapy

Feet that are fully corrected can be held in bivalved casts or forefoot abduction shoes attached to a Denis-Browne bar. The mother performs eversion and dorsiflexion exercises at each diaper change. She should be carefully instructed not to dorsiflex the forefoot, but to let it be carried by the dorsiflexion of the hindfoot. The forefoot is stretched into abduction daily, however.

The patient is seen regularly by the orthopaedist during the first 2 or 3 years. If the foot begins to lose mobility, it is promptly placed in long leg plaster casts and wedged out into full correction. Short let casts cannot fully control the forefoot adduction or the equinus.

SEVERE OR RECURRENT CLUBFEET

In the arthrogrypotic or spastic cerebral palsy patient, the clubfoot deformity is more severe. Due to neuromuscular deficit or imbalance, recurrence is likely. Experience has shown that in the arthrogrypotic patient, an astragalectomy (talectomy) done at an early age will have the best change of yielding a peranent correction. Furthermore, if done at an earlier age (under 12 months), there may be adaptive remodeling between the mortise and calcaneus, such that a corrected, pain-free, stable foot results (Fig. 4.49).

sule is then incised. The posterior tibial tendon attachments to the sustentaculum tali and spring ligament are cut, and the spring ligament is detached from the sustentaculum tali (Fig. 4.48 *G*).

When the foot is then everted, the subtalar joint is exposed, permitting release of the superficial layer of the deltoid ligament. The deep portion inserting into the body of the talus is preserved.

Further subtalar release involves the bifurcated (Y) ligament extending from the calcaneus to the lateral border of the navicular and medial border of the cuboid. Turco advocates releasing the talocalcaneal interosseus ligament, but we feel that this is wrong. If done, a complete subtalar dislocation may occur as a late sequela.

The navicular is then correctly reduced onto the head of the talus. The os calcis must have been released both anteriorly and posteriorly to correct the heel deformity completely.

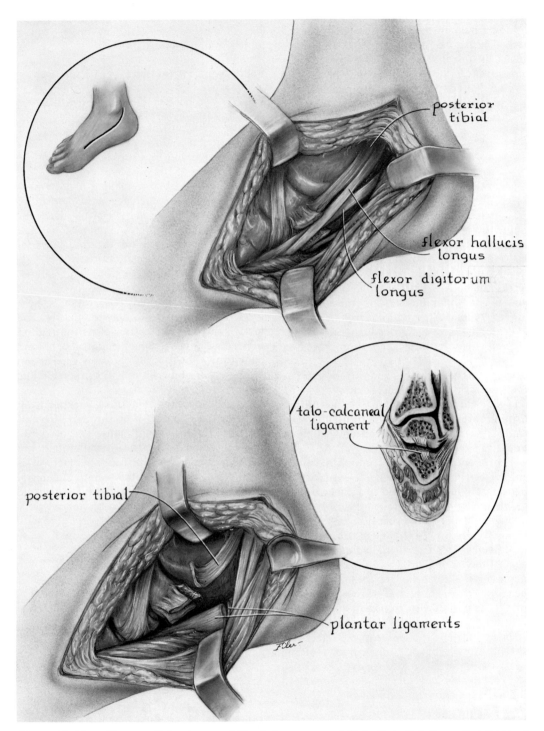

Figure 4.49. The medial release of Bost, Larsen, and Schottstadt follows the lines of the old Ober ligamentous procedure and is the basis of the still more complete procedures as described by Turco.

In myelomeningocoel or severe spastic cerebral palsy, the clubfoot is also quite resistant to permanent correction. Repetitive serial casting with good intermittent correction, followed by relapse, is not uncommon. Failed repetitive casting followed by a well performed Turco procedure with subsequent failure may mean that either tendon transfers or an astragalectomy is indicated.

Astragalectomy

Menelaus suggested that astragalectomy overcomes some of the inadequacies of soft-tissue release in severe, fixed deformity. This is due to the resection of the "spacer" across which the contracted soft tissues and abnormal muscles act. Astragalectomy creates relatively lax soft tissues to allow adequate correction of both equinus and varus deformities. It is an operation that is not necessary for congenital talipes equinovarus.

Whitman used this procedure for a variety of paralytic deformities, reporting on it first in 1901.

Menelaus used as his indications for talectomy (1) badly deformed equinovarus feet, (2) very rigid feet, and (3) multiple disabilities making prolonged standing unlikely. The usual age at operation is 3 years and is limited to the age group of 1–5 years.

The operation is done through a curved anterolateral incision. The ankle subtalar and midtarsal joints are opened and the ligaments divided. The talus is grasped with a towel clip and rotated as the soft tissue is stripped from it (Fig. 4.50). The heel cord may be lengthened. The lateral malleolus may abut against the lateral surface of the os calcis—if necessary the tip of the lateral malleolus may be removed. The os calcis is thrust posteriorly in the ankle mortise to maintain the heel contour.

The low lateral malleolus may project sufficiently to warrant trimming, thus avoiding pressure in the shoe. After operation, a plaster cast is applied for 6 weeks—ankle in neutral, heel corrected into valgus.

Recurring Clubfeet below Age 5

Wedging casts are resorted to in this period to restore full correction. These feet presumably once were fully correctable and readily tend to wedge out. The forefoot adduction is wedged across the midtarsal area. Equinus is corrected by wedges at the level of the ankle joint and not below it.

ANTERIOR TIBIAL TRANSPLANT

Recurrence of deformity in apparently well corrected feet may be due to peroneal weakness or imbalance between the anterior and posterior tibia and the peroneals (Fig. 4.51).

As emphasized by Garceau and Manning, if supination occurs on active dorsiflexion, a lateral anterior tibial transplant may be necessary to prevent recurrence of the deformity. The usual age period when the need for transplantation becomes apparent is 4–6 years. The foot should be corrected by serial casts prior to transplantation.

The anterior tibial tendon, when transplanted to the lateral side of the foot (base of the fifth metatarsal), has been found to be a weak dorsiflexor and to function poorly. The usual procedure is to transplant the tendon to the base of the second metatarsal or second cuneiform. This position preserves the action of the anterior tibial as a dorsiflexor while weakening it as a supinator.

The anterior tibial tendon is detached from its insertion and drawn up through a second incision into the calf. It is then rerouted into the common extensor sheath and brought out on the dorsum of the forefoot. Here it is attached to the base of the second metatarsal through a drill hole or trap door. It is sutured firmly onto the dorsal periosteum after pulling the tendon tip through the drill hole with a Keith needle attached to the suture holding the tip.

POSTERIOR TIBIAL TRANSPLANT

Owing to results with the anterior tibial transplant that did not completely satisfy our service, we have turned to the posterior tibial transplant, which has given improved performance as to both correction and function.

In many resistant clubfeet, the posterior tibial tendon appears taut and when released allows correction that had not been possible previously. While operating through the medial incision, the surgeon can also perform a capsulotomy at the navicular talar joint and release the medial structures that hold the hindfoot in inversion. A second incision is made on the medial aspect of the calf running

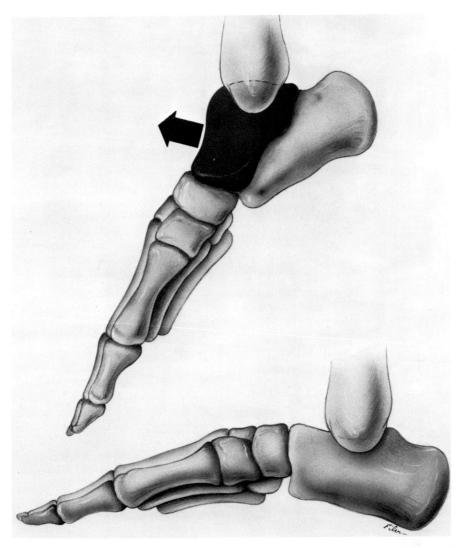

Figure 4.50. Diagrammatic representation of the talectomy with positioning of the os calcis in the ankle mortise.

proximal from just above the medial malleolus. The posterior tibial tendon can be found just beneath the great toe flexor. The neurovascular bundle is carefully avoided. A linear incision into the interosseous membrane is made from a point at which tibia and fibula come so close together that anything further in that direction is impractical for about 2 inches. The tendon is then passed through this opening into the anterior compartment and distal to an incision made over the base of the second cuneiform. The tendon is not long, but usually just reaches the metatarsal if it has been thoroughly mobilized before

detachment. Occasionally it is necessary to attach it proximally to this position. The tendon, once attached at its resting length, holds the foot in good position. A long leg cast is applied for 6 weeks.

Rocker-bottom Foot

Rocker-bottom foot is a product of inappropriate casting. The foot has, for practical purposes, been overstretched in the midtarsal region. This results in a prominent cuboid area that becomes the point of weight bear-

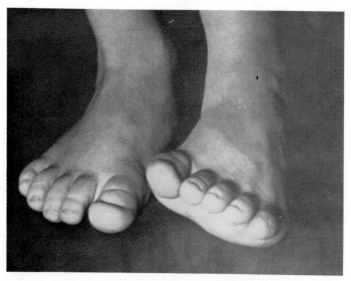

Figure 4.51.   Recurring clubfoot with dorsiflexion in inversion. This foot has unbalanced muscle power controlling it, and recurrence can be expected with growth. Either brace control of operative restoration of muscle balance is necessary.

ing, with resultant callus and disability. There are at least four ways this foot can be produced: (1) pushing the forefoot up out of equinus before the hindfoot equinus is corrected; (2) slipping of the foot up into the cast so that the forefoot must be pushed up; (3) walking on a foot with uncorrected equinus; (4) dorsiflexing the forefoot in exercises.

This tendency in the foot is very difficult to correct, and the foot must be recasted for a considerable period. The forefoot is pushed back down into equinus until it is lined up with the hindfoot in the cast. The foot is then brought up as a unit until it is corrected.

When the foot cannot be corrected because of persistent equinus of the hindfoot, a heel cord lengthening and ankle capsulotomy posteriorly may be necessary. It is usual also to insert a wire into the posteriosuperior angle of the os calcis to control its position. The wire is incorporated into the cast (see congenital vertical talus).

At 6 weeks the cast is removed, but still further holding in plaster may be necessary for perhaps 2 or 3 months, with cast changes at approximately 3-week intervals.

Uncorrected Clubfeet after Age 5

It is apparent by the age of 5 that considerable fixed bony deformity can be present in the uncorrected or severe, relapsed clubfoot. Recurrence may occur despite aggressive repetitive casting, an adequate Turco procedure, and/or tendon transfers (Figs. 4.52 and 4.53). Furthermore, children with recurrence may occasionally be referred for treatment; and, although it is difficult to determine the nature of the initial casting or surgery, nevertheless fixed bony deformity is now present.

In these individuals, the principles of Dilwyn Evans are most helpful. Evans advanced the concept of visualizing the foot as medial and lateral columns. In the congenital clubfoot, the medial column is too short due to the hypoplastic, medially deviated talar neck. Shortening the lateral column thus balances the foot. This lateral column shortening could be performed either by enucleating the cuboid or performing a shortening calcaneocuboid fusion (Fig. 4.54). This laterally based wedge osteotomy may also be oriented slightly anteriorly or plantarly, depending upon whether supination or pronation of the forefoot would require correction as well. In the relapsed clubfoot, forefoot supination is generally present, and the wedge must be anterolaterally based.

In combination with this, it is sometimes necessary to perform a plantar and medial soft-tissue release. The plantar ligament, if tight, may be released subcutaneously by

either a small meniscotome or with a #15
scalpel blade. Care should be taken to stay
plantarly and on the anterior border of the
calcaneus to avoid neurovascular structures.
The talonavicular, naviculocuneiform, and
cuneiform-first metatarsal joints may also require release so that the midfoot may swing
around as the lateral wedge is closed.

TRIPLE ARTHRODESIS

When the child is past the age of 12, a
triple arthrodesis may be considered as a
means to provide permanent bony correction.
If done unilaterally before the age of 12,
continued growth of the contralateral foot
will result in a significant discrepancy in shoe

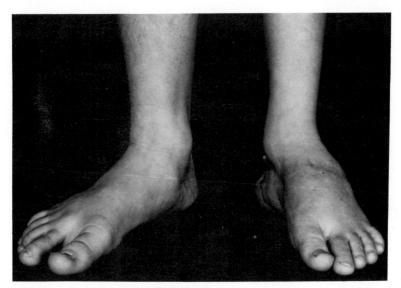

Figure 4.52. This child is 6 years of age and has had two Turco procedures and two
Heyman-Herndon procedures. These procedures were technically well done. The severe
atrophy of the left calf is a clue as to why there is marked recurrence.

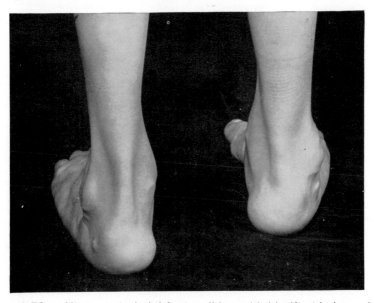

Figure 4.53. Uncorrected clubfoot walking with hindfoot in inversion.

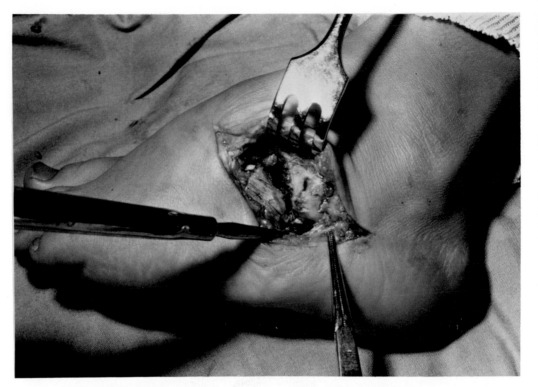

Figure 4.54. The Dilwyn-Evans procedure consists either of cuboid enucleation or a wedge arthrodesis across the calcaneocuboid joint.

size. The Hoke arthrodesis has been shown to be quite adequate in obtaining permanent correction. Appropriate wedges should be removed to correct hindfoot varus, equinus, and forefoot adduction. Further principles in the performance of a triple arthrodesis are illustrated in the section on Charcot-Marie-Tooth disease.

Overcorrected Clubfoot

One of the risks in extensive clubfoot surgery is that the release is more than necessary, producing a marked pes valgus. Overcorrection of the navicular on the talus will produce forefoot pronation. Excessive subtalar release will produce subtalar dislocation with severe hindfoot valgus (Fig. 4.55). Harris views and standing lateral roentgenograms will determine whether the child's excessive pes valgus is due to midfoot or hindfoot overcorrection (Fig. 4.56).

The treatment here may be difficult at best (Figs. 4.57–4.59). High-top, straight-last shoes with a medial arch or navicular-cookie will

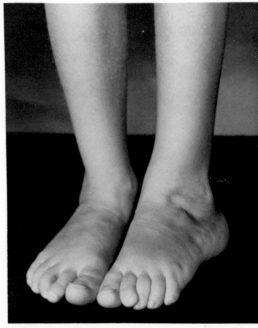

Figure 4.55. Severe, disabling hindfoot valgus after a Turco procedure, performed to the letter of the original description.

be adequate treatment if the deformity is in the midfoot. Hindfoot valgus is a more difficult problem to manage. If Harris views clearly define that there is subtalar dislocation, the correction must be achieved through bony surgery. Previous attempts by this author to reconstruct the interosseous ligament, holding the correction with a Steinman pin, were unsatisfactory. Therefore, it was necessary to perform the Chambers procedure, levering the calcaneus under the talus. In our hands, this has resulted in permanent correction. Should relapse occur, however, an extraarticular subtalar arthrodesis in the manner of Grice would be necessary.

METATARSUS VARUS

In pediatric orthopaedic practice, two variations of a common deformity, metatarsus varus (also called "metatarsus adductus") are seen. In the first, there seems to be purely forefoot adduction, with the arch and hindfoot appearing normal. In the second form of this deformity, the foot has the appearance of a serpentine or "Z-like" deformity with adducted forefoot, flattened longitudinal arch, and valgus hindfoot.

The first form of metatarsus varus has also been termed a "third of a clubfoot," emphasizing that the deformity lies only in the adducted forefoot. These feet are easily corrected by serial casting, and the etiology of this type of forefoot adduction is probably associated with the "uterine packing" phenomenon (Figs. 4.60–4.62).

The second form of this deformity is more complex, and its etioligy is less well understood. There seems to be no sex-related variation. The condition may be unilateral but is often bilateral. There is often a tendency to turn the unaffected foot out. In anatomic

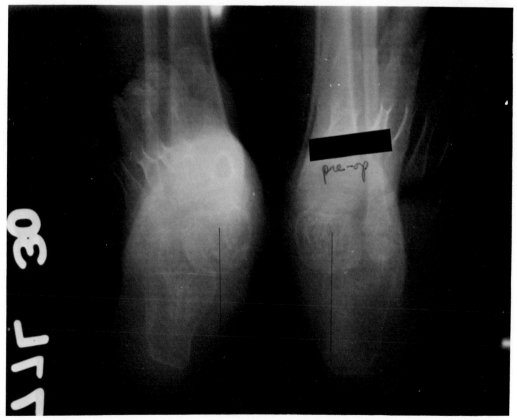

Figure 4.56.   The Harris views of the patient from Figure 4.55 illustrating the subtalar dislocation caused by sectioning the talocalcaneal interosseus ligament.

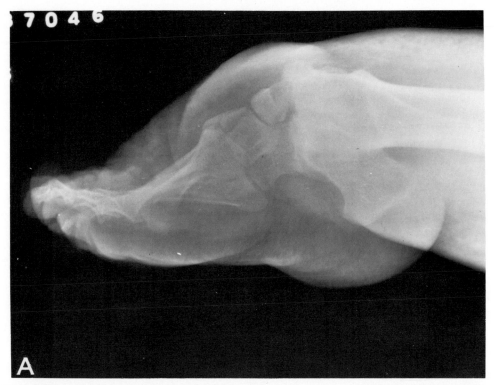

Figure 4.57. (*A–C*) Untreated equinovarus foot in 30-year-old woman. Fixed equinus and inversion are shown with secondary holding of the bone shapes. The persistent external torsion of the fibula and tibial relationships is clearly evident in the anteroposteior view of the ankle.

studies, it seems as though a muscle imbalance may be primary in producing this second Z-foot deformity. An anomalous insertion of the tibialis posterior onto the medial aspect of the navicular has been well documented by Browne and Paton. The anomalous insertion causes the tendon to act as an adductor, not a plantar-flexor-supinator. Hence, the production of forefoot varus, loss of the arch, and secondary hindfoot valgus.

Clinical Picture

The deformity is present at birth. An important clinical distinction between the two variations of it should be made. Sometimes the forefoot can readily be pulled into a normal alignment with the hindfoot by passive motion. In a few such instances, the everting muscles of the baby's foot can be stimulated to active contraction, and the foot is thus partially corrected. The baby's foot tends to follow, rather than to pull away from the stimulating finger that strokes it. The second and less common variety cannot be passively corrected and constitutes a true deformity. It is important to make this distinction as a basis for treatment.

There is usually an accompanying internal torsion of the tibia that accentuates the "turned-in" appearance of the foot. The patients often make their first appearance for treatment at the age of 2 or 3 months. At that time the foot has become troublesome because it has failed to improve, owing either to the patient's sleeping on the abdomen with feet turned in (in the case of a mobile foot) or to the foot's being of a fixed variety.

Treatment

MOBILE FOOT

Because it is not desirable to change the baby's sleeping habits, the simplest method of getting the foot in good position

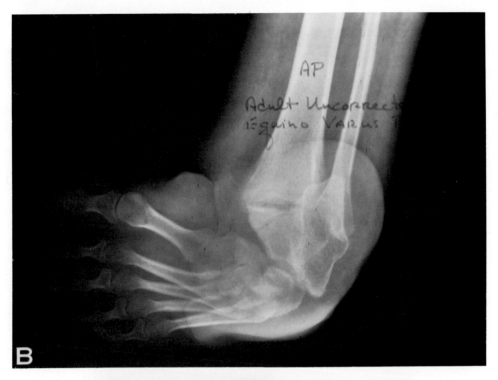

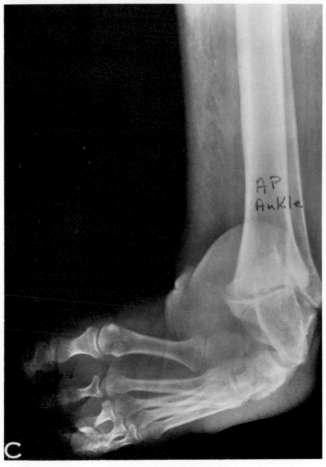

Fig. 4.57 (*B*** and ***C***)**

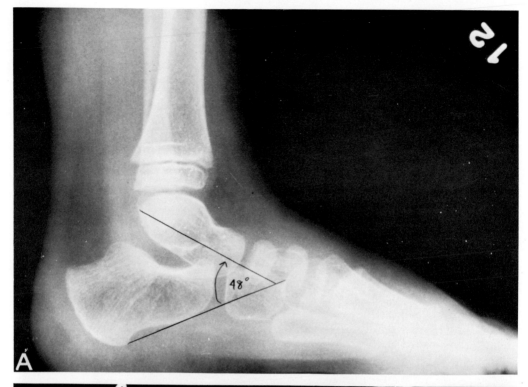

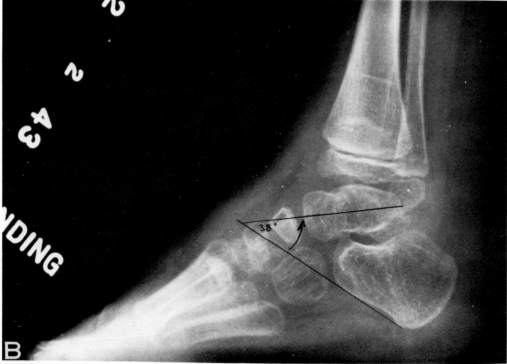

Figure 4.58. Comparison of the normal foot with treated clubfoot of the same patient (girl, age 5). (*A*) Lateral normal foot. (*B*) The external torsion normally present in clubfoot deformity is accentuated by the obliquity of the hindfoot to the x-ray. This also results in

during sleep is to use reversed shoes on a Denis-Browne bar. The shoes are placed on the bar in about 45 degrees of external rotation. While the baby is awake, reversed shoes or forefoot abduction shoes without the bar are used to avoid a tendency to develop genu valgus.

In addition, at each diaper change, the mother holds the hindfoot and carries the forefoot into abduction with the other hand. She thus lines the foot up in normal position and stretches the structures of the medial side of the foot. The usual time needed to procure

correction is 4–6 months. When walking starts, straight-last shoes are used, as there is a tendency to recurrence.

There will occasionally present an infant with initial forefoot adduction that does not correct easily. After several weeks of passive stretching have been unproductive, serial casting should be started. As there is no mid- or hindfoot deformity associated with this first deformity, forefoot adduction alone is addressed. The cast may either be changed weekly or applied one week and wedged the next (Fig. 4.63). Overcorrection well past neu-

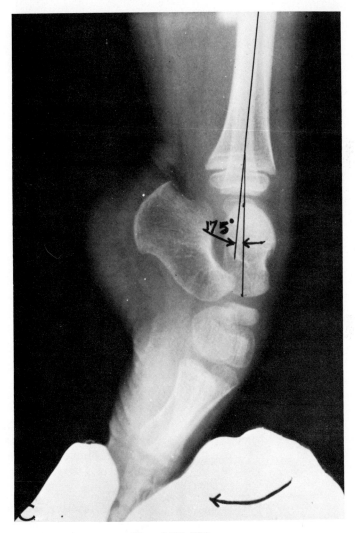

Fig. 4.58 (C)

a flat-topped appearance of the astragalus. The os calcis is in calcaneus, the forefoot in relative equinus, the navicular deformed. The x-ray is a true lateral of the forefoot. This is maximum dorsiflexion for this foot. (C) The normal foot is supple when plantar flexed,

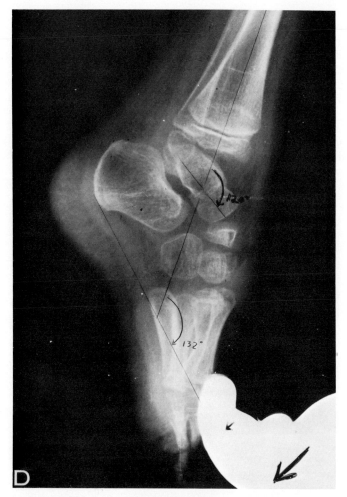

Fig. 4.58 (D)

and motion takes place equally in the forefoot and ankle joint. (D) The old equinovarus foot has limited eccentric motion at the ankle joint as the astragalus hinges out of it in plantar flexion. The forefoot achieves most of the plantar flexion.

tral should be achieved (20–30 degrees), and the Denis-Browne bar with reversed-last shoes and intermittent passive stretching by the mother should be a part of the postcasting treatment (Fig. 4.64).

FIXED FOOT

Despite the "Z-deformity," these feet will also respond well to serial casting followed by the Denis-Browne bar and passive stretching exercises. The cast may be applied as a single unit, using tincture of benzoin as an assist in preventing the cast from being kicked off by the infant. If necessary, a long

leg cast with the knee bent may be applied. The forefoot adduction is gently corrected, but at the same time the hindfoot is manipulated into varus. As in the flexible foot, casting is continued until overcorrection is achieved (Fig. 4.63).

Operative Treatment

In the serpentine or Z-foot deformity, there is frequently a marked tendency to recur. This is particularly noted when the child stands, and it indicates that prolonged follow-up is necessary. If there is recurrence more

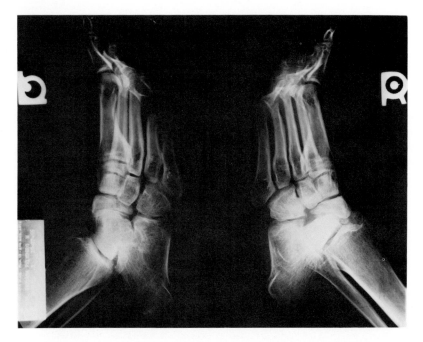

Figure 4.59. Aseptic necrosis of the body of the astragalus resulting from resection of the anterior portion for equinovarus foot deformity. An osteotomy of the astragalus corrects the deformity but cannot be done without the risk of necrosis.

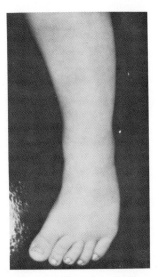

Figure 4.60. Positional metatarsus varus correctable by passive manipulation.

than twice after successful overcorrection with serial casting, it is apparent that the deformity is resistant and that further recasting will probably be fruitless. Furthermore, this recurrence would imply that there is an anomalous posterior tibialis insertion; there-fore, this must be addressed. Operative reduction is indicated.

The Heyman-Herndon procedure has been shown to provide satisfactory reduction. Our only modification of this procedure is to inspect the posterior tibialis insertion and to transfer it plantarly, if indicated. We prefer to perform the metatarsal-cuneiform release through three longitudinal incisions (Fig. 4.65). The medial first incision should be centered anteromedially over the first metatarsocuneiform joint and extend long enough to allow mobilization of the tissues. This is to allow for inspection of the posterior tibialis tendon as well as release of the capsule of the first and second metatarsocuneiform joints. The second incision is centered between the second and third metatarsocuneiform joints, and the last incision is between the fourth and fifth. Dissection should be subperiosteal, elevating and protecting the dorsal neurovascular structures with either a joker or small periosteal elevator. The dorsal capsule and intermetatarsal ligament at each joint should be released sharply in one cut with a #15 scalpel. Repetitive, inadequate cutting will damage the articular surfaces and result ultimately in producing a stiff foot. The plantar capsule should be released by blunt pressure

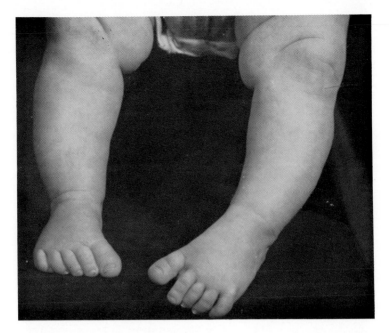

Figure 4.61. The patient's right forefoot deviates medially, forming a metatarsus varus. The left foot is carried medialward by internal torsion of the tibia, while the knee points forward.

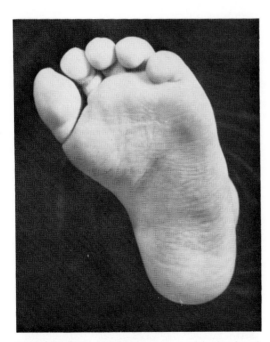

Figure 4.62. Forefoot varus with the heel in neutral position in metatarsus varus. This can be demonstrated as positional by applying passive correction and achieving a normal relation between forefoot and hindfoot.

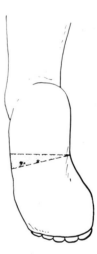

Figure 4.63. Correcting forefoot adduction by wedging cast.

with a small periosteal elevator. Plantar release with a scalpel should be avoided in order to protect the hidden plantar neurovascular structures. Care should be taken to ensure that the correct interval at the metatarsal cuneiform joints is being released. It is quite easy to lose orientation and erroneously perform a cuneiform-tarsal release in such a small foot.

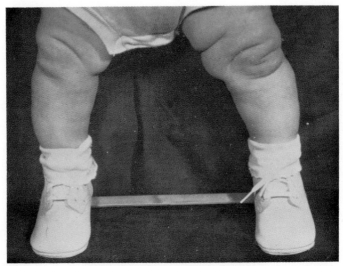

Figure 4.64. A bar holding the feet forward tends to correct internal torsion of the tibia and holds a corrected metatarsus varus in straight alignment.

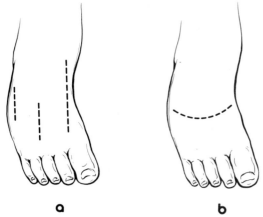

a b

Figure 4.65. Two approaches for the operative corrections of metatarsus adductus consist of either three longitudinal incisions (a) or a long transverse approach (b). The transverse incision compromises venous drainage and risks skin slough and/or damage to neurovascular structures.

Once the midfoot release is complete, the forefoot is held in overcorrection and a smooth K-wire driven up the first metatarsal and through the first cuneiform, navicular, and talus. At the time the wire is driven up, in addition to the forefoot correction, an assistant should attempt to put pressure on the talonavicular joint in an effort to create an arch. If necessary, the posterior tibialis position may be corrected either before or after the correction with the K-wire.

This procedure is also reported using a long transverse incision across the foot (Fig. 4.65). In the author's opinion, this approach should be discouraged. The transverse incision compromises venous drainage and predisposes either to skin slough or prolonged distal edema. Furthermore, the transverse incision, if inadvertently carried too deep, may transect neurovascular structures that run perpendicular to the incision.

The Heyman-Herndon procedure should be considered only for patients under the age of 5. The likelihood that there will be corrective cartilage remodeling is high, and a stiff, painful foot will not occur. After age 5, remodeling potential diminishes, and it is better to consider proximal metatarsal osteotomies as a means of providing correction. These may be performed through the same dorsal approach as described for the Heyman-Herndon procedure. The osteotomies should be performed either with a reciprocating saw or with an osteotome. A Hall drill should not be used, as the heat generated will predispose to later nonunion.

COMBINATION OF POSITIONAL METATARSUS VARUS OF ONE FOOT AND CALCANEAL VALGUS OF THE OTHER

This is a frequently seen positional deformity in infants. The child appears to be deviating to one side; some refer to this abnormality as skiing to one side.

The positional element of the metatarsus varus deformity can be recognized by the fact that the forefoot can readily be pushed into proper alignment with the hindfoot. The opposite foot at birth was pushed up against the tibia; it can readily be brought into proper alignment, but it resumes a calcaneous position on release of pressure.

The infant usually perpetuates the deformity by sleeping on his stomach with the feet in this position.

Treatment consists of the use of a Denis-Browne bar attached to shoes to control the deformity. The shoe for the metatarsus varus is sold as a so-called "prewalker"; that is, the toe of the shoe is open. The last is built with forefoot abduction to carry the forefoot into a corrective position. It is turned outward 45 degrees on the bar. The calcaneus foot is treated with a prewalker type shoe with a regular last, or with a straight last if a regular one cannot be obtained. This shoe is turned inward 45 degrees. The total effect of this apparatus is to hold the feet in positions that deviate in directions opposite to the deviations seen in the examination. This apparatus is usually worn for 4 months during all sleeping hours, night and day. In waking hours, the bar only is removed. The shoes remain on except during the hour of the bath, which is at 10 or 11 a.m. in most families.

METATARSUS ATAVICUS (MORTON'S FOOT)

In the metatarsus atavicus anomaly, described by D. J. Morton, the first metatarsal is excessively short. Its length is usually less than that of the second and third. This defect results in excessive pressure and pain under the second metatarsal head. There is a tendency to pronate the foot in order to put the head of the first metatarsal into a weight-bearing position. Feet pronated for this reason should be supported by a prolongation of a longitudinal arch pad beneath the first metatarsal to procure weight bearing. If conservative therapy is unsuccessful, an oblique or dorsal wedge osteotomy of the second metatarsal may be performed to diminish second metatarsal pressure.

METATARSUS PRIMUS VARUS (BUNIONS)

Bunion is a lay term used to describe the medial bony prominence at the base of the great toe. There are various etiologies associated with the formation of bunions. Hereditary factors seem to be prominent, with approximately two-thirds of those presenting for surgery having a prominent family history. Certain African and Indochinese tribes seem to have a predominant incidence of bunions, despite the fact that they never wore shoes. Gender also seems to be related to the formation of bunions, with females predominant. Clearly, the wearing of high heels or ill fitting shoes is closely associated.

A multitude of other factors is also associated, such as neurogenic disorders (stroke, spastic cerebral palsy, etc.), a long first ray, an amputated second toe, etc. However, in the pediatric population, bunions are predominantly hereditary in etiology.

Clinical Appearance

The patients are usually female and have a parent or close relative with an identical problem. The great toe is in valgus, and there is a prominence at the first metatarsal head. Generally the foot is narrow, elongated, and pronated (Fig. 4.66). This pronation accentuates the hallux valgus, particularly at push-off during walking or running. Providing support under the medial arch will diminish the valgus force on the great toe and improve alignment (Fig. 4.67).

In addition to the pronation of the foot, the great toe itself is pronated, and on active extension or flexion of the toe, the long hallus tendons may be observed to be "bowstrung" laterally.

Hardy and Clapham serially followed a large adolescent population, noting that as hallux valgus progressed, metatarsus primus varus occurred. It would appear that as the great toe is pushed into valgus (either due to a long first ray, pronation of the foot, or muscle imbalance), once the proximal phalanx is subluxed, the extensor and flexor tendons act as abductors, increasing the deformity. With flexion and extension, they act to lever out the first metatarsal (Fig. 4.68). The repetitive varus pressure produces meta-

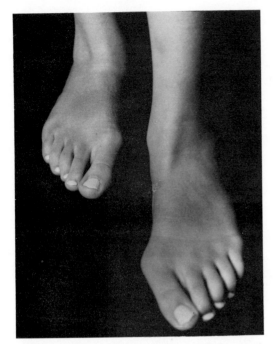

Figure 4.66. Severe hallux valgus and metatarsus primus varus in a 12-year-old female. The foot is narrow, the first ray elongated, the arch collapsed, and the great toe pronated.

tarsus primus varus with secondary remodeling at the first metatarsal cuneiform joint. Thus, the "bunion" deformity is created (Fig. 4.69).

Roentgen Appearance

The management of bunions should be undertaken only after a careful assessment of the entire appearance of the foot during gait, the roentgenographic characteristics, the age of the patient, and the degree of progression and symptoms.

Roentgenographically, the foot must be assessed from the standing anteroposterior view and the axial sesamoid view (Fig. 4.70). The standing anteroposterior will delineate the degree of hallux valgus, metatarsus primus varus, and secondary first metatarsal cuneiform changes. The axial sesamoid view will determine whether there is first metatarsal pronation and the degree to which the sesamoids are subluxed or dislocated. The first ray may be excessively long in relation to the second (predisposing to the bunion) or

short (altering the operative considerations). The first metatarsophalangeal joint may be excessively rounded (predisposing to rapid progression) or it may be slightly squared, indicating that further progression is unlikely.

Treatment

Early prevention would be ideal, but bunions are generally seen only after they have occurred. When a patient presents with a bunion deformity, it is helpful to ask if other family members have bunions as well, particularly questioning as to the appearance of family members in the adolescent age group. Early recognition of this deformity before hallux valgus progresses to the extent of subluxation can give the physician a chance at preventive management.

As illustrated in Figure 4.67, the use of support under the arch significantly diminishes the valgus moment on the great toe. Further, the use of a great toe spacer in combination with the arch support will assist in medializing the great toe, preventing the "bowstrung" force of the long tendons that

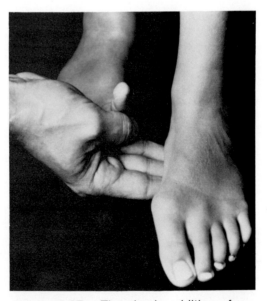

Figure 4.67. The simple addition of medial arch support diminishes the valgus moment applied to the great toe. Medial arch supports, a great toe spacer, and open-toed shoes would assist greatly in preventing further progression of this deformity.

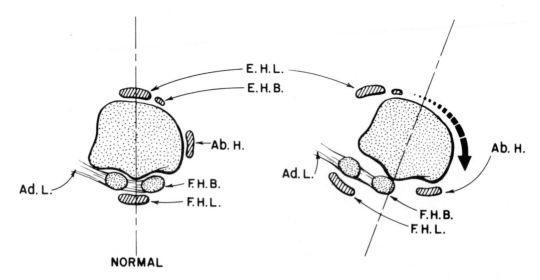

NORMAL

E.H.L. EXTENSOR HALLUCIS LONGUS	**F.H.L.** FLEXOR HALLUCIS LONGUS
E.H.B. EXTENSOR HALLUCIS BREVIS	**Ad. L.** ADDUCTOR LONGUS
F.H.B. FLEXOR HALLUCIS BREVIS	**Ab. H.** ABDUCTOR HALLUCIS

Figure 4.68. A diagrammatic illustration of the effect of first ray pronation in the muscular balance. As the abductor is rolled inferiorly, there are no muscular structures to balance the valgus forces.

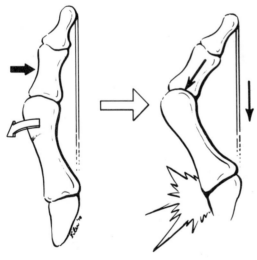

Figure 4.69. The proposed method of production of hallux valgus and metatarsus primus varus. Mechanical factors (tight shoes, a long first ray, pronation, etc.) produce hallux valgus. Each time the bow-strung hallux tendons contract, a varus moment is generated, levering the first metatarsal medially. Secondary remodeling occurs at the first metatarsocuneiform joint.

would further increase the hallux valgus. Lastly, the use of wide or open-toed, low-heeled shoes should be encouraged to prevent the mechanical enhancement of this deformity. If there is already marked subluxation of the great toe and prominent metatarsus primus varus, these conservative means will probably not be effective in preventing further deformity.

Operative management is undertaken when irreducible deformity is present and painful symptoms of recurrent bursitis persist over the medial first metatarsal head prominence. Surgery is directed toward the specific anatomic deformity.

SILVER PROCEDURE

This procedure was originally described by David Silver in 1923. It specifically addresses the medial prominence or "bunion." In the adolescent, it should not be used when there is metatarsus primus varus or hallux valgus. It should only be performed in the rare patient who presents with an isolated medial exostosis but otherwise no structural problems.

The incision should be centered medially over the first metatarsophalangeal joint. It extends carefully down through the subcutaneous tissues (identifying and protecting the digital sensory nerves), bursae, and capsule to the bones. The capsule is reflected anteriorly and posteriorly to fully expose the exostosis. Using a sharp osteotome, the exostosis is excised, being careful not to remove too much and inadvertently split the metatarsal shaft. The edges are smoothed with a rongeur, and the capsule is reapproximated in a "pants-over-vest" fashion with absorbable suture. Care is again taken not to incorporate a digital nerve in the closure. A soft, compressive dressing is applied, and protected weight bearing is allowed as tolerated.

AKINS PROCEDURE

The Akins procedure is designed to correct the bunion deformity associated primarily with irreducible hallux valgus but no metatarsus primus varus. It is, in essence, a medially based wedge osteotomy of the proximal first phalanx, in combination with a Silver bunionectomy. The osteotomy should be performed with a small oscillating or reciprocating saw. During the exposure, the flexor hallucis brevis is identified, and the osteotomy is performed just distal to its insertion. Upon removal of the bony wedge, the hallux valgus is reduced and a smooth K-wire driven down the distal and proximal phalanx (retrograde if necessary) to secure the reduction. As the metatarsophalangeal joint is easily visualized, the K-wire may be driven exactly up to, but not through, the phalangeal articular surface.

The closure is in the fashion described by David Silver, with the abductor hallucis tendon reefed dorsally to assist in preventing recurrence. The postoperative dressing should be either a short leg walking cast with a rubber stopper that will assist in preventing push-off at the great toe, or a bulky, soft compressive dressing. At 4 weeks the pin may be removed, but a great toe spacer should be used for an additional 6 weeks.

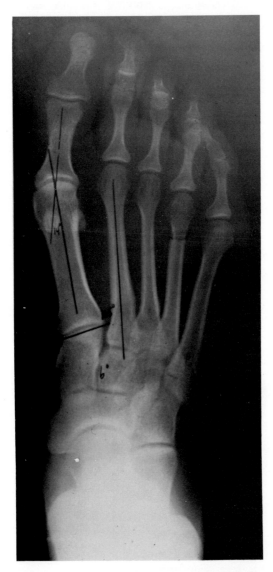

Figure 4.70. The standing anteroposterior roentgenogram of a normal foot illustrates the measurements of concern in assessing the "bunion" patient. The degree of hallux valgus is determined by the first metatarsophalangeal angle. The degree of metatarsus primus varus is determined by either the intermetatarsal angle or the second metatarsocuneiform angle. The roentgenogram must be weight bearing.

MITCHELL OR WILSON PROCEDURE

Various distal, first metatarsal procedures have been developed, designed to correct both hallux valgus and metatarsus primus varus. These have been described as pegged, notched, interlocking, sliding, etc. The Wilson and Mitchell procedures are the most commonly used. In our experience, bunion patients with a long first ray, sedentary patients, and patients with pronation of the foot will benefit from these procedures. This is because the first ray is effectively shortened, diminishing the later mechanical impingement of shoes and the valgus moment at the great toe during push-off if the foot is pronated.

The Wilson procedure and its variants are generally a distal or mid first metatarsal oblique osteotomy designed to allow the first metatarsal to shorten on itself and angulate laterally to correct metatarsus primus varus. A Silver bunionectomy and capsular reefing correct hallux valgus.

A modification of this procedure has been to perform the osteotomy approximately at the midpoint of the first metatarsal (Fig. 4.71). A wedge of bone based laterally is removed. The base of the wedge faces toward the second metatarsal and should be sufficient to fully correct the deformity when the wedge is closed. This correction is held by some form of internal fixation, as the deformity otherwise will readily recur in the cast. We have placed drill holes through the cortex on either side of the operative defect and held the closure by wire sutures. Transferring the adductor tendon in addition greatly increases the surgery in this relatively small area and has not been found necessary if the osteotomy is done far enough distally on the metatarsal.

The correction obtained can be seen in Figure 4.71. The obliteration of the space between the first and second metatarsal heads and the realignment of the great toe secondary to this correction is evident. A short leg cast is necessary for 6 weeks.

The Mitchell osteotomy has also been shown to be very effective in obtaining permanent correction. In our experience, in those patients with failed previous bunion surgery or severe pronation of the foot, the Mitchell procedure, if carefully done, will be successful. The complications of hallux elevatus, hallux varus, and painful secondary lateral metatarsalgia may all be avoided, provided the surgery is technically precise, not too much bone is removed, and patients with preoperative length discrepancies are avoided (Figs. 4.72 and 4.73 A and B).

The Mitchell procedure involves the identical medial approach to the first metatarsophalangeal joint. Using a Hall drill, dorsal cuts are made as indicated in Figure 4.72 and the distal head then translocated laterally. Although Mitchell advocated excising the medial bunion, in our experience the lateral translation of the distal head buries this prominence. The corrected position must be held either with nonabsorbable stay sutures through drill holes in the metatarsal or with smooth K-wires. The capsular closure is in

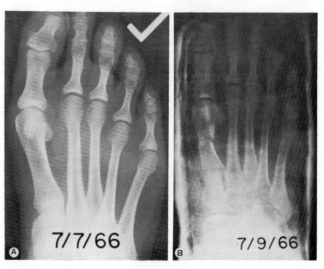

Figure 4.71. (A) Preoperative roentgenogram showing the deviation medially of the first metatarsal and hallux valgus, with the space between the first and second metatarsal head. (B) Postoperative correction of the first metatarsal by osteotomy. The great toe no longer is in a deformed position, as the first metatarsal has been aligned with it. A wire suture holds the osteotomy closed.

MITCHELL OSTEOTOMY

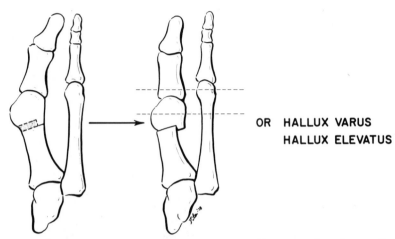

OR HALLUX VARUS
HALLUX ELEVATUS

Figure 4.72. The Mitchell bunionectomy is performed by resecting the medial rectangle of bone (*shaded area*) and laterally displacing the distal ray. Lack of attention technically to precision surgery may lead to length discrepancies, hallux varus, or hallux elevatus.

the manner of Silver. A short leg walking cast is applied, completely covering the toes. Pressure is exerted as this cast hardens so that the great toe is held in alignment with the lateral toes, and a walker is applied in such a way that push-off occurs with this rubber heel rolling over, not with pressure on the distal aspect of the foot. After 6 weeks, the cast is removed, and the patient begins walking with an arch support and a great toe spacer for an additional 6 weeks.

PROXIMAL OSTEOTOMY OR LAPIDUS PROCEDURE

Many authors have advanced the thesis that the primary defect in "bunion" patients is maldevelopment at the first metatarsal-cuneiform joint. This defect supposedly represents an atavistic throwback to the prehensile foot of the ape. The resultant medial deviation at the first metatarsal-cuneiform joint causes a medial protrusion of the first metatarsal with secondary hallux valgus.

As pointed out in the introductory comments on bunions, there are a large number of well documented etiologies. Further, it has been aptly illustrated by DuVries and Hardy and Clapham that in adolescents and adults hallux valgus occurs first, followed by metatarsus primus varus. It should be remembered, however, that although the debate may be endless as to the role of proximal or distal

forces that produce this deformity, all bony deformities must be reduced or abnormal alignment will recur.

The Lapidus procedure or the proximal first metatarsal osteotomy, in combination with a Silver bunionectomy, will provide correction, provided that certain principles are adhered to. In our experience, the arthrodesis of the first and second metatarsocuneiform joints seems more a salvage procedure than a reconstructive one, and we prefer not to perform it. Nevertheless, the modifications described for the proximal osteotomy procedure are quite applicable to the Lapidus as well.

The proximal osteotomy should not be performed in individuals with pes valgus and narrow feet, because in our experience it may fail due to a tendency to accentuate the midfoot collapse. Furthermore, in the long, narrow foot, the valgus moment at the great toe during push-off is considerable, also predisposing to recurrence. In the wider foot with a pronated great toe but satisfactory arch, this procedure will yield excellent results.

The operation is performed through a long medial incision, running from the medial base of the first metatarsal to the proximal phalanx. If excessive hallux valgus is present, an Akins procedure may be performed. A Silver bunionectomy is followed by a proximal, closing metatarsal osteotomy, performed with an oscillating saw or osteotome

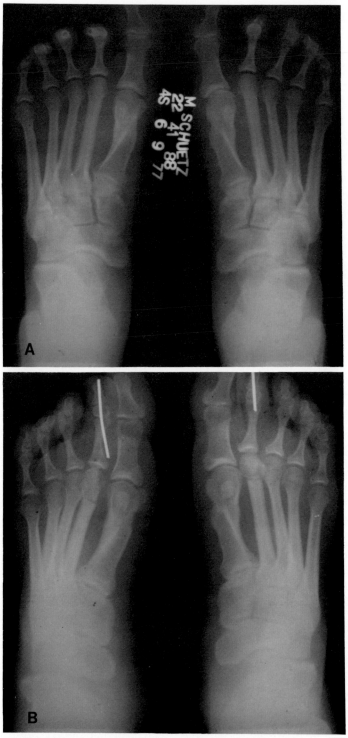

Figure 4.73. (*A*) This 14-year-old female is 1 year post-Mitchell bunionectomies. She has an excellent cosmetic result, but an excessive length discrepancy between the first and second metatarsal was created, in addition to hallux elevatus. She has bilateral, severe, second metatarsalgia and secondary second hammer toes. (*B*) A bilateral, second, proximal interphalangeal fusion was performed in addition to a second metatarsal wedge osteotomy. If it is apparent preoperatively or intraoperatively that there will be a significant length discrepancy, a second metatarsal (proximal) osteotomy should be done prophylactically.

after predrilling. A Hall drill may be used, but overheating of the bone margins must not occur or a nonunion will result. The laterally based wedge of bone is easily removed from the medial side, and the first ray derotated if necessary until the pronated great toe is at neutral. Crossed smooth K-wires hold the correction, and closure is after the fashion of Silver. A short leg walking cast is worn for 6 weeks, after which the smooth K-wires are removed. The patient then walks with an arch support and great toe spacer for an additional 6 weeks.

The essence of this procedure may be incorporated into the Lapidus procedure, if so desired. The Akins procedure and derotation of the first ray can each be performed in combination with the arthrodesis, if necessary. Proximal opening osteotomies alone, in our experience, have been fraught with difficulties (Fig. 4.74). If there is significant, uncorrected pronation of the first ray, even though the initial osteotomy is successful, the bowstrung tendons will cause a recurrence of hallux valgus. Later, secondary metatarsus primus varus will result. In addition, if the osteotomy is performed in a "greenstick" fashion, leaving the lateral cortex intact, or if the graft is too small, graft resorption will occur with recurrence of deformity.

The essential in bunion surgery is to recognize predisposing factors and the anatomic components of the deformity, as well as to retain a flexible approach during surgery so that appropriate permanent correction is attained.

CAVUS FEET

The characteristics of cavus feet—high arched feet with equinus of the forefoot, reducible claw toes, and a calcaneous position of the hindfoot—are readily recognized clinically. This foot without a very severe deformity can produce severe disability. It is very rarely seen below the age of 3.

Etiology

Such a foot brings to mind a triad of neurologic diagnoses as possible underlying causes. The first is an anomaly of the lumbosacral spine with tethering cord adhesions interfering with foot function. The resultant muscular imbalance is thought to result in the cavus foot. A previous attack of poliomyelitis may result in muscular imbalance. Weakness of dorsiflexors with the posterior tibial still present may result in this situation. Such degenerative neurologic conditions as Friedreich's ataxia or Charcot-Marie-Tooth disease may underlie this foot deformity. It is important to recognize that chronic neurologic disturbance may exist and to take appropriate steps to diagnose it.

Clinical Appearance

These youngsters are usually recognized in the 7 to 14-year age group. The changes in the foot by this time are well established. The

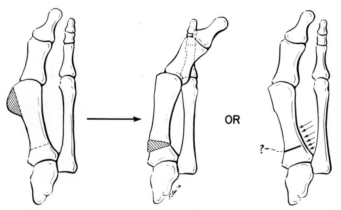

Figure 4.74. The proximal osteotomy is fraught with pitfalls. If the proximal correction is satisfactory but the distal correction of hallux valgus is inadequate, the great toe will return to valgus, again levering medially the first metatarsal. If the osteotomy is left intact laterally, a greenstick effect is exerted, causing graft resorption.

usual complaint is deformity, which is noted by the parents. Symptoms in this age group are rare. Calluses beneath the metatarsal heads or over the proximal interphalangeal joint may be the presenting complaint.

Suspicion of the foot deformity is aroused by equinus of the forefoot in non-weight bearing. Confirming factors are hyperextension deformity of the metatarsophalangeal joints and flexion deformity of the interphalangeal joints, which results in claw toes. These toes are subluxated dorsalward on the metatarsal heads. The os calcis is not in equinus but in a calcaneous or dorsiflexed position; it thus gives rise to the high arch. Passive elevation of the forefoot in this age group results in straightening of the toes (Fig. 4.75 A and D).

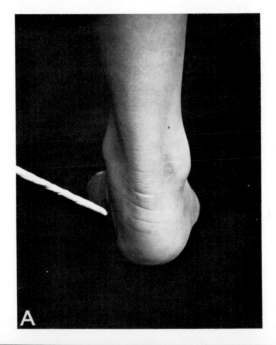

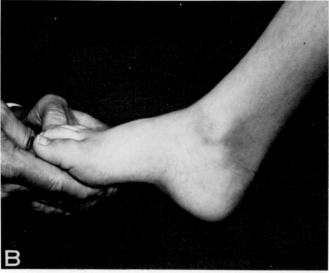

Figure 4.75. Demonstration of the hindfoot-forefoot relationships in cavus feet. (*A*) The hindfoot is in varus and related to the ankle, which is in external rotation. The forefoot is abducted. (*B*) When the forefoot is held up, the cavus deformity is partially masked. (*C*)

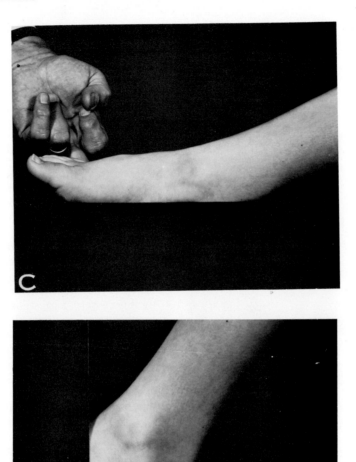

Fig. 4.75 (C and D)

Covering the hindfoot makes the equinus deformity of the forefoot apparent as a direct continuation of the tibia. (*D*) Covering the forefoot with a black sheet makes the relative lack of equinus of the hindfoot apparent—actually the os calcis is in calcaneus.

Depending on the duration and severity of the deformity, there may be thinning and atrophy of the fat pads over the metatarsal heads so that they may readily be palpated. Calluses may form over these bony processes. The plantar fascia may be palpated as a tight contracted band on attempted correction of the forefoot and may limit full correction (Fig. 4.76).

Diagnosis

The large percentage of these patients presenting with cavus feet have a mild, bilateral deformity, and no underlying pathologic etiology will be discovered. Asymmetric or a unilateral cavus foot should be cause for suspicion. The initial examination should include an inspection of the back for skin

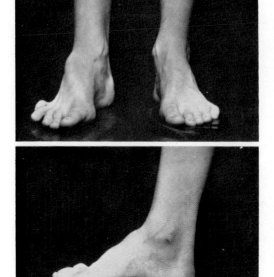

Figure 4.76. Cavus feet (note equinus of forefoot in relation to hindfoot).

markers, as well as a single, anteroposterior lumbar roentgenogram. Further diagnostic studies, such as electromyography or a myelogram, would not be indicated unless abnormalities were noted on the initial inspection. Tomograms of the lumbar spine or a fascicular, sural nerve and muscle biopsy may be necessary if occult neurogenic disorder is suspected.

Treatment

Conservative treatment consists of passive stretching of the plantar fascia by dorsiflexion of the forefoot and flattening of the medial arch. The toes are brought down from their subluxated position on the dorsum of the metatarsal heads, and the interphalangeal flexion deformity is passively stretched.

A Jones bar pad is either worn as an inner sole, where it is most efficient, or built into the sole of the shoe. This pad, to be corrective, must be placed so that its elevation is directly behind the metatarsal heads. In the still pliable foot, this elevation restores the toes to their rightful position. The shoe aids in holding them down. A supplementary arch support may also be of assistance if the pa-

tient is complaining of posterior tibialis tendonitis symptoms (Figs. 4.77 and 4.78).

Operation is considered in the presence of progressive deformity in a conservative regime and must be performed before the fat pads beneath the metatarsal heads have atrophied.

Either of two soft-tissue procedures may be considered if the metatarsal pads have not atrophied and if the claw toes are reducible. The tendon transfers of "flexors-into-extensors" is quite satisfactory in increasing the toe support distally and reducing deformity. Another procedure is the transplantation of the long extensor tendons to the metatarsal necks. The short extensor tendons are detached at their insertion into the proximal phalanx and sewn into the stumps of the insertion of the long extensors (Figs. 4.78 and 4.79). If necessary, a capsulotomy of the metatarsophalangeal joints is done on the dorsum. An accessory bit of surgery that is sometimes necessary is a division of the plantar fascia. This is done just forward of the origin of the fascia from the os calcis.

The most medial incision is used for the great toe. Two tendons are approached through each of the other two incisions. The result of too few incisions is unnecessary retraction at the expense of the vitality of the skin edges. Smooth K-wires should be inserted down each toe and across the metatarsophalangeal joint to provide stability while healing occurs. The feet should be casted, and the K-wires may be removed after 3 weeks.

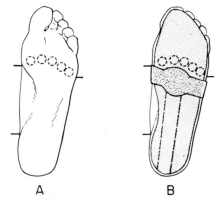

A   B

Figure 4.77. Tracing of pad with Jones bar to elevate forefoot. The transverse bar is felt covered with leather. The *dotted lines* indicate the position of a corset to impart stiffness to the pad.

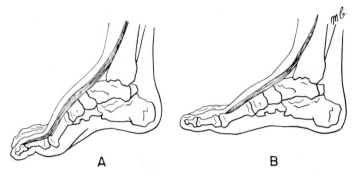

A   B

Figure 4.78. Effect of moving long extensor of toes back to metatarsal neck to correct equinus of forefoot and allowing toes to drop down to correct dorsiflexion of the proximal phalanx.

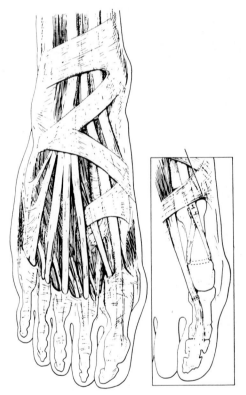

Figure 4.79. Detail of insertion of the long extensor tendon into the metatarsal neck, with insertion of the short extensor tendon into the stump of longus.

When bony deformity is fixed and severe, three different structural procedures may be considered. A midfoot dorsal wedge osteotomy in combination with a plantar fascia release will correct pronounced forefoot equinus. If there is marked hindfoot calca-

neus and varus, a Dwyer or crescentic calcaneal osteotomy may be performed, also in combination with a plantar fascial release.

Lastly, a triple arthrodesis is sometimes used for correction of severe deformity. This procedure is usually performed when there is severe neurogenic cavoequinovarus deformity. Clawing of the toes can be partially reduced by the shortening effect of this procedure. In the severely deformed, rigid foot, visualization is extremely important. If the triple arthrodesis is performed through a single lateral incision, it will soon be apparent in this marked cavoequinovarus foot that the medial talonavicular joint is a significant distance from the lateral incision. Thus, the incision must extend adequately. We prefer a long, anterolateral longitudinal incision to preserve postoperative venous drainage, and thus reduce swelling and pain (Figs. 4.80 and 4.81).

A second point of consideration is that of choosing the plane of osteotomies when performing the fusions. Dilwynn Evans' principle of visualizing the foot as medial and lateral columns is particularly helpful. In this cavoequinovarus foot, there must be significant shortening laterally at the calcaneocuboid joint. In addition, the talonavicular osteotomy must be based dorsolaterally to bring the equinus forefoot superiorly as well as laterally. We prefer to perform the operation in a manner similar to the Hoke-type triple arthrodesis, but the Lambrinudi may also be used if forefoot equinus is severe. Staples are optional. Finally, as there is significant bone bleeding from six cut surfaces, a compression dressing with a plaster splint is applied at the end of the case. In 3 days,

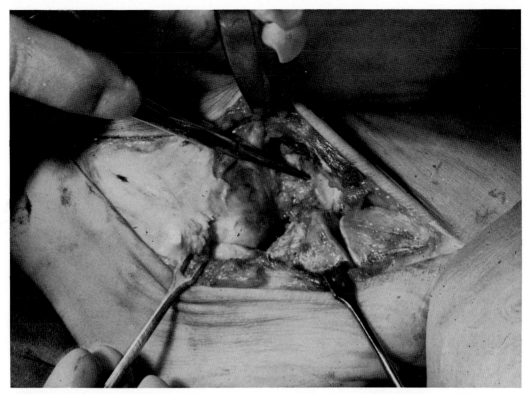

Figure 4.80. An intraoperative photograph of the left foot, illustrating the excellent visualization of the subtalar, calcaneocuboid, and talonavicular joints, using the anterolateral longitudinal approach. The hemostat points to the talonavicular joint.

this is removed, and the first short leg cast is applied for 6 weeks of non-weight bearing. A second, walking cast is then applied for a final 4–6 weeks, depending upon alignment of the triple and the degree of healing. Permanent, satisfying correction of the cavoequinovarus deformity can be achieved following these principles.

VASCULAR DISORDERS (OSTEOCHONDROSES)

Köhler's Disease

Köhler's disease is a condition causing pain and swelling in the forefoot. The roentgenogram reveals abnormal density of the navicular bone (Fig. 4.82). Involved in this way, the navicular can be compressed if it is not protected. Unfortunately this condition, which is quite rare, is often confused with the normal fragmentary ossification of the

navicular, which is not associated with symptoms.

Normal ossification of the navicular from multiple centers occurs in the 3- to 6-year-old age group. Cases showing increased density of the navicular consistent with Köhler's disease usually occur past this stage in the 6- to 10-year age group.

ETIOLOGY

This condition is usually thought of as secondary to circulatory interference. The reason for this change is not clear. It is related presumably to other lesions such as Kienböck's disease, Frieberg's disease of the second metatarsal head, or avascular necrosis of other tarsal bones such as the cuneiforms or cuboid.

CLINICAL PICTURE

The patient complains of foot pain that tends to be continuous rather than intermittent, as in the case of foot strain. There is tenderness over the area occupied by the navicular bone. Thickening and even frank swelling may be noted in this area. When the condition is active, limping and a tendency to walk on the lateral side of the foot are noted.

ROENTGEN FINDINGS

The disease can be accurately diagnosed by roentgenogram. Confusion with normal ossification of the navicular can be avoided once it is realized that the navicular normally arises from at least three separate centers of ossification in the 3- to 6-year age group. These centers coalesce rapidly to form one center. When one overlies another, an appearance of increased density is sometimes given. In Köhler's disease, the navicular or a portion of it exhibits increased density and then fragments. The radiolucent areas finally heal in to form normal-appearing bone.

While it is going through the dense stage, the navicular may become narrowed and compressed if the patient has been weight bearing.

TREATMENT

The patient is taken off weight bearing. A protective plaster cast and crutches are used, usually for several months. Before weight bearing protected with crutches is begun, the areas of density should be repaired and the soft-tissue thickening relieved. Full weight bearing is gradually achieved as the lesion heals.

Freiberg's Disease

Although patients with pain beneath the second metatarsal head and with roentgenographic evidence of deformity of the head of

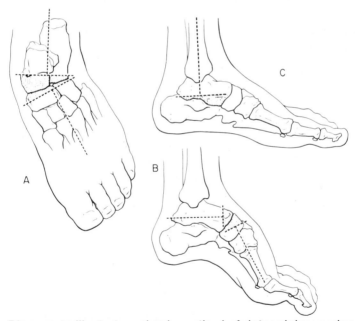

Figure 4.81. Diagram to illustrate a simple method of determining wedge resections in triple arthrodeses to correct the deformity. The *long dotted lines* illustrate the axis of forefoot and hindfoot as in (*A*). All cuts in the forefoot side are made at right angles to the forefoot axis. All cuts on the hindfoot side are made at right angles to the hindfoot axis. All cuts should come out at the apex of the triangle at the junction of cartilage of the joint surface of bone. In this way, no more bone will be removed than is absolutely necessary, and a normal-looking foot will be maintained. In (*C*), the talar cut is made in relation to the axis line of the tibia. The os calcis cut, based posteriorly, will follow the line of the subastragalar joint but will still bear the axis of the os calcis in mind. Triple arthrodeses ordinarily require 8 weeks in a long leg plaster cast followed by several weeks in a short leg walking cast before fixation is terminated. Crutches are usually required for at least 4 weeks thereafter.

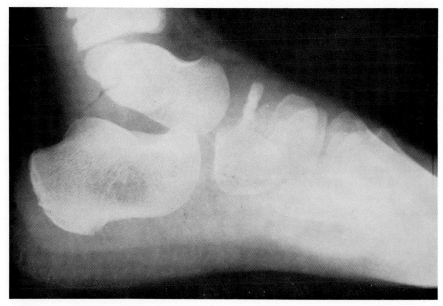

Figure 4.82. Roentgenogram of compressed and dense navicular in Köhler's disease with associated soft-tissue swelling.

the second metatarsal are often first seen as adults, the onset of this disease is in adolescence. The disease seems to be an aseptic necrosis of the epiphyseal area of the second metatarsal occurring about the time of epiphyseal line closure (Fig. 4.83). There is often a history of chronic trauma caused by such activities as ballet dancing. The disorder is much more common in female patients, and it is not uncommon to note that the second ray is quite long relative to the first and third.

Although Freiberg's disease was originally noted to occur predominantly at the second metatarsal head, it is not uncommon to see isolated involvement of other metatarsal heads, including the first.

CLINICAL PICTURE

There is a complaint of pain with use in the region of the second metatarsal head. Swelling about the area is appreciated by palpation and is often visible. Tenderness may be acute.

ROENTGEN FINDINGS

The epiphyseal area is originally dense; then rarefied areas appear at the base of the metatarsal head, and irregular replacement follows so that the density is eventually completely removed. If, during this period, the

area is unprotected, the joint surface becomes flattened. This deformity is a permanent, residual one. In the great toe, hallux rigidus is a common sequela.

TREATMENT

When seen at the onset of the disease, the youngster should be immobilized in a walking plaster cast molded to bring the pressure of weight bearing behind the metatarsal heads. After the swelling has subsided, a carefully molded foot plate is worn so that the metatarsal head does not take weight directly. The elevation of the plate in the midmetatarsal area must be sufficient to accomplish this and can be checked by lateral roentgenogram of the foot in the shoe. A Jones metatarsal bar in the sole of the shoe may be an additional safeguard. Once deformity has occurred, the metatarsal head cannot be reconstituted. Persistent pain may lead to resection of the proximal portion of the proximal phalanx in order to procure a new joint.

PAINFUL HEELS IN CHILDREN

Pain located at the superior angle of the os calcis is a common childhood complaint in the 6- to 12-year-old age group. The causes of such complaints are varied (Figs. 4.84–4.88).

There is also a common occurrence in the teenage group wherein a painful callus and underlying bursa arise. In slang terms this condition has been designated "pump bumps" and is very common when the wearing of a loafer style shoe dependent on a tight fit is in vogue.

An excessive prominence of the posterior superior angle of the os calcis predisposes to the development of this bursa, which can become very painful. The tight upper ridge of the heel counter sliding back and forth over this prominence is the cause. To remove it, either the bony prominence must be re-moved surgically or the design of the heel counter changed.

Obviously, the latter alternative is preferable. The stiff support of the heel counter may be removed or careful attention paid to procuring a shoe with a heel counter of sufficient height that its superior reinforced edge is above the bone prominence.

Operative Treatment

In the child with severe recurrent heel pain due to prominence of the posterior calcaneal angle, surgery may be necessary. When this is done, the posterior angle is removed with-

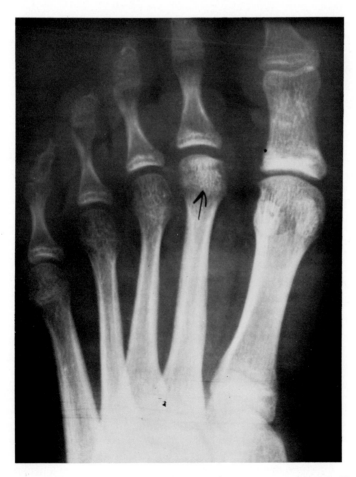

Figure 4.83. Anteroposterior view of the foot in a 12-year-old girl. Flattening of the surface of the second metatarsal head (*arrow*) has already taken place. There is increased density distally and a line of rarefaction proximal to it as vascular penetration takes place.

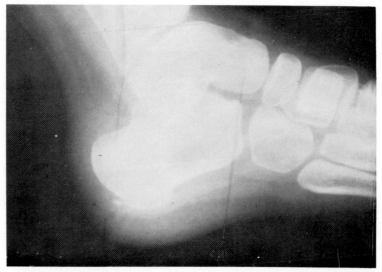

Figure 4.84. Aseptic inflammatory swelling at the junction of Achilles tendon and os calcis.

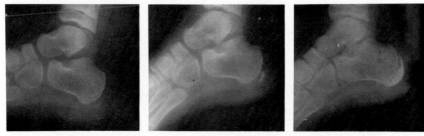

Figure 4.85. The normal development of the os calcis includes a dense stage of the apophysis; (*left*) 4½ years; (*center*) 5 years; (*right*) 8 years.

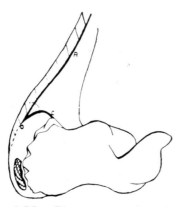

Figure 4.86. Diagram emphasizing the angle made by the junction of the Achilles tendon and the os calcis. This angle is obscured by inflammatory swelling at the heel. Angle *AOC* is formed by the junction of the Achilles tendon and the superior surface of the os calcis.

out destroying the attachment of the tendo achillis.

Stress Fractures

Another cause for painful heels in children is a stress fracture of the calcaneal apophysis (Fig. 4.89). A history of intense involvement in athletics is usually elicited, particularly in sports such as basketball or gymnastics, where there is repetitive shock absorption. Usually there is no tenderness in the Achilles tendon, nor in the retrocalcaneal bursal region. Direct pressure over the posterior calcaneus will reproduce symptoms. Treatment should consist of rest, a heel pad, and casting, if necessary. These stress fractures should not be confused with so-called "Sivers disease," which was erroneously thought to rep-

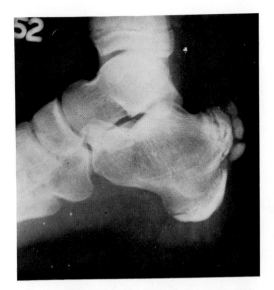

Figure 4.87. Congenital duplication of the apophysis of the os calcis. As a result of the excessive superior prominence, a bursa formed over it and secondary ossification developed within it. Clinically this resulted in a marked form of the syndrome known as "pump bumps."

resent avascular necrosis of the calcaneal apophysis (Fig. 4.90).

Achilles Tendonitis

Another diagnosis to consider in the child with painful heels is Achilles tendonitis. This is generally quite rare in this age group. There may be an associated retrocalcaneal bursitis, but there is distinct pain on direct pressure upon squeezing the Achilles tendon. Resisted plantar flexion reproduces symptoms, and frequently there will be a history of a previous blow to that region. Treatment should consist of rest, anti-inflammatory agents, and a heel lift. Casting may be instituted if necessary.

CONGENITAL ANOMALIES

Before considering obvious structural maldevelopment, it is necessary to consider normal, benign variations. In the developing foot, ossification is frequently irregular and

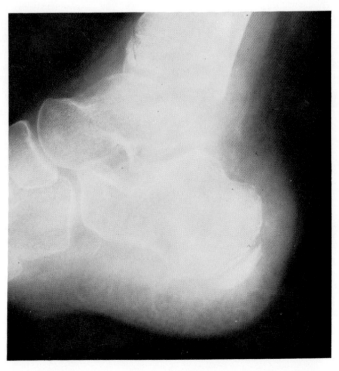

Figure 4.88. Inflammatory swelling about the heel in osteomyelitis of the os calcis. This marked inflammation obscures angle AOC as shown in Figure 4.32.

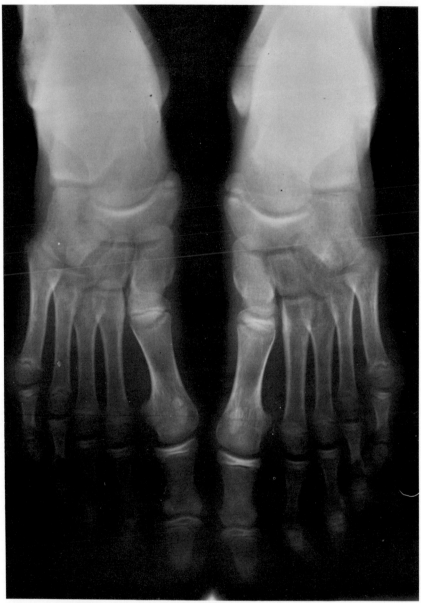

Figure 4.89. This individual presented to an emergency room with complaints of ankle pain. An anteroposterior roentgenogram of the feet revealed the bilateral accessory naviculars, the bipartite sesamoids, and the os vesalium. These were normal, asymptomatic variations in bony development.

separate ossification centers and rudimentary bones may or may not coalesce. This can result in some difficulty in determining whether bony changes seen in a suspected injury are normal variations or, in fact, represent an acute fracture (Fig. 4.89). The os sustencaculum, os trigonum, os vesalium, accessory navicular, and bi-, tri-, and quadripartite sesamoids are frequent anatomic variations. Exostoses, as well, are not uncommon. They may represent the reossification of an avulsed ligament, one of multiple hereditary exostoses, or an isolated phenomenon. The subungual exostosis is the most common isolated benign growth (Fig. 4.91). It arises most commonly on the dorsal aspect of the first distal phalanx. Frequently, it is asymptomatic and discovered only by accident. Excessive growth will result in a protrusion through the nailbed, chronic irritation, and pain. Operative excision will result in a complete cure.

The variety and complexity of congenital foot anomalies makes classification difficult at best. Most commonly, there is abnormal development associated with the metatarsals or toes, more rarely the tarsal bones. Many deformities, such as absent toes or length discrepancies in toes or metatarsals, require little or no treatment (Fig. 4.92).

Overlapping Fifth Toes

The fifth toe, when structurally overlapped, is held in place by a tight skin fold and a shortened tendon. This deformity is frequently familial. The condition is often bilateral, and accompanying radial angulation of the distal phalanx of the fifth fingers is not uncommon (Fig. 4.93).

In mild degrees of the condition, the toe may be strapped in place with adhesive for many months with the possibility of some success. When the fifth toe is well up over the fourth, however, conservative methods will not correct the deformity. Surgical correction is indicated because the condition has a tendency to cause a soft corn to develop between the fourth and fifth toes and a callus overlying the dorsum of the fifth. Correction includes a Z-plasty in the line of the short skin segment, lengthening of the extensor tendons, and a capsulotomy of the metatarsophalangeal joint. At the conclusion of surgery, the toe should lie naturally in normal position without having to be splinted.

Occasionally it is necessary to perform bony work to correct the overlap, particularly if there is a midphalangeal "delta deformity." One of two procedures may be considered. For the fifth toe, the Ruiz procedure consists

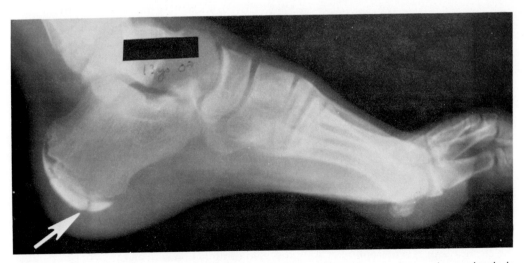

Figure 4.90. An athletically aggressive aolescent with an open calcaneal apophysis is prone to stress fractures. This 13-year-old basketball player had exquisite pain at the plantar heel (*arrow*). There were no plantar fascia or Achilles tendon symptoms. (Reproduced with permission from McMaster: *Principles of Scholastic and Collegiate Sports Medicine*, Baltimore: Williams & Wilkins, 1980.)

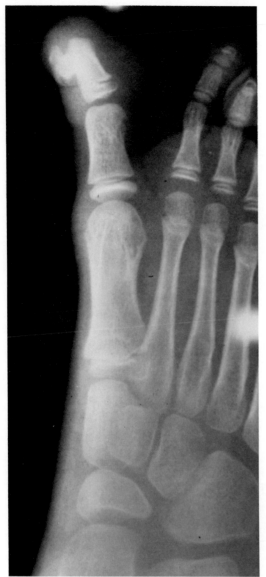

Figure 4.91. A subungual exostosis in a 7-year-old male.

fusion is necessary. The osteotomy or removal of appropriate bone is performed through a dorsal incision. Fixation is with a retrograde smooth K-wire.

Supernumerary Digits

There will occasionally present one or more rudimentary toe buds. These, by and large, represent nothing more than soft-tissue "tags." They may be removed merely by the application of a strangulating, absorbable suture-ligature. The dried tag and ligature will generally fall off within a week, and only a Bandaid is necessary.

Occasionally, there will be associated anomalies in the metatarsals as well (Fig. 4.94). A rudimentary metatarsal may be present, or there may be two phalanges articulating with one metatarsal. If necessary, the rudimentary metatarsal may be excised as well, or the lateral phalanx should be excised. Shoe wear will be facilitated by the lateral excision.

Multiple Tarsal Anomalies

There is a great deal of variation in midtarsal and hindfoot anomalies. It is better to consider them from a functional standpoint than to attempt an impractical anatomic classification. These foot deformities should be classified according to whether or not the patient has a functional foot, a dysfunctional foot that can nevertheless fit plantigrade into a shoe, or, finally, a dysfunctional foot that interferes with shoe wear, balance, and support (Figs. 4.95 and 4.96). Treatment is then planned accordingly. The patient in Figure 4.95 is such an example. On the right the patient has congenital absence of the fibula and multiple tarsal bones and rays. As the foot is dysfunctional and will prohibit shoe wear, a definite Syme's procedure is the best approach on the right.

The left side has a foot of normal appearance, but two rays are absent, as is the fibula, in combination with an early congenital tibial pseudarthrosis. Here, although the foot appears as though it could function, the proximal anomalies will undoubtedly prohibit this, and multiple surgical procedures may be necessary merely to maintain an aligned limb

of a proximal phalangectomy, combined with soft-tissue shortening. A longitudinal, plantar oval or "race track" of skin is removed, and the phalanx is removed from this incision. The closure is in reverse, approximating the distal to proximal edges, in effect shortening the toe.

If there is a delta deformity in the middle phalanges of the middle toes, creating impingement, an osteotomy or interphalangeal

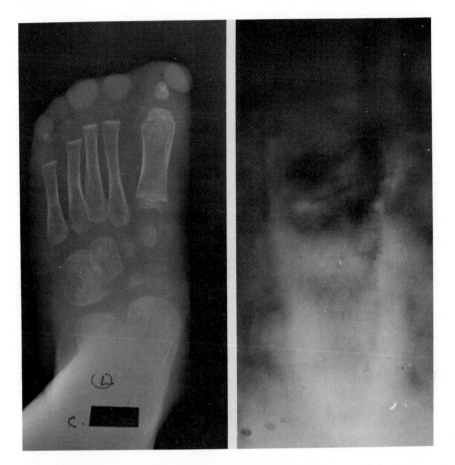

Figure 4.92.   This 8-year-old presented with congenital absence of the toes and metatarsalgia. The cholesterol crystal force plate study revealed increased pressure under the metatarsal region, secondary to the absence of toe support.

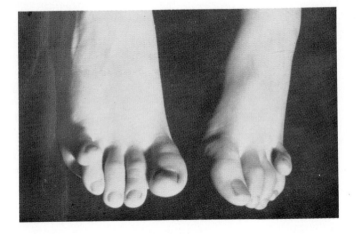

Figure 4.93.   Fifth toes overlapping bilaterally—a fixed congenital deformity. Pulling the toe laterally reveals the contracture of the skin on the dorsum of the foot.

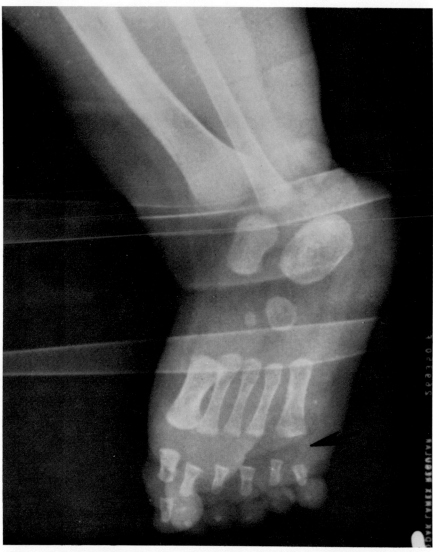

Figure 4.94.   This 6-month-old infant presented with a supernumary digit and a double articulation. Excision of the sixth toe and the lateral half of the metatarsal was performed.

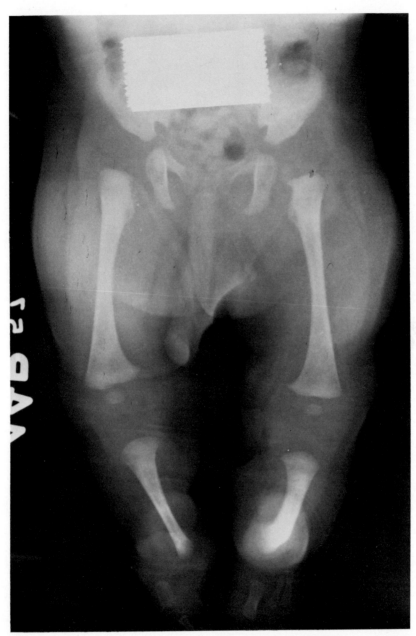

Figure 4.95. This infant presented with bilateral congenital absence of the fibula, a left congenital bowing of the tibia, and absent or coalesced tarsal bones. A right Syme's and left below-knee amputation was performed at 6 months of age.

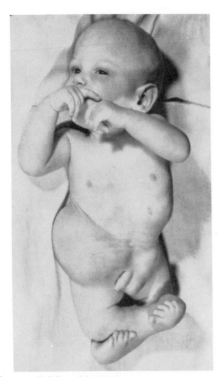

Figure 4.96. Multiple congenital anomalies with abdominal wall hernia, absence of cord below the twelfth dorsal vertebra, and equinovarus deformities. Paralytic feet such as these are exceedingly difficult to correct. Once corrected, bracing is necessary to hold the correction as the child grows.

and plantigrade foot. Therefore, a definitive below-knee amputation is the treatment of choice.

References

1. Akin, O. F.: The treatment of hallux valgus—a new operative procedure and its results, *Med. Sent., 33:* 678, 1925.
2. Beckham, C., Diamond, R., and Greenlee, T.: The role of movement in the development of a digital flexor tendon, *Am. J. Anat., 150:* 443, 1977.
3. Bell, J. F., and Grice, D. S.: Treatment of congenital talipes equinovarus by modified Denis-Browne split, *J. Bone Joint Surg., 26:* 799, 1944.
4. Bleck, E.: Congenital clubfoot: pathomechanics, radiographic analysis, and the results of surgical treatment, *Clin. Orthop., 115:* 119, 1977.
5. Bleck, E., and Berzins, U.: Conservative management of pes valgus with plantar flexed talus, flexible. *Clin. Orthop., 122:* 85, 1977.
6. Bost, F. C., Schottstaedt, E. R., and Larsen, L. J.: Plantar dissection, and operation to release the soft tissues in recurrent and recalcitrant talipes equinovarus, *J. Bone Joint Surg., 42A:* 151, 1960.
7. Bratberg, J., and Scheer, G.: Extra-articular arthro-desis of the subtalar joint: a clinical study and review, *Clin. Orthop., 126:* 220, 1977.
8. Brockman, E. P.: Modern methods of treatment of clubfoot, *Br. Med. J., 2:* 572, 1937.
9. Browne, R., and Paton, D.: Anomalous insertion of the tibialis posterior tendon in congenital metatarsus varus, *J. Bone Joint Surg., 61B:* 74, 1979.
10. Clark, M., D'Ambrosia, R., and Ferguson, A.: Congenital vertical talus; treatment by open reduction and navicular excision, *J. Bone Joint Surg., 59A:* 816, 1977.
11. Coleman, S., Steeling, F., and Jarrett, J.: Pathomechanics and treatment of congenital vertical talus, *Clin. Orthop., 70:* 62, 1970.
12. *DuVries Surgery of the Foot,* Ed. 4, St. Louis: C. V. Mosby, 1978.
13. Evans, D.: Relapsed clubfoot, *J. Bone Joint Surg., 43B:* 722, 1961.
14. Garceau, G. J., and Manning, K. R.: Transplantation of the anterior tibial tendon in the treatment of recurrent congenital clubfoot, *J. Bone Joint Surg., 29:* 1044, 1947.
15. Giannestras, N.: *Foot Disorders,* Ed. 2; Philadelphia: Lea & Febiger, 1973.
16. Giannestras, W.: Flexible valgus flatfoot resulting from naviculocuneiform and talonavicular sag: surgical correction in the adolescent. In *Foot Science,* pp. 67–105, Philadelphia: W. B. Saunders, 1976.
17. Hardy, R., and Clapham, J.: Hallux valgus; predisposing anatomic cause, *Lancet, 1:* 1180, 1952.
18. Harris, R. I., and Beath, T.: Hypermobile flat foot with short tendo achillis, *J. Bone Joint Surg., 30A:* 116, 1948.
19. Harris, R. I., and Beath, T.: Etiology of peroneal spastic flat foot, *J. Bone Joint Surg., 30B:* 624, 1948.
20. Heyman, C., Herndon, C., and Strong, J.: Mobilization of the tarsometatarsal and intermetatarsal joints for the correction of resistant adduction of the fore part of the foot in congenital clubfoot and congenital metatarsus varus, *J. Bone Joint Surg., 40A:* 299, 1958.
21. Hsu, L.: Valgus deformity of the ankle resulting from fibular resection for a graft in subtalar fusion in children, *J. Bone Joint Surg., 54A:* 585, 1972.
22. Isaacs, H., Handelsman, J., Badenhorst, M., and Pickering, A.: The muscles in clubfoot—a histological, histochemical, and electron microscopic study, *J. Bone Joint Surg., 59B:* 465, 1977.
23. Kite, J. H.: Congenital talipes equinovarus, *J. Bone Joint Surg., 39A:* 282, 1957.
24. Kite, J. H.: Congenital metatarsus varus, *J. Bone Joint Surg., 49A:* 388, 1967.
25. Lapidus, P.: Operative correction of the metatarsus varus primus in hallux valgus, *Surg. Gynecol. Obstet., 58:* 183, 1934.
26. Lapidus, P.: Spastic flat foot, *J. Bone Joint Surg., 28:* 126, 1946.
27. Lovell, W.: The non-operative management of the congenital clubfoot, Presented at the Annual Dillehunt Lecture, Portland, Oregon, 1977.
28. Lusted, L. B., and Keats, T. E.: *Atlas of Roentgenographic Measurements,* Ed. 2; Chicago: Year Book Medical Publishers, 1967.
29. Menelaus, M. B.: *The Orthopaedic Management of Spina Bifida Cystica;* Edinburgh: E. & S. Livingstone, 1971.
30. Menelaus, M. B.: Talectomy for equinovarus deformity in arthrogryposis and spina bifida, *J. Bone Joint Surg., 53B:* 468, 1971.
31. Mitchell, L., Fleming, J., Allen, R., Glenney, C., and

Sanford, G.: Osteotomy-bunionectomy for hallux valgus, *J. Bone Joint Surg., 40A:* 41, 1958.

32. Osmond-Clark, H.: Congenital vertical talus, *J. Bone Joint Surg., 38B:* 334, 1956.

33. Puluska, D. Ankle valgus after the Grice subtalar stabilization, *Clin. Orthop., 59:* 137, 1968.

34. Silver, D.: The operative treatment of hallux valgus, *J. Bone Joint Surg., 5:* 225, 1923.

35. Simons, G. External rotational deformities in clubfeet, *Clin. Orthop,* 176: 239, 1977.

36. Smith, W., Hunter, S., and Whatley, J.: The tibialis posterior—a dynamic support of the plantar arch, Presented at the Annual Meeting of the American Orthopaedic Foot Society, February 21, 1979.

37. Thomason, J.: Treatment of congenital flat foot, *J. Bone Joint Surg., 28:* 787, 1946.

38. Turco, V. J.: Surgical correction of resistant clubfoot, *J. Bone Joint Surg., 53A:* 477, 1971.

39. Turco, V.: *Surgical Treatment of Resistant Clubfeet,* American Academy of Orthopaedic Surgeons, Instructional Courses, Dallas, 1978.

40. Whitman, R.: The operative treatment of paralytic talipes of the calcaneus type, *Trans. Am. Orthop. Assoc., 14:* 178, 1901.

41. Williams, P., and Menelaus, M.: Triple arthrodesis by inlay grafting—a method suitable for the undeformed valgus foot, *J. Bone Joint Surg., 59B:* 333, 1977.

CHAPTER 5

The Knee

It is well to mention at the outset that knee pain in children may not be a symptom of pathology centered at the knee. Hip joint pathology frequently gives rise to knee pain. Foot strain may sometimes seem to rise to knee symptoms.

Lesions of the knee in children include entities such as osteochondritis dissecans, discoid meniscus, and Osgood-Schlatter disease. Popliteal cysts or Baker's cysts cause swelling posteriorly at the knee. Monarticular arthritis, a rheumatoid-like lesion, occurs most commonly at the knee. Foreign bodies sometimes give rise to a chronic swelling at the knee. Septic arthritis and tuberculous synovitis are not uncommon.

POSITIONAL DEFORMITIES

Apparent Bowlegs

The infant with an almost constant flexion of the hips and knees·can give an appearance of bowleggedness to the family. The internal tibial torsion that accompanies this flexion accentuates the appearance because it turns the soft tissues lateralward and the foot inward (Fig. 5.1). If the examiner hides the foot with one hand and pulls the soft tissues of the calf medialward and then fully extends the knee, it can be appreciated that the knee actually gives a position of valgus to the tibia. The tibia is straight, and it is safe to tell the family that, by the age of 3 years, the youngster will actually be somewhat knock-kneed.

It must also be noted that when the infant first stands, the hips are in external rotation while the foot is straight or turned in, and the apparent bowleggedness is thus further accentuated (Fig. 5.2). Because of the wide-based stance of infancy, the viewer situated in front of the child actually sees the medial aspect of the flexed leg. Telling the family this in advance helps to allay their fears.

Aside from prescribing corrective shoes, the physician should refrain from treating the infant. He should persuade everyone concerned to wait for growth to occur. One often suspects that the hardest principle to observe in raising children is that of allowing them to grow out of difficult stages, whether the difficulty is physical or psychologic.

The internal tibial torsion results in a varus facing of the ankle joint. Secondarily, the child must pronate when he attempts to stand. During this period, shoes with Thomas heels and ⅛-inch inner heel wedges to carry the foot in line with the ankle joint are important. They prevent overstretching of the ligament of the medial side of the foot.

Uterine Packing Syndrome

The name that is given this bowing deformity of the lower extremities implies that the etiology is known. It has been thought that this particular deformity was the result of intrauterine crowding because of its spontaneous tendency to correct and a lack of associated anomalies.

CLINICAL FINDINGS

It is important to distinguish just what deformity is included in this syndrome. Clinically, a varus bow of the distal tibia and fibula is evident. The lower leg is not the only site of involvement, however, for the thigh may exhibit an isolated bow. The lower leg and thigh deformities do not ordinarily occur together.

ROENTGEN APPEARANCE

The important diagnostic feature is readily evident on the roentgen film of the lower extremities (Fig. 5.3). Both tibia and fibula are bowed symmetrically at the same level. There is no associated abnormality of the bone such as increased density or widening

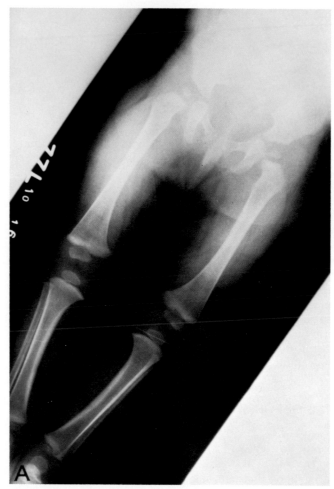

Figure 5.1. The difference in position of the tibia relative to the femur is apparent when standing in children with positional tibia vara. (*A*) Recumbent film shows accentuated medial cortex on tibia. Epiphyseal growth centers are normal. (*B*) On weight bearing, the knee joint opens up laterally due to the tilt of the tibia medialward. The foot pronates secondarily.

of the cortex to obscure the medullary canal. Such narrowing of the medullary cavity as may occur is only that brought on by the physical deformation. The curve of the bow is rounded, not angular.

TREATMENT

The most important aspect of treatment is accurate recognition of the condition. Once the physician is certain of the diagnosis, it is fundamental to understand that active use of the limb will correct the deformity. Casts or braces are not indicated. If the limb is left free and the infant allowed full activity, the deformity will correct itself over the first year of growth.

Developmental Genu Valgum

Valgus at the knee is a natural and normal phase of development. Although often present at birth, it is masked by internal torsion of the tibia and flexion at the knee and hips in the first 2 years of life. When internal torsion of the tibia is combined with a wide and externally rotated stance of the lower extremities, the child may appear to have bowlegs. After walking starts, by holding the

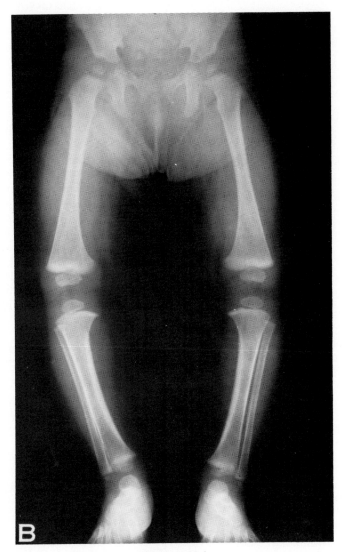

Fig. 5.1 (*B*)

legs straight and rotating the knee so that it faces forward, one can appreciate the true genu valgum (Fig. 5.4).

Developmental valgus at the knee is most marked in the age group of 2–5 years. It has a natural tendency to improve, except in children who are the victims of underlying growth disturbances. Some valgus remains into adult life owing to the medial deviation of the femur from its lateral position at the side of the pelvis.

Valgus at the knee of this type is recognized by its symmetry. It rarely exceeds 20 degrees at each knee. Its presence in children 2–5 years old is to be expected.

An x-ray of the knee helps to separate from the group with symmetric valgus those rare individuals who have an underlying disease affecting growth, such as rickets. Asymmetric or unilateral valgus demands a thorough search for the underlying cause.

TREATMENT

Pronated feet often accompany the genu valgum. Medial arch pads combined with ⅛-inch inner heel wedges are indicated in an attempt to keep the heel inverted and to prevent the development of further valgus (Fig. 5.5). These simple measures often seem

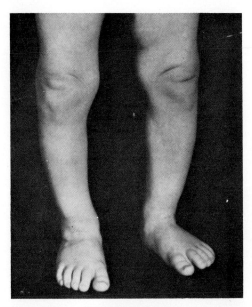

Figure 5.2. Stance with tibia vara—external rotation at the hips, internal tibial torsion with medial inclination of the ankle joint, and secondary pronation of the feet to bring the foot flat on the floor and straight ahead.

but a small obstacle to put in the path of the obvious stress of weight bearing. It is perhaps fortunate that improvement is in most cases naturally indicated. Osteotomy for the correction of symmetric developmental valgus has not been indicated in our experience. Braces with built-in correction that bends the knee over a medial pad seem to us nothing but a means of crowding an emotional disability on top of a normal difficulty of growth.

OSTEOCHONDRITIS DISSECANS

Osteochondritis dissecans is known in adults, but, in the presence of intermittent disability at the knee, it must be considered in children. It is most common in males, at least one-third of the cases are bilateral, and it has a tendency to be symmetric. The lateral aspect of the medial femoral condyle is the most common site (Fig. 5.6) although rarely it can occur in the lateral condyle and in the patella. Osteochondritis dissecans occurs at the ankle, hip, and elbow, but it is so frequent at the knee that it is rarely though of at other

joints prior to roentgenogram. It has not been reported below the age of 4 and may be confused with irregular ossification of the condyle in young children.

Pathology

From the pathologic point of view, the lesion appears to be an aseptic necrosis of the subchondral bone for a variable, but usually quite shallow, depth. The cartilage is not primarily involved, but becomes so when its underlying support is weakened (Fig. 5.7). It is possible on viewing the lesion to find that the articular cartilage is intact and yet the typical roentgenographic changes are present. The cartilage overlying the lesion secondarily develops fibrillation and cleaves from the cartilage areas that are well supported by normal subchondral bone. The fragment that

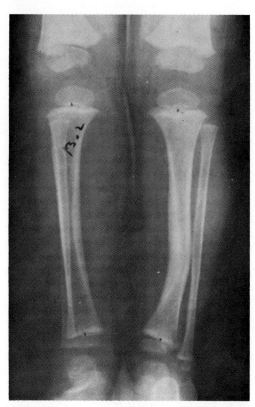

Figure 5.3. Intrauterine packing syndrome. There is no abnormality at either metaphysis of the tibia, and the bowing is gradually straightening out with growth and full activity.

separates includes subchondral bone and cartilage.

Etiology

It is assumed that the lesion develops because of localized interference with the blood supply to the area. The lesion has been likened to that which would occur if a small area of a hollow sphere were indented and then allowed to spring back into place. If the lesion is allowed to heal on a conservative regime, it does so by creeping substitution. The etiology is not clear, but trauma seems to be the initiating factor.

Clinical Picture

Most characteristic perhpas is the intermittency of the symptoms. Recurrent pain at the knee is the presenting complaint, and there is a further history of clicking, giving way, and intermittent swelling at the knee. If a fragment has become detached, previous mild symptoms may be unnoticed in the acute and sudden onset of pain and swelling at the knee.

Depending on the duration of symptoms, a variable degree of atrophy of the thigh may occur. Such atrophy reflects the disability that the patient has undergone. Fluid may be

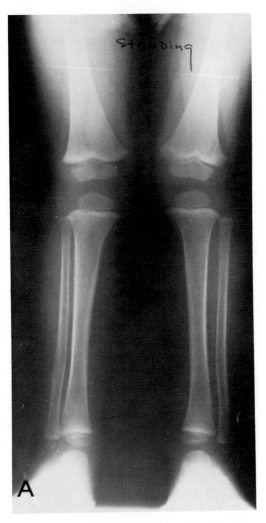 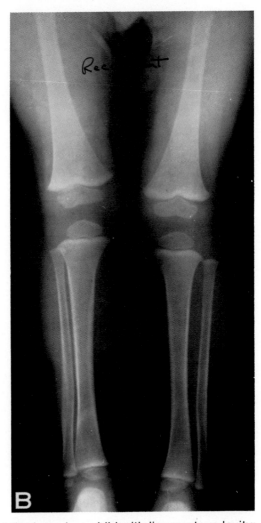

Figure 5.4. The effect of weight bearing at the knee in a child with ligamentous laxity: (A) weight bearing, (B) recumbent. Valgus is apparent on standing.

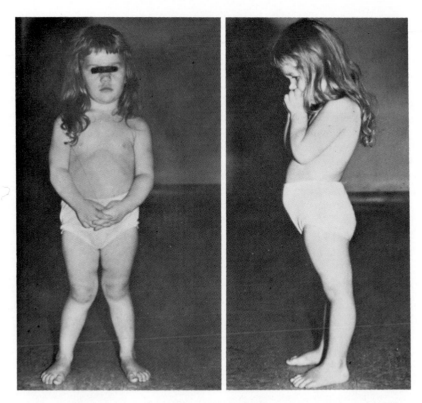

Figure 5.5. (*Left*) Developmental genu valgum with fairly severe deformity. The child stands with pronated feet as well. Surgery is not indicated at this age, but the feet should be supported with medial arch pads and medial heel wedges in the shoes. (*Right*) Lateral view of a child with developmental genu valgum. The hyperextended knees are seen. The general posture is typical of a child with excessive ligamentous laxity.

noted in the knee, but diagnostically most pertinent is localized tenderness on the lateral aspect of the medial condyle (Fig. 5.8). The intermittent symptoms may be the only reason for clinical attention, for there may be no signs of apparent disability.

Roentgen Findings

There is involvement of the subchondral bone. A radiolucent line separates a small dense fragment of this bone from the parent area. A minimal amount of reactive bone may be found about the lesion. The lesion may not be clearly visualized in the usual anteroposterior view of the knee. A so-called "tunnel" view—taken posteroanteriorly—with the knee flexed approximately 30 degrees is helpful in throwing the area most commonly involved into relief. When the patella is involved, a tangential view of it may be helpful. Irregular ossification of the medial condyle is

a normal finding in the 2- to 6-year old age group.

Treatment

Green and Banks[1] have called attention to the fact that the lesion may be treated conservatively with a non-weight-bearing regime with good results. Such treatment, which uses a non-weight-bearing splint or brace, involves a healing period of approximately 4–6 months and perhaps longer. The opportunity it offers of achieving an intact articular surface makes this conservative regime the treatment of choice, as compared to surgical excision, which of necessity leaves a cartilage defect. For patients under 10, in whom detachment is unlikely, this is the treatment of choice.

Operative treatment has been frequently advocated and is followed by good results. It has the advantage of requiring a shorter pe-

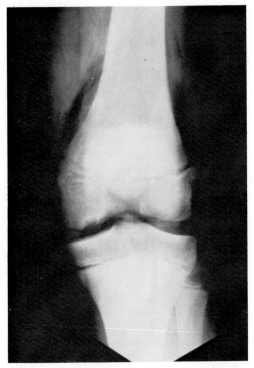

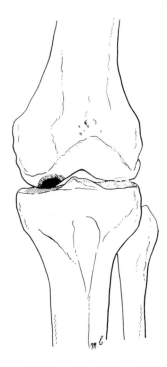

Figure 5.6. Air injection of the knee reveals a defect in the medial femoral condyle with a fragment loose in the center of the joint.

Figure 5.8. Diagram of characteristic site of osteochondritis dissecans slightly toward the lateral aspect of the medial femoral condyle.

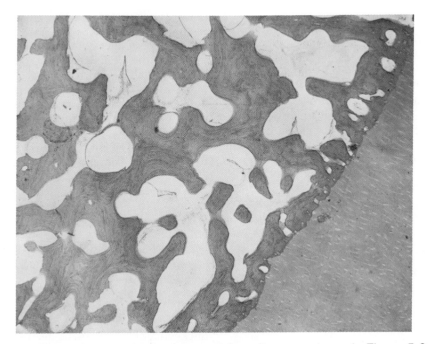

Figure 5.7. Photomicrograph of a fragment from the case shown in Figure 5.6 shows dead bone and articular cartilage.

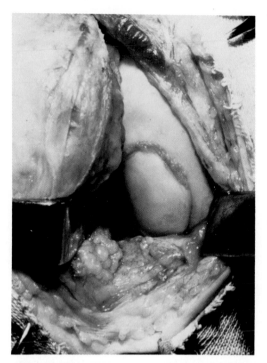

Figure 5.9. A large osteochondritic fragment involving the lateral surface of the medial condyle. Fragments of this magnitude are seen in the older age group, in this case at 16 years.

riod of convalescence—usually about 6 weeks. If the fragment of subchondral bone and cartilage has become detached, its removal is indicated. If it is still partially attached, the lesion, when visualized, can be readily eased from the surrounding bone. A cleavage plane of fibrous tissue exists between the fragment and the parent bone.

When the cartilage is completely intact, the area of subchondral weakness can be recognized by palpation and by a slight grayish discoloration. The lesion is cored out so that it has smooth edges and so that no unattached cartilage or bone remains. Drilling the base of the lesion may result in unwelcome exuberant repair; it is not recommended.

Actual detachment of a separate fragment is so rare below age 10 that operative therapy is ordinarily done in the teenage group (Fig. 5.9).

Reference

1. Green, W. T., and Banks, H.: Osteochondritis dissecans in children, *J. Bone Joint Surg.*, 35A: 26, 1953.

DISCOID MENISCUS

Congenital "discoid" meniscus is a lesion of the cartilaginous meniscus of the knee occurring primarily in the lateral meniscus.

Normal Development

It has been stated that the meniscus originally consists of a complete disc. Kaplan[1] disputed this as a result of his fetal dissections, stating that the meniscus assumes its adult form immediately on differentiation of the structure. The intermediate zone between the femur and tibia that appears early in embryologic development is called the intermediate disc. The disc does not break up into two separate discs, according to Kaplan, but directly into two semilunar menisci. The theory that the central portion of the originally disc-shaped structure wears away thus becomes untenable. Normally (in humans) both the lateral and the medial meniscus are attached to the tibia both anteriorly and posteriorly on the intercondylar ridge.

Etiology

Dissection of animals enabled Kaplan to point out that none of the animals has a discoid meniscus except those in which the lateral meniscus normally is not attached posteriorly to the tibia, but instead continues via the ligament of Wrisberg to attach posteriorly to the lateral face of the medial femoral condyle (meniscofemoral ligament). Knees in animals are adapted to the flexed position, whereas, in humans, knees are used primarily in extension. The lateral meniscus in anthropoids is almost completely circular, but never discoid.

In humans, lack of attachment of the lateral meniscus to the tibia is an anomaly that leaves the ligament of Wrisberg the sole posterior attachment. In extension, this short ligament fails to allow the meniscus to glide forward. As extension takes place, the lateral meniscus is pulled into the intercondylar area. Persistent action of this type wears a groove in the center of the cartilage as the meniscus is drawn into the joint. Secondary thickening of the meniscus due to hyperplasia and the formation of fibrocartilage results in a deeper than normal cartilaginous meniscus with a ridge on either side of the groove (Figs. 5.10 and 5.11). The original depth of the meniscus is not greater than normal, but development and use of the knee secondarily results in increased apparent depth.

Clinical Picture

Classically, as emphasized in the literature, the primary complaint is a "snapping knee," In the early years of childhood such complaints are vague indeed, and the diagnosis is usually not made until the eighth or ninth year. By this time the displacement of the cartilage that occurs as the knee is extended results in a very audible "clunk" in the knee, and an anterior prominence can be felt when the "clunk" is heard. The motion of the cartilage can be palpated anteriorly at the joint line. Older children may complain of a "giving way" of the knee. Rarely there may be episodes of swelling at the knee, and fluid may be palpable on examination. The author has never seen this lesion in the medial meniscus. It is a rare condition usually found only once a year in a large children's orthopaedic service. As time goes on, the symptoms are sufficiently severe to curtail the youngster's activities.

Treatment

Excision of the disc is justified on the basis of the abnormal mechanics it introduces at the knee. The recovery period following such an excision is greatly shortened if the youngster has been taught quadriceps-setting exercises prior to surgery. It is difficult to teach these exercises immediately after the operation when the child has a painful knee.

Kaplan,[1] in his excellent article, pointed out that an abnormal meniscus of the lateral joint compartment in children, compared to the same lesion in adults, is difficult to excise. He recommended making two incisions: a posterior one to divide the meniscofemoral ligament of Wrisberg, and an anterolateral one. The posterior incision needs to be really posterior if it is going to be done at all. Coming down on the lateral head of the gastrocnemius, the operator, standing posterior to the biceps tendon, retracts it. The joint is entered, and the posterior attachment via the meniscofemoral ligament is divided. To compromise by remaining lateral and anterior to the biceps tendon results in poor visualization of the ligament. The anterolateral excision is simple and usual. An attempt to remove the meniscus by means of an anterior approach alone is unsuccessful be-

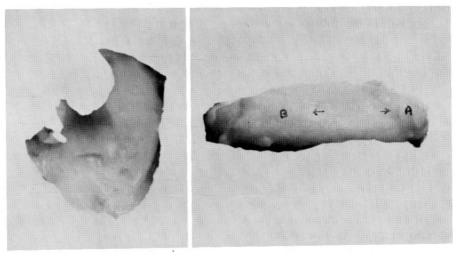

Figure 5.10 (*Left*). Discoid lateral meniscus with ridge due to fibrocartilaginous hypertrophy beginning at the periphery.

Figure 5.11 (*Right*). Lateral view with free edge of the meniscus toward the reader. A ridge forming both anteriorly (*A*) and posteriorly (*B*) can be discerned.

cause the usual more proximal posterior attachment is not present and because the posterior meniscofemoral attachment cannot be visualized when the anterior incision alone is made.

Crutch walking is begun when the foot can be lifted from the bed while the knee is extended. Full activity is allowed in the presence of full motion and a strong quadriceps and in the absence of swelling at the knee. The approximate period of convalescence for a child is 6 weeks.

References

1. Kaplan, E. B.: Discoid lateral meniscus of the knee joint; nature, mechanism and operative treatment, J. Bone Joint Surg., 39A: 77, 1957.
2. Smillie, I. S.: The congenital discoid meniscus, J. Bone Joint Surg., 30B: 671, 1948.

OSGOOD-SCHLATTER DISEASE

Osgood-Schlatter disease, a disease of adolescence, causes pain anteriorly at the knee. Osgood first called attention to the enlargement of the tibial apophysis in 1903. The entity is best understood when thought of as a tendinosis, rather than as an apophysitis, however. Hughes notes that the common feature by roentgenogram is calcification within, or enlargement of the ligamentum patellae. The disease is self-limited and runs a 2- to 3-year course. The age of incidence is from 10–16 years. It is slightly more common in males, and unilateral cases occur twice as often as bilateral ones.

Etiology

A history of an extremely rapid growth spurt in the year preceding the onset of symptoms is to be expected. One suspects that the increased soft-tissue tension produced by very rapid growth causes abnormal stress at the apophysis of the tibia. Such stress is directly transmitted by the ligamentum patellae. There is a resultant swelling of the tendon at its insertion and, secondarily, an irregular ossification. Changes very similar to those caused by Osgood-Schlatter disease can be produced in the rat by shortening the patellar tendon. The disease in humans ceases with fusion of the apophysis to the

parent bone, if it is still active when this fusion occurs. Growth plays an important part in the etiology by producing abnormal stress at the tibial apophysis. It is possible that trauma to the tibial tubercle may also produce such stress.

Clinical Picture

The history reveals that the discomfort is experienced with activity and decreases with rest. Sports which involve much running and jumping are particularly likely to produce exacerbations of the disease. A rapid growth spurt is common in the year preceding onset. Discomfort and swelling are located anteriorly in the region of the tibial apophysis. There is not swelling that involves the joint itself. Thickening and enlargement of the tibial tubercle are characteristic (Fig. 5.12).

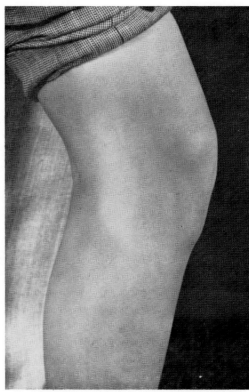

Figure 5.12. Swelling in the area in which the patellar tendon inserts into the tibial tubercle in a case of Osgood-Schlatter disease.

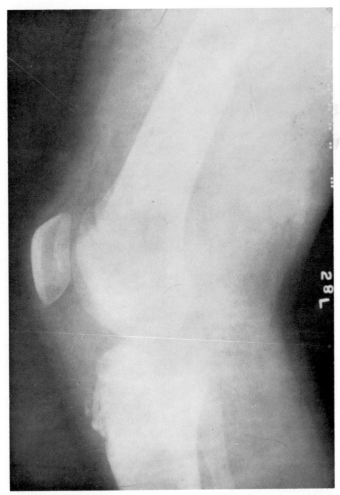

Figure 5.13. Swelling at the patellar tendon insertion and fragmentation of the tibial apophysis, as seen by roentgenogram. The soft-tissue reaction seen here is characteristic of Osgood-Schlatter disease.

Careful palpation reveals tenderness at the point of insertion of the tendon into the bone, but not over the apophysis itself. Extreme flexion is painful. Atrophy of the quadriceps is not remarkable unless the symptoms have been severe.

Roentgen Findings

In males, the apophysis ordinarily appears at the age of 11 and fuses with the parent epiphysis at 15. It is most hazardous to base the diagnosis on irregular ossification of the apophysis because this kind of irregularity may be part of normal development. The one constant finding is swelling of the tendon shadow where the tendon inserts into the bone (Figs. 5.13 and 5.14). The swelling frequently obliterates the angle formed by the tendon and the bone. In some cases adventitious ossification may proceed into the tendon itself.

Treatment

The discrepancy in functional length between soft tissue and bone may take 2–3 years to adjust. If the abnormal stress of soft tissues disappears, the symptoms may cease even before fusion of the apophysis with the parent bone takes place. When the symptoms are severe, rest is enforced by strapping the

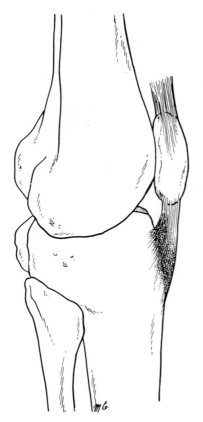

Figure 5.14. Diagram of the area of swelling in Osgood-Schlatter disease. The swelling of the distal portion of the patellar tendon appears to precede the bony changes.

knee with adhesive. If necessary, a walking plaster cast in the form of a cylinder may be applied.

Voluntary limitation of activities may often be obtained in this age group, particularly when the relationship between activity and symptoms is pointed out to the patient and his or her parents. The patient may remain ambulatory but should abstain from sports, running, and long walks. The relationship between activity and symptoms is a very direct one and is readily appreciated by the patient once it is pointed out. Limitation of activity is usually necessary for a period of only approximately 6 months. Once the functional length of the soft tissues has caught up with that of the bone, the patient can enter into full activity with impunity. Hydrocortone injected into the swollen area may give symptomatic relief in cases of acute inflammation.

Thickening and enlargement of the apophysis persist even after the disease heals and symptoms subside. The enlargement itself may be a source of discomfort in kneeling that persists after the disease is no longer active.

POPLITEAL CYSTS

Popliteal cysts have also been named "Baker's cysts." Baker[1] in 1877 described cases of swelling in the popliteal space and thought that perhaps they were herniations of the knee joint space that had been chronically distended by fluid. Faucher, in 1856, had described 11 dissected specimens under the impression that they represented distension of bursae located in the region of the medial head of the gastrocnemiosemimembranosus bursa that had become filled with fluid as a result of chronic irritation.

These cysts are not uncommon in children, for about one-third of the cases occur in the 1- to 15-year age group. They are most common in males (by a ratio of 2:1) and are ordinarily unilateral. The etiology of these cysts in adults may be quite different from that in children. Most children have a history of no previous effusion or symptoms at the knee when the cyst is discovered.

Clinical Picture

The complaint, in children, is the swelling itself. There are no symptoms of the knee joint dysfunction. In the adult, these cysts are often associated with osteoarthritis. The symptoms referable to the knees are usually based on the arthritis, and these symtpoms are due to the arthritis itself.

Because it is very difficult to palpate the popliteal area, the physician may often be misled into believing that a cyst exists. In general, when one does exist, there is no doubt. The swelling tends to lie distal to the knee crease and on the medial side of the posterior aspect of the knee (Figs. 5.15–5.17).

Roentgen Findings

The x-ray picture should be of help in confirming the clinical impression. A

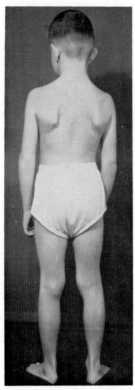

Figure 5.15. Popliteal cyst, posterior view.

smoothly outlined swelling of fluid density is present in the popliteal space and can be noted particularly in contrast with the picture of the other knee. The fact that the cysts are rarely bilateral is of great help.

Treatment

Excision is recommended in the usual case. Wilson et al.[2] dissected the gastrocnemi-osemimembranosus bursa in 1938 and pointed out the anatomic relationship of this bursa to the popliteal cyst (Fig. 5.18). Invariably there is an intimate attachment of the bursa to the tendinous portion of the medial head of the gastrocnemius and semimembranosus muscles, requiring a partial resection of these structures in order to maintain the cyst wall. The cysts often communicate with the knee joint capsule through an opening on the proximal portion of the medial condyle beneath the medial head of the gastrocnemius. Wilson stated that this connection was found in 15 of 21 operated cysts and in 17 of 30 anatomic specimens of the bursa.

Examination of the cyst walls after removal reveals fibrous thickening, areas of retained hemosiderin, and areas of metaplasia into cartilaginous and osteoid elements.

References

1. Baker, W. M.: On the formation of synovial cysts in the leg in connection with disease of the knee joint, St. Barth. Hosp. Rep., 13: 245, 1877.
2. Wilson, P. D., Eyre Brook, A. L., and Francis, J. D.: A clinical and anatomical study of the semimembranosus bursa in relation to popliteal cyst, J. Bone Joint Surg., 20: 963, 1938.

MONARTICULAR ARTHRITIS

Monarticular arthritis consists of chronic synovial thickening. The joint fluid findings are similar to those in rheumatoid arthritis but are limited to one joint. The anomaly may occur at other areas, such as the ankle, hip, and elbow but is so characteristic at the knee that it is fully described in this chapter (Fig. 5.19). The age group affected is not well defined, but most cases occur between 5 and 10 years of age. The disease is slightly more common in females.

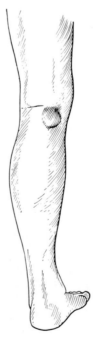

Figure 5.16. Diagram of popliteal cyst location—medial posterior aspect of knee, inferior to knee crease.

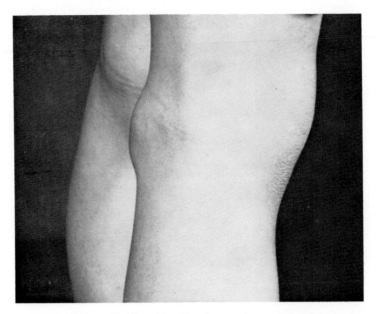

Figure 5.17.   Popliteal cyst, lateral view.

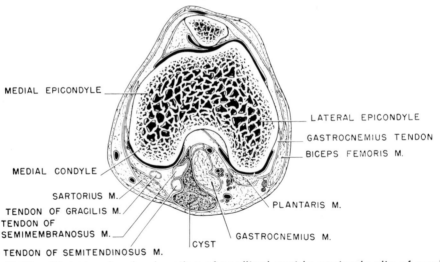

MEDIAL EPICONDYLE

LATERAL EPICONDYLE

GASTROCNEMIUS TENDON

BICEPS FEMORIS M.

MEDIAL CONDYLE

SARTORIUS M.

TENDON OF GRACILIS M.

TENDON OF
SEMIMEMBRANOSUS M.

PLANTARIS M.

GASTROCNEMIUS M.

CYST

TENDON OF SEMITENDINOSUS M.

Figure 5.18.   Diagram showing location of popliteal cyst in anatomic site of semimembranosus bursa. (Redrawn from P. D. Wilson, A. L. Eyre-Brook, and J. D. Francis: Clinical anatomical study of semimembranosus bursa in relation to popliteal cyst, *Journal of Bone and Joint Surgery, 20:*963, 1938.)

Etiology

The etiology is very closely related to that of rheumatoid arthritis—so closely that some cases under observation are noted to develop other involvement. Imperceptibly, thickening and fluid develop at other joints and obtain the more typical rheumatoid distribution. Aspiration of fluid from the joint reveals cellular chemical changes similar to those found in rheumatoid arthritis. Nonetheless, this entity is very frequently limited to one joint and remains so. Amelioration of symptoms is possible with intelligent care.

Clinical Picture

The child presents chronic swelling of the knee often of several weeks' or months' duration (Fig. 5.20). Pain is not a prominent feature, but a limp is usually noted by the parents. The knee reveals synovial thickening, and fluid in the suprapatellar pouch produces a ballottable patella and a fluid wave in examination. There is increased heat and moderate tenderness of the anatomic area occupied by the joint. The knee lacks 10–20 degrees of full extension. Full flexion is also limited. There is palpable and measurable atrophy of the quadriceps.

Laboratory Findings

Laboratory work reveals an increased sedimentation rate and occasionally a mild leukocytosis. Aspiration of the joint may reveal a considerable elevation of polymorphonuclear cells, and the total cell count may reach 3,000–4,000 cells per mm^3. The joint sugar may be depressed in relation to the blood sugar taken at the same time—that is, by more than 20 mg/100 ml. A positive tuberculin test (in the absence of a clear-cut clinical differentiation from tuberculosis) may necessitate biopsy of the joint to establish the diagnosis.

Treatment

The child often walks with a knee flexion contracture (Fig. 5.21). This position of strain in weight bearing does not help a low grade condition of this type to clear. Traction is often advisable to secure full extension. Bi-valved plaster casts may be used with non-weight-bearing exercises to secure the same result.

Rest is still the therapy of choice for monarticular arthritis, although Hydrocortone injected into the joint may be of some help. Absolute rest from weight bearing is achieved by means of a bivalved cast or a removable splint holding the knee just off full extension.

It is important that the parents understand the chronicity of the lesion. The child is usually at rest for 4 months and gradually resumes weight bearing (with crutches) in the following 2 months. Signs of recurrence of fluid are regularly sought, and the sedimentation rate is checked.

The joint, handled tenderly and slowly, responds first by losing its fluid and thereafter by a gain in the range of motion, loss of heat, and subsidence of most of the synovial thickening. Some slight thickening may remain. Rest during the early months includes complete bed rest, and a home teacher should be arranged for if the patient is of school age.

A careful and gradual resumption of activity of the joint is usually rewarded by complete cure, except in those cases that pass gradually over into rheumatoid arthritis.

FOREIGN BODY KNEE

A picture very similar to that of monarticular arthritis is sometimes seen in a patient with a history of marked trauma in the

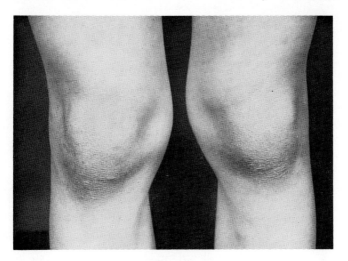

Figure 5.19. Swelling of the suprapatellar area due to synovial thickening and fluid.

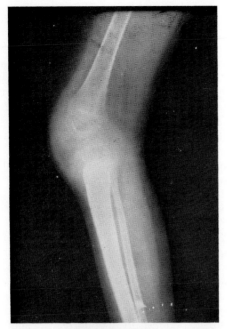

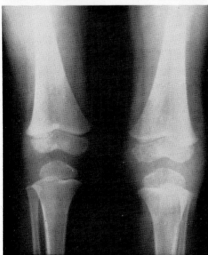

fluid often contains an unusual amount of fibrin clot.

Incision into the joint reveals a large fibrin clot filling the suprapatellar pouch. This knee may require synovectomy of the accessible portions of the joint to effect a cure. The synovectomy must be followed by traction and physiotherapy, including range-of-motion exercises and active exercises of the quadriceps musculature, to effect a good result. Synovectomy should not be undertaken

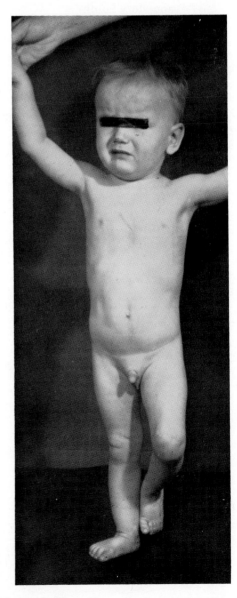

Figure 5.20. Lateral and anterior view of knee in monarticular arthritis. There is thickening of the capsular shadows about the joint and posterior subluxation of the tibia.

months immediately preceding consultation. The trauma is such that pieces of glass, wood, cinders, or clothing might have been driven into the knee (Fig. 5.22).

The patient has a unilateral chronic, swollen knee. X-ray may reveal small bits of foreign body, but often it does not. The joint

Figure 5.21. Knee flexion contracture in ambulant child.

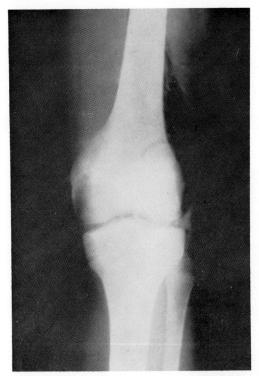

Figure 5.22. Air arthrogram of knee with pieces of glass present laterally and in the femoral notch.

until it has been demonstrated that removal of the fibrin clot and accessible foreign material will not effect a cure.

SEPTIC ARTHRITIS OF KNEE

Septic arthritis is not as common in the knee as in the hip because the metaphyseal area of the knee is nto enclosed within the joint.

Etiology

When acute, it is most often blood borne—a complication of a severe childhood septicemia. In patients below the age of 1, the most likely etiologic agent is the Streptococcus; the older age group is more often involved with the Staphylococcus. Direct involvement of the knee by foreign bodies following puncture wounds gives rise to a low grade type of septic arthritis that is frequently a puzzling diagnostic problem.

Clinical Picture

The acute septic knee gives rise to apprehension, pain at the knee, elevated temperature, and increased pulse—the signs of sepsis. The swollen joint is extremely tender to palpation. The knee is held in a flexed position, and there is marked hamstring spasm. Swelling is most apparent in the region of the suprapatellar pouch.

JOINT FLUID FINDINGS

Aspiration reveals a white, cloudy to thick, purulent fluid. Cells usually number more than 4,000 per mm^3, and almost all of them are polymorphonuclear. Smear with a Gram stain frequently reveals the organism.

The fluid clots on standing; it contains increased protein and frequently clumps of fibrin. The joint sugar is depressed more than 20 mg/100 ml below the blood sugar taken at the same time.

Aspiration is performed from the lateral side into the suprapatellar pouch just proximal to the upper pole of the patella (Fig. 5.23). A needle (at least 19 gauge and preferably 18 gauge) such as that used for spinal puncture is most valuable. The aspiration is likely to be more successful if pressure is exerted on the joint and the fluid is milked out rather than withdrawn by suction. Chemotherapeutic agents in appropriate concentration may be inserted into the joint after aspiration. Both anaerobic and aerobic cultures should be made of joint fluid. In a small percentage of joints, the suprapatellar bursa does not communicate with the joint space, and aspiration must be done into the joint space on either side of the patella at its lower pole.

Treatment

The patient is made comfortable by traction in line with the flexion deformity of the knee. Such traction is most simply accomplished by means of both a sling under the knee and a foot strap; this method is called split Russell traction.

Following aspiration, chemotherapy of the sort indicated for the suspected organism is instituted. As a rule the symptoms tend to subside rapidly. Intra-articular insertion of

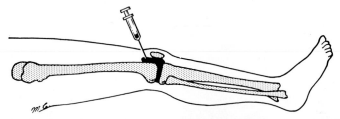

Figure 5.23.   Aspiration of knee from suprapatellar pouch. In a small percentage of cases, the pouch does not communicate with the knee joint itself.

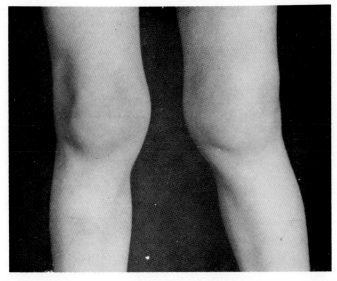

Figure 5.24.   Synovial tuberculosis of the knee. The normal anatomic outlines proximal to the patella have been obliterated by swelling of the suprapatellar pouch on the right.

the chemotherapeutic agent may be continued. In some cases the suprapatellar pouch and joint remain thick and boggy. The temperature continues to hover at a slight elevation, and the sedimentation rate remains elevated. It may be necessary to drain the joint if symptoms do not rapidly subside. Incision into the joint reveals it to be filled with fibrin clot. Once the joint is emptied, the synovia is repaired with plain catgut. A catheter for the instillation of appropriate chemotherapy may be left in place, but the remainder of the wound is repaired per primam. The expected course is subsidence of symptoms.

TUBERCULOSIS OF KNEE

Tuberculosis at the knee in childhood occurs in a typical form which must be differentiated from other causes of chronic joint effusion.

Etiology

The disease is metastatic to the knee following primary involvement of the lung and is due to the tubercle bacillus originally described by Koch in 1882.

Pathology

It is most common for the synovia to be involved initially (Figs. 5.24 and 5.25). Rarely the epiphysis of either the femur or tibia is first involved, and the synovia is involved secondarily. In the typical early case the synovia, which is markedly redundant, tends to fill the joint space. There is an increased amount of joint fluid. The synovia tends to have a grayish discoloration, but when viewed at operation under tourniquet, it appears plum colored. Tubercle formation is usually not visible in the gross but is seen microscopically (Fig. 5.26). The articular cartilage appears uninvolved, although this appearance may be deceptive. The portions that are involved are usually covered with adherent synovial membrane.

It should be remembered that tuberculosis has a tendency to extend subchondrally, leaving the cartilage relatively uninvolved but separated from the subchondral bone by underlying granulation tissue. Rheumatoid arthritis, on the other hand, extends suprachondrally, covering the cartilage with pannus.

In late cases there is extensive involvement of the ligamentous structures. The result is great disorganization of the joint. Such progression of the disease leaves little hope for preservation of the joint as a functioning structure. There is ordinarily a history of exposure to an individual suffering from tuberculosis or a record of previous involvement, which may include tuberculous glands or meningitis, as well as disease of the lungs.

Clinical Picture

It is usual to see the patient after swelling of the knee has been noted for several months. Pain is not a prominent feature in synovial tuberculosis seen at the knee.

Palpation reveals a plastic type of protuberance in the suprapatellar region. Areas in which the synovia can be palpated are thickened and tender. A fluid wave can often be demonstrated. There is usually a flexion contracture of the joint.

The tuberculin test is positive. Where the disease is suspected, it is best to begin testing with a dilution of 1:100,000. The sedimentation rate is elevated, and the white blood cell count, although not markedly elevated, frequently reveals a lymphocytes-to-monocytes ratio of well over 5 or 6:1.

Aspiration of the joint reveals white cells ranging from about 1,000 to 2,000 per mm^3 and preponderantly polymorphonuclear. The fluid is slightly cloudy to turbid and may contain flecks of fibrin. The joint sugar is usually more than 20 mg/100 ml lower than a blood sugar count taken at the same time.

Roentgen Findings

There is a shadow of water density filling in the suprapatellar pouch area and rounding out the normal anatomic shadows of the joint (Fig. 5.25). Signs of chronicity are apparent in the demineralized bone. In cases of fairly long duration, the joint space is narrow. Rarely an area of bone destruction may be seen in the epiphysis. However, areas of bone destruction may usually be seen in the subchondral region running linearly.

Treatment

The absolute rest of joints that has been enforced on tuberculous patients since the disease was first recognized remains a dominant treatment to the present day. Joint fusion was developed to aid in obtaining complete rest and healing of the disease. Such fusions save the epiphyseal discs, but in children they sometimes cause progressive de-

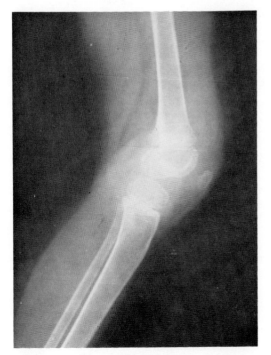

Figure 5.25. Thickened capsular shadows and filling of suprapatellar pouch area with shadows of soft-tissue density in synovial tuberculosis of the knee.

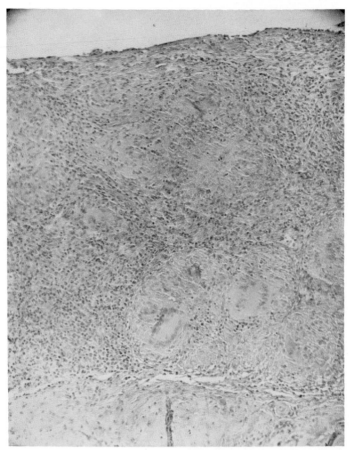

Figure 5.26. Synovial tuberculosis of the knee. The joint surface is at the top; tubercle formation, mononuclear phagocytes, lymphocytes, and giant cells are seen below.

formity at the knee. The soft bone in this area allows considerable flexion to develop.

A unilateral hip spica is necessary to secure rest for the knee and should be applied after biopsy is performed. Biopsy is usually necessary to confirm the diagnosis. The current tendency is to try to preserve knee motion under the cover of the chemotherapy of tuberculosis. There is no reason to abandon rest as a principle, however, and to do so leads to recurrences of the disease.

The spica is bivalved and fixed with canvas straps; the leg is removed from it twice daily for exercise. The usual duration of treatment with chemotherapy and apica is 7 months for synovial disease of the knee. Synovectomy of the knee results in considerable impairment of motion and, in view of the excellent possibility of healing tuberculosis

of the knee in childhood, is not thought necessary.

Chemotherapy allows a period of conservative therapy to be shortened and results in greater likelihood of obtaining a cure and a functioning joint. Traction can be used as an adjunct to rest in a bivalved spica to obtain motion at the knee once the disease is controlled. There should be a normal sedimentation rate and restoration of a normal lymphocyte-monocyte ratio. The resumption of weight bearing should be gradual; it should be delayed for a 6-month period after chemotherapy and the cessation of signs of activity of the disease. During these 6 months, the patient may walk in a non-weight-bearing splint. Afterward, progress may be made in the absence of signs of recurrence to partial and finally full, weight bearing. The patient should have 90 degrees of flexion and full extension of the knee and a good quadriceps before weight bearing is resumed.

References

1. Bosworth, D. M., Della Pietra, A., and Farell, R. F.: Streptomycin in tuberculosis bone and joint lesions with mixed infection and sinuses, *J. Bone Joint Surg.*, *32A*: 103, 1950.
2. Hughes, F. S., Mardis, R. E., Dye, W. E., and Tempel, C. W.: Combined intermittent regimens in the treatment of non-miliary pulmonary tuberculosis, In *Transactions of the Tenth Conference on Chemotherapy of Tuberculosis*, Washington Veteran's Administration—Army-Navy, p. 67, 1954.

CONGENITAL DISLOCATION OF THE KNEE

This is an apparent congenital deformity consisting of a subluxation of the tibia anteriorly on the femur and a hyperextension of the knee (Fig. 5.27).

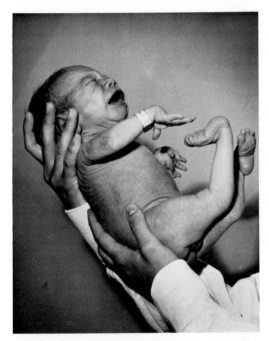

Figure 5.27. The hyperextended position of both knees is evident in this infant. Genu recurvation may actually include dislocation of the tibia in relation to the femur and secondary changes in the soft tissues. This infant has evident hand and foot deformities as well.

There is some confusion as to whether this is an intrauterine positional deformity or a true congenital deformity (Fig. 5.28). In some cases, usually unilateral ones, anterior subluxation is not marked and correction is readily and permanently obtained. More commonly, however, the deformity occurs in both knees. The incidence of breech presentation in cases of congenital dislocation of the knee is well above the expected 4% of the population. Associated dislocation of the hip has occurred in 50% of some series. An occasional patient has multiple deformities involving the upper as well as the lower extremities.

Deformities of the condyles of the femur and tibia appear to be secondary changes seen in older infants, but not evident, at least by roentgenogram, in the newborn.

In a 25-year period Curtis and Fisher[1] reported 16 patients with resistant congenital hyperextension of the knee who were admitted to Newington Children's Hospital. In the same period there were 650 cases of congenital dislocation of the hip.

In resistant cases the principal obstacle to reduction is a tight anterior capsule and contracted quadriceps mechanism.

Clinical Picture

The positional type does not reveal any fibrotic feel in the quadriceps area. The quadriceps readily responds to gentle stretching and active exercise. Progressive flexion casts may be necessary to regain flexion. Even though it does regain flexion, it is necessary to hold the knee in 90 degrees of flexion for a 6-week period in early infancy to prevent a recurrence of the hyperextended position. Once stabilized, there is no tendency toward recurrence of the hyperextended position, since the quadriceps is not involved in a fibrotic process.

Those with fibrosis of the quadriceps, loss of suprapatella pouch space, and more severely lateral dislocation of the patella represent a more difficult treatment story.

Other musculoskeletal deformities are common—of 11 patients reported by Curtis and Fisher, 7 were felt to have arthrogryposis multiplex congenita, 10 had congenital dislocation of the hip, and 7 had congenital foot deformities. Other organ systems were not involved.

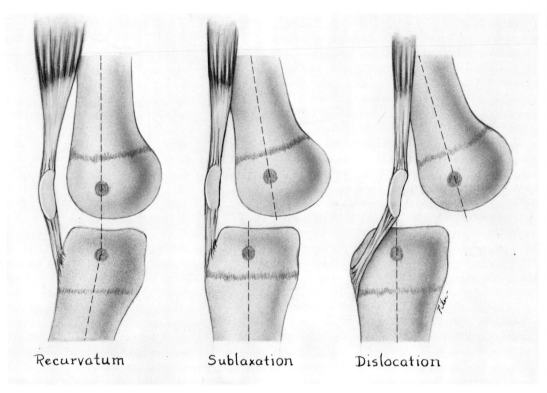

Recurvatum　　　Sublaxation　　　Dislocation

Figure 5.28. Congenital hyperextension of the knee runs the gamut from a positional deformity to actual dislocation and a fibrous remnant of the quadriceps tightly binding down the deformity.

A tight extensor mechanism with fibrous replacement of the quadriceps is a virtually constant finding in the operative cases. This occurs predominantly in the lateral portion of the muscle. Displacement of the entire quadriceps mechanism and patella occurred to the lateral side in over one-half of the cases operated by Curtis and Fisher.

Treatment

Repeated use of flexion casts that bring the knee joint into corrective flexion at each application is usually a successful method of reduction.

If the more resistant cases after at least 90 degrees of flexion are obtained it is important to hold the knee in a flexed position over a 3-month period. The cast may be bivalved for active exercise of the quadriceps and hamstrings, but never allowing hyperextension.

Kirschner wire traction may be necessary in some cases to achieve a conservative reduction. Should the more conservative methods fail, an open reduction that frees the anterior capsule, replaces the quadriceps mechanism over the anterior aspect of the knee, and where necessary lengthens the quadriceps is a desirable procedure (Fig. 5.29). It is desirable before secondary deformities of the proximal tibial and distal femoral epiphysis occur.

Even after open reduction, however, a holding period of many months is important to avoid ligamentous instability—not only in the plane of flexion, but also laterally and medially.

Niebauer and King[3] have described lengthening of the patella ligament and quadriceps and advancement of the insertion of the anterior cruciate ligament in the tibial plateau.

References

1. Curtis, B. H., and Fisher, R. L.: Congenital hyperextension with anterior subluxaticn of the knee, *J. Bone Joint Surg.*, *51A*: 255, 1969.
2. Leveuf, J., and Pais, C.: Les dislocations congenitles du genou, *Rev. Orthop.*, *32*: 313, 1946.

3. Niebauer, J. J., and King, D. E.: Congenital dislocation of the knee, *J. Bone Joint Surg.*, 42A: 207, 1960.

GENU VALGUM

It is important to know that children pass through a stage of fairly marked genu valgum in the process of growth and development. This natural "deformity" is most noticeable about age 2; it becomes less noticeable with increased height by the age of 6. Because of the natural tendency toward improvement, surgical correction is not indicated in this age period.

The lateral condyle of the femur normally bears the most weight in the human. Valgus is a normal position of the knee and is built into the normal femur. The distance between the femurs at the hips is greater than the distance between the knees. Intrinsic valgus corrects for this discrepancy and results in apparently straight limbs.

In the younger age groups, pronation of the feet is frequently present as well. In some, pronation reflects a loose ligamentous structure which can be demonstrated at wrist and elbow by hyperextension. Roentgenogram examination may reveal that the valgus is greater in weight bearing than in recumbency in these children.

Treatment

In the 2- to 6-year age group, treatment consists of increasing medial arch support in order to invert the heel, separate the knees, and shift pressure from the lateral to the medial femoral condyle.

Where the valgus is marked, use of a longitudinal arch support and a ⅛-inch inner heel wedge with a prolongation of the medial heel (Thomas heel) seems a puny effort in relation to the deformity. High shoes will increase the efficiency of this apparatus somewhat, and rarely a long leg brace with a

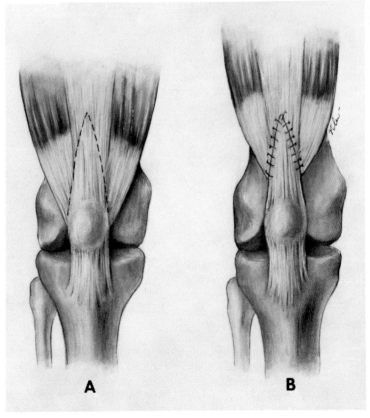

Figure 5.29. Lengthening of the quadriceps to allow reduction of the tibia on the femur and knee flexion by achieving increased length.

medial pad at the femoral condyles and a built-in overcorrection to the knee may be indicated. We are concerned here not with a pathologic growth distrubance but only with a normal stage of development, and bracing is usually too limiting to the child for the slightness of the condition.

Surgical Correction

Surgical correction of a genu valgum may be indicated, for example, in cases of unilateral genu valgum secondary to trauma or to a growth abnormality such as may occur in achondroplasia or Ollier's disease. Poliomyelitis may be implicated by the development of contracture laterally at the knee.

Trauma includes scarring laterally at the knee when the soft tissues have been lost owing either to traumatic avulsion or to burns. The scar may have a stapling effect that hinders the rate of growth laterally at the epiphyseal line compared to that of the medial aspect.

There are some clinical considerations in determining whether the correction should take place above or below the knee.

The desirable end result is an anatomic alignment of the plane of the ankle and that of the knee joint (Fig. 5.30). Both planes should then be at right angles to the weight-bearing line. When the deformity has taken place principally in the distal femur, in which case the plane of the knee joint is oblique, correction should take place in the distal femur. When the deviation takes place in the proximal tibia, the plane of the knee joint is unaffected, but the plane of the ankle joint is oblique on weight bearing. Here correction must be done in the proximal tibia to ensure the desired result.

Roentgenograms of both knee joint and ankle joint are important in evaluating the individual case.

Inasmuch as the abnormality seldom occurs in only one place and often includes a rotary deformity as well, wedge resections are seldom used. A transverse cut of the bone results in an unstable situation that is difficult to place accurately in plaster. Incidentally, a single hip spica, not merely a long leg cast, is necessary to be certain of maintaining position.

A dome-shaped or telescoping V osteotomy gives more stability and increases the

bone surface available for healing. It also allows correction in more than one plane. When the osteotomy is done in the tibia, the fibula must always be divided to allow accurate correction.

RECURRENT DISLOCATION OF PATELLA

A good illustration of the effect of body mechanics and growth on the production of disease is afforded by the entity known as recurrent dislocation of the patella. The patella may be dislocated at birth and may remain dislocated unless it is surgically corrected. Simple dislocation may follow trauma. Recurrent dislocation is a result of an

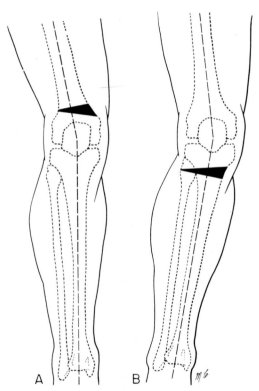

Figure 5.30. Diagrams illustrating that valgus may arise above (*A*) or below (*B*) the knee joint. The location of the anomaly determines the area selected for surgical correction, because it is desirable to have both the plane of the knee and that of the ankle at right angles to the straightened weight-bearing line.

abnormal direction of pull of the quadriceps muscle and may or may not be accompanied by other structural abnormalities which render dislocation easy. It is twice as common in females and tends to be familial.

Etiology

To produce a recurrent dislocation, the quadriceps musculature—which contains the patella in the manner of a sesamoid bone—must, when contracted, tend to pull the patella laterally (Figs. 5.31 and 5.32). The factors that bring about a lateral force rather than a force running straight through the condyles of the femur include structural abnormalities which carry the patella tendon insertion in a lateral direction. This is true in genu valgus and in external rotation of the tibia. Both of these structural deviations may result from abnormal growth secondary to unequal muscle pull, as in poliomyelitis, or from congenital anomalies of the lower legs.

Absence of the vastus medial from whatever cause, underdevelopment of the lateral condyle of the tibia, failure of the intercondylar groove to form—these all aid in the production of dislocation. An unusually long patellar tendon allowing the patella to lie above the intercondylar groove also promotes lateral displacement.

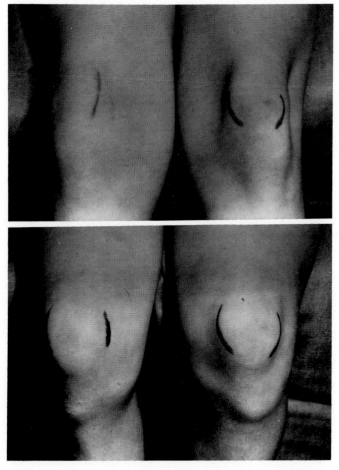

Figure 5.31 (*Top*). As this 10-year-old extends the knee, the knee to the reader's left exhibits lateral displacement of the patella—an abnormal mechanism giving rise to damage of the opposing cartilaginous surfaces.

Figure 5.32 (*Bottom*). With flexion, the patella is drawn back into the intercondylar notch.

Mechanism

For functional purposes the quadriceps musculature may be visualized as contracting in a straight line between the origin of the rectus femoris or the anterior inferior spine of the ilium and the insertion of the quadriceps via the patellar tendon into the tibial tubercle or apophysis. This line should run directly between the condyles of the femurs in the intercondylar groove. Either valgus or external rotation of the tibia in relation to the knee may carry the tibial tubercle lateralward (Fig. 5.33). When the patient is unusually long limbed, even a small lateral displacement may produce lateral motion of the patella.

The lateral condyle of the femur ordinarily provides a bony hindrance to lateral movement of the patella. The vastus medialis and the medial capsule provide a ligamentous hindrance. Underdevelopment of the lateral condyle, paralysis or absence of the vastus medialis, and laxity of the medial capsule eliminate these check reins. Any, all, or none of these features may be present.

A patella tendon that allows the patella to ride above the intercondylar notch eliminates the lateral condyle as a buttress in preventing lateral dislocation and may be a contributing mechanism.

Clinical Picture

The child is usually more than 6 years old and tends to be in the early adolescent group. A period of rapid growth of the extremities often precedes the development of the condition. The rather tall, long legged, early adolescent girl with genu valgum of moderate severity is the typical subject.

The dislocation is usually not seen. The child is brought to the physician because of recurrent pain or swelling at the knee. The actual dislocation which occurs when the knee is flexed ordinarily reduces itself when the knee is extended. The history usually contains several episodes of difficulty. These are most likely to occur after periods of prolonged sitting, for example, when the child has been entertained. On arising, inability to straighten the knee is noted, and the displacement of the patella may actually be appreciated, although often it is not.

When the patient is seen within 48 hrs of the dislocation (Fig. 5.34), the knee usually

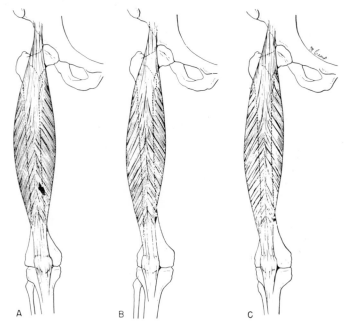

Figure 5.33.　The line of quadriceps pull. (*A*) Normal, (*B*) valgus at the knee, (*C*) external rotation of the tibia. Lateral displacement of the patella tendon insertion tends to carry the patella laterally on contraction of the quadriceps.

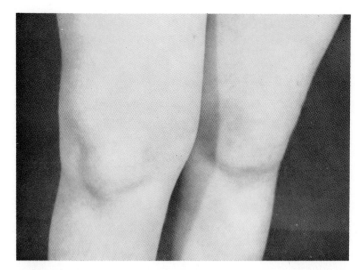

Figure 5.34. Dislocated patella in 6-year-old girl. The *apparent* patella prominence is due to a fat pad. The *actual* prominence can be seen above and lateral to it.

contains fluid. The medial capsule of the knee in the parapatellar area is tender. Atrophy of the thigh is variable and dependent on the degree of previous disability.

A helpful sign of diagnosis, whether the child is seen immediately after the dislocation or many months later, is acute apprehension on an attempted lateral displacement of the patella. When the knee is extended and the quadriceps relaxed, passively pushing the patella over the lateral condyle of the femur gives rise to acute apprehension as the patient feels the patella about to slip out of control.

Structural abnormalities are noted. A mild valgus position of the tibia results in considerable lateral displacement of the tibial tubercle in a tall, long limbed child. There may be external rotation of the tibia, again with lateral displacement of the tibial tubercle.

When the patient is seen at a time well removed from the acute episode, examination of the knee while the patient is sitting and the knee is flexed 90 degrees is frequently very revealing. As the knee is extended, the patella may be seen to sublux laterally. Now, when the knee is flexed, the patella first has to track over into the intercondylar groove. This movement is accompanied by a palpable, and often audible, clicking, from which damage to the opposing cartilaginous surfaces may be inferred. Pressing the patella so as to rub it against the femur frequently reveals crepitus secondary to the cartilage changes.

Destruction of the patella and the condylar surface has been seen to be secondary to recurrent dislocation of the patella so often that surgical correction of the mechanism is urged as a preventive measure against further trauma.

Roentgen Findings

The anteroposterior view of the knee may reveal dislocation of the patella, if it is present (Fig. 5.35). A tendency of the reduced patella to ride more lateralward than usual and valgus at the knee may be noted. A lateral film may reveal the patella to be proximal to, or at the superior edge of, the femoral condyles. A view taken tangential to the condyles to show the intercondylar notch and the relation of the patella to it may reveal dislocation or underdevelopment of the lateral condyles (Fig. 5.36).

Treatment

The fundamental aim in treatment is to correct the line of pull of the quadriceps so that it runs through the intercondylar area. Because a lateral force produces the dislocation, it follows that correction of this force will result in a cure of the condition (Fig. 5.37 A-C).

The reasons for attempting cure are alleviation of episodes of discomfort, production

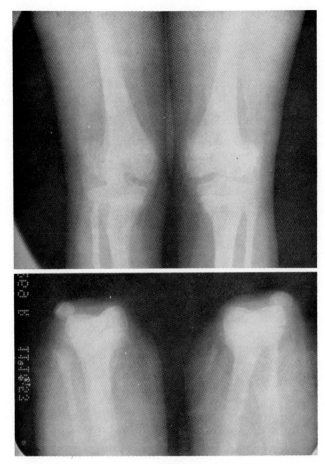

Figure 5.35.   Roentgenogram of bilateral dislocated patellae. Anteroposterior view (*top*) and view with ray directed tangential to the patellae as the knee is flexed (*bottom*).

of normal function, and protection of the undersurface of the patella from further injury. Chondromalacia of the patella seen in later life often gives a history of recurrent or chronic dislocation of the patella in childhood.

The treatment may be complicated by the patient's age. Before the age of 14 in girls and 16 in boys, interference with the growing apophysis forming the tibial tubercle may give rise to growth deformity. After this age, the mechanical line of pull of the quadriceps can readily be corrected by transference medialward of the patellar tendon insertion. The age of election for surgery for any individual patient varies.

In the young age group, when the recurrent dislocations are frequent and productive of fluid in the knee, temporizing measures may have to be undertaken. However, to prevent the development of chondromalacia of the patella in the "teenage" period, an attempt at surgical correction may be made in young patients, even though the results are not as satisfactory as those of moving a bone and the attached tendon in the later age group.

In the child with the epiphyseal line still open, the incision is made laterally above the patella and is brought medialward below the patella to cross the tibial tubercle and to extend far enough to allow for easy reimplantation. The tight lateral capsule, as well as the fascia, is divided over the distal vastus lateralis. The infrapatellar fat pad is exposed, and the patellar tendon is delineated. The tendon is skinned from the tibial tubercle area in such a way as to leave some of its fibers still covering the tubercle. Great care must be taken to avoid scarring or damaging the cartilage of the tubercle, which is continuous with the epiphyseal line. The distal end of the patellar tendon is sewn subperiosteally just distal to the epiphyseal line. The fact that there is some slack in the patellar tendon when it is in full extension allows this. It is not wise to try to advance the tendon further than just beyond the line, however, as to do so would secondarily put considerable pressure on the cartilage surfaces related to the patella. A cylinder cast that holds the knee extended is worn for 6 weeks.

Green[1] has advocated extensive reconstruction of the quadriceps mechanism in relation to its pull on the patella. This includes division of the lateral insertion and advancement of the insertion medially of the vastus medialis.

It is, of course, preferable to wait for closure of the epiphyseal line at the proximal tibia to perform the operation. In such a case, the incision is again lateral and curves medialward over the tibial tubercle. The patellar tendon is separated from the infrapatellar fat pad. The area of the patellar tendon insertion is outlined by drill holes, and a bone block having a superior edge approximately ⅛ inch above the beginning of the insertion is removed. Drill holes now outline the bed into which this bone block is to be placed. This bed is tilted so that its long axis lies in line

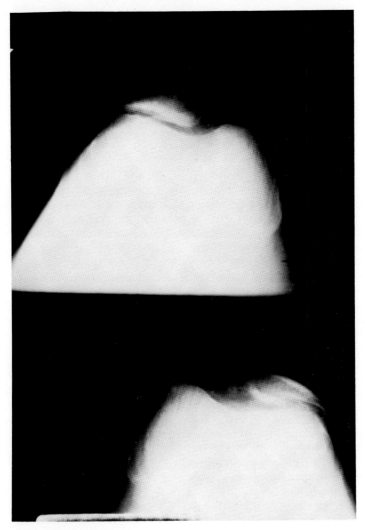

Figure 5.36. The lateral riding patella leads to patellofemoral arthritis. The narrowing of the joint space, sclerotic and irregular subchondral bone are evident in the skyline roentgenogram of the patellofemoral joint (45-year-old male).

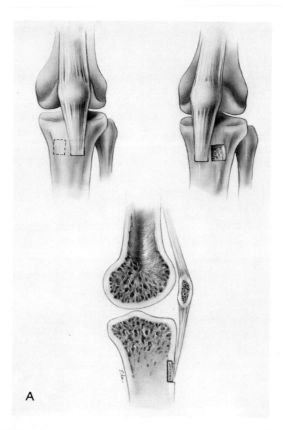

Figure 5.37. (A) Changing the line of the quadriceps pull and the patellar tendon alignment requires some careful attention to significant details in order to be successful. When done for dislocating patella, the bone block should never be advanced. The bed into which the patella tendon and its attached bone block from its point of insertion is put is immediately adjacent to the site of the original insertion. The new bed is angled slightly to avoid torque in the tendon. Lateral bands are divided as high as need be to allow the patella tendon to pull in a direct line with the quadriceps. The proximal cortex of the new bed is undercut with a curette to allow a projection superiorly of the bone block attached to the patella tendon to go beneath it. When the fascia and tendinous insertion of the pes anserinus is then sewn back over, the block and patella tendon are firmly held without the need of screw fixation. (B) Anteroposterior and (C) lateral view of the proximal tibia with bone block fashioned for a patellar tendon transplant visible. Note that patella is not advanced; block is sunk beneath cortical level and angled in line with the patella tendon pull.

with the expected pull of the patellar tendon. This position brings the superior lateral corner of the bed close to the area from which the first bone block was removed. No attempt is made to advance the patellar tendon unless it is excessively relaxed. The superior lip of the new bed is cleared infracortically by a curette so that the bone block can be hooked under it. A single screw is inserted through the center of the bone block, and the block is now securely held. A cylinder cast supported by straps running over the contralat-

eral shoulder is worn for 6 weeks. Quadriceps-setting exercises are used while the patient is in the cast. Active motion and quadriceps exercises are begun as soon as the cast is removed.

Elevation of the Tibial Tubercle

It did not take too long in the practice of orthopaedic surgery to find out that in doing

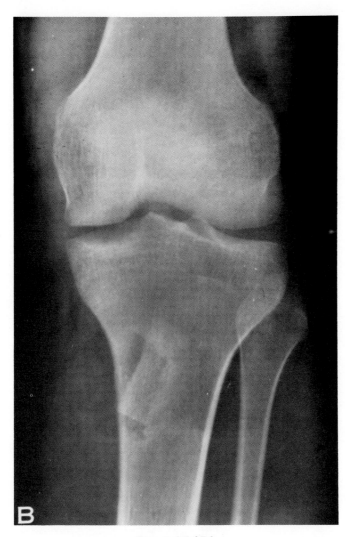

Fig. 5.37 (B)

any version of the Hauser procedure the patella tendon insertion should not be advanced
distally. It took longer to realize that insertion
of the tendon block beneath the cortex of the
tibia might increase patellofemoral pressure
and increase the hazard of chondromalacia
patellae. Maquet pointed out that displacement of the tibial tubercle forward would
decrease the force vector at the patellofemoral joint.

In the past few years we have devised a
modification of Maquet's procedure to both
elevate the bone to which the patella tendon
is attached and to move the insertion medially (Fig. 5.38).

It is very important that the incision be
transverse at the level of the tibial tubercle
rather than longitudinal. This will avoid closing the tissue with tension—a situation that
could cause a slough over the tibial tubercle.
A long thin bone sliver is raised for about
1½–2 inches. When elevated it backs distally
and can readily be moved medially. A bone
block ½-inch square is removed from Gur-
dey's tubercle herewith the anterior portion
of the insertion of fascia lata. This block is
placed beneath the raised cortical segment to
hold it elevated ½ inch and in its medial
position. A cylinder cast is then applied,
which remains on for 6 weeks.

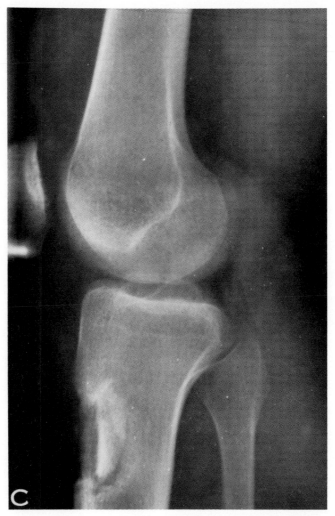

Fig. 5.37 (C)

References

1. Green, W. T.: Recurrent dislocation of the patella; its surgical correction in the growing child, *J. Bone Joint Surg.*, *47A*: 1670, 1965.
2. Goodfellow, J., Hungerford, D. S., and Zindel, M.: Patello-femoral mechanics and pathology. I. Functional anatomy of the patello-femoral joint, *J. Bone Joint Surg.*, *58-B*: 287, 1976.
3. Goymann, V., and Müller, H. G.: New calculation of the biomechanics of the patellofemoral joint and its clinical significance, In *The Knee Joint: Recent Advances in Basic Research and Clinical Aspects*, pp. 16–21, International Congress Series No. 324; Amsterdam: Excerpta Medica, 1974.
4. Kaufer, H.: Mechanical function of the patella, *J. Bone Joint Surg.*, *53A*: 1551, 1971.
5. Murray, J. W. G.: The Maquet principle; its application in severe chondromalacia patellae, patellofemoral and global knee osteoarthritis, Orthop. Rev., *1*: 29, 1976.
6. Pauwels, F.: *Biomechanics of the Normal and Diseased Hip*; Berlin: Springer, 1976.
7. Reilly, D. T., and Martens, M.: Experimental analysis of the quadriceps muscle force and patello-femoral joint reaction force for various activities, *Acta Orthop. Scand.*, *43*: 126, 1972.

LARSON-JOHANSSON DISEASE (OSTEOCHONDRITIS OF PATELLA)

The lower pole of the patella normally has an accessory ossification center. However, there is a syndrome of pain, swelling of the site of origin of the patella tendon from the patella, and local tenderness at this site. It occurs principally in boys running through

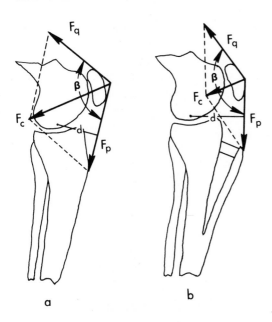

Figure 5.38.   The reduction of total patellofemoral contact force (F_c) by means of anterior tibial tubercle elevation. The resultant quadriceps tension vector (F_q) and patellar tendon vector (F_p), obtained by the parallelogram rule, can be seen to decrease because the angle β is increased and because the patellar tendon moment arm d is decreased.

the age groups of 7–14 years. It is most often bilateral, but can occur unilaterally or be considerably more symptomatic on one side. Larson and Johansson separately described this disease in 1921.

Activity increases symptoms and rest relieves them. Although painful on occasion there is no implication of destruction of the infrapatellar surface as a result of continued activity. It acts in the manner similar to Osgood-Schlatter disease but at the proximal rather than the distal end of the patella.

As the accessory center fuses with the parent bone, the symptoms subside.

Roentgen Findings

The normal infrapatella ossification center is linear, regular, and separated from the patella by a thin, dark line. When the area is the seat of Larson-Johansson disease, the proximal pole of the patella tendon exhibits swelling of the soft-tissue shadow outlining it. There may be irregular ossification extending out into the center of the tendon area (Fig. 5.39).

Treatment

Explanation to the parent and child is an important form of therapy. The symptoms are ordinarily not severe enough to justify cast immobilization. Although the symptoms will subside with immobilization, they can be expected to recur with activity until approximately age 15 or when fusion of the accessory patella center is complete.

OSTEOCHONDROMA OF DISTAL FEMORAL EPIPHYSIS

Osteochondroma of the distal femoral epiphysis is rare, but it is a serious problem for a growing child who develops progressive deformity of the knee because of it.

The growth of the osteochondroma can effect the condyles to produce asymmetry—most often to cause progressive valgus deformity.

The mass of the osteochondroma destroys the overlying articular cartilage and produces secondary cupping in the opposing tibial condyle.

On physical examination crepitus-limited flexion and usually a valgus deformity are present at the knee (Fig. 5.40).

Treatment

Early, before growth has proceeded to extensive deformity, the mass can be partially

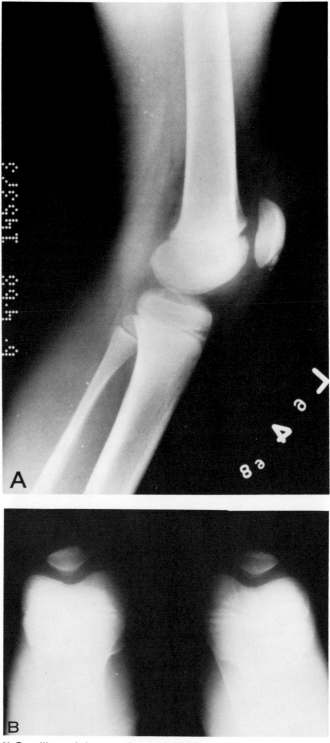

Figure 5.39. (*A*) Swelling of the proximal end of the patella tendon as it arises from the patella in Larson-Johannson disease. There is some irregular ossification extending out into the center of the tendon shadow from the accessory center at the lower pole of the patella (*B*) Normal irregular ossification of the projecting anterior surface of the patella as ossification becomes complete and the accessory center forms at the lower pole of the patella.

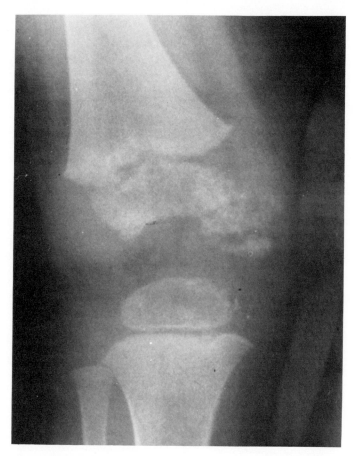

Figure 5.40. The distal femoral epiphysis has lost its normal shape, and the subchondral bone that should be running continuously around it is interrupted. Irregular, disorganized bone fills the mass projecting from the epiphysis and produces a valgus deformity of the knee.

removed. The condyle is shaped to conform to the expected volume and shape of the condyle normally. The reshaping should be sufficient to restore normal alignment to the leg.

This will leave some laxity in the collateral ligaments, and the alignment of the limb must be preserved long enough to allow growth to compensate for this.

A cylinder cast holds the limb for 3–4 weeks. Thereafter daily active motion is carried out and the limb is aligned in a double weight brace. The knee hinge allows free flexion and extension.

After several years, when the knee is sta-ble, the brace is discontinued. However, the child is followed throughout the growth period because further growth of the osteochondroma may cause a recurrence of the deformity. The procedure may have to be repeated.

As an adult the knee obviously does not have a normal surface and the tibial surface has developed some adapative deformity.

The alignment of the leg remains sufficiently good that ambulation without a brace is possible. One expects that the knee will develop traumatic arthritis as the years go by, but this can be dealt with in a knee with adequate stock to support a prosthetic device.

CHAPTER 6

The Hip

CONGENITAL HIP DISEASE

Primary congenital dislocation of the hip without any associated nerve or muscle lesion is one of the most common congenital malformations. It can be found in the newborn child if looked for specifically within the first few days of life (Figs. 6.1 and 6.2). The instance has been variously reported as from 1–15 per 1,000 live births. This instance would be consistent with that found in Europe and in the United States. It is more common among the Navajo Indians in North America, and it may be simplistic to say that this is because they swaddle their young. It is relatively rare among Negroes and Chinese. It cannot be clearly related that carrying the infant on the hip with legs spread is the feature that reduces the incidence.

Abduction splints are not found among these races. It may be that the abduction is accomplished more slowly and gracefully. There is no question that there is an increased instance of breeched presentations among those children having congenital dislocation of the hip (17–20%) as compared to the normal instance of 2–4%.

Two surveys have investigated the relationship of social class to congenital dislocation of the hip. No effect of the social environment was noted in either investigation in terms of uncovering late diagnosis of the disease. Upper social class patients have an increased instance of neonatal congenital dislocation of the hip, and there is an increased proportion of siblings in these families compared with lower income groups. A significantly greater number of children with this deformity are born during the winter months than during the summer. There has been no real explanation for this, but it has been pointed out by Wynne-Davies.

We have been able to divide children with dislocation of the hip in its various forms, exclusive of those with neurologic disease, into three types:

1. *Neonatal Type.* Dislocation is found with the femoral head separated from its seat in the acetabulum by a tight iliopsoas and capsular constricture. This is by far the most common. It is important to realize that this type has all the elements that it should have for a normally constituted joint with a fully formed acetabulum, a normal capsule, a normal ligament, and a normal femoral head. Secondary changes in these structures result from the position in which the femoral head is maintained relative to the acetabulum (Fig. 6.3).

2. *Dislocation Associated with Lax Ligaments.* In this type the hip slides in and out of the acetabulum due to excessive distensibility of the capsule; and if the life style of the infant is such as to promote dislocation, the incidence of this type can go up. It is relatively rare compared to the first type and occurred once in 45 incidences of congenital dislocation of the hip in our series. It should be emphasized again that all the elements that the hip joint should have are present in this type, including acetabulum, labrum, femoral head, and ligamentum teres capsule.

3. *Teratologic Dislocation.* The important distinction here is that there has been a definite intrauterine disturbance at the time of formation of the hip joint, and some portion of the hip joint is actually missing at birth. This may include any of the elements of the proximal third of the femur and may include various portions of the acetabulum including complete failure of the acetabulum to form. This type is exceedingly rare and is often associated with other extremity anomalies.

The very noticeable limp due to weakness of the hip abductors when the hip is unstable has been with mankind since the first civilizations. Hippocrates (460–370 B.C.) wrote:

There are persons who, from birth or from disease, have dislocations outward of both thighs;

285

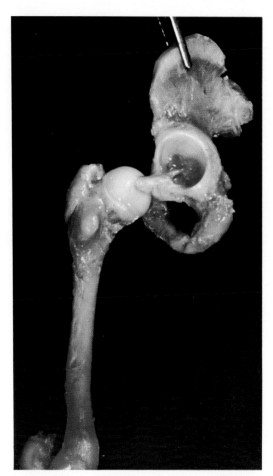

Figure 6.1. The normal hip is well formed at birth. The acetabulum is not shallow at birth but a deep, rounded cartilaginous cup. The femoral head is a section of a perfect sphere and fits congruously within the acetabulum.

in them, then, the bones are affected in a like manner, but the fleshy parts in their case lose their strength less; the legs, too, are plump and fleshy, except that there is some little deficiency at the inside, and they are plump because they have the equal use of both legs, for in walking, they totter equally to this side and that.

An enlightened medical community has succeeded in recent years in recognizing states which predispose to dislocation and, thereby, has greatly reduced its incidence. Hart[21,22] has emphasized the preventive nature of treatment undertaken within the first year of life in order to form an adequate hip joint in an individual who might otherwise develop dislocation of a previously dysplastic

hip joint. Hart has also shown that the end result of an uncorrected subluxated hip may be degenerative arthritis in adult life (Figs. 6.4 and 6.5).

Dislocation may be present at birth, but it also may occur in the first years of development. Dysplasia or presubluxation may be the first indication of abnormal mechanical forces that may eventually result in dislocation. The work of Hart, of Hass, and of the Italian orthopaedic surgeons such as Putti,[39] Scaglietti, and Poli[36] has been responsible for the recognition of anomalies of the hip other than frank dislocation.

Gill,[19,20] Crego and Schwartzmann,[11] and others have noted that the age at which treatment is begun may be correlated with the excellence of the end results in terms of percentages. The percentage of failure rises with the age of the patients at initial treatment.

The sex incidence of congenital dislocation in various reported series has varied from 81–87% females. Hass stated that female in-

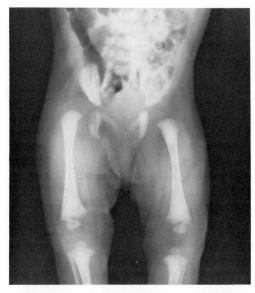

Figure 6.2. Dislocation of the hip present at birth can be easily missed on roentgen examination. An increased slant to the acetabulum when present as the only sign means little. The femoral head rides in the lateral one-third of the acetabulum without riding upward, and signs of this location should be looked for. An attempted abduction x-ray is helpful.

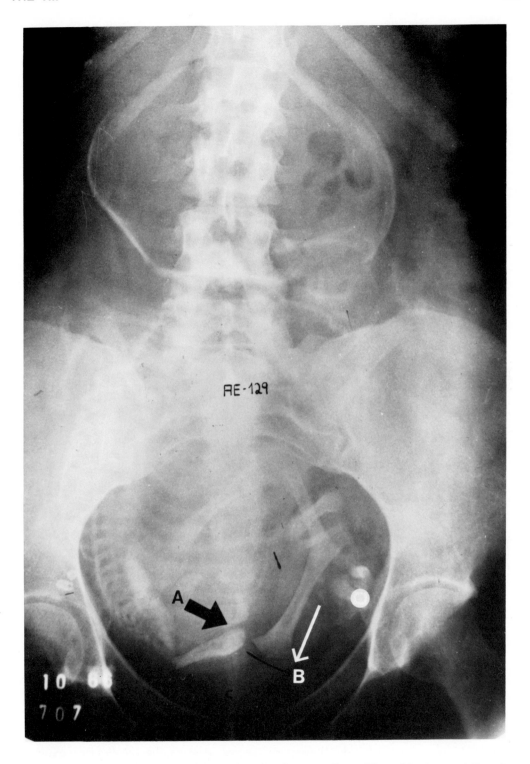

Figure 6.3. The *black arrow* points to the triradiate cartilage. The *white arrow* delineates the position of the proximal femur. The hip joint thus outlined reveals a dislocation of the hip with the fetus in the breech position. (Reproduced with permission from A. Campos Da Paz, Jr.: Congenital dislocation of the hip in the newborn, *Italian Journal of Orthopaedics and Trauma, 2:* 261–268, 1976.)

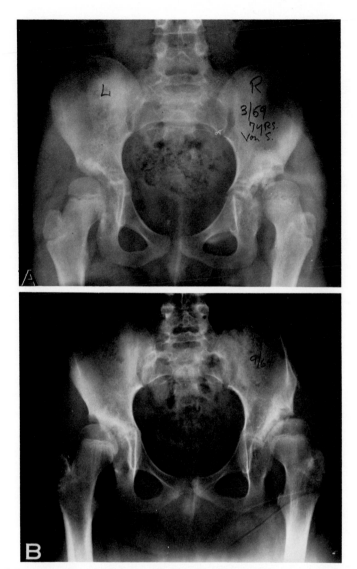

Figure 6.4. A femoral head located in the lateral third of the acetabulum leads to early osteoarthritis and will not get better with use but instead will regress. (*A*) Seven-year-old girl with previously treated congenital dislocation of the hip. The lateral position of the femoral head and secondary acetabular cysts are seen. (*B*) Despite attempts at repair of the acetabulum, the femoral head has progressed still further.

fants are affected 6 times as frequently as males. Unilateral dislocations are twice as common as bilateral ones, when frank dislocation is spoken of (Fig. 6.6). When various forms of hip dysplasia are included, however, the incidence of bilateral involvement, particularly in the age group under 1 year, is more nearly equal to that of unilateral difficulty.

Congenital dislocation of the hip becomes extraordinarily frequent in some areas. Lo-

calities have been reported in France, Holland, and Italy—the northern provinces of Italy, for example—in which the incidence of the disease seems to be greatly increased. It seems, however, that the disease is exceptionally rare among Negroes. In Asiatic countries, where the mother characteristically carries her child balanced on her hip with its legs in abduction, the incidence of poor hip development is much reduced.

Congenital dislocation of the hip is a poor term for a lesion that often begins with the hip fully formed, but with the femoral head laterally displaced, and further pathology developing as a result of this position.

Etiology

A review of the many scholarly attempts to determine the etiology of congenital dislocation of the hip leads to the conclusion that there is not just one but many causes of this condition.

The possibility that primary acetabular dysplasia is the cause has been supported by many. It has been thought that the posterior superior, buttress-like acetabular roof may genetically be prevented from forming. This does not fit the pathology that we have observed.

The femoral head originally must have been in relationship to the acetabulum, because the joint develops as a cleft in the primordial cell block. Embryologic studies by Strayer revealed that this cleft does not become complete until the embryo reaches the 35-mm stage. Joint clefts have formed, how-

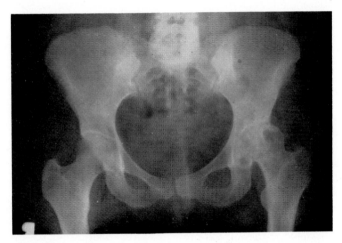

Figure 6.5.   Old uncorrected subluxation of the hip with degenerative changes.

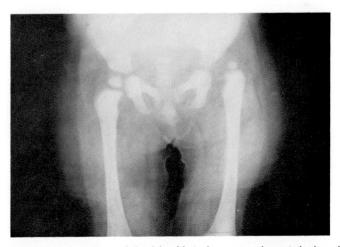

Figure 6.6.   Unilateral dislocation of the hip. Note increased acetabular slant, diminished size of the epiphyseal growth center, lateral and superior position of the femur, and anteversion as shown by the externally rotated position of the proximal femur in relation to the anteroposterior view of the distal femur.

ever, even in the absence of the distal bone. It is obvious that, although the cleft may develop as the result of primary differentiating factors, the later development of the joint becomes more and more subject to other factors.

Badgley,[2] beginning with the 8-mm embryo, reviewed the embryologic development of the hip joint (Figs. 6.7 and 6.8). The following comments are drawn from his article. Only nerves and vessels are added from the trunk to the original limb bud in its development. At the stage of 14.8 mm, the predestined site of the hip joint can be seen as a dense accumulation of mesenchymal cells. These undifferentiated mesenchymal cells are still present at the 25-mm stage between the femoral head and acetabulum. The capsular structures and glenoidal labrum have begun to form.

At the 33-mm stage, the ligamentum teres has appeared, and the joint space is completely differentiated. The glenoid labrum is prolonged over the head of the femur. The limb bud has developed during this period in marked abduction, which is decreased considerably by the time the 58-mm embryo is reached. During this developmental period, the limb bud is also undergoing rotation.

It seems reasonable to assume that, up to the point of innervation of the musculature of the limb, development of the joint is predestined. As Badgley pointed out, delay in rotation of the limb bud or in innervation of the muscles at a period of rapid embryologic growth may produce alterations in the development of the acetabulum or in the head and neck of the femur. Adaptive changes to malposition can occur in intrauterine as well as in postnatal life. Breech births have been noted frequently to be the subjects of adduction contractures at the hip joint.

Underdevelopment of the limbus may encourage dislocation of the hip. The cartilaginous acetabulum and limbus cover the femoral head at birth. Elongation of the capsule, allowing subluxation and dislocation, has been mentioned as a contributing factor by Howorth.

Anteversion, which may be the result of inward rotation of the limb bud as an angle of 90 degrees is traversed to bring the patella forward, is a factor in poor presentation of the femoral head to the acetabulum. It may be the one of the adaptive changes responsible, at least in part, for dislocation. The hip, developing in the flexed position and extending after birth, is aided in its tendency toward dislocation by the anteversion. Anteversion is more evident after conventional treatment than at birth.

Dislocation of the hip sometimes occurs in association with other anomalies, such as clubfeet, clubhands, metatarsus varus, and arthrogryposis. That dislocation may not be present at birth and yet develop, presumably through the stages of dysplasia to subluxation to actual dislocation, has been noted by many (Fig. 6.3). Such hips may, however, already have joint development changes that allow dislocation such as displacement laterally into the outer third of the acetabulum.

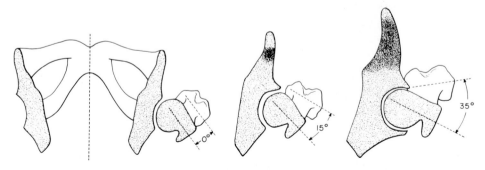

Figure 6.7. Development of the normal hip joint, viewed from the rear and as if the femur were flexed 90 degrees. Note the progressive deepening of the acetabulum as the limb bud changes from a lateral to a parallel position. There is progressive development of anteversion from 0 degrees at 3 months to 35 degrees at birth. (Redrawn from C. E. Badgley: Etiology of congenital dislocation of hip, *Journal of Bone and Joint Surgery, 31A:* 352, 1949.)

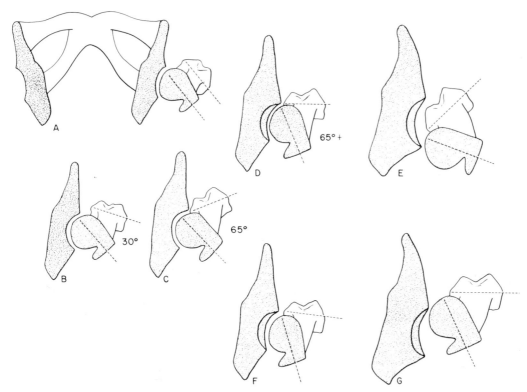

Figure 6.8. Development of congenital dislocation of the hip and acetabular dysplasia. (*A*) The 35-mm fetus without anteversion of the femur. (*B* and *C*) Development of normal and then excessive anteversion. (*D* and *E*) Progressive dislocation with increasing anteversion and lack of normal pressure resulting in acetabular dysplasia. (*F* and *G*) Development of anterior dislocation. There is delay in proper timing of the rotation of the head into the acetabulum with both anterior and posterior dislocation, as illustrated in the series from *D–G*, so that at no time does it actually point into the acetabulum. Depending on the degree of the developmental error, either dysplasia or dislocation may be the result. (Redrawn from C. E. Badgley: Etiology of congenital dislocation of hip, *Journal of Bone and Joint Surgery, 31A:* 353, 1949.)

The development of dislocation after birth is similary due to many factors. The classic direction of dislocation is said to be posterior, although McCarroll and Crego[31] stated that primary anterior dislocation of the hip occurs in approximately one-fifth of the cases. The presence of an adducted position of the femur relative to the pelvis, with a myostatic contracture of the adductors maintaining this position, stands out from a clinical point of view. Enlargement of the ligamentum teres and of the Haversian pad of fat lying in the acetabulum depths has been implicated but appears secondary to the lateral position.

The acetabulum seems to have the ability to respond to correct seating of the femoral head within it and is slow to develop when these forces are not transmitted to it. Anteversion, as well as adduction, of the femur is important in this regard.

Weight bearing is regarded by some as a factor influencing a hip that is subluxated toward dislocation.

The forces of heredity may be instrumental in delaying rotation of the limb or its innervation and, as such, may accomplish the sequence of events outlined by Badgley. However, this is difficult to prove. Many factors seem to play a part in producing congenital dislocation of the hip.

Mechanics of Iliopsoas

This discussion of etiology has included all types of dislocated hips from so-called dysplasia to the teratologic dislocation, excluding neurologic dislocation. It should be emphasized, however, that despite the fact that the acetabular index may appear slanted excessively by x-ray, the reader should bear in mind that he is looking only at the ossification. In the normal hip at birth the cartilage components of the acetabulum form a deep cup just as in the adult, and it may be very misleading to assume nonexistence of these components from viewing the ossification alone. Position obviously plays an important role in etiology—witness the increased incidence in breech births, in higher social class environments, and in winter months. These factors may lend some credence to the fact that the heavily swaddled child has no opportunity to spontaneously correct the dislocation that is present at birth.

The author's own feeling heavily implicates a positional contracture of the iliopsoas and occasionally the hypertrophy of this muscle as a cause of congenital dislocation of the hip. The hip forms fully in all its components in this disease. The flexed intrauterine position may allow the femoral head to wander into the lateral third of the acetabulum. The iliopsoas is not stretched with growth and tends to lie medial to the femoral head. The infant is born with the hip flexion contracture. As the youngster extends the hip in the first 6 weeks of life, if the femoral head is lying deep in the acetabulum rather than in the outer third, the iliopsoas will stretch, and the youngster will have a normal hip. If it happens to be slightly laterally displaced, further progression of the pathology of congenital dislocation of the hip may be expected to take place with medial migration of the iliopsoas tendon. If not diagnosed in the neonate, it may go on to the frank dislocation with which we are familiar. McKibbin[32] has shown that with a contracted iliopsoas the hip cannot be seated in extension.

The importance of the iliopsoas contracture as an etiologic factor in congenital dislocation of the hip helps to explain the influence of life style in terms of swaddling the baby because that increases the incidence of congenital dislocation of the hip.

Of all the factors that have been reviewed here, the iliopsoas seems to us to be by far the most prominent in effecting what is otherwise a normal hip (Figs. 6.9–6.11). The other factor which may be of importance is the excessive laxity of the ligaments, allowing the femoral head to lie easily in the lateral third of the acetabulum (Figs. 6.12–6.17). We have seen no evidence for enlargement of the ligamentum teres (Figs. 6.18–6.21), the filling of the acetabulum with soft tissue of various types, or failure of the limbus to develop

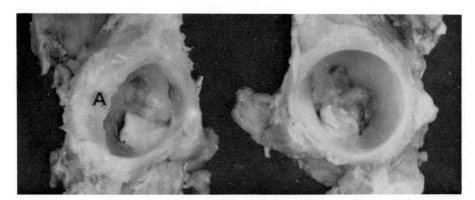

Figure 6.9. View of the acetabulum from child with dislocated hip on the *left* and, for contrast, the normal side on the *right*. On the *left* the limbus or cartilaginous rim has been pressed toward the acetabulum. This is the result of forcibly abducting the hip without correcting the tight iliopsoas contracture. As a result, the limbus, by being pushed in, appears enlarged (*A*) and partially obscures the acetabulum. The femur must be pulled down by traction in line with the trunk before being abducted to avoid the production of this pathology. Forcible abduction without correction of the iliopsoas leads not only to deformity of the acetabular rim, but also to degeneration of the cartilage of the femoral head, which is the seat of this localized pressure.

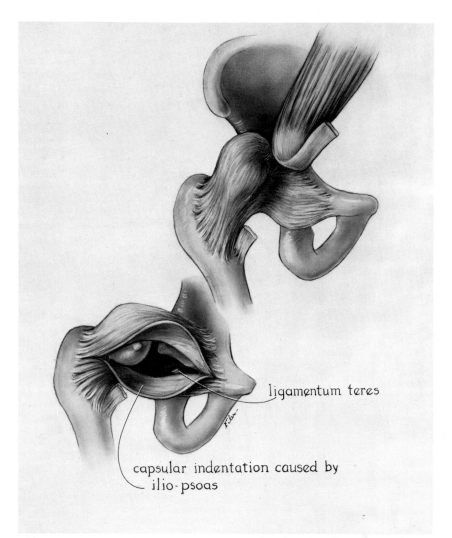

ligamentum teres

capsular indentation caused by
ilio-psoas

Figure 6.10. Drawing of the capsular defect caused by the iliopsoas. As the capsule is drawn up, the opening for reduction of the femoral head is reduced.

(except in teratologic dislocation). Bear in mind in considering etiology that all elements of the hip are fully formed at birth in this disease.

Acetabular Index

If one uses the acetabular index as the sole feature of determining that a hip is dysplastic, one will be markedly misled. This has been emphasized by Caffey, and it is perfectly possible for a normal youngster with normal hips to have an acetabular index as recorded by our usual measurements of over 40 degrees and to develop the hips normally. When this occurs, it is usually bilateral. It is more important to appreciate the develop-

ment of the outer third of the acetabulum than it is to appreciate the slanting edge to the ossification center of the ilium that is forming the acetabulum. When one measures this ossification one has not measured the actual formation of the acetabulum, which is cartilaginous in infancy and cannot be seen. The outer third of the acetabulum can be contrasted with the inner third and, when the outer third slants in relation to the inner third, this is significant.

Severin[42,43] has reported a means of measuring the acetabular angle that was originally devised by Hilgenreiner (Fig. 6.22). This generally accepted and simple method serves to emphasize the importance of the acetabular obliquity in congenital dislocation of the hip. Kleinberg and Lieberman reported the angle

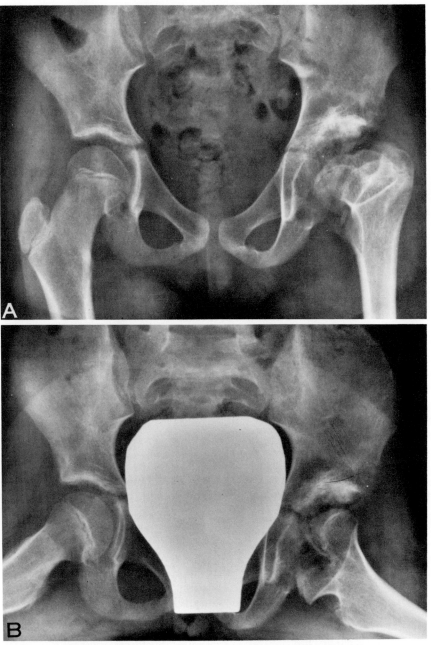

Figure 6.11. Forcible abduction on the acetabular rim can result in an apparent two-headed femur. In (A) the femoral neck is short, the head height diminished. In (B) the deep cleft between the two segments of the head is clearly evident.

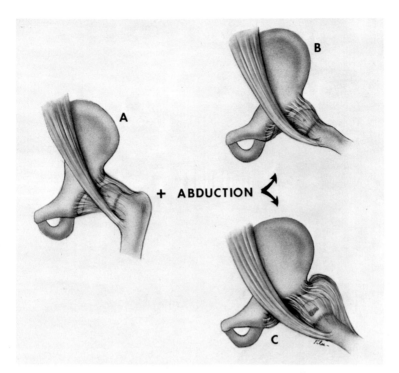

Figure 6.12. Abduction of an improperly seated femoral head yields either acetabulum deformity (*A*) or femoral head deformity (*B*).

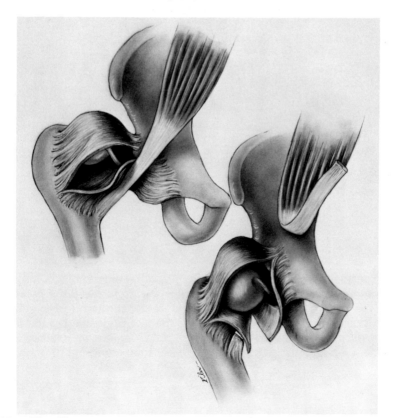

Figure 6.13. The iliopsoas in hip dislocation pulls the inferior capsule across the acetabulum, effectively blocking the placement of the femoral head with the joint. The capsule can be easily mistaken for fibrous tissue in the depths of the acetabulum.

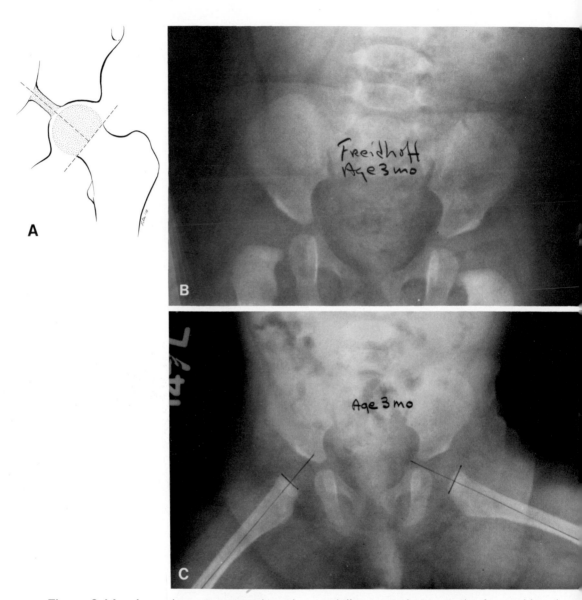

Figure 6.14. A good way to recognize minor malalignments between the femoral head and acetabulum that may be very significant clinically. (*A*) Erect a perpendicular from a line drawn at the proximal metaphysis. It should center through the triradiate cartilage. (*B*) The anteroposterior roentgenogram reveals the lateral position of the femur and the absence of the ossification center. (*C*) The lines make obvious the malalignment with the axial line on the left riding up the acetabulum rather than centering through the triradiate cartilage.

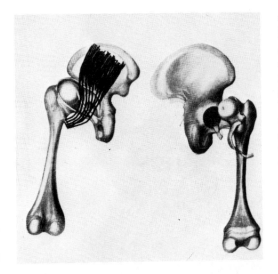

Figure 6.15. Ludloff's article in the 1912 edition of the *American Journal of Orthopedic Surgery* contained this illustration comparing the normal and the dislocated hip. On the dislocated side the iliopsoas muscle and tendon have been drawn in. Many of the features of the pathology of dislocated hip have been drawn in—the capsule drawn up by the iliopsoas, the acetabulum bent up in its outer one-third, etc.

to be 27.5 degrees at birth and 20 degrees between ages 1 and 2. The normal acetabular angle is considered to be 23–25 degrees, and any greater measurement is taken as indicating abnormality, particularly in the patient more than 6 months of age. A line is drawn between the tips of the ilia at the triradiate cartilage in the depth of the acetabulum. A second line drawn from the tip of the ilium to the outer edge of the acetabulum creates the angle known as the acetabular index. The significance of an acetabular index that is apparently higher than normal is easily misinterpreted.

Remember that it is the outer third of the acetabulum that is significant in congenital dislocation of the hip. Caffey's study of children constituting a well child population helps to bring this out. A higher than normal index occurred with infants who were shown as they developed in later life to have had normal hips. It is true that children with dislocation in the older age group will have deficiency of ossification of the lateral third. This is secondary to the cartilage deformity that develops in this disease, but one cannot use the high acetabular index as the sole feature on which a diagnosis of dislocation of

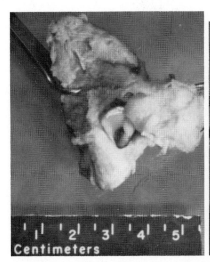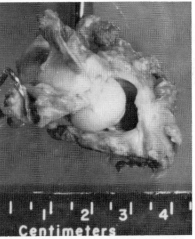

Figure 6.16 (*Left*). Dislocated hip in newborn infant; capsule opened from the anterior and superior aspects. The cartilage of the acetabulum, instead of shelving over the femoral head, is opposed to an enlarged ligamentum teres that intervenes between the cartilage and the femoral head. Here the femur has been displaced from the acetabulum.
Figure 6.17 (*Right*). The normally developed hip—contralateral side of same patient. The head has been detached from the joint. The cartilage of the acetabulum runs horizontally and shelves out over the femoral head.

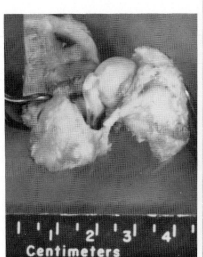 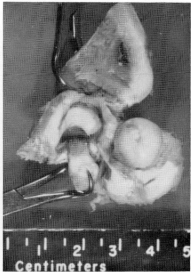

Figure 6.18 (*Left*). The dislocated hip. The enlarged ligamentum teres has been partially torn from its insertion. The acetabulum runs vertically rather than horizontally. An enlarged limbus was not seen. The inability to seat the femoral head without division of the inferior capsule is quite evident.

Figure 6.19 (*Right*). The lower clamp is attached to the ligamentum teres, which has been pulled inferiorly. The joint space for acceptance of the head is minimal, the acetabulum is vertical, and the capsule tents across the joint just inferior to either end of the acetabular cartilage.

the hip is based. The diagnosis must also rest on other features of acetabular development, such as irregular ossification in the outer third, alteration of the head of the femur to the acetabulum, the delayed development of the capital femoral epiphysis, and then finally, of course, on physical examination as well. In this regard we have found it most helpful to have an anteroposterior roentgenogram made with the hips in neutral, and another one with the hips abducted, which helps bring out the malalignment of the femur in relation to the acetabulum. This will not occur in the presence of high acetabular indexes if the hips are normally located.

C-E Angle

Wiberg has established an objective method of evaluating the position of the femoral head in relation to the acetabular roof. The measurement is called the C-E angle (center of the capital femoral epiphysis to the lateral edge of the acetabulum).

A line is drawn from the center of the head of the femur to the lateral edge of the acetabulum. This line forms an angle with a vertical line running through the center of the head. A transparent circular protractor placed on the x-ray film so that its central point is at the center of a circle enclosing the head of the femur readily enables this angle to be read.

The angle is less than normal when either the acetabular roof is underdeveloped or the femoral head is laterally displaced. It is helpful in determining both acetabular dysplasia and subluxation of the femoral head.

Severin[42,43] gave figures for this angle based on a study of 136 children between 6 and 13 years. He believes that a C-E angle of less than 15 degrees is definitely pathologic, of 15–19 degrees equivocal, and of more than 20 degrees is consistent with normal development.

Anteversion

Anteversion may be defined as the relation of the long axis of the femoral neck to a line drawn through the femoral condyles in the coronal plane (Figs. 6.23 and 6.24).

Anteversion at birth is approximately 25 degrees but it has a tendency to decrease with growth to 5–15 degrees. The anteversion normally present is approximately 15 degrees, and it is associated with about 45 degrees of internal rotation in flexion at the hip joint. When anteversion is increased, internal ro-

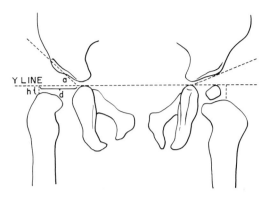

Figure 6.22. Measurement of the acetabular angle by the method of Hilgenreiner. The *Y line* connects the triradiate cartilages. *Line h* indicates the tendency of the diaphysis to ride superiorly as compared with the normal position on the other side. *Line d* indicates the lateral displacement from the acetabular floor. (Redrawn from V. L. Hart: *Congenital Dyplasia of the Hip Joint and Sequelae in the Newborn and Early Postnatal Life*, p. 39; Springfield, Ill.: Charles C Thomas, 1952.)

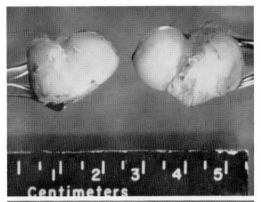

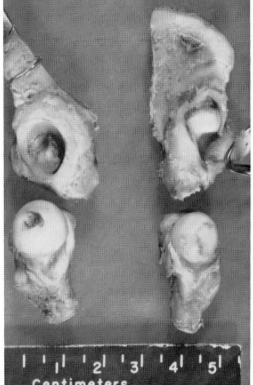

Figure 6.20 (*Top*). View of superior aspect of femoral head, neck, and greater trochanter showing deformity of head on left and increased anteversion.

Figure 6.21 (*Bottom*). Comparison of normal hip (*left*) and dislocated hip (*right*) with enlarged ligamentum teres on the right hip pulled laterally.

tation is correspondingly increased. Thus excessive anteversion may permit internal rotation as great as 90 degrees.

Anteversion of the femur is recognized by the fact that a roentgenogram of the hip taken with the knees straight ahead reveals the hip to be in external rotation. It is differentiated from valgus of the femoral neck by the fact that the height of the femoral head is not increased over the trochanter. A roentgenogram taken with the femur in internal rotation is also helpful in differentiating anteversion from valgus.

Anteversion of the femur may play a part in poor development of the acetabulum after the femoral head has been placed in the acetabulum. In internal rotation the femoral head is placed well beneath the overhanging roof of the acetabulum. With the limb in the neutral position and the knee pointing forward, anteversion of the femur tends to bring the femoral head to the anterior lip of the acetabulum and to cause the femur to subluxate outward.

Relation of Hip to Spine

Routine spinal x-rays of patients suspected of congenital dislocation of the hip are illu-

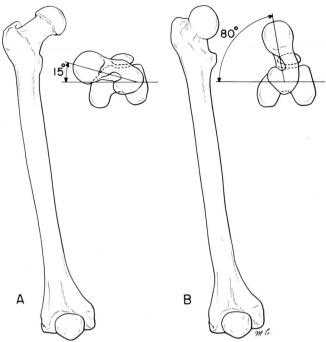

Figure 6.23. Anteversion of the femur illustrated diagrammatically as the relation between the axis of the neck and the axis of the femoral condyles. In the anteroposterior view, the anteverted femoral neck appears shortened and straightened in relation to the shaft.

minating. Two types of spine curvature are often revealed.

1. Curvature of the Spine Secondary to Adduction Contracture of the Hip. The patient, when aligned in the anatomic position for the roentgenograms, develops a pelvic tilt as the result of the adduction contracture. The pelvis is "high" on the adducted side, and there is a secondary curve in the low lumbar area to compensate for this tilt and to align the occiput with the pelvis.

2. Primary Curvature of the Spine. This curve is a total curve involving the entire spine in a single long curve. It results in a tilted pelvis and an adducted position of the hip. Clinically, affected babies will have a limitation of lateral bend in the direction correcting the curve. There may or may not be an accompanying adduction contracture of the hip. Primary spinal curve is presumably the result of position in utero.

When there is no adduction contracture, the hip may be quite well developed by x-ray, which accounts for the baby who is thought to have a congenital hip problem; and yet little is revealed by roentgenogram.

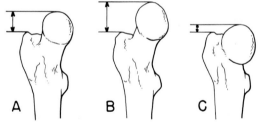

Figure 6.24. Anteversion (*A*), valgus (*B*), and varus (*C*) of the femoral neck can be differentiated in the anteroposterior view by the relative height of the femoral head above the greater trochanter.

The thigh folds are often asymmetric in such a child.

When there is an adduction contracture, the hip is usually underdeveloped; i.e., there is an increased slant to the acetabulum and a delay in mineralization of the growth center of the proximal femoral epiphysis. Improvement of such a hip is markedly aided by trunk-stretching exercises at the hip. Failure to correct the trunk curve delays return of the hip to a normal appearance by x-ray.

There are various forms of underdevelopment of the hip. In the first year of life the hip may not develop into the stable, functioning joint that it should be. This may be owing to actual congenital deformity or to neurologic conditions, but much more commonly it is owing to a persistent adduction and anteversion of the hip. The earlier such abnormal stresses are recognized, the easier it is to correct the hip and to promote its further growth.

The various stages of failure of the hip joint to develop may be designated as: (1) the dysplastic hip, (2) the subluxated hip, and (3) the dislocated hip (Fig. 6.25). The relationship between the underdeveloped hip joint and malum coxae senilis in later life has been pointed out by Hart.[22] The severe disability that degenerative arthritis of the hip may impose on the adult makes the goal of normal hip development in the child a very worthwhile one to pursue.

DYSPLASTIC HIP

The mother frequently brings the child with dysplastic hip for inspection because she has noted difficulties with one of the legs while placing diapers on the child. The dysplastic hip is recognized clinically by asymmetry of the thigh folds, an adduction contracture of the hip, and an apparent shortening of the leg (Figs. 6.26–6.28). The infant is examined for an adduction contracture in recumbency. In this position, the thighs are flexed 90 degrees and then abducted. A limitation of full abduction is very evident by this examination.

A persistent adducted position of the femur relative to the pelvis may be due to a contracture of the adductor muscle group. The adducted position may, however, be secondary to an elevation of one side of the pelvis and a curvature of the spine.

The adducted position results in apparent shortening of the extremity. The hip appears more prominent laterally on the involved side. The knee and popliteal creases are at different levels. The inguinal fold is deepened on the involved side so that the labia are partially hidden by it.

Roentgen Signs

The acetabular roof has an angle greater than 25 degrees. The hip is not markedly displaced either laterally or superiorly. There is usually recognizable anteversion of the femur. A delay in development of the hip joint is evident. The ossification center for the femoral head is late in appearance. Ossification of the acetabular roof and closure of the ischiopubic juncture are delayed.

Treatment

The treatment attempts primarily to eliminate the adducted position of the femur relative to the pelvis. The inability of the trunk to bend equally to both sides, if present, must be corrected by stretching exercises.

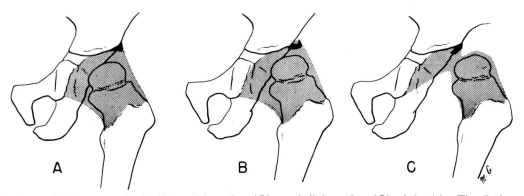

Figure 6.25. Dysplasia (*A*), subluxation (*B*), and dislocation (*C*) of the hip. The limbus in subluxation is pushed superiorly against the ilium; in dislocation the femoral head may press the limbs inferiorly into the acetabulum.

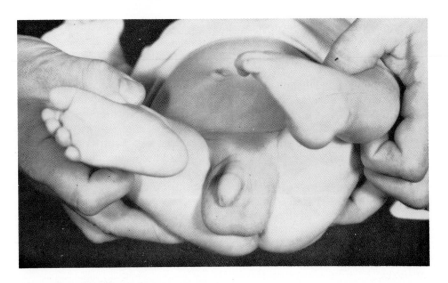

Figure 6.26. On attempted abduction in flexion, an adduction contracture strated, particularly on the right.

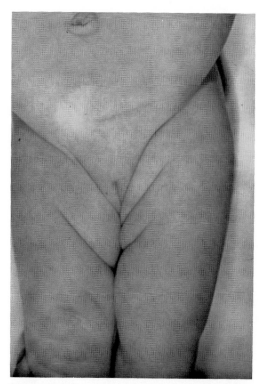

Figure 6.27. Inguinal fold obscuring labia on the involved side. Note the asymmetric folds.

We no longer use abduction splints either of plastic or of soft felt. Even in the normal hip there is a significant incidence of avascular necrosis (3–6%) and pressure effect on the epiphyseal line such that it starts off as a minimal disability and becomes a severe one through treatment. Abduction exercises done by the mother do not hold the hip in the abducted position and are used instead. The bulk of the ordinary diaper is sufficient abduction with which to treat this condition. The child's own activity will tend to stretch this final contracture. If all of these persist, the child has been underdiagnosed, and there actually is a dislocation of the hip with the hip lying in the lateral third of the acetabulum. For this condition a more radical treatment approach is indicated.

SUBLUXATED HIP

Subluxation of the hip, both as a stage in the development of dislocation and as an individual entity, has been studied by Hart,[21,22] who noted that the subluxated state, if not treated, may not progress to dislocation but that it remains, along with an underdeveloped, slanting acetabular roof and a tendency of the femoral head to progress still further laterally and superiorly in the joint.

In this condition the acetabular roof again has a marked slant that is greater than the usually acceptable angle of 25 degrees. The appearance of the epiphyseal growth center is delayed. This hip is distinguished from the dysplastic hip, however, in that it rides laterally in the joint to the point of actual dislocation. These criteria form a triad enunciated by Putti[39] that enables determination of the so-called "preluxation" state (Fig. 6.29).

From the pathologic point of view, the head of the femur may have pressed the cartilaginous rim or limbus of the acetabulum upward and toward the ilium. As brought out by Leveuf,[24] the limbus may remain attached in this position and be a serious detriment to the formation of the acetabular roof.

The subluxated hip, so-called, is but one stage of the disease of congenital dislocation of the hip. The hip is lying in the lateral third of the acetabulum and abduction x-rays bring out the malalignment of the femur in relation to the triradiate cartilage centrally in the acetabulum. These children are those who have not walked, but because of the lateral position of the femoral head are developing increasing changes consistent with dislocation as a result of this position. These changes include pressing the cartilaginous rim or flattening of the femoral head opposite this area. The outer third of the acetabulum is often underdeveloped so far as the ossification center is concerned in the ilium. As compared to so-called dysplasia it is quite evident that the hip rides laterally in the lateral third of the acetabulum, and the abduction x-ray will bring this out. The ossification center of the femoral head is delayed in its appearance and development. Because subluxation is actually

the first stage of dislocation, if untreated the development of the joint can be expected to be abnormal and become more evident with later roentgenograms as the skeleton matures.

We believe it is very important to treat this condition fully and radically. By x-ray there is lateral displacement of the femoral shaft in relation to the ilium. A line drawn through the center and neck no longer points toward the center of the triradiate cartilage and the depth of the acetabulum. Clinically there are often asymmetrical thigh and buttock folds. Prominence of the trochanter on the involved side and the adduction contracture can be demonstrated. Palpation of the femoral head beneath the femoral artery and just below the inguinal ligament may still give some feeling of fullness due to the fact that lateral dislocation is not marked at this stage.

Treatment

If the abduction film on a child of this type fails to reveal that the femur sits normally in relation to the acetabulum, then a Pavlik harness may be used. This harness allows considerable activity by the child without keeping the legs in fixed abduction. A line drawn through the femoral neck should transect the triradiate cartilage. If it does not do so when the hip is abducted, those measures must be undertaken to accomplish correction

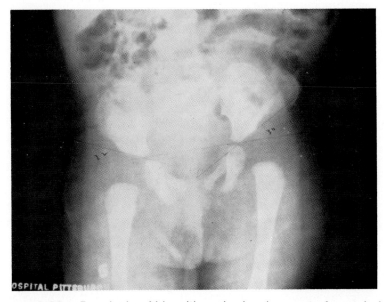

Figure 6.28. Dysplasia of hip with underdevelopment of acetabulum.

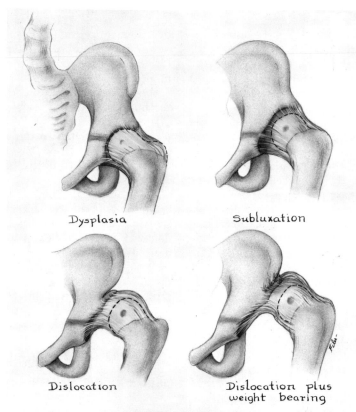

Figure 6.28.1. Diagram of the features of dysplasia, subluxation, dislocation, and dislocation plus ambulation. In dysplasia, the hip is actually centered in the acetabulum but forces are at work preventing the development of the hip from equaling the other side. The most common situation is a positional trunk contracture at birth elevating the pelvis on one side and adducting the hip. In subluxation, the hip is not truly centered in the acetabulum but lies in the lateral third and is beginning to make a plastic impression on both the cartilage of the acetabulum and of the hip. In dislocation, the hip is not centered—a line running centrally up the femoral neck will not bisect the triradiate cartilage. The lateral one-third of the acetabulum is permanently deformed either by pressing the limbus up along the ilium or, if the leg has been maintained abducted, it could press the limbus inward. The cartilage of the femoral head is fibrillated and deformed. Ambulation causes the femoral head to progress superiorly, causing the formation of a groove in the lateral cartilage of the acetabulum.

of these findings by x-ray. We no longer use simple abduction as a means of accomplishing this because of the high morbidity accompanying the use of fixed abduction devices. Traction in line with the trunk may pull the iliopsoas sufficiently to allow it to stretch and not form a limitation when the hips are abducted. This is primarily true in the youngster with relaxed ligaments, and in these individuals the correction of the abduction x-ray is so quick and easy that it is no problem. For the rest, however, division of the iliopsoas tendon and underlying capsule, which will be discussed under the treatment of dislocation of the hip, is recommended. It is rec-

ommended because the pathology is actually that of a dislocated hip without the development of marked cartilage deformity, and the factor preventing normal seating of the femoral head must be quickly corrected.

PATHOLOGY AND RECOGNITION OF CONGENITAL DISLOCATION OF HIP

The clinical recognition of congenital dislocation of the hip is confused by the fact that an adduction contracture and asymmetrical thigh folds can exist in infants with normal hips. It is further confused by fascial snaps, clicks, or jerks in the region of the hip. These may occur as a result of tight tendons snapping over bony prominences; medially, the likely culprit is the iliopsoas; laterally, the tensor fascia lata.

The frank jolt of a truly dislocated hip during abduction in flexion (described by Ortolani) does not occur in all dislocated hips; when it does occur, the entire examination is usually classic and the dislocation frank.

There are two parts to the pathology of congenital dislocation of the hip. One is the fact that it exists at birth. The second is the deformity that develops with growth as a result of the dislocated position of the femur relative to the acetabulum.

The pathology of dislocation of the hip at birth reveals the importance of the iliopsoas muscle in providing a fundamental contracture that causes the femoral head to ride with pressure on the lateral third of the acetabulum. The femoral head has not risen ceph-

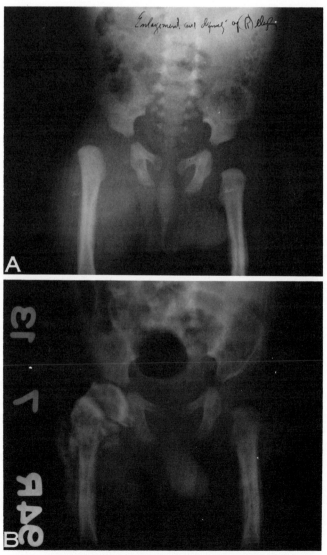

Figure 6.29. (A) Apparent dislocation of the hip accompanied by soft-tissue swelling. (B) The arthrogram outlines the callus surrounding a birth fracture with displacement of the femoral shaft, but a located femoral head.

alad, but only laterally. The cause of this lateral position is the block to full medial seating of the femoral head found by tight hypertrophied iliopsoas and secondarily the capsular contracture.

The inferior capsule is pulled up by the iliopsoas tendon to cover between 40 and 50% of the acetabulum. There is no way in which the dislocated hip examined on the autopsy table could be seated without pressure on this deformed capsule.

At birth the femoral head is deformed to accommodate to the pressure coming from a medial direction. The cartilage of the femoral head does not reveal any fibrillation at first but if the hip has undergone treatment—particularly casted in abduction—this evidence of pathology may exist.

The capsule is not abnormally thickened, but the capsular deformity is permanent in nature.

In a study of 240 hips of 120 stillborn infants and dead newborn infants, Stanisavjevic and Mitchell found 2 dislocated hips and 3 subluxated. In 9 of their normal hips a click or Ortolani's sign was noted as the thighs were abducted. This was found to be produced by the interposition of an unusually large ligamentum capitis femoris in 4 and by sliding of the iliopsoas tendon over an enlarged iliopectineal bursa in 5. In the abnormal hips, hypertrophy of the iliopsoas tendon was found in every instance.

The hip, when dislocated, lies superior to the acetabulum and separates the gluteus medius and minimus from the ilium. The cartilaginous limbus forming the rim of the acetabulum lies inferior to the femoral head. The limbus is often indented by pressure from the head. It is normally largest posteriorly and superiorly. The capsule is stretched so that it continues to enclose the head in its position distant from the acetabulum. There tends to be a constriction of the capsule between the head and the acetabulum. This constriction is the result of pressure from the iliopsoas tendon. The capsule is often adherent, at least in part, to the ilium, where it is held against the bone by the pressure of the head. It may also be adherent inferiorly where it tents across the acetabulum.

Anteversion of the femur of some degree is a virtually constant accompaniment. Normal anteversion at birth is about 25 degrees; it decreases with growth to about 15 degrees.

The acetabulum may be filled by an enlarged Haversian fat pad. The ligamentum teres, which is greatly elongated in actual dislocation, may appear hypertrophied.

In late dislocations the head may lose its round full shape, become flattened in the area pressed against the ilium, and assume a more conelike appearance. The cartilage of the head may become pitted and fibrillated.

Clinical Picture

The patient is usually a female with inability to abduct the hip. This is often noted by the mother when she puts on the diaper. Some asymmetry of the thigh and buttock folds may also be noted. Apparently shortening of the leg on the affected side is a frequent complaint.

The adductors are apparently short in relation to the other musculature about the hip when the hip is dislocated. This is best demonstrated with the leg in 90 degrees of flexion at the hip when abduction is attempted. Whereas infants with normal hips can usually achieve 45 degrees or more of abduction, those with subluxed or dislocated hips are limited to 20 degrees or less. However, the real obstacle to reduction is the iliopsoas.

The buttock fold tends to be higher on the side of the adducted hip than on the unaffected side, and the thigh folds beneath it are frequently asymmetric. There is some apparent shortening of the side involved, and a high pelvis can be demonstrated on that side by palpating the anterior superior spines of the ilium. The inguinal fold runs into the labia so that it appears smaller on the involved side.

With actual dislocation, the femoral head is absent from its normal position beneath the femoral artery just distal to the inguinal ligament (Fig. 6.30). The trochanter is unduly prominent (Fig. 6.31) and lies above Nélaton's line, which connects the anterosuperior spine and the tuberosity of the ischium (Fig. 6.33). In unilateral dislocation, Galeazzi's sign is positive; when the femurs are flexed to 90 degrees, one knee, owing to the shortening of the thigh with dislocation, lies below the level of the other (Fig. 6.32). Internal rotation is usually increased to 70 degrees or more owing to anteversion of the hip. The "sign of the jerk" is the click that is felt when the

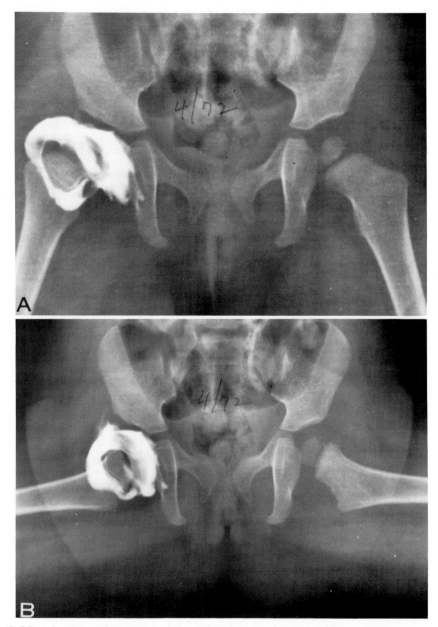

Figure 6.30. In the arthrogram of the laterally placed femoral head, the groove in the capsule formed by the iliopsoas tendon is seen. (*A*) Anteroposterior, (*B*) lateral.

thigh is abducted in flexion and the femoral head slides over the acetabular rim. The adductors must be relaxed to elicit this click, which may be felt on both exit and entry in the dysplastic acetabulum.

When the dislocation is bilateral, the perineum is widened. It may be possible to detect telescoping of the hip by applying traction with one hand while the other grasps

the pelvis and, with a finger, palpates the trochanter.

X-rays reveal the hip to have slipped superiorly in relation to the acetabulum and Shenton's line, therefore, to be discontinuous. Shenton's line is formed by the inferior border of the neck and the superior border of the obturator foramen. Discontinuity of it, when it is the only finding, is not a reliable

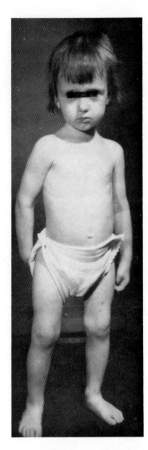

Figure 6.31. Child, age 2, with bilateral dislocation of the hips, wide perineum, and prominent trochanters.

of the hip abductors; of these the principal one is the gluteus medius (Fig. 6.34). Shortening of the functional length of the muscle results in weakness.

When the patient stands on one leg, inability of the abductors to elevate the pelvis on the opposite side results in a positive Trendelenburg's sign. The pelvis on the opposite side drops (Fig. 6.36). This can be made quite apparent by marking the posterior superior spines of the ilium before the test is performed.

This inability to elevate the pelvis results secondarily in inability to clear the opposite leg on walking. In order to clear the leg when walking, the patient compensates for the abductor weakness by bringing the body weight over and beyond the femoral head. This allows the lateral trunk musculature to aid in elevating the pelvis.

Such a gait, which transfers the trunk over the involved hip with each step, results in a medius limp. If both hips are involved, the trunk is transferred first over one hip and then over the other. The symmetry of such a gait makes it less noticeable than the gait in cases of unilateral involvement and accounts for the fact that, among children who are not found to have hip dislocation until they are walking, unilateral is discovered earlier than bilateral involvement.

sign of hip difficulty, but as an adjunct finding, it aids in the interpretation of the x-rays. The dislocation may have begun either anteriorly or posteriorly. Acetabular views of the hip reveal the anterior or posterior relation to the acetabulum. The signs of underdevelopment of the joint and proximal femur previously discussed are also present.

In so-called unilateral dislocation, the contralateral hip is worthy of study. A roentgenographic study by DiPrampero[14] has brought some interesting facts to light in this regard. Of 200 patients with unilateral dislocation, subluxation or dysplasia of the hip on the contralateral side was found in 108 cases.

Signs Due to Weakness of Hip Abductors

The displacement upward of the femur and the lack of a stable joint result in weakness

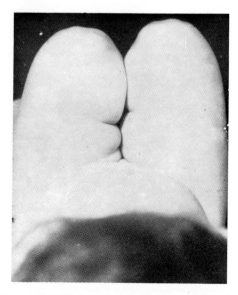

Figure 6.32. In unilateral dislocation, flexion of the thighs to a right angle may reveal shortening on sighting along top of knees (Galeazzi's sign).

Differential Diagnosis

Inasmuch as the adducted position of the femur relative to the pelvis is responsible for most of the clinical signs that make us suspect dysplasia, subluxation, or dislocation of the hip, it is helpful to review other conditions, of which there are a surprisingly large number, that might cause the same adduction. All of these conditions, of course, have other characteristics that allow differentiation. They are listed here in an order that suggests their relative incidence.

The attempt to adduct the hip on either flexion or extension may reveal a limitation in this plane. Such a limitation could be due to:

1. Voluntary resistance, which can be overcome by thoroughness and persistence in examination.

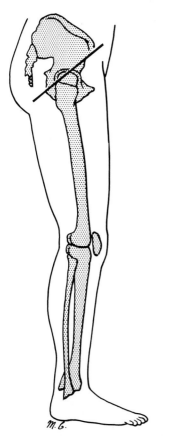

Figure 6.33. Diagram of Nélaton's line, which runs from the anterior superior spine of the ilium to the tuberosity of the ischium. In dislocation, the greater trochanter is palpated above this line.

2. Spina bifida, with weak hip abductors and adduction contracture, which develops with persistent maintenance of the adducted position.

3. Hip joint infection—pyogenic, tuberculous, luetic, etc.—which also limits motion in other places.

4. Obstetric trauma—contusion, fractures of the epiphyseal area, or dislocation—which may result in resistance to abduction while the hip is tender.

5. Chondrodystrophy—Morquio's syndrome or Hurler's syndrome—which may limit abduction but also cause other obvious stigmata.

6. Scurvy or rickets, which may result in painful limbs and limited motion (scurvy occasionally is associated with the reverse of this—a flaccid pseudoparalysis).

7. Developmental coxa vara with deformity of the femoral neck, which apes congenital dislocation well on examination, but is unusual before the age of 4 (in this condition, the femoral head is still in the acetabulum and there is no telescoping).

8. In newborns, the limitation of full extension at the hip and knee that is present at birth and with which limitation of abudction is associated (the examiner should be able to abduct each hip 20 degrees, however).

9. Cerebral palsy with spastic paralysis, which characteristically causes a stretch reflex in the adductors that limits abduction.

10. Still's disease (rheumatoid arthritis involving the hips in children), which limits motion in other places as well as abduction.

11. Poliomyelitis, from which an adduction contracture may develop, although an abduction contracture is more usual.

12. Congenital scoliosis, which may result in an elevation of the pelvis on one side and an adducted position of the hip, but which is ordinarily not associated with an actual limitation of motion of the joint.

The age of the patient when he is presented for treatment largely determines both the severity of the treatment and the prognosis of its effects. An awareness of the condition on the part of the medical community results in early presentation of the patient for treatment and is preventive medicine in the highest sense of the word. Throughout treatment, tightness of the iliopsoas muscle must be overcome. It is more important than adductor tightness.

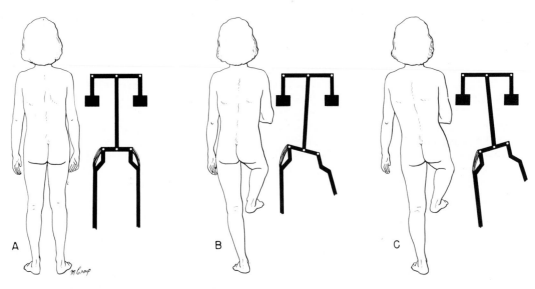

Figure 6.34. Signs of weakness of the gluteus medius such as may be associated with congenital dislocation of the hip. (*A*) Normal standing. (*B*) Dropping of pelvis of contralateral side when standing on affected leg. (*C*) Compensation for weakness when walking by shifting center of gravity of trunk in order to elevate pelvis on opposite side.

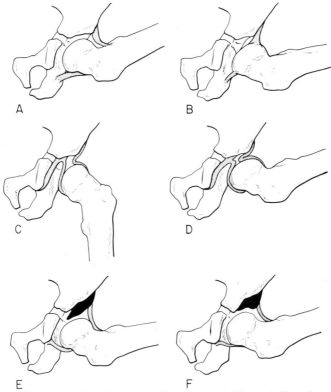

Figure 6.35. Possible obstacles to reduction include: (*A* and *B*) adherent capsule, (*C* and *D*) capsule lining the joint with hourglass constriction. This hourglass constriction follows from pressure of the overriding iliopsoas tendon. (Redrawn from V. L. Hart: *Congenital Dysplasia of the Hip Joint and Sequelae in the Newborn and Early Postnatal Life*, p. 48; Springfield, Ill., Charles C Thomas, 1952.)

TREATMENT OF CONGENITAL DISLOCATION OF HIP UNDER AGE 2

Rationale: Both closed and open reductions of the dislocated hip in infancy have well recognized complications in the form of avascular necrosis of the ossification center of the femoral head, necrosis of the epiphyseal plate, and stiffness of the hip.

Avascular necrosis and cessation of growth of the proximal femoral epiphysis are two of the major complications of conservative treatment (Fig. 6.40). Massie[28] (1951) reported abnormal epiphyseal changes in 75% of 62 dislocated hips after closed reduction. Of these abnormalities 72% were found to be troublesome. Bost and associates[4] found that 52% of 112 hips were involved. Ponseti[38] (1966) found changes in 46.2% of 173 hips treated by closed reduction. Massie and Howorth[29] (1951) and Judet (1958) reported a higher incidence of these changes after closed as compared to open reduction. The lower

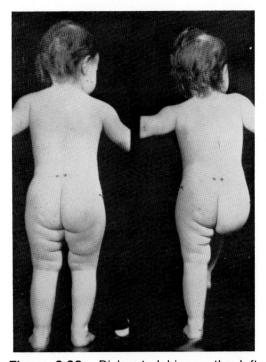

Figure 6.36. Dislocated hip on the left with high buttock fold, asymmetric thigh folds, prominent trochanter, and positive Trendelenburg. The opposite side of the pelvis drops when the patient stands on the affected leg.

incidence of epiphyseal changes after open reduction can be explained by the release of soft tissues necessitated in the surgical exposure and the consequent elimination of constricting pressure.

Nicholson and associates in 1954 demonstrated by angiography performed in children postmortem that the frog leg position interfered with arterial filling of the medial and lateral circumflex and the profunda femoris arteries. Ogden (1973) demonstrated in anatomic specimens that the limbus as a projecting edge entered the angle at the base of the neck between it and the trochanteric epiphysis. This shut down the lateral epiphyseal vessels in the abducted position.

At the American Academy of Orthopaedic Surgeons meeting in 1972, Gage and Winter reported 6 cases of avascular necrosis of the normal hip in 154 patients treated for congenital dislocation. Hoyt reported the lowered incidence of avascular necrosis following preliminary traction. Less extreme positions are helpful in reducing the incidence of complications. Wilkinson and Carter found that the femoral head appeared to be fragmented and deformed in 24 of 108 patients after using neutral rotation in a plaster cast or a Denis-Browne harness.

The use of abduction splints causes sufficient difficulty if the hip is kept abducted to negate their use (Fig. 6.41). There is considerable variation in the definition of a dislocated hip amongst various authors. Von Rosen[47] used the Ortolani click as a diagnostic test and reported that all of 31 hips became stable in an abduction-lateral rotation splint and only 3 failed to have a normal appearance at follow-up. If the dislocation is defined as those in whom the femoral head has moved to the lateral third of the acetabulum, the abduction must confront soft-tissue obstacles interfering with vascularity in the abducted position even when the femur is flexed rather than fully extended.

Because the iliofemoral approach can be expected to leave some residual stiffness of the hip, a surgical approach must be used which relieves the soft-tissue obstruction without leaving a residual limitation of motion. After the iliofemoral approach Scaglietti and Calandriello found normal motion in only 50 of 171 hips followed for 6 months to 10 years.

The importance of the tight iliopsoas and the capsule as the seat of soft-tissue obstruction to seating of the femoral head is stressed.

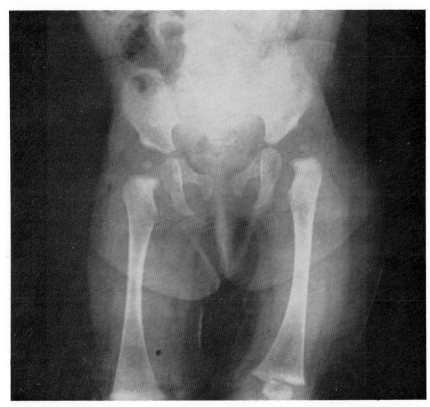

Figure 6.37. Further development of congenital hip disease with riding upward of the femur.

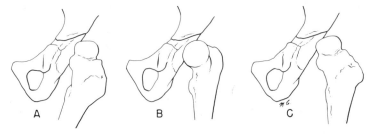

Figure 6.38. Some of the causes of poor seating of the femoral head in the acetabulum. (*A*) Adduction, (*B*) anteversion, (*C*) improper alignment.

Because this can be relieved simply through a medial adductor approach, we have used this surgical relief as the first stage of treatment for infants below age 2. Over age 2, further development of the pathology with growth and/or unsuccesful treatment necessitate further measures and a different approach.

Median Adductor Approach

A medial incision in line with the posterior margin of the adductor longus is used. The patient is supine with the hip flexed 90 degrees and abducted, a position that brings out the abduction contracture of the unreduced hip (Figs. 6.42 and 6.43).

A straight incision is made along the course of the adductor longus distally from the iliac crease. After division of the deep fascia, the approach goes posterior to the adductor longus, separating it from the adductor magnus and gracilis by blunt dissection. The adductor magnus with the obturator nerve lying on it is then exposed. The dissection thereafter proceeds posterior to the adductor brevis, where the lesser trochanter is readily palpated. Any precapsular fat can now be pushed medially so that the iliopsoas tendon is readily visualized. A curved hemostat is inserted beneath the tendon, which when divided transversely retracts superiorly. Fat can then be pushed superiorly off the anterior capsule so that the hourglass constriction along the former course of the tendon is seen. A retractor can now be passed along the anterior surface of the capsule and superior to the femoral head. The capsule can then be incised along the axis of the femoral neck, the incision proceeding medially and anteriorly far enough to allow the femoral head to be brought into the empty acetabulum, where it is in view. When the head is located, the capsular incision is spread and cannot be closed. The adductors, however, fall back together and the skin edges are readily approximated. After reduction, both hips are held in 10–20 degrees of internal rotation, 30 degrees of abduction, and 10 degrees of flexion.

When the spica cast is applied, it must be molded on the dislocated side to maintain medially directed pressure over the trochanter to keep the head in the acetabulum. The dislocated position creates a pocket into which the femur will fall by gravity unless this is done. The adduction contracture present when the hip was dislocated vanishes with reduction. It is not necessary to divide the adductors, nor is it necessary to remove soft tissue from the acetabulum. The extent of the deformity of the acetabulum can readily be evaluated by palpation during the operation.

It is evident that this procedure removes the obstacle to reduction without pressure but does nothing to alter the deformed cartilage acetabulum except to relieve the pressure of the femoral head on it. The door to the acetabulum is opened, but the roof must still form. Recovery of the cartilage is possible once the mechanical forces acting on it are changed. If the pressure is not relieved in children over 2 months of age, this deformity becomes progressively more serious with advancing age so that, in children more than 2 years old, secondary changes have occurred with capsular adherence to the ilium above the acetabulum as well as to the inferior half of the acetabulum. The operation is used in children in the newborn period and up to 2

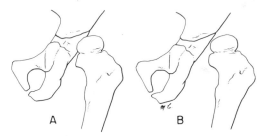

Figure 6.39. Undercorrected subluxation tends to progress, not to regress.

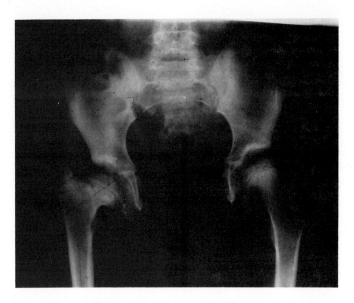

Figure 6.40. Avascular necrosis and growth arrest of the capital femoral epiphysis secondary to treatment—overgrowth of the trochanteric epiphysis occurs secondarily.

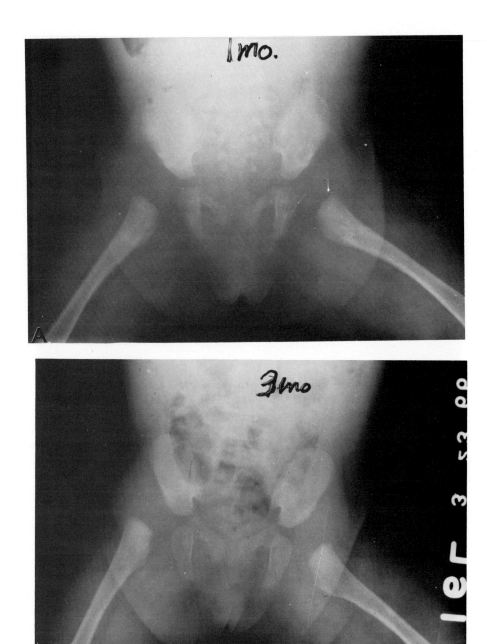

Figure 6.41. Series of roentgenograms in an infant girl from age 1 month to age 3 years, 9 months. (*A*) At 1 month of age, a line drawn along the femoral shaft deviates from the triradiate cartilage. (*B*) This is still more marked at age 3 months. (*C*) The patient was treated with preliminary traction and abduction cast and readily located. (*D*) At age 9 months the ossification center appears delayed. (*E*) At age 3 years, 9 months, bone is ossifying irregularly and with diminished height—secondary to an interruption of the blood supply to the capital femoral epiphysis.

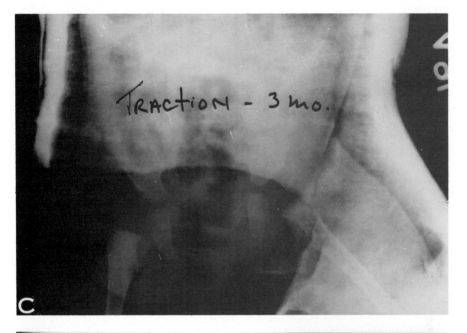

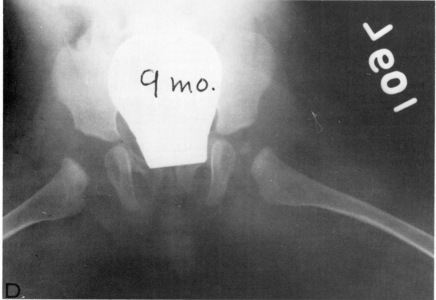

Fig. 6.41 (*C* and *D*)

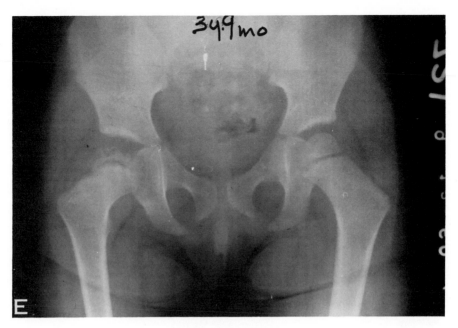

Fig. 6.41 (E)

years of age with success, provided the hip is immobilized in the functional position of 30 degrees of abduction, 10–20 degrees of internal rotation, and little or no flexion for at least 4 months after the operation.

Evaluation of Reduction

Roentgenograms of the hip should include anteroposterior and acetabular views, and review of them should be exceptionally discerning. Failure to find a perfect reduction in both views should result in open reduction, but this is seldom necessary in the infantile group.

Some infantile hips readily reduce when the patient is under anesthesia, but forceful maneuvers should never be used to achieve this result.

Most patients with dislocated hips have excessive anteversion, which prevents normal seating of the femoral head when the knee is foreward and the limb in line with the trunk. With infants less than 6 months old, there is no need to rush into an anteversion osteotomy, because there is great opportunity for corrective growth in the period of rapid growing that they are in. Once the infant is past

this early period, the need for osteotomy may be demonstrated by a comparison of roentgenograms of the hip taken anteroposteriorly while the hip is abducted and neutrally rotated with films taken in internal rotation and abduction (Fig. 6.44). Such a comparison may reveal the femoral head to point out of the joint in neutral rotation and to be in perfect alignment in internal rotation. When osteotomy is necessary, it should not be delayed.

Despite the apparent ease of treating hips in early infancy, difficult cases are found and careful roentgenographic examination must be made in order to produce a well developed joint with the femoral head in normal position (Fig. 6.45).

In evaluating end results it is frequently not appreciated that the femoral head is damaged in varying degrees when the child first presents for treatment. The head may be flattened from pressure against either the acetabular rim or the ilium. The cartilage of the femoral head may also be fibrillated. The shape of the femoral head may not be fully appreciated for several years when the ossification center finally begins to form. It frequently begins ossification eccentrically and may form from a number of separate centers. This irregular ossification has been inter-

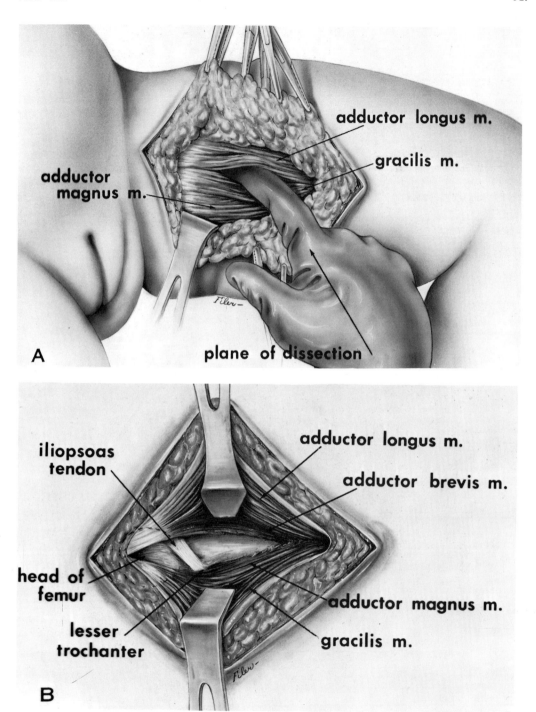

Figure 6.42. (*A*) Diagram of the medial adductor approach to the hip. This differs from the Ludloff approach in that the adductor longus and brevis are carried superiorly. (*B*) Finger dissection readily palpates the lesser trochanter—the gracilis and adductor magnus are inferior. There will frequently be some fat lobules about the capsule which must be pushed aside to visualize it and the iliopsoas tendon. (*C*) The iliopsoas tendon and the inferior capsule are divided. The iliopsoas will ascend superiorly—the capsule once opened cannot be brought together with the hip in its located position. (*D*)

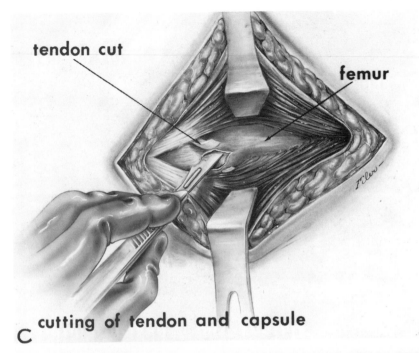

C

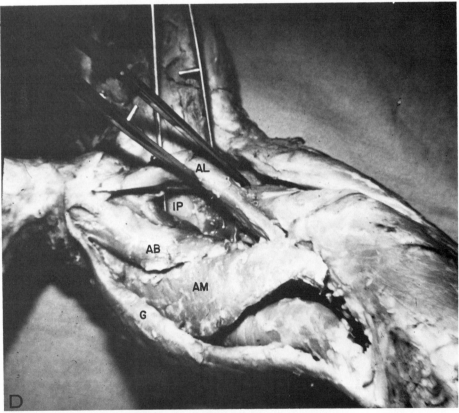

D

Photograph of the anatomy of the median adductor approach by John Ogden. (*AL*, adductor longus; *IP*, iliopsoas tendon; *AB*, adductor brevis; *AM*, adductor magnus; *G*, gracilis.) The superior forceps are on either side of the iliopsoas muscle as it descends to the lesser trochanter.

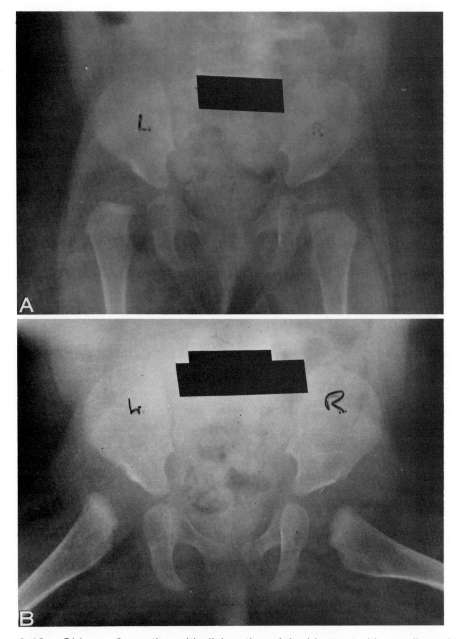

Figure 6.43.   Girl, age 6 months, with dislocation of the hip treated by median adductor approach. (A) Anteroposterior view shows lateral riding of femoral shaft on left. (B) Abduction anteroposterior view emphasizes the lateral riding femoral shaft. No ossification center is visible on the left for the capital femoral epiphysis. (C) At a period of 4 months postoperative, the ossification center for the epiphysis of the femoral head is ossifying well. (D) At 2 years postoperative, the hip is developing well with minor irregularities in ossification of the acetabulum secondary to the old dislocation and deformation of the acetabular cartilage (anteroposterior view). (E) Abduction (anteroposterior view) revealing alignment of femoral shaft to the triradiate cartilage.

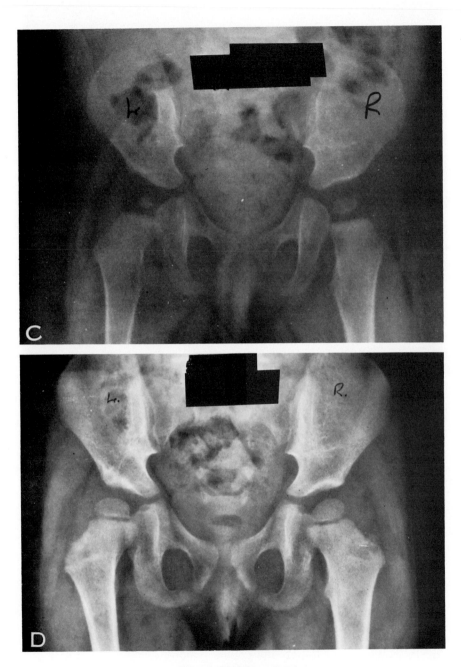

Fig. 6.43 (*C* and *D*)

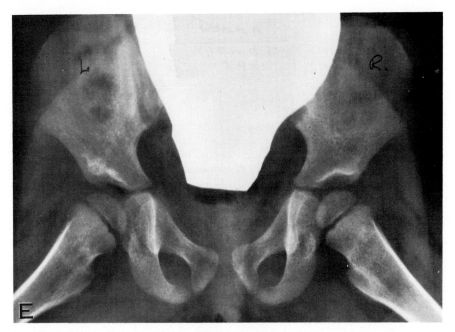

Fig. 6.43 (E)

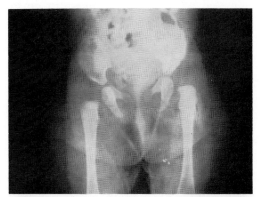

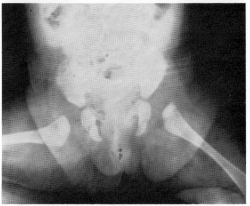

Figure 6.44.   Subluxation of hip; note malalignment on abduction.

preted as aseptic necrosis although there is no pathologic proof that this is true. The same can be said for delayed ossification of the femoral head. This may not actually be aseptic necrosis but rather a reflection of the abnormal physical forces which have been placed on the femoral head in the past.

An additional aid in determining the adequacy of reduction when it is questionable consists of contrast injection. Approximately 3 ml of an appropriate contrast medium to which the patient is not sensitive and which does not irritate the joint can be inserted into the joint cavity. The approach can be lateral to the femoral artery and anterior, or beneath the femoral artery through the hip adductors.

The dye gives most information if it is inserted just prior to reduction and films are taken. After the hip has been reduced, the position of the limbus can be determined as well as the presence of soft tissue in the joint.

Closed Reduction

If traction and closed reduction are the surgeon's choice then traction should be continued sufficiently long to allow an easily closed reduction. The percentage of hips considered for open reduction can be expected to rise if the use of force is limited and criteria for reduction are exact.

After closed reduction, the hip is placed in a plaster hip spica that holds the involved side to the foot and the uninvolved side to the knee. At the end of 6 weeks, the long side of the cast is shortened to the knee so that rotation of the hip is possible. Such spicas usually last 2–3 months before the child outgrows them. When to discontinue the spicas is a matter of judgment based on a study of x-rays showing the progress of the hip. The ancetabular roof should develop into the normal range, and the epiphyseal growth center should appear. The ability of the acetabular roof to respond to the femoral head placed in normal position within it usually continues, at least in part, to age 4.

While in the cast the patient is kept on a Bradford frame, which eases the care of the child and keeps the cast clean. The frame has an opening beneath the genitalia and is kept at a slight downward slant so that urine will not run into the cast but into the bedpan beneath the frame.

Closed reduction, when it is done, should only be done gently. Bost et al.[4] gave the incidence of aseptic necrosis of the femoral head following closed reduction as 12% of reductions done in the first year of life, 59% in the second year, and 62% in the third year. Aseptic necrosis following hip reduction does not always run the protracted course sometimes associated with Legg-Perthes disease.

TREATMENT OF DISLOCATED HIP AT AGE 2–4

In this group skeletal traction and open reduction of the hip become the treatment for the majority, rather than the minority, of patients. These youngsters are often affected bilaterally, for a unilateral dislocation presents more obvious physical signs in the gait and is, therefore, recognized earlier. Because these children have been walking for some time, a considerable upward displacement of the hip is likely. Telescoping of the hip as a physical sign is more easily elicited in this group than in any other.

It becomes more important than ever to pull the femoral head into a position opposite the acetabulum (Fig. 6.46). From this position, regardless of the mode of therapy, it can be placed in the acetabulum with relative ease if there is no obstruction (Fig. 6.47). The efficiency of the traction becomes very important. A well leg spica to hold the child in place is necessary, with skeletal traction on the femur (Figs. 6.48 and 6.49).

In this age group, some hips can be replaced by closed reduction so that there is perfect alignment—the centers of the head and neck point directly toward the triradiate cartilage—and no persistent widening of the joint.

The majority of youngsters over 2 have developed changes in the capsule, in the

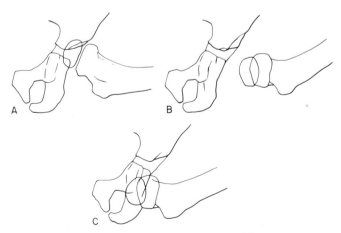

Figure 6.45. Incorrect positions following reduction. (*A*) Femoral head posterior to the acetabulum, (*B*) too great lateral displacement remaining, (*C*) femoral head inferior to the acetabulum in the region of the obturator foramen. (Redrawn from J. Hass: *Congenital Dislocation of the Hip*, p. 167; Springfield, Ill.: Charles C Thomas, 1951.)

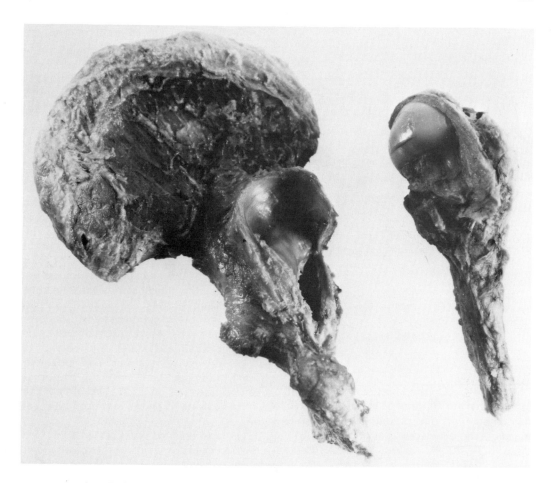

Figure 6.46. Deformity of the acetabulum resulting from malalignment of the femoral head affects the outer third of the acetabulum. Arthrogryposis as an underlying etiology reveals this deformity in its extreme as in this 5-month-old female. The outer third of the acetabulum laterally forms part of what has been termed a false acetabulum. The remaining acetabulum is below the deformed pertion. (Reprinted with permission from J. A. Ogden and H. L. Moss: Pathologic anatomy of congenital hip disease, In *Progress in Orthopaedic Surgery*; Berlin: Springer Verlag, 1978.)

shape of the head, and in adherence of the capsule to the acetabulum, so that a perfect reduction is not obtainable. Probably the most important barrier to a reduction is the iliopsoas tendon (Fig. 6.47). Open reduction is necessary to correct these difficulties. The surgeon should be aware that he will have to carry his dissection to the medial side of the ilipsoas or he will not adequately visualize the acetabulum.

Iliofemoral Incision

An anterior iliofemoral or Smith-Peterson incision is often used. The cartilaginous apo-physis of the ilium is carefully spared as the gluteus group is removed from the ilium by subperiosteal dissection. The cartilage apophysis of the ilium is elevated from the bony ilium and packed medially. The dissection must be carried to the medial border of the iliopsoas. Dividing the iliopsoas tendon and retracting the muscle proximally reveals the femoral nerve. This nerve must be visualized, because the true acetabulum lies beneath it. The lateral third of the acetabulum, which is deformed in these cases, can be mistaken for the true acetabulum (Figs. 6.50 and 6.51). The femoral head, on opening of the capsule, is found to have varying degrees of fibrillation of the cartilage and flattening of the surface

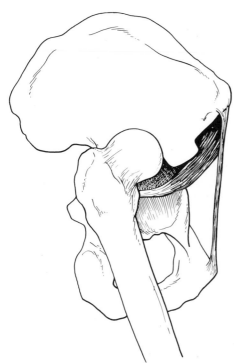

Figure 6.47. Constriction of the hip joint capsule by the tendon of the iliopsoas in dislocated hip riding superiorly. This is a major obstacle to reduction, and traction in line with the trunk is necessary to overcome it—not in abduction. (Redrawn from J. Hass: *Congenital Dislocation of the Hip*, p. 70; Springfield, Ill.: Charles C Thomas, 1951.)

in a position of extreme internal rotation, the capsule tends to be wound about the neck, constricting the circulation to the femoral head. Such a position may be responsible for aseptic necrosis of the femoral head after open reduction.

Anteversion Osteotomy

Osteotomies to correct anteversion are only done in the presence of excessive internal rotation at the hip. When done in the subtrochanteric region, a Steinmann pin is first placed in the femoral neck to hold the hip in internal rotation (Fig. 6.52). The distal fragment is then rotated until the knee joint is in line with the anatomic position of the body. When the patient stands with the knee joint pointing straight ahead, the hip is in internal rotation by comparison with its previous position. Excessive internal rotation is no longer possible. The use of osteotomy to correct anteversion is a matter of judgment in each individual case since the degree of anteversion varies in each. Osteotomy can also be performed in the supracondylar region.

Hips that tend to redislocate after open reduction need correction of the factor allowing the redislocation. An acetabular shelf or buttress may have to be built and anteversion, if a factor, corrected at a later date.

Treatment of Primary Anterior Congenital Dislocation

McCarroll and Crego[31] emphasized primary anterior dislocation of the hip as constituting 22.5% of a series of congenital dislocations of the hip. Such dislocations may be the result of rudimentary development of the anterior portion of the acetabulum or of a tendency of the acetabulum to face foreward and thereby to diminish the anterior buttress in relation to the head. Dega, in a review of 100 fetal specimens, noted that the angle of foreward inclination of the acetabulum was 29.5 degrees.

McCarroll advocates for this condition preliminary skeletal traction followed by attempted closed reduction. Should the closed reduction be unsuccessful, open reduction is in order. While an effort has been made to form either a shelf or buttress at the anterior

opposed to the ilium. The capsule is adherent to the side of the ilium and needs dissection to be brought down to the level of the actual acetabular rim. The psoas muscle may run across the joint in a manner preventing reduction and may need lengthening or transplantation to be removed as an obstacle. The hourglass constriction of the capsule will be formed just beneath it. The femoral nerve will be found just medial and superior to the iliopsoas. The hip usually appears most stable in internal rotation.

The femoral head, when placed in the acetabulum, is held in the postion which is most stable. The capsule is repaired in this position.

A spica is applied and bivalved postoperatively at 3 weeks, and gentle, active, guided exercises to obtain further internal rotation and abduction are begun. If the hip is placed

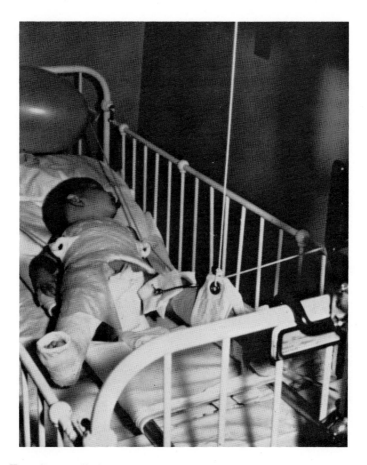

Figure 6.48. Traction preliminary to reduction of a dislocated hip. A well leg spica is used with eyelets so that the cast can be tied to the Bradford frame. A pin is placed through the femur and traction is axial in line with the trunk, not in abduction, which forces the femoral head against the ilium. The lower leg is supported by a sling underneath the proximal tibia and adhesive traction to the calf.

margin, the results have not been entirely satisfactory. The innominate osteotomy developed by Salter seems to be an excellent answer for this condition.

Salter's Osteotomy

Robert Salter[40] in 1962 described a method of overcoming frank dislocation or subluxation of the femoral head in children over 18 months old. This method used an osteotomy of the innominate bone extending into the sciatic notch (Fig. 6.53). The fragment was then rotated, with the pubic joint used as a hinge, to redirect the angle of the acetabulum without changing its shape. Pemberton in 1958 had reported an osteotomy of the ilium which was hinged on the triradiate cartilage. Salter's method had considerable appeal because it changes not the shape of the joint but its location in relation to the femoral head.

The hip is exposed through a Smith-Petersen anterior iliofemoral approach. The ilium is exposed both medially and laterally, and the osteotomy is carried out in a straight line from the anterior inferior iliac spine to the sciatic notch. A Gigli's saw is first passed through the sciatic notch, and the bone is cut toward the operator. A full thickness graft is removed from the anterior part of the ilium and trimmed in the shape of a wedge, the base of which is equal to the distance between the anterior superior and the anterior inferior spines. If open reduction of the frankly dislocated hip is necessary, it is carried out as a

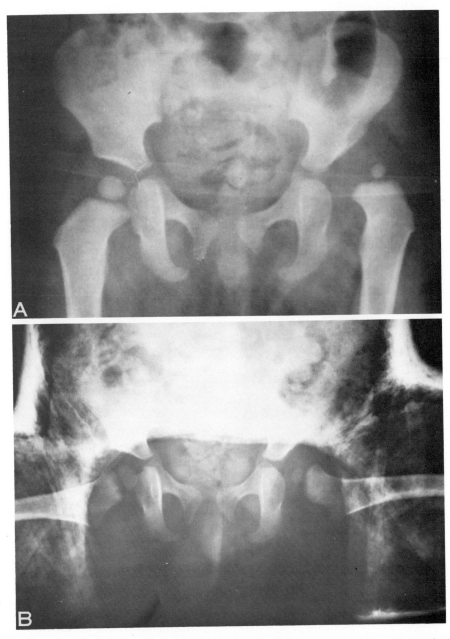

Figure 6.49. Dislocated hip at age 6 months treated by abduction-cast method. (*A*) Dislocation on right with lateral displacement of the shaft and smaller ossification center. (*B*) Abducted in cast in located position. (*C*) Anteroposterior view 10 years later with diminished head height slanting acetabulum. (*D*) Lateral view with diminished height of capital femoral epiphysis and delay in ossification anteriorly.

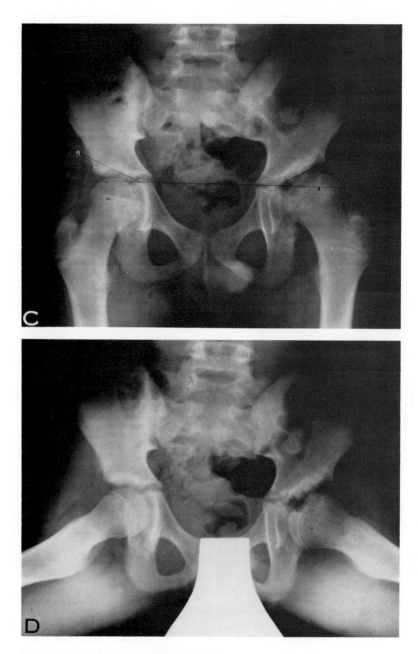

Fig. 6.49 (*C* and *D*)

first step of the procedure, and obstructing bands of adipose tissue are removed. The abnormal facing of the acetabulum can usually be appreciated at this time.

The principle of this procedure is to ensure that a reduced subluxation or dislocation previously stable only in abduction and flexion is made stable in the position of function. This stabilization allows early weight bearing once the osteotomy has healed.

The patient is immobilized in a unilateral hip spica that holds the hip in slight abduction, flexion, and internal rotation for 6 weeks.

TREATMENT OF DISLOCATED HIP AFTER AGE 4

Dislocated hips in this age group have a poor prognosis, so far as development of the hip is concerned, after a mere replacement in the acetabulum, even when the replacement is done openly. The joint must be maintained in abduction for many months, and frequently there is little or no improvement in the acetabulum itself.

Here again Salter's osteotomy offers great promise, but other procedures which may be used are described here. They have the disadvantage of changing the shape of the acetabulum rather than its relationship to the femoral head.

An acetabular osteotomy has been helpful in cases in which the femoral head is centered laterally in a shallow and slanting acetabulum. Anteversion of a fairly marked degree is usually still present in such cases.

Osteotomy of Acetabulum

It is most important in this procedure, as in the Colonna[7,8] operation or acetabular

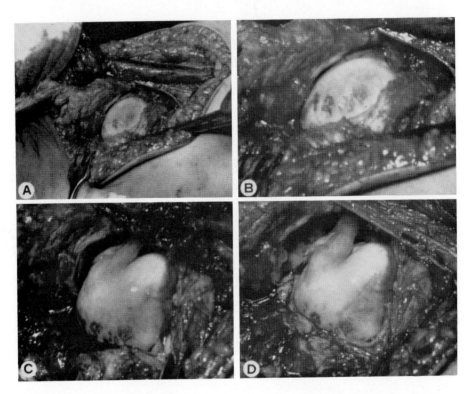

Figure 6.50. (A) The iliopsoas muscle and tendon have been released and retracted superiorly. Branches of the femoral nerve can be seen coursing just above the femoral head. The anterior superior iliac spine projects to the reader's left and the limb extends to the reader's right. The capsule is seen on the femoral head as it nestles in the false acetabulum. (B) A close-up of the femoral head reveals the damaged cartilaginous surface. (C) The femoral head has been retracted slightly from the false acetabulum revealing the acorn shape of the head, the result of persistent pressure in an abnormal position. The false acetabulum frequently leads the operator astray at this point. The elongated ligamentum teres can be seen disappearing into the depths of the wound. The capsule has been striated after having been divided superiorly. It is pulled to the reader's right. (D) Persistence in obtaining good exposure reveals the true acetabulum as a dark shadow just to the right of the false acetabulum. The ligamentum teres disappears into it. The apparent acetabular rim to the left is related to the false acetabulum only and not the actual acetabulum, the lines of which can be seen coursing over it underneath the femoral nerve branches.

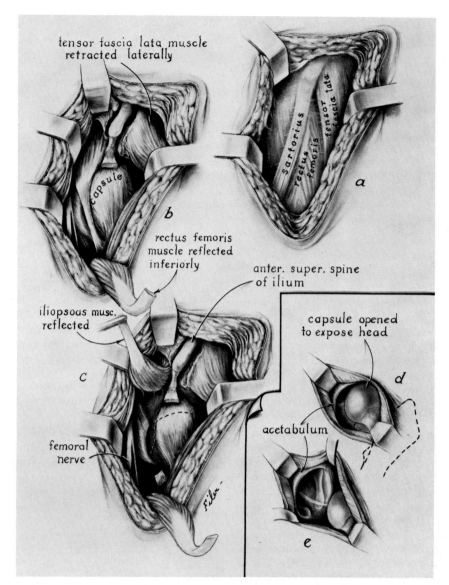

Figure 6.51. The iliofemoral approach exposing both the anterior ilium and the hip joint. It must be carried medially enough to visualize the femoral nerve by retracting or dividing the iliopsoas muscle and tendon.

shelf procedure, that the femur be pulled down by skeletal traction so that it is well centered in the area normally occupied by the acetabulum. This means a displacement of several centimeters distally from the previous position of the femoral head. Success in all these procedures is possible only if the pressure of the femoral head against the reconstructed area is relieved (Fig. 6.54). In order to achieve the required displacement, excellent mechanical efficiency of the traction

is necessary. A well leg, single spica is applied to secure good countertraction. A wire or pin is passed through the distal femur, and traction is applied through this pin by means of a horseshoe clamp holding the pin. The traction is directly in line with the trunk so that it pulls against the iliopsoas, which must be lengthened if the head is to be seated in its normal position.

Traction usually requires between 3 and 4 weeks. When operation is performed, a trac-

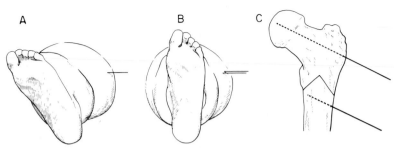

Figure 6.52. Anteversion osteotomy. (A) The leg is internally rotated for the desired degree of correction, and a Steinmann pin is placed in the proximal fragment. (B) The bone is divided, and the distal fragment is rotated until the knee is upright; a second pin is inserted in the distal fragment parallel to the first. (C) Anterior view of the final situation with parallel pins in place and incorporated in plaster.

tion table is used and traction is applied. The proximal two-thirds of a Smith-Peterson incision is used without stripping the ilium medially. The cartilage apophysis covering the iliac crest is also left intact. After the glutei are stripped from the ilium subperiosteally, the capsule is visualized. It is attached well above the actual acetabular rim and is stripped down by sharp dissection. A small linear incision is made into the joint to make certain of the location of the acetabular rim and the femoral head. The previous location of the head, now uncovered by its downward excursion, is adequately visualized. A curved osteotomy line is begun around the acetabular rim deep within the joint, but exterior to it and within the bone. This entire area is now pried down so that it covers the femoral head, which is held in internal rotation and abduction. A triangular space is now opened up by the descent of the articular flap. A suitable graft is taken above and posterior to the ilium, which may be very thin in areas so that care must be taken to avoid complete penetration. The bone is packed into the defect, which is held open by a periosteal elevator. Once completed, the new acetabular rim should be very close to the femoral head, and the femoral head should no longer be visible. After wound closure a spica is applied to hold the leg in abduction and internal rotation. An osteotomy of the distal femur is often necessary 1–2 weeks later to bring the knee out of anteversion and into a neutral position. After a total of 8 weeks, the spica is removed for active exercise at both hip and knee. A period of recumbency is now necessary for a further 8 weeks following which motion is well developed and partial weight

bearing with crutches is begun. It is usually possible to discard the crutches 6 months after the operation itself. Pemberton has described a very complete osteotomy of the ilium just above the acetabulum in order to develop an adequate mold for the femoral head.

Acetabuloplasty

Where the fundamental feature of the pathology of the dislocation that remains is a misshapen acetabulum, a direct surgical approach on this feature is possible (Fig. 6.55). Redirecting the acetabulum by iliac osteotomy by the method of Salter, Pemberton, or Chiari does not fully answer this problem since the acetabulum remains enlarged and flattened in its lateral third. In a sense this is the residual of the so-called subluxation, which in reality is an intra-acetabular dislocation with the lateral third hollowed out and pressed back by the femoral head.

As a clinical problem the hip often appears only minimally displaced. However a gluteus medius lurch and positive Trendelenberg test are common accompaniments. Internal rotation is often increased by residual anteversion of the femur.

OPERATION

There are two stages necessary to secure a successful result for this procedure.

First Stage. Skeletal traction is used with a Steinmann pin placed through the distal femoral metaphysis. A well leg spica incorporates the other lower extremity and trunk.

Traction is continued until there is a definable space between acetabulum and femoral head. The femoral head should be drawn down sufficiently to bring the femur into a normal relationship with the original medial third of the acetabulum. There is now sufficient space to pry down the outer one-half of the acetabulum and have it stay down without pressure from the femoral head.

Second Stage. The case is removed; the pin may remain in place covered with sterile drapes to provde a convenient means of putting traction on the leg during the operation.

The patient is positioned three-fourths of the way up on the opposite side, because it is necessary to see the posterior as well as the anterior portion of the acetabulum.

An anterior iliofemoral approach is used going well posteriorly. The capsule is divided from the lateral edge of the acetabulum after running an anterior incision in the capsule in line with the femoral neck.

The portion of acetabular cartilage bent superiorly is clearly seen once traction is applied to the femur. This acetabular cartilage must be brought down in symmetrical fashion around the relocated femoral head.

To accomplish this, an incision into the ilium is begun just superior to the acetabular cartilage and carried anteriorly and posteriorly in rounded symmetric fashion staying outside the acetabular cartilage, but carrying the osteotomy deep enough to carry the deformed portion of the head. A periosteal elevator keeps it pried down as the subchondral bone is backed by graft from the ilium. This maintains the lateral one-half of the acetabulum in its new position (Fig. 6.56). Traction is maintained on the femur as the child has a long leg spica applied. The unoperated thigh is encased to the knee. The case remains on for 6 weeks.

After x-rays to verify graft incorporation, the child is started on range-of-motion exer-

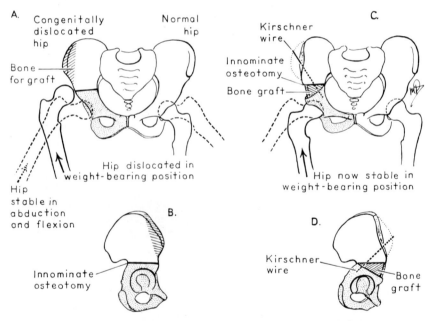

Figure 6.53. The principle of the innominate osteotomy. A Gigli's saw is inserted in the sciatic notch and drawn forward to the anteroinferior spine. The distal fragment hinged at the symphysis pubis can now be tilted by opening the osteotomy anteriorly and laterally. This carries the acetabulum over the femoral head so that a stable hip is achieved once the osteotomy is healed. It is not necessary to wait for acetabular development to allow the patient to begin weight bearing. If the hip is frankly dislocated, an open reduction is carried out at the same operation, prior to the osteotomy. (Reproduced from R. B. Salter: Innominate osteotomy in the treatment of congenital dislocation of the hip, *Journal of Bone and Joint Surgery*, 43B: 524, 1961.)

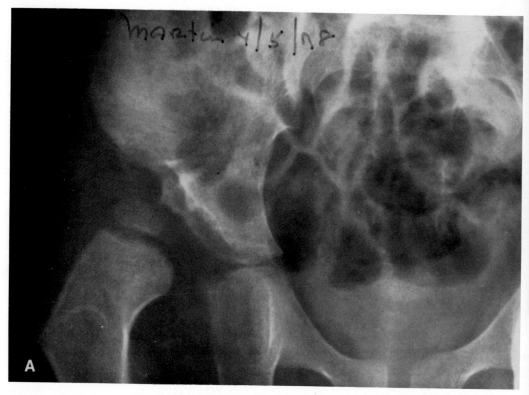

Figure 6.54. (*A*) Deformity of the acetabulum is shown with pressure deformation of the lateral third. (*B*) Deformity of the acetabulum has to be corrected by a Chiari type of osteotomy. The osteotomy must begin at the junction of the true acetabulum and the deformed outer third. When the osteotomy is correctly positioned and the hip reduced, a very satisfactory acetabulum is formed. (*C*) Looking into the acetabulum one sees the pressed upward deformity of the outer third of the acetabulum. At *A* the femoral head is located in the outer third above the ridge created by this deformity. In *B* the femoral head

cises. Although crutches are used for ambulation, no weight bearing is permitted for a minimum of 3 months. A three-point type of gait with crutches is used to encourage use of the hip joint in the gait.

Other Procedures

There are several other procedures for developing the joint to the point at which the hip is maintained in position. Colonna has developed an operation for the dislocated hip in the age group of 4–8 years (Fig. 6.57). After preliminary traction has placed the hip opposite the acetabulum, an open reduction is performed. In this procedure, the joint capsule is carefully dissected free of the ilium and surrounding structures. The acetabulum is curetted so that a deep and adequate cavity is produced. In this process, the acetabular

cartilage is removed, and the cartilage line at the junction of pubis, ischium, and ilium is visualized.

The capsule, which was left attached at the base of the neck, is sewn at its open end so as to enclose the femoral head. The head and enclosing capsule are then replaced in the joint.

The patient is kept in a cast for 4 weeks thereafter. Following this period, motion is begun at the hip in flexion, abduction, and internal rotation with traction. There follows a very gradual and carefully guarded return to full weight-bearing.

If traction preliminary to operation has brought the head opposite the acetabulum so that it is not forced into the newly made joint, the procedure usually produces a good result.

A third procedure to create an adequate joint consists of building an acetabular shelf (Fig. 6.58). This procedure is of value also in

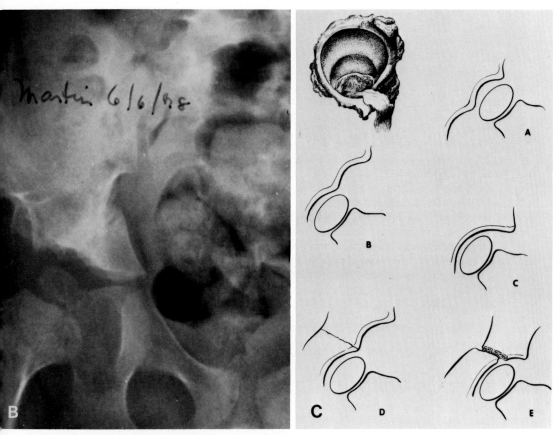

is located, hopefully the response of the acetabulum would be reconstitution of the outer third (C). If this does not occur (D), the acetabular deformity can be corrected by a modified Chiari osteotomy with medial displacement as is diagrammed (E). The osteotomy has to begin inside the acetabulum to accomplish correction of the deformity.

treatment of the subluxated hip that is progressing to further subluxation. The insertion of a shelf may be enough to produce stability and prevent progression. Again, to ensure a good result, the hip must be pulled down by traction.

At operation the femoral head should lie opposite the acetabulum. In Ghormley's[18] procedure the anterior iliac crest and acetabular margins are exposed by a lateral hip incision. The capsule is kept intact and bone chips are turned down over the head from the ilium, leaving a bony notch. The anterior superior spine and anterior portion of the ilium are freed subperiosteally. This section of the ilium is then osteotomized on a level. The leveled edge of this bone graft is then placed into the supra-acetabular groove. Traction is maintained for 8 weeks with the patient in a spica to the ankle. Crutch walking is then permitted. When the procedure is

being done for a hip drawn down opposite the acetabulum, failure to recognize the true acetabular rim at operation may be a pitfall. Not infrequently the capsule is turned up on the ilium and adherent to it. The capsule frequently has to be dissected from the ilium until the true rim is reached. Occasionally, as suggested by Anderson and Bickel, the capsule may be opened and the acetabular margin visualized.

Variations of the method of building an acetabular shelf have been described by Alber, Gill,[19,20] Phemister, and Lowman. Both tibial grafts and sections of the ilium may be used as grafts after the superior, posterior, or anterior portions of the acetabulum are pried down over the femoral head by osteotomy.

There remains a small group of patients, who are becoming quite rare in recent times, in the older age group with a severely dislocated hip that is well removed from the original acetabulum. These hips cannot be pulled down by traction to a point opposite the acetabulum. Here the general aim is to secure greater stability fofor the hip and thus to aid elimination of the medius limp.

Exercises to develop greater strength in the gluteus medius are used. When the dislocation is bilateral, these patients are perhaps best left alone. When it is unilateral, some stabilizing procedure is often used. Such a procedure is the building of a shelf with the hip brought to a position just above the acetabulum, after the suggestion of Dickson.[13] Osteotomies have been devised by Lorenz and Schanz which procure increased bony support by displacement of the proximal portion of the distal fragment medially. In the case of the Lorenz osteotomy, there is an actual placing of the shaft in acetabulum (Fig. 6.59).

Criteria of Reduction

Clinical criteria of reduction are:

1. The prominence of the trochanter is diminished.

2. The femoral head is palpated beneath the femoral artery one finger's breadth below the inguinal ligament.

3. The previously extending knee no longer extends.

X-ray criteria include:

1. There is no widening of the joint space.

2. The line through the center of the femoral neck and head runs through the center of the triradiate cartilage in all views.

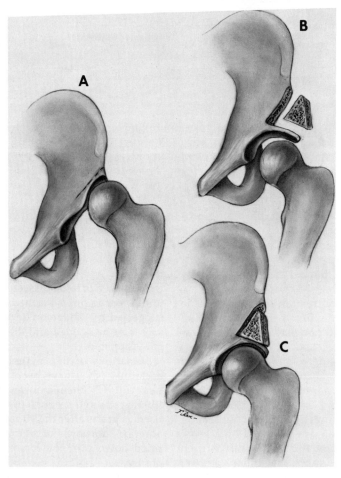

Figure 6.55.   Acetabuloplasty prying down the lateral one-half of the acetabular rim in order to reshape the acetabulum.

NEUROGENIC DISLOCATION OF HIP

Such hip dislocations occur following both spastic and flail paralysis of the lower extremities. The underlying etiologic factor is often a combination of events associated with each form of difficulty.

A principal factor in association with spastic paralysis is the persistent adducted position. Shortening of the adductors with use, and reinforcement of the adducted position with growth, may cause the limbs gradually to bend superiorly and the femoral head to ride out. Such a dislocation is aided by valgus of the femoral neck and uncorrected anteversion (Fig. 6.60).

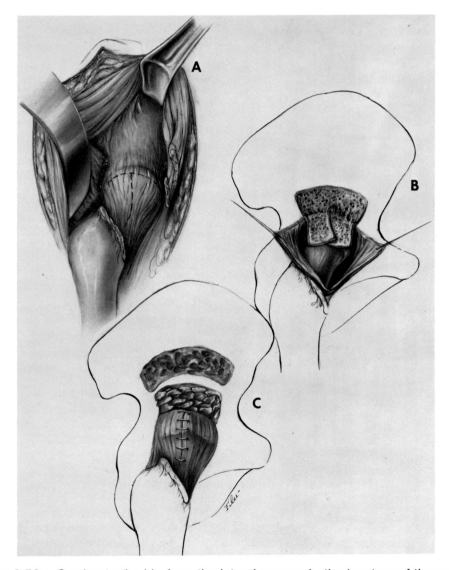

Figure 6.56. Coming to the hip from the lateral approach, the juncture of the capsule and acetabular rim can readily be visualized. (*A*) The lateral one-third to one-half of the acetabulum is turned down liberally and as far anterior and posterior as possible (*B*). Bone chips are used (*C*) to hold the reshaped portion of the acetabulum in its new position.

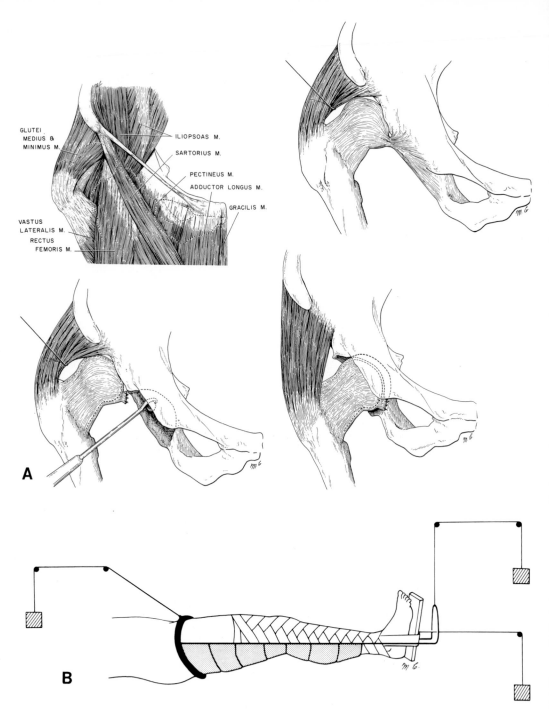

Figure 6.57. (*A*) (*Top left*) In a capsular arthroplasty developed by Colonna, the intact capsule is exposed by a Smith-Peterson incision. (*Top right* and *bottom left*) The acetabulum is refashioned by curetting, and the femoral head enclosed in the capsule is placed within the new joint. By preliminary traction, the femoral head was brought down opposite the acetabulum so that it could readily be reduced. (*Bottom right*) The femoral head enclosed in the capsular sac is in place in the newly fashioned acetabulum (Redrawn from P. C. Colonna: Congenital dislocation of the hip, *Instructional Course Lectures: American Academy of Orthopaedic Surgeons*, 8: 175, 1951.) (*B*) Traction applied to the hip to bring it down to a point opposite the acetabulum. Efficient countertraction is necessary to achieve results. Skeletal traction on the femur may be used.

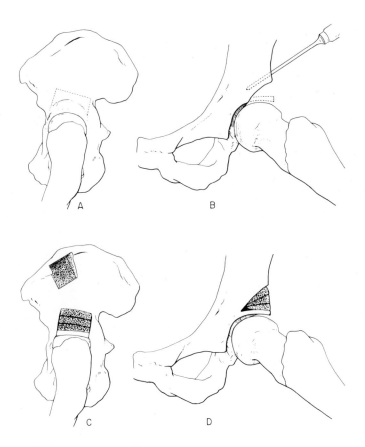

Figure 6.58. There are many methods of performing a shelf procedure to stabilize the femoral head in the true acetabulum. The operation basically pries down ilium and outer portion of the acetabulum and maintains the shelf in position by a bone graft, which may be taken from the ilium. (Redrawn from J. Hass: *Congenital Dislocation of the Hip*, p. 288; Springfield, Ill.: Charles C Thomas, 1951.)

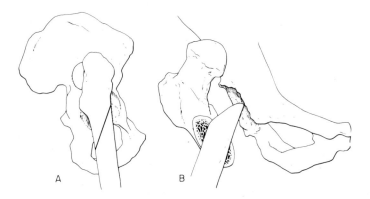

Figure 6.59. Osteotomy may be used to increase stability in a dislocated hip of long standing. In the Lorenz osteotomy, the shaft of the femur is displaced into the acetabulum. (Redrawn from J. Hass: *Congenital Dislocation of the Hip*, p. 295; Springfield, Ill.: Charles C Thomas, 1951.)

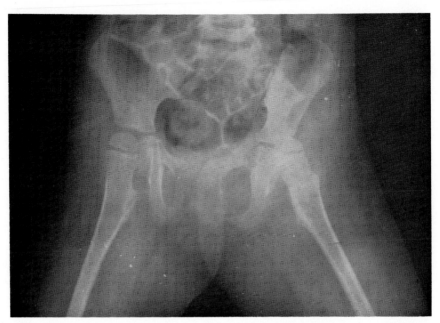

Figure 6.60. Neurogenic dislocation on right with excessive anteversion and valgus in both hips.

In flail paralysis, valgus of the femoral neck with non-weight bearing is a very common finding. Uncorrected anteversion of the femur may accompany it. One is hard put to weigh properly the relative importance of valgus and anteversion in any one case. In poliomyelitis, where the muscles may not be completely flail and contractures may arise, these may also play a part. The tightness of the fascia lata with contracture in abduction is important because it results in a flexed position with the hip in neutral. Extension then tends to drive the hip posteriorward and over the acetabular rim. Poor seating of the femoral head due to valgus or anteversion aids the progress of the hip laterally. Again, however, the condition must usually be accompanied by factors such as anteversion or valgus to result in actual dislocation. The tightness of the iliopsoas when a flexion contracture is present is a major factor in neurogenic dislocation.

Neurogenic dislocations are seen particularly in connection with myelomeningocele, cerebral palsy, or poliomyelitis. Further discussion will occur under those headings.

Treatment

Maintenance of an abducted position helps to counteract the progression of the femoral head toward dislocation. It also aids in reinforcing reduction, once this has been achieved. The forces which originally drove the femur into a dislocated position must be corrected, however, to guard against recurrence. Keeping the patient in plaster spicas over the years may be too costly from the point of view of mental and physical health, and other means must be sought.

In the presence of a well developed acetabulum, correction of anteversion and valgus by femoral osteotomy may be all that is necessary (Figs. 6.61 and 6.62). In cases in which the acetabulum is deficient, shelf procedures to create a stable abutment may be indicated. Levering down the acetabular rim and blocking it in position will be successful only if the hip has been pulled down by traction so that it is not exerting a strong pressure on the reconstructed area.

This procedure has been described in the preceding section. The innominate osteotomy also described in the preceding section may well answer the requirements here better than any other procedure when an acetabulum that covers the femoral head is desired. It has the advantages of maintaining congruity of acetabulum in relation to the femoral head, of requiring a relatively short convalescence, and of bringing about an immediate change in the stability of the hip.

The preliminary of achieving reduction is essential. The hip can be tested for stability at the time of open reduction through a Smith-Peterson approach. The line of the osteotomy runs from the sciatic notch to the anterior inferior spine and is done with a Gigli's saw. A graft is removed from the anterior portion of the iliac crest. It is trimmed to the shape of a wedge, the base of which is equal to the distance between the anterosuperior and anteroinferior spines.

The distal segment is shifted forward, downward, and outward so that the osteotomy site opens up anterolaterally. The wedge-shaped graft is fitted into this opening. A Kirschner wire is inserted across the osteotomy site and through the graft; it is buried in the subcutaneous fat as the skin is closed. Salter found displacement of the distal fragment (which is hinged on the symphysis pubica) easier when the femoral head was dislocated at the time. He recommends retaining the limbus by wide exposure and reduction of the femoral head deep to it, and he warns against backward or inward displacement of the distal segment. The patient is placed in a hip spica in a position of slight flexion, slight abduction, and slight medial rotation. The spica remains in place for 6 weeks, after which the patient actively exercises to regain muscle function. When this goal is achieved, partial weight bearing is

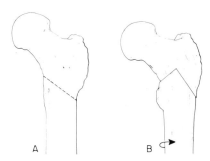

Figure 6.62. A type of osteotomy for anteversion which also corrects valgus and is of special help in neurogenic dislocation.

allowed for several weeks, and full weight bearing follows.

Other methods of treating neurogenic dislocations, including Mustard's iliopsoas transplant are discussed under "Spina Bifida Syndrome."

References

1. Adams, F.: *The Genuine Works of Hippocrates*, London, 1849.
2. Badgley, C. E.: Correlation of clinical and anatomical parts leading to a conception of the etiology of congenital hip dislocation. *J. Bone Joint Surg., 31A:* 341, 1949.
3. Barlow, T. G.: Early diagnosis and treatment of congenital dislocation of the hip, *J. Bone Joint Surg., 44B:* 292, 1962.
4. Bost, F. C., Hagey, H., Schottstaedt, E. R., and Larsen, L. J.: The results of treatment of congenital dislocation of the hip in infancy. *J. Bone Joint Surg., 30A:* 454, 1948.
5. Bradford, E. H.: Treatment of congenital dislocation of the hip, *Boston Med. Surg. J., 108:* 73, 1883.
6. Bradford, E. H.: Congenital dislocation of the hip—results of treatment at the Boston Children's Hospital, *Am. J. Orthop. Surg., 7:* 57, 1909.
7. Colonna, P. C.: An arthroplastic operation for congenital dislocation of the hip—a two stage procedure, *Surg. Gynecol. Obstet., 63:* 777, 1936.
8. Colonna, P. C.: Arthroplasty of the hip for congenital dislocation in children. *J. Bone Joint Surg., 29:* 711, 1947.
9. Compere, E. L.: The shelf operation for congenital dislocation of the hip, *Am. J. Surg., 43:* 404, 1939.
10. Crego, C. H., Jr.: Preliminary skeletal traction in the treatment of congenital dislocation of the hip, *South. Med. J., 26:* 845, 1933.
11. Crego, C. H. Jr., and Schwartzmann, J. R.: Follow-up study of the early treatment of congenital dislocation of the hip, *J. Bone Joint Surg., 30A:* 128, 1948.
12. DeNuce, M.: Luxation congenitale de la hanche; operation de Hoffa, *Rev. Orthop., 1s.4:* 108, 1893.
13. Dickson, F. D.: The shelf operation in the treatment of congenital dislocation of the hip. *J. Bone Joint Surg., 17:* 43, 1935.
14. DePrampero, A.: Morfolojia radiohica dell'ance cosi detta sana nella lussazione congenita laterale, *Chir. Orgi. Mov., 25:* 1, 1939.

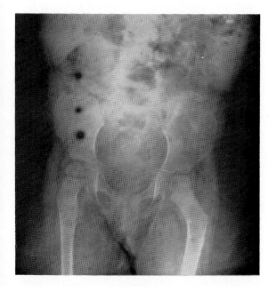

Figure 6.61. Anteversion osteotomy on right to aid in keeping femoral head in normal relation acetabulum.

15. Frejka, B.: Prävention der angeborenen Juftörren-burg durch das Abduktionspolster, *Wien. Klin. Wochenschr., 91:* 523, 1941.

16. Gage, J. R., and Winter, R. B.: Avascular necrosis of the capital femoral epiphysis as a complication of closed reduction of congenital dislocation of the hip; a critical review of twenty years experience at Gillette Children's Hospital, *J. Bone Joint Surg., 54-A:* 373, 1972.

17. Galeazzi, R.: Esiti fontani della crura incrimenta della lussazione congenita dell'anca, *Arch. Ortop., 32:* 191, 1915.

18. Ghormley, R. K.: Use of the anterior superior spine and crest of the ilium in surgery of the hip joint. *J. Bone Joint Surg., 13:* 784, 1931.

19. Gill, A. B.: Plastic construction of an acetabulum in congenital dislocation of the hip. *J. Bone Joint Surg., 17:* 48, 1935.

20. Gill, A. B.: The end results of early treatment of congenital dislocation of the hip, *J. Bone Joint Surg., 30A:* 442, 1948.

21. Hart, V. L.: Primary genetic dysplasia of the hip with or without classical dislocation. *J. Bone Joint Surg., 24:* 753, 1942.

22. Hart, V. L.: *Congenital Dysplasia of the Hip Joint and Sequelae;* Springfield, Ill: Charles C Thomas, 1952.

23. Hoyt, W. A., Jr., Weiner, D. S., and O'Dell, H. W.: Congenital dislocation of the hip: an investigation into the efficacy of pre-manipulative traction—the prevention of aseptic necrosis of the hip, *J. Bone Joint Surg., 54-A:* 1799, 1972.

24. Leveuf, J.: Primary congenital subluxation of the hip, *J. Bone Joint Surg., 30A:* 875, 1948.

25. Lorenz, A.: La riduzione della lussazione congenita dell'anca, *Arch. Ortop., 14:* 1, 1897.

26. Ludloff, K.: Zur blutigen Einrenkung der angeborenen Hüftluxation, *Z. Orthop. Chir., 22:* 272, 1908.

27. Ludloff, K.: The open reduction of the congenital hip dislocation by an anterior incision, *Am. J. Orthop. Surg., 10:* 438, 1913.

28. Massie, W. K.: Vascular epiphyseal changes in congenital dislocation of the hip, results in adults compared with results in coxa plana and in congenital dislocation without vascular changes, *J. Bone Joint Surg., 33-A:* 284, 1951.

29. Massie, W. K., and Howorth, W. B.: Congenital dislocation of the hip, *J. Bone Joint Surg., 33A:* 171, 1951.

30. Mau, H., Dörr, W. M., Henkel, L., and Lutsche, J.: Open reduction of congenital dislocation of the hip by Ludloff's method, *J. Bone Joint Surg., 53-A:* 1281, 1971.

31. McCarroll, H. R., and Crego, C. H., Jr.: Primary anterior congenital dislocation of the hip, *J. Bone Joint Surg., 21:* 648, 1939.

32. McKibbin, B.: Action of the iliopsoas muscle in the newborn, *J. Bone Joint Surg., 50B:* 161, 1968.

33. Mitchell, G. P.: Problems in the early diagnosis and management of congenital dislocation of the hip, *J. Bone Joint Surg., 54B:* 1972.

34. Muller, G. M., and Seddorn, H. J.: Late results of treatment of congenital subluxation of the hip, *J. Bone Joint Surg., 35B:* 342, 1953.

35. Nélation, E.: *Elements de pathologie chirurgicale edit,* Vol. 3, p. 328; Paris: Pean, 1874.

36. Poli, A.: Contributo alla cura precoce della lussazione congenita dell'anca, *Arch. Ortop., 52:* 749, 1936.

37. Ponseti, I.: Causes of failure in the treatment of congenital dislocation of the hip. *J. Bone Joint Surg., 26:* 775, 1944.

38. Ponseti, I. V.: Nonsurgical treatment of congenital dislocation of the hip, *J. Bone Joint Surg., 48A:* 1392, 1966.

39. Putti, V.: Early treatment of congenital dislocation of the hip, *J. Bone Joint Surg., 11:* 798, 1929.

40. Salter, R. B.: Innominate osteotomy in the treatment of congenital dislocation and subluxation of the hip, *J. Bone Joint Surg., 43B:* 518, 1961.

41. Scaglietti, O., and Calandriello, B.: Open reduction of congenital dislocation of the hip. *J. Bone Joint Surg., 44B:* 257, 1962.

42. Severin, E.: Arthrography in congenital dislocation of the hip. *J. Bone Joint Surg., 21:* 304, 1939.

43. Severin, E.: Contribution to knowledge of congenital dislocation of the hip joint; late results of closed reduction, *Acta Chir. Scand., 84:* Suppl. 63, 1941.

44. Smith, W. S., Coleman, C. R., Olix, M. L., and Slager, R. F.: Etiology and congenital dislocation of the hip; an experimental approach to the problem using young dogs, *J. Bone Joint Surg., 45A:* 491, 1963.

45. Somerville, E. W.: Results of treatment of 100 congenitally dislocated hips, *J. Bone Joint Surg., 49B:* 258, 1967.

46. Stanisavljevic, S., and Mitchell, C. L.: Congenital dysplasia, subluxation, and dislocation of the hip in stillborn and newborn infants; an anatomical-pathological study, *J. Bone Joint Surg., 45A:* 1147, 1963.

47. von Rosen, S.: Diagnosis and treatment of congenital dislocation of the hip joint in the newborn, *J. Bone Joint Surg., 44B:* 284, 1962.

48. Wilkinson, J. A.: A post-natal survey for congenital dislocation of the hip, *J. Bone Joint Surg., 54B:* 40, 1972.

DEVELOPMENTAL COXA VARA

Developmental coxa vara has been related to the congenital short femur by Golding.[3] It is not unusual to find the two coexisting. Congenital coxa vara results from anomalous ossification of the proximal femur. The deformity thus produced gives rise to a medius type limp and to marked limitation of abduction, which, when bilateral, is especially disabling.

The lesion results in progressive deformity. Abnormality of the gait does not ordinarily become noticeable before the age of 3 or 4. Thereafter, the gait difficulty caused by the mechanical abnormality of the proximal femur is increasingly noticeable.

There is a gradually decreasing amount of anteversion of the femur as the coxa vara increases. When the varus is well established, retroversion is the rule (Fig. 6.63).

There is no hereditary or familial incidence.

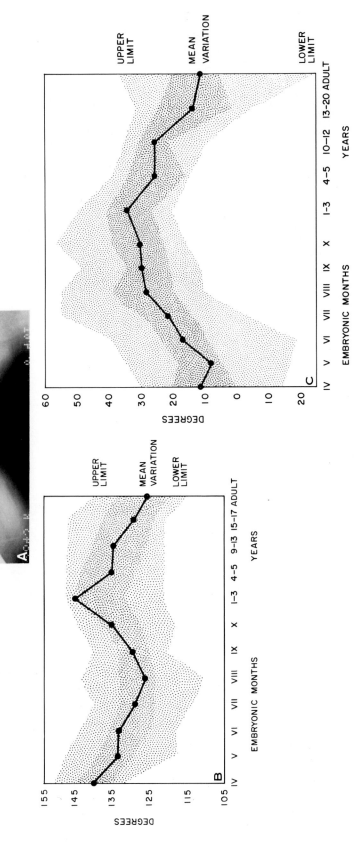

Figure 6.63. (A) Retroversion is a prominent feature of coxa vara. (B) Variation of femoral torsion with age. (C) Variation of the neck-shaft angle with age. (B and C are redrawn from T. von Lanz and A. Mayet: Die Gelenkkor per des Menschlischen Huft gelenkes in der Progredienten Phase Ihrer Unwegiglen Ausforming, *Zeitschrift fur Anatomie und Entwicklungsgeschichte, 117:317, 1953.*)

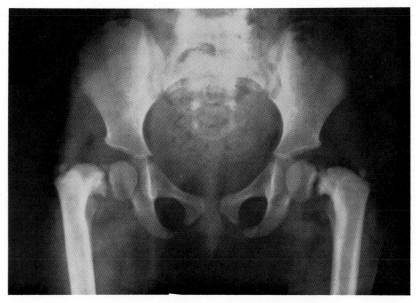

Figure 6.64. Bilateral developmental coxa vara. Note widened epiphyseal line and filling in of inferior neck angle with triangular area of ossification.

The deformity is more commonly unilateral (3:1) but, when bilateral, tends to be symmetrical (Figs. 6.64 and 6.65). The condition affects both sexes equally. Other anomalies are not ordinarily present helping to differentiate the condition from congenital short and bowed femora, which frequently are associated with other anomalies.

Roentgen Findings

The usual angle formed by the femoral neck with the shaft of the femur is 135 degrees. Some change in the direction of increasing varus is always present, and if the patient is first seen between the ages of 4 and 7, the neck of the femur usually forms a right angle with the shaft. The area occupied by the epiphyseal line is usually wide in the young age group. This increased area of radiolucency apparently results from the epiphyseal line plus a gap just distal to it, which occasionally branches away from it as it nears the base of the neck. A triangular segment of bone is thus isolated, as emphasized by Le Mesurier.[4]

In later cases the area occupied by the epiphyseal line becomes quite thin, irregular, and fragmented. The neck appears shorter than it is normally expected to be. The line tends to close prematurely. It becomes evi-

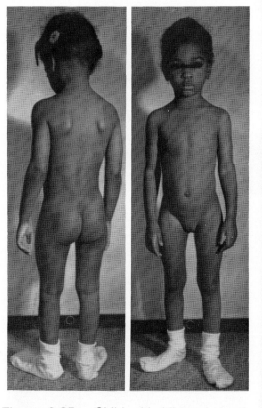

Figure 6.65. Child with bilateral development coxa vara and clinical signs of widened perineum and prominent trochanters.

dent that there is a decreased rate of growth at this line.

The trochanteric epiphyseal line appears to be normal.

Clinical Picture

The child is brought to medical attention because of a waddling gait due to the medius limp. The limp is progressively more noticeable as the age of the child advances. Pain is not a symptom.

The limitation of abduction is most strikingly effective on the hip motion itself, because the other planes of motion are usually less affected, except in cases of severe deformity. There is a positive Trendelenburg when the patient stands on the involved side. With weight bearing, the trunk shifts over the involved hip in order to clear the opposite leg and to elevate the pelvis, and this movement gives rise to the gait associated with weakness of the gluteus medius. The trochanter is above Nélaton's line. The condition may be confused with dislocation of the hip on physical examination, for actual disloca-

tion is a much more common lesion. The femoral head is palpated in normal position. Telescoping, however, cannot be elicited in coxa vara. Shortening to measurement would depend on the degree of coxa vara present.

Course

If the case is untreated, progressive deformity of the femoral neck-to-shaft relationship to at least a right angle can be expected, and more often there is an an even more severe change in the direction of varus (Fig. 6.66).

Because premature closure of the epiphyseal line is the rule, it is unusual to see progression after the age of 12. Once the line is closed, the neck is composed of bone of apparently normal tissue.

Pathology

There has not been a good opportunity to study the actual pathology involving the femoral neck. Study of the x-ray picture yields

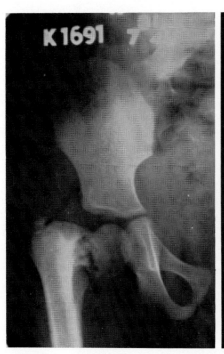 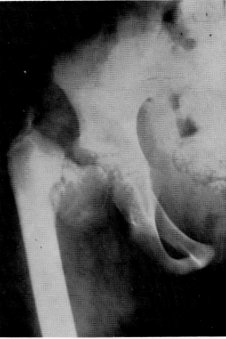

Figure 6.66. Progression in developmental coxa vara. There is an 8-year interval between the roentgenogram on the *left* and that of the same hip on the *right* with marked increase in deformity.

the principal information about the disease. It is presumed to be a form of anomalous ossification of the proximal third of the femur (Fig. 6.67).

Treatment

Traction has not been shown to affect the deformity. The treatment chosen depends on the degree of deformity at the time the patient is first seen, the amount of growth left, and the gap present in the femoral neck.

EARLY CASES

Where the deformity present is compatible with good function of the hip and further progression can be expected, attention may be directed to attempting to gain rigid fusion of the epiphyseal line. Le Mesurier[4] has advocated both nailing with a Smith-Peterson nail inserted across the gap and actual bone grafting. Bone grafts may be inserted from the lateral cortex and passed up the femoral neck. Patients treated in this manner should be followed through the growth period thereafter, because continued growth of the trochanteric epiphysis may still result in sufficient varus deformity to need osteotomy.

LATE CASES

An abduction osteotomy which obtains adequate correction does not give an absolutely perfect hip so far as motion is concerned, but it results in improvement in gait and abduction at the hip (Figs. 6.68–6.71). Where the condition is bilateral, such improvement may be essential. The osteotomy is done just below the level of the lesser trochanter through a lateral incision.

Haas (1933) and White (1946) and more recently Macewen and Shands[5] have used an oblique trochanteric osteotomy to correct this condition (Fig. 6.68). The oblique osteotomy is performed in a coronal plane. If the oste-

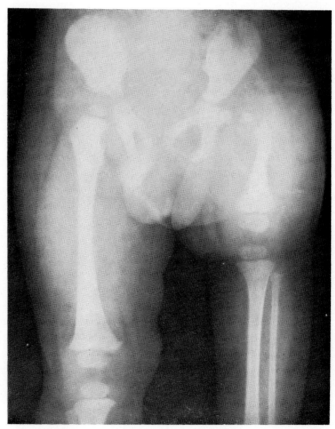

Figure 6.67.　Congenital short femur and developmental coxa vara in combination.

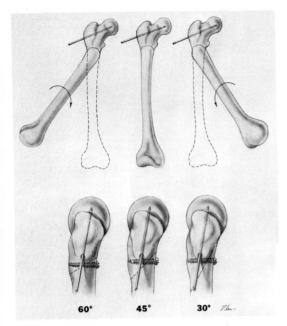

Figure 6.68. An oblique intertrochanteric osteotomy of the proximal femur can accomplish various combinations of changes in neck-shaft angle and anterversion or retroversion rotational correction. The degree of obliquity determines the amount of correction of rotation that can be obtained in relation to angulation. Because in most cases the change in angulation desired is greater than that needed for rotation, a cut approaching the axis of the femoral shaft is used as in the drawing at 30 degrees. *Above,* the abduction of the distal fragment produces internal rotation of the fragment and an increase in the neck-shaft angle. To the *right, above,* adduction of the distal fragment produces external rotation of the distal fragment and a decrease in the neck-shaft angle. (Redrawn from G. D. MacEwen and A. R. Shands, Jr.: Oblique trochanteric osteotomy, *Journal of Bone and Joint Surgery, 49A:* 345, 1976.)

otomy runs obliquely from the anterior surface of the femur distally and posteriorly and the distal fragment abducted it will correct coxa vara and retroversion. Inasmuch as retroversion is the most common accompaniment of the condition, this is the cut most often used. A screw is placed across the osteotomy line to stabilize the fragments. A Steinmann pin progressing through the femoral neck stabilizes the proximal fragment

and protrudes through the skin to be incorporated in the plaster. The pin should be introduced to the femoral neck through the skin, not through the wound.

Borden et al.[2] reported on a technique of subtrochanteric osteotomy end to side which was fixed with an infant-size blade plate (Fig. 6.69). The plate is present at an angle of 140 degrees. The lateral cortex of the proximal fragment is placed in apposition to the end of the distal fragment. The plate is inserted parallel to the neck prior to accomplishing the osteotomy. It is preceded by a guide wire fixing the capital femoral epiphysis.

The osteotomy position to bring the plate to the lateral cortex of the distal femur is accomplished by traction. It has not been necessary to do an adductor myotomy. There is need for a second procedure to remove the plate and screws. Length is increased by this procedure; the blade is carefully inserted below the trochanteric epiphysis to avoid injuring this growth structure.

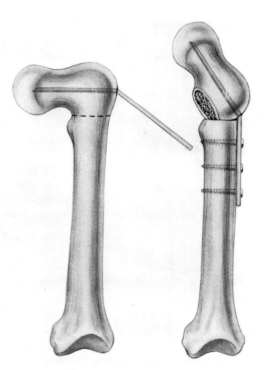

Figure 6.69. Correction of coxa vara in children is difficult to acheive and to hold. One alternative proposed by Borden used a small blade plate and an end-to-side position when the proximal fragment was tilted up.

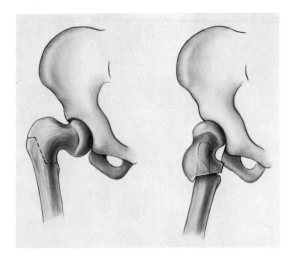

Figure 6.70. Amstutz devised a type of osteotomy to correct coxa vara using intrinsic carpentry to hold the position. The lateral cortex is extended into the trochanteric area as a spike to hold the valgus position when it is inserted into the medullary cavity of the femoral neck.

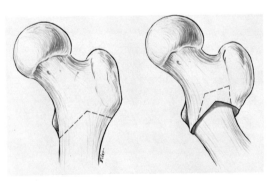

Figure 6.71. The telescoping V osteotomy offers another means of achieving intrinsic stability.

Good healing is obtained before the cast is removed, and the hip is then mobilized with the aid of traction and exercises.

References

1. Barr, J. S.: Congenital coxa vara, *Arch. Surg.*, 18: 1909, 1929.
2. Borden, J., Spencer, G. E., and Herndon, C. H.: Treatment of coxa vara in children by means of a modified osteotomy, *J. Bone Joint Surg.*, 48A: 1103, 1966.
3. Golding, F. E.: Congenital coxa vara, *J. Bone Joint Surg.*, 30B: 161, 1948.
4. Le Mesurier, A. B.: Developmental coxa vara, *J. Bone Joint Surg.*, 30B: 595, 1948.
5. Macewen, G. D., and Shands, A. R.: Oblique trochanteric osteotomy, *J. Bone Joint Surg.*, 49A: 345, 1967.

SLIPPED CAPITAL FEMORAL EPIPHYSIS

The essence of slipped capital femoral epiphysis is a mechanical change from normal of the relationship of the femoral neck to the capital femoral epiphysis (Figs. 4.72–4.75). The anomaly occurs primarily in adolescents.

The results of treatment in cases in which a minimal change has taken place are better than those in cases of marked change in the relationship. An early diagnosis is thus of great value.

The usual age range is 10–17 years; females, by virtue of their approximately 2-year advancement in skeletal maturation, are seen in the early years of this range. Rarely,

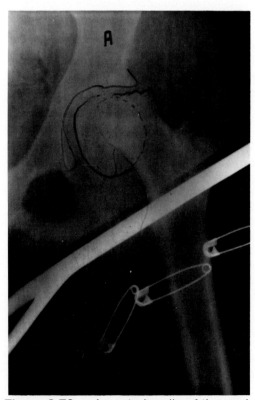

Figure 6.72. An anterior slip of the capital femoral epiphysis in relation to the femoral shaft is unusual, but possible. When it occurs it is usually acute and traumatic.

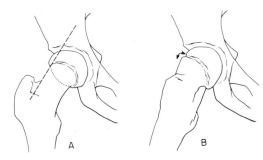

Figure 6.73. Diagram of the normal relation of the capital femoral epiphysis to the extension of a line drawn along the superior aspect of the neck. (*A*) Anterior view, (*B*) lateral view. (Redrawn from the *American Journal of Roentgenology, Radium Therapy, and Nuclear Medicine,46:* 386, 1951.)

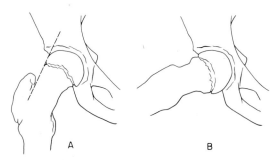

Figure 6.74. Diagram of slip visible in the anteroposterior view only. No slip is seen in the lateral view. (Redrawn from the *American Journal of Roentgenology, Radium Therapy, and Nuclear Medicine, 46:* 386, 1951.)

cases are seen in even younger children. The disorder is much more common in males (5: 1), and bilateral cases occur in approximately 20% of those affected. Klein et al.[4] stated that x-ray signs of bilateral involvement exist in 40%, even though clinical symptoms may be confined to one side only.

Etiology

Two general body types are frequently involved by this disease. One is the so-called Fröhlich type, in which there is female fat distribution and underdevelopment of the genitalia; the other is the type of the thin individual whose extremities are long and whose adolescent growth has been very rapid. Approximately one-half of the patients

with this disease fall into one or the other group.

The epiphyseal line in the femoral neck is perhaps more subject to a shearing type of stress than any other. Although it is perhaps possible to visualize the onset and progress of the disease on the basis of shearing stress on this line alone, it is as yet unproved that this is sufficient evidence.

An endocrine basis for this disease is suggested by the growth abnormalities. Both growth hormone and sex hormone affect the rate of proliferation of cartilage cells at the epiphyseal plates, which, in turn, may exert a profound effect on the rate of skeletal growth.

Harris tested the shearing force necessary to detach the proximal tibial epiphysis from the shaft in rats. In growth hormone-treated rats with epiphyseal plates thickened principally in the layers of proliferating and maturing cartilage cells, a lesser than normal average force was required. In estrogen-treated rats with thinner plates at the epiphyseal line, a greater average force was necessary than that required in the normal controls.

Although all epiphyses presumably react to endocrine changes, the placement of the proximal femoral epiphysis, which subjects it to shearing stress, may cause this area to become involved to the exclusion of others.

Ghormley and Fairchild[2] emphasized the fact that the epiphyseal plate changes from a horizontal to an oblique position during preadolescent and adolescent periods.

In view of the lack of clear-cut evidence for endocrine factors, some favor the idea

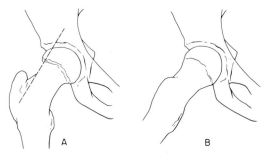

Figure 6.75. Diagram of slip recognizable in the lateral view only. (Redrawn from the *American Journal of Roentgenology, Radium Therapy, and Nuclear Medicine, 46:* 386, 1951.)

that trauma taking place at this point of low resistance to shearing stress is the only etiology.

Pathology

Irritation of the hip joint results in edema and hyperemia in the synovia. In the earliest stage of slipped epiphysis these changes, plus some perivascular lymphocytic infiltrations and villous formation, are all that are noted. In the cases of actual slipping, the epiphysis is not completely detached from the neck but remains attached by periosteum and fibrous tissue. The epiphyseal disc remains attached to the head, the slipping taking place in the more distal layers. The epiphysis is downward and posterior to the neck, which slips forward and upward. The angles between neck and epiphysis tend to fill in with callus. The articular cartilage appears normal. The bluish fibrous tissue covering that part of the neck formerly contiguous with the epiphyseal line is smooth and glistening and tends to hide the true location of the epiphyseal line. During a period of several years, the head and neck gradually form a bony union incorporating the epiphyseal line. Late changes in this disease reveal a firm, sclerotic, and thickened capsule and conversion of the callus at the inferior angle of the epiphysis to bone.

Clinical Picture

The typical patient has noted pain in the hip, thigh, or knee, often for several months, and has developed an antalgic limp. Because the hip capsule may not always be markedly irritated, it is not uncommon for the patient to have a history of low grade symptoms of considerable duration.

If the symptoms and the limp are acute, one suspects a slip that has caused the neck and shaft to rotate outward and upward in relation to the head.

On examination the appearance of the patient may be so typical as to allow suspicion of the diagnosis on sight. A large frame, heavy thighs, underdeveloped genitalia, and external rotation of the leg point to the slipped epiphysis. When the thigh is flexed, the leg tends to ride into external rotation and frequently cannot be brought to neutral.

If the hip is irritated, other motion is also limited and a hip flexion contracture is present. If hip irritation is minimal, the patient may actually have increased hyperextension consistent with the degree of slip.

When slipped femoral epiphysis is suspected, the patient should leave the examining room in recumbency, since further slip complicates treatment and jeopardizes the end result.

Roentgen Signs

The earliest manifestation of slipping consists of widening of the epiphyseal line and irregular demineralization of the area immediately adjacent to it (Figs. 6.76 and 6.77). The capsular shadow is rounded and more prominent than normal.

Klein et al.[4] have emphasized the fact that a line drawn along the superior surface of the neck to the outer edge of the acetabulum normally leaves the lateral angle of the head outside it. Medial slipping can be detected in the anteroposterior view of the hip when the head is not transected by this line but lies within it. Posterior slipping, in which the change in relationship is more obvious because the axis of the neck leaves the epiphysis, is detected in the lateral view. A generalized atrophy or demineralization of the head and neck may be apparent.

The epiphysis does not always lie both posterior and medial to the neck. In the anteroposterior view in Klein's cases, a medial slip was apparent in only 68%. In the lateral view of these cases, posterior displacement was evident in 98%. In speaking of the degree or distance of slip, the lateral view is ordinarily used.

Treatment

Treatment begins immediately upon suspicion of the diagnosis (Table 6.1). The external rotation maneuver performed on the x-ray table to procure the lateral view should be gently and not forcibly done. Once the diagnosis is made, the patient is placed in traction in abduction, and an internal rotation strap is added to his thigh. A considerable improvement in the range of hip motion can often be obtained by traction prior to operation.

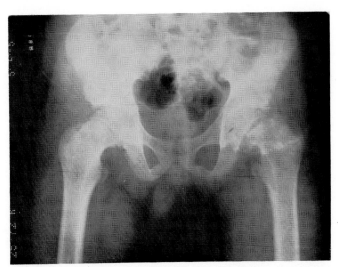

Figure 6.76.   A well defined epiphyseal slip with widened epiphyseal line and a build-up of bone beneath the head on the inferior neck on the right are seen.

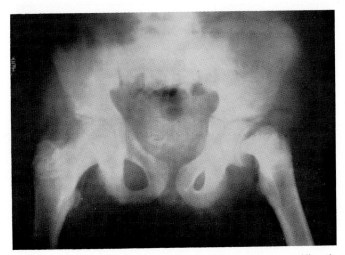

Figure 6.77.   Acute slip of the femoral epiphysis without ossification at the inferior neck.

Slipped epiphysis of minimal degree may be treated conservatively by a plaster spica and immobilization of the hip until the epiphyseal line is obliterated. The immobilization should be interrupted by periods of traction to maintain good hip motion.

Internal fixation in situ is generally thought to be preferable. There is a generally accepted rule that displacement of 1 cm or less can be internally fixed in situ. A minimal slip of this type is compatible with good function of the hip if no further slip occurs.

Fixation in situ is done through a lateral proximal femoral incision in a manner similar to that used in treating transcervical fractures of the hip in the adult. A cassette is placed beneath the hip, and a second portable x-ray machine is placed under the contralateral thigh and aimed so as to take a lateral view of the neck with the anterior superior spine of the ilium in the direct line of the rays. The first machine is moved over the hip for the anterior posterior view when necessary. Accurate and firm fixation with the device

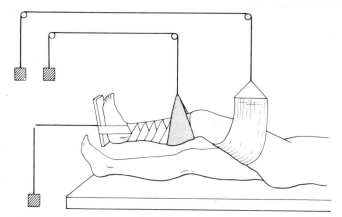

Figure 6.78. The use of the internal rotation strap aids in reducing the external rotation contracture. The adhesive is kept from pulling on the lateral side of the leg by felt placed between it and the skin.

Table 6.1
Treatment of Slipped Capital Femoral Epiphysis

Possible Method	Possible Disadvantage
Mild	
Pin in situ	Projection into joint
	Aseptic necrosis
Transcervical epiphysiodesis	Poor placement in relation to epiphyseal line
Open epiphysiodesis	Opening joint
Moderate	
Pin in situ	Late treatment
Open epiphysiodesis accompanied by preliminary manipulation	Add osteoplasty or Southwick osteotomy
Severe	
Osteotomy through epiphyseal line	Aseptic necrosis
Epiphysiodesis with later correction of deformity by osteotomy or osteoplasty	Aseptic necrosis, creation of deformity to correct initial deformity
Base of neck osteotomy	Needs internal fixation
Cuneiform osteotomy	Aseptic necrosis
Acute	
Preliminary manipulation under anesthesia	Aseptic necrosis
Pin in situ	

placed well into the femoral head is necessary.

If a nail of the triflanged Smith-Peterson type is used, it should have an especially sharp point, and the possibility of displacing the head in the process of driving in the nail should be borne in mind. If a screw is used, the head should be fixed by an external wire in the process of insertion so that rotation of the head does not result in further displacement. It is possible that the impaction produced by a screw at the epiphyseal line will result in earlier fusion (Fig. 6.80). In general, the insertion of one or two screws is preferable to the use of a nail or pins.

The use of grafts of the match stick type placed across the epiphyseal line has been advocated by Howorth[3] to hasten closure of the line.

Approximately 1 out of 4 cases of slipped epiphysis seen is afflicted by a severe degree of slipping and by reposition of the epiphysis in relation to the neck (Fig. 6.81). It is necessary to procure a functioning hip which will not degenerate later into the marked limitation brought on by arthritic changes.

A very few patients with severe cases have an acute history. There is no rounding of the corners of the neck or build-up of callus about the slipped epiphysis by x-ray in cases of acute slip (Fig. 6.82). When the slip has been associated with acute trauma, it is sometimes possible to manipulate the hip with internal rotation and abduction of the lower extremity. When gentle manipulation is successful, the hip may be nailed in situ. The remaining cases of acute slip require open arthrotomy for correction of the mechanical derangement and internal fixation.

SOUTHWICK BIPLANE OSTEOTOMY

Southwick[5] has noted that if the capital femoral epiphysis has left its anatomic position by 30 degrees or more in any one plane, the function of the hip will be seriously affected. He has devised a method of correction that leads to accurate restoration of the position of the slipped capital femoral epiphysis through an osteotomy at the level of the lesser trochanter.

The physical examination of the patient is used to aid in determining the degree of correction required. If the normal hip flexes to 130 degrees and the affected hip to but 70 degrees with no external rotation, a 60 degree correction of posterior tilt would be required. A similar estimate of the limitation of abduction is made. These estimates are used in conjunction with the x-ray measurement.

Anteroposterior films are obtained with the hip in neutral positions (Fig. 6.83). A frogleg lateral view is taken with the hip in maximum abductor and external rotation with the knees flexed and the feet facing each other while their lateral surfaces rest on the table. Measurements are made on the films to determine the varus deformity and degree of posterior tilting. A tin template bent at 90 degrees to wrap around the femur and giving both the anterior and lateral osteotomy outline is made. The more bone that is removed, the more shortening will occur—it should be as little as possible and with exact accuracy as to the angles.

As the wedge of bone is removed, a flat surface will be left on both upper and lower fragment (Fig. 6.84). The osteotomy wedge need not occupy the entire transverse diam-

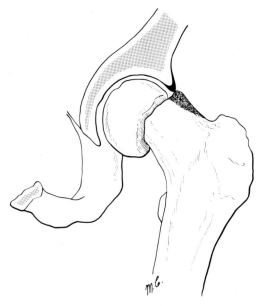

Figure 6.79.   In this diagram of subluxation existing with slipped epiphysis of the proximal femur, the abutment of the uncovered neck against the acetabular rim is emphasized. Considerable improvement in cases of old healed slips in a malunited position may be gained by surgical excision of the *shaded area*, as emphasized by Heyman.

eter of the bone; the remaining bone can be divided transversely. Sufficient bone should be removed, however, to provide broad bony contact. Tilting of the osteotomy site by more than 60 degrees shortens the femur excessively. The osteotomy is closed bringing the cut bony surface together. Southwick holds his osteotomy in position by multiple pins inserted through a pin-holding device into the proximal and distal fragments. Plates may be used. A plaster spica is also necessary after this preliminary support is applied. The cast ordinarily holds the patient for 8 weeks. The epiphyseal line is normally fused by the time the osteotomy is healed.

The operation is done through a lateral incision exposing the anterolateral aspect of the femoral shaft at the level of the lesser trochanter. The iliopsoas tendon is released. The anterolateral edge or corner of the femoral shaft is marked with an osteotome. Another orientation mark is made at right angles to the first at the level of the lesser trochanter. This mark is transverse to the femoral shaft. The template is superimposed in relation to

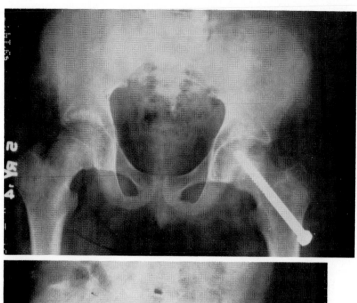

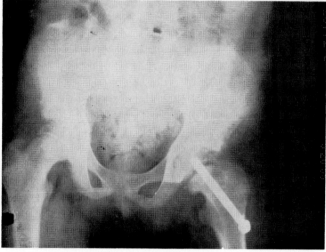

Figure 6.80. (*Top*) Slipped femoral epiphysis treated by screw fixation on the right, and apparently normal hip on left. (*Bottom*) Same patient 4 months later with filling in of the epiphyseal line on the right, but widening and radiolucency of the epiphyseal line developing on the left.

these orientation and transverse marks. The appropriate outline is marked with an osteotome. It will lead to a laterally based wedge looking at the anterior surface of the femur and an anteriorly based wedge looking at the lateral aspect.

A Steinmann pin is inserted to control the proximal femur prior to making the biplane osteotomy cuts.

WEDGE OSTEOTOMY AND KLEIN PROCEDURE

The hip may be approached anteriorly through the Smith-Peterson incision, as ad-

vocated by Klein et al.,[4] or posteriorly through a Gibson incision.

The displacement of the epiphysis may be corrected by a wedge osteotomy of the neck. Another method concentrates on the area of the epiphyseal line. This area is divided without removal of a wedge, and the neck is slid back into place beneath the epiphysis.

The first method results in shortening of the neck and thereby relieves stress on the stretched neck vessels. The fact that this method does not interfere with the retinaculum of Weitbrecht and maintains circulation to the femoral epiphysis has been noted by Green. The second method has produced

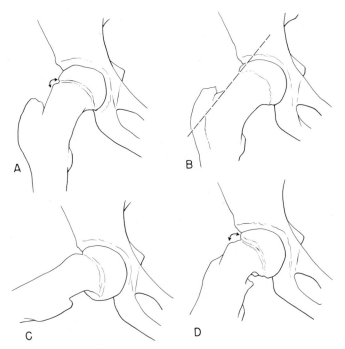

A B

C D

Figure 6.81. Measurement of the amount of slip is made along the arc of slip, as indicated by the *arrows* in the anteroposterior views (*A* and *B*) and lateral views (*C* and *D*).

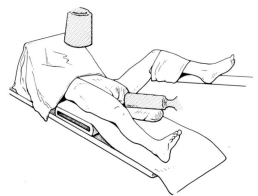

Figure 6.82. Equipment to procure roentgengrams of the hip is necessary when treating slipped epiphysis operatively. Films must be taken in two planes. The placement of the tube for anteroposterior and lateral views is shown. (Redrawn from A. Klein et al.: *Slipped Capital Femoral Epiphysis*; Springfield, Ill.: Charles C Thomas, 1953.)

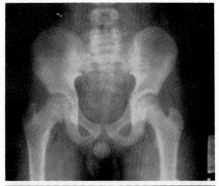

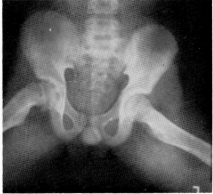

excellent results in the cases treated by Klein et al.[4] When a wedge of bone has been removed prior to replacement of the head, an absolute anatomic reduction cannot be reacquired.

Figure 6.83. Slipped epiphysis, anteroposterior and lateral roentgenograms. Displacement is visible in the lateral view.

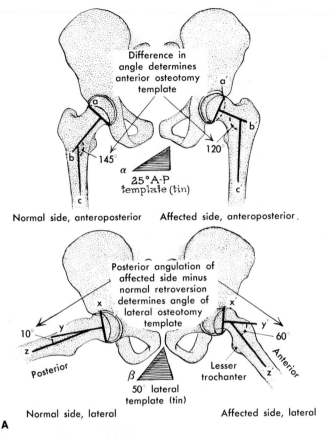

Figure 6.84. Southwick has devised a biplane osteotomy accurately designed to correct the degree of malalignment of the capital femoral epiphysis to the femoral shaft in two planes. (*A*) Diagram of the calculations for the template guiding the osteotomy, (*B*) Operative site. (*C*) Wedge removed at operative site. (*D*) Placement of internal fixation. (Reprinted from W. O. Southwick: Osteotomy through the lesser trochanter for slipped capital femoral epiphysis, *Journal of Bone and Joint Surgery, 49A:* 807, 1967.)

The operation, whether it is performed through an anterior or posterior approach with or without the removal of a wedge, has certain underlying principles.

These include gentle handling of the epiphysis and maintenance of the blood supply to it (Fig. 6.85). Both the internal and external femoral circumflex arteries provide branches running up to the femoral neck. The posterior, superior, and inferior portions of the capsule are particularly important. The capsule should be divided parallel to the lip of the acetabulum and next to it. A further incision should be made only if it is absolutely necessary and should split the capsule in line with the femoral neck so that there is as little interference as possible with the blood supply.

After the head is divided from the neck, the reduction is carried out with the aid of a bone skid and is followed by internal fixation from the lateral cortex of the femur.

Postoperative Treatment

The patient is placed in traction until the postoperative discomfort and muscle spasm have subsided. When the hip can be moved freely, the patient is allowed partial weight bearing with crutches. Fusion of the epiphysis is noted in 2–8 months after open reduction and in 6 months to 2 years following nailing in situ. Once the epiphysis has fused, the internal fixation apparatus is removed.

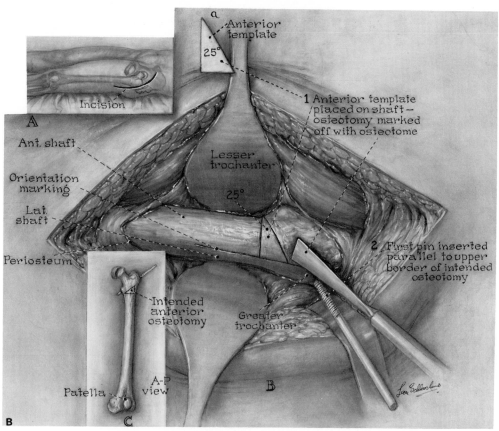

A

Incision

B

Ant. shaft

Orientation marking

Lat. shaft

Periosteum

a Anterior template

25°

1 Anterior template placed on shaft — osteotomy marked off with osteotome

Lesser trochanter

25°

2 First pin inserted parallel to upper border of intended osteotomy

Greater trochanter

Intended anterior osteotomy

Patella

A-P view

C

B

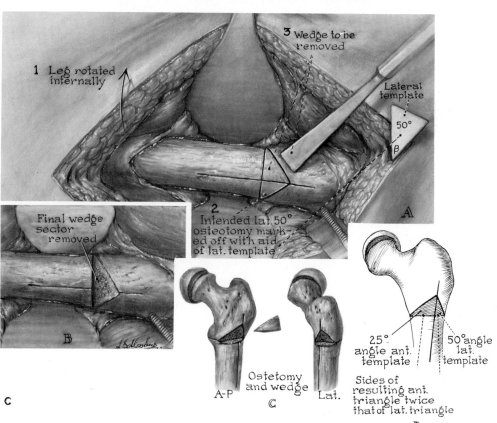

1 Leg rotated internally

3 Wedge to be removed

Lateral template

50°

β

2 Intended lat. 50° osteotomy marked off with aid of lat. template

Final wedge sector removed

B

A

Ostetomy and wedge

A-P   Lat.

C

25° angle ant. template

50° angle lat. template

Sides of resulting ant. triangle twice that of lat. triangle

D

C

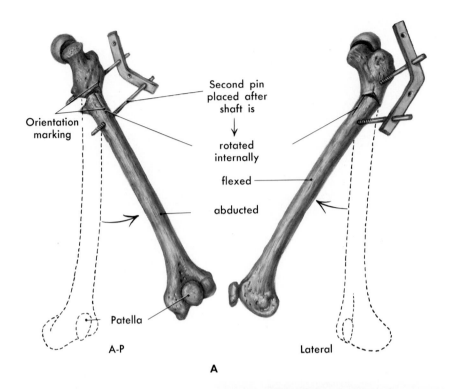

Orientation marking

Second pin placed after shaft is

rotated internally

flexed

abducted

Patella

A-P

Lateral

A

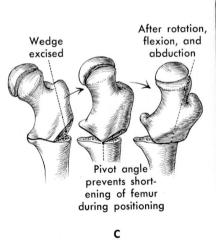

Wedge excised

After rotation, flexion, and abduction

Pivot angle prevents short-ening of femur during positioning

C

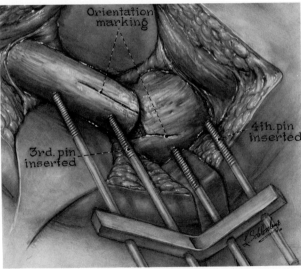

Orientation marking

3rd. pin inserted

4th. pin inserted

D

Fig. 6.84 (D)

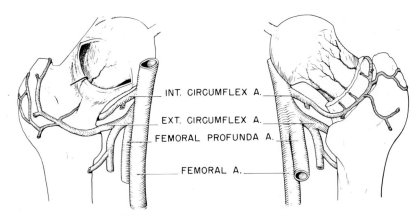

INT. CIRCUMFLEX A.

EXT. CIRCUMFLEX A.

FEMORAL PROFUNDA A.

FEMORAL A.

Figure 6.85.   Diagram of the anatomy of the circulation to the proximal femoral epiphysis. Note the transverse division of the capsule proximally (acetabular side) does not
jeopardize the circulation.

The possibility of involvement of the contralateral side must be constantly kept in
mind, and nailing in situ must be performed
if the diagnosis is made. Postoperative films
should always include both hips. Involvement of the other hip usually takes place
within the first 1½ years after the initial diagnosis, but may not occur until 2 or more
years later.

The results following nailing in situ for
minimal slips are excellent. The results following open reduction are good if the basic
requirements of care are well attended to.
These requirements include sparing the vascular supply to the epiphysis during the operation, anatomic repositioning, and early
mobilization.

The development of aseptic necrosis of the
head threatens a successful result. Such complications are rare, but they occur in all series.
Badgley reported three instances in 75 hips.
The initial displacement may predetermine
aseptic necrosis regardless of the method
used and the care taken in handling the case.

Cartilage Necrosis

Narrowing of the hip joint cartilage space
as seen by x-ray is a complication of slipped
epiphysis. It occurs in approximately 10% of
the cases. It seems to be related to a severe
synovitis of the hip accompanying the disease. Clinically it is manifest by markedly
limited motion in all planes and by muscle
spasm and pain. It can result in a severe hip
disability. Not all cases are irreversible, however. Some will recover a considerable portion of the joint space and joint function if

followed on a conservative, non-weight-bearing regime with preliminary traction.

For the others the disease represents a
severe complication. It can be seen after both
minimal and severe slips of the capital femoral epiphysis. Recent evidence suggests that
protrusion of the fixation pin may play a part
in the etiology.

References

1. Ferguson, A. B., and Howorth, M. B.: Slipping of the
   upper femoral epiphysis, *J.A.M.A., 97:* 1867, 1931.
2. Ghormley, R. K., and Fairchild, R. D.: Diagnosis and
   treatment of slipped epiphysis, *J.A.M.A., 114:* 229,
   1940.
3. Howorth, M. B.: Slipping of the upper femoral epiphysis. *J. Bone Joint Surg., 31A:* 734, 1949.
4. Klein, A., Joplin, R., Reidy, J., and Hanelin, J.:
   Slipped Capital Femoral Epiphysis; Springfield, Ill.:
   Charles C Thomas, 1948.
5. Southwick, W. O.: Osteotomy through the lesser
   trochanter for slipped capital femoral epiphysis. *J.
   Bone Joint Surg., 49A:* 807, 1967.
6. Waldenstrom, H.: On necrosis of the joint cartilage
   of epiphysiolysis capites femoris, *Acta Chir. Scand.,
   67:* 936, 1930.
7. Wilson, P. D.: Treatment of slipping of the upper
   femoral epiphysis with minimal displacement. *J.
   Bone Joint Surg., 20:* 379, 1938.

SYNOVITIS OF HIP*

Acute synovitis of the hip is one of the
most common orthopaedic conditions seen

---

* This section, "Synovitis of Hip," is reprinted from
A. B. Ferguson, Jr.: Synovitis of the hip and Legg-Perthes
disease, *Clinical Orthopaedics, 4:* 180, 1954, by permission of J. B. Lippincott Company.

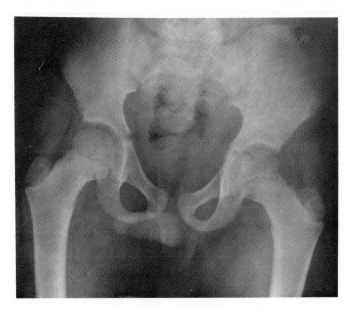

Figure 6.86.   Synovitis of the hip. The outline of the capsular shadows is rounded and increased in width on the *right*; the normal straight outline is seen on the *left*.

(Fig. 6.86). It is an inflammatory conditon of the hip of short duration, relieved by rest. It looms in the forefront of every differential diagnosis of childhood limp. Although this condition is so common, it seldom has been described. It is related to Legg-Perthes disease in that it is potentially preliminary to it.

A review of the cases admitted to the Children's Hospital (Pittsburgh) over the last 4 years reveals that the age distribution is very similar to the 3- to 10-year-old group found in coxa plana. Occasionally, a case as old as 12 may be seen. Four of 5 cases are males.

Acute synovitis of the hip is sometimes so mild that its symptoms attract little attention; sometimes it is so severe that it is mistaken for a septic hip joint. Occasionally, cases are recognized by roentgenogram only as synovitis which go on to develop the typical changes of coxa plana.

Etiology

Very frequently, there is a history of respiratory illness from 10 days to 3 weeks prior to the onset of hip symptoms. The relationship of these predominantly streptococcal infections to the inflammatory changes of the hip is not clear. When trauma looms large in the history, the presence of free blood in the joint is postulated. Occasionally, this has been confirmed by aspiration. Despite this occasionally clear implication, it is apparent that no single etiologic agent exists; whether or not such a joint is an allergic manifestation is uncertain.

Clinical Features

The patient is typically a male about the age of 5. Pain usually begins at the knee in the previous 24 hr. The pain tends to become more localized at the hip as the disease progresses. Frequently, the temperature at the height of the symptoms is as high as 101F, occasionally, 103F. However, the leukocytes ordinarily are not increased. The failure of an increase in the leukocytes aids in differentiating the condition from a septic hip when the temperature is high. The sedimentation rate may be slightly elevated.

Motion of the hip always is limited. There is temporary flexion contracture and limited rotation, particularly internal rotation in flexion, together with limited abduction. Palpation of the hip joint reveals both anterior and posterior tenderness.

Roentgen Findings

There are two definite x-ray findings. The most obvious of these is swelling of the capsular shadows about the hip (Fig. 6.87). The

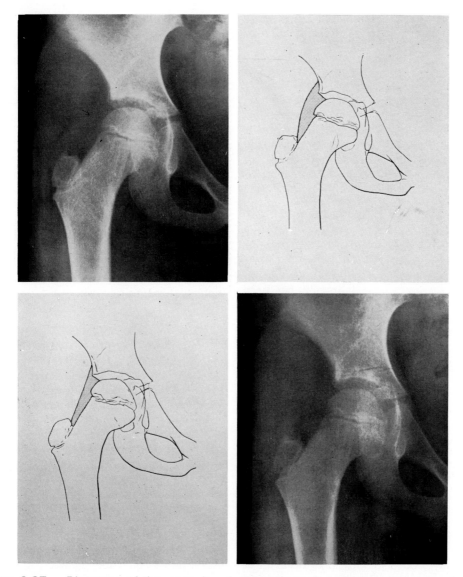

Figure 6.87.   Diagrams of the capsular shadows from the accompanying roentgenograms. (*Top*) The hip is that of a patient with symptoms and signs of synovitis with bulging
capsular shadow. (*Bottom*) The hip is normal.

rounded, increased prominence of the capsular shadows about the hip is seen best
superiorly and laterally. Accompanying this
is a minimal widening of the hip joint. Although slight and often found only by measurement, still it is commonly seen. Widening of the hip joint space is recognized more
easily in the medial inferior portion of the
joint. The anteroposterior view of the hip is
most instructive. There are no bone changes
suggestive of coxa plana.

Differential Diagnosis

The hip inflamed because of tuberculous
involvement has a chronic history which
acute synovitis does not have. Septic involvement of the hip must be differentiated by the
more definite signs of sepsis—elevation of
the white count and shift to the left. Aspiration may be necessary but in practice rarely
turns out to be so. Other possible underlying
causes of inflammation of the hip, such as

rheumatic fever or rheumatoid arthritis, are evident on general physical examination or future course.

Treatment

The inflammation about the hip tends readily to subside when weight bearing is eliminated. Traction in line with the flexion contracture is the most certain method of obtaining rapid subsidence of symptoms. Although relief from pain is almost immediate, it usually takes from 36–72 hr to regain full motion at the hip. Failure to regain full motion at the hip within 4 or 5 days leads to a suspicion that a more serious etiology underlies the condition.

The patient usually is given 1 week of nonweight bearing after full motion has been regained to guard against recurrence. Recurrences lead to a suspicion of coxa plana.

LEGG-PERTHES DISEASE**

Although synovitis of the hip may be preliminary to coxa plana, aseptic necrosis of the proximal femoral epiphysis may start without any previous difficulty at the hip (Fig. 6.90). It is known variously as Legg-Perthes disease, osteochondritis deformans coxae juvenilis, or coxa plana. The condition may be defined as a disease of the hip limited by age group and largely by sex; it results in changes in the femoral head apparently secondary to a loss of adequate vascular supply. Its duration is self-limited, but its course may result in irreversible mechanical impairment of the hip. The age group runs predominantly from 3–10 years old, with occasionally a case as old as 12. As in synovitis of the hip, the disease occurs predominantly in males (80%). Although Legg-Perthes disease can be bilateral, it is most often unilateral (90%).

The past few years have greatly increased our knowledge and understanding of the etiology and pathology involved in a vascular

---

** Parts of this section, "Legg-Perthes Disease," are reprinted from A. B. Ferguson, Jr.: Recent advances in understanding Legg-Perthes disease, *Orthopaedic Survey*, *1*: 307, 1978, by permission of Williams & Wilkins Company.

insult to the femoral head in both children and adults. The segmental nature of the necrosis involving one segment of the femoral head in both Legg-Perthes disease and idiopathic aseptic necrosis in the adult has been shown pathologically by superselective injection techniques, by radioisotope inspections, by surgical specimens, and experimentally. The branch of the lateral epiphyseal artery that appears to be involved—supplying the central segment of the head—could be injured by stress within the femoral head. Engineering studies to demonstrate the area where tensile compressive and shear stress develop in the femoral head were made to explain the segmental nature of the disease. Many past contributions to the literature have shown features that tie in well with the developing picture of the etiology and pathology of aseptic necrosis.

Significance

The National Center for Health Statistics reported that in the United States in 1972, 10.8 of 100 functionally limited persons referred to the cause of their loss of mobility as being due to impairments of the lower extremities and hips. Symptoms due to arthritis and rheumatism were reported by 22.2 persons and, for contrast, 8.7 persons reported heart disease. Legg-Perthes disease currently affects 25,000 boys and 6,000 girls between the ages of 3 and 14 years in the United States.

There has been no consensus in the past as to the etiology of the vascular insult to the hip—trauma, infection, genetic predisposition, synovial effusion, and most recently internal vascular occlusion have all been implicated. The wide range of treatment modalities has included subtrochanteric and innominate osteotomy, cancellous bone grafts, muscle pedicle transplants, medication, absolute bed rest, cast immobilization in abduction, and several brace designs.

Much of the failure to achieve a consensus as to treatment has arisen because of the confusion as to etiology, pathology, and the basic biomechanical factors involved. These same biomechanical factors are implicated in adult aseptic necrosis, and an improved basic understanding offers hope for improved therapeutic regimens.

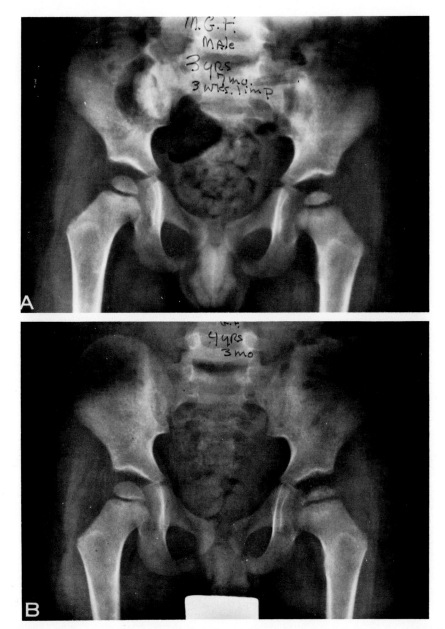

Figure 6.88. Boy, age 3 years, 7 months, with growth arrest of the capital femoral epiphysis on the reader's right (*A*). In (*B*) 8 months later, demineralization of the epiphysis has occurred. (*C*) Growth restoration is evident 14 months after onset; (*D*) 25 months after onset, the epiphysis is restored.

Past Contributions

Molloy and MacMahon[33] have estimated that idiopathic aseptic necrosis of the femoral head affects 1 in 750 boys and 1 in 14,000 girls. That the underlying necrosis is caused by interruption of blood supply can at least be agreed upon. The injection studies of Trueta[45] established that the lateral epiphyseal artery constituted the sole blood supply to the area that is involved in aseptic necrosis, although Salter and Bell,[40] using pigs, pro-

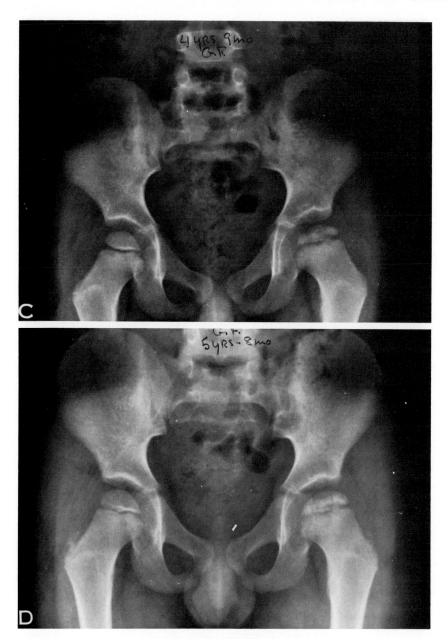

Fig. 6.88 (*C* and *D*)

duced a condition that strongly resembled Legg-Perthes disease by occluding the femoral head blood supply. Robichon and co-workers[38] ligated the femoral neck of piglets and were able to produce in addition to the avascular necrosis of the femoral head the shortening and widening of the femoral neck seen in the growing child after vascular insult to the head.

In the past the nature of the initial vascular insult remained unknown. A number of workers have identified retarded skeletal maturation in growing patients subject to this disease. Girdany and Osman[20] reported this high incidence and along with the study by Weiner and O'Dell,[48] their report tends to shape the child with Legg-Perthes disease as one who is short but with average or above

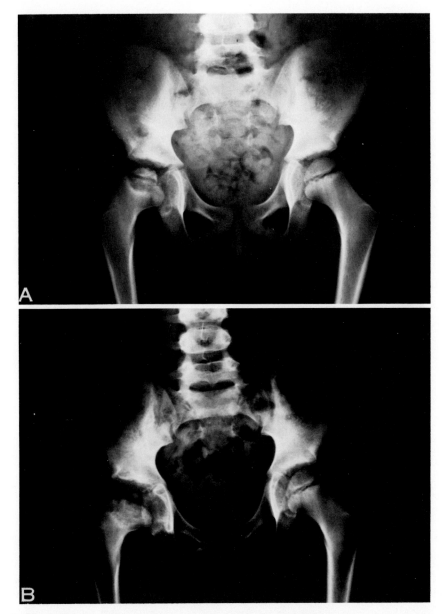

Figure 6.89. (A) Growth arrest and metaphyseal demineralization followed by bone resorption in (B).

average weight. Fisher[18] identified a higher than expected family incidence as well. Fluid pressure elevation due to synovitis may play a part in disturbing the blood supply. Gledhill and McIntyre[21] pointed out that the syndrome of transient synovitis was quite distinct from these cases occasionally seen clinically associated with Legg-Perthes disease.

Caffey[5] pointed out one of the early roentgenographic features, correctly designating the development of the separation between the subchondral bone and the underlying injured segment as being due to a fracture (Fig. 6.91). The compression of the epiphyseal center by the subchondral bone with central flattening resulted in the disappearance of this radiolucent line in a 2- to 4-month interval. Our own work[15] has shown that the lateral epiphyseal artery courses through the region of elevated shear stress in the femoral

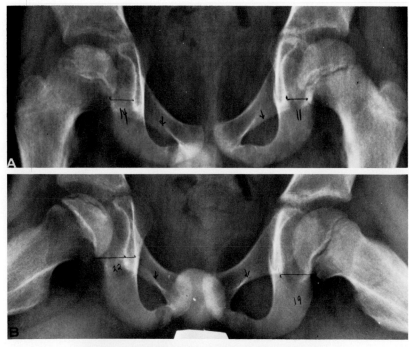

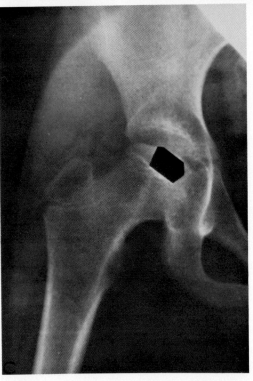

Figure 6.90. (*A*) Onset of Legg-Perthes disease, with growth arrest and central involvement. (*B*) Lateral view reveals fracture of living peripheral (cortical) bone from the present avascular bone as described by Caffey (on *left*). (*C*) Later roentgenogram from anteroposterior view, blocking out dead central segment which has collapsed. The living bone laterally is evident and uninvolved.

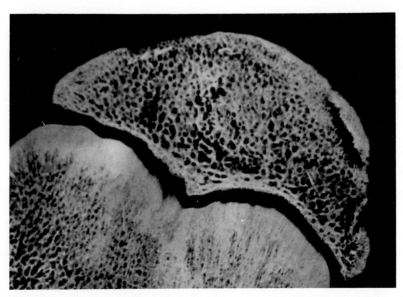

Figure 6.91.   The fracture of living cortical bone segment from the avascular central segment. (Courtesy of Robert Clark, M. D.)

head and is highly vulnerable to mechanical load elevations. The recording of elevated shear stress when the hip is in a position analogous to abduction points out the possibility for injury.

Catterall[9] divided the patients with Legg-Perthes disease into four groups and pointed out that the first two of these with milder involvement had a good prognosis for future use of the hip, the latter two having a very poor outlook for the use of the hip in adult life with the later development of arthritis. Differences between the first two groups and the latter two revolved around several significant features. Loss of height of the femoral head could be endured provided the lateral portion of the head did not project beyond the lateral edge of the acetabulum. Some flattening that would occur over the central segment could be endured with a marked tendency in childhood to remodeling once full motion has been reobtained. By contrast the groups that did not remodel satisfactorily and did go on to further difficulty not only had loss of height of the femoral ossification center, but also lateral projection of the lateral segment of the head beyond the lateral edge of the acetabulum, thus allowing pressure to occur directly on the involved segment and leading to still further mechanical dissolution of the hip joint as a functioning entity. It was not possible to agree with one of Catterall's

statements, however, and that is that a patient did not progress from one of the first two groups into the third or fourth group. Our own work[15] has shown many individuals, followed serially, in whom that occurred.

Katz[27] made some important observations with a series of patients treated conservatively. He found that the prognosis was most favorable in younger patients and that neither the duration of symptoms nor the duration of therapy was related to the prognosis. The development of subluxation and pressure seemed to be a dominant cause of deformity. Somerville[42] heavily emphasized containment of the femoral head within the acetabulum so that the femoral head could be molded into proper shape as reossification occurred. Containment has become a very important goal to achieve. Petrie and Bitenc[34] emphasized the attainment of this goal with the use of ambulatory abduction casts. Catterall,[9] Ferguson,[17] and Salter[39] all emphasized the importance of preventing the lateral extrusion of the vascular lateral segment accompanying the acetabulum.

Two authors have shown that there is no particular advantage in recumbent treatment as compared to other forms of therapy for this disease. These studies by Cumming[11] and by Catterall[9] will spell the death knell for the long term bed rest treatment of this disease. The current favorite therapy is to allow full activity and at the same time apply devices that ensure that the femoral head remains contained. Petrie and Bitenc[34] used their 45 degree abduction plaster cast. Bobechko[2] developed a dynamic brace and Harris and Hobson[23] devised a forced abduction-flexion internal rotation splint. The difficulties in maintaining the splint at maximum efficiency in the face of active ambulatory activity led to some emphasis on surgical repositioning of the femoral head. Canale and co-workers[8] recommended their innominate osteotomy to achieve this surgical repositioning. There was significant improvement in patients, provided the disease was not already so old and so healed that no possibility for improvement remained. Somerville[42] and Ferguson[17] have both emphasized subtrochanteric osteotomy, because it has the advantage of producing a vascular blush to the proximal femur in addition to repositioning the head for purposes of better coverage. Gower and Johnson[22] observed that the degree of deformity demonstrated by x-ray at the time of healing correlated strongly with the likelihood for later development of degenerative arthritis.

Improvement of treatment will arise from better understanding of the nature of idiopathic aseptic necrosis as regards both pathology and biomechanical degradation.

One Vascular Insult or Multiple Vascular Insults

McKibbin and Ralis[32] felt that the slow progress of healing and the deformation that takes place deserved consideration of more than one vascular insult. Freeman and England[19] and Zahir and Freeman[49] produced a picture in the dog closely resembling human Legg-Perthes disease with a second interference with the blood supply. This gave a pathology to the femoral head which was segmental in nature with the central segment involved. The medial and lateral segments were still vascular. Trueta[45] suggested that the slow progress was due to mechanical collapse which might interfere with the vascularization of the central segment. Salter and Bell[40] felt that the slow progress of deformation of the head was due to biologic plasticity of the cartilage of the head. The variation from adult aseptic necrosis in the childhood

disease seems due to the large amount of cartilage comprising the femoral head (and the consequent deformation and recovery possibilities) and of course the presence of the epiphyseal line giving relatively weak support to the area beneath the epiphyseal line.

Pathology

FIRST STAGE

Salter[39] has pointed out the apparent growth arrest that occurs in the ossification center for the femoral head when a vascular insult has occurred. At this time the general increase in density evident radiologically leads to a concept that the entire femoral head is involved. This concept soon vanishes, however, as the child is followed by serial roentgen examinations. A slight loss of sphericity of the head occurs centrally, and a radiolucent line described by Caffey[5] appears just below the subchondral bone overlying the central segment. We know from examining adult femoral heads at this stage that this radiolucent line represents a fracture of vascular subchondral bone from the injured segment. It is followed by convolution of the cartilage of the weight-bearing portion of the femoral head superior to the fovea. These cartilage ridges outline the area under which the subchondral bone has lost support and leaves a well defined smooth surface to the femoral head both medially and laterally; this covers segments of the femoral head which remain well vascularized. Synovitis of the hip joint accompanies the development of this central flattening and the convolution of the cartilage over it. Lang[28] published a postmortem photograph in 1932 of the femoral head subject to Legg-Perthes disease, showing the convolutions identical in extent to those seen in adult aseptic necrosis. In the adult we have many specimens detailing this change in femoral heads removed in the process of reconstruction of the hip joint. Until lateral protrusion occurs either in the child or the adult there is still some possibility for recovery of an adequate hip joint.

SECOND STAGE

In the child two mechanisms may occur to produce lateral extrusion. One is concentric

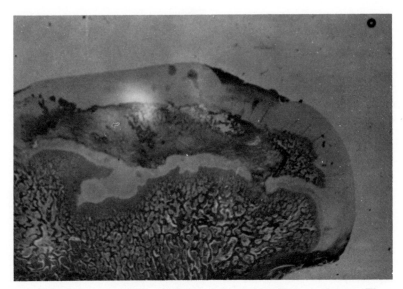

Figure 6.92. The dead segment centrally replaced by fibrous tissue. The periphery is vital and living bone. The cartilage is overgrown.

cartilage overgrowth—an overgrowth that may not only involve the articular surface, but may spill over, cascading down the femoral neck. The second mechanism is lateral shifting of the lateral viable segment beyond the lateral edge of the acetabulum—a process that appears to take place at the junction of the epiphyseal line and metaphysis and is akin to an epiphyseal fracture. Some have felt this lateral protruding bone is due to new bone formation, but there is little evidence for this concept and no periosteum to generate it. In the adult with aseptic necrosis the lateral viable segment does not shift position relative to the neck, but the central segment as it collapses allows the lateral edge of the acetabulum to come inside the lateral viable bone, leaving it projecting to interfere with attempted abduction of the hip.

The collapse of the central segment produces mechanical disruption of the epiphyseal line, as noted by both Haythorn[25] and Ponseti.[35] The stimulus to fibrous tissue invasion of the dead segment which is now fractured on all sides and surrounded by fibrous tissue appears to be the collapse of either the epiphyseal line in the child or the area marking the old epiphyseal line in the adult.

THIRD STAGE

Once the later stages of the pathology are evident the disruption of the anatomy be-

comes so severe that the original segmental nature of the process is hard to discern.

The flattening of the central segment becomes severe, and originally viable lateral and medial segments become subject to mechanical pressure, further flattening the femoral head. An end product of this flattened femoral head is the secondary adaptation of the acetabulum to it in an irregular manner to coincide with the convolutions of the femoral head. This adaptive congruity is a late change due to mechanical pressure. Motion of the hip must now be mechanically limited over and above that secondary to synovitis with resulting muscle spasm.

Pathologic Specimens from Patients with Legg-Perthes Disease

If allowance is made for the abundance of cartilage in the childhood femoral head, it is amazing how similar are the gross pathologic specimens examined in both Legg-Perthes disease and aseptic necrosis in the adult.

When collapse of the involved central segment occurs, it does so with depression of the overlying articular cartilage and convolution of the cartilage at the edge outlining this segment. The medial and lateral areas are maintained until late progress of the disease. The fibrous invasion into the involved central area is evident, as well as the hyper-

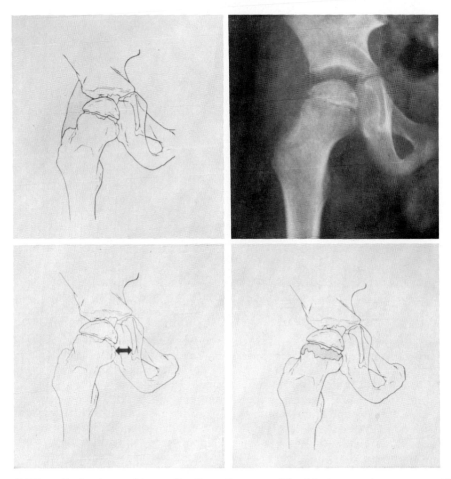

Figure 6.93. Early signs of Legg-Perthes disease of the hip by roentgenogram. Bulging capsular shadows, increased density of epiphysis, widened joint space, and demineralized metaphysis adjacent to the epiphyseal line are shown.

trophy of both the medial and lateral blood supply to produce this activity. McKibbin and Ralis[32] noted the slowness of the repair in this center segment. It is apparent that considerable interference with the process of repair can occur with mechanical change in the outline of the femoral head and with lateral displacement of the lateral segment. Cartilage is thickened markedly but ossification is diminished at the area where it would normally be found. The thickened bony trabeculae in the area of fractured and disrupted bony trabeculae were believed by McKibbin and Ralis[32] to be evidence for early vascular insult to the area and later secondary insults. Cartilage proliferation has continued when endochondral ossification has stopped.

Close examination of the specimens reveals, however, that cartilage proliferation continues principally medially and laterally. There is no evidence of new ossification centers arising laterally.

The two cases described by Jensen and Lauritzen[26, 29] were similar. Synovitis or evidence of old synovitis was not in evidence. The central involved segment is the site of the fibrous-vascular invasion. The cartilage hypertrophy is very much in evidence but there are no new centers of bone formation, the lateral-appearing bone formation in the head progressing as the central portion flattens. There is a change in direction of the lateral portion of the epiphyseal line as it bends inferiorly. As the epiphyseal line loses continuity centrally, granulation tissue forms and fibrous tissue begins to occupy the center segment, with resorption of dead and thickened trabeculae.

Blood Supply to the Central Segment of the Femoral Head

Both Claffey[7] and Brodetti,[3] working with injection studies, showed the branching of the lateral epiphyseal artery as it entered the femoral head to supply a lateral, a central, and a medial segment. Claffey showed how internal fixation devices could interfere with the blood supply to the central segment.

Théron[44] used a delicate superselective injection technique to delineate the area where the vessels were cut off in 18 cases of idiopathic aseptic necrosis. The segmental nature of the involvement was again confirmed as the stump of the vessel could be visualized in the lateral area of the head-neck junction where it was cut off. Théron also showed dilation of the medial vascular supply to continue the vascularity to this portion of the femoral head. The importance of Théron's demonstrations is great, because this was the first time segmental interruption of the lateral epiphyseal vessel had been shown in connection with idiopathic aseptic necrosis.

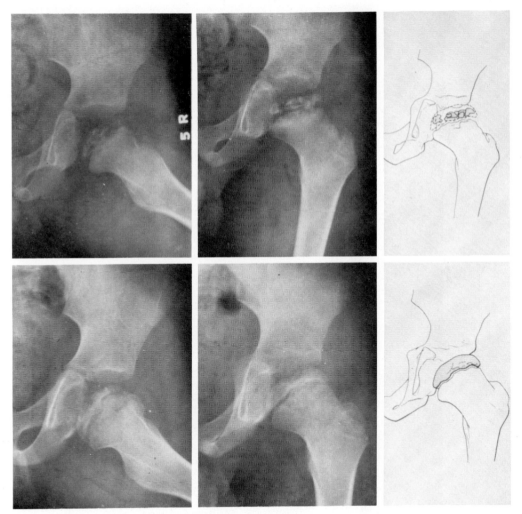

Figure 6.94.   Prediction of expected result in coxa plana from the roentgenogram when first seen. The predicted flattened outline of the head is diagrammed at *top right.* (*Bottom*) The follow-up roentgenogram of the same case and accompanying diagram.

The studies of Crock[10] showed in injected and cleaned specimens the normal nature of the blood supply to the femoral head in various age groups. The segmental nature of the supply from branches of the lateral epiphyseal vessel is beautifully shown in his demonstrations.

Trueta and Amato[46] showed that if the vessels supplying the epiphyseal plate were interrupted the plate cells proliferated and the plate broadened as occurs in Legg-Perthes disease, the nourishment of the plate depending on epiphyseal vessels and endochondral ossification depending on the metaphysial blood supply.

The sum of the various injection studies showing the vascularization of the proximal femoral epiphysis in children is as follows: The artery accompanying the ligamentum teres supplies a small segment of subchondral bone over the central portion of the femoral epiphysis. The diaphyseal artery diminishes in importance in the 5- to 10-year age group, with the main supply coming from the lateral epiphyseal artery. The inferior and anterior retinacular arteries fail to pass the plate in

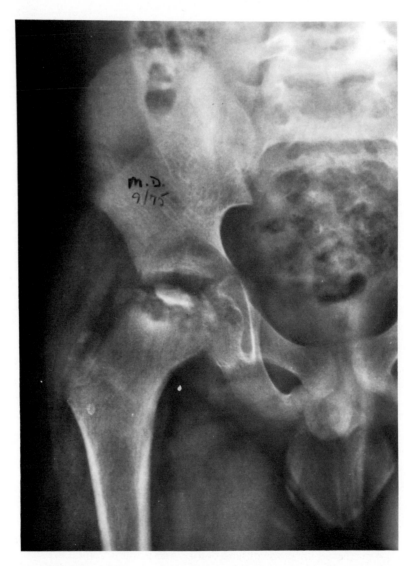

Figure 6.95. Late Legg-Perthes involvement with central involved segment down on epiphyseal line with secondary metaphyseal involvement. The lateral viable segment has been extruded beyond the lateral acetabular margin.

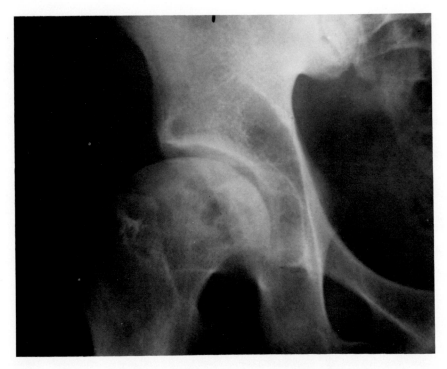

Figure 6.96. Old Legg-Perthes involvement in the adult, with widening of head and neck and central radiolucent area remaining.

most cases. This leaves the posterior-superior retinacular artery (lateral epiphyseal artery) to shoulder the main burden of blood supply. Immediately on entering the epiphysis it divides into a lateral branch and posterior medial branch, the main branch continuing to supply the segment which is central and involved in both Legg-Perthes disease and idiopathic aseptic necrosis.

Disturbance of venous outflow from the metaphysis of the femoral neck was observed by Suramo and co-workers[43] in the fragmentation stage of Legg-Perthes disease. This does not tie in well with the pathology of Legg-Perthes disease, because no evidence of venous dilation has been observed. In our own attempts at interosseous venogram in the metaphysis we observed rapid outflow and we felt that we were on the wrong side of the epiphyseal line to demonstrate any possible obstruction which could be assumed to be relevant.

Stress within the Femoral Head

Brown,[4] working in our laboratory, has developed a computerized analysis of the femoral head. This was based on testing over 200 cubed sections of the femoral head in order to determine the variation of the structure of the femoral head from a similar shape composed of homogenous material. Application of pressure by the Instron machine gave values which were used to construct the model. The femoral head unit was outlined by minute force transducers applied to the femoral head. This work (to be published elsewhere) became very interesting relative to aseptic necrosis when it was shown that the development of tensile stress laterally and compressive stress medially within the femoral head-neck specimen also gave rise to the development of significant shear stress when the femoral head and neck were placed in the varus position. This would be analogous to jumping onto the extended lower limb when the hip was in abduction—a fairly common incident in healthy children. Further studies in progress may still further delineate the effect of stress within the femoral head as a means of interfering with the blood supply to the central segment.

Surgical Treatment of Aseptic Necrosis in Child and Adult

Our own experience with surgery for aseptic necrosis in both the child and the adult

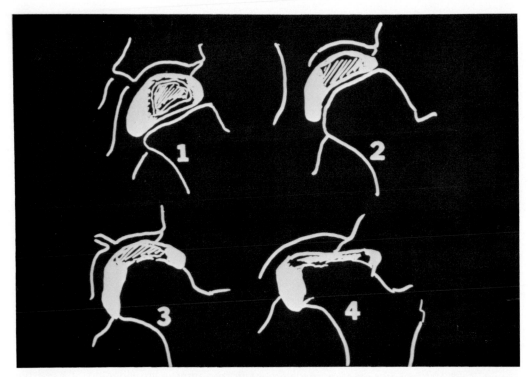

Figure 6.97. Although inspired by Catterall's division of Legg-Perthes involvement into four groups related to prognosis, this diagram is more an interpretation than a literal transcription. The outlook is good in groups 1 and 2. In group 1 the sphericity is maintained, as is most of the height of the epiphysis, with no lateral protrusion of the ossific nucleus. In group 2 there is no protrusion laterally beyond the acetabulum, but the height of the epiphysis has been further diminished and some flattening has occurred. Groups 1 and 2 are at risk, but if there is no further progression a good result with spherical remodeling can be expected. Groups 3 and 4 lose sphericity to an extent leading to adult symptoms. In group 3 lateral protrusion has occurred without severe flattening and loss of height. In group 4 the lateral protrusion is further accentuated by central crush leading to severe diminution in height and flattening. The lateral segment of the femoral head is displaced laterally. Adaptation of the acetabulum to the incongruous fit of the femoral head within it can be expected. If the patient when first seen is in group 1 or 2, then every effort must be extended to avoid progression to group 3 or 4.

has been limited to proximal femoral osteotomy. The use of innominate osteotomy to procure coverage of the lateral segment represents an alternate approach with both advantages and disadvantages. The use of surgery has greatly awakened interest as more is learned about this disease because of the possibility of continued ambulation while the femoral head is protected in its regenerating phase.

Howard Steel showed that there was an effect on healing of the femoral head sub-jected to vascular insult even when no mechanical change in the position of the fragments was involved. He osteotomized the proximal femur without mechanically rearranging the fragment and showed acceleration of the healing phase.

This has been our own experience, although we have added a 15–20 degree tilt into a varus position in order to get the viable lateral segment beneath the lateral edge of the acetabulum in a walking position. A vascular blush of the proximal segment is clearly

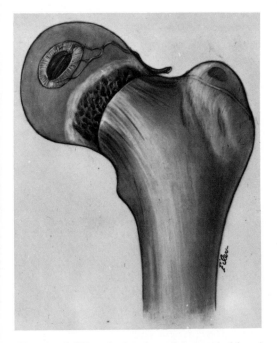

Figure 6.98. Lateral epiphyseal blood supply to ossific nucleus of femoral head dividing into medial, lateral, and central branches.

forward) of having the lateral segment displace lateralward beyond the lateral edge of the acetabulum. The more severe degrees of deformity can sometimes be brought into a contained position within the acetabulum by adding varying degrees of flexion to the proximal fragment.

Internal fixation that is trustworthy is a necessity, because our experience with external pin fixation has not been good. In addition, in the childhood group we have added a spica cast for 6 weeks to guard against excessive activity in this early phase of healing. Full activity has been allowed with return of full motion at the hip and demonstrated healing of the osteotomy line. There has been no progression of deformity as a result of this full activity. This is not a paper on the detailed follow-up of osteotomy for aseptic necrosis, but the possibilities for recovery and revascularization are excellent in the childhood group and diminish with age. This is

evident by the clear delineation of the avascular central segment after the osteotomy is performed in the region just proximal to the lesser trochanter. This has given us additional information of value, because it has exposed the clear involvement of the central segment even when the initial roentgenogram did not make this clear. This has led to the realization that when the slightest flattening occurs over the central segment, then isolation of this segment by fracture from the surrounding living bone has already occurred. The disappearance of the radiolucent line described by Caffey[5] after 4 months in serial x-ray examination is accounted for by the crushing down of the superior subchondral bone against the avascular segment.

Our experience with osteotomy over the past 10 years has taught us several important lessons. The osteotomy should be performed as soon as flattening occurs superiorly even in slight degree, because this indicates that a crush fracture has already taken place. Certainly the head is at risk (from this point

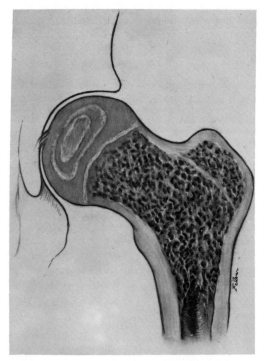

Figure 6.99. Growth arrest of ossific nucleus occurring in young age group below age 4, with resumption of growth resulting in head within a head sign remarked on by Robert Salter.

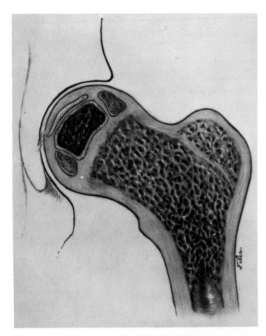

Figure 6.100. Involvement in an older child with Legg-Perthes disease. The central segment is involved; the medial and lateral segments and superior subchondral bone segment still have blood supply.

a situation which is to be expected, given the tissue viability of both age groups.

Conservative Treatment

The initial discussion of treatment relates to the early stages of the disease.

The primary treatment of Legg-Perthes disease revolves around the principle of containment. By containment is meant achieving location of the acetabular rim outside the femoral head. No matter what ultimate method we are going to choose to maintain this position, we are first going to have to achieve abduction of the hip.

FIRST GOAL

A full range of motion of the hip joint must be obtained by alleviating both synovitis and muscle spasm. Do not let a child go with limited hip motion. This leads to local pressure of the lateral third of the acetabulum on the femoral head and collapse and deformity at the junction of the living and dead bone.

To achieve a full range of motion, rest is certainly necessary and traction may have to be added. Traction carries with it the connotation of relieving muscle spasm, protecting the hip. This cannot be done by pulling on the hip in extension (as for instance by Buck's extension, which is not traction). Traction must be in line with the deformity of contracture. In these cases there is often a flexion contracture of the hip of 45 degrees or more. This requires, at minimum, a sling beneath the proximal end of the tibia (Russell's traction) often accompanied by a pillow beneath the thigh. The traction must be alive—i.e., watched and changed as the muscle relaxes to gradually bring the hip out of deformity. In Legg-Perthes disease the limited motion may persist beyond the economic feasibility of maintaining the child in the hospital in traction. Do not be afraid of insisting on bed rest and a home-bound instruction (teacher) program for 3 months before embarking on your ultimate therapy of containment.

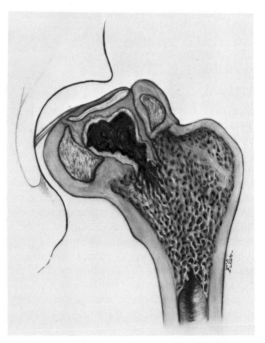

Figure 6.101. Diagram of late progression in Legg-Perthes disease. The central segment has crushed in toward fracturing the epiphyseal line. The lateral segment has shiften lateralward, and extrusion of the head relative to the acetabulum brings about a difficult treatment situation.

Arteries of the
ligament of the head

Superior ascending branches
of the arterial ring of the
femoral neck

Arterial ring of the
femoral neck

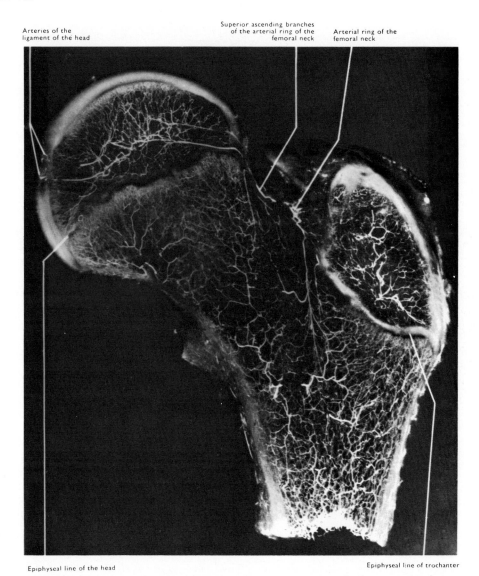

Epiphyseal line of the head

Epiphyseal line of trochanter

Figure 6.102. The blood supply to the femoral head in childhood demonstrated by injection study of Henry Crock of Melbourne. Note branch going to center of the femoral head. (Reproduced with permission from H. V. Crock: *The Blood Supply of the Lower Limb Bones in Man*; London: Livingstone, 1967.)

The full range of motion having been achieved, there are a number of therapy choices.

1. Full Activity and Full Weight Bearing. This is only feasible if the early stage is clearly over and there is minimal involvement of the femoral head so that obviously live bone is available for weight bearing and the head is naturally contained due to failure of the widening of the femoral neck and head to develop. This is most often true in younger children below age 6. If this program is embarked on, it pays to recheck the child at 6-week intervals in the early phase to make certain that synovitis and limited motion do not develop.

2. Abduction Cast (Petrie and Cruess). The application of an abduction spica followed by containment of the femoral head wholly within the acetabulum gives excellent

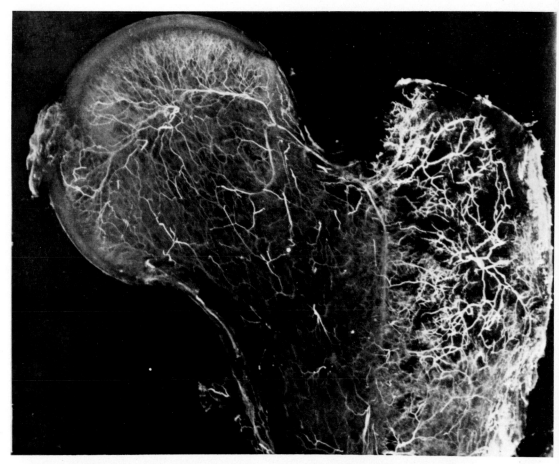

Figure 6.103. Blood supply to the femoral head in the adult. Note central branch of lateral epiphyseal going to central segment of femoral head. (Reproduced with permission from H. V. Crock: *The Blood Supply of the Lower Limb Bones in Man*; London: Livingstone, 1967.)

results in terms of preventing further deformity. It has disadvantages. It is hard to walk with crutches in an abduction spica. That the kids do merely proves how wonderful children are and what good athletes they can become, given a difficult task. The spica obviously limits motion—this is an undesirable feature because local pressure may occur causing fibrillation of cartilage. The results as reported speak for themselves, however.

At Newington Children's Hospital, the inevitable immobilization of plaster has been relieved by a bivalved plaster simulation of the abduction spica. This is removable for non-weight-bearing exercise, including swimming. This obvious advantage is countered by the fact that it is difficult for this apparatus to stand up to crutch walk-

ing—no matter what the fastenings holding the two halves together.

3. Abduction Splint. There are two types: the ball joint abduction splint used in Toronto by Babechko and the tripod extension of a patten bottom splint (Tachduan). Of the two, the ball joint abduction splint answers most of the biomechanical analysis eliminating weight-bearing pressure more firmly than the patten bottom splint modification.

How difficult it is for any material, including steel, to stand up to the activities of a child is evidenced by the ball joint abduction splint—it will fail in the face of a boy's activities although it may stand up forever in a Chevrolet cap. There is more freedom, there is hip motion, it is still difficult to get around, but it has some advantages over the spica.

4. Patten Bottom Splint. Holding the foot 3 inches off the ground with a cork elevation of the shoe on the uninvolved side does not prevent adduction of the hip and, therefore, failure of containment. It has the advantage of stretching out tight musculature by making a single lever arm of the leg (no knee hinge), but in the process excessive pressure on the femoral head must occur.

The extension of the patten bottom splint to prevent adduction by holding the splint abducted through a weight-bearing tripod attached on the medial side of the splint answers some of the objections to the splint.

The patten bottom splinting allows the child to enter into the programs of children his own age, an important advantage for his emotional and intellectual growth. Prolonged non-weight-bearing treatment in an institu-

tion is mentioned at this point only to be condemned.

Development of Osteoarthritis

There have been many studies attempting to determine the late occurrence of osteoarthritis after Legg-Perthes disease. Because the conclusions tend to vary, one is forced to emphasize a consensus of these results to try to establish a useful working hypothesis. In general it can be said that where sphericity of the femoral head is lost osteoarthritic changes will follow; this is equally true in adult aseptic necrosis. In the child the enlargement of the head due to concentric growth of cartilage may result in extrusion from the acetabulum, but this will have a

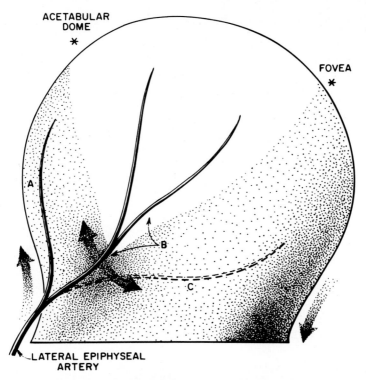

B – CENTRAL BRANCH ARTERY AT RISK AND THE AREA
OF THE FEMORAL HEAD THAT IT SUPPLIES

Figure 6.104. Diagram of femoral head outline illustrating the stress distribution secondary to pressure at the acetabular dome (tensile stress occurs laterally and compressive stress occurs medially) accentuated by progressive varus. Shear stress develops in the region of the course of the branches of the lateral epiphyseal artery to the femoral head. These shear stresses may (by trabecular fracture within the femoral head) cause loss of blood supply to the central segment.

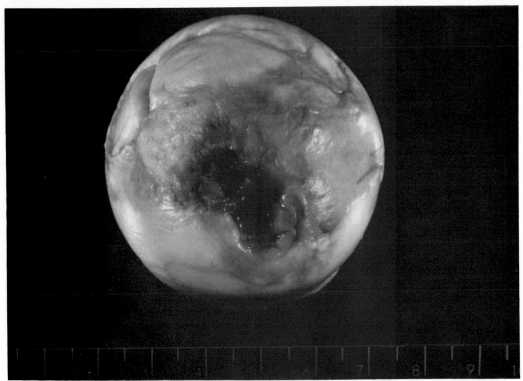

Figure 6.105. Looking directly at the fovea in an adult hip specimen with aseptic necrosis. The cartilage surface shows the convoluted edge of the depressed central area which outlines the extent of the involvement of the central portion of the femoral head.

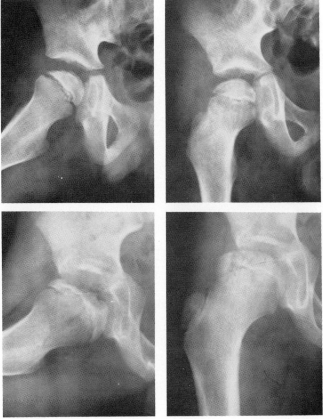

Figure 6.106. Development of coxa magna from early coxa plana.

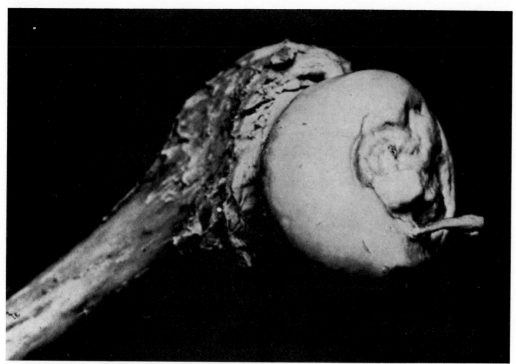

Figure 6.107.   Illustration of the femoral head in Legg-Perthes disease, published by Lang[28] in 1932. Note the similarity of the distribution of the depressed cartilage area in this 12-year-old child to the similar area in the adult. (From *Journal of Bone and Joint Surgery 14:* 563–573, 1932.)

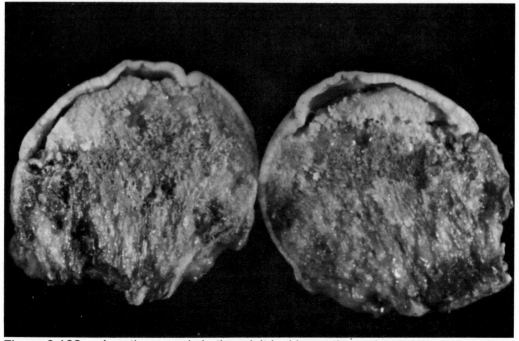

Figure 6.108.   Aseptic necrosis in the adult looking at the surface of the femoral head divided in the coronal plane. The illustration shows the fracture of the overlying cartilage and subchondral bone from the central involved segment. This gives rise to the radiolucent line noted in the roentgenogram in both aseptic necrosis and Legg-Perthes disease.

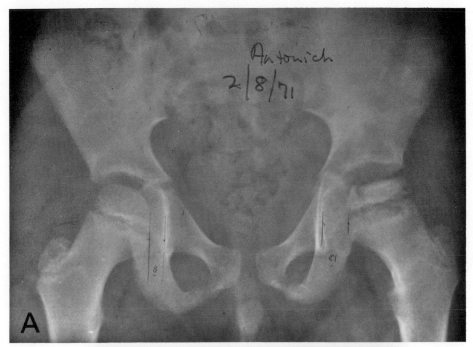

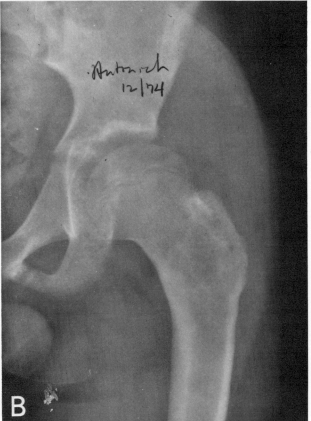

Figure 6.109. (*A*) Severe early involvement in Legg-Perthes disease with crushing of central segment and secondary metaphyseal involvement. (*B*) Three-year follow-up varus osteotomy.

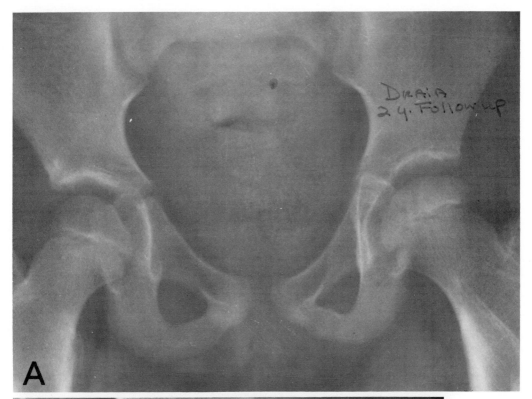

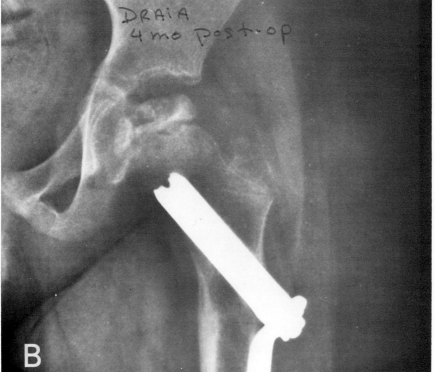

Figure 6.110. (A) Four-month postoperative roentgenogram after varus osteotomy with central segment involvement clearly evident following vascular blush after osteotomy. (B) Two-year follow-up after varus osteotomy in Legg-Perthes disease.

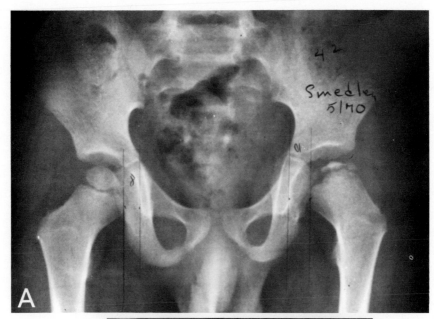

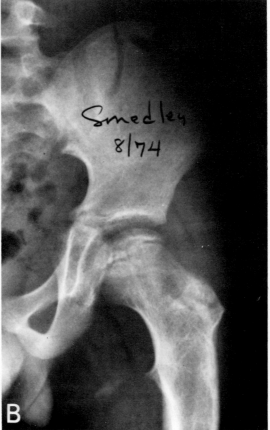

Figure 6.111. (*A*) Severe femoral head involvement in a child 4 years, 2 months old with crushing of central segment. (*B*) Four-year follow-up after osteotomy.

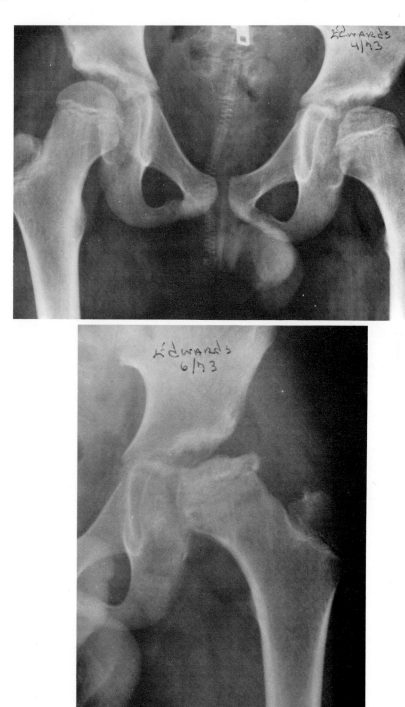

Figure 6.112. Rapid collapse of central segment of the femoral head. (*Top*) April 1973: fracture line beneath subchondral bone over central segment. (*Bottom*) June 1973: collapse with lateral projection of uninvolved segment. This rapid progression shows the emergency nature of the necessity for containment of the lateral segment within the acetabulum.

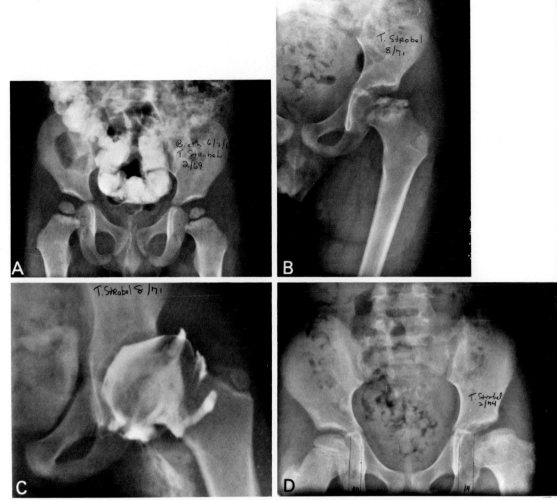

Figure 6.113. Metaphyseal involvement with severe crush of femoral head. (*A*) Early Legg-Perthes disease in a 3-year-old. The segmental nature of the involvement is not as clear in the relatively small ossific center of this age group. (*B*) At 2-year follow-up with center crush affecting epiphyseal line and the development of radiolucent areas in the metaphysis filled with fibrous tissue. (*C*) Arthrogram outlining central crush and lateral movement of lateral segment. (*D*) Follow-up 5 years later with diminished height and loss of sphericity.

surprisingly low incidence of osteoarthritis, provided the head remains spherical and the acetabulum congruous.

Early follow-up series such as that of Waldenstrom[47] showed that, despite the small number of normal hips in 45 untested cases, the patients were functioning surprisingly well. In Ratliff's series[37] only 10% evidenced major osteoarthritis 17 years later.

Trueta (clinical note) found that osteoarthritis coincided with deformity and incongruity.

Danielsson and Hernborg[12] found patients with problems only when they fell into the group with deformity and restriction of motion; the most severe osteoarthritis occurred in patients with the most severe deformity.

Eaton[14] and Sanders and MacEwen[41] both defined with exactness the possibility of osteoarthritis developing later, a radius variation of less than 3 mm apparently being compatible with useful life of the hip joint throughout the patient's active years.

Acetabular Osteotomy. It occurred to Robert Salter that changing the acetabulum relative to the femoral head and answering the principle of containment was achievable by doing the iliac osteotomy that he devised.

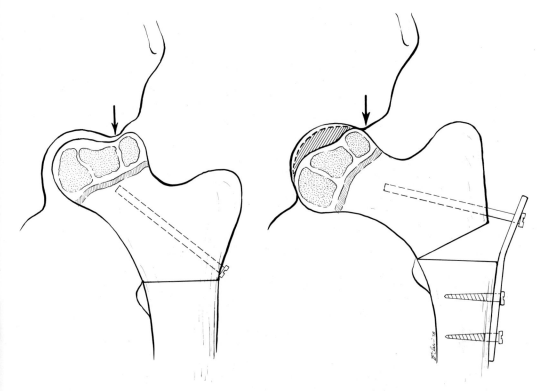

Figure 6.114. Osteotomy of the proximal femur in Legg-Perthes disease when there is considerable deformity is difficult. The lateral prominence must be contained within the acetabulum. If this cannot be accomplished by abduction and internal solution, it may be aided by flexion. If necessary the proximal fragment may be left in flexion when the fixation is applied.

It is an important means of containing the femoral head and permitting the child full activity.

The prerequisite is enough abduction to bring the femoral head wholly within the acetabulum. At a youngish age (over 10), there are secondary problems with the anatomic distortion secondary to iliac osteotomy.

There is no point in this osteotomy of the ilium if the acetabular rim cannot fully slide over the femoral head. Make sure this can occur before you start. The technique of a Salter osteotomy is fully described elsewhere. If you are not a consummate orthopaedic surgeon who can do this osteotomy easily, do not start down this road.

If well done, the results can be excellent. Containment as a principle is observed, motion is quickly regained, and full activity is permitted. Once again, if this is not true, the operation should not have been done in the first place. The wholly contained hip with a good rim of living bone at the edge of the

femoral head should sustain itself without the development of further deformity.

Missing will be the hematologic blush secondary to femoral osteotomy; gained is no varus—no limp—no necessity to regain valgus with growth.

Excision of Lateral Aspect of Femoral Head. This is occasionally referred to as bumpectomy—a term that seems too unprofessional for a textbook.

The problem is serious. The hip cannot be abducted and wholly contained within the acetabulum due to projection of a squashed or deformed lateral aspect of the femoral head projecting beyond the acetabulum.

If the motion is otherwise normal including rotation and abduction and the patient is older—over 10—you have a candidate for this procedure whom you can help. If you are going to remove this lateral projection, make sure you are going to do it completely. This requires good exposure, not necessarily iliofemoral. The posterior approach is useful,

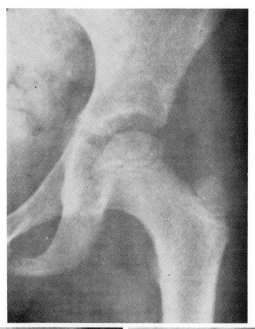

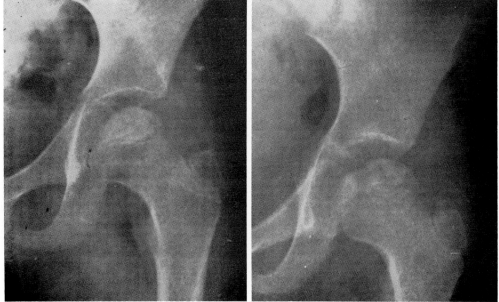

Figure 6.115.   Legg-Perthes disease in a patient who first presented late in the disease. Time interval: 2 years.

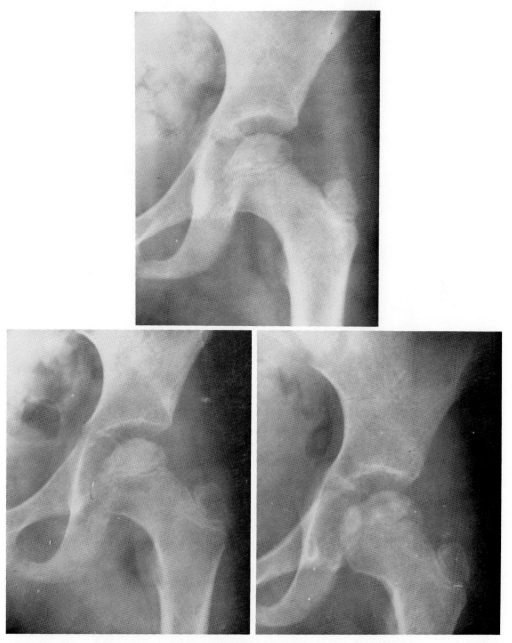

Figure 6.116. Legg-Perthes disease in patient who was first seen early in the course of the disease. Time interval: 1 year.

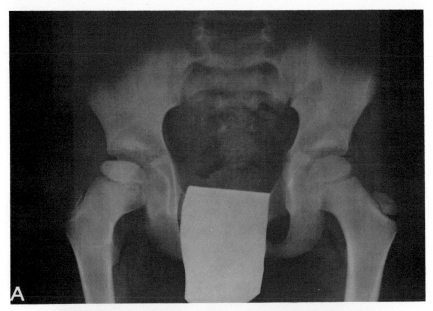

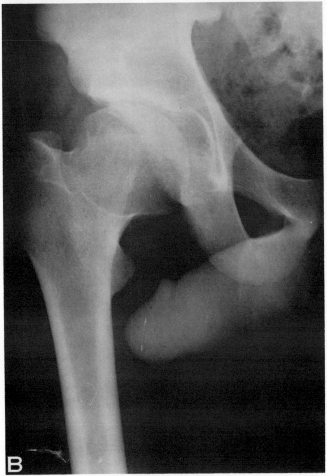

Figure 6.117. Follow up in Legg-Perthes disease. (*A*) Boy first seen at age 6 with growth arrest and collapse of the central segment of the femoral head. (*B*) Anteroposterior view 15 years later with diminished head height and rounded outline. At this time the boy had become a prominent college basketball player who complained of an aching hip after each game. (*C*) The lateral view is more revealing as to the cause of symptoms with a small anterior projection at the junction of the femoral head and neck.

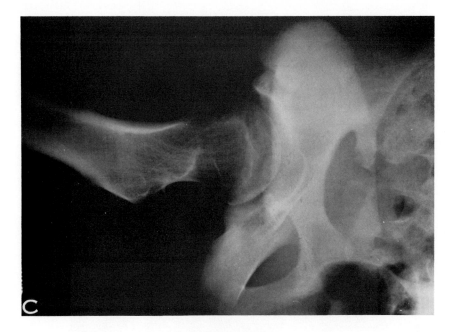

Fig. 6. 117 (C)

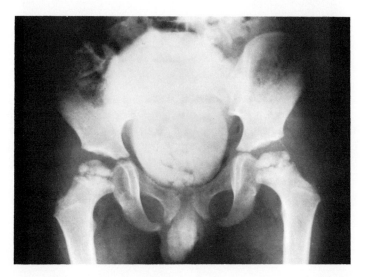

Figure 6.118.   Irregular ossification of both hips simulating Legg-Perthes disease. No clinical limitation of motion of the hips was apparent.

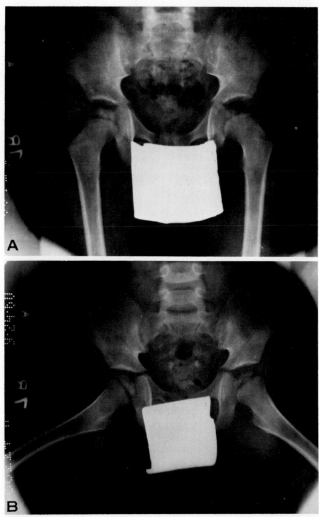

Figure 6.119.   A case of epiphyseal dysplasia showing of the salient roentgen features. (*A* and *B*) Anteroposterior and lateral views of the hips show irregular ossification of the femoral heads without soft-tissue swelling, bilateral. (*C*) The lower leg shows diminished height medially of the distal tibial epiphysis. (*D*) Delay in mineralization of the lateral proximal humeral epiphysis and of the small bones of the wrists.

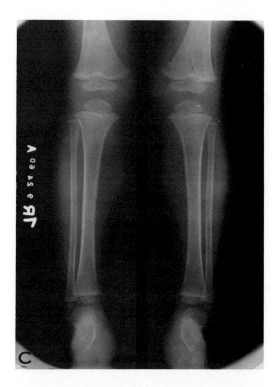

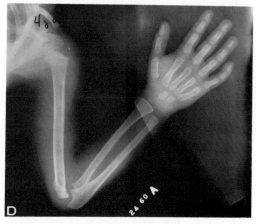

Fig. 6.119 (C and D)

as the lateral aspect of the head is readily visualized and all projections of the femoral head that limit motion can be readily visualized.

This is rewarding compared to the preoperative state. Do not expect too much out of it—the hip will not regain full motion, but the immediate preoperative limitation will be relieved.

SUMMARY

The lateral and slightly posterior placement of a hip nail can result in localized segmental avascular necrosis. The interruption of the lateral epiphyseal artery gives a picture of involvement which is consistent in both Legg-Perthes disease and in aseptic necrosis in the adult.

Containment becomes a principle in treatment that can be achieved. With evident fracture and hopefully before lateral epiphyseal fracture of the viable segment has occurred, containment must be achieved so healing can occur. If the head and neck begin to widen, osteotomy is indicated. If containment can be done some other way—as by bracing—then it may be indicated as well. There is a vascular flush that occurs with osteotomy that may be of some help in addition to the positioning. The rapidity with which serious changes can occur is evident in following serial films. If fracture is present the patient is already at risk to develop lateral extrusion due to epiphyseal fracture; it takes about 2 months for this to occur. Further attempts at abduction in walking in this situation still further laterally extrudes the viable fragment and compresses the dead central fragment.

References

1. Bobechko, W., and Harris, W. R.: Radiographic density of avascular bone, *J. Bone Joint Surg., 42B:* 626, 1960.
2. Bobechko, W. P.: The Toronto brace for Legg-Perthes disease, *Clin. Orthop, 102:* 115, 1974.
3. Brodetti, A.: The blood supply of the femoral neck and head in relation to the damaging effects of nails and screws, *J. Bone Joint Surg., 42B:* 794, 1960.
4. Brown, T. D., and Ferguson, A. B.: The development of computational stress analysis of the femoral head, *J. Bone Joint Surg., 60A:* 619, 1978.
5. Caffey, J.: The early roentgenographic change in coxa plana; significance of pathogenesis, *Am. J. Roentgenol., 103:* 620, 1968.
6. Calvé, J.: Sur ine forme particulure de pseudo-coxlelgie grefee sur des deformations coracteristiques de l'extremite superiure du femier, *Rev. Chir., 30:* 54, 1910.
7. Claffey, T. J.: Avascular necrosis of the femoral head, *J. Bone Joint Surg., 42B:* 802, 1960.
8. Canale, S. T., D'Anca, A. F., Cotler, J. M., and Snedden, H. E.: Innominate osteotomy in Legg-Calvé-Perthes disease, *J. Bone Joint Surg., 54A:* 25, 1972.
9. Catterall, A.: The natural history of Perthes' disease, *J. Bone Joint Surg., 43B:* 37, 1971.
10. Crock, H. V.: *The Blood Supply of the Lower Limb Bones in Man;* London: Livingstone, 1967.
11. Cumming, W. J.: A review of 100 cases of Legg-Calvé-Perthes syndrome treated by recumbency, *J. Bone Joint Surg., 49B:* 386, 1967.
12. Danielsson, L. G., and Hernborg, J.: Late results of Perthes' disease, *Acta Orthop. Scand., 36:* 70, 1965.
13. Dolman, C. L., and Bell, H. M.: The pathology of Legg-Calvé Perthes disease, *J. Bone Joint Surg., 55A:* 184, 1973.
14. Eaton, G. O.: Long term results of treatment in coxa plana, *J. Bone Joint Surg., 49A:* 1031, 1967.
15. Ferguson, A. B., and Howorth, M. B.: Coxa plana and related conditions at the hip, *J. Bone Joint Surg., 16:* 781, 1934.
16. Ferguson, A. B., Jr.: The pathology of Legg-Perthes disease and its comparison with aseptic necrosis, *Clin. Orthop., 106:* 7, 1975.
17. Ferguson, A. B., Jr.: The pathology and treatment of Legg-Perthes disease, *Pediatr. Ann., 5:* 113, 1976.
18. Fisher, R. L.: An epidemiological study of Legg-Perthes disease, *J. Bone Joint Surg., 54A:* 769, 1972.
19. Freeman, M. A. R., and England, J. P. S.: Experimental infarction of the immature canine femoral head, *Proc. R. Soc. Med, 62:* 431, 1969.
20. Girdany, B. R., and Osman, M. Z.: Longitudinal growth and skeletal maturation in Perthes disease, *Radiol. Clin. North Am., 6:* 245, 1968.
21. Gledhill, R. B., and McIntyre, J. M.: Transient synovitis and Legg-Calvé-Perthes disease; a comparative study, *Can. Med. Assoc. J., 100:* 311, 1969.
22. Gower, W. E., and Johnson, R. C.: Legg-Perthes disease—long term follow-up of thirty-six patients, *J. Bone Joint Surg., 53A:* 759, 1971.
23. Harris, W. R., and Hobson, K. W.: Histological changes in experimentally displaced upper femoral epiphyses in rabbits, *J. Bone Joint Surg, 38B:* 914, 1956.
24. Harrison, M. H. M., Turner, M. H., and Nicholson, F. J.: Coxa plana, *J. Bone Joint Surg., 51A:* 1057, 1969.
25. Haythorn, S. R.: The pathological change found in material removed at operation in Legg-Calvé-Perthes disease, *J. Bone Joint Surg., 31A:* 599, 1949.
26. Jensen, O. M., and Lauritzen, J.: Legg-Calvé-Perthes disease—morphological studies in two cases examined at necropsy, *J. Bone Joint Surg., 58B:* 332, 1976.
27. Katz, J. F.: Conservative treatment of Legg-Calvé-Perthes disease. *J. Bone Joint Surg., 49A:* 1043, 1967.
28. Lang, F. J.: Osteo-arthritis deformans contrasted with osteo-arthritis deformans juvenilis, *J. Bone Joint Surg., 14:* 563, 1932.
29. Lauritzen, J.: The arterial supply to the femoral head in children, *Acta Orthop. Scand., 45:* 724, 1974.
30. Lauritzen, J.: Legg-Calvé-Perthes disease; a comparative study, *Acta Orthop. Scand. Suppl., 159:* 23, 1975.
31. Legg, A.: An obscure affection of the hip-joint, *Boston Med. Surg. J., 162:* 202, 1910.
32. McKibbin, B., and Ralis, Z.: Pathological changes in a case of Legg-Perthes disease, *J. Bone Joint Surg., 56B:* 438, 1974.
33. Molloy, M. K., and MacMahon, B.: Incidence of Legg-Perthes disease (osteochondritis dissecans), *N. Engl. J. Med., 275:* 988, 1966.
34. Petrie, J. G., and Bitenc, I.: The abduction weight bearing treatment in Legg-Perthes disease, *J. Bone Joint Surg., 53B:* 54, 1971.
35. Ponseti, I. V.: Legg-Perthes disease; observation and pathological changes in two cases, *J. Bone Joint Surg., 38:* 739, 1956.
36. Ponseti, I. V., and Cotton, R. L.: Legg-Calvé-Perthes disease; pathogenesis and evolution, *J. Bone Joint Surg., 43A:* 261, 1961.
37. Ratliff, A. H. C.: Pseudocoxalgia—a study of late results in the adult, *J. Bone Joint Surg., 38B:* 498, 1956.
38. Robichon, J., Desjardins, J. P., Koch, M., and Hooper, C. E.: The femoral neck in Legg-Perthes disease—its relationship to epiphyseal change and its importance in early prognosis, *J. Bone Joint Surg., 56B:* 62, 1974.

39. Salter, R. B.: Experimental and clinical aspects of Perthes disease, *J. Bone Joint Surg.*, *48B:* 393, 1966.

40. Salter, R. B., and Bell, M.: The pathogenesis of deformity in Legg-Perthes disease—an experimental investigation, *J. Bone Joint Surg.*, *50B:* 436, 1968.

41. Sanders, J. H., and MacEwen, G. D.: A long term follow up on coxa plana at the Alfred I. DuPont Institute, *South. Med. J.*, *62:* 1042, 1969.

42. Sommerville, W. W.: Perthes disease of the hip, *J. Bone Joint Surg.*, *53B:* 639, 1971.

43. Suramo, I., Puranen, J., Heikkinen, E., and Vuorinen, P.: Disturbed patterns of venous drainage of the femoral neck in Perthes disease, *J. Bone Joint Surg.*, *56B:* 448, 1974.

44. Théron, J.: Superselective angiography of the hip, *Radiology*, *124:* 649, 1977.

45. Trueta, J.: The normal vascular anatomy of the femoral head during growth, *J. Bone Joint Surg.*, *39B:* 358, 1957.

46. Trueta, J., and Amato, V. P.: The vascular contribution to osteogenesis. III. Changes in growth cartilage caused by experimentally induced ischaemia, *J. Bone Joint Surg.*, *42B:* 571, 1960.

47. Waldenstrom, H.: On coxa plana: osteochondritis deformans coxa juvenilis, Leggs disease, Maladie de Calvé, Perthes Krankheit, *Acta Chir. Scand.*, *55:* 577, 1923.

48. Weiner, D. S., and O'Dell, H. W.: Legg-Calvé-Perthes disease; observation on skeletal maturation, *Clin. Orthop.*, *68:* 44, 1968.

49. Zahir, A., and Freeman, M. A. R.: Cartilage changes following a single episode of infarction in the capital epiphysis in the dog, *J. Bone Joint Surg.*, *54A:* 125, 1972.

50. Zamansky, A. P.: The pathology and pathogenesis of Legg-Calvé-Perthes disease, *Am. J. Surg.*, *4:* 169, 1928.

EPIPHYSEAL DYSPLASIA

This condition has two elements of importance. First, the epiphysis may be deformed sufficiently that secondary arthritic changes develop, particularly at the hip. Second, the epiphyseal changes may be confused with other anomalies, such as Legg-Perthes disease. Epiphyseal dysplasia may occur as an isolated epiphyseal change or in the form of multiple abnormalities involving particularly the proximal humerus, the distal femur and tibia, and the proximal femoral epiphysis.

It is common for mineralization of the epiphyses to be delayed by arbitrary standards, such as those of Todd. Such delay, visualized at the wrist by roentgenogram, often amounts to a 3- to 4-year deficiency. A familial incidence, visualized by roentgenogram in the parents and siblings, is not uncommon with epiphyseal deformities.

The patients with multiple ossification centers forming their epiphysis vary from those with a normal cartilage anlage for the epiphysis to those in which the anlage is already malformed and as ossification progresses this is evident on roentgen examination and is evident by physical malformation or limited motion.

Other variables are various mesoectodermal disturbances that could be associated in various combinations and possibly be so severe as to leave the child with a very limited outlook. It is exceedingly hard to conceive of each of these variations as a clear-cut entity, but to give the reader a concept of the variations involved the classification of Bailey follows:

MULTIPLE EPIPHYSEAL DYSPLASIA CONGENITA

Type I.	Normal stature.
Type II.	Short stature, saddle nose deformity.
Type III.	Short stature, saddle nose, upper limb rhizomelia.
Type IV.	Short stature, saddle nose, upper and lower limb inequality in leg lengths, scoliosis, rhizomelia, ectodermal changes, intelligence changes.
Type V.	Same as above plus mental retardation, failure to thrive, and early death.
Type VI.	Atypical cases.

The cases are few, but those classified as Type V are the most common and are often reported as Conradi's disease.

Clinical Picture

The youngster is usually short in stature and often among the shortest 10% according to the growth chart. Other outward signs are usually conspicuous by their absence unless gross skeletal deformity at the knee or ankle is evident. In the older age groups, there may be signs of hip disease, such as limited motion in internal rotation, abduction, and flexion and possibly a hip flexion contracture.

Often there are no complaints, the condition being incidentally noted on the roentgenogram after trauma or other disease calls for examination.

Roentgen Findings

The spectrum varies from the mild multiple ossification centers in a normally formed epiphysis to those with deformities of the epiphyseal ends of the bones that gradually become evident with growth. There is often delay in appearance of the ossification centers and restriction of growth in the epiphysis may become clearly evident (Fig. 6.119).

Instability of the atlanto-axial joint may be evident in infancy in the severely affected.

At the wrist, delayed mineralization of the carpal bones is noted. The lateral portion of the proximal humeral epiphysis may be deficient in size by comparison with the medial humeral head. At the hips, the condition appears to be trying to create two femoral heads, and the acetabulum mirrors this contour. Slight degrees of the deformity, causing a central depression in the head, are most common. Relatively minor forms consist of only delayed mineralization of the proximal femoral epiphysis with irregular ossification of the epiphysis. It is this type that is frequently confused with Legg-Perthes disease. The roentgenogram appearance, however, is not accompanied by signs of limited motion at the hips. The lateral portion of the distal femoral epiphysis is often deficient in height when compared with the medial portion. At the distal tibial epiphysis, a similar type of deformity gives the epiphysis a triangular shape, and the deficiency frequently exists in the lateral portion.

Treatment

For many patients no treatment is indicated or of value. These youngsters have full joint motion and, except for a short stature, are unremarkable. Youngsters are seen who already have limited hip motion and considerable femoral head deformity. The joint space, however, is usually still well maintained. Although the need for reconstruction seems inevitable, it is usually not indicated in childhood. Periods in traction and recumbency to attempt to improve motion at the hips may be indicated. Osteotomy at the knee may be necessary in the presence of gross deformity.

Perhaps most important is the necessity for distinguishing this condition from the conditions loosely termed osteochondritis.

References

1. Bailey, J. A.: Forms of dwarfism recognizable at birth, Clin. Orthop, 76: 150, 1971.
2. Christiansen, W. R., Lin, R. K., and Berhaut, J.: Dysplasia epiphysialis multiplex, Am. J. Roentgenol., 74: 1059, 1955.
3. Elsbach, L.: Bilateral hereditary microepiphyseal dysplasia of the hips, J. Bone Joint Surg., 41B: 514, 1959.
4. Fairbank, H. A. T.: Dysplasia epiphysialis multiplex, Br. J. Surg., 34: 225, 1947.
5. Fairbank, T.: An Atlas of General Affections of the Skeletal System; Edinburgh: E. S. Livingstone, 1951.
6. Freiberger, R. H.: Multiple epiphyseal dysplasia, Radiology, 70: 379, 1958.
7. Jackson, W. P. U., Hanelin, J., and Albright, F.: Metaphyseal dysplasia, epiphyseal dysplasia, diaphyseal dysplasia, and related conditions. II. Multiple epiphyseal dysplasia, Arch. Intern. Med., 94: 886, 1954.
8. Litchman, H., and Chirls, M.: Dysplasia epiphysialis multiplex, Bull. Hosp. Joint Dis., 1957.
9. Silverman, F. N.: A differential diagnosis of adrondroplasie, Radiol. Clin. North Am., 6: 223, 1968.

CHAPTER 7

Congenital Orthopaedic Conditions

HEMIHYPERTROPHY

Hemihypertrophy is uncommon in the pure form that its name implies. Most of the youngsters that will be seen with this condition actually have involvement of only one limb to any marked degree. Lower extremity involvement is much more common than upper. There is no evidence of any hereditary transmission, and the distribution between the sexes is equal. General involvement rather than increased length of the limb is the eventual clinical problem.

Birthmarks and evident involvement of the vascular system in terms of venous enlargement are evident early in life. Mental deficiency, an involvement in 15–20% of the cases, may be the presenting complaint. It is evident that the bone is only mirroring the general enlargement of the soft tissues rather than being the eccentric devil at the core of the syndrome. The growth centers do appear earlier than usual in the involved limb, however. There is excessive reaction of the sebaceous and sweat glands. The hair is usually thickened. Varices appear early. Many anomalies have been described in association with the abnormal enlargement of the limb, such as clubfeet, congenital heart disease, polydactylism, and even Wilms' tumor. Hypertrophy of one of paired organs may occur.

Wagner originally described the condition in 1839. He was describing a case with enlargement of the lower extremities associated with lipomas and telangiectasia. There was also a tongue enlargement. Hemiatrophy is not a problem in clinical differentation because it is secondary to neurologic conditions such as lesions of the postcentral gyrus.

In Ward's classification of the varying forms of this condition, "segmented" refers to a digit or ray; "crossed" to involve one limb or side with a ray or digit involved on the other side; and hemihypertrophy includes the more common partial hypertrophy involving principally the lower extremity. So little is known of the etiology that it is hardly worthwhile to repeat the speculations.

Treatment

The syndrome of hemihypertrophy has involved following the child throughout the growth period. The initial vascular studies, such as arthrograms and interosseous venograms, have been disappointing in their failure to reveal an abnormality. Obviously frank arteriovenous fistulas and massive hemangiomas are treated early. Although increased blood flow is clearly evident in increased warmth of the extremity, it must occur beyond the major vessel level.

The length problem is rarely one that cannot be handled at the appropriate time by simple epiphyseal arrest. Much more troublesome are the enlarged soft tissues. This often becomes so severe that excision of subcutaneous tissue is indicated. We have not ventured beyond a third of the circumference of the extremity in doing this and have leveled the edges of our excised mass to avoid a sudden concavity in the calf. The deep fascia is exposed and the deep layer of the subcutaneous tissue is excised gradually, progressing around the limb. Defatted skin laid down on the calf fails to achieve the cosmetic improvement that is the objective.

Local Giantism

Enlargement of a digit or ray is a total enlargement of the finger or toe and may or may not include the metacarpal or metatarsal. It may accompany the syndrome of hemihypertrophy. In the finger, epiphyseal arrest of the phalanges may be indicated relatively early. In the toes, excision of the proximal phalanx is a worthwhile procedure if done early in the child's life where the size of the digit clearly indicates shoe-fitting problems. Where the whole ray is involved, amputation of the entire segment digit and metatarsus may be indicated to achieve a workable foot. In the hand, wedge resection of the soft tissue to narrow the digit or ray may have to be done early to preserve the finger and prevent enlargement to the point of interference with function. Wedge resection may also be necessary in the foot for the same reason.

Other Causes of Limb Enlargement

ARTERIOVENOUS FISTULA

The congenital type is usually clearly evident at birth. The thrill or bruit associated with it is diagnostic. It is continuous but accentuated by systole. Seldom does the fistula present for the simple one-connection excision; rather, extensive fistulas, with multiple arteriovenous connections which prove difficult to resect, are found.

The acquired arteriovenous fistula in our own experience has been iatrogenic. Knee surgery in childhood is particularly productive. The acquired type initially goes through a clinical syndrome of arterial insufficiency, and gangrene of the limb could result. Later, as collateral circulation and hypervascularity occur, venous insufficiency could result, with varicose veins, edema, pigmentation, and ulcers.

HEMANGIOMAS

The types of hemangioma most likely to occupy the orthopaedist's attention and lead to limb enlargement are those of relatively massive signs involving muscle. The capillary hemangioma involving skin, which though prominent at birth tends to regress and can occasionally be hastened in that course with judicious applications via the dermatologic route, is not ordinarily associated with a growth problem. The massive cavernous hemangioma is a resection problem of no mean magnitude on occasion. Division through the center of the hemangioma can lead to massive blood loss as if one had opened into the general circulation. It is usually readily controlled, the area being overlapped on itself and sewn. However, the real excision problem when the hemangioma has proved invasive is how much to resect without interfering with muscle function. Because this is individualized, no statement of treatment, no matter how beautifully done, could possibly encompass it all.

There are no thrills or bruit with hemangiomas. Venous dilation as age progresses, increased skin temperature, and an occasional mass are seen. It is stated that the hemangioma is painless, but it has been found by the author to be a significant answer to unexplained limb pain with local tenderness and occasional calcification in the muscle mass by x-ray—giving the diagnosis. These phleboliths have a soft, rounded calcific density that is characteristic.

Hemangiomas may be more destructive than they would initially appear. They may result in fibrosis and contracture of muscles that markedly interfere with their function. Hemangiomas ordinarily do not enlarge after 18–20 years of age.

LYMPHATIC ABERRATIONS

The onset of lymphatic praecox and Milroy's disease is a nebulous, poorly defined area. Certainly it is seen in children. There is no early indication of vascular involvement. The limb is enlarged by a pitting edema with a smooth skin. There is accompanying tissue hypertrophy both of the soft tissues and bone. Later varices appear, and also lymphangitis and cellulitis, in about 10% of the youngsters.

The symptoms are those of increased weight of the limb, but not pain due to the invasion of other anatomic structures.

At this writing, treatment is not efficient or curative. We have started elastic support early on recognition of edematous involvement of the limb and have reason to think that this has controlled the development of a massive elephantiasis as these children have achieved adult life.

LYMPHANGIOSARCOMA

This is a rare condition that has resulted in amputation of the limb in our experience.

NEUROFIBROMA

There is no question that neurofibromatous involvement of a limb can cause massive enlargement of a limb. The only question is, how does it do it? Is it merely excessive blood supply to the epiphyseal side of the epiphyseal line or is it direct neural control or lack of control? Ectodermal dysplasia leading to excessive tissue is associated with neurofibromatosis. There is often a familial history. All the secondary phenomena of excessive blood supply to the limb may result, particularly when the limb is dependent. A lesion arising in bone has still to be proven; a lesion involving bone has been reported. Excision of involved tissue leads to improvement. There comes a time when excision of tissue with peripheral nerve involvement will lead to a loss of function. Which way the decision lies, then, is a matter of the individual case and the anatomic area involved. May the surgeon choose wisely and well.

Strangely enough, there are gains to be made by excision of the tissue with nerve involvement, which may be nothing more than endoneural involvement initially. This frequently leads to arrest of the condition, at least in the area attacked.

EHLERS-DANLOS SYNDROME

This syndrome is characterized by hyperextensibility of the joints and skin. Because this phenomenon may reach proportions that are intriguing from a popular point of view, it is an ancient disease in terms of recognition. Persons with the syndrome have frequently been exhibitionists. The anomaly was described in 1682 by Job van Meckeren of Amsterdam, who told of a Spaniard who could easily pull the pectoral skin on the right side of his body to his left ear. Ehlers of Denmark noted the excessive mobility of the joints in 1901, and Danlos described the subcutaneous tumors that may accompany this syndrome.

Clinical Picture

Hyperelasticity of the skin is striking and hypermobility of the joints accompanies it. Less well known is fragility of the vessels, which may be so marked that repair after trauma is jeopardized. When the skin is lacerated, sutures may not hold well, and large, gaping wounds from relatively superficial injuries are not uncommon. Ligating of the vessels has been a clinical problem.

A few people with this syndrome complain of cyanotic changes in the fingers and toes with cold weather and of a phenomenon like Raynaud's. The laxity of the ligaments and the brittleness of the skin and vessels may lead to clinical complications. Symptoms related to flat feet are not uncommon. The clavicle may be abnormally mobile, but these patients are obviously not good candidates for repair of subluxating joints.

The disease may be inherited as a simple autosomal dominant trait.

The pathologic change may be a failure of development of an intermeshing network of collagen bundles. The expected finding of a larger than normal amount of elastic fibers has not been substantiated. An increase in elastic tissue is a very relative determination, however.

Treatment

Support of the feet and measures based on the individual patient's complaints are the orthopaedic treatment. There is no available cure of the disorder.

References

1. Hass, J., and Hass, R.: Arthrochalasis multiplex congenita, *J. Bone Joint Surg.*, 40A: 663, 1958.
2. McKusick, V. A.: *Heritable Disorders of Connective Tissue*; St. Louis: C. V. Mosby, 1960.
3. Sutro, C. J.: Hypermobility of the bones due to "overlengthened" capsular and ligamentous tissues: cause for recurrent intro-articular effusions, *Surgery*, 21: 67, 1947.
4. Tschemogobow, A.: Cutis laxa, Mhft. Prakt., *Dermatologica, 14:* 76, 1892.

PROXIMAL FEMORAL FOCAL DEFICIENCY (CONGENITAL SHORT FEMUR)

If this deformity is termed proximal femoral phocomelia, there needs to be an understanding of the numerous possible variations. There may be simple shortening of the femur with or without bowing. The bowing is often accompanied by a skin dimple at the height of the bow. The short femur may be accompanied by coxa vara with a large segment of the femoral neck unossified or with full ossification, an epiphyseal line of normal width, and the deformity only. The proximal one-third to one-half may be absent. The acetabulum may be absent or rudimentary.

There are many variations of congenital short femur (Figs. 7.1 and 7.2). The disorder varies from a femur that approximates its counterpart on the opposite side of the body to a limb in which only a rudimentary portion of the femur remains and the knee approaches the inguinal fold. The calf is usually surprisingly well formed, although the tibia may be somewhat shorter on the affected than on the normal side. No bilateral case is known to the author.

Heredity seems to play no part in the development of the anomaly. Cases are not infrequent in a children's orthopaedic clinic.

In addition to the obvious shortening, the deformity most obviously needing correction

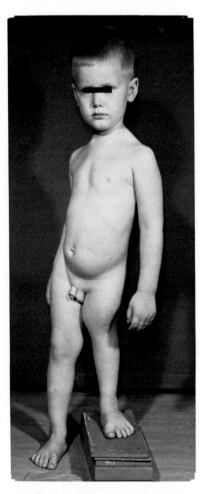

Figure 7.1. Congenital short femur.

is the flexed, abducted, and extremely rotated position of the thigh. The ankle is often close to the knee joint—a reflection not only of shortening, but contracture. The fibula is frequently absent on the affected side. Aitkin[1] reported a 70% incidence.

Clinical Picture

The deformity is noted at birth. Examination reveals the discrepancy of leg lengths in which the lower leg plays only a minor part. The patella has a great tendency to be rudimentary, and it is often dislocated laterally.

Coxa vara deformity, which is sometimes associated with the disorder, may cause the trochanter to ride above Nélaton's line. A hip flexion deformity is frequently found. Muscular function is ordinarily sufficient to stabilize the joint at hip and knee.

The picture in females is distressing. There is a refusal to wear skirts or any form of clothing that reveals the deformity. Males can more readily cover the deformity and engage in normal activities. Unfortunately, the lesion seems to be more common in females.

A portion of the distal femur is always present. Since by age 2 1/2 the ossification of the capital femoral epiphysis will be recognizable, it should be possible to proportionate fairly accurately regarding limb length from then on. A constant growth ratio between the normal and abnormal limb occurs in 9 of 10 cases.

Prior to 2 years of age, the delay in ossification may render a clear recognition of the type of anomaly involved in the proximal femur difficult.

Classification

Amstutz and Wilson[2] have classified five distinct types of this anomaly (Fig. 7.3).

TYPE I

Type I is the combination of bowing of the femoral diaphysis and involvement of the proximal femur with a nonprogressive coxa vara. There is medial femoral cortical sclerosis. Delay in ossification of the capital femoral epiphysis leads to confusion with dislocation of the hip. The shaft is laterally displaced by the bowing.

TYPE II

The area between the capital femoral epiphysis and the femoral shaft is occupied by a cartilaginous anlage—multiple ossification centers often appear in this area. The varus is progressive. A subtrochanteric pseudarthrosis may persist.

TYPE III

The acetabulum is present, and ossification of the capital femoral epiphysis is naturally delayed. The proximal femoral nonossified gap between epiphysis and femoral shaft is marred with the obvious necessity of considerable varus of the rudimentary cartilaginous

anlage. Ossification of this area is usually complete by 6 years. The proximal femoral shaft is bulbous.

TYPE IV

There is severe alteration of the proximal femur, and the proximal end of the distal femoral shaft tapers sharply. The shaft is not as laterally displaced as in the first two types, leading to a suspicion of a very rudimentary connection between the capital femoral epiphysis and the femoral shaft. Proximal impaction of the femoral shaft occurs because of weakness in this area of persisting pseudarthrosis. The acetabulum becomes dysplas-

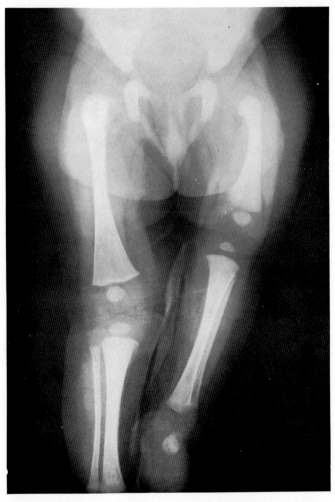

Figure 7.2. The short femur and relatively unaffected tibia and fibula are seen. The unossified portion of the proximal femur at the base of the neck on the involved side contains femoral head and varus neck.

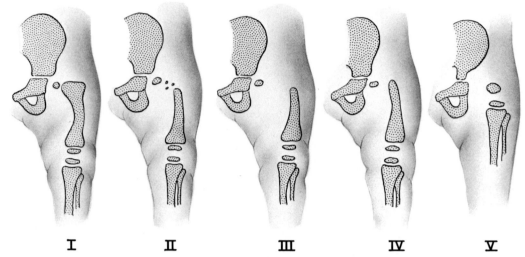

I   II   III   IV   V

Figure 7.3.   The five distinctive types of involvement in the deformity known as proximal femoral focal deficiency according to Amstutz and Wilson. (*I*) Involvement of the proximal femur in a nonprogressive coxa vara. (*II*) A cartilaginous enlage between the capital femoral epiphysis and femoral shaft. (*III*) A nonossified gap between epiphysis and femoral shaft with considerable lateral displacement of the femoral shaft and of necessity varus. (*IV*) Severe alteration with tapering of femoral shaft and proximal impaction—a very rudimentary connection. (*V*) The acetabulum and capital epiphysis are not present.

tic as this alteration continues with lack of functional stress.

In one series the inhibition of growth averaged 64% in this group. Further migration and contractures can increase this figure with regard to functional shortening.

TYPE V

In this type the acetabulum and capital femoral epiphysis are not present. There is a poorly formed iliac projection just above the level of the acetabulum. The obturator foramen is spherical. Bilaterality may be present in this group.

Associated lower leg anomalies occurred in 50% of Types III and IV and to a lesser degree in Types I, II, and V. This may result in still further leg length inequality, leading to additional clinical considerations.

Treatment

The severity of the defect justifies radical measures, particularly in the female. In cases in which the ankle of the short leg is only slightly higher than that of the normal leg, an appropriate epiphyseal arrest can be performed at the proper time.

When the ankle of the short leg seems likely finally to be more nearly opposite the knee than the ankle of the normal leg, the best approach may be to secure an ankle at the level of the sound knee.

There is a fundamental approach to the anomaly. Dissatisfaction with the conservative approach arises from the fact that a prominent feature of the clinical picture is the flexed, abducted, and externally rotated position of the thigh. Bracing, whether a socket, ischial weight bearing, or platform with double uprights for weight bearing through the foot, encourages the continuance and growth in this position (Fig. 7.6). This leaves the limb quite lateral to the trunk weight-bearing line. Progressively the deformity becomes more difficult to fit with a brace both cosmetically and functionally.

It becomes important, then, to establish the elements of the proximal femur that are available and then to get the femoral shaft aligned beneath or close to the weight-bearing line descending from the capital femoral epiphysis. Bracing them becomes cosmetically and functionally easy. Growth that exists contributes to the longitudinal axis.

As King[8] has emphasized, a simple skeletal lever must be achieved. If an acetabulum is

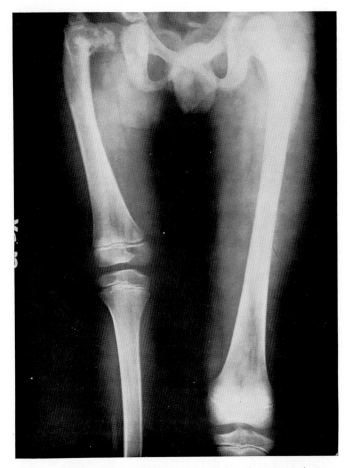

Figure 7.4.   Congenital short femur and developmental coxa vara.

present, a capital femoral epiphysis exists and will eventually ossify.

Each must be individually assayed. A simple subtrochanteric osteotomy may suffice, or several fragments may have to be aligned.

The first phase of treatment then consists of aligning the femoral shaft below the capital femoral epiphysis.

The second phase, once alignment, a good hip, and thereafter adequate bracing have been achieved, is to ponder the problems of growth and relative alignment of ankle and knee.

No matter what will be done later, attention to the hip joint and femoral shaft alignment is the first order of business. Soft-tissue release alone both at hip and knee has failed repeatedly—this is principally because bracing reconstitutes the deformity. King has demonstrated the importance of producing a single skeletal lever and the use of an intramedullary rod.

Leg lengthening is not a feasible alternative in this anomaly. The mechanical problems are too great, and the knee takes too much abuse.

Knee arthrodesis is a frequently necessary procedure, depending on the shortening involved. In severe shortening, knee arthrodesis is a necessary part of the rebuilding of an amputation stump that is adequate.

The aim below the hip joint seems by consensus to be to produce an amputation stump that provides improved function and cosmesis. The collective Shriner's Hospital experience summarized by Westin supports this approach. The equinus deformity of the foot does not aid the condition, being too difficult to camouflage in a prosthetic device. Rotational operations of the Van Nes type

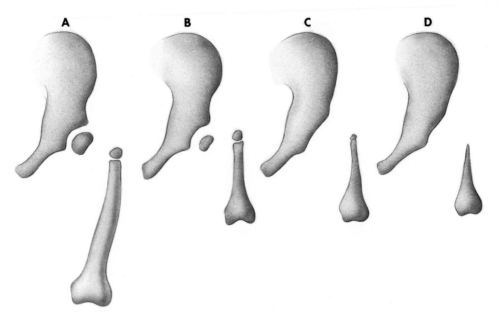

Figure 7.5. Aitken's classification of proximal femoral focal deficiency.

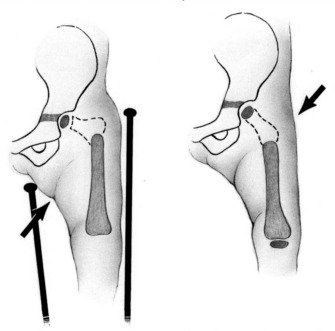

Figure 7.6. Effect of bracing of ischial weight-bearing type in anomalies associated with congenital short femur may be to promote lateral displacement of the femur. Alignment of the leg beneath the weight-bearing line is needed.

have not been sufficiently successful to justify their use.

The Syme's type of amputation at the level of the opposite knee when possible seems to be a very successful answer.

Where little is left of the femur, the proximal end of the tibia can be placed in the acetabulum after excising the short femoral fragment. An acetabulum must exist for the procedure to result in shaping of the proximal tibia with growth.

Valgus osteotomy of the hip is useful where sufficient ossification of the deformed proximal end of the femur is present.

The prosthesis should be designed for end bearing with a total-contact socket.

References

1. Aitken, G. T.: Proximal femoral focal deficiency: definition, classification, and management, Paper presented at a Symposium on Proximal Femoral Focal Deficiency, Washington, D.C., June 1968, Washington, D.C., National Academy of Science, 1969.
2. Amstutz, H. C., and Wilson, P. D.: Dysgenesis of the proximal femur (coxa vara) and its surgical management, *J. Bone Joint Surg.* 44: 1, 1962.
3. Babb, F. S., Ghormley, R. K., and Chatterton, C. C.: Congenital coxa vara, *J. Bone Joint Surg.,* 31: 115, 1949.
4. Bevan-Thomas, W. H., and Millar, E. A.: A review of proximal focal femoral deficiencies, *J. Bone Joint Surg.,* 49:1376, 1967.
5. Fixsen, J. A., and Lloyd-Roberts, G. C.: The natural history and early treatment of proximal femoral dysplasia, *J. Bone Joint Surg.,* 56: 86, 1974.
6. Golding, C.: Congenital coxa vara and the short femur, *Proc. R. Soc. Med.,* 32: 641, 1939.
7. Golding, F. C.: Congenital coxa vara, *J. Bone Joint Surg,* 30: 161, 1948.
8. King, R. E.: Some concepts of proximal femoral focal deficiency, Paper presented at a Symposium on Proximal Femoral Focal Deficiency, Washington, D.C., June 1968.
9. Mital, M. A., Masalawalla, K. S., and Desai, M. G.: Bilateral congenital aplasia of the femur, *J. Bone Joint Surg.,* 45: 561, 1963.
10. Morgan, J. D., and Somerville, E. W.: Normal and abnormal growth at the upper end of the femur, *J. Bone Joint Surg.,* 42: 264, 1960.

CONGENITAL ABSENCE OF FIBULA (PARAXIAL HEMIMELIA (FIBULA))

The work of Thompson, Strant, and Arnold[4] has caused a reevaluation of the treatment of this anomaly and a better understanding of it.

The disorder exhibits either complete or partial absence of the fibula. Associated with it are shortening of the extremity, various degrees of anterior bowing of the tibia, and anomalies of the foot (Fig. 7.7).

Clinical Picture

The shortening of the lower extremity, which is evident at birth, is usually too great to be sufficiently corrected by either lengthening of the involved extremity or epiphyseal arrest of the opposite extremity. The

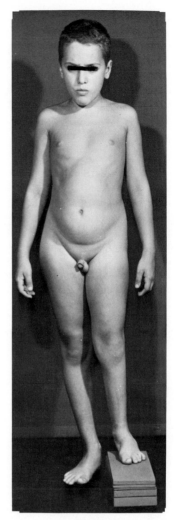

Figure 7.7. Absent fibula with associated shortening.

discrepancy between the two legs often reaches 5 inches.

Kruger and Talbott,[3] in a study of 62 instances of absent fibula, found that a 3-inch length discrepancy occurred in the vast majority of cases, with those cases having hypoplasia of the femur being subject to still further shortening. Femoral shortening of ½–4 inches occurred in 65%. There was an inverse relationship between leg length discrepancy and absence of metatarsal rays.

The average discrepancy at age 1 was 2 inches and at age 8 had increased to 5½ inches.

The anteriorly bowed tibia is often accompanied by a skin dimple anteriorly at the height of the bow. The bowing increases the discrepancy and occurs at the junction of the middle and distal thirds (Fig. 7.8).

The foot is in an equinovalgus position. One or more of the metatarsal rays are usually missing. There is a tendency for the foot to subluxate laterally as growth progresses. The condition is bilateral in 30% of the cases.

Pathology

The important element in this anomaly is the heavy fibrous band attached to the interosseous membrane and apparently representing the vestigial fibula.

Although the tibia is bowed, in most cases the medullary canal is present and of reasonable width for the bone. The talus and os calcis are often fused, and various other bones may be fused with them to the extent that there may be a single midtarsal bone mass. The appearance of ossification centers is delayed, and one or more metatarsal rays may be absent.

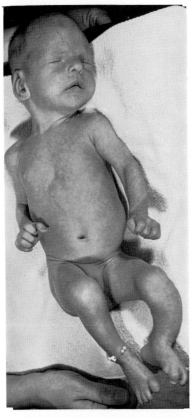

Figure 7.8. Congenital absence of the fibula with anterior angulation of the tibia.

Treatment

Preliminary assessment of the deformity is made in terms of the length of the extremity. Marked shortening leads to a guarded prognosis for the usefulness of the extremity.

Early excision of the tight fibrous lateral band has been found by Thompson et al. to give the bowed tibia a tendency to straighten spontaneously with growth. It also aids in correcting the equinus. Wedging or repeated use of corrective casts may be necessary to align the foot well under the tibia so that normal weight bearing can occur.

A shoe or a metal post elevation is usually necessary when weight bearing is begun. In addition, we have often found it necessary to add a leather gauntlet laced up the calf with lateral steel uprights in order to keep the foot under the tibia. Osteotomy of the tibia may be necessary to correct the bow and to put the foot in a weight-bearing position. Coventry and Johnson[2] noted no difficulty in the healing of the bone in such cases.

Early ankle fusion done with injury to the distal tibial epiphyseal line may be necessary to keep the foot located correctly.

At age 5, a decision to keep the foot on some sort of patten bottom appliance in order to equalize leg length or to amputate usually has to be made. If amputation is chosen, a Syme's type procedure is preferred because it permits the use of plantar heel skin for weight bearing. The stump that results is a very satisfactory one because, in this type of case with the associated shortening, it usually falls at midcalf level and thus permits a cosmetically excellent prosthesis.

When a Syme's amputation is done in a growing child, the problem of keeping the heel pad correctly located over the end of the tibia is a difficult one. Great care must be taken at the time of operation to fix the heel pad and to eliminate such future deformity as too tight tissues on one side. We usually keep the child in a cast that holds the tissues in a correct position for 6 weeks following such a procedure as a means of eliminating future difficulty.

References

1. Aitken, G. T., and Frantz, C. H.: The juvenile amputee, *J. Bone Joint Surg.*, *35:* 359, 1953.
2. Coventry, and Johnson, E. W.: Congenital absence of the fibula, *J. Bone Joint Surg.*, *34A:* 941, 1952.
3. Kruger, L. M., and Talbott, R. D.: Amputation and

prosthesis as definitive treatment in congenital absence of the fibula, *J. Bone Joint Surg.*, *43A*: 625, 1961.

4. Thompson, T. C., Strant, L. R., and Arnold, W. D.: Congenital absence of the fibula, *J. Bone Joint Surg.*, *39A*: 1229, 1957.

ABSENT TIBIA (PARAXIAL HEMIMELIA (TIBIA))

Absence of the tibia may be partial or complete; usually some remnant remains proximally.

The lower leg is shortened not only by the absence of the tibia, but also by the fact that the fibula lies more proximal than it normally does at the knee and may be subluxated laterally at the foot. Tarsal anomalies in various combinations are the rule rather than the exception. Anterior bowing as in absence of the fibula is not a feature.

Tibial dysplasia is extremely variable in its presentation. There may be complete absence of cartilage and bone. More frequently an osteocartilagenous anlage of the proximal tibia is present (Fig. 7.10). Basing "absence" on radiographic criteria may be quite misleading. Figure 7.10 shows an allegedly absent tibia. No knee or ankle joints were present. This probably represents an early stage of the type of tibial "absence" that develops an ossification center when the child is several years old.

Tibial dysplasia results in significant shortening of the lower leg. The length inequality may be compounded by subluxation or dislocation of the fibula at knee or ankle. Bowing of the fibula is infrequent. Variable tarsal, metatarsal, and phalangeal abnormalities frequently are present. Decreased stresses at the knee joint may lessen growth of the distal femoral physis.

Treatment

Amputation with all its attendant growth problems should not be rushed into. Rather, every effort should be made to develop a leg

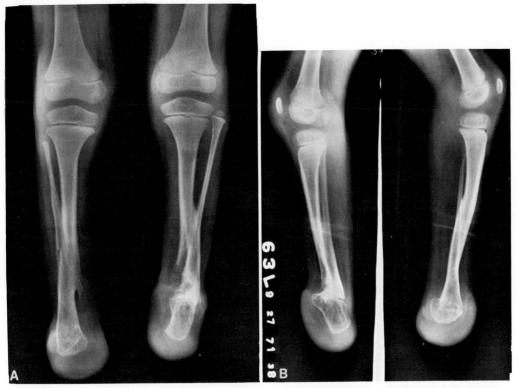

Figure 7.9. Rebuilding in congenital absence of the tibia with cross union to fibula—amputation and union of os calcis to end of hypertrophied fibula. (*A*) Anteroposterior view, (*B*) lateral view.

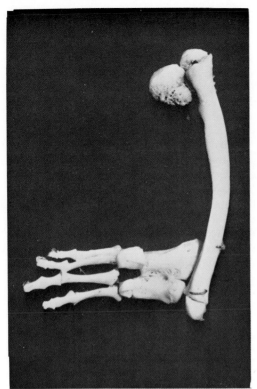

Figure 7.10. Absent tibia and associated anomalies of the tarsal bones. A remnant of tibia remains.

below the knee which, if unsatisfactory in its entirety, can be used as the stump for a below-knee prosthesis and can thus increase function.

The fibula can be transplanted to the proximal portion of the remaining tibia. Hopefully, this portion will be sufficient to provide a good functional knee. Inasmuch as hypertrophy of the transplanted fibula, which is desired, usually occurs to a remarkable degree, the operation should be performed as soon as sufficient bone to permit union has developed in the proximal tibial remnant. The shape of this remnant is usually such that the fibula is most directly under the femur when a long oblique cut in the fibula is opposed to the medial side of the remnant.

Where there is no remnant of tibia, the fibula can be moved directly under the intercondylar notch into a surgically created pocket and held there by the fibrous tissue which represents the only vestige of the tibia.

At the distal end, the fibula may be inserted into a distal tibial remnant, the astragalus, or the os calcis.

The surgery has to bring bone to bone and

not fibula to cartilage portions of the remnant. Because of this requirement, the operation may have to be deferred. The treatment has to be greatly individualized to suit the variations of this anomaly.

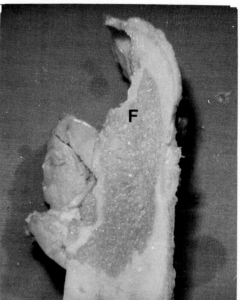

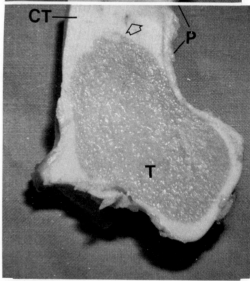

Figure 7.11. Complete absence of tibia demonstrating distal femoral epiphyseal (*F*) and talar (*T*) ossification centers, no knee or ankle joints, and a dense cartilaginous tibial anlage (*CT*). A perichondrium (*P*) was found only on the anterior portion. The *arrow* indicates a small focus of ossification. A relatively normal fibula, dislocated at both knee and ankle, was also present. (Courtesy of John Ogden, M.D.)

After union is secured, exercises for the knee, including both quadriceps and ham strings, are important. A laced leather cuff, long leg brace with a free knee hinge is usually worn for the first several years, during which the bone is developing, in order to protect it against fracture.

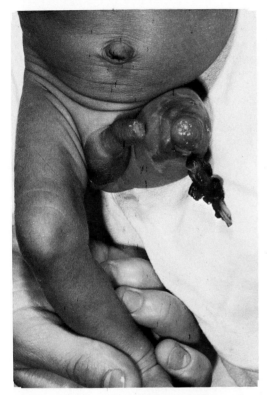

Figure 7.12. Congenital amputation (hemimelia). The necrotic tibia and fibula are still attached to the thigh stump.

CONGENITAL AMPUTATIONS AND CONSTRICTING BANDS

So called "congenital amputations" exist as a single anomaly. The part involved may be a digit or the major portion of an extremity (Fig. 7.12). It has been felt that these amputations may be a further extension of constricting bands, which eventually disturb the vascular system or a part. Streeter[1] believes that they are primary germ plasm defects.

Constricting bands, which have been noted most commonly in the lower leg, may exhibit varying degrees of severity (Fig. 7.13). The usual clinical picture is that of a tight fibrous band about the bone through which—in an incredibly small area—pass nerves, blood vessels, and tendons. The distal part of the extremity often is enlarged and has a woody edema. After intrauterine amputations, the necrotic portion may remain attached.

Treatment

The treatment of the amputation consists in preventing deformity by active and passive exercise and by splinting. Such measures vary with the part involved. Bracing is usually accomplished with an appropriate socket and a double upright, jointed prosthesis rather than with an anatomic-appearing prosthesis, until growth is finished.

The constricting band can be very satisfactorily excised if it is not all handled at once. Approximately a third of the circumference is done at one sitting. The incision is made

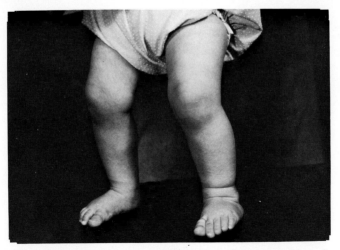

Figure 7.13. Mild degree of constricting band that needs no treatment.

on the external surface, where the skin folds initially come together, rather than deep in the crevice, so that the scar remains at skin level and does not indent. Dissection must be meticulous, as there is no room to spare. Some superficial adipose tissue distal to the band may also have to be excised at a later date.

Reference

1. Streeter, G. L.: Focal deficiencies in fetal tissues and their relation to intra-uterine amputations, p. 126, In *Contributions to Embryology*, Publication 414; Washington, D.C.: Carnegie Institute, 1930.

CLEIDOCRANIAL DYSOSTOSIS

Cleidocranial dysostosis is a hereditary defect in skeletal development that causes absence of the clavicles or aplasia of these bones to the degree that they are rudimentary (Fig. 7.14). Associated defects include an increase in the transverse diameter of the skull due to delayed union of the sutures, delayed dentition, delayed ossification of the pubis, deformities of the metacarpals and metatarsals, and absence of bones other than the clavicles.

The clavicles may be represented by a fibrous cord. The patients may be short owing to a decrease in the longitudinal growth of long bones. Not only may the teeth be delayed in development, but loss of deciduous teeth may be delayed. Other skeletal variations, such as genu valgum, coxa vara, and scoliosis, may be noted.

Clinical Picture

The usual clinical picture is that of involvment of the clavicles and bones of the skull. The sutures are widened at birth, the fontanels gape, and the clavicles are absent. The picture may vary, and various combinations of defects may be present. The shoulders can be brought together anteriorly owing to the absence of the clavicles, and the upper portion of the thorax is narrowed and flattened.

The patient is symptomless. Motor function, for the most part, is not interfered with, and the patient is not handicapped.

Treatment

Treatment is ordinarily not indicated. Should deformity produce disability, it is corrected according to the needs of the individual.

CONGENITAL POSTERIOR ANGULATION OF TIBIA WITH TALIPES CALCANEUS

It is rather rare for children to have a posterior and medial bowing of the tibia and

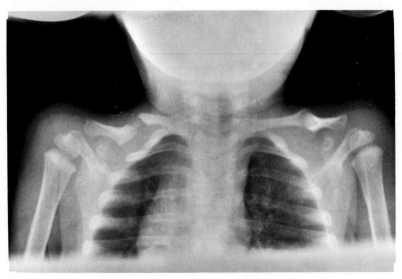

Figure 7.14.   Bilateral congenital pseudarthrosis of the clavicle.

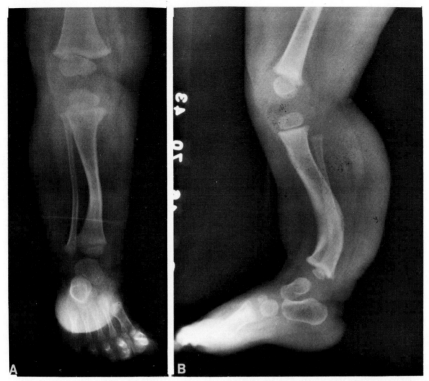

Figure 7.15. Posterior angulation of the tibia with shortening. (*A*) Anteroposterior view, (*B*) lateral view.

fibula at the junction of the middle and lower thirds (Fig. 7.15). Associated with this deformity have been a severe talipes calcaneus and tightness of the anterior muscles of the lower leg and triceps surae. A dimple is frequently found over the point of maximal bow, and the limb is short.

Treatment

In infancy, bivalved plaster casts are used to hold the foot in plantar flexion once the initial tightness anteriorly has been overcome by corrective casts. When the child starts walking, a long leg, double upright brace with an anterior strap to limit dorsiflexion is used, In the series of Heyman, Herndon, and Heiple,[2] this conservative approach was sufficient to correct the deformity (Fig. 7.16).

Osteotomy for correction has been reported to result in healing of the tibia without incident. There is also a growth problem; epiphyseal arrest of the normal tibia at the appropriate time is indicated if the growth discrepancy is a clinical problem.

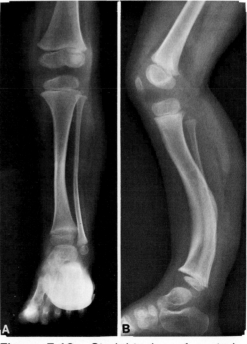

Figure 7.16. Straightening of posterior angulation of the tibia with 2 years of growth. (*A*) Anteroposterior view, (*B*) lateral view. No brace is used.

References

1. Badgeley, C. E., O'Connor, J. J., and Kudner, D. F.: Congenital kyphoscoliotic tibia, *J. Bone Joint Surg., 34A:* 349, 1952.
2. Heyman, C. H., Herndon, C. H., and Heiple, G. H.: Congenital posterior angulation of the tibia with talipes calcaneous; a long term report of 11 patients, *J. Bone Joint Surg., 41A:* 476, 1959.
3. Miller, B. F.: Longitudinal posterior bowing of the tibia in childhood, *J. Bone Joint Surg., 33B:* 50, 1951.

RADIOULNAR SYNOSTOSIS

This rare congenital defect is usually noted in children of 3 or 4 years, but it is seldom appreciated in infancy. Only when increasing demands for function are made is the deficit recognized. The lack of ability to pronate and supinate is masked by rotation at the shoulder and by flexion combined with radial or ulnar deviation at the wrist (Figs. 7.17 and 7.18).

The fusion between radius and ulna involves the proximal portion of these bones and may occasionally be associated with radial head dislocation.

Treatment

Whether anything should be done or not is often debatable. The forearm is in slight to moderate pronation, and it functions quite well by adaptation. It can be improved, however, if permanent pronation-supination motion of significant degree can be obtained and actively used.

It is possible to gain a good range of motion (that is 50–60 degrees of both pronation and supination) passively. The proximal radius is resected, and then (most important) the interosseous membrane is divided along the ulna from one end to the other. This second step is necessary because the disability includes a soft-tissue defect as well as the bony anomaly so evident by x-ray (Figs. 7.19 and 7.20).

Gaining active motion to maintain the range obtained passively requires further procedures. The best motor for supination appears to be the extensor carpi radialis longus transplanted to the ventral side of the wrist. For pronation, the radial flexor can be transplanted dorsally.

If the disability is to be attacked at all, several operations are necessary, and, as with

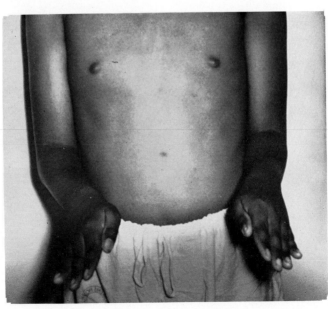

Figure 7.17. In radioulnar synostosis, some apparent pronation is developed at the wrist.

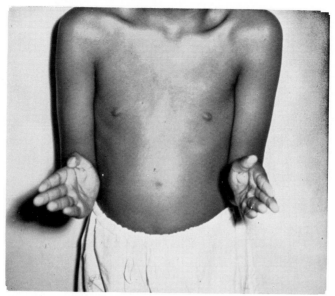

Figure 7.18. The patient shown in Figure 7.17 brings the hands to neutral in apparent supination.

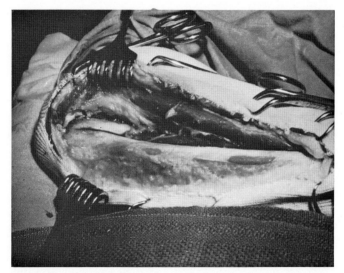

Figure 7.19. Operation for radioulnar synostosis has exposed the entire edge of the ulna, which is seen inferiorly. The radius united to the ulna is visualized to the reader's left.

many motions for which an eventual involuntary pattern of use is desired, they are best done in the early childhood years. The desire to begin early, however must be tempered by judgment of the child's ability to comprehend and to train the transplant actively; most children need to be at least 6 years old.

MILROY'S DISEASE

Although often thought of as the congenital lymphedema of feet and hands noted at birth, Milroy's disease actually is more commonly first noted at puberty. It is also termed

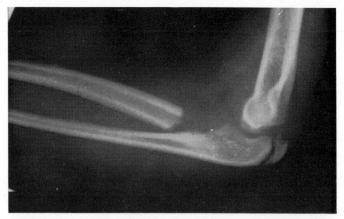

Figure 7.20. Postoperative photograph of radioulnar synostosis after excision of proximal radius and area of union with the ulna; the interosseous membrane has also been divided at its ulnar attachment.

"hereditary trophedema." Just when a brawny type of edema in the extremities for which there is no evident cause is Milroy's disease and when it is merely congenital lymphedema is by no means clear; neither is it clear that there is any marked difference between the entities.

Clinical Picture

A silent onset is typical. Puberty is the usual period of occurrence. The edema often first appears about the ankle and gradually extends up the calf and down into the foot. It is often unilateral. The edema is not soft, and it pits only after prolonged firm pressure. After the edema has existed for a considerable period, fibrotic changes take place in the subcutaneous tissues and secondary skin changes appear. Episodes of lymphangitis may occur.

There is no evident cause, such as a tumor or a mechanical lymphatic obstruction, for chronic edema.

The etiology is unknown.

Treatment

An elastic stocking is usually used from the time of first diagnosis onward. Later, plastic reconstructive procedures, including excision of the subcutaneous areas, may be used in cases in which deformity or loss of function justifies them.

CONGENITAL DISLOCATION OF RADIAL HEAD

This is a rare anaomaly which has been reported in the past to be a familial trait. In our own series, it has occurred as an isolated anomaly in an otherwise normal child who had no familial history of the disability.

Clinical Picture

The dislocation may be either anterior or posterior. Increased length of the radius in relation to the ulna is quite apparent, as the radius grows past the lateral condyle either superiorly or inferiorly (Fig. 7.21). Limitation of extension has always been present, and occasionally there is limitation of flexion as well. The usual age group seen is that between 5 and 9 years. The prominence of the radial head produces a deformity at the elbow.

Treatment

The anomaly may be disregarded. Function is limited but compatible with most tasks that have to be performed in life.

If parent and child are not satisfied with the appearance and function, some improvement can be gained, although absolutely normal function does not seem attainable. As a

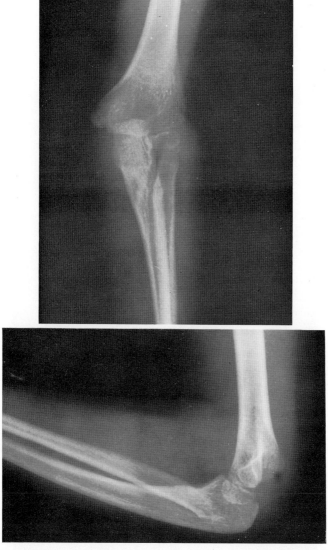

Figure 7.21. Preoperative roentgenograms of congenital dislocation of the radius. The length of the radius carries it past the capitellum, and the radial head is underdeveloped.

result of prolonged loss of articulation between the radial head and the capitellum, the radial head is deformed somewhat in the manner of a dislocated femoral head which has lain up against the ilium for years.

A segment of the radius sufficiently large to allow the proximal radial fragment to be reduced is removed distal to the orbicular ligament (Fig. 7.22). The head is spikelike and flattened on one side. The cut surfaces of the radius are now opposed. A thin Kirschner wire or Steinmann pin is driven through the humeral condyle and down the center of the proximal and distal fragments of the radius to hold them in position. The orbicular ligament is maintained intact. The wire or pin is removed after 3 weeks, but the arm is maintained in a long arm cast with the elbow at right angle flexion until union is affected. The proximal fragment must be rotated at operation so that it will not slide by the capitellum with further growth (Fig. 7.23). Great care must be taken to guard the radial nerve during this procedure.

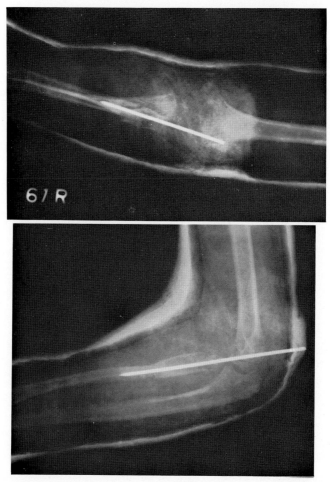

Figure 7.22.   A segment of the radius has been removed, and the proximal fragment has been reduced in relation to the capitellum. The proximal and distal radial fragments are aligned on a pin in a natural relation to the capitellum. The shortening of the radius allows the reduction.

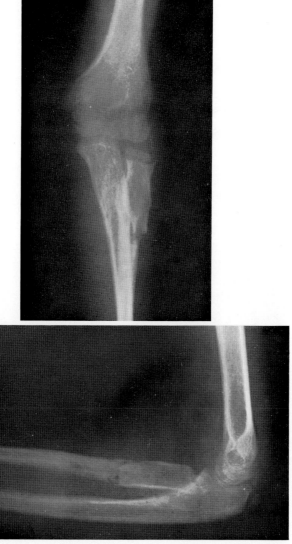

Figure 7.23. Postoperative views on cast removal show the new relation of the radial head to the capitellum.

References

1. Abbott, F. C.: Congenital dislocation of radius, *Lancet, 1:* 800, 1892.
2. McFarland, B.: Congenital dislocation of the head of the radius, *Br. J. Surg., 24:* 41, 1936.

ULNAR-DEFICIENT EXTREMITY

Ulnar deficiency (or absence) is much less frequent than radial absence. Characteristically, there are bowing of the radius, ulnar deviation at the wrist, reduction of the carpal bones (by synostosis or actual absence), and reduction in the number of metacarpal/phalangeal rays (Fig. 7.24). Three significant variations may be found at the elbow: (1) normal or near normal radiohumeral joint, (2) radiohumeral synostosis (if an ossified portion of the deficient ulna is present, it is usually fused to the radius and/or the humerus), and (3) dislocation of the radiohumeral joint.

The amount of ulna present by roentgenogram may be misleading, because, unlike absence of the radius, the nonossified portion of the ulna is often present as a large fibrocartilaginous band that may insert onto the distal radius and/or carpus. This band creates a tethering effect that produced and accentuates radial curvature, abnormal development of the distal radial growth plate, deviation of the wrist, and radiohumeral joint abnormalities. In the radial clubhand, the resultant deformity is mainly determined by eccentric muscle pull. In contrast, the resultant deformity of the ulnar-deficient extremity is significantly determined by this fibrocartilaginous remnant of the distal ulna.

Initial treatment should be directed to exploration and resection of this fibrocartilaginous band. This will lessen the incidence of

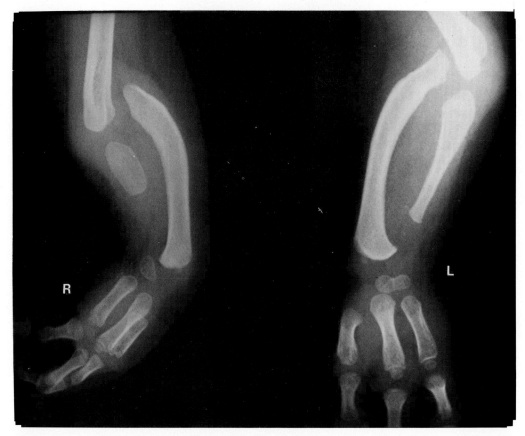

Figure 7.24. Ulnar-deficient extremity. The bilateral ulnar deficiency illustrates the variable presentation. The ulna on the right was not radiologically visible for more than 3 years. Note the dislocated proximal radius, curvature of the radius, and ulnar wrist deviation.

the aforementioned deformities. Creation of a one-bone forearm is often the treatment of choice.

NAIL-PATELLA SYNDROME (OSTEO-ONYCHODYSTROPHY)

This inherited disturbance of mesodermal and ectodermal tissue is transmitted by an autosomal dominant gene.

The patellae are hypoplastic or absent. The radial heads are dislocated, limiting elbow motion, and iliac horn formation is common. There may be a hereditary nephropathy resulting in significant renal impairment in adult life.

References

1. Beals, R. K., and Eckhardt, A. L.: Hereditary onycho-osteodysplasia (nail-platella syndrome); a report of 9 kindreds, *J. Bone Joint Surg., 51A:* 505, 1969.
2. Darlington, D., and Hawkins, C. F.: Nail-patella syndrome with iliac horns and hereditary nephropathy, *J. Bone Joint Surg., 49B:* 164, 1967.
3. Duthie, R. B., and Hecht, F.: The inheritance and development of the nail-patella syndrome, *J. Bone Joint Surg., 45B:* 259, 1963.

CHAPTER 8

Defective Formation of Bone

Chondrodysplasia and chondrodystrophy are terms which are often used loosely without exact definition. In this chapter they are interpreted as follows: *chondrodysplasia* is defective formation of bone from cartilage resulting in relatively permanent defects in the bone structure; *chondrodystrophy* is defective formation of bone from cartilage altering the size or contour of the bone but not resulting in permanent defects in the bone structure.

These definitions exclude transformation in formed bone—osteitis fibrosa of parathyroidism, benign giant cell tumor, and benign aneurysmal bone cyst—and complete or partial absence of cartilage—hemivertebra, incomplete segmentation of vertebrae (congenital fusion), and cleidocranial dysostosis. Also excluded are effects on formed bone and on growth rate of affections of tissues about bone, as osteopsathyrosis, myelomuscular disturbances, and neurofibromatosis, and conditions resulting from stress developed by resistance of soft tissues to elongation by the growing bones, as in developmental or "congenital" coxa vara, developmental genu valgum, and developmental genu varum (Blount's disease, the Blount-Barber syndrome, or osteochondrosis deformans tibiae).

CHONDRODYSTROPHIES

Chondrodystrophia Fetalis (Achondroplastic Dwarfism)

Chondrodystrophia fetalis (achondroplastic dwarfism) begins in fetal life and is often demonstrably familial. Diminished production of growth cartilage and relatively prompt conversion of cartilage to bone cause the growth discs to be grossly and roentgenographically thin. The tubular bones are short, and often somewhat distorted, but adequately wide (Fig. 8.1). The face is flat and the nose small and saddle shaped, but the vault of the skull is voluminous. The trunk is long relative to the short extremities; this is an obvious difference from Morquio's syndrome, in which the trunk is short. There is no effective treatment for the systemic condition. Orthopaedic treatment is rarely necessary but, if osteotomy is contemplated for correction of deformity, union of bone fragments follows the pattern for normal bones.

Morquio's syndrome is a systemic disease in which chondrodystrophy is a feature. It is mentioned here to point out that the dystrophy affects chiefly the formation of bone from vertebral and articular cartilage. Because metaphyseal bone formation is less disturbed, the limbs are relatively long and the trunk relatively short. In spite of these characteristics, an exact pattern of roentgenographic bone changes is not to be expected because the degree of chondrodystrophic change varies greatly from case to case and the dysfunctioning cartilage may also produce permanent defects in bone structure (chondrodysplasia), usually central type defects, in the epiphyses and metaphyses.

Local Chondrodystrophies

Chondrodystrophy may occur locally in a restricted area or in a single bone. Some examples follow.

In developmental dorsolumbar round back, a vertebra near the dorsolumbar junction, usually the twelfth dorsal or first lumbar, may be deficient in development at its anterior superior quadrant and its anterior surface. This deficiency may occur as an incidental feature in a systemic chondrodystrophy such as Morquio's syndrome, but it is not infrequent as an isolated lesion. In the latter case, deformity begins in infancy or shortly thereafter with development of rounded dorsolumbar kyphos greater than

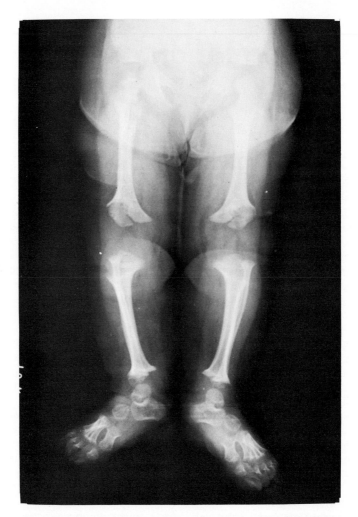

Figure 8.1.   Short and broad bones with abnormal outline in chondrodystrophy.

the normal postural dorsolumbar round back of infancy. The deficiency of the vertebra is clearly evident and characteristic in the lateral roentgenogram. Two adjacent vertebrae may be affected. The deformity tends to progress for a few years and then to decrease and improve. Reversion toward normal development may be aided by encouraging the prone and restricting the erect posture. When deformity is great, recumbency in a posterior plaster shell or other apparatus maintaining moderate extension relative to the kyphos should be used to assure earlier and adequate recovery from the developmental deficiency.

Developmental valgus (or varus) of a phalanx is characterized by moderate shortness of the phalanx and angulation of its distal articular plane transversely relative to its proximal articular plane. The middle phalanx

of a finger is the usual site of the deformity, but other phalanges, and more than one phalanx, may be affected. The condition is often demonstrably familial and gene controlled. In at least one family it is regarded as evidence of relationship. It may be detectable at birth but usually is not recognized until bone development is well advanced. The deformity does not reverse itself in the later stages of growth, but the writer has not yet seen a case in which any treatment seemed advisable.

Delayed conversion of cartilage to bone is a descriptive phrase applicable to those rare cases in which the rate of formation of cartilage is normal but its conversion to bone is delayed. The result is an unusual depth of the growth disc; the writer has seen, for example, cases in which the apophyseal disc of each ulna measured 1 inch in the axial diameter. The condition has been observed only as a local chondrodystrophy, and the cases are too few to demonstrate familial occurrence. Because no symptoms or deformities develop, the anomaly is disclosed only incidentally by roentgenogram. No treatment is necessary.

It should be noted here that, in pituitary gigantism, cartilage is produced with increased rapidity and converted to bone at a relatively normal rate, to result in abnormally long bones and roentgenographically normal growth discs; and that, in cretinism, the production of cartilage and its conversion to bone are equally slowed so that the bones maintain a normal roentgenographic appearance but take an abnormally long time to reach a given stage of development. These chondrodystrophic features of the diseases cause no noteworthy orthopaedic problems.

Premature union of an epiphysis may cause shortness of one or more metacarpal or metatarsal bones in pseudohypoparathyroidism, clubfoot, spina bifida, and paralysis of the lower extremity occurring before the fourth birthday. This condition is a form of local chondrodystrophy secondary to abnormality of adjacent soft tissues. In some instances it may be an inherited trait. The shortness is seldom recognized before the eighth birthday. The adjacent phalanx may also be affected. Treatment to correct the shortness is not necessary. Partial premature union of an epiphysis following destruction

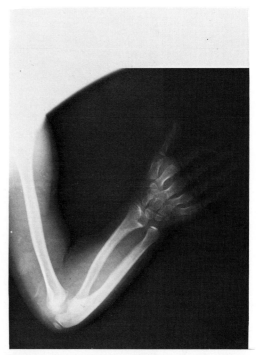

Figure 8.3. Forearm and hand with deformity, broadening of distal radius, and shortened metacarpals.

of cartilage by injury or inflammation is not chondrodystrophy.

CHONDRODYSPLASIAS

The important factors in the production of permanent defects of bone structure by defective conversion of cartilage to bone during growth are as follows.

1. One or more of the many possible predisposing factors or exciting causes of such defective formation of bone must have been present. Among these are:
   a. Normal probability that not all cell divisions will have a normal result.
   b. Increased probability of conversion defects when cartilage is older, when it grows more rapidly, or when it approaches completion of ossification. These factors make conversion defects rarer in infancy and more common in adolescence; some are not fully developed until after the pediatric age period. These factors also do much to account for the facts that conversion defects are most

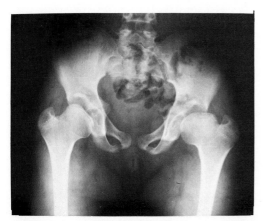

Figure 8.2. Hip joints such as these in chondrodystrophic patient may later become the site of degenerative arthritis. The tendency to appear as a femoral head duplication is evident.

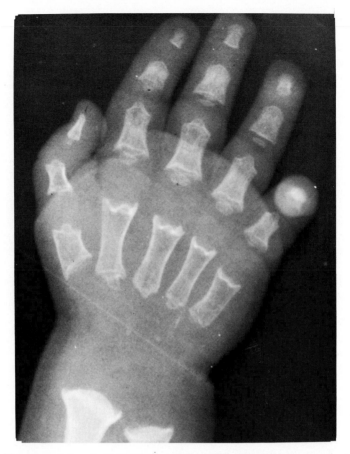

Figure 8.4. The hand in chondrodystrophy. Note irregularity in metaphyseal area adjacent to the epiphyseal line and short, broad phalanges.

common at the distal metaphysis of the femur, which is the most rapidly growing metaphysis, that epiphyseal bone formed more slowly from articular cartilage is less subject to defects, and that the portion of a long bone formed from fetal cartilage, which is young and which grows little after it begins its conversion to bone, is seldom the site of conversion defects.

c. Tension at the attachment of fibrous tissue to cartilage resulting from growth of the bone, especially rapid growth.

d. Hemorrhage or faulty development of vascular buds at the area of conversion of cartilage to bone.

e. Either hemorrhage or blebs adjacent to the conversion area.

f. Localized injury of the conversion area.

g. Familial tendencies or gene-controlled factors affecting development, as in multiple enchondromas of the hands or in diaphyseal aclasia.

h. Endocrine disturbances affecting development as in cretinism, parathyroidism, polyglandular dystrophy, or Albright's disease.

i. Affections of neighboring tissues which alter the nutrition of bone and cartilage, as in Morquio's syndrome, gargoylism, and generalized neurofibromatosis.

j. Any other condition that disturbs the nutrition or functioning of cartilage or adjacent bone.

2. Material that is not bone is formed at the affected area. The material may be

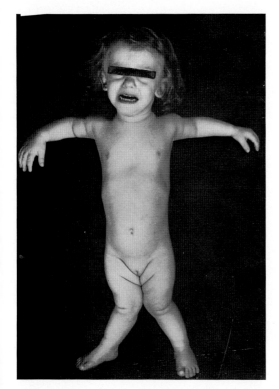

Figure 8.5. Achondroplastic dwarf with extremities that are short relative to the trunk.

calcareous without bone structure, or it may be cartilage or fibrous tissue. Fibrous tissue may contain giant cells or cystic areas; it may form one large cyst. The defect may contain a mixture of the materials mentioned. For most types of defect, there is no constant relation between the predisposing or causative factor and the character of the material in the defect.

3. The defective material is left behind in situ as the bone grows in length. The axial length of the defect is thus determined by the time during which defective conversion of cartilage to bone continues and the rate of growth in that time. A defect that still extends to the cartilage at the time of examination is a continuous defect, whereas one that has become separated from the cartilage by reversion to normal bone formation is an intermittent defect.

4. The defective material is not altered by the normal remodeling process in the shaft of a long bone, nor is it subject to Wolff's law. The extent to which the defect interferes with these processes depends chiefly upon whether the defect occupies or approaches the periph-

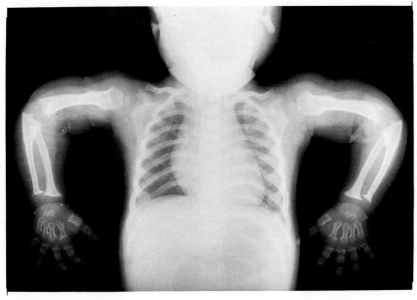

Figure 8.6. Upper extremities in chondrodystrophia fetalis (achondroplastic dwarf). Note that the trunk is relatively unaffected.

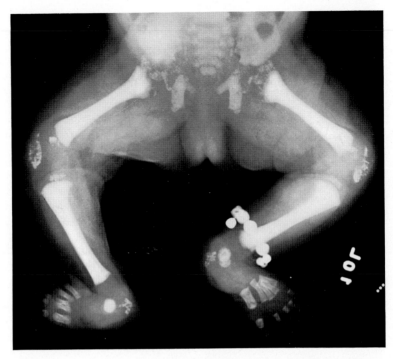

Figure 8.7. Chondrodystrophia multiplex congenita with multiple ossification centers in the epiphyses.

ery of the bone and, to a lesser degree, upon the breadth and length of the defect and the number of defects.

5. The defective material does not tend to exhibit autonomous growth. A cyst may accumulate more fluid and become larger and more rounded with resorption of adjacent bone. A sufficiently broad defect may increase slightly in breadth owing to compression in the axial diameter by soft tissues that resist elongation by the growing bone. A cartilaginous defect may retain some of its physiologic capacity to produce cartilage and bone and may express that capacity if it is stimulated by repeated motion or trauma. These are not autonomous growths. Conversion defects practically never exhibit autonomous tumorous growth except in the few cases that develop secondary malignancy or the rare cases that develop large osteochondromata.

6. Because conversion defects are often symptomless, they may attract notice only incidentally by roentgenographic examination late in life, but they are formed during the growth period and are detectable in increasing frequency up to the end of adolescence.

7. The great number of differences in appearance and character of conversion defects that may result from different combinations of the factors that have been mentioned is further augmented by variation in the number and distribution of the defects and by combinations of different defects. The possibilities seem infinite.

A few of these defects, which are seen sufficiently often to appear to represent types, are discussed below. They are classified as peripheral, submarginal, or central defects at articular, metaphyseal, or fetal cartilage.

Peripheral Conversion Defects

SINGLE PERIPHERAL METAPHYSEAL CHONDRODYSPLASIA

In single peripheral metaphyseal chondrodysplasia (exostosis, osteoma, osteochondroma), a portion of cartilage derived from the epiphyseal disc becomes separated at the periosteal attachment (Fig. 8.9). The separated portion remains in situ in the periosteum, and its radial distance from the center of the bone remains constant as it is left behind by growth at the metaphysis. If the separation begins sufficiently early in life, the eventual site of the cartilage defect may be several inches from the metaphysis. The defect preserves the underlying bone while adjacent bone is remodeled, so that it soon appears as though there were a projection of bone with cartilage at its crest. The projection is directed away from the near metaphysis because resorption on the far surface of the exostosis is accelerated owing to traction on the periosteum created by metaphyseal growth. The projection has the usual pencil type appearance in cases in which the defect became intermittent shortly after it began, but a broader, table type projection is developed when the duration of formation of the defect was longer. The radial projection of the exostosis may be increased slightly by physiologic activity of the cartilage cap, which produces some cartilage and bone. In cases in which such activity causes the mass

to be bulbous, it may be called an osteoma if it is practically entirely bony, an osteochondroma if bone and cartilage are obviously present. These distinctions and the diagnosis are usually made roentgenographically.

No autonomous tumorous growth has been mentioned in the preceding description. Usually there is none. Occasionally, the radial projection of the mass beyond its metaphyseal site is great enough to justify the suspicion that some autonomous growth has occurred, and in rare instances an osteochondromatous mass several inches in diameter may eventually develop.

These defects are innocuous and require no treatment except that a mass in an exposed position, where it is subject to repeated irritation or traumatism from external sources or by movement of tissues over it, may be removed by surgical excision at its base for the purpose of relieving discomfort or annoyance and as prophylaxis against secondary malignancy, which eventually occurs with some frequency in such irritated lesions. This treatment is definitely advisable when an exostosis on a rib is subject to friction by an adjacent rib in breathing.

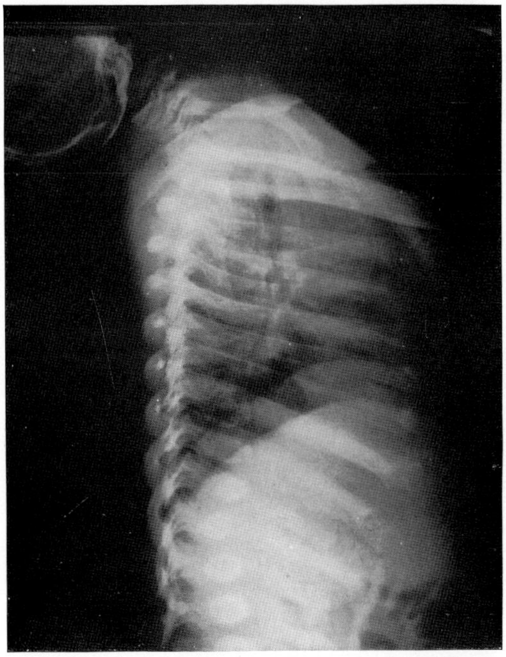

Figure 8.8. The spine in chondrodystrophy with increased anteroposterior diameter of the vertebrae and bony deformity.

MULTIPLE PERIPHERAL METAPHYSEAL CHONDRODYSPLASIA (DIAPHYSEAL ACLASIA)

Multiple peripheral metaphyseal chondrodysplasia (diaphyseal aclasia, multiple cartilaginous exostoses, hereditary deforming chondrodysplasia, Ehrenfried's disease) is a roughly symmetric, bilateral production of metaphyseal exostoses (Figs. 8.13–8.15). The long bones and ribs are principally involved, but other bones may also be affected. Each exostosis develops and may be treated as described above for single exostosis. The condition is demonstrably familial, and it affects male more often than female patients. Central metaphyseal defects of various types may be detectable in some cases.

Selected cases exhibit various degrees of relative prominence of peripheral, as opposed to central, defects and of bilateral, as opposed to unilateral, distribution. They make it impossible to define exactly the limits of diaphyseal aclasia as compared to Ollier's disease.

UNILATERAL MULTIPLE PERIPHERAL AND CENTRAL METAPHYSEAL CHONDRODYSPLASIA (OLLIER'S DISEASE)

Unilateral multiple peripheral and central metaphyseal chondrodysplasia (unilateral dyschondroplasia, Ollier's disease) is characterized by extensive unilateral involvement of metaphyses by an assortment of narrow and broad central and submarginal continuous defects (see below); the defects are mostly cartilaginous, but some are fibrous, and sometimes they are peripheral (Figs. 8.16–8.18). In the older portion of the affected area, which is formed before the metaphysis becomes completely involved, axial striae representing thin lines of relatively normal ossification between defective areas may be seen. The long bones of the lower extremity and the ilium are most commonly affected. Occasionally both sides of the body are af-

fected, and cases intermediate between Ollier's disease and diaphyseal aclasia are encountered. Cartilage in defects within the bone may undergo nodular calcification as life advances, and in Ollier's disease this calcification may begin to appear early, even in childhood, and may falsely suggest a relationship to some form of calcinosis. When the metaphysis is completely involved throughout its breadth, the defective tissues are unable to overcome completely the resistance of soft tissues to elongation by the growing bone, and growth in length becomes deficient. This axial compression results in some lateral bulging of the defective tissue at the metaphysis; the epiphyseal disc develops over the bulged tissue, and the metaphysis thus becomes abnormally wide. The same process may result in angular deformity when involvement is less complete toward one aspect of the metaphysis. The defective formation of bone cannot be controlled. Cor-

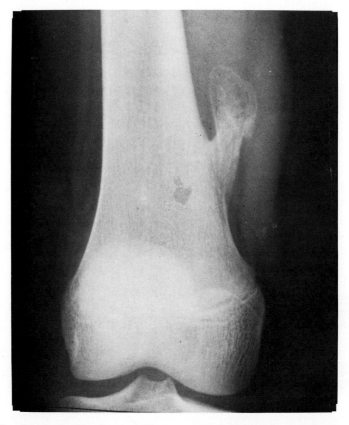

Figure 8.9. The single exostosis—cartilage capped, remodeled at the base. The lesion and the bone supporting it are not remodeled, a characteristic of chondrodysplasia.

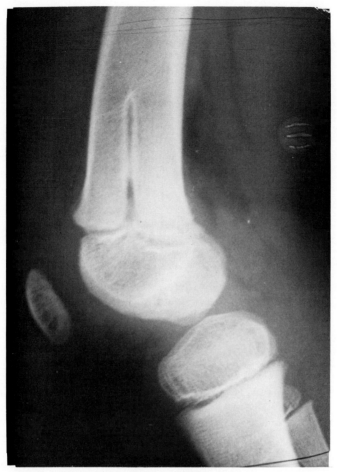

Figure 8.10. Traumatic chondrodysplasia—linear defect in the bone laid down from the epiphyseal line arose at the site of insertion of a Kirschner wire.

rection of angular deformity by osteotomy may be expected to result in normal union of bone fragments. Shortness of one leg may be compensated for partially by stapling at epiphyseal disc in the opposite leg at an appropriate time, or later a bone in the opposite leg may be shortened surgically by removal of a section.

PERIPHERAL EPIPHYSEAL CHONDRODYSPLASIA

Pheripheral epiphyseal chondrodysplasia produces separation of a cartilaginous conversion defect from articular cartilage at the site of attachment of fibrous tissue near the epiphyseal disc (Fig. 8.19), and the plaque of cartilage becomes increasingly separated from its area of origin by growth of bone epiphyses at the joint until its position is nearly opposite the center of articulation. Motion at the joint producing friction and stress at the cartilage defect stimulate its physiologic capacity to grow, and a mass 1 or 2 cm in diameter may result. Such cartilage is slow to ossify, but it eventually does ossify centrally and cartilage usually persists at its surface.

The intermittent peripheral epiphyseal defect (sesamoidoma, benign bone-forming tumor) thus forms a cartilaginous or bony mass in fibrous tissue at a joint and suggests an unusual sesamoid bone. The mass is rarely recognized before it ossifies. As many as 4 or 5 such masses may be present at a joint, most commonly at the knee or ankle. The condition is innocuous and may be ignored unless

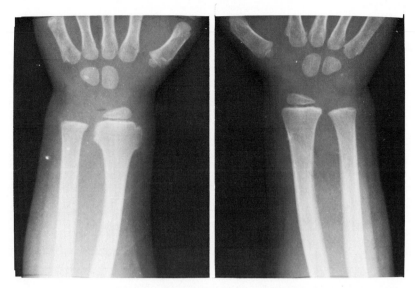

Figure 8.11. Failure to remodel in defective formation of bone from cartilage. Note persistent boxlike metaphysis on left compared with remodeled metaphysis on right.

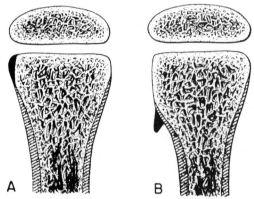

Figure 8.12. Diagram of the formation of exostosis, which, with its cartilage cap, is not subjected to remodeling as is the uninvolved bone around it.

mechanical interference with motion makes surgical removal advisable.

The continuous peripheral epiphyseal defect maintains continuity of cartilage between the defect and the epiphysis as the defect gradually becomes more displaced by growth of the two epiphyses. The asymmetric condylar mass thus formed distorts the joint in angular deformity, which increases as the mass increases. Because of such deformity, the patient is apt to be seen early, before the cartilage at the defect ossifies. Roentgenogram then suggests the presence of a space-occupying mass in the peripheral portion of the joint with corresponding angulation at the joint and underdevelopment of the adjacent aspects of the epiphyses to conform to the mass. No reactive phenomena are visible in adjacent bone or soft tissues. The knee is most commonly affected. When the patient is seen in this stage, osteotomy through the shaft of the bone for correction of the angular deformity is not advisable because it does not restore normal conformation at the joint or prevent further development of deformity. On the other hand, surgical treatment by paring off the adventitious cartilage sufficiently to approach normal conformation at the joint is feasible, and it has proved satisfactory in the 2 cases thus treated under the writer's observation; the joint remained stable, deformity did not increase appreciably, and there was no stimulation of tumorous growth of the remaining cartilage. Later in life, when physiologic ossification has developed in the cartilage mass, treatment is less satisfactory. At that time, reshaping the distorted epiphysis is not feasible because a cartilaginous surface cannot be maintained, and the condition may not justify such radical procedures as insertion of an internal prosthesis or fusion in corrected alignment; restoration of alignment by osteotomy through the shaft of one of the bones is, therefore, the only treatment commonly justifiable, and it leaves a distorted joint operating in an abnormal plane. Obviously, it is important to recognize and treat these patients early, when the best results may be obtained.

Submarginal Conversion Defects

Submarginal metaphyseal chondrodysplasia is defective formation of bone from cartilage situated within the bone but sufficiently near the periphery to be brought to the surface eventually as the defect is left behind by the growing metaphysis and the remodeling process causes the bone to become narrower. The defect may be recognized early, when it is still entirely within the bone at the metaphyseal area, or late, when

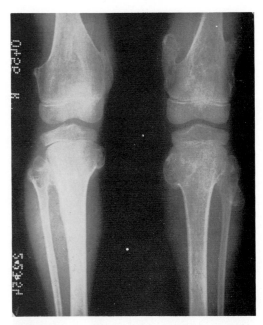

Figure 8.14. Multiple cartilaginous exostoses of distal femur and proximal tibia.

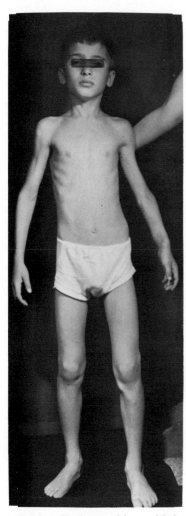

Figure 8.13. Patient with multiple cartilaginous exostoses involving the metaphyseal areas of the long bones.

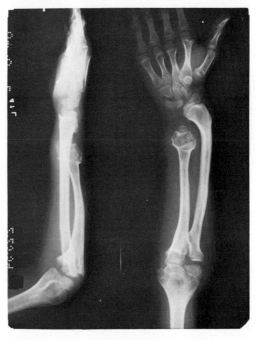

Figure 8.15. Multiple cartilaginous exostoses with short ulna.

it is entirely at the surface of the remodeled narrow portion of the shaft, but it is most characteristic in the intermediate stage, when it is partly within the bone and partly at the

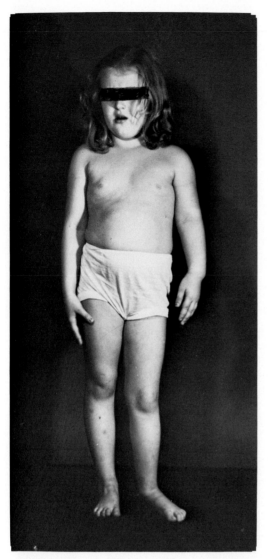

Figure 8.16. Ollier's dyschondroplasia with unilateral deformity.

surface and the perforation of the cortex is parallel to the long axis of the bone but oblique to the flared portion of the cortex, which it perforates. Submarginal defects may be broad enough to involve the peripheral or central areas, or they may be accompanied by other defects in those areas. A thin line of cortex visible roentgenographically may be preserved over the defect by inhibition of remodeling, and a thin calcareous wall may be formed about the defect by processes of accommodation in the adjacent bone structure. The diameter of the defect varies with the breadth of the defective formation at

different times during the period of continuity so that the sides of the defect may appear wavy or even scalloped.

BENIGN NONOSTEOGENIC FIBROMA

Benign nonosteogenic fibroma is typically submarginal metaphyseal chondrodysplasia (Fig. 8.20). The writer has not yet seen a case in which there was histologic or roentgenographic evidence that the lesion was the site of autonomous tumor growth or a case in which continued observation without surgical interference demonstrated increase in size of the lesion except by continued formation of defective material at the metaphysis. The material at the defect is spindle cell fibrous tissue (Fig. 8.21); giant cells and foam cells may be present. The condition is innocuous, is usually discovered incidentally by roentgenogram, and requires no treatment, although biopsy and more extensive surgery are often done. If symptoms are present, they can safely be assumed to be due to some other condition, such as injury at the neighboring joint.

Calcareous submarginal chondrodysplasia is present when the contents of a submarginal defect are calcareous. The calcific material does not have trabeculated or cortical bone structure, and it appears amorphous in the roentgenogram, in which it is readily visible because of its great density. Such defects of moderate length are frequently observable in adolescence and later, especially in bones of the feet and in the fibula. They may widen the cortical area peripherally or narrow the medullary canal endosteally, or both, depending upon their breadth and situation relative to the radius of the bone and the remodeled area of the bone. They are innocuous and symptomless, and they require no treatment.

MELORRHEOSTOSIS

Melorrheostosis is calcareous submarginal chondrodysplasia that has developed in the metaphyseal and fetal areas along one aspect of a bone or succession of bones in a limb and that tends to correspond with a somatic segment. It has been identified in childhood but usually does not attract attention until later, when pain appears, motion becomes limited, and calcification may develop in soft tissues about the joints. The periosteum tends

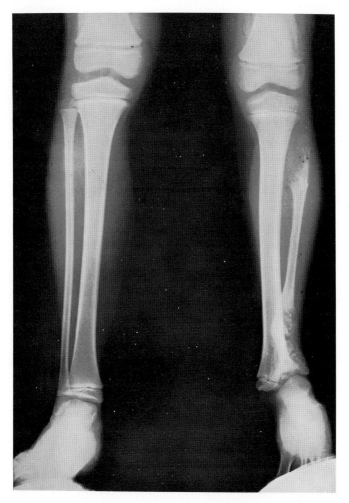

Figure 8.17. Ollier's disease: unilateral chondrodysplasia. Note defects in structure of bone that is laid down.

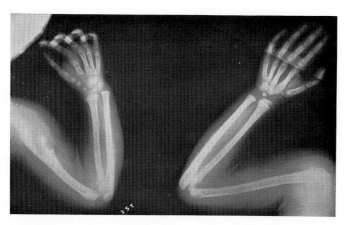

Figure 8.18. Roentgenogram of upper extremity in unilateral chondrodysplasia with involvement of long bones and metacarpals.

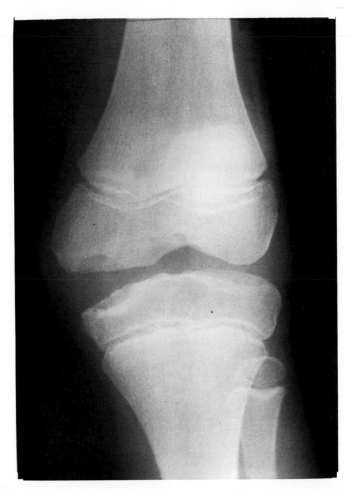

Figure 8.19.   Epiphyseal osteochondroma involving medial condyle of the femur.

to adhere to the calcific mass, and pain is probably the result of stress exerted by tissues attaching to the periosteum. The pain is relieved by rest. No other treatment is necessary. Prognosis is good in that the condition is self-limited and symptoms do not become marked.

Cartilaginous submarginal (and central) chondrodysplasia is characterized by the presence of cartilage throughout most or all of the defect. This character of the material is often not identifiable until the tissue is examined, but it is suggested roentgenographically when the defect is eccentrically situated in the bone, irregularly rounded, and not elongated axially, and it is indicated in the adult when characteristic nodular calcification has developed in the cartilage of the defect. These defects are innocuous and symptomless unless they are in exposed sit-

uations where contusion or periosteal stress can excite physiologic activity of the cartilage.

A small cartilaginous defect situated centrally in the medullary tissue where it does not deprive the bone of an appreciable amount of trabeculation is not detectable in the child but becomes recognizable in the adult, usually after age 30, when nodular calcification occurs within it.

A cartilaginous defect in the submarginal area brought to the surface of the cortex beneath the periosteum by the remodeling process may be too small to be detectable but may exhibit physiologic activity of the cartilage and formation of subperiosteal chondroma in adolescence or later.

A small cartilaginous conversion defect in fetal cartilage or early in metaphyseal growth is the probable source of the rare benign myxoma of bone of infancy.

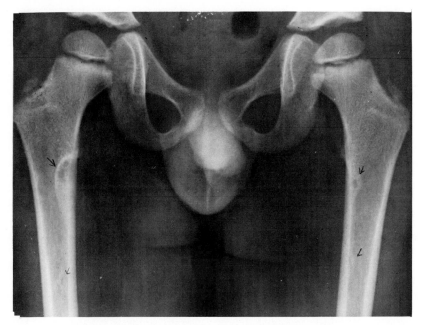

Figure 8.20. Submarginal metaphyseal chondrodysplasia (benign nonosteogenic fibroma) in the proximal femur bilaterally.

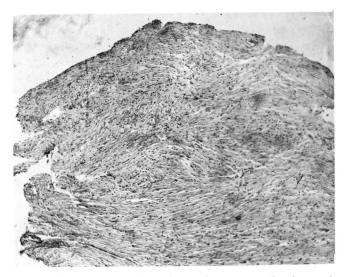

Figure 8.21. Fibrous tissue removed at biopsy from area of submarginal metaphyseal chondrodysplasia.

The broad central cartilaginous defect (benign central chondroma) may be encountered in childhood but usually does not attract attention until later. A bone of the hands, feet, or ribs is commonly affected. The lesion is usually eccentric, and the thin cortical line at its surface may undulate instead of presenting a smooth fusiform outline. Its treatment is the same as that for other broad central defects (q.v.), and it may not be distinguished from them until tissue is examined.

MULTIPLE ENCHONDROMAS

Multiple enchondromas of the hands constitute submarginal and central chondrodysplasia, which is apparently gene controlled. The feet may also be affected. The defects are mostly submarginal and cartilaginous, but tiny peripheral exostoses may be seen and some central fibrous or cystic defects may appear on tissue examination. The conversion defects are visible roentgenographically early in life (some may form from fetal cartilage), and they continue to form or to be added to throughout most of the period of metaphyseal growth of the bones of the hands. Physiologic activity of the cartilage persists, probably because of the more or less constant use of the hands, and the cartilage masses tend to enlarge and may become quite big in relation to the size of the bones of origin. Individual masses that interfere with function or become tender owing to repeated pressures may be removed surgically, and the resulting cavity in the bone, if any, may be filled with bone chips. Incomplete removal of a particular mass should be avoided if possible.

Central Conversion Defects

Central chondrodysplasia develops conversion defects in the area of the bone which is not brought to the surface by the remodeling process. The defects may be single or multiple, broad or narrow, long or short, calcareous, noncalcareous, or mixed. When the breadth of the bone occupied by a defect or by a number of defects is sufficient, the operation of Wolff's law preserves enough bone about the defect to meet stresses normally applied to it and thus inhibits remodeling and presents the appearance of "expansion" of the cortex. The cortex over such an area seen roentgenographically is thin and smoothly fusiform in shape, except that rigid material (cartilage or calcareous material) in the defect may cause the outline to be wavy. Such "expansion" is the hallmark of the large central defect.

Pyle's disease (Fig. 8.22) presents roentgenographic evidence of "expansion" toward the ends of the long bones (dumbbell bones) owing to multiple noncalcareous defects which are individually too small to be visible. A similar condition may affect a single metaphyseal area symmetrically or eccentrically. The condition is symptomless and innocuous, and it requires no treatment.

Single, broad, central noncalcareous defects in metaphyseal chondrodysplasia (osteitis fibrosa circumscripta, bone cyst, central chondroma) present roentgenographically a conspicuous area of deficient bone structure usually oval in shape but with a transverse limit toward the epiphyseal cartilage if they are continuous or only recently intermittent. "Expansion" of the cortex is present to the degree necessitated by the size and position of the lesion. The position of the lesion in the long axis of the bone depends upon the length of the bone at the time the lesion began to form. It takes more than a year of defective bone formation to form a sizable lesion, and years may pass before the lesion attracts attention. The condition is therefore rarely encountered before the age of 4, and its frequency increases thereafter. The material in the defect is not positively identifiable before tissue examination, but the roentgenogram suggests cartilage when the lesion is eccentric or its outline undulant and fibrous tissue if the lesion is well separated from the metaphysis and symmetric—the cyst tends to fracture before much separation from the metaphysis is achieved.

Broad central defects may be of mixed type and may contain some structureless calcareous material. They may also present a great variety of bizarre appearances on roentgenographic examination.

A variation of the broad central defect occurs in cases in which the defect becomes intermittent shortly after its onset. This kind of development produces only a thin plane of defective material, which is left behind by the growing metaphysis. The thin defect is not visible roentgenographically until remodeling narrows the cortex to the diameter of the defect, and then a thin transverse break in the continuity of the cortex is visible. Transverse fracture occurs spontaneously at such a defect, and if the defect does not extend completely across the bone, it may be completed by trivial injury. The writer believes that this type of defect is the commonest cause of "spontaneous" fracture precisely in the transverse plane in childhood and early adolescence.

Broad, central calcareous defects in metaphyseal chondrodysplasia (marble bones, osteopetrosis) exhibit roentgenographically a transverse dense area of structureless calcareous material toward the ends of the shafts.

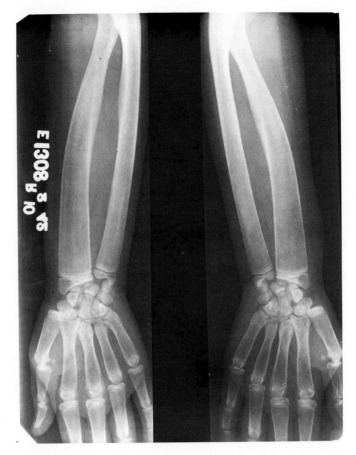

Figure 8.22. The forearm and hand in Pyle's disease.

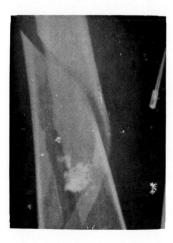

Figure 8.23. Central chondrodysplasia calcified in the adult. (From A. B. Ferguson, Jr.: Calcified medullary defects in bone, *Journal of Bone and Joint Surgery*, 29: 598, 1947.)

When the axial extent of the defects is not great, the condition is symptomless and requires no treatment. When the condition begins early in life (Albers-Schönberg disease), the abnormal bone formation is generalized and may involve bone derived from fetal as well as from metaphyseal cartilage. Little room remains for medullary tissue, and anemia and activity of accessory hematopoietic organs develop. Blindness and deafness may result from faulty development of the skull. Predisposition to the disease is probably due to a gene-controlled Mendelian recessive character. Blood chemistry and bone chemistry are essentially normal. Patients exhibiting the condition in infancy usually die young, but those with later onset and sufficient medullary tissue in the bones have a good prognosis. The bones are subject to fracture, which may be treated as similar fractures in normal bone. No other treatment

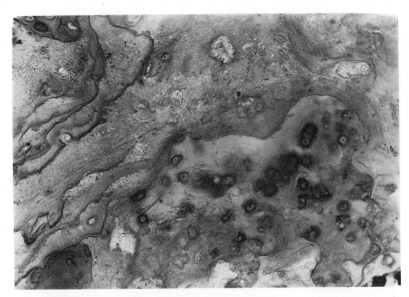

Figure 8.24.   Calcified cartilage matrix removed from specimen taken from patient shown in Figure 8.23. (From A. B. Ferguson, Jr.: Calcified medullary defects in bone, *Journal of Bone and Joint Surgery, 29:* 598, 1947.)

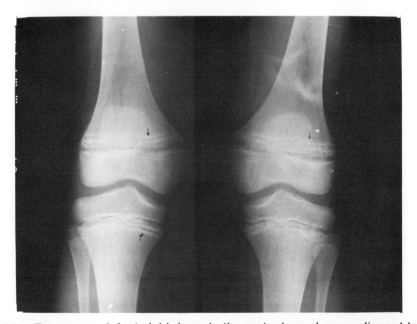

Figure 8.25.   Transverse defects laid down in the metaphyseal area adjacent to the epiphyseal line.

is useful except medical supportive treatment to combat anemia.

Multiple, small, central calcareous conversion defects of chondrodysplasia (osteopoikilosis) are usually systemically distributed in the epiphyses and, toward the end of the growth period, in the metaphyses. The de-

fects are irregularly rounded and rarely over 5 mm in diameter. They are symptomless and require no treatment. The prognosis is excellent although the defects are permanent.

Single, small, central calcareous conversion defects form single dense nodules, visible roentgenographically, which have often been described as bone whorls and as osteocle-rosis. The calcaneus, talus, and proximal fe-mur are common sites. The lesions are in-nocuous and should be ignored.

Small, noncalcareous, central metaphyseal conversion defects, which have been men-tioned in association with other defects (Ol-lier's disease, Pyle's disease, etc.), may not deprive the bone of enough structure to be visible individually in the roentgenogram. They may be visible individually, however, if adjacent bone forms a calcareous limiting wall about them. Such a defect is indicated when a small circular area of deficient bone structure is outlined roentgenographically by a thin circular calcareous wall and there is no reaction in adjacent tissue. The defect is com-mon in the femoral neck. It requires no treat-ment but should be observed over a period of time, rather than subjected to immediate biopsy, in order to confirm its innocuous character.

Defective bone formation may occur along the surface of epiphyses in Morquio's syn-drome and in association with chondrodys-trophy, spina bifida, and other conditions, but articular cartilage does not form noncal-careous defects (visible within the epiphysis) as often as does metaphyseal cartilage. Be-cause it grows more slowly, the epiphysis is less subject to defective formation, and for the same reason, the defect must continue for a longer time in order to achieve a size which is recognizable unless it is outlined by a calcareous ring as described above. Other single noncalcareous epiphyseal defects, if visible, are apt to occupy a considerable por-tion of the epiphysis and to produce a bizarre effect. Lack of symptoms, lack of reaction in adjacent tissues, and a tendency of the sides of the defect to be straight and parallel to the direction of growth identify the defect in the roentgenogram. No treatment is necessary.

The vertebrae are subject to noncalcareous conversion defects at their upper and lower surfaces (commonly called Schmorl's nodes) (Figs. 8.27 and 8.28). They may be detected by roentgenogram in midchildhood as an early defect producing a shallow indentation of the ossified surface of the vertebra. If such a defect is followed through the growth pe-riod, it will be observed to increase in depth exactly as bone is added to the vertebral surface by growth, the sides of the defect remaining perpendicular and the base paral-lel to the surface until late adolescence or later, when the defect may become somewhat rounded by adjustment of adjacent bone to it. One or more such defects can be found in most spines in adolescence and later. They

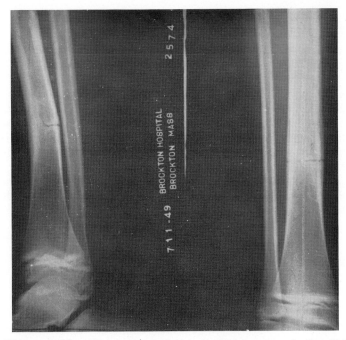

Figure 8.26. Transverse "stress" type fracture in the tibia.

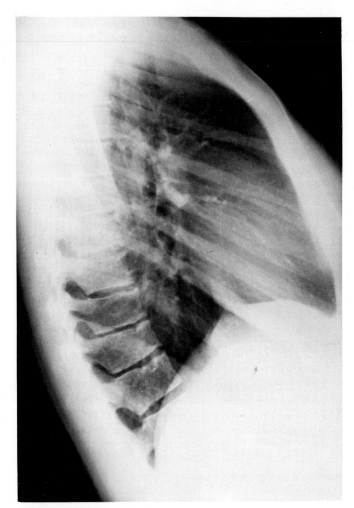

Figure 8.27. Developing Schmorl's node, a form of chondrodysplasia. (See Fig. 8.28 for the progressive development of the lesion with growth.)

are ordinarily symptomless and can be ignored, but occasionally the developmental disturbance affects the cartilage more extensively and the underdeveloped disc may be thin owing to deficiency of cartilage and nucleus pulposus. In the lumbar area, where normal motion is considerable, such a lesion may produce local ache after activity because of the poor mechanical action of the joint.

GARGOYLISM

Gargoylism (Hurler-Pfaundler syndrome, dysostosis multiplex, lipochondrodystrophy) is a disease of uncertain etiology which is

sometimes familial. It begins to become apparent in the first year of life, or soon thereafter, when there is evidence of mental retardation, infantilism, and dwarfism. The skin becomes coarse and thick, and the corneas may be cloudy. Potbelly, hepatomegaly, and splenomegaly develop. Hydrocephalus is frequent. The neck is usually short, dorsolumbar round back is present, and mobility of the joints is impaired, especially in the spine and hands. Lipoid deposits are found in some cases (but not in all) in the liver, spleen, lymph nodes, cornea, brain, and pituitary gland, and the sella turcica is enlarged. The central portion of the long bones, especially in the hands, tends to be bulbous; roentgenographically this suggests disturbance of accretion and resorption in formed bone rather than defective formation of bone cartilage. In the presence of such widespread disease, chondrodystrophic changes appear relatively minor and incidental. They are of the type seen roentgenographically in Morquio's syndrome but are less marked. They consist of developmental dorsolumbar round back, shortness of long bones, distorted metaphyses, and underdeveloped epiphyses. The changes in the long bones are most evident in the distal portion of the upper extremity. There is no effective treatment for the condition, and no orthopaedic treatment is advisable except the use of an extension frame or similar apparatus for inhibition or improvement of the round back.

ACHONDROGENESIS

Achondrogenesis is a lethal variety of short limbed dwarfism that may be mistaken for neonatal achondroplasia. Most are stillborn or die shortly after birth due to respiratory insufficiency. Crown-rump length may be only mildly reduced, but limb shortening is severe. The femur may be little more than an inch in length.

The roentgenographic findings include a normal skull, retarded rib development, absent sternal ossification, severely retarded cervicothoracic spine ossification with re-

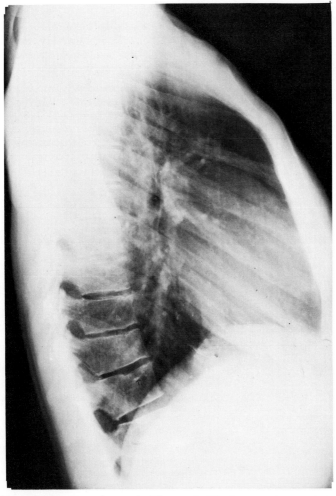

Figure 8.28. Same patient as shown in Figure 8.27, 2 years later. Note that edges are straight and the bottom flat and that the node has increased in depth and become well marked in the vertebra. A similar defect is beginning in the vertebra just above.

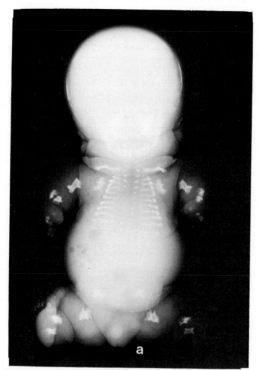

Figure 8.29. *(a)* Roentgenogram of stillborn with achondrogenesis. Note normal skull and clavicle development, but severe retardation of the axial skeleton and significant shortening and metaphyseal flaring of the appendicular skeleton.

tarded to absent ossification of the lumbosacral spine (in contrast to congenital absence of the lumbosacral spine, cartilage precursors are present), increased interpedicular distances, and marked retardation of long bone formation with metaphyseal flaring (Fig. 8.29a).

Of most significance are the alterations in normal epiphyseal/endochondral bone formation. The integrity of the articular cartilage is lost. There is extensive periosteal erosion of the peripheral chondroepiphysis. There is excessive vascularization of the chondroepiphysis with loss of normal cartilage canal patterns. In the growth plate there are focal areas of more orderly patterns of ossification juxtaposed to much larger sections of immature and disorganized growth plate (Fig. 8.29b).

This disorder is probably an inherited biochemical abnormality affecting matrix production or elaboration (one report described a twin pregnancy, one normal child and one with achondrogenesis). It is interesting that thiourea-induced hypothyroidism and thallium administration in chick embryos produce a similar histologic picture (Fig. 8.29c). It is postulated that thyroxin normally maintains chondroepiphyseal integrity by controlling the rate of erosion and resorption of cartilage and playing a role in synthesis or

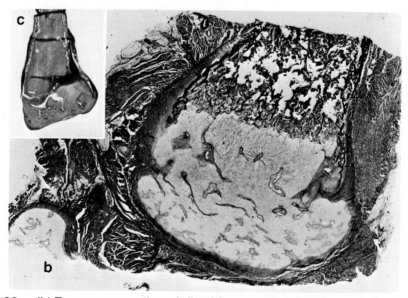

Figure 8.29. *(b)* Transverse section of distal femur with achondrogenesis. Ossification is proceeding relatively normally, but the structures of the growth plate and chondroepiphysis are severely disrupted. *(c)* Thiourea-treated proximal tibia from a chick showing increased vascular invasion of the epiphysis.

deposition of acid-mucopolysaccharide-protein complexes into the matrix.

BY JOHN OGDEN, M.D.

HUMERUS VARUS

Humerus varus is an infrequent deformity that may be found in association with hypothyroidism, mucopolysaccharidosis, rickets, and osteomyelitis. It is being recognized more frequently in children with thalassemia. However, the majority of cases probably occur as a result of birth trauma (usually breech delivery, with the involved arm caught over the head) or a shoulder injury in a very young child.

The major clinical problem is shortening of the arm. The forearm and hand are usually normal. Unfortunately, the length discrepancy is often not appreciated until early adolescence, when a significant deformity is already present. The difficulty of recognition until early adolescence makes close follow-up in the young, birth-injured child imperative. The average shortening in 7 cm. Abduction is generally restricted, but other glenohumeral motions are usually retained.

The diagnosis is characteristic by roentgenographic examination (Fig. 8.30). The head is in marked varus and is usually flattened. The greater tuberosity may be higher than the

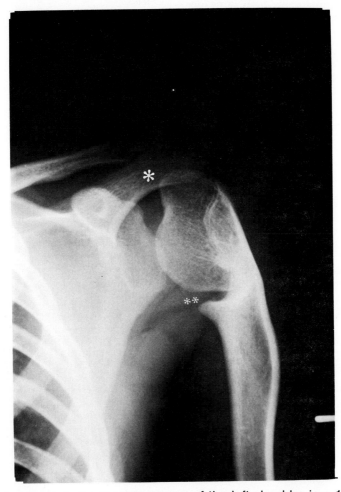

Figure 8.30. Anteroposterior roentgenogram of the left shoulder in a 12-year-old boy with humerus varus complicating a fracture during birth. Note particularly the proximal/medial direction of the greater tuberosity (*) and the apparent metaphyseal defect (**). The growth plate above this "defect" is crossed by a bony bridge.

articular portion of the humeral head. The epiphysis is parallel to the longitudinal axis of the humerus, rather than transverse or oblique. Premature fusion may occur. The medial (inferior) portion of the growth plate has a sclerotic region of bone bridging epiphysis and metaphysis. The medial cortex of the metaphysis appears to have a large defect.

The mechanism of injury in most cases is damage to the medial side of the growth plate, severely limiting its capacity for normal longitudinal growth, while the lateral portion continues to grow at a relatively normal rate. Trueta produced a similar deformity in rabbits by damaging the perichondrium. As the humeral head is progressively tilted into varus, sections of the articular cartilage begin to appose metaphyseal bone. Articular cartilage, during much of longitudinal bone development, is not capable of ossification and thus will present a block to a significant bony bridge between epiphysis and metaphysis. The "defect" in Figure 8.30 is thus filled with articular cartilage "overgrown" by the widening metaphysis. With closure of the growth plate, the articular cartilage undergoes biochemical changes that allow closure of the "defect."

Treatment should be offered only to the symptomatic individual. Epiphyseodesis will lessen the risk of fracture of the long metaphyseal fragment. Realignment osteotomy may improve motion, but only at the expense of some degree of further shortening of the arm. Most cases do not require treatment.

BY JOHN OGDEN, M.D.

Reference

1. Trueta, J.: Role of the vessels in osteogenesis, *J. Bone Joint Surg.*, *45B*: 402, 1963.

CHAPTER 9

Metabolic and Generalized Orthopaedic Conditions

HISTIOCYTOSIS X

A solitary eosinophilic granuloma or multiple granulomas in bone and soft tissue, comprising Hand-Schüller-Christian disease and Letterer-Siwe disease, have been considered different manifestations of the same disease process by Tauber (1941), Malloy (1942), and Lichtenstein[6] (1953). Lichtenstein used the term histiocytosis X.

Clinical Features

Cheyne estimated the incidence of this condition as 1:2,000,000 per year. It is most common in the first 4 years of life and equally distributed between the sexes. Approximately one-half the patients will clearly recover. Of those who die, the course is rapidly progressive within 4 years and the vast majority of these come from the infantile group. The age of onset carries a prognostic significance.

Just under 10% will have no detectable bony lesions. Lymph node involvement alone is entirely compatible with survival, but with involvement of the liver one-half of the patients have died. Progressive anemia leads to a poor prognosis. Petechiae and hemorrhage internally seem to play a part in this anemia. Massive marrow replacement is also seen. The lungs may be involved, leading to fibrosis and cysts. About 25% of the patients will have a rash not unlike seborrheic dermatitis.

The skull, femur, and spine are the most common sites of skeletal involvement.

Roentgen Features

The spine lesion is one of the causes of vertebral plana or "Calvé's disease." The involvement tends to be in the posterior portion of the vertebrae but progresses to occupy most of the body; as it does, the body is compressed, loses height, and can become wafer thin.

When a lesion is in a bone it can occupy the metaphysis or diaphysis and only rarely the epiphysis. It is totally lucent within the area it occuppies; through destroyed cortex it becomes radiologically visible. The edge is smooth rather than grossly destructive.

The amount of reaction about the lesion is variable from slight to moderate. A considerable amount of periosteal reaction can occur.

Histologic Features

The histiocyte-containing eosinophilic cytoplasm is the characteristic cell, with a variable infiltration of eosinophilic leukocytes in addition. These are contained in a granuloma with blood vessels running into the lesion from the periphery.

In Letterer-Siwe disease, the histiocytes are smaller with paler cytoplasm and tend to resemble reticulum cells.

The histocytes accumulate in a cellular lipid. The cholesterol content of the tissues is only raised in the region of these cells, representing a change in cellular metabolism. In Hand-Schüller-Christian disease, the cells are markedly swollen.

When the histiocytes are proliferating and accumulating cholesterol, the eosinophils and blood vessels may be less prominent.

References

1. Abt, A. F., and Deneholz, E. J.: Letterer-Siwe's disease: splenohepatomegaly associated with widespread hyperplasia of nonlipoid-storing macrophages; discussion of the so-called reticulo-endothelioses, Am. J. Dis. Child., 51: 499, 1936.
2. Avery, M. E., McAfee, J. G., and Guild, H. G.: The course and prognosis of reticuloendotheliosis of bone, Am. J. Med., 22: 636, 1957.

3. Christian, H. A.: Defects in membranous bones, exophthalmos, and diabetes insipidus; an unusual syndrome of dyspituitarism, *Med. Clin. North Am., 3:* 849, 1920.
4. Green, W. T., and Farber, S.: Eosinophilic or "solitary granuloma" of bone, *J. Bone Joint Surg., 24:* 499, 1942.
5. Lichtenstein, L.: Eosinophilic granuloma of bone, *Arch. Pathol., 37:* 99, 1944.
6. Lichtenstein, L.: Histiocytosis X, *Arch. Pathol., 56:* 84, 1953.
7. Lichtenstein, L., and Jaffe, H. L.: Eosinophilic granuloma of bone, *Am. J. Pathol., 16:* 595, 1940.
8. Oberman, H. A.: Idiopathic histiocytosis, *Pediatrics, 28:* 307, 1961.
9. Thanhauser, S. J., *Lipoidoses,* Ed. 3; New York: Grune & Stratton, 1958.

GAUCHER'S DISEASE

Gaucher's disease[3] has been known since its description in 1882. It was thought originally to be a neoplasm. Cushing and Stout[1] in 1926 reported a case involving the hip and causing a marked collapse of the proximal femur and acetabulum. With this case in a woman of 33, the disease was first recognized to involve the bone. It represents a rare familial disorder of lipoid metabolsim in which kerosin is deposited in the reticulum cells of the reticuloendothelial system. These cells, which have a typical appearance, are called Gaucher cells, and they may appear in the spleen, liver, lymph nodes, and bone marrow. The disease is most common in Jewish patients. Symptoms are usually noted in childhood and adolescence, but the disease is chronic and only slowly progressive.

The most common area of bone involvement is the lower femur, which is involved in about two-thirds of the cases, and the hip is second in frequency (Fig. 9.1).

According to Schein and Arkin,[5] the skeletal changes are due to infiltration and replacement of the bone trabeculae by kerosin-containing reticulum cells. This infiltration results in linear radiolucent areas that give the bone a characteristic mottled appearance. The cortex tends to become thinned and the bone to be slightly but not markedly expanded in the metaphyseal area. The expansion is fusiform rather than lobular. Secondary changes may occur, particularly at the hip, where the femoral head may collapse or undergo aseptic necrosis (Figs. 9.2 and 9.3). Pathologic fracture of the femoral neck and a tendency to coxa vara, as well as vertebral involvement and collapse, also occur.

These bone changes in a patient with splenomegaly, hepatomegaly, secondary anemia, hemorrhages, and brown pigmentation of the skin result in the diagnosis of Gaucher's disease. The suspicion can be confirmed by bone marrow biopsy.

Treatment

The care of these skeletal lesions consists of measures to relieve pain and to prevent

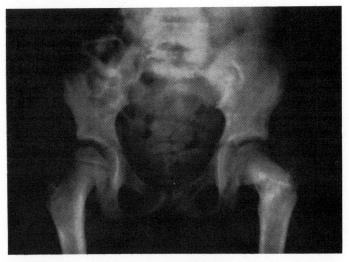

Figure 9.1. The femoral neck can be weakened to such an extent that a coxa vara deformity gradually develops in Gaucher's disease.

deformity. Bed rest is indicated during periods of acute symptoms. The hip joint and femoral neck lesions must frequently be kept from the hazards of weight bearing and subsequent deformity by non-weight-bearing splints or, when indicated, by plaster spicas. In the carefully followed case, regeneration of the femoral head and development of more normal bone structure has been observed. Aseptic necrosis of the femoral head has apparently been caused by infiltration of the femoral neck.

References

1. Cushing, E. H., and Stout, A. P.: Gaucher's disease, with report of a case showing bone disintegration and joint involvement, Arch. Surg., 12: 639, 1926.
2. Davies, F. W. T.: Gaucher's disease in bone, J. Bone Joint Surg., 34B: 454, 1952.
3. Gaucher, P. C. E.: De L'epithelioma primitif de la rate, hypertrophie de la rate sans leucémie, These de Paris, 1882.
4. Milch, H., and Pomeranz, W.: Bone changes in Gaucher's splenomegaly, Arch. Intern. Med., 61: 793, 1938.
5. Schein, A. J., and Arkin, A. M.: Hip joint involvement in Gaucher's disease, J. Bone Joint Surg., 24: 396, 1942.
6. Vaughan-Jackson, O. J.: Gaucher's disease with involvement of both hip joints (case report), J. Bone Joint Surg., 34B: 460, 1952.
7. Wood, H.: Gaucher's disease with pseudocoxalgia, J. Bone Joint Surg., 34B: 462, 1952.

MUCOPOLYSACCHARIDOSES

McKusick has divided the mucopolysaccharidoses into five recognizable states growing out of the cases that have previously been grouped together as Hurler's syndrome. In addition to the urinary mucopolysaccharidoses, metachromatic granules may be found in circulating lymphocytes stained with toluidine blue.

MPS Type I (Hurler's Syndrome)

Type I is inherited as an autosomal recessive disease, with death occurring at less than 10 years from respiratory infection or cardiac failure. It is marked by progressive mental deterioration, lumbar gibbus, stiff joints, chest deformity, rhinitis, clouding of the cornea, enlarged liver, "gargoyle face," short neck, broad hands with stubby fingers, and splenomegaly.

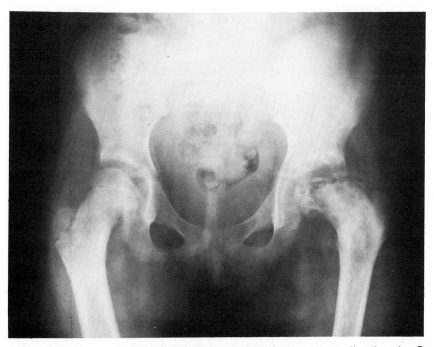

Figure 9.2. Aseptic necrosis of the femoral head as a complication in Gaucher's disease.

ROENTGEN FINDINGS

The findings are those of various aspects of osteochondrodystrophy. In the hands the fifth metacarpal shows this most severe involvement with a hypoplastic terminal phalanx. The proximal phalanges are broadened, as are the metacarpals, and both are short.

The vertebrae tend to irregularity—some with beaking. In the dorsolumbar region, a kyphos may be present with a deficiency of the anterosuperior corner of the supporting vertebrae. The intervertebral spaces may be widened.

The diaphysis of the long bones is thickened, possibly wavy, and with the metaphyseal ends slanted to accommodate coxa valga and genu valgum.

LABORATORY FINDINGS

Evidence of chondroitin sulfate B (dermatan sulfate) in the urine is the major finding. Heparitin sulfate is increased, but less so. An acid-albumin turbidimetric test is a suitable scanning device.

MPS Type II (Hunter's Syndrome)

Type II is thought to occur through an X-linked recessive inheritance. The clinical picture is similar to that of Type I, but less severe. Mental deterioration is slower, and lumbar gibbus does not occur. Clouding of the cornea is not clinically evident. Patients often live to the 30s, with precocious osteoarthritis of the head of the femur, pes cavus,

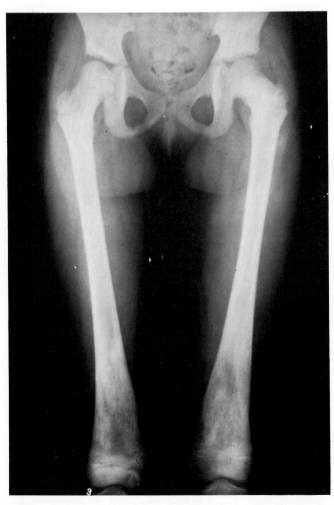

Figure 9.3. Involvement of the distal femur in Gaucher's disease.

congestive heart failure, thickened coronary arteries, or pulmonary hypertension. The skin may be grooved, ridged, or nodular. It occurs in 1:200,000 births, X-ray and pathologic features are as for Type I; urinary dermatan sulfate and heparitin sulfate are critical laboratory findings.

MPS Type III (Sanfilippo's Syndrome)

Type III is inherited as an autosomal recessive disease of severe mental retardation but relatively less severe somatic changes. The intellect deteriorates so that by school age retardation is evident; by the teens it is marked. Clouding of the cornea does not occur. Hepatosplenomegaly is only slight or moderate. Stiffness of the joints is less severe than in Types I or II. Patients may live to the fourth decade. X-rays show minor changes, as in the anterior part of the lumbar vertebrae. The incidence is 1:200,000. An increase in urinary heparitin sulfate is the fundamental metabolic defect.

MPS Type IV (Morquio's Syndrome)

Type IV is inherited as an autosomal recessive disease. Patients show strikingly dwarfed (truncal) stature, knock-knees, enlarged wrists, misshapen hands, pigeon breast (sternal kyphos), short neck, semi-crouching stance, broad mouth, and frequent hernias. Neurologic symptoms may occur from spinal cord and medullary compression; spastic paraplegia is frequent, with respiratory paralysis occurring in late stages. Intelligence may be normal or mildly impaired. All patients, should they reach sufficient age, show corneal opacities and such cardiac manifestations as aortic regurgitation.

Early x-rays of the spine resemble those seen in Type I mucopolysaccharidosis. Later, flattened vertebrae plus osteoporosis can be seen. Late films also show changes in femoral heads and characteristic skeletal lesions. It occurs in 1:40,000 births. Increased keratosulfate in the urine is the fundamental defect.

MPS Type V (Scheie's Syndrome)

In this autosomal recessive inherited disease, the intellect is impaired little or not at all. Stiff joints, clawhands, excessive body hair, retinitis pigmentosa, and corneal clouding may be seen. Stature is normal or low normal; the carpal tunnel syndrome with increased collagenous tissue is frequent, as is aortic regurgitation. Psychosis is seen. X-ray features are unremarkable, but skin, cornea, and conjunctiva show the same histologic changes as observed in Type I mucopolysaccharidosis. The rate of occurrence is unknown. There is increased urinary dermatan sulfate.

MPS Type VI (Maroteaux-Lamy Syndrome; Polydystrophic Dwarfism)

Occurring through autosomal recessive inheritance, this type shows the chief abnormality of growth retardation, noted at age 2–3 years. Stunting of both the trunk and the limbs is usually present, as well as genu valgum, lumbar kyphosis, and anterior sternal protrusion. There is face abnormality, hepatosplenomegaly is usual, and bony abnormalities are severe. Corneal opacities develop fairly early. Cardiac mainfestations are not seen.

X-ray features show long bones with irregular metaphysis and epiphysis slightly deformed, particularly the head of the femur, which may be fragmented, and the upper end of the humerus, which is hatchet shaped. The distal end of the radius and ulna is oblique, the carpal and tarsal ossification centers are hypoplastic. The vertebral bodies have reduced height. The first lumbar and last dorsal vertebrae are wedge shaped and posteriorly displaced. Pathology, prevalence, and metabolic defect are as for Type V mucopolysaccharidosis.

References

1. Dorfman, A., and Matalin, R.: The Hurler and Hunter syndromes, Am. J. Med., 47: 691, 1969.
2. Fratantoni, J. C., Hall, C. W., and Neufeld, E. F.: Defect of Hurler's and Hunter's syndromes. II. Faulty degradation of mucopolysaccharides, Proc. Natl. Acad. Sci. U.S.A., 60: 699, 1968.
3. McKusick, V. A.: The nosology of the mucopolysaccharidoses, Am. J. Med., 47: 730, 1969.
4. McKusick, V. A., Kaplan, D., Wise, D., Hanley, W., Suddarth, S., Sevick, M., and Maumanee, A.: The genetic mucopolysaccharidoses, Medicine, 44: 445, 1965.
5. Muir, H.: The structure and metabolism of mucopolysaccharides (glycosaminoglycans), and the

problem of mucopolysaccharidoses, *Am. J. Med., 47:*
673, 1969.
6. Rubin, P.: *Dynamic Classification of Bone Dysplasias:* Chicago: Year Book Medical Publishers, 1964.

EOSINOPHILIC GRANULOMA

One of the considered diagnoses of a cyst-like lesion of bone is eosinophilic granuloma. Such a lesion totally destroys the central area that it occupies. It is most common in the skull but is often seen as an isolated lesion of the long bones. It may be a forerunner of similar lesions of the skeleton, which may be combined with visceral lesions to form the entity known as Hand-Schüller-Christian disease. It is much more common in children than in adults (Figs. 9.4 and 9.5).

Pathology

Farber has studied this disease extensively and has concluded that the so-called eosinophilic granuloma represents one variant of a more basic disease process grouped under the general heading of xanthoma. The lesion is a granuloma which appears gelatinous and reddish-yellow on gross examination. Microscopically there are numerous large mononuclear phagocytes with granular to finely vacuolated cytoplasm. Numerous eosinophils are a prominent feature. They may form evident clumps, or they may be scattered diffusely. The more mature granulomas have

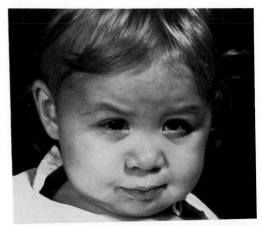

Figure 9.5. The same patient as in Figure 9.4, 4 weeks after roentgen therapy of the granuloma.

large, vacuolated mononuclear cells rather than eosinophils.

Roentgen Findings

The contour of the individual lesions is variable in outline but tends to be either oval or round. They are totally destructive; that is, no bone remnants are contained within the area outlined by the lesion (Fig. 9.8). The cortex is not expanded, but it may be destroyed. The edge of the lesion usually appears well outlined and benign; but in some lesions, particularly those in the skull, it is minutely spiculated. The reaction in bone surrounding the lesion consists of minimal increased deposition of bone rather than marked sclerosis.

The lesions are most common in the skull and ribs. Flat bones are predominantly involved. When the bones of an extremity are involved, the area closest to the trunk is the most frequent site. Involvement of the distal end of the extremities is virtually unknown. There is no particularly predominant site within the long bones.

Clinical Picture

In some reported series, the lesion has been more common in males. The symptoms relate to the area of involvement. Minimal pain and swelling prominent enough to be readily seen are features that bring the patient to the physician. When an area of the skull is in-

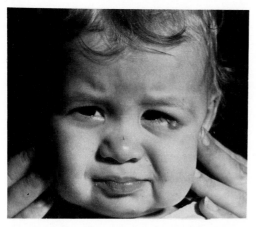

Figure 9.4. Granuloma involving lateral portion of lower eyelid (eosinophilic granuloma).

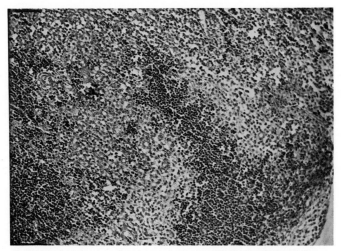

Figure 9.6. Eosinophilic granuloma with dark-staining eosinophils distributed over the background of the pale-staining histiocytes.

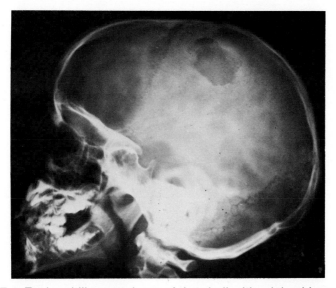

Figure 9.7. Eosinophilic granuloma of the skull with minimal bony reaction.

volved, swelling is present, often with pain. The swelling is soft and not particularly tender to palpation. Unilateral exophthalmos or periorbital swelling may result from lesions in this area. Long bone involvement is more likely to cause pain.

There is little evidence of generalized illness when the patient is first seen. Loss of weight and anorexia follow multiple severe areas of involvement. The laboratory findings are not remarkable. Lichtenstein and Jaffe noted an eosinophilia in from 4–10% of their cases. There may be a mild leukocytosis. The

calcium, phosphorus, phosphatase, total protein, and blood cholesterol are usually normal.

Differential Diagnosis

Cystic lesions of the bone must be considered. These include solitary bone cyst, giant cell tumor, and benign growth defects. Solitary bone cyst is associated with the epiphyseal line, appears to be derived from it, and is not subject to remodeling. Giant cell tumor

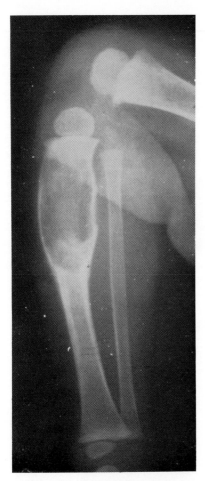

Figure 9.8. Eosinophilic granuloma of the tibia revealing cystlike appearance and total destruction.

The differentiation from solitary bone cyst may be impossible except by biopsy.

Treatment

The initial or most accessible lesion is biopsied, and diagnosis follows correlation of the patient's examination, laboratory data, history, and gross and microscopic findings. The rapidity with which lesions can appear, and also disappear with treatment, is impressive.

Once the diagnosis is established, the choice between curettage and roentgen therapy depends upon the location of the lesion. Both methods are very efficacious in removing the individual lesions. In areas where other structures, such as epiphyseal lines and ovaries may be affected by roentgen therapy, curettage is favored. The accessibility of the lesions and the gravity of the procedure involved are other considerations.

The course of the patient cannot be predicted at the outset. New lesions may appear while the original lesions are being treated. As long as the entity is confined to bone, the prognosis is good. The ever present possibility of Hand-Schüller-Christian disease should, however, prompt a guarded outlook.

RESISTANT RICKETS AND OTHER DISORDERS OF CALCIUM AND PHOSPHATE METABOLISM

BY ROBERT KLEIN, M.D.

Patients with resistant or refractory rickets constitute a problem which is so common that all orthopaedic surgeons dealing with children should be conversant with the disease and its manifestations (Fig. 9.9). Indeed, in most pediatric clinics, cases of ordinary vitamin D deficiency rickets constitute only about one-half of the total number of cases of rickets. Unless patients with refractory rickets are discovered early, they become severe orthopaedic problems. In a 5-year span, 6 cases of renal rickets and 3 cases of hepatic rickets were seen. At the same time, there were 20 cases of vitamin D deficiency rickets. There is no point in applying orthopaedic treatment to patients with resistant or other forms of rickets until the metabolic disease is brought under complete control.

occurs in the early adult age group. Growth defects are usually linear rather than rounded and are not associated with bone reaction.

Osteomyelitis, tuberculosis, and syphilis should be borne in mind. Osteomyelitis is accompanied by clinical and laboratory evidence of infection. When eosinophilic granuloma involves a vertebra, to differentiate it from tuberculosis by roentgenogram may be quite difficult because the abscess shadow associated with tuberculosis may be duplicated by this lesion. Compere has pointed out that eosinophilic granulomas produce the picture of Calvé's disease in the vertebra.

Lesions such as Ewing's tumor and leukemia are ordinarily characterized by an infiltrating type of destruction rather than by the total destruction of an eosinophilic granuloma. Multiple myeloma is an adult disease.

Therefore, before refractory rickets is discussed as a clinical entity, it is important that the metabolic changes in this and related diseases be considered. No mention of the x-ray changes or the appearance on histologic section of the various forms of rickets will be considered in this chapter, because it is, in general, correct to state that neither gives sufficient evidence to determine etiology. "Rickets is rickets" when studied by these methods. In patients with vitamin D deficiency rickets, rickets associated with total renal failure, rickets associated with renal tubular disease, and hepatic rickets, therefore, the metabolic and clinical changes must be understood so that the proper diagnosis can be made and adequate therapy carried out.

Some Metabolic Changes in Rickets

The growing infant deprived of any extra-dietary source of vitamin D and kept from sufficient sunlight to manufacture his own vitamin D develops rickets as evidenced by x-ray, clinical, and histologic changes. His serum phosphate is low, and his serum calcium is usually normal or only slightly depressed. Serum phosphatase is very high.

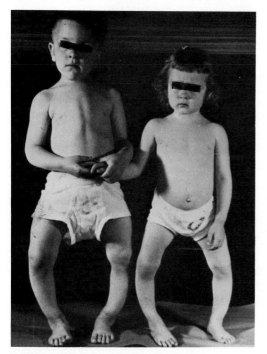

Figure 9.9. Siblings with bowing of the tibia in resistant rickets.

Actually his bone phosphatase is also high, but this is not of diagnostic importance. He absorbs calcium and phosphate poorly from the intestinal tract and excretes excessive amounts of phosphate in the urine in the face of low serum phosphate values. When the diagnosis is made and he is in a steady state, the magnitude of his phosphate excretion is not absolutely large. The excretion is, however, relatively great in view of his low serum phosphate level. His tubular resorption of phosphate per 100 ml of glomerular filtrate is low. He has an increased aminoaciduria, a decreased citric aciduria, and a depressed citric acid level in his blood. When he is given vitamin D in therapeutic doses, usually less than 5,000 units per day, the first response is increased tubular resorption of phosphate. This, coupled with the increased absorption of calcium and phosphate, from the gut, leads to an elevated serum phosphate level. The administration of vitamin D also returns the aminoaciduria to normal and elevates the blood citric acid level and the citric acid excretion.

Action of Vitamin D and Parathyroid Hormone

It has been suggested recently that vitamin D acts in this instance by inhibiting directly or indirectly the secretion of parthyroid hormone. This theory explains most of the known facts, but not all of them; it requires ancillary postulations for whose validity there is no evidence at the present time. In any event, when extremely large doses of vitamin D are given to normal subjects or to patients with hypoparathyroidism, the vitamin seems also to have a direct renal effect. It increases the renal excretion of phosphate. This action causes a lowering of serum phosphate and, coupled presumably with increased absorption from the gut, leads to an elevation of the serum calcium both in patients with hypoparathyroidism and in normal persons intoxicated with vitamin D. Thus, vitamin D has two different actions at different dosage levels. In ordinary therapeutic doses, the vitamin increases the tubular resorption of phosphate and lessens its excretion. In high doses, of the order of magnitude of 100,000 units or more per day, it increases the renal excretion of phosphate. In addition, the administration of vitamin D at both dosage levels leads to an increased absorption of calcium from the gut.

Parathyroid hormone may elevate serum calcium by directly causing its release from bones. Vitamin D may act in a similar manner, although it has not been proved to do so. Agents lowering serum phosphate tend to raise serum calcium. The lowering of serum phosphates lowers the product of calcium and phosphate ions, and more calcium and phosphate are released from the bone until the point of saturation is once more reached. This is an oversimplified theory that has value chiefly as a didactic device. In any event, both parathyroid hormone and massive doses of vitamin D lower serum phosphate by increasing phosphate excretion, and they raise serum calcium. Both of these agents, in excessive amounts, lead to hyper-

calcemia and intoxication. The clinical aspects of vitamin D intoxication will be discussed subsequently.

Action of Vitamin D in Refractory Rickets

There is no evidence, at present, to show whether the patient with vitamin D-refractory rickets has any other defects in metabolism beyond a quantitative inability to respond normally to the usually required doses of vitamin D. On the other hand, there is no proof that he responds to a large dose of vitamin D in the same fashion as a normal patient responds to small doses of vitamin D. The one bit of evidence against this latter possibility is the response of the patient with vitamin D-refractory rickets when he is given

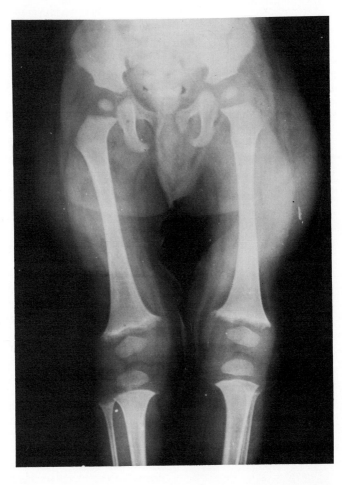

Figure 9.10. Rachitic changes of the distal femoral epiphyseal line. This area, which is subject to most active growth, may be the only one to show changes and the last to regress.

a sufficient amount of vitamin D. His rickets heals, but his serum phosphate still remains lower than normal, although it does rise above the pretreatment level. This response might be explained by postulating a dissociation between the two mechanisms of vitamin D action in the patient with resistant rickets. The patient with vitamin D-refractory rickets may require a much larger dose of vitamin D to benefit from the ordinary antirachitic action. At the same time, however, he may require no more than the normal subject to obtain the direct renal effect of the vitamin, which is the phosphate-losing action. Therefore, with the large doses used to heal his rickets, the effect upon calcium absorption goes on normally, but the increased phosphate resorption, which would ordinarily take place, is partially counteracted by the directed renal phosphate-losing action of vitamin D in massive doses.

Renal Phosphate-losing Rickets

Other diseases that have some of the same metabolic features as refractory rickets include the De Toni-Fanconi syndrome, in which there is hyperphosphaturia, hyperaminoaciduria, glycosuria, and albuminuria. This is basically a disease of the renal tubules that, like other related syndromes, causes an acidosis often accompanied by the secretion of an alkaline urine. The other renal tubular diseases are difficult to separate from each other and from the De Toni-Fanconi syndrome. There is a considerable argument about whether the syndrome of cystinosis is a universal concomitant of the De Toni-Fanconi syndrome, occurs as part of it sometimes, or is an entirely separate syndrome. The relationship of the De Toni-Fanconi syndrome to the other renal tubular diseases producing rickets is vague. These other diseases have been characterized by Gardner as having renal base-losing lesions produced by a defect either in the resorption of bicarbonate or in the ammonia-forming mechanism. These syndromes sometimes are associated with loss of much fixed base including calcium in the urine. They are characterized by a depressed serum pH and the secretion of an alkaline urine. Patients with these syndromes vary greatly in the number of symptoms had and the combinations in which these symptoms occur. They may show all

the signs of the De Toni-Fanconi syndrome, including the acidosis, phosphaturia, aminoaciduria, albuminuria, glycosuria, polyuria, and often the inability to resorb bicarbonate or the failure to manufacture ammonia, or they may show any combination of these symptoms and be classified under various eponyms.

The aminoaciduria in these diseases and the changes in citirc acid metabolism also tend to disappear with the administration of vitamin D. Vitamin D decreases the phosphaturia, but complete healing of the rickets frequently occurs only after large amounts of fixed base have also been given to reduce the acidosis. In general, the rickets in these patients is not so severe as to require orthopaedic care. Perhaps this is because many of the patients die early with uremia. It is more likely, however, that the rickets is mild because the children grow very poorly and very slowly; rickets does not often become apparent in the child who does not grow. However, these children do suffer from osteomalacia, as does the nongrowing adult who is on a diet poor in calcium and is deprived of vitamin D and sunlight over a long period of time. Milkman's syndrome may occur in the later stages of these diseases, but it occurs more frequently in patients with the syndrome to be described next.

Renal Phosphate-retaining Rickets

Patients with a diagnosis of "renal rickets" contrast with those whose rickets is associated with a tubular defect. This group of patients is made up of individuals with chronic renal failure of diverse etiology. They present all the classic signs of chronic renal failure. They have the continuing acidosis and a retention of nitrogenous products marked by a high blood urea nitrogen or nonprotein nitrogen. In addition, they have a high serum phosphate due to depressed glomerular filtration. This is frequently accompanied by a lowered serum calcium. This situation stimulates a relative or secondary hyperparathyroidism, and in a certain number of these patients, the calcium is maintained at normal levels. Coincident with this, these patients develop signs of rickets. The excess parathyroid hormone apparently causes the release of calcium and phosphate from the bones, which leads to a failure to calcify osteoid and prevents the orderly change of growing cartilage to bone. This failure is characteristic of rickets. The acidosis contributes to the leaching of calcium from bone. Furthermore, there may be an excessive loss of fixed base, including calcium, in this condition, which also contributes to the development of the rickets.

Rickets associated with renal tubular defects such as the De Toni-Fanconi syndrome, frequently progresses to chronic renal failure. It is then impossible to distinguish from members of the group usually characterized as "renal rickets." The nomenclature is difficult and at times confusing. However, a diagnosis of "renal rickets" usually implies rickets associated with chronic renal failure and signs of uremia in greater or lesser degrees. On the other hand, patients with specific tubular defects have no elevation of nonprotein nitrogen or of blood urea nitrogen and do not exhibit the signs of renal failure until late. The syndromes should perhaps be regrouped as renal phosphate-losing rickets and renal phosphate-retaining rickets or according to some similar classification. Admittedly there would be an overlap between the groups due to the phosphate-losing patients who develop uremia.

Hypercalcemia

Nearly all of the changes of vitamin D intoxication are duplicated by hyperparathyroidism. The latter seems to present a higher incidence of gross renal calculi and bone rarefaction, but this may merely be a question of chronicity. When large doses of vitamin D are given by error or for their pharmacologic action on the kidney, and there is an overdose, the first sign associated with hypercalcemia is usually anorexia followed by constipation. Polyuria, accompanied by polydipsia, occurs very early. The specific gravity of the urine is low, and if the child is very small or for some reason fluid cannot be ingested, dehydration may supervene. Nausea occurs early. As the toxic symptoms progress, there are vomiting and signs of nervous system change, accompanied by irritability, lethargy, and extreme flaccidity of the muscles. Apparently, there is actual relaxation of the ligaments because these children frequently have hyperextendable joints in addition to

flaccidity. As the disease progresses, metastatic calcification may occur. Further signs of renal damage are produced, which may result from calcification of the kidney parenchyma, although presumably the earlier renal changes are merely a further manifestation of the pharmacologic, or direct toxic, action of the high doses of vitamin D upon the kidney. The renal damage may be manifested by an elevated blood nonprotein nitrogen, but this elevation, in part, may be due to the dehydration that occurs. The skin becomes sallow and pale and mottles readily. At times it is dry and coarse. Metastatic calcification occurs elsewhere throughout the body. It is apparently easily found just beneath the conjunctival tissues by slit-lamp examination.

Hypercalcemia may also be produced by immobilization of even the normal child or adult. The child, of course, is less likely to be immobilized unless he is actually in a cast or some other restraining device. However, even the comparative immobility of enforced bed rest will lead to a release of calcium and phosphate from the bones of the normal individual. This may at times be great enough to produce a hypercalcemia sufficiently severe to cause symptoms. Renal stones may be produced by the attendant hypercalcemia.

Refractory Rickets

Refractory rickets is an inherited disease. In the clinic of Children's Hospital at Pittsburgh, three generations of several families are being followed. The disease can be traced back in these and other families for several more generations. This kind of incidence is common in all such clinics. There are, of course, instances in which no previous manifestations of refractory rickets can be found. If the disease is not recognized in the parent, the children are often considered to have rickets of the usual variety, and indeed, when first seen, they are not distinguishable in any way from patients with vitamin D deficiency rickets. When they are then treated for this condition with the usual dose of vitamin D, however, no response is obtained and the rickets progresses to severe deformity.

It is important to arrest the disease in female patients before deformities of the pelvis are so great as to make delivery impossible except by cesarean section. In the older generations, the usual story is that the mother who was affected has had several cesarean sections. If the disease is not recognized, osteotomies are frequently performed for the correction of the deformity of the leg, but vitamin D is not administered except in small doses. The osteotomies heal well and the immediate results are good, but unless the rickets is controlled, the deformities recur as severely as before. It is imperative that the diagnosis be made early so that deformities can be prevented. If deformities have already occurred, the disease must be brought under control before reparative surgery is performed.

If, when the patient is first seen, he is about 1 year of age, there is no way to distinguish refractory from vitamin D deficiency rickets. The physical findings in both conditions are the same, as are the chemical findings of a normal or slightly low serum calcium, a low phosphate, and an elevated phosphatase. One is suspicious of the refractory disease when the patient with rickets is several or more years of age. Suspicion is confirmed when the patient fails to respond to the ordinary therapeutic dose of vitamin D. At this time it is necessary to consider the various types of rickets that do not respond to the usual treatment. These are genetic refractory rickets and the rickets of the various renal diseases. (Chronic hepatic disease and spruelike syndromes can also cause rickets, but the etiology should be apparent whenever the rickets occurs and will not be considered here.)

Renal function should be investigated first. Simple urinalysis is exceptionally helpful in these diseases. The patient with the De Toni-Fanconi syndrome has albuminuria and glycosuria, although the latter is not constantly present and repeated specimens must be analyzed. The specific gravity of urine in all these diseases tends to be low and somewhat fixed. Inasmuch as the normal obligatory urinary solute excretion, coupled with the low specific gravity, characteristically produces polyuria, an accurate measurement of urinary output is helpful. Where this is not possible, measurement of fluid intake is useful. At times, the polyuria and polydipsia are enough to cause these patients to be diagnosed as suffering from diabetes insipidus. The excretion of alkaline or nearly neutral urine in the presence of systemic acidosis is practically pathognomonic of one of these renal tubular

diseases, even if more sophisticated measurements, such as estimations of the ability to form ammonia or of bicarbonate resorption, cannot be done. Therapeutic responsiveness is of no help in distinguishing between the various renal tubular diseases and genetic refractory rickets. Both will respond to high doses of vitamin D, although the renal disease may require the additional administration of various alkalies.

When the diagnosis of genetic refractory rickets has been made, the treatment should be carried out with large doses of vitamin D given by mouth, although it can be administered intramuscularly. Unless there is some failure or difficulty in gastrointestinal absorption such as occurs in the celial syndrome, there is no reason why vitamin D should not be given by mouth. Because the required dose of vitamin D may be anywhere between 50,000 and 1,000,000 units per day, the initial dose is chosen arbitrarily. A dose near the lowest end of the therapeutic range should be used, of course. It has been our custom to start with either 50,000 or 100,000 units a day, depending upon the size of the child. If there is no response as evidenced by rising serum phosphate or falling serum phosphatase, or later by roentgen evidence of healing of the rickets, the dose is raised. We check the serum calcium, phosphate, and phosphatase values at least once a month and at the same time do a routine urinalysis plus a Sulkowitch test on the urine. An increasing Sulkowitch response should be a warning of hypercalcemia and is a help to avoiding serious signs of vitamin D intoxication. Healing occurs in the absence of a normal serum phosphate. Usually the serum phosphate is maintained just over 3 g per 100 ml. This is higher than in the untreated patient but lower than in the normal growing child. Apparently, this level of serum phosphate represents a balance between the pharmacologic effect of vitamin D in huge doses—that is, phosphate excretion—and the more physiologic effect of small doses of vitamin D in the normal child—that is, the increased tubular resorption of phosphate. When rickets is controlled, the serum calcium value rises to normal, if it has been slightly low, and the serum phosphatase falls within the normal range. It is difficult, at times, to maintain healing of the rickets without permitting a small amount of hypercalcemia. The patient with controlled refractory rickets usually has higher serum calcium than he had before treatment; frequently it is at the top of the normal range or just above.

The goal in the treatment of refractory rickets is to find a dose of vitamin D that is large enough to maintain healing of the rickets and yet does not produce enough hypercalcemia to cause symptoms. In our clinic the average well controlled patient with refractory rickets has a normal serum phosphatase but a calcium that averages 11 g, and a phosphorous just slightly more than 3 g, per 100 ml. The slight hypercalcemia which he may occasionally have gives no symptoms. He eats well, gains weight, and in general looks much healthier than before. His color is improved. Although these patients begin to grow more rapidly after they are treated, even the treated patient tends to grow less rapidly than normal, and as adults they tend to be short. However, they are not as dwarfed as the grotesque untreated patient with this disease. The excessive lordosis and potbelly of rickets disappear with treatment, and, as growth continues, the visible and reparable stigmata of rickets disappear.

If treatment is carried out late, when the child is in a period of slow growth, not all of the bony deformities disappear under vitamin therapy. Patients who are not seen during the period of rapid growth, then, are the ones who require osteotomy and other surgical care. One statement that must be taken with a grain of salt is that these patients can never grow to a normal height. In this clinic, all of the patients were diagnosed after some deformity was visible, and they had already lived beyond the rapid phase of growth of the first 2 years of life; yet the possibility remains that their eventual height will be normal if they were treated early enough.

When these patients are brought in for osteotomy, the vitamin D therapy should be stopped; if it is not, immobilization tends to give them hypercalcemia, which may produce serious kidney damage. After the osteotomy, the patient should be mobilized as soon as possible. Exercises, or as much motion as possible, should be carried out even when the child is in bed in a cast. Renal stones in these patients are avoidable.

After such a patient has been controlled for a period of time, the dosage required usually is fairly stable. Fluctuations occur, however, with changes in the rate of growth, with changes in diet, and perhaps with variations in the amount of sunlight to which the patient is exposed. Until the dosage is well stabilized, these patients should be seen at least once a month for at least 1 year. The interval between visits may then be steadily increased until they are seen only once or twice a year, if good rapport is maintained with the family and if the family can be relied upon to report any changes early. After growth is stopped, the administration of vitamin D may be cut, probably entirely, without any real harm. Further bony deformities will not develop, although some degree of osteomalacia will exist. However, it has been our habit to give a large but reduced dosage of vitamin D to our adult patients. We have no evidence of the value of this treatment.

SCURVY

BY ROBERT KLEIN, M.D.

The incidence of scurvy in pediatric practice, like that of congenital syphilis, has become minimal. The very rarity of these diseases in some ways makes them important to the pediatric orthopaedic surgeon. Just as undiagnosed cases of congenital lues are referred to him because of the pseudoparalysis that the disease induces, so the patient with scurvy may be erroneously considered to have primary bone or joint disease because of his refusal to sit or stand and because of the attending bony tenderness. When these diseases were more common, they were less likely to be misdiagnosed and referred to orthopaedic care. With the widespread use of orange juice and ascorbic acid pills or drops, the few cases of scurvy seen are the result of ignorance or neglect.

The most common cause of scurvy in our experience has been the boiling of orange juice; the second most common cause has been iatrogenic. The doctor has, usually mistakenly, supposed that the baby's eczema is due to the orange juice ingested. The mother is told not to give the orange juice, but adequate provision for its replacement by ascorbic acid is not made. Breast milk ordinarily contains an adequate amount of ascorbic acid unless the mother has been on a deficient diet herself. Cow's milk contains approximately one-fourth as much vitamin C as human milk, and after pasteuriziation the content falls even lower.

The disease occurs most often in children between the ages of 6 months and 1 year. Scurvy should be considered by the orthopaedic surgeon when he is asked to see an infant in the latter half of the first year of life who refuses to stand or perhaps to sit, evidences tenderness in his legs, or keeps his legs drawn up in a frog leg position. As the disease progresses, the areas of tenderness may be swollen. These areas usually are the ends of the long bones. The specific symptoms are caused by the subperiosteal hemorrhages that these infants have much more often than hemorrhage elsewhere (Fig. 9.11). Typical petechiae may be seen on the skin. Orbital hemorrhage occurs on rare occasions. Very rarely is there any bleeding from the gums, probably because of the paucity of teeth at this age. The gums are said to be swollen at times and sore, but we have not observed this condition. The symptoms of bone pain are also produced by the infractions that occur around the epiphyses. As the disease progresses, the patients develop beading at the costochondral junctions, which is very difficult to distinguish from the beading of rickets. In the best defined and well advanced cases, the beading is much sharper and firmer, and frequently it is tender.

Once the diagnosis is considered, there usually is no trouble in establishing it. On close questioning a history of the lack of intake of vitamin C is usually obtainable, even though the mother may have thought that she was giving it. The differential diagnosis from trauma must be made, although everyday trauma probably is the cause of the infractions and some of the hemorrhages that children with scurvy have. However, in the patient with scurvy, these changes are produced by a much less severe trauma than that needed to produce the same changes in a normal child. Moreover, the normal child who has undergone trauma usually does not have symmetric lesions.

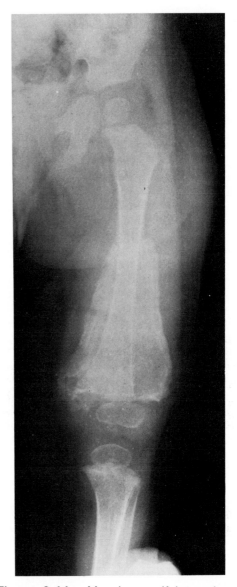

Figure 9.11. Massive ossifying subperiosteal hemorrhage in scurvy. Halolike epiphyses are seen.

The pseudoparalysis that some of these patients have suggests poliomyelitis, but its true nature is usually easily ascertained. The painful swellings about the joints may suggest osteomyelitis, suppurative arthritis, or even some rheumatoid process. However, these patients are much younger than patients with a rheumatoid disease usually are. The symmetric diffuse distribution of the scorbutic lesions helps rule out most of these processes. Scurvy is frequently accompanied by elevation of temperature, which also might suggest infection. However, leukocytosis does not usually occur in uncomplicated scurvy. The pseudoparalysis seen in congenital lues usually occurs at a younger age and is accompanied by other manifestations of syphilis. The distribution of the lesion in infantile cortical hyperostosis is unlike that of scurvy; the former lesion involves the mandible, clavicle, and ulna chiefly. There is no hemorrhage, and the x-ray is diagnostic of this syndrome.

Finally the roentgen appearance of the bones should confirm the diagnosis of scurvy. The most dramatic changes on x-ray are those of early healing when new bone begins to form beneath the elevated periosteum. The periosteum itself is, of course, invisible on x-ray. At times the new bone has suggested bony tumor. More important for clinical diagnosis is the ground glass appearance of the long bones due to the atrophy of the trabeculae. The cortex is thin, and the zone of provisional calcification shows increased density beneath which is a zone of rarefaction. Infractions occur at the epiphyseal line, and actual displacement of the epiphyses is occasionally seen. Calcification is seen in the form of spurs that extend out from the epiphyseal line where the periosteum is attached.

There are various tests that prove the diagnosis of ascorbic acid deficiency. Perhaps the best of these is the measurement of ascorbic acid content of the buffy coat of centrifuged blood.

Treatment of the disease, which is simple, requires the administration of ascorbic acid. Very rarely is any local treatment of the extremities needed. The normal contours of the bones may not be seen by x-ray for many months, or even for a year, if the subperiosteal bone formation has been great. The subsidence of symptoms with treatment is very rapid and very dramatic (Fig. 9.12).

HEMOPHILIA

BY RONALD HILLEGASS, M.D.

History and Incidence

Although the inherited condition which we recognize as hemophilia was described in the

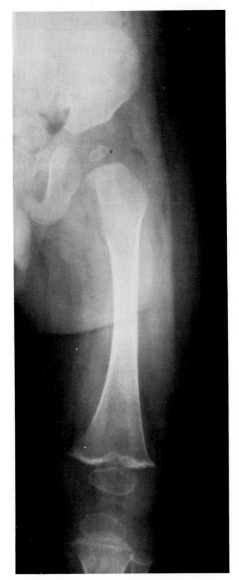

Figure 9.12. Healing 1 year later of the same femur seen in Figure 9.22.

Talmud, the term hemophilia was first used in 1828 by Hopff, a student of Johann Schönlein of Wurzburg. He used this term to describe an inherited condition which resulted in prolonged bleeding following an injury. Hemophilia has since been specifically identified to result from a specific disorder in the clotting mechanism of blood. The most frequent disorder is a deficiency in Factor VIII (AHF) which occurs in approximately 85% of hemophiliacs. This is also called Type A hemophilia. Type B hemophilia occurs in approximately 15% of patients and results from a deficiency of Factor IX (PTC) of the clotting mechanism. This is also called Christmas disease. Both Type A and Type B hemophilia are sex-linked recessives. In addition, some people feel that Factor XI (PTA) deficiency is also a type of hemophilia, or Type C. This may occur in either males or females. Von Willebrand's disease also has a deficiency Factor VIII. This disorder has an increased bleeding time, a decreased platelet efficiency, and is present in both males and females. The male has the defect in the clotting mechanism in Factor VIII and Factor IX deficiency. The female serves as the carrier for this sex-linked recessive condition. Cases have been reported in a female who has inherited the recessive trait from both her parents.

The incidence of hemophilia is approximately 8:10,000 live births, or 1:3,000–4,000 live male births. It is estimated that there are between 5,000 and 7,000 severe hemophiliacs in the United States. The importance of this is apparent when clinical evidence of arthritis is present in 89% of hemophiliacs by the age of 10.

Etiology

The patient has a genetic inability to manufacture the appropriate clotting protein, a β-globulin. Bennet and Huehns[3] described three types of deficiency. The first is no biologic activity and no Factor VIII type protein. The second condition is no biologic activity but normal amounts of a Factor VIII type protein. The third mechanism is a low level of Factor VIII activity with a normal amount of a Factor VIII type protein. Absence of a significant level of the protein clotting factor results in a hemophiliac condition.

Clinical Picture

The patient with hemophilia usually presents with prolonged bleeding from either a relatively minor injury or a surgical procedure or has spontaneous bleeding. This may be overt bleeding or may be a hemarthrosis or bleeding into the soft tissue. Prolonged and frequent bleeding into the joint may result in changes similar to those seen with degenerative arthritis. The involved joint may be painful and have a limited range of mo-

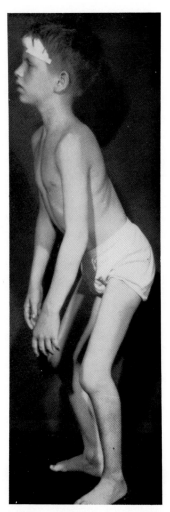

Figure 9.13. Knee flexion contractures in patient with hemophilia.

tion. The joints most frequently affected are the knees, the elbows, and the ankles. Pseudotumors may occur from bleeding around the periosteum (Fig. 9.14), and neurologic deficit may occur following pressure on a nerve from soft-tissue bleeding. The severity of bleeding is dependent on the amount of clotting factor present in plasma. If this is less than 1% of the normal level, the patient has severe hemophilia that is manifested by frequent spontaneous bleeding into the joints and soft tissues. With a level of 1–5%, moderate hemophilia is present with less bleeding and fewer chronic articular changes. When the level reaches 5–30%, the hemophilia is mild and spontaneous hemorrhages are rare.

Diagnosis

The diagnosis is suspected when there is a history of spontaneous or traumatic inappropriately excessive bleeding. If this is accompanied by a family history of hemophilia and the patient is a male, the diagnosis is more likely. Laboratory investigation must be conducted by someone who is familiar with the clotting mechanism. Only in the most severe cases is the blood clotting time prolonged and abnormal. It may be normal with a very small percentage of clotting factor. The kaolin-cephalin clotting time is a more sensitive test for Factor VII or Factor IX deficiency. It is positive for moderate and severe deficiencies of Factors I, V, VIII, IX, X, XI, and XII. In routine coagulation studies, a thromboplastin generation test (one-stage prothrombin time) may be the best method to diagnose hemophilia. This may be present with a deficiency of Factor V and with a thrombocytopenia. The most refined test is the identification of the percentage of the plasma level of a specific factor. This can be readily done for both Factors VIII and IX.

Diagnosis by radiologic methods is nonspecific for hemophilia. Boldero and Kemp[4] in 1966 emphasized this. They listed three different types of x-ray changes which may be present. The first type occurs as a result of hemorrhage into the joint cavity. The second type occurs as a result of immobilization and from the reactive hyperemia which may follow hemorrhage. The third type are changes that occur in specific areas. Hemorrhage may result in a distention of the joint cavity. When this becomes more chronic, synovial thickening may be present. Subarticular erosions, reduction of the cartilage space, and collapse of the subchondral bone may be noted. Cystic changes and osteophytes will ultimately occur (Figs. 9.15 and 9.16).

With loss of mobility and hyperemia, muscle wasting and bone atrophy occur. The trabecula pattern becomes lattice-like. Osteoporosis develops and frequently Harris lines are present. Enlargement of the epiphysis develops as a result of hyperemia.

Certain anatomic areas have demonstrated changes that are considered characteristic of hemophilia. The two most frequently noted are squaring of the lower pole of the patella (Fig. 9.16) and widening of the intracondylar notch of the distal femur. However, both of these may occur with other conditions, especially juvenile rheumatoid arthritis.

As the disease progresses and the joint becomes destroyed and contractures occur, deformities of the joint may develop. Frequently there is posterior subluxation of the tibia at the knee (Fig. 9.17). Premature closing of the epiphyseal plate occurs. Bony ankylosis is occasionally noted.

Pathology

The pathology within the joint is a result of hemorrhage with an inflammatory reaction. This causes proliferation of the synovium. A synovial hemosiderosis may develop because of the phagocytosis of the synovial cell. Fibrin becomes adherent to the synovial surface as the disease progresses. Subsequently, intrasynovial adhesions may develop. These decrease the size of the joint cavity and joint motion. Cartilage fibrillation develops, and the cartilage subsequently becomes destroyed. Hoaglund[8] was able to produce these changes in the laboratory. Stonyen described three types of tissue changes found in hemophilia. The first is a hypertrophic change which is angiomatous with vascular

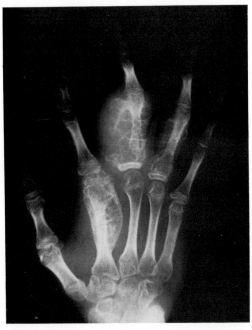

Figure 9.14. Pseudotumor formation in hemophilia.

proliferation. Subsequently a hypertrophic synovitis is present which is pigmented from a deposit of iron from phagocytosis. Finally, the synovium is hypertrophied and there is much fibrous material in the synovium. The synovial tissue undergoes involution with fibrosis. Ultimately, there may be pieces of cartilage and bone contained within the synovium.

The articular cartilage changes are similar to those seen in joints with degenerative arthritis except that they tend to be more diffuse. Initially there is a granular change in the cartilage surface with fibrillation and pitting. Erosion of the cartilage surface is finally noted. This is secondary to the chronic inflammatory process and enzyme destruction. Bone cysts ultimately develop which communicate with the joint and are lined by synovial tissue.

Treatment

The basic aspect of treatment is the replacement of the deficient clotting factor. Until 1965, plasma was used for this. It was noted that fresh frozen plasma was needed and that serum did not contain the deficient factor. Prolonged storage of plasma resulted in the destruction of Factors VIII and IX. In 1965, Factor VIII was isolated as a cryoprecipitate of plasma. It can be stored at −20 to −30°C. The remainder of the plasma may be used for other blood products. The availability of this material reduces the problem of overload of cardiovascular system which developed when plasma was used for replacement. Cryoprecipitate does not contain Factor IX. In addition, the potency is variable, which makes replacement more difficult.

More recently, other types of precipitates have been developed. These have the advantage of being stable at −4° and may be stored in a dried fashion. In addition, they have a known potency for a particular dose. However, they are more expensive. Factor XI is also available as a concentrate.

The cryoprecipitate used for Factor VIII replacement normally has 125–140 units per bag. The concentrates have 250 units per bottle. The Konyne replacement for Factor IX has 500 units per bottle. One unit is equal to the amount of AHF or PTC in 1 ml of fresh normal plasma. This can be used to calculate the replacement. Factor VIII has a half-life of approximately 12 hr, and Factor IX has a half-life of approximately 18 hr.

For an acute early hemarthrosis, a hematoma in a nonhazardous area, or external bleeding, a single dose of factor replacement sufficient to bring the level to 30% of the normal plasma volume is usually sufficient to control the hemorrhage. If more is needed, it should be given every 6 hr for the first 24 hr and then every 8 hr. Factor IX replacement may be given every 8 hr for 24 hr and then on a 12-hr program. For more severe bleeding, a hemarthrosis that has developed more than 12 hr previously, or hematuria, the level should be raised to greater than 40%. Also, a level of greater than 40% is indicated when surgery is to be performed. With severe joint bleeding, the replacement may be necessary for 2–4 days. For a fracture, it is usually advisable to give factor replacement for at least 3 days. With major surgery, 10–14 days of therapy may be indicated. With deep soft-tissue operations, this may need to be extended. In addition, when a physical therapy program is being initiated following surgery or immobilization, it may be necessary to replace the factor to prevent a hemarthrosis from developing.

It should be noted that there is a risk of hepatitis at any time that blood products prepared from poor plasma are used. Therefore, a recurrent testing program for Australian antigen may be advisable.

Approximately 10% of people who have a deficiency of Factor VIII and have had replacement therapy develop an antibody to their replacement factor. This is a 7S-immunoglobulin (IgG) and acts as an inhibitor. This may be suspected when a patient fails to improve with a dose of factor replacement that is normally effective. Medical judgment must be exercised in treating a patient with this problem. Our approach has been to replace the factor with a very high dose and to treat the patient with steroids during this period. In this situation, factor replacement is used only if there is a significant threat to the patient's life or to the possible loss of a limb. More frequently, when this problem is present and a patient suffers a bleeding episode, he is treated by immobilization alone.

Pain is a frequent problem with a bleeding episode in hemophilia. It should be emphasized that aspirin is contraindicated. It impairs platelet function and may cause and prolong a bleeding episode. Any aspirin-con-

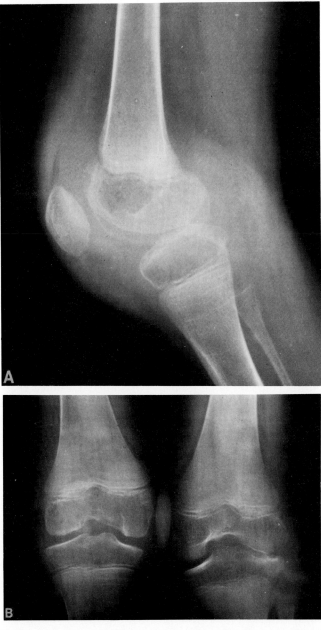

Figure 9.15. Changes in knee of 9-year-old boy with hemophilia. (*A*) Note marked synovial hypertrophy. (*B*) Anteroposterior view shows early enlarged epiphysis of left femur, hyperemia with increased radiolucency of epiphysis, irregularity of subchondral bone, and early cyst formation of left lateral femoral condyle. Note widened intracondylar notch. (*C*) Lateral view of left knee showing bony fusion 3 years later. Contour of epiphyses is still visible. (*D*) Anteroposterior view of left knee at age 15. Well organized bony fusion. (*E*) Lateral view of left knee at age 15 demonstrating bony fusion. Note absence of ''squared'' patella.

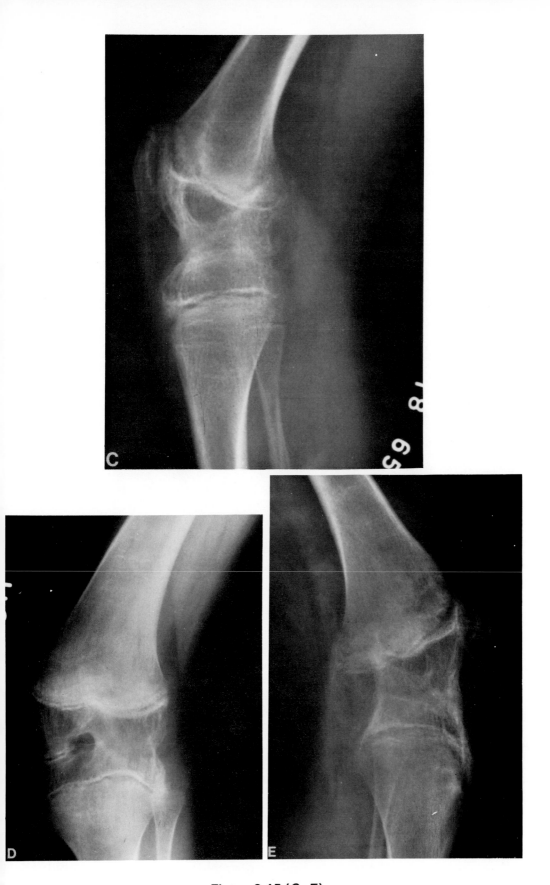

Figure 9.15 (C–E)

463

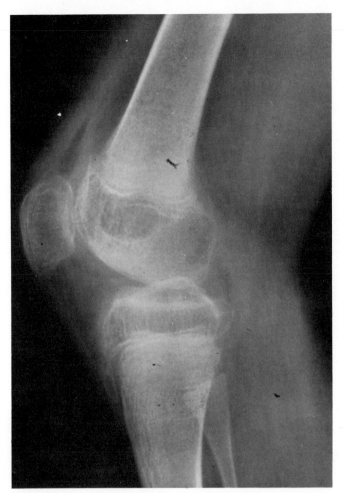

Figure 9.16. Lateral view of knee in 13-year-old hemophiliac. Note the "square" appearance of the lower pole of the patella.

taining product should be avoided. Other adjuncts of therapy, such as immobilization, aspiration, and steroids, will be discussed under the specific problems.

Specific Problems

ACUTE HEMARTHROSIS

The clinical features of an acute hemarthrosis are swelling, pain secondary to the distention of the joint, warmth as a result of the bleeding into the joint, and loss of motion. Frequently, the patient will have observed symptoms such as an aching sensation or stiffness prior to the onset of these more familiar characteristics. The treatment program must stop the bleeding and eliminate

the pain. Ultimately, the joint function must be maintained and restored, and an effort should be made to eliminate chronic joint changes. As has been observed in our clinic recently, the early factor replacement is the most critical single feature in achieving these objectives. Early factor replacement maintains good joint function and minimizes the therapeutic effort. In a study of Ali et al.,[1] 72% of 39 patients treated at the onset of their bleeding episode returned to full activity in less than 1 week; 52% of 44 patients who were not treated initially within the first 8 hr were unable to return to full activity for more than 2 weeks. In following these patients, 1 of 39 had joint deformities if treated early, compared to 1 of 7 who did not have early factor replacement. The efficacy of early factor replacement has been demonstrated. It

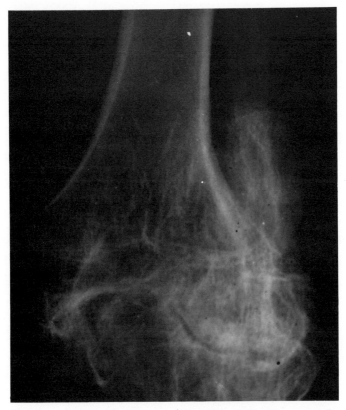

Figure 9.17. Severe destruction in 31-year-old adult. Knee subluxed and without normal configuration.

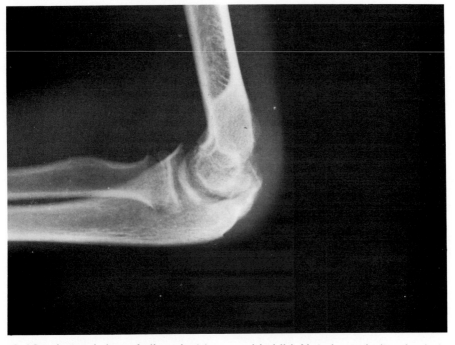

Figure 9.18. Lateral view of elbow in 11-year-old child. Note irregularity of subchondral bone and radiolucency in metaphyseal region as a result of hyperemia.

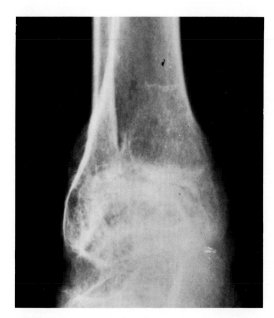

Figure 9.19. Ankle showing severe destructive changes as adult. Note loss of cartilage at tibiotalar joint and bony fusion at talofibular joint.

allows the patient to resume early activity and minimizes chronic joint deformities.

In our clinic, many of the patients are on a home program for factor replacement. The patient or parents have been instructed in the intravenous administration of the factor. At the earliest sign of bleeding into a joint, the clinic is notified and a consultation is obtained with the physician. If the physician feels that it is appropriate, the factor may be given at home. This early replacement has resulted in fewer chronic problems from an acute hemarthrosis.

Immoblization is a second essential aspect of treatment. Splinting the joint decreases the metabolic demand and allows for more rapid resorption of the hemarthrosis. It also decreases the amount of pain the patient experiences. The immobilization is done initially in the position of comfort. Complete splinting is continued for approximately 24–36 hr or until the severe pain has subsided. The splinting should continue while effusion and warmth are present in the joint except for range-of-motion exercises, which should be performed 3–4 times a day. Splinting may be discontinued when the warmth and effusion have subsided and a previous range of motion has been obtained. At that time, full activity

may be allowed. If the patient had a limited range of motion at the time of onset of the acute hemarthrosis, it may be advisable to continue splinting for the weight-bearing joints and to use night splints for a few additional weeks.

Aspiration represents a controversial adjunct of therapy. In our clinic, aspiration is performed only if the joint is markedly painful. It is rarely done. If aspiration is to be attempted, the patient must be additionally treated with factor replacement. A theoretical argument for aspiration is that, by diminishing the amount of blood within the joint, there is less material to be phagocytized and, therefore, the breakdown products and lysosomal release with its cell destruction of the joint cartilage are mininized. In addition, the pressure within the joint, which can also cause cartilage destruction, is minimized. The arguments against aspiration are that bleeding will tend to occur even after the joint is aspirated and that there is increased trauma to the patient and a risk of infection.

The application of ice to the joint at the time of the acute hemarthrosis may have a beneficial effect; we use this in the first 24–36 hr.

Steroids have been suggested for use on either a local or systemic basis. The evidence that this significantly alters the course is inadequate at the present time. The local injections have a risk of infection. Systemic steroids have other potential problems, and because their efficacy has not been adequately demonstrated, these are not used at the present time in our clinic.

Hyaluronidase injected into the joints has been advocated. This is not being done at the present time.

It should be emphasized again that aspirin is contraindicated as an analgesic in hemophilia. Despite a continued warning, it is not infrequent that aspirin is used by the unwary in caring for the hemophiliac patient.

MUSCLE AND SOFT-TISSUE BLEEDING

After hemarthrosis, bleeding into the muscle and soft tissue is the second most common problem encountered in caring for the hemophiliac patient, With an acute bleed episode into muscle or soft tissue, the treatment is similar to that used in an acute hemarthrosis. Early factor replacement is indicated. Immobilization should also be used. This should be done in a position of comfort. Subsequently, the splinting should be corrected to prevent the development of a joint contracture. Aspiration is not indicated. Fibrosis of the muscle may occur as a result of bleeding within the muscle tissue. This may result in a muscle which has diminished excursion and power. Other problems which occur with acute bleeding in the soft tissue are nerve involvement, a compartmental syndrome, and a pseudotumor.

Nerve involvement is most likely secondary to external pressure on the nerve. This usually results in neuropraxia which takes 2–3 weeks to recover. Occasionally axonotmesis may occur, which requires 6–12 months to repair. The bleeding causes a sudden increase in pressure on the nerve. It frequently starts a day or two following the onset of bleeding. The femoral nerve is most commonly involved, although the median, ulnar, and tibial nerves have also been reported to be affected. Compartmental syndromes may occur, although they are rare despite the frequency of massive soft-tissue bleeding. They most frequently occur as a Volkmann's ischemia of the forearm or in the anterior or posterior compartments of the calf. These may develop rapidly and, if they occur, can require a surgical fasciotomy to prevent muscle necrosis. This may represent a surgical emergency in the treatment of hemophilia.

A pseudotumor may develop as a result of bleeding under the periosteum or occasionally within the bone substance itself. This results in pressure on the bone and the surrounding soft tissue. The clinical picture of this may cause it to mimic a sarcoma or osteomyelitis. Progressive enlargement may occur and ultimately result in skin necrosis, ulceration, infection, and hemorrhage. The x-ray picture shows bone destruction with a surrounding soft-tissue mass (Fig. 9.20). Peripheral sclerosis is seen rarely. The initial treatment of a pseudotumor is factor replacement and immobilization. If the patient does not respond, surgical incision and drainage are indicated.

CHRONIC SYNOVITIS AND ARTHRITIS

Despite ideal therapy, many patients develop chronic synovitis and changes similar to those of degenerative arthritis. Steroids have not been shown to be helpful in this problem. Radiation therapy, which has been tried, may allow malignant degeneration. Results are accumulating which favor the use of synovectomy for chronic hemophiliac synovitis (Storti et al.[14,15]. Many of these have been shown to have no recurrence on a 3-year follow-up. It should be emphasized that synovectomy in a child is a difficult procedure because it does require the patient to participate in the rehabilitation. This is often difficult for a child with a painful joint following surgery.

Joint contractures are frequently present. Serial cast correction with a Quingel or wedging cast may be used. Precautions should be taken to restore the gliding motion of the joint. Frequently the tibia is subluxed posteriorly on the femoral condyle and may be hinged in its subluxed position. Significant contractures may require posterior capsulotomy in an effort to get the knee in a weight-bearing position. It should be emphasized that a joint in the lower extremity must be in a position to bear weight.

The degenerative arthritis changes which occur in the hemophiliac may be treated as degenerative arthritis in other areas. Most of the treatment will be performed on the adult rather than a child. It should be noted that arthrodesis must be considered very carefully because of the potential problem of arthritic changes in other joints. An arthrodesis may increase markedly the stress placed on another diseased joint. With good control of the clotting mechanism, surgery may be performed in a hemophiliac as it is on a patient with degenerative joint changes. The increased risk of bleeding should not be a contraindication to surgery which can maintain or restore joint function to the patient. It should be emphasized that in the rehabilitation following surgery factor replacement may be necessary to prevent a recurrent bleeding episode.

Leg length evaluations should be performed in children who have chronic synovitis. The premature epiphyseal closure on one side may result in a leg length discrepancy which may aggrevate arthritic changes at a later date.

Preventive Treatment

With the advent of home factor replacement and the ability to treat an acute hemarthrosis earlier, the need for bracing has de-

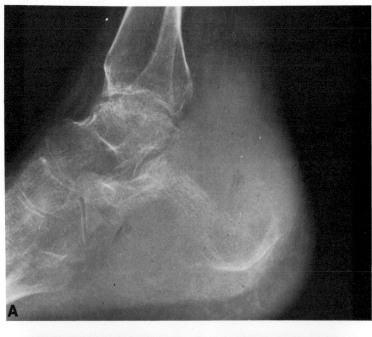

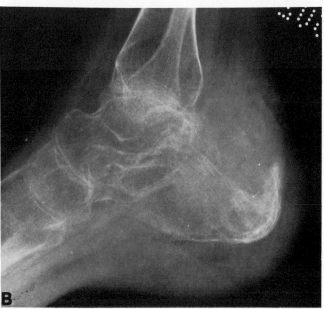

Figure 9.20. Progression of pseudotumor cyst of os calcis. (A) Sixteen-year-old boy. Note marked soft-tissue component; (B) 3 months later. Soft-tissue component notably decreased; (C) and (D) 6 months later, after onset noted in (A); (E) 2 years after (A).

creased. Bracing still is indicated in children who are subjected to repeated trauma and who lack the maturity to assist in caring for their joint function. It may also be indicated for children who have developed a chronic joint problem where it is felt that surgery is not indicated at the present time and protection is necessary. However, bracing is being used less frequently with the availability of early factor replacement.

A good physical therapy program must be emphasized. These people have a tremen-

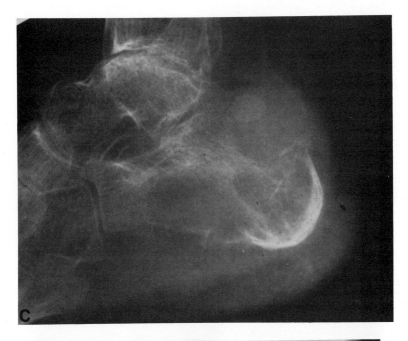

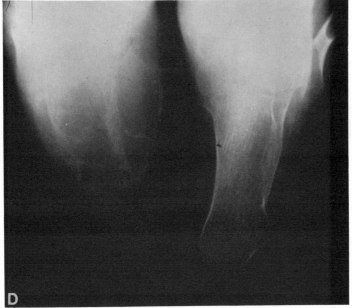

Figure 9.20 (*C* and *D*)

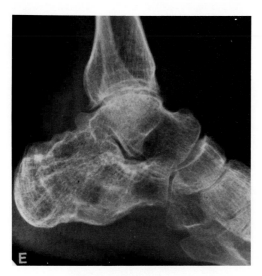

Figure 9.20 (E)

dous need for maintaining good muscle function to help protect a joint. Development of a good quadriceps muscle has, without question, eliminated the frequency of acute hemarthrosis.

Inasmuch as hemophilia represents a deficiency in a distinct clotting factor, the ideal treatment program would allow for replacement of this on a routine basis such as is used in managing a diabetic patient with insulin. At the present time, this is an expensive procedure. It has been tried in a number of centers. These patients are able to lead a full life with normal physical and psychologic development. The patient is more likely to attend a regular school and participate in gainful employment. The joints remain better than those which are treated only when they have a bleeding episode. Analysis of this type of treatment has shown that it is less expensive than treatment of a hemophiliac only when he has a bleeding episode. It minimizes the requirement for hospitalization and intensive therapy. The ultimate cost to society could be reduced if this type of treatment is made available.

References

1. Ali, A. M., Gandy, R. H., Britten, M. I., and Dormandy, K. M.: Joint hemorrhage in hemophilia; is full advantage take of plasma therapy? Br. Med. J., 3: 828, 1967.
2. Bennett, B., and Ratnoff, O. D.: Detection of the carrier state for classic hemophilia, N. Engl. J. Med., 288: 342, 1973.
3. Bennet, E., and Huehns, E. R.: Immunologic differentiation of three types of hemophilia and identification of some female carriers, Lancet, 2: 956, 1970.
4. Boldero, J. L., and Kemp, H. S.: The early bone and joint changes in hemophilia and similar blood dyscrasias, Br. J. Radiol., 39: 172, 1966.
5. Dallman, P. R., and Pool, J. G.: Treatment of hemophilia with factor VIII concentrates, N. Engl. J. Med., 278: 199, 1968.
6. Day, A. J.: Orthopaedic management of hemophilia, In American Academy of Orthopaedic Surgeons Instructional Course Lectures, Vol. 20, pp. 15–19; St. Louis: C. V. Mosby, 1971.
7. George, J. N., and Breckenridge, R. T.: The use of Factor VIII and Factor IX concentrates during surgery, J.A.M.A., 214: 1673, 1970.
8. Hoaglund, F. T.: Experimental hemarthrosis; the response of canine knees to injections of autologous blood, J. Bone Joint Surg., 49A: 285, 1967.
9. Kasper, C. K., Dietrich, S. L., and Rapaport, S. I.: Hemophilia prophylaxis with Factor VIII concentrate, Arch. Intern. Med., 125: 1004, 1970.
10. Kisker, C. T., Perlman, A. W., and Benton, C.: Arthritis and hemophilia, Semin. Arthritis Rheum., 1: 220, 1971.
11. Rabiner, S. F., Telfer, M. C., and Fajardo, R.: Home transfusions of hemophiliacs, J.A.M.A., 221: 885, 1972.
12. Rudowski, W. J., and Ziemski, J. M.: Extensive surgical procedures in patients with hemophilia, Surg. Gynecol. Obstet., 135: 571, 1972.
13. Seeler, R. A.: Hemolysis due to anti-A and anti-B and Factor VIII preparations Arch. Intern. Med., 130: 101, 1972.
14. Storti, E., Traldi, A., Tosatti, E., and Davoli, P. G.: Synovectomy; new approach to hemophiliac arthropathy, Acta Haematol, 41: 193, 1969.
15. Storti, E., Traldi, A., Tosatti, E., and Davoli, P. G.: Synovectomy in haemophiliac arthropathy, Schweiz. Med. Wochenschr., 100: 2005, 1970.
16. Van Creveld, S.: Prophylaxis of joint hemorrhages in hemophilia, Acta Haematol., 45: 120, 1971.

RHEUMATOID ARTHRITIS IN CHILDREN

Children with severe metabolic disease due to rheumatoid arthritis become a problem in the maintenance of life. Enlargement of the liver and spleen, anemia, and severe malnutrition are overriding problems here. The functioning of their extremities often becomes a secondary problem in their care. However, good principles in the maintenance of joint function can be followed simultaneously with their general medical care so that the child who survives the onslaughts of a metabolic disturbance is not left hopelessly deformed and crippled for activity in life. In the care of the whole child, the concept that the musculoskeletal system is part of that whole child is often ignored. From the following description of rheumatoid arthritis, which is commonly seen in children without marked metabolic disturbance, the principles of maintenance of function, prevention of deformity, and rehabilitation may be employed in treating the child with metabolic disease as well.

Age and Sex Incidence

The average age at onset in our series was 5.7 years, but synovitis began in one child age 6 months and the oldest was 15 years. Whether the onset led to monarticular, oligoarticular, or eventually was polyarticular arthritis, the average age at onset was 5.9 years, 5.8 years, or 5.9 years—all very similar.

On the other hand, patients who would be classified as having Still's disease were significantly different, with an average age at onset of 2.0 years, ranging from 1–4 years of age.

There was no female predominance of the type evident in rheumatoid arthritis in the adult. The entire series was divided into 54.7% female and 45.3% male. Only the oligoarticular group had a 2:1 female ratio.

Mode of Onset

Although 50.5% of the patients were found at onset to have involvement of a single joint, only 8.6% remained with a single joint in the course of their disease (Table 9.1). Of those who began with two or three joints (31.6% of the total) affected, few members progressed to further involvement and remained finally at 27.4%. Only 15.4% of the total group began with four or more joints and systemic signs. However, this group progressed to involve 59.4% of the total with polyarticular involvement.

Where the mode of onset differed from the final outcome, the change took place in the first 3 months (Table 9.2).

Systemic Manifestations

Systemic manifestations often preceded the joint symptoms by many months. Fever, rash, fatigability, malaise, anorexia, weight loss, iritis, lymphadenopathy, and splenomegaly all represented systemic involvement. Subcutaneous nodules were found in 2 patients, as compared to approximately 20% found in adults.

Fatigue, malaise, anorexia, and weight loss tended to be closely associated with the magnitude of the fever in the children in this series. These manifestations are rarely seen in the monarticular group and only occasionally in the oligoarticular group. Lymphadenitis was found in 30 patients and only in those whose involvement was severe with multiple joints or Still's disease. One patient with polyarticular involvement and who was operated on for acute appendicitis had marked mesenteric lymphadenitis. Splenomegaly was found only in those who were severely ill. Fever was present in more than 80% of all patients early in the disease; 47% had low grade to moderate fever (37–40°C),

Table 9.1
Spectrum of Disease in 117 Arthritic Patients

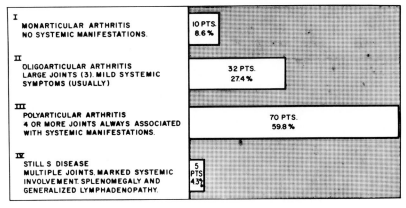

Table 9.2
Joints Involved within 3 Months of Onset

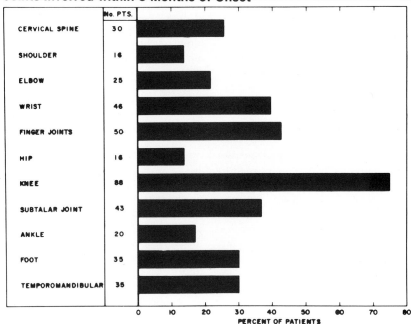

	No. PTS.
CERVICAL SPINE	30
SHOULDER	16
ELBOW	25
WRIST	46
FINGER JOINTS	50
HIP	16
KNEE	88
SUBTALAR JOINT	43
ANKLE	20
FOOT	35
TEMPOROMANDIBULAR	35

PERCENT OF PATIENTS

and 36.8% had marked febrile episodes over 40°C. The fever was intermittent. In monarticular involvement, fever was absent in 60% of the cases. Febrile episodes progressed in frequency to involve 100% of the cases of Still's disease.

Rash was present in 32.5% of all the patients in the series at onset. Good has described the rash as being characteristically a nonpruritic, erythematous, macular or slightly maculopapular eruption of the trunk, neck, or extremities. None of the monarticular patients had a rash.

Rheumatoid Arthritis without Metabolic Involvement

This type of arthritis seen in children has been designated "pauciarticular arthritis" by Green. The majority of affected children are less than 4 years of age. The involvement in the presence of generally good health varies from one to several joints. The anomaly affects females almost twice as commonly as males. The duration of joint swelling varies from several months to many years and averages approximately 3 years.

Clinical Picture

A well child notes pain and swelling of gradual onset about a major joint, most commonly the knee. Almost half of the children are affected in only one joint. In addition to the knees, the ankles, elbows, and hips are commonly involved (Fig. 9.21). Two- and three-joint involvement is almost as common as single-joint involvement. In children with multiple-joint involvement, the wrists and subtalar joints also become sites of the disease.

The joint is warm and painful, and its motion is limited in all planes to varying degrees, according to the acuteness of the synovial inflammation.

Fluid is readily palpated in those joints that are easily available, such as the knee, ankle, and wrist. It is readily aspirated with a small-gauge needle, such as a No. 22 or 23, and it appears slightly cloudy. The polymorphonuclear cells are markedly increased over the normal 6% of the total cell count; they form the principal cell. The total white cell count is usually at least several thousand. The mucin is of only fair quality when it is precipitated with acetic acid. The joint fluid content

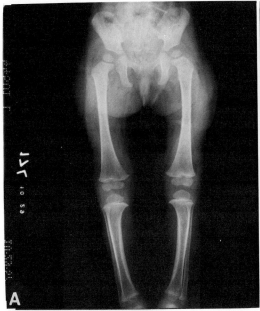
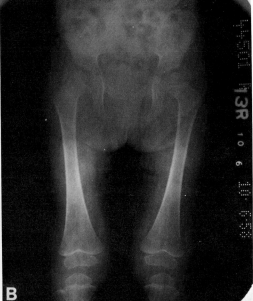
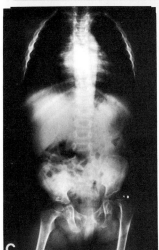
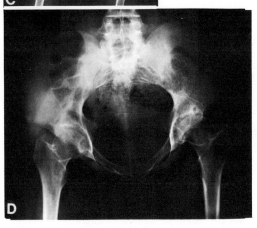

Figure 9.21. (*A*) Onset of multijoint arthritis principally involving both hips and knees. (*B*) Diminished density of the bone about the major joints and extensive soft-tissue swelling 1 year later. (*C*) Subluxation of the hip with continued involvement 2 years later. (*D*) Osteoarthritis secondary to the onset of rheumatoid arthritis, 10 years later. Narrowing of the joint cartilage space and a cyst of the acetabulum are seen.

of sugar is usually approximately 20 mg below the blood sugar level.

The sedimentation rate is moderately elevated (Table 9.3). The latex fixation test is usually negative, as are tests for the febrile agglutinins. The C-reactive protein test may be positive.

Children who pass to full fledged metabolic rheumatoid arthritis usually do so in the first 6 months after the onset of the initial joint swelling. This is a rare occurrence.

Treatment

Once the presence or absence of metabolic disease has been determined, the problem becomes one of keeping the child a functioning individual in the home and at school and, at the same time, protecting and maintaining the function of the joint until the disease has run its course.

Rest usually brings the joint to a stable condition without tenderness, heat, or fluid in 2–4 months. Thereafter, increased activity may irritate the joint once again, and a considerable period, often of several years' duration, passes before the child can resume full normal activity. Bed rest alone takes the child out of normal contacts, and absolute fixation of the limb leads to myotatic contracture. Cortisone therapy is a two-edged sword; it quiets the joint but leads to metabolic complications. The undeformed child having full motion of the joint and attending school and home activities, yet keeping the

joint at rest, seems to represent the ideal solution. To attain any success with the rest portion of this program, one must use a bivalved cast that the child can remove to exercise the limb, yet still be contained on a rest regime. Prior to establishing all phases of the child's life as fully as possible, those features of his joint disease which may limit his activity permanently must be overcome. Injection of the joint with Hydrocortone or similar substances has not been of permanent value in our cases; usually the fluid in the joint recurs after several weeks.

CORRECTION OF DEFORMITY

Traction is indicated to overcome deformity and restore motion. The initial traction must be applied in line with the deformity if muscle spasms are to subside. As the spasms subside, the joint is brought progressively further and further into a corrected position. As motion is regained, that portion of the joint limited by muscle spasm is overcome. The spasm that remains is due to myotatic contracture, or occasionally to actual intra-articular adhesions or deformity. A common situation complicating the correction of knee flexion contractures is posterior subluxation of the tibia; in this situation, although the leverage action of the lower leg allows rotation about the knee joint axis, the hamstrings prevent the gliding of the tibia forward with extension. Active contractions of the limb musculature are encouraged while the child is in traction.

Table 9.3
Erythrocyte Sedimentation Rate (Corrected)

TYPE	No. PATIENTS	NORMAL ↑20mm/h	SLIGHTLY ELEVATED 20-30mm/h	MODERATELY ELEVATED 30-40mm/h	MARKEDLY ELEVATED ↑40mm/h
MONARTICULAR ARTHRITIS	10	4 (40 %)	4 (40 %)	2 (20 %)	0
OLIGOARTICULAR ARTHRITIS	32	11 (34.4 %)	8 (25.0 %)	3 (9.4 %)	10 (31.2 %)
POLYARTICULAR ARTHRITIS	70	15 (21.4 %)	22 (31.4 %)	25 (35.7 %)	8 (11.4 %)
STILL'S DISEASE	5	0	1 (20 %)	2 (40 %)	2 (40 %)
ALL PATIENTS	117	30 (25.6 %)	35 (29.9 %)	32 (27.4 %)	20 (17.1 %)

To overcome the most rigid portion of the contracture, several possible regimens are now used:

1. The child may be placed in warm water. The limb is floated, and active guided motion is used to achieve further joint range and increased muscle function. In the intervals between these baths, the child remains in traction.

2. A bivalved cast is made at the point of maximal possible correction of the joint. The limb is removed from the cast several times daily for active guided motion, during which the child usually lies on his side so that the arm is supported against the pull of gravity and the insecurity and consequent muscle spasm it engenders. As correction is gradually accomplished, a new bivalved cast, taking up the amount of correction achieved, is made.

3. For the last few degrees of correction, wedging type casts may be used. They are the least preferable mode of therapy because the joint is fixed during this period and pressure on cartilaginous surfaces may be great. They are sometimes necessary in resistant situations, but they should be used for no longer than several weeks. Following the cor-

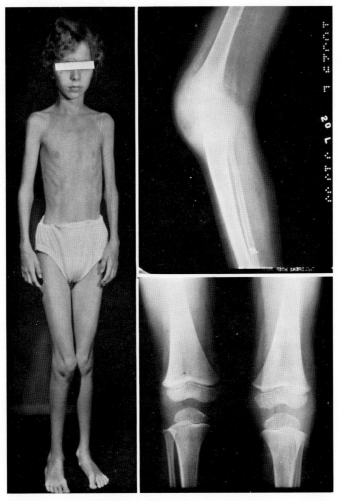

Figure 9.22 (*Left*).   Rheumatoid arthritis originally with systemic symptoms. The residuals of the disease for this patient are limited motion at the major joints and foot deformities. Bilateral limitation of motion at the hip produces a particularly disabling gait.
Figure 9.23 (*Right*).   Swelling limiting the outline of the knee joint capsule in rheumatoid synovitis of the knee.

rection of deformity, a bivalved cast to maintain the correction is made.

BIVALVED CAST ROUTINE

Once the joint has regained full motion and is no longer deformed, the bivalved cast ensures lack of weight bearing and is a mode of controlling the child's activity at home. It is removed at least twice daily for ½-hr periods. During this time, the child remains recumbent but carries the joint through a full range of motion and actively uses the flexor and extensor muscles without resistance.

With crutches and bivalved casts, the child may leave bed, attend school and home activities, and see his friends. Once the inflammation has completely subsided—that is, when there is no evidence of heat, tenderness, or fluid and the sedimentation rate has returned to normal—removal of the cast may be considered. It is usually well to be ultra-conservative in order to avoid recurrence.

Once the child has been 1 month without the bivalved cast and with no evidence of recurrence, partial weight bearing with crutches is begun. A three-point gait is used for involvement of a single extremity and a four-point gait when both extremities are involved. If during the next interval between visits to the physician (usually 4 weeks) there is no recurrence, activity is increased partially and the crutches are discarded. During another period, the joint muscles are exercised on a progressive resistance routine in order to overcome atrophy.

Synovectomy in Childhood—Rheumatoid

The children who are brought to the point of consideration of synovectomy are principally those who have failed to respond to conservative therapy and whose general physical condition seems unaffected by the disease.

The major joint under consideration for synovectomy is the knee. In general the involvement in other joints is minor. Considerable soft-tissue thickening is evident at the knee, and the soft-tissue component is major compared to the fluid distension of the joint.

Anxiety in both the child and parents is apparent, as the swelling has persisted despite non-weight bearing with repeated substance and recurrence.

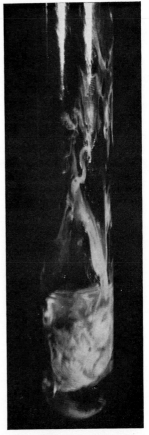

Figure 9.24. Mucin of good quality precipitates as a soft, well formed clump of material that does not break up into shreds.

When the synovectomy is performed, a definite plan of action must be outlined to the parents. A gentle manipulation is often necessary at 3 weeks postoperatively, and, when done, 90 degrees of flexion should be achieved.

The synovectomy is done anteriorly, removing the suprapatellar pouch. The child is immobilized in a long leg plaster cast for 10 days and then placed in split Russell traction (Fig. 9.25). At 3 weeks, if 90 degrees of flexion have not been achieved, a gentle manipulation under anesthesia is done. The traction is continued for 1 week, followed by a bivalved cast with the knee in 10 degrees of flexion. The child is sent home with the cast removed twice daily for flexion and extension exercises. After several months this can be discontinued, but partial weight bearing with crutches persists until the swelling at the knee subsides on both flexion and weight bearing.

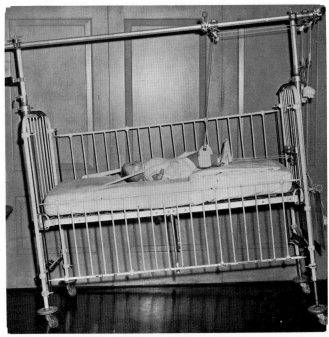

Figure 9.25. Here a manikin is used to illustrate split Russell traction in line with the deformity. Note that the foot of the bed is elevated for countertraction and that perineal straps aid in maintaining the position of the child. The knee sling is under the proximal tibia to prevent posterior subluxation as the flexion deformity is decreased. The sling is pulled at a posterior angle of about 20 degrees. A foot board prevents the weights from catching on the bed. A rubberized bumper on the head upright prevents damage to hospital walls.

An operated joint such as this, once a good functional joint is achieved, is not the seat of a recurrence of rheumatoid arthritis.

Regimen of Therapy

A review of 117 patients has been carried out (Figs. 9.26–9.31). The methods of treatment for the patients of this series could be divided into six categories. Of these 50% were seen medically only, 30% were seen chiefly by orthopaedic surgeons, and 20% had a combined approach. The more mild the disease the greater the tendency to be followed by the medical clinician, whereas the more severely affected patients tended to be followed by orthopaedic surgeons alone or with their medical colleagues. The conservative orthopaedic approach consisted of traction, active exercises, the use of splinting, and crutches. Fifty per cent of all patients received either salicylates alone or salicylates with conservative orthopaedic measures. Sixteen patients received no treatment after their initial diag-

nosis. The other regimens of therapy were almost equally distributed between those receiving corticosteroids (13.7%), undergoing synovectomy (11.1%), or synovectomy and debridement (10.2%).

Comparison of Therapy

If all 117 patients are grouped together, the trend to more aggressive treatment of the more severely involved is evident.

No treatment was the regimen received by 16 patients. Their natural history was quite similar. Predominantly they had oligoarticular or polyarticular involvement. Many were severely ill and became well after a 1- to 6-month period. Fifteen of these patients were in the excellent or good category at follow-up.

Of 32 patients receiving only salicylate therapy, 19 had excellent or good results and 13 poor.

Salicylates combined with orthopaedic

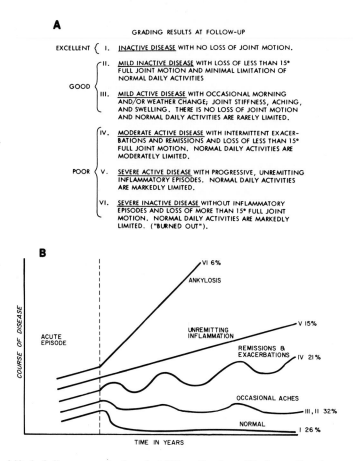

Figure 9.26. (*A*) A follow-up study of 117 patients with juvenile rheumatoid arthritis with an average follow-up of 8.3 years used the criteria and classification listed. The study was done by Stanley Kampner, M.D. (*B*) Course of rheumatoid disease.

care, in the more severe types of disease, were the therapy of 25. Fifteen were classified as having excellent or good results, and 10 patients had a poor end result.

Long term corticosteroid therapy was given to the more severely involved patients, and the end results showed little improvement.

Of 16 receiving corticosteroids only, 3 had good results, with 13 in the poor category. Of the 13 poor results, 11 continued to have florid disease. The only death in this series was a child treated with corticosteroids for 2 years who died with an overwhelming infection.

In patients who had severe involvement with frequent inflammatory episodes or progression in remitting disease, there were 13 who underwent synovectomy and 12 who had synovectomy and debridement.

Thirteen of the 15 patients in the synovectomy group had an excellent or good result, and 5 of the 12 patients in the synovectomy and debridement group who had a similar outcome spoke well for these procedures, but the only individuals with a Grade VI result were also from those surgically treated. With conservative or medical regimen of therapy, there were only Grade IV and Grade V included as a poor end result.

Surgical intervention seems to have no middle ground, having either a very good or very poor end result.

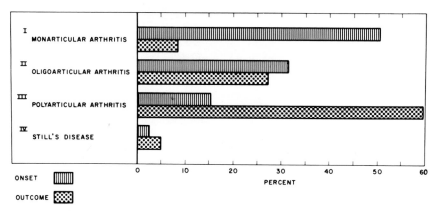

Figure 9.27. A study of this bar graph reveals that, although a large number of patients started out with monarticular arthritis, a large number soon went on to multiple joint involvement. And those who started with polyarticular arthritis were soon joined by others from the group with a minimal number of joints involved.

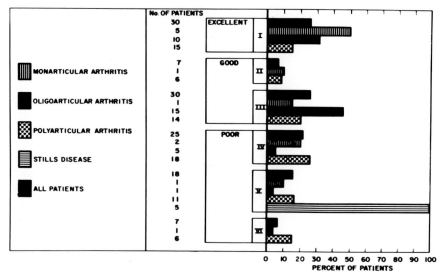

Figure 9.28. The patients with monarticular arthritis tended to have good to excellent recovery, whereas those with polyarticular arthritis and Still's disease tended to end up in the poor category.

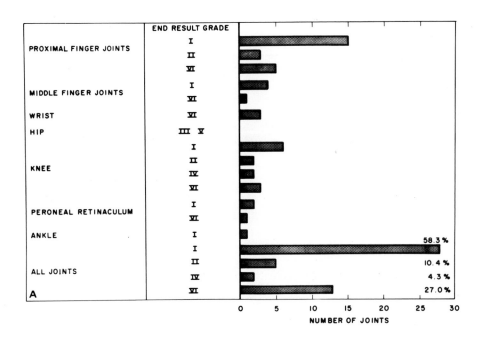

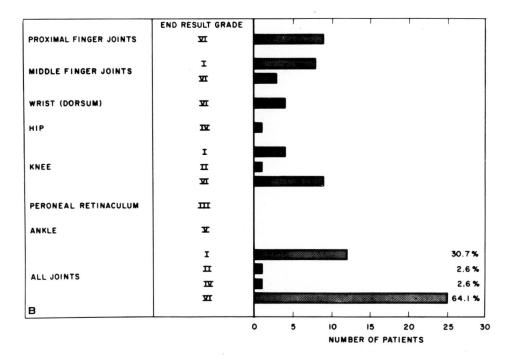

Figure 9.29. (*A*) Patients having synovectomy alone got considerably more relief from the surgery than those patients having synovectomy and debridement (*B*) obviously necessitated by considerable joint destruction.

No. PATIENTS	TYPE	PATIENTS TREATED	I 30	II 7	III 30	IV 25	V 18	VI 7
10	MONARTICULAR ARTHRITIS	0 / 0%						
32	OLIGOARTICULAR ARTHRITIS	1 / 3.1%			1			
70	POLYARTICULAR ARTHRITIS	12 / 17.1%		1	1	2	8	
5	STILL'S DISEASE	3 / 60%					3	
117	ALL PATIENTS	16 / 13.7%	0	1	2	2	11	0
			EXC.	GOOD		POOR		

Figure 9.30. Patients treated with corticosteroids had little else in the way of therapy and ended up largely in the poor category.

No. PATIENTS	TYPE	PATIENTS WITH NO TREATMENT	I 30	II 7	III 30	IV 25	V 18	VI 7
10	MONARTICULAR ARTHRITIS	1 / 10%				1		
32	OLIGOARTICULAR ARTHRITIS	6 / 18.7%	4	1	1			
70	POLYARTICULAR ARTHRITIS	9 / 12.9%	4		5			
5	STILL'S DISEASE	0 / 0%						
117	ALL PATIENTS	16 / 13.7%	8	1	6	1	0	0
			EXC.	GOOD		POOR		

Figure 9.31. Patients having no therapy ended up quite well and were almost exclusively in the excellent to good category. They obviously appeared to need less clinically, but some had polyarticular involvement.

References

1. Bywaters, E. G. L., and Ansell, B. B.: Monarticular arthritis in children, Ann. Rheum. Dis., 24: 116, 1965.
2. Calabro, J. J., and Marchesano, J. M.: The early natural history of juvenile rheumatoid arthritis; a 10-year followup of 100 cases, Med. Clin. North Am., 52: 567, 1968.
3. Cassidy, J. T., Brody, G. L., and Martel, W.: Monarticular juvenile rheumatoid arthritis, J. Pediatr., 70: 867, 1967.
4. Edstrom, G.: Rheumatoid arthritis and Still's disease in children; survey of 161 cases, Arthritis Rheum., 1: 497, 1958.
5. Edstrom, G., and Gedda, P. L.: Clinic and prognosis of rheumatoid arthritis in children, Acta Rheum. Scand., 3: 129, 1957.
6. Eyring, E. J.: Synovectomy in juvenile rheumatoid arthritis, J. Bone Joint Surg., 53A: 638, 1971.
7. Fink, C. W., Baum, J., Paradies, L. H., and Carrell, B. C.: Synovectomy in juvenile rheumatoid arthritis, Ann. Rheum. Dis., 28: 612, 1969.
8. Griffin, P. P., Tachdjian, M. O. and Green, W. T.: Pauciarticular arthritis in children, J.A.M.A., 184: 23, 1963.
9. Kampner, S. L., and Ferguson, A. B., Jr.: Juvenile rheumatoid arthritis; disease course and comparison of therapeutic regimens, J. Bone Joint Surg., 53A: 1029, 1971.
10. Kampner, S. L., and Ferguson, A. B., Jr.: Efficacy of synovectomy in juvenile rheumatoid arthritis, Clin. Orthop., 88: 94, 1972.
11. Laaksonen, A. L.: A prognostic study of juvenile rheumatoid arthritis; analysis of 544 cases, Acta Paediatr. Scand., 166 (Suppl.): 1966.
12. Lindbjerg, I. F.: Juvenile rheumatoid arthritis; followup of 75 cases, Arch. Dis. Child., 39: 576, 1964.
13. Ragan, C.: Intermittent hydrarthrosis, In Arthritis and Allied Conditions, Hollander, J. L. (ed.), pp. 755–758; Philadelphia: Lea & Febiger, 1966.
14. Steinbrocker, O., Traeger, C. H., and Batterman, R. C.: Therapeutic criteria in rheumatoid arthritis, J.A.M.A., 140: 659, 1949.
15. Still, G. F.: On a form of chronic joint disease in children. Med. Chir. Tr., 80: 47, 1897.
16. Sury, N.: Rheumatoid Arthritis in Children: A Clinical Study; Copenhagen: Munksgaard, 1952.

17. Wissler, V. H.: Subsepsis allergica, *Helv. Paediatr. Acta,* 13: 405, 1958.

GENERALIZED AFFECTIONS

Fibrous Dysplasia

Fibrous dysplasia is a disease entity which may involve one or many bones. It may be combined with abnormal pigmentation of the skin, precocious sexual development, and early skeletal maturation. Still other endocrine-based abnormalities may be present, and there may be various combinations of effects and areas of bony involvement in any one case.

The disease seems to be a developmental defect. It is most common in childhood but may occur in adults; the adult lesion tends to be monostotic. It is a widespread anomaly of skeletal development that ranks next to multiple exostoses in incidence. It is more common in the female.

CLINICAL PICTURE

The disease may exist in various forms from the clinical point of view. It seems possible to divide it into three general types.

I. Involvement of Single Bone. The lesion is usually insidious in its onset unless a weight-bearing bone is involved, in which case it may lead to pain and limp. Rib, clavicle, maxilla, tibia, or femur have all been involved in this monostotic form, which comprises approximately one-third of the reported cases (Fig. 9.32). Limitation of joint motion may be present should areas such as the femoral neck be involved. Expansion of the bone and local tenderness may be evident on examination. A pathologic fracture may first bring the patient to medical attention.

II. Lesions in Several Bones. Skin pigmentation of the café au lait type may or may not be present. About 35% of the 90 cases in the literature summarized by Lichtenstein and Jaffe[1] showed a noticeable cutaneous pigmentation.

III. Multiple Lesions. Pigmentation of the skin and precocious puberty mark these cases, which represent the most severe form of the disease. Cases in which the lesions tend to remain unilateral may be regarded as less severe than those in which the lesions are widespread. The more severe forms are found in very young children and infants, and involvement of the skull is common. This form of disease may lead to serious deformities and crippling, and there may be repeated pathologic fractures in the past history.

Only the female seems to be subject to precocious puberty with this disease. Rarely, hyperthyroidism has also been found to accompany the bone lesions. The laboratory findings have usually been within normal limits except that the serum alkaline phosphatase has occasionally been elevated beyond that expected for the age.

ROENTGEN FINDINGS

Areas of decreased density appear in the bone (Figs. 9.33 and 9.34). The involved area has a ground glass appearance which decreases the contrast with the surrounding bone and aids in distinguishing the lesion from a single bone cyst. The lesion spares the epiphyses.

With growth the cortex may become attenuated and expanded. As involvement becomes more generalized, the entire long bone reveals the thinned cortex and fine trabeculae somewhat reminiscent of osteogenesis imperfecta. There may be bone deformity secondary to previous fractures. Generalized involvement of the bone, rather than localized cystlike areas, may become the most striking feature. Rapid extension of the condition is not characteristic. Indeed many localized lesions have been observed to be dormant for years.

Sclerosis of any marked degree about the lesions is not characteristic. In the generalized disease, the base of the skull may appear sclerotic, however. There is, in addition, replacement of normal contrasting bone by areas of "ground glass" appearance in varying portions of the remainder of the skull.

PATHOLOGY

Lichtenstein and Jaffe[1] have been responsible for clarifying the pathology of this condition under the heading fibrous dysplasia. When a localized lesion is approached surgically, the cortex overlying it is frequently found to be eroded from the medullary side and more vascular than normal.

The contents of the area consist of a firm, compressible tissue that is generally whitish but has occasional red specks. The tissue is primarily connective tissue that is perhaps gritty to cut if bone formation is prevalent within it; it occasionally contains areas of cartilage. This tissue may form virtually all of the medullary portion of the bone (Fig. 9.35). Rarely, some cystic softening of this tissue may be encountered.

Microscopically such tissue is composed of small, spindle-shaped cells in a loose and whorled arrangement. The cellularity varies considerably. Scattered irregularly in this tissue may be primitive osseous elements formed by metaplasia of the connective tissue. This osseous tissue is atypically calcified or frankly osteoid. The tissue tends to be avascular except in highly cellular areas. Small islands of hyaline cartilage may also be found. The presence of the cartilage foci aids the certainty of the diagnosis.

TREATMENT

Although the disease, particularly in severe forms, tends to begin in infancy and childhood, it is the general rule that the patient will survive into adulthood. A surgical attack of an isolated lesion with curettage and replacement of the area with bone chips is ususlly followed by eradication of the lesion. In the more florid and widespread form of the disease, surgery is reserved for those lesions which by location or extent are a source of clinical trouble. In widespread areas, as pointed out by Strassburger, Garber, and Hallock, the repair process may fall before the spread of the lesion, and the bone chips may be resorbed.

Isolated lesions may be attacked for diagnosis, but it should be remembered that, with

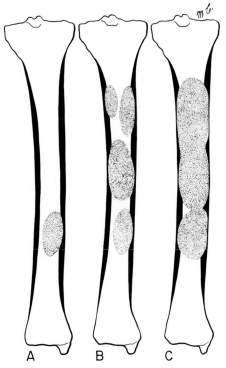

Figure 9.32. The development of fibrous dysplasia in bone. In (A) and (B), the single lesion is followed by multiple foci. At (C) the lesions have coalesced to give the scalloped appearance of the cortex that is characteristic of fibrous dysplasia.

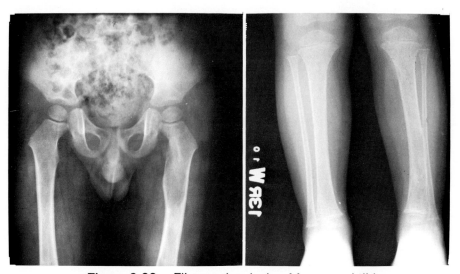

Figure 9.33. Fibrous dysplasia of femur and tibia.

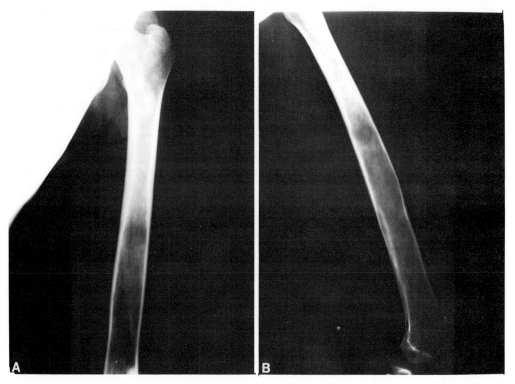

Figure 9.34. Appearance of the femur in a 35-year-old woman. Femur shows multiple foci, widened medullary canal, and is scalloped. (*A*) Anteroposterior view of proximal femur; (*B*) lateral view of distal femur.

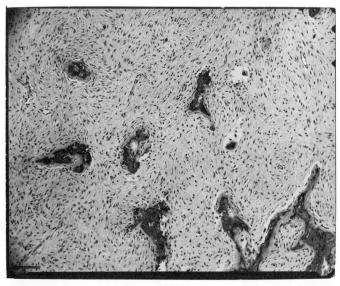

Figure 9.35. Replacement of medullary cavity contents in bone by proliferating fibrous tissue and osteoid in fibrous dysplasia.

cessation of growth, the lesion appears to diminish in activity and to become dormant.

Reference

1. Lichenstein, W., and Jaffe, H.: Fibrous dysplasia of bone, Arch. Pathol., 33: 777, 1942.

Osteopetrosis

This condition was described by Albers-Schönberg in 1904. It is characterized by a homogeneous opacity of the bones, obliteration of the marrow cavities, and a tendency toward loss of trabecular structure. The bones may be abnormally fragile. An accompanying myelophthisic anemia is the rule.

The disease is rare and has been found in both male and female. There is a strong familial tendency. It has been found in fetuses as well as in children and adults. The cause is unknown.

The disease in childhood is progressive, and anemia, hemorrhage, and infection usually lead to an early fatal outcome. Some cases run a more benign course, and with adulthood the disease tends to become stationary. According to Nussey, the condition is benign when it is inherited and malignant when there is consanguinity of the parents.

The children tend to be retarded in all phases of development, and a degree of dwarfism is usually present. In addition to the anemia, optic atrophy, deafness, and facial or ocular palsy are often found. The blood chemistry does not show any characteristic changes, although the serum calcium is occasionally raised. Analysis of the bones indicates an increased calcium and phosphorus content.

Cohen[1] reviewed the pathology of this disease and found all bones of the skeleton affected. Membranous bones showed changes analogous to the changes of cartilaginous ones. Cartilage cell columns continued to mature, but there was a disturbance of the normal sequences of resorption of the primary spongiosa. Thus there appeared to be a great quantity of unresorbed cartilage matrix upon which the usual process of deposition of bone and osteoid continued even though the matrix was not resorbed.

Fractures heal at an unusually rapid rate, but there is marked delay in the remodeling sequences associated with growth (Figs. 9.36 and 9.37). There is no tubular marrow cavity. The cartilage and bone matrix appear well calcified, but there are large areas of osteoid formation. Cohen noted that the transverse lines in the metaphyses of osteopetrosic bone were fractures in various stages of healing.

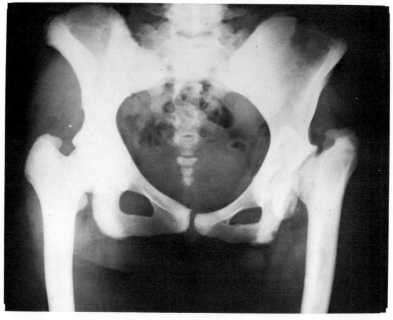

Figure 9.36.   Osteopetrosis with pathologic fracture of the femoral neck.

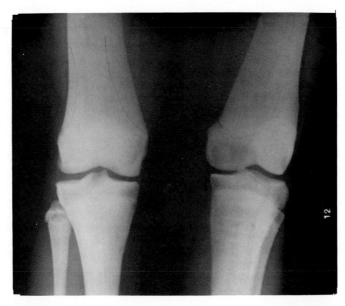

Figure 9.37. Osteopetrosis in which remodeling of the metaphyseal areas of the femur and tibia is hindered.

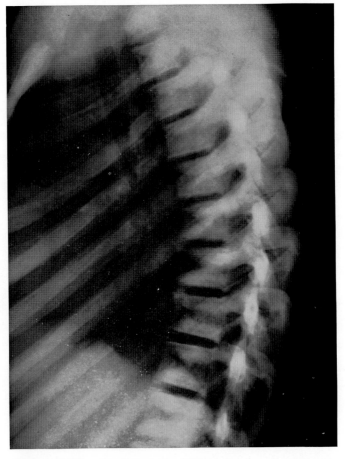

Figure 9.38. Involvement of the spine in osteopetrosis.

By x-ray the bones appear to have an increased opacity and loss of structure within their outline (Fig. 9.38). The metaphyses show a failure of remodeling that makes them clubbed or boxelike. Transverse dense lines are frequently apparent, and they occasionally separate metaphysis from diaphysis. The skull shows an increased density that is most marked at the base.

The bones appear solid on cross section and gray-white in color. No fatty marrow is seen. The trabeculae are increased in number and thickness. Some nodules of cartilage may persist among the trabeculae. As Cohen suggests, the delay in remodeling results in the formation of chondro-osseous complexes and the absence of a marrow cavity, and it may also account for the clubbed metaphyses.

The treatment involves around aid for the every present anemia, which may vary in severity and be characterized by exacerbations and remissions. The child with exceptionally fragile bones is frequently seen with fractures. The duration of immobilization should be shorter than that normally used. No cure for the fundamental condition is known.

References

1. Cohen, J.: Osteopetrosis: case report, autopsy findings, and pathological interpretation; failure of treatment with vitamin A, *J. Bone Joint Surg.*, *33A:* 923, 1951.
2. Kramer, B., Yuska, H., and Steiner, M.: Marble bones. II. Chemical analysis: Albers-Schoenberg disease (marble bones), report of a case and morphologic study, *Am. J. Pathol.*, *23:* 755, 1947.
3. VanCreveld, S., and Heybrock, N.: On Albers-Schoenberg disease (marble bones), *Acta Paediatr.*, *27:* 462, 1939.

OSTEOGENESIS IMPERFECTA

The most severe form of this rare disease occurs prenatally and may cause fractures and deformities to develop in utero. A second and less severe form appears postnatally and causes mechanical weakness of the bones and blue sclerae. The disease affects both sexes but is slightly more common in females (Fig. 9.39).

While the outlook for survival is poor in the hereditary prenatal case, an individual infant may survive many months even with a very severe case. Patients with milder cases may survive into adult life. A tendency to improve is frequently seen. Postnatal cases may have only an occasional fracture and a

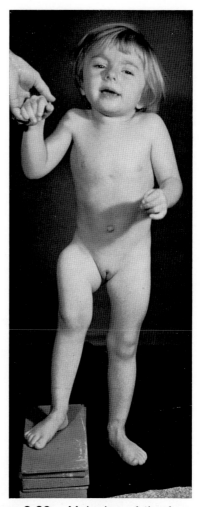

Figure 9.39. Malunion of the femur and secondary shortening of the limb in osteogenesis imperfecta.

full life expectancy, although severe cases are seen in this group also. The etiology is unknown. The inheritance is a Mendelian dominant.

Bauze's Classification

Bauze summarized his findings in 42 patients and divided them into three categories. In the mild category (22) there was no long bone deformity. In the moderate category (3) there was mild long bone deformity. There were 17 cases in the severe category with severe long bone deformity.

MILD

The family history is prominent. The age of onset averaged 3½ years but ran from 1–25 years. Females were 3 times more affected than males. Fractures were relatively infrequent, averaging 8.

Ligamentous laxity was common. All had blue sclerae. Deafness was common, but scoliosis and dentinogenesis imperfecta were uncommon.

Fractures were few and late in appearing, and disability was virtually nonexistent.

SEVERE

The family history is uncommon. Few had blue sclerae, but most of the patients developed scoliosis. The disability was severe, deafness was uncommon, and dentinogenesis imperfecta was common.

The fractures appeared early and were frequent. Males predominated. The average age of onset was 15 months, but ran from birth to 11 years. Hyperplastic callus was seen only in this group.

Collagen Deficiency. If one continues the categorization into those with mild deformity and those with severe deformity and disability, some interesting observations could be made relative to collagen. In the mild group, the amount of collagen was depressed, accounting for the blue sclerae in this group. The stability of the structural collagen as distinct from soluble collagen was normal in the mild group. The severe group exhibited a normal amount of collagen (few blue sclerae) but with very unstable cross linkage of the structural collagen.

Clinical Picture

Another name for this disease, fragilitas ossium, gives a clue to its dominant clinical characteristic. It is the fractures of the skeleton that bring the patient to medical attention

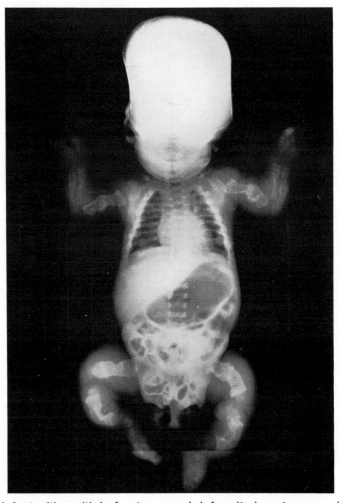

Figure 9.40. Infant with multiple fractures and deformity in osteogenesis imperfecta.

(Fig. 9.40). The relaxation of the joint capsules and the blue sclerae that frequently accompany the condition are noted secondarily. The musculature is frequently loose, elastic, and diminished in volume.

Osteosclerosis may occur in patients who survive into adult life. According to Bickel et al.,[1] it most commonly accompanies the hereditary type of the disease. Otosclerosis has also been found in adults who have blue scleritis without evidence of bone fragility.

Victims of the more severe cases exhibit diminished growth to the point of dwarfism. The skull is unusually broad and has prominent occipital and parietal bosses. The teeth in childhood are poorly calcified and translucent. Blood chemistry values have not been found of diagnostic value.

Pathology

The most striking finding on bone section is the sparse distribution and the thin, frail nature of the bone trabeculae. The cortex is poorly formed. The trabeculae are frequently osteoid (Fig. 9.41). Islands of cartilage are seen, and the medulla is in part fibrous or fat containing. The number of osteoblasts is frequently deficient.

Roentgen Findings

The mild group exhibits a minor modeling defect of the long bone. By contrast the severe group has bones that are obviously severely affected by their environment. This results in a host of patterns all part of a severe functional defect. Some bones are wide with wide medullary canals and thin cortices. Others end up with needle thin wavy bones with the cortex there but the medullary canal by contrast still thinner to result occasionally in only a thin radiolucent line representing the medullary cavity. Cystic metaphyses are seen giving rise to a soap bubble appearance. In this group massive wads of hyperplastic callus are seen.

The most common type of bone seen is thinned and has a diminished trabeculation and slender cortices. Various degrees and

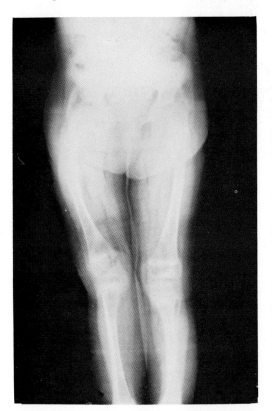

Figure 9.41. Older child with thin cortices in fragilitas ossium (osteogenesis imperfecta) and with fracture of femoral diaphysis.

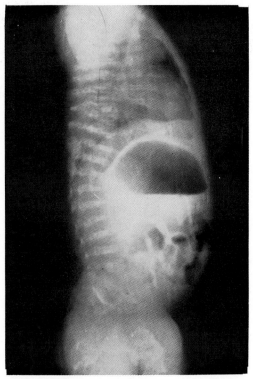

Figure 9.42. Compression of vertebrae in osteogenesis imperfecta.

types of deformity, depending on the past history, may be seen. Many transverse lines are present in the metaphysis. The ossification of the skull is imperfect and patchy. The fibula may be a mere thin line. The vertebrae may be compressed and biconcave owing to the pressure of the interventing vertebral discs (Figs. 9.42 and 9.43).

Fairbank[3] has differentiated a type in which the major long bones are short and widened but still have excessively thin cortices. Fractures, as well as the deformity, are frequently seen.

Healing of Fracture

The fractures in general tend to heal, although nonunion and delayed union have been seen. Some patients tend to put out a very hyperplastic callus containing a "chondroid tissue."

Treatment

The physician must tread a delicate line in treating fractures in victims of this disease. Prolonged immobilization leads to further atrophy of bone and the resultant hazard of further fracture in convalescence. Insufficient immobilization leads to bowing, which is per-

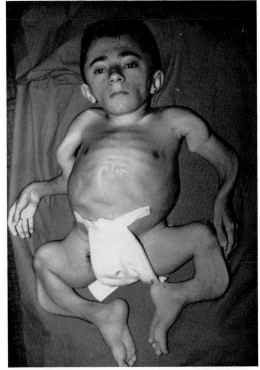

Figure 9.44. Osteogenesis imperfecta in an adult. These completely disabling deformities speak for themselves. Great effort is justified to prevent a patient from arriving at such a minimal functional opportunity in life.

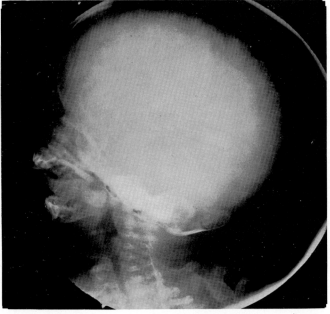

Figure 9.43. Skull with wormian bone pattern visible in fragilitas ossium (osteogenesis imperfecta).

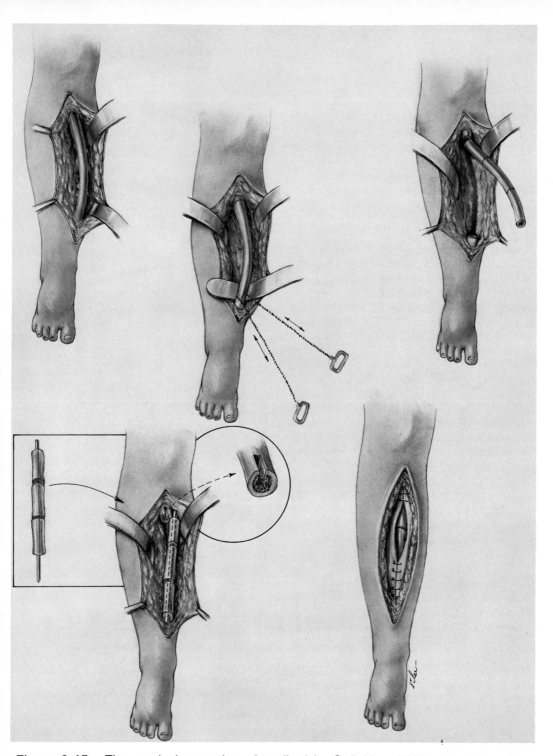

Figure 9.45. The surgical procedure described by Sofield and Millar is designed to maintain activity in patients with osteogenesis imperfecta who have severe deformity. The bowed bone represents an engineering structural weakness additionally predisposing to fracture. Correction of the tibia with excessive bowing is illustrated. (Redrawn from H. A. Sofield and E. A. Millar: Intramedullary fixation of deformities of the long bones, *Journal of Bone and Joint Surgery, 41A:* 1372, 1959.) The bowed tibia is stripped of its periosteal cuff, keeping it intact. The diaphysis is then divided at either end and made into segments. When the metal rod is placed through these segments, it is possible to insert its projecting tip into the distal medullary canal. In order to place it proximally and still maintain length, it is often necessary to make a small slot in the cortex of the proximal metaphysis. The projecting tip proximally can then be lain into the medullary canal.

mitted by the soft callus. Because muscle tone is generally poor, for children who are relatively inactive and light in weight the time of immobilization can be shortened without interfering with alignment. Healing in deformity almost inevitably results in refracture.

Medical measures undertaken with a view toward providing a stronger and better calcified skeletal system have proved of little avail.

Sofield and Millar[6] reported in 1959 on 80 operations involving 22 patients with severe deformity of the long bones caused by osteogenesis imperfecta. The age of the patients, in the main, was between 2 and 8 years. The procedure followed since 1948 seems to be a great aid in preventing recurring fractures and in procuring mobilization of the patient.

According to this technique, a subperiosteal exposure of the shaft of the long bone involved is made (Figs. 9.45 and 9.46). An osteotomy at the proximal and distal metaphyses follows, and the shaft is removed. The shaft is then divided into the smallest number of fragments that can be threaded on a straight metal rod. It is not necessary to keep the fragments in order because they serve as a scaffolding to hold the periosteum in the shape of the new bone to be formed. The projecting end of the rod is bent to prevent migration, and the distal end approaches the distal epiphyseal line. It is often necessary to insert the rod in retrograde fashion, thread on the fragments, and then drive it into the distal metaphyseal fragment. The periosteum is closed over these fragments as completely as possible. The limb is then immobilized in plaster for approximately 6–8 weeks.

As the child grows, it is common for the distal epiphysis to become well removed from the end of the rod. A longer rod may have to be inserted to prevent refracture, which has occurred distal to the rod.

Anyone who has struggled to attain weight bearing for these children and to rehabilitate them among children of their own age group appreciates the breaking of the vicious cycle of discouraging periods of non-weight bearing, fracture, and further atrophy of the bone. Our own experience with this procedure has borne out Sofield's list of its advantages: (1) the frequency of fractures is reduced, and pain is diminished; (2) deformities are corrected; and (3) normal use, particularly of weight-bearing extremities, is achieved.

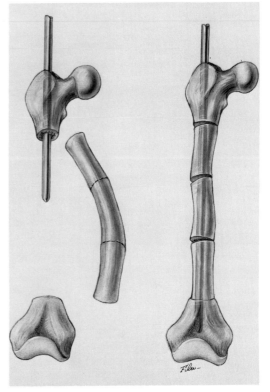

Figure 9.46. In the femur the bowing is similarly straightened by dividing into segments. The metal rod can be driven retrograde fashion into the proximal segment, and then the additional segments are placed on the rod. The rod is further driven into the distal segment.

References

1. Bickel, W. H., Ghormley, R. K., and Camp, J. D.: Osteogenesis imperfecta, *Radiology,* 40: 145, 1943.
2. Fairbank, H. A. T.: Osteogenesis imperfecta, *Proc. R. Soc. Med.,* 23: 1263, 1930.
3. Fairbank, H. A. T.: Hyperplastic callus formation with or without evidence of fracture in osteogenesis imperfecta, *Br. J. Surg.,* 36: 1, 1948.
4. Fleming, B. L., Radasch, H. E., and Williams, T.: Osteogenesis imperfecta, *J. Bone Joint Surg.,* 19: 725, 1937.
5. Pelner, H., and Cohen, J. N.: Osteogenesis imperfecta tarda, *Am. J. Roentgenol.,* 61: 690, 1949.
6. Sofield, H. A., and Millar, E. A.: Fragmentation, realignment, and intramedullary rod fixation of deformities of the long bones in children (a 10-year appraisal), *J. Bone Joint Surg.,* 41A: 1371, 1959.
7. Wright, P. B., Gernstetter, S. L., and Greenblatt, R. B.: Therapeutic acceleration of bone age in osteogenesis imperfecta, *J. Bone Joint Surg.,* 33A: 939, 1951.
8. Wyatt, T. C., and McEachen, T. H.: Congenital bone dysplasia (osteogenesis imperfecta) associated with

lesions of the parathyroid glands, *Am. J. Dis. Child.,* 43: 403, 1932.

OSTEOPATHIA STRIATA

At this writing 6 cases have been described in the literature, 3 in one family. Occasionally osteochondromas have been found accompanying this anomaly, which is principally a radiographic finding.

Voorhoeve described the radiographic findings in 1924. The linear streaks appearing in the bone are not easily explained because they involve the metaphysis and diaphysis but also extend through into the epiphysis. The cortex appears normal. The striated appearance appears to be a thickening of the medullary trabeculae in long streaklike aberrations (Fig. 9.47). If there is abnormality of the cortex, it is hidden from the x-ray view.

Attempts to relate this condition to other conditions such as osteopoikilosis and Engelmann's disease do not seem well founded either from a radiographic or clinical point of view.

There are no symptoms, and this condition must be classified as a skeletal anomaly not affecting either the shape, form, or function of the skeleton.

Reference

1. Hurt, R. L.: Osteopathia striata, *J. Bone Joint Surg.,* 35B: 89, 1953.

MAFFUCCI'S SYNDROME (MULTIPLE CARTILAGE TUMORS ASSOCIATED WITH HEMANGIOMAS OF THE EXTREMITY)

In Maffucci's original patient, whom he described in 1881,[4] there were multiple bony hard masses of the forearm found in a 40-year-old woman. Hemangiomas overlaid these masses but were not necessarily in direct association with them. This patient ultimately died of the consequences of a malignant transformation of a tumor of the scapula.

Patients involved with the lesions associated with this syndrome tend to be of short stature with the principal involvement occurring in the hands and feet. The bones involved become so riddled with cartilage growth that the remaining bony septa fracture easily, leading to deformity. An important secondary complication is malignant transformation to chondrosarcoma—an incidence of 14 of 75 cases (18.6%) when reviewed by Elmore and Cantrell.[2] There is no evidence of a genetic or familial control. It is well established that mothers with this involvement can give birth to normal children.

In children who will ultimately develop Maffucci's syndrome no abnormality is noted at birth. There is no sex predilection. Sometime prior to adolescence, nodules of bony involvement of the extremities may occur in an irregular and asymmetrical manner. A unilateral involvement is slightly more frequent than bilateral.

After the second decade the tumor growth becomes quiescent unless transformation occurs.

A complication of the clinical course is the easy fracturing of a heavily involved bone.

X-ray Examination

The roentgenogram can reveal patchy areas of calcification associated with hemangiomas in the soft-tissue masses. The bony involvement is quite different than that seen in Ollier's disease. In that disease the cartilage areas tend to be linear and progress down the metaphysis from the epiphyseal line. The long bones are shortened with widened flaring metaphyses.

In Maffucci's syndrome the areas of cartilage involvement are rounded, involve a given area of the bone completely, and break through the cortex to give rise to a tumerous growth forming a mass which is quite distinct. These areas are multiple and not related in so obvious a fashion to the epiphyseal line. The peripheral location of the most marked involvement—the small bones of the hand and feet—is striking, with involvement progressively less frequent toward the trunk, although any one mass of cartilage may reach a large size.

Pathology

The cartilage masses in the bone are gray-white, shiny, and discrete with occasional

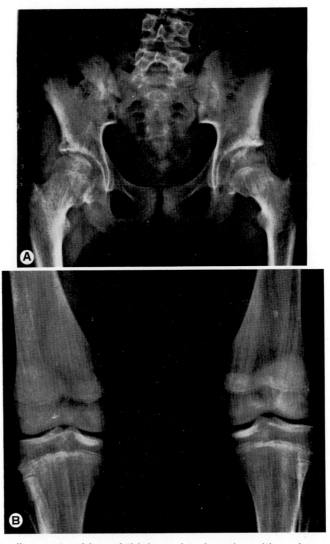

Figure 9.47. The linear streaking of thickened trabeculae although most prominent in the metaphysis at the hip (*A*) and knee (*B*). The appearance gives rise to the designation osteopathia striata.

joining into large sheets. The cartilage is very cellular and disorganized in its arrangement of cells. The hemangiomas are cavernous in type with phlebectasia and frequent thromboses.

Treatment

Recognition of fractures with minimal trauma should be part of the education of the patient so that treatment may avoid deformity. Masses are removed that are unsightly or heavily involving a bone to the point of making its integrity precarious. Malignant transformation is common enough to warrant frequent surveillance. Occasionally masses and deformity that are sufficiently gross to warrant amputation may present when the patient is first seen.

References

1. Bean, W. B.: Dyschondroplasm and hemangiomata (Maffucci's syndrome), *A. M. A. Arch. Intern. Med.*, *102:* 544, 1958.
2. Elmore, S. M., and Cantrell, W. C. Maffucci's syndrome, *J. Bone Joint Surg.*, *48A:* 1607, 1966.
3. Johnson, T. L., Webster, J. R., and Sippy, H. J.: Maffucci's syndrome, *Am. J. Med.*, *28:* 866, 1960.
4. Maffucci, A.: Di un coso di encondroma ed angioma multiple. Contribuzioni ala genesi embrionale dei tumor movimento, *Med. Chir.*, *25-3:* 399, 1881.

CHAPTER 10

Affections of Muscle

PSEUDOHYPERTROPHIC MUSCULAR DYSTROPHY

Pseudohypertrophic muscular dystrophy, a progressive condition of loss of muscle function, is seen quite commonly in orthopaedic clinics. It is a primary myopathy. The cases are often hidden among patients reporting because of flat feet.

The disease is often familial, and its frequent incidence in male siblings is familiar. The onset usually takes place before the age of 6. The weakness is symmetric and progressive, and it is featured by enlargement of muscle groups, most strikingly those of the calf (Fig. 10.1). At the same time, or slightly later, atrophy about the shoulder girdle may be noted.

Its incidence was reported as 4 per 100,000 for North Carolina.

The Duchenne type occurs almost entirely in males and the onset is usually in the first 4 years of life—coming into clinical notice at about that time. The transmission is sex-linked recessive, and the mutation rate is high. Landouzy and Déjérine[6] described muscular dystrophy of the facial, pectoral, and shoulder-girdle muscles. Erb[5] reported a condition with limb-girdle dystrophy and little or no facial involvement. The latter two types occur in both sexes.

The onset of the facioscapulohumeral type may arise symptomatically from early childhood to late adult life. Transmission is by an autosomal dominant gene. Involvement may be very mild. The limb-girdle type occurs in both sexes with an onset of symptoms usually in the first 3 decades of life.

Pseudohypertrophic muscular dystrophy is often familial and has a frequent incidence in male siblings. The weakness is symmetric and progressive and is featured by enlargement of muscle groups, most strikingly those of the calf. Mild cases may be found first presenting because of flat feet.

Etiology

The theory that there is an underlying involvement of the central nervous system has not been substantiated. A familial history can usually be obtained. The muscle defect causing the atrophy is unknown, but it is conceded to be hereditary.

Progressive muscular dystrophy is an inherited disease with various modes of transmission, but spontaneous occurrence accounts for approximately one-third of the cases. There are various disturbances of the enzyme systems concerned with muscle metabolism, but it is not clear that they are primary.

Clinical Picture

The onset is insidious, and the symptoms are first noted in the 3–7 age group. That the patient is weak is usually not appreciated by the family. Difficulty in climbing stairs, easy fatigue, or flattening of the arch of the foot may be a complaint.

The pseudohypertrophic type is more common in males. The feet are pronated, and contracture of the gastrocnemius is noted early in the development of the disease. Difficulty in the gait, such as stumbling and frequent falls, is noted. The calves are enlarged and have a doughy feel on palpation, not the hard feel of normal muscle. The child placed on the floor arises by aiding extension of the knee by the quadriceps with the hand. He then extends the hips by pushing further on the thigh.

Atrophy of the shoulder girdle, particularly the pectorals, may be noted on palpation. Muscle test reveals diminished muscle power, particularly in the quadriceps and proximal limb muscles, until late in the disease.

The facioscapulohumeral type of Landouzy-Déjérine is marked by early involve-

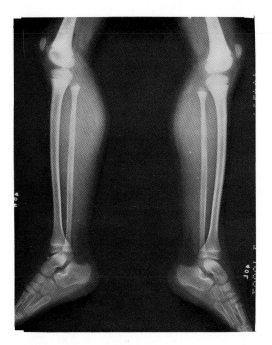

unit potentials, many of which become polyphasic and of short duration. No fibrillation potentials are seen. Nerve conduction velocities are normal.

On palpation the hypertrophic muscles feel firm and rubbery. The atrophic muscles are often difficult to feel on account of the overlying fat. The involvement of the muscles is symmetric. Abnormal movements are not present, and fibrillary twitchings of the muscles occur only rarely. Pseudohypertrophy may precede atrophy, or atrophy may develop in muscles never hypertrophied.

The sensory examination is normal, and there are no sphincter disturbances. The deep reflexes may be lost early in the course of the disease or they may persist in atrophied muscle. Cutaneous reflexes are preserved and the plantar responses are usually flexor.

Figure 10.1. Roentgenogram of the calf enlargement with streaks of fat density. Enlargement is limited initially to the area of the calf.

ment of the muscles of the face, which gives a masklike, dull expression. Expression remains about the eyes longer than elsewhere in the face, although difficulty is experienced in closing the eyes. The lower lip hangs down and out. Atrophy of the shoulder girdle and arms is marked. Later there is involvement of the pelvic girdle.

In the juvenile scapulohumeral form of Erb,[5] atrophy of the shoulder girdle is the first form (Fig. 10.2). The onset is later than that of the early childhood type; the disease begins in pseudohypertrophic muscular dystrophy (Fig. 10.3) and usually occurs in the teen-age group. The reflexes are absent in muscle that are severely involved.

Late forms of muscular dystrophy with pelvic girdle atrophy shows a gluteus maximus and medius limp. Scoliosis and trunk weakness are found and are progressive, even in those patients confined to a wheelchair.

There is also an increase in the amount of creatine secreted in the urine. The electromyogram is of considerable value in diagnosis. The pattern of voluntary effort recorded by means of concentric needle electrodes is characterized by a disintegration of motor

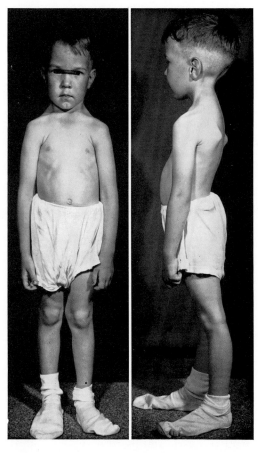

Figure 10.2. Scapulohumeral form of muscular dystrophy.

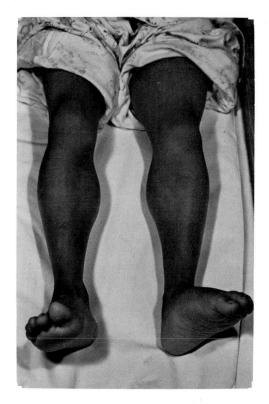

Figure 10.3. Enlargement of the calves in pseudohypertrophic muscular dystrophy.

Serum Enzymes in Muscular Dystrophy

The diagnosis of muscular dystrophy has been helped recently by serum enzyme studies, notably creatine kinase and aldolase. Of these the most striking is creatine kinase; this is particularly true in the Duchenne type of muscular dystrophy.

Creatine kinase is present primarily in skeletal muscle, and reversibility transfers a phosphate group from creatine phosphate to adenosine diphosphate. The average normal level is 2 units (per mole of creatine formed per hour per milliliter of serum). Values have ranged up to several hundred units in muscular drystrophy. The evidence points to an abnormality of metabolism as the cause of the leakage of this enzyme according to Ebashi, Toyokura, Momoi, and Sugita[4] in 1959.

Female carriers of the Duchenne type of dystrophy have also been found to have elevated levels. The proportion showing an elevated serum aldolase has been smaller.

The enzyme aldolase is present in most tissues and is a catalytic agent in one of the steps of glucose breakdown, namely, the splitting of fructose 1,6-diphosphate. Although normally found at levels less than 10 Bruns units, figures over 100 have been found. Principal values are found early in the disease, with lesser values found as the disease progresses. Less marked values have been found in adult dystrophy. A rise has been reported in polymyositis and dermatomyositis, but only rarely and low in neuromuscular disease.

Both these enzymes offer a nice distinction between neural atrophy and primary myopathy.

Pearson[8] found a rise before clinical signs of weakness were evident. He also found evidence of widespread histologic changes before the clinical disease was evident.

Increased serum levels of aldolase, creatine phosphokinase (CPK), lactic dehydrogenase, phosphohexoisomerase, and transaminase have been reported. Serum enzyme levels, especially CPK, are most consistently elevated in the early stages of the Duchenne variety of muscular dystrophy. Detection of the disease in the preclinical stage of Duchenne's dystrophy can be made by determination of the serum enzymes, and detection of the carrier state in unaffected females is manifested by an increase in the serum CPK and aldolase.

Pathology

The essential muscle changes are similar in all types of dystrophy. The gastrocnemius in a marked case of hypertrophy looks fatty. The muscle color varies from pale grayish to yellowish.

There is considerable variation in fiber size, fatty replacement, and connective tissue invasion of the muscle. Swelling of the fiber is apparently the first change.

Sarcolemmic nuclei are increased in number and may be increased in size. In some forms of dystrophy, the nuclei may occupy a central position in the fiber. Denny-Brown[3] has noted that the biopsy site, if rebiopsied 10–14 days later, exhibits such degenerative changes as loss of myofibrils without evidence of regeneration of muscle buds. In later cases vascular and granular degeneration of the fibers is found. Changes in sensory and motor nerve fibers are not seen. Changes late in the disease are relatively minor and do not point toward a neural atrophy.

Differential Diagnosis

Progressive muscular dystrophy must be distinguished from the diseases of infancy and childhood which are accompanied by muscular wasting (Table 10.1). The atypical adult-onset cases must be distinguished from diseases of adult life accompanied by muscular wasting.

Infantile muscular atrophy is recognized by its onset in infancy, the presence of fibrillations, and the rapidly fatal course.

Myotonic muscular dystrophy is distinguished from the cases of muscular dystrophy of relatively late onset by the absence of pseudohypertrophy and by the presence of myotonia, cataracts, testicular atrophy, and early baldness.

Peroneal muscular atrophy may be confused with the rare cases of progressive muscular atrophy with an unusual degree of atrophy in the distal portion of the extremities, especially the legs. The presence of cutaneous sensory loss or impairment of the proprioceptive senses should establish the diagnosis of peroneal muscular atrophy.

Amyotrophic lateral sclerosis is distinguished by the extensive degree of atrophy in the distal parts of the extremities, the fibrillary twitchings, hyperactive reflexes, and by the absence of hypertrophy.

In infectious polyneuritis the muscular weakness may occasionally be greatest in the girdle muscles. The acute onset of the symptoms, the increased cerebrospinal fluid protein, and the subsequent regression of symptoms establish the diagnosis.

Pseudohypertropy of the muscles may occasionally be seen with syringomyelia, but other features should leave no doubt about the diagnosis.

The differential diagnosis between myositis or dermatomyositis and progressive muscular dystrophy can be made by biopsy of the affected muscles.

Treatment

A specific treatment to stop the progress of the disease has not been found. Various medications have been thought helpful, at least for periods in the patient's course. These include glycine taken by mouth and subcutaneous injections of epinephrine and pilocarpine. a-Tocopherol (vitamin E) has been found to inhibit the creatinuria in some of these patients. A program of resistive exercises for key muscles, such as the gastrocnemius, quadriceps, and gluteus maximus, has been helpful, providing the course is periodically interrupted to allow the patient's interest to freshen.

There is no treatment which has been known to be effective in arresting the course of the disease. Obesity, of course, should be prevented by dietary measures.

In the absense of curative medical therapy, management by the orthopaedist should include:

1. Strengthening muscles where possible.
2. Preventing or correcting contractures to ensure *full* use of available *strength* and *function.*

Table 10.1
Progressive Muscular Dystrophies

Diagnostic Criteria	Duchenne	Facioscapulohumeral	Limb Girdle
Age at onset	Childhood	Adolescence	Early or late
Sex	Male	Either	Either
Pseudohypertrophy	Common	Rare	Uncommon
Initial distribution	Pelvic girdle	Shoulder girdle	Either
Involvement of face	Rare	Always	Possibly never
Rate of progression	Relatively rapid	Slow (abortive)	Intermediate
Contractures and deformity	Common	Rare	Occasional
Inheritance	Sex-linked recessive	Dominant	Either

3. Bracing (after correction of deformities) to extend the length of the ambulatory period.
4. Surgery to correct contractures and deformities as well as to remove deforming forces.

With regard to contractures, it is best to prevent rather than to treat contractures. Spencer[11, 12] advocates a program of stretching and night splinting. The contractures that occur first and are usually most severe are those of the heel cord and iliotibial band followed later by equinovarus deformity secondary to the strong pull of the frequently normal or near normal posterior tibial muscle.

Gucker has found that frequently light plaster shells will prevent contractures of the knees and heel cords if they are used for prolonged periods when the deformities are first diagnosed.

A combination of surgery followed by bracing shortly before or after a patient ceases to walk can preserve ambulation, on the average, for 4 or more years. Crutches have not been useful in prolonging ambulation because of weakness of the shoulder depressor muscles.

Spencer[11, 12] has found a typical pattern of muscle weakness when the patient is about to stop ambulation. The quadriceps have dropped to fair minus on manual muscle testing. However, the plantar flexors continue to be good for an exceedingly long time. The evertors are fair minus, and the dorsiflexors and anterior tibials remain fair.

Stretching exercises are particularly necessary for the gastrocnemius. The tendency toward contracture is marked and provides an additional handicap to the already overburdened patient. Tenotomy of the tendo achillis is rarely necessary to release such a contracture. Bivalved night casts that hold the limb in the corrected position may be an aid to prevention.

Prolonged periods of bed rest must be avoided because they further weaken the patient. Muscle biopsy of the gastrocnemius, when done to confirm the diagnosis, should be followed by use of a protective splint and by early weight bearing to prevent contracture.

The iliotibial bands are corrected by a low Yount fasciotomy in which a large rectangular section of the iliotibial tract is excised, including a section of the lateral intermuscular septum down to the linea aspera of the femur.

The equinus contractures are corrected by a closed Achilles tenotomy. Open tenotomy contributed to prolonged postoperative disability of the patient with increasing disuse atrophy. After a transverse tenotomy the correction is held by applying the cast with as much dorsiflexion and eversion of the ankle as can be obtained.

To prevent recurrence of the equinus deformity and to correct varus deformity, the posterior tibial tendon is transferred to the third cuneiform through the interosseous membrane.

The principal factor in loss of independent ambulation is progressive muscle weakness. However, loss of independent ambulation often occurs prematurely due to contractures. Another major factor leading to premature loss of ambulation is obesity which, with diet, can be controlled.

Eventually, even surgery and braces cannot maintain ambulation. The wheelchair becomes a necessity. Eventually, seat belts, folding desks, and an electric-power chair may be necessary. For patients confined to a wheelchair, Spencer believes that measures that might help to prevent or lessen scoliosis include (1) light plaster jackets, (2) corsets, (3) standing tables, and (4) Rodpri braces.

Respiratory function always deteriorates as the disease advances until vital capacity measures little more than tidal volume. Acute respiratory arrest is the common course. Even a common cold may cause the patient to succumb.

The dystrophic process inevitably involves the myocardium with enlargment of the heart and electrocardiographic abnormalities. Practically, there is no indication for treatment until symptoms occur. Chronic cardiac failure with either pulmonary or peripheral edema is the case. Friedberg reports that in 12 muscular dystrophy patients at rest cardiac catheterization was essentially normal, but during exercise revealed the typical findings associated with congestive heart failure.

References

1. Adams, R. D., Denny-Brown, D., and Pearson, C. M.: *Diseases of Muscles* New York: Paul B. Hoeber, 1953.
2. Danowski, T. S., and Fetterman, G.: Muscular dys-

trophy history, clinical status, muscle strength and biopsy findings, *J. Dis. Child,* 91:326, 1956.

3. Denny-Brown, D.: The nature of muscular diseases, *Can. Med Assoc. J,* 67:1, 1952.

4. Ebashi, S., Toyokura, Y., Momoi, H., and Sugita, H.: High creative phosphokinase activity of sera of progressive muscular dystrophy patients, *J. Biochem. (Tokyo),* 46:413, 1959.

5. Erb, W. H.: Uber die "juvenile form" der progressiven Muskelatrophia; ihre Beziehungen zur sogenannten Pseudohypertrophie der Muskeln, *Dtsch. Arch. Klin. Med,* 34:464, 1884.

6. Landouzy, L., and Déjérine, J.: De la myopathie atrophique progressive; Myopathie sans neuropathie, débutant d'ordinaire dans l'enface, par la face, *Rev. Méd,* 6:81, 253, 1885.

7. Miller, W.: Management of muscular dystrophy, *J. Bone Joint Surg,* 49A:1205, 1967.

8. Pearson, C. M.: Serum enzymes in muscular dystrophy and certain other muscular and neuromuscular diseases. I. Serum, glutamic, oxalacetic transaminase, *N. Engl. J. Med,* 256:1069, 1957.

9. Pearson, C. M.: Histopathological features of muscle in the preclinical stages of muscular dystrophy, *Brain,* 85:109, 1962.

10. Siegel, et al.: Subcutaneous lower limb tenotomy in the treatment of pseudohypertrophic muscular dystrophy, *J. Bone Joint Surg,* 50A:1437, 1968.

11. Spencer, G.: Orthopedic care of progressive muscular dystrophy, *J. Bone Joint Surg,* 49A:1201, 1967.

12. Spencer, G.: Bracing for ambulation in childhood progressive muscular dystrophy, *J. Bone Joint Surg,* 44A:234, 1962.

13. Vignos, J.: Maintenance of ambulation in childhood muscular dystrophy, *J. Chronic Dis,* August: 273, 1960.

DERMATOMYOSITIS

This is a rare, highly disabling disease whose activity leads to marked contractures. When it involves muscles of respiration and deglutition, it may lead to a fatal outcome. The activity of the disease is marked by a nonsuppurative inflammation of striated muscles that is usually accompanied by skin lesions.

Etiology

Attempts have been made to implicate parasitic, viral, and bacterial agents, but they have not been substantiated. No definite nutritional disturbance has been found. The disease has been grouped with so-called "collagen diseases," such as scleroderma.

Clinical Picture

The onset is usually insidious and marked by weakness and chronic fatigue. The development of limb stiffness and muscle pain follows these initial symptoms. Dermatomyositis may eventually cause considerable weakness, which is usually irreversible if extensive. The muscle soreness leads to flexion contractures of the joints.

A low grade fever is present at some time in the course of the disease. The skin of the face may be involved early in the disease. The extremities tend to become wasted and to feel brawny and inelastic. Shiny or scaly skin tends to be drawn tightly over bones and atrophied muscles. The atrophy is extensive.

A fatal termination, if the disease follows that course, usually takes place in the first 2 years, the disease thereafter tending to become quiescent.

Pathology

A biopsy of skin, subcutaneous tissue, and muscle taken in continuity from one area may be helpful in establishing the diagnosis. Early changes show edema of subepithelial tissues and collections of polymorphonuclear leukocytes in both skin and muscles. The leukocytes are mainly eosinophils. Later, foci of lymphocytes and monocytes are seen, particularly at the junction of fascia and muscle. Muscle necrosis may be seen. In the late stages, atrophy with disappearance of muscle fibers without inflammation is usual.

Treatment

The measures to combat the disease are centered upon prevention of deformity and compensation for muscle weakness. Periods of rest in the corrective position and bivalved casts, if the tendency to deformity is great, are essential. Use of casts must be balanced by periods of exercise out of casts during the day. To correct an existing deformity, traction, splints, corrective operations, and stretching by active and passive manipulation may all be necessary.

Improvement is characterized by increase in muscle strength, decrease in fever, if present, subsidence of skin lesions and muscle soreness, and gain in body weight. Active exercises of a resistive type may be given when the muscles are no longer sore.

Medication has ranged from hormones, including adrenocorticotropic hormone, to vitamin E. Results have not been encouraging, but occasionally there is a suggestive improvement which is difficult to evaluate because of the tendency toward spontaneous remission.

ARTHROGRYPOSIS MULTIPLEX CONGENITA

This disease of uncertain etiology was first described by Otto in 1841. The unfortunate youngster frequently has multiple deformities of the extremities, although the trunk is relatively unaffected. Rosenkranz named the disease "arthrogryposis" because of the curved joints it causes but "amyoplasia congenita" is a more popular term among the pathologists. The condition is best thought of as involving principally the muscles, which may be represented by only a few undeveloped fibers. It is not progressive. Meade, Lithgow, and Sweeney have delineated the features of its clinical course very well in their series, which included 12 patients followed into adulthood. Mental retardation is not a feature. Clubfeet, clubhands, and dislocated hips are common forms of involvement. The joints are fixed, and their motion is extremely limited.

Etiology

Various forms of intrauterine compression have been thought to be the primary cause of the thin, atrophic limbs. The joint limitation has sometimes, however, been attributed to intrauterine arthritis, but there is no evidence for this etiology in the clinical cases seen. The skeletal muscles have not developed in the involved area, and Middleton[5] has suggested that the primitive myoblast failed to mature. That the muscle picture is secondary to disease of the central nervous system has seemed plausible to other authors, who noted degeneration of anterior horn cells, and intrauterine poliomyelitis has been postulated as the underlying factor. The cause of what is often a very severe clinical picture is not clearly known, however.

Clinical Picture

The outline of the involved extremity is often cylindrical and lacking muscle prominences and normal skin creases. Any extremity or any joint area, or any combination of extremities and joint areas, may be involved. Most often all four extremities are affected (Fig. 10.4). Even though the joints are contracted, some motion is usually possible, although it may be small in degree. This motion is painless, free, and often greater in the passive range than in the active.

The extremities feel softer than normal and are conical in shape. The picture of the entire body reveals equinovarus feet, clubhands, dislocated hips, and knee and elbow contractures. The disease is suspected, however, in cases of more discrete lesions, such as the equinovarus foot with a thin calf at birth or a congenital contracture of the knee or elbow.

Roentgen Picture

Roentgen studies reveal the contracture or an associated deformity. The muscle shadows are nothing more than thin strands of water density that run through the extremity, which appears to consist largely of fat (Fig. 10.5). The joint space is unaffected, except when a condition such as a dislocated hip is associated with the disorder.

Pathology

Adams, Denny-Brown, and Pearson,[1] in their text, point out that, in one of their cases of hip flexion contracture due to this disease, the flexors of the hip were well developed but the extensors were atrophied. Their finding lends some credence to a neurologic etiology. Some muscles cannot be found at all in the masses of fatty tissue; others are represented by occasional, rudimentary, pale pink

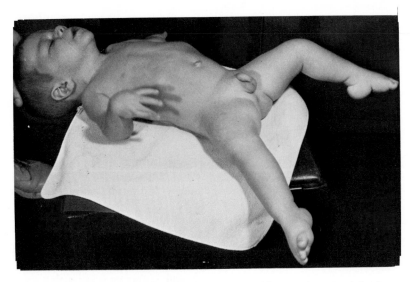

Figure 10.4.   Contractures of the hands, feet, and knees in amyoplasia congenita.

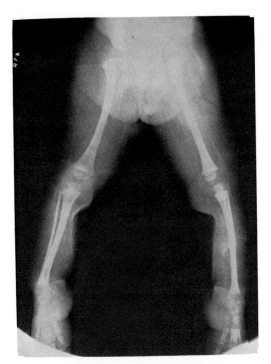

Figure 10.5.   Roentgenogram revealing thin strands that represent muscular tissue running through shadows of fat density in the leg in a case of arthrogryposis.

fibers. The smallness of the muscle fibers seen is noteworthy. Degeneration of muscle fibers is not a marked finding. The joints themselves are unaffected; their cartilaginous surfaces appear normal. It is apparent that the cause of the limited motion and contractures lies in the soft tissues. In the cord, the anterior horn cells are markedly reduced in number, and in some areas they may be completely absent. Mead et al. have been impressed by the increased fibrosis about the joints and the lack of loose areolar tissue under the skin.

Treatment

Correcting the contracture and increasing the range of motion are exceedingly difficult. Some gain can be achieved by slow, patient application of plaster casts that hold the limb in a correcting position. The gain is important because it is frequently great enough to enable ambulation in a reasonable position. Surgical correction is not as rewarding as the surgeon might hope, because the inelastic skin, vessels, and nerves prove to be limiting factors. It is sometimes indicated (Fig. 10.6) and necessary, however. The range of passive motion achieved is greater than the patient can handle actively, but, as in clubfoot, it is a nonetheless necessary achievement for satisfactory ambulation. Bracing is usually necessary to hold the correction, in view of the lack of active muscle power. The foot must be brought to a weight-bearing position, or a rocker-bottom deformity may result.

When the hip is dislocated, the soft tissues frequently hold it rather rigidly in abduction and flexion. In some cases the deformity must be accepted; however, a conservative attempt at reduction is always justified, and, when this fails, an open reduction should often be attempted. Traction, which is helpful in patients with a congenital dislocation but good soft tissues, is of little avail against the rigid structures present in this disease.

The knees may be fixed in a range of flexion deformity or occasionally in hyperextension. Quadriceps action often seems to be absent, and bracing is frequently necessary.

At the elbow, a rather rigid extension deformity is frequently a problem, and flexion of one elbow is often desirable. Passive flexion can be achieved by capsulotomy, but active flexion is usually absent.

At the wrist, there is usually a flexion deformity which does not respond to conservative attempts at correction. Absence of dorsiflexion power is a common finding. Surgical correction in the older age group frequently includes fusion to hold the wrist for better function, but each patient must be individually evaluated in terms of what function is present.

Little can be done for the rather rigid tapering fingers, except the thumb, in which the adductor web can frequently be lengthened to gain function. Because the patients have had to confront the problem since

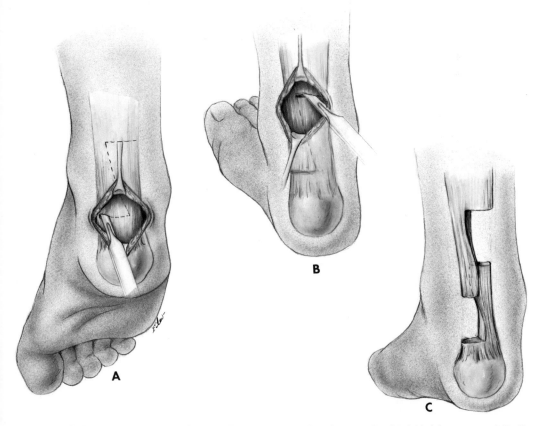

Figure 10.6. Lengthening the tendo calcaneus by the method of Kuhlmann and Bell. There is a short transverse incision made above the insertion of the tendon into the os calcis. The foot is plantar flexed, and a medial transverse incision is made. As the foot is dorsiflexed, the long limb of the Z is made in an oblique fashion through the center of the tendon. The fibers are separated rather than divided. The length of the cut is ½–1 inch as needed. With dorsiflexion, the posteriolateral portion of the tendon is divided by retracting the superior margin of the skin incision. The tendon is not sutured; the skin incision is closed.

birth, there is frequently more function in the hands than the extent of the contractures would lead one to anticipate.

References

1. Adams, R. D., Denny-Brown, D., and Pearson, C.: *Diseases of Muscle*, Ed. 2; New York: Paul B. Hoeber, 1962.
2. Brandt, S.: A case of arthrogryposis multiplex congenita, *Acta Paediatr.*, *34:* 365, 1947.
3. Ealing, M. I.: Amyoplasia congenita causing malpresentation of the fetus, *J. Obstet. Gynaecol. Br. Emp.*, *51:* 144, 1944.
4. Gilmour, J. R.: Amyoplasia congenita, *J. Pathol. Bacteriol.*, *58:* 675, 1946.
5. Middleton, D. S.: Studies on prenatal lesions of striated muscle as a cause of congenital deformity, *Edinburgh Med. J.*, *41:* 401, 1934.

MYOSITIS OSSIFICANS (CIRCUMSCRIPTA)

The formation of bone in heterotypic fashion in muscle occurs most commonly in the quadriceps and brachialis muscle groups and exhibits two distinguishing clinical features: (1) an association with the age group of 16 and 17 years and (2) trauma or repeated trauma.

Myositis ossificans circumscripta must be distinguished from myositis ossificans progressiva, a familial disease which progresses to "turn the man to stone" as motion is lost at joints and in the chest wall to the point of inhibiting respiratory function and threatening life. The involvement here is related to

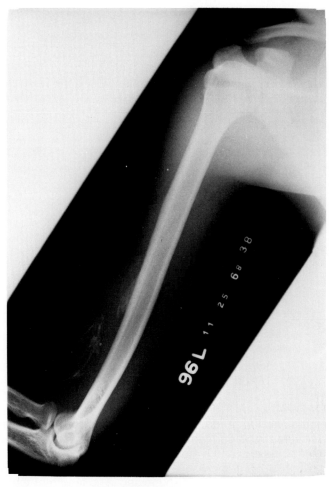

Figure 10.7. Blocker's exostosis. Irregular bone formation within the brachialis muscle with swelling of the muscle and soft tissues about.

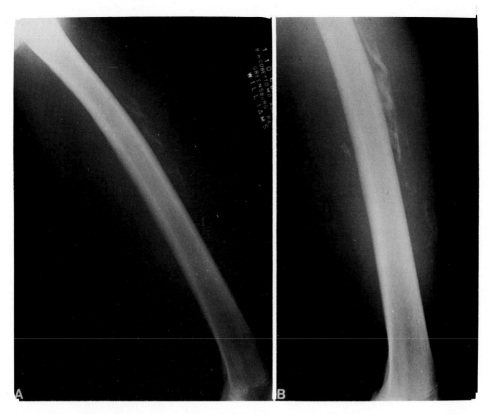

Figure 10.8. The irregular formation of bone in the quadriceps muscle in a 17-year old boy after a football injury. The bone is separate from the underlying femur. There are irregular projections into the muscle belly itself. (*A*) At the end of football season; (*B*) 6 weeks later. An ossifying hematoma would have a smooth outline and be closely adherent to the underlying femur. A tumor would present a rounded mass rather than a poorly defined inflammatory swelling and would not have the irregular extension through the muscle.

tendons and ligaments. In the isolated form, the lesion is solitary and related to muscle, including the collagenous supportive tissue of the involved muscle.

It is also necessary to distinguish an ossifying hematoma from myositis ossificans. This is not developed in irregular extending fashion into the body of the muscle, but has a smooth exterior wall. It is closely related to the bone and does not continue to proliferate in a tumorous fashion as does myositis in its early phases. This type of ossification is not limited by age group as is myositis. There are also various forms of heterotype bone formation occurring in paraplegia, following burns, and after massive trauma around joints involving the capsule in an ossifying repair reaction.

Clinical Picture

The patient is usually male and in the 16 to 17-year-old group. The athletic activity of the individual is prominent in the history, and a major contusion is often remembered at the onset. Thereafter, repeated blows seem to be suffered in the same area as tenderness and swelling become apparent. The biceps-brachialis area gives rise to a progressively more tender swelling known as a "blocker's exostosis" (Fig. 10.7). The quadriceps in mid-thigh progressively enlarges, is markedly tender, and ability to flex the knee is progressively restricted (Fig. 10.8). The early stages may be complicated by vigorous stretching therapy to get the joint motion back, which only results in increasing swelling and progressive limitation.

Pathology

In the early stages there is definite inflammation about the lesion which appears to be a hematoma and necrosis secondary to muscle tear and contusion, but such an initial inflammatory response will be resorbed and the inflammation will subside normally. In myositis ossificans (circumscripta) there is a definite cellular proliferative response. There is metaplasia of the collagen into osteoblasts and chondroblasts. The formed bone is normal in appearance. There may be viable muscle cells persisting in the areas of osteoblastic proliferation. At the periphery the cellular activity is more a reaction than neoplastic. There are three definite zones of maturity in the area of myositis rather than the uniform cellular proliferation of an osteosarcoma. The cells are more regular.

Treatment

Initially the inflammation should be allowed to subside. Physical therapy at this juncture in any form—electrical, manual, or stretching—can keep the activity of the lesion alive. The motion of the limb should be carried out by the patient alone within the range which is pain free. As the swelling and tenderness subside, the active range of motion may be gradually increased. If treatment has been vigorous initially there may be a large bony mass form. This begins with indistinct outline next to the bone but not attached to it and extending through the muscle belly and along septal planes. Over a 3- to 4-month period it gains a regular, distinct outline and appears as mature bone.

At this juncture one does not palpate heavily swollen tissues about the bony lesion.

Where the limitation of motion is apparently permanent, surgical excision of the bony mass may be considered. Where operated on at the correct stage the muscle separates readily from it and a space between the bony mass and the adjacent bone may be found. Hematoma formation is minimized by clean surgery and keeping the limb at rest for 10 days before guarded active motion is started by the patient. Full motion will be regained unless bone formation again takes place.

Reference

1. Aegerter, E., and Kirkpatrick, J. A.: *Orthopaedic Diseases*, Ed. 2, pp. 345–346; Philadelphia: W. B. Saunders, 1963.

PERSISTENT ADDUCTED FEMURS (POSITIONAL)

A contracture apparently due to intrauterine position causes a number of infants to be seen in the office practice of orthopaedic surgery (Fig. 10.9). These children have many of the physical signs associated with subluxated or dislocated hips. Hip roentgenograms reveal the adducted position of the hip, but there is a normal acetabulum, a normal lo-

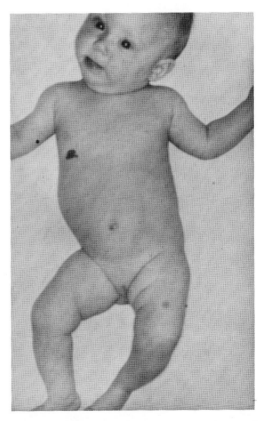

Figure 10.9. Adduction contracture of the hip. Note the tendency to lie in a total curve as well.

cation of the femoral neck in relation to the triradiate cartilage, and often a normal development of the ossification center of the femoral head (if present). Occasionally this ossification center is smaller than the one on the opposite side.

These infants are normally seen in the first 6 months of life. The birth history is usually normal.

Physical Examination

Asymmetric thigh folds often first call attention to the condition. The infant examined as to total posture is found to lie with the pelvis high on the adducted side and with a total curve of the spine correcting for the adduction. The head and neck tend to assume a posture in line with this spinal curve. When turned on the stomach, the infant maintains this position. It is even possible to be fooled into the recognition of a positive Galeazzi's sign if the position of the pelvis is not carefully compensated for when the thighs are flexed.

Treatment

It is necessary to aid the patient to overcome the adduction contracture despite the fact that much of the normal infant's daily routine stretches these muscles. Adductor stretching with the thighs flexed is taught to the mother. Holding the legs abducted with double diapers for approximately 3 months is all that is ordinarily necessary to overcome this positional disability. Forced abduction should be avoided.

CHAPTER 11

Benign and Malignant Tumors of Bone

BENIGN TUMORS IN CHILDHOOD*

Benign tumors involving bone tend to have a cystic appearance. The area involved is generally totally lytic and the juncture of tumor with bone is smooth rather than having the irregular, finely spiculated edge of active destruction seen in malignancy. A discussion of simple bone cyst and osteoid osteoma is included here solely to aid in their differentiation, because they are not true tumors.

Giant cell tumor is included here, but it is neither truly benign nor characteristically a childhood lesion. Its presence at the far end of the scale as a cystic, invasive, locally recurrent, and occasionally frankly malignant tumor which can occur in the late teenage group makes it necessary to include it.

The difficulty in deciding when a lesion is an osteogenic fibroma and when an osteoid osteoma, as the less characteristic form of the two merge, illustrates some of the difficulties with this group of conditions.

OSTEOGENIC FIBROMA AND OSTEOID OSTEOMA

Attempts have been made to identify a lesion as ossifying fibroma or benign osteoblastoma. The cases fade imperceptibly into the osteoid osteomas and appear to be one edge of the spectrum of this condition. As in osteoid osteomas there is no evidence that the lesion has the power of autonomous growth, and it has many of the elements of

repair. The use of the terms "fibroma" and "osteoma" is unfortunate.

The age group and location of ossifying fibroma is identical with that of osteoid osteoma. They occur roughly from age 6 to age 26. It is true that they may rarely be found beyond this span. The principal incidence is in the late teens. As one might expect in a process which may represent prolonged repair under difficulty, males are heir to the condition twice as often as females.

Pain, worse at night and relieved by salicylates, is a characteristic feature. Clinically, the low grade, insidious nature of the lesion results in a history of many months' duration before being seen, and atrophy of the involved limb is usually marked and common. It is very wise clinically to suspect osteoid osteoma or osteogenic fibroma when atrophy is present and a history of prolonged pain exists with little else in the way of a clinical finding to guide the orthopaedist to the lesion. A careful search of the roentgenogram, making sure the suspected bone is entirely covered, is then indicated. Local tenderness exists over the lesion if it can be found.

In osteoid osteoma there may be very little evidence on the film of the lesion early in its course. In those cases likely to be interpreted as osteogenic fibroma the lesion is more fluid and large, giving rise to still a third term, giant osteoid osteoma. Some of the cases of giant osteoid osteoma coming into our experience have eventually turned out to be osteosarcoma.

As in so many lesions in bone the diagnosis is based on the clinical course, roentgen findings, and view of the microscopic section rather than on the microscopic pathology alone.

---

* Reprinted in part from A. B. Ferguson, Jr.: Benign tumors of bone in childhood, *Pediatric Clinics of North America,* 14:683, 1967.

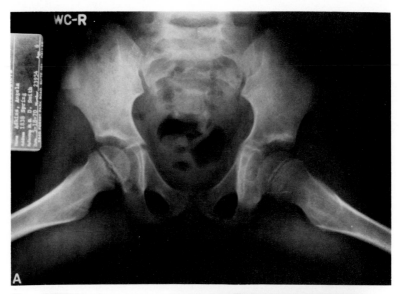

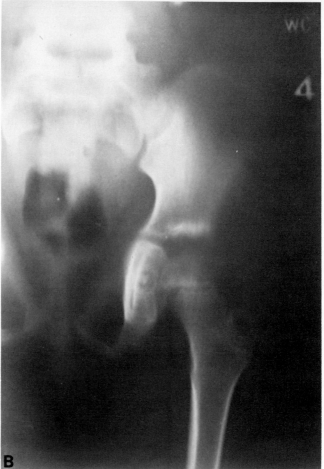

Figure 11.1. (*A*) Osteoid osteoma of the acetabulum in a 6-year-old girl. In the inferior acetabulum a rounded radiolucent area with central dense nidus is visible to the reader's right. The cartilage joint space of the affected hip is widened. (*B*) The tomogram brings out the details of the lesion. There is a shell of sclerosis about the nidus, and the central density is irregular.

Roentgen Findings

The lesion occurs principally in the diaphysis and is eccentric or cortical. Once this is said it is appropriate to add that lesions have been found in the small bones of the hand, foot, vertebra—in the posterior elements, sacrum, ilium, and, rarely, in the epiphysis. For osteoid osteoma the nidus is radiolucent and small, occasionally with some flecks of calcific density within it (Fig. 11.1). Around it, as the lesion develops, new bone may form from both the endosteum and periosteum. This eventually gives rise to considerable sclerosis and localized, axial thickenings of the diaphysis on one side. The ossifying fibroma could be described as having a more central location and less sclerotic reaction.

Pathology

The area occupied by the essential process is sharply delineated from the surrounding bone. It is rather dark reddish brown and cuts with a gritty feel. The bone around it is dense when the location is cortical; where it lies in anatomic areas that are principally cancellous, the bony reaction is thinner and less noticeable.

On microscopic section, there are areas of osteoid in the center of the lesion. The cells are principally fibroblasts lying in a loose vascular matrix. Denser osteoblasts line the spicules of osteoid and are about bony spicules at the edge. There is not fat and no hematopoietic marrow.

The ossifying fibroma or osteoblastoma varies only in size and, being larger, has less sclerotic reaction. The basic elements are the same with giant cells being perhaps more evident in the large lesion. These are consistent with the giant cells of repair rather than turnover. The lesion may be quite cellular with large numbers of fibroblasts and osteoblasts in some areas. Osteoid formation is still a prominent feature, although mineralization of this material may be quite sparse.

Treatment

The treatment consists of an en bloc excision of the nidus. Because of the difficulty of identifying the nidus beneath the bony reaction about it, an intelligent approach is to perform the surgery using x-ray marker films while the bone is exposed so that the involved area is removed with certainty.

When a fair sized block of bone has been removed the surgeon must support the skeleton in plaster while repair fills in the area. This process is ordinarily rapid and complete without evidence of disturbing tumorous bone formation. Should this occur, it is well to review the entire case, including the pathologic section, to make certain the diagnosis is correct and that the lesion has not been underinterpreted.

Although some of these lesions have eventually proved to be osteosarcoma, it is usually

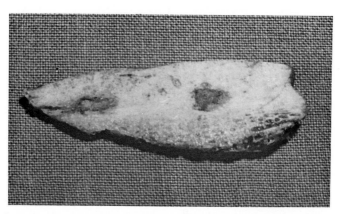

Figure 11.2. Specimens of cortex involved with lesion diagnosed as osteoid osteoma. Note that there are two separate and distinct nidi. This example helps to support contention that this is not a true tumor.

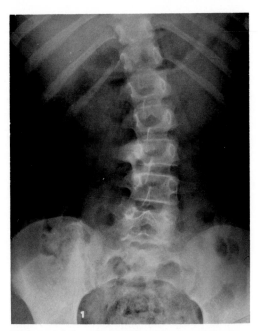

Figure 11.3. Osteoid osteoma of the lumbar spine. The enlargement of the pedicle and transverse process at the third lumbar vertebra is easily seen. The scoliosis is secondary to protective muscle spasm guarding this painful lesion.

apparent on final review that the features of tumor were there from the onset.

There is little to suggest that osteoid osteoma or ossifying fibroma (benign osteoblastoma) are tumors and a great deal to suggest that they represent repair which has been interfered with in some way. Some of the lesions have been reported as eventually healing themselves after a prolonged course.

References

1. Dahlin, D. C., and Johnson, E. W., Jr.: Giant osteoid osteoma, *J. Bone Joint Surg.,* 36A:559, 1954.
2. Jaffe, H. L., and Lichtenstein, L.: Osteoid-osteoma; further experience with this benign tumor of bone, with special reference to cases showing lesion in relation to shaft cortices and commonly misclassified as instances of sclerosing non-suppurative osteomyelitis or cortical-bone, *J. Bone Joint Surg.,* 22:645, 1940.
3. Lichtenstein, L.: Benign osteoblastoma; category of osteoid- and bone-forming tumors other than classical osteoid osteoma, which may be mistaken for giant-cell tumor or osteogenic sarcoma, *Cancer, 9:* 1044, 1956.

NONOSTEOGENIC FIBROMA (BENIGN CORTICAL DEFECT)

There is little real evidence that nonosteogenic fibroma differs materially from so-called benign cortical defects. The more extensive involvement of the cortex leads to the use of the term "fibroma," particularly where no osteoid is seen on microscopic section. In neither of these lesions is there any evidence that the process is neoplastic. A conversion defect seems to be the nature of the pathology, with the tissue laid down by the epiphyseal line failing to be converted to bone. The metaphyseal area is the only area involved—or at least only that area of the bone derived from the epiphyseal line as compared to the original fetal bone segment.

To understand the development of this process, which is usually seen as an incidental roentgen finding, it is important to remember a fundamental of x-ray interpretation. For the pathologic process to be seen on the x-ray film at all, the cortex must be involved, otherwise the x-ray density of the cortex hides the abnormalities within it. The bone is analogous to a metal pipe, the wall of which must be thinned or a hole drilled through it in order to appreciate on a roentgen film that something has occurred within it.

Thus this lesion could occur in the medullary cavity and be unnoted. Consequently it is thought of as primarily a cortical lesion because this involvement results in its being seen.

Large lesions obviously do involve the medullary canal as well as the cortex. These are relatively rare and may come to clinical attention because of pathologic fracture. A benign cortical defect is generally regarded as asymptomatic.

Following the lesion in time sequence as the child grows, one finds that it goes through a fairly characteristic sequence. It is first seen as the metaphysis undergoes tubulation. As age progresses, more and more of the lesion appears. The epiphyseal line by this time has laid down additional bone, and the lesion consequently is still further exposed as it occupies a position closer to the diaphysis.

The lesion is linear. The long axis is parallel to the long axis of the bone and has a thin cortical wall at its edge. Either the anteroposterior or lateral view confirms its eccentric cortical position. It is important to remember that more of the lesion may exist than is seen by x-ray. As growth progresses the lesion may disappear roentgenographically at the diaphyseal end, and more of the cortical defect appears at the epiphyseal end. The lesion itself may have existed throughout in its original form. The roentgenographic visibility of the lesion varies with its position in the metaphysis.

The age span when the lesion is seen is roughly from 4–14 years. Time from first being noted roentgenographically to disappearance varies from 2–5 years. It disappears entirely or leaves a small area of sclerosis at its site as it reaches a portion of the metaphysis where remodeling of the involved bone is complete.

The commonest bone involved is the femur, particularly the medial posterior distal metaphysis (Fig. 11.4). The medial proximal third is also common. Any area that is formed of bone laid down by an epiphyseal line can be a site.

It is obvious that the epiphyseal line is these patients over a large or small portion of its surface lays down tissue which, rather than being converted to bone, becomes fibrous tissue. It then, as a result of the bone's undergoing tubulation, appears to the roentgen film viewer. There is no evidence of expansion—the lesion is never wider than the epiphyseal line.

Pathology

A thin layer of cortical bone is often seen about the lesion, although, when biopsied, portions of the lesion are usually exposed without bone covering. It is yellow white in color, soft, and fibrous. There is no osteoid, but occasionally some of the collagen areas appear hyalinized. The lesion cuts without a gritty sensation. The cells are spindle-shaped fibroblasts with fairly minimal collagen production. Occasionally there are some large pale cells which give rise to the thought (when these are plentiful) that this is a xanthoma. Occasional giant cells are seen among the fibroblasts; their nuclei are small. Hemosiderin deposits have been noted.

Treatment

Because the lesion is largely asymptomatic, the most important treatment is to recognize it. Peculiar anatomic locations can occasionally cause the lesion to be implicated as a cause of pain with muscle pull, etc., but there does not seem to be much justification for this thought. The lesion may be biopsied if it is necessary to make the diagnosis in children who are complaining of pain in the area without other evident cause. Where it is large enough to cause a pathologic fracture, removal of the tissue and bone grafting are ordinarily successful (Fig. 11.5).

References

1. Caffe, J.: *Adv. Pediatr,* 7:13, 1955.
2. Ponseti, I. V., and Friedman, B. J.: Evolution of metaphyseal fibrous defects, *J. Bone Joint Surg,* 31A:582, 1949.

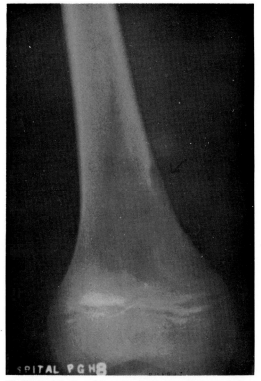

Figure 11.4. The typical medial femoral cortical defect of nonosteogenic fibroma.

OSTEOCHONDROMA

The relationship between nonosteogenic fibroma and osteochondroma can be recognized if one dwells on one essential feature,

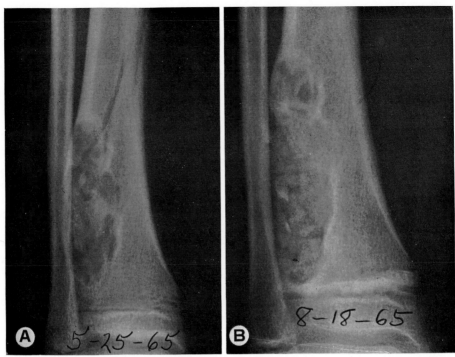

Figure 11.5. Nonosteogenic fibroma involving a sufficient amount of the bone to allow fracture. The lesion is linear, convoluted, metaphyseal, and smooth walled and does involve the cortex of the distal tibia. (*A*) Distal tibia at the time of fracture; (*B*) 3 months later after healing of the fracture and bone grafting.

i.e., the process which gives birth to each. At first we had fibrous tissue as the product of the metabolism and degradation of the epiphyseal line, visible when its location was cortical. Now we have cartilage left as the product of the maturation of the epiphyseal line and left, due to some fault as yet unknown, to live as cartilage rather than being converted to bone. Again, if its location is cortical, many changes will be obvious; but, if its location is central, it may exist unrecognized by our prime detector, the x-ray film. It may be true that cartilage with the ability to grow following its isolation from the epiphyseal line exists only as a product of the cells at the periphery. There, for a moment, epiphyseal, metaphysis, and epiphyseal line join. These cells indeed are peculiarly reproductive. Cartilage which has been found centrally in bone has been particularly acellular and consists principally of matrix.

A peculiarity of products of the epiphyseal line—be they fibrous tissue, cartilage, abnormal bone, or any percentage mixture of these ingredients—is their failure to respond to the remodeling so characteristic of the normal metaphysis as it narrows into the diaphysis (Fig. 11.6). This abnormal degeneration of material other than normal bone by the epiphyseal line can be designated chondrodysplasia. An osteochondroma with peripheral cartilage based on bone which is not subject to remodeling and with ability of the cartilage to resume growth is a form of chondrodysplasia.

Experimental Osteochondroma

True osteochondromas were produced in the laboratory by D'Ambrosia and Ferguson.[1] Articular cartilage transplants and transplants in which the polarity of the epiphyseal line was reversed did not give rise to true osteochondroma formation. A true osteochondroma occurred almost uniformly when all elements of an epiphyseal line were transplanted in a definite polarity (Figs. 11.7 and 11.8). There was a direct communication of the medullary cavity of the rabbit's tibia into

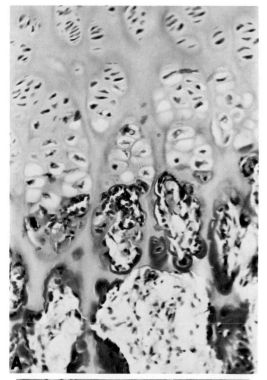

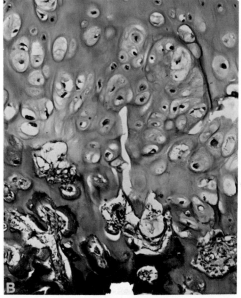

Figure 11.6. (*A*) Normal human epiphyseal line at the junction of blood vessels and the cartilage cell columns as bone formation begins. (*B*) Cartilage cap of osteochondroma. The slight disorganization and irregular lineup of the cartilage cells is evident but so, too, is the basic similarity to the epiphyseal line.

the medullary cavity of the osteochondroma, and modeling of the metaphysis occurred in characteristic fashion about the lesion.

There have been many theories about the origin of these cartilage-capped bony lesions. Virchow suggested in 1891 that a portion of the epiphyseal line for reasons unknown became separated from the parent tissue. Muller (1913) suggested that the cartilage cap found from the "cambium layer" of the periosteum. Keith (1920) felt that the osteochondroma was made possible by a defect in the periosteal ring surrounding the growth zone (aclasis). Geschickter and Copeland (1949) emphasized tendon attachments pulling on local accumulations of embryonic connective tissue as a starting point for these tumors. The laboratory creation of the tumors and the importance of polarity of the epiphyseal line in the successful creation support the thought that their origin is an offshoot of the epiphyseal line separated traumatically in the isolated osteochondroma or by genetic code in multiple exostoses.

Clinical Picture

The osteochondroma is the commonest bone tumor of childhood. Although any one tumor in a patient with multiple lesions may be similar to a tumor occurring as an isolated instance, it is quite evident that more than just the development of the tumor is involved in the patient with multiple lesions (Fig. 11.9). In hereditary multiple exostoses there is a strong tendency for a familial involvement (80%). Males are heirs to the condition 3 times as often as females and seem to be the chief carriers of the syndrome.

The effect on growth is profound in the patient with multiple cartilaginous exostoses, and it is exceedingly typical for the ulna and fibula to be short in relation to the radius and tibia. This results in curving of the radius, producing a wrist deformity similar to Madelung's and occasional dislocation of the radial head (Figs. 11.10 and 11.11). The extremities are short, the patient is short, and the long bone involvement is very evident in both the upper and lower extremities. Involvement is fairly symmetric.

There is little reason to call this disease diaphyseal aclasis because it is primarily a disease of the metaphysis and epiphyseal

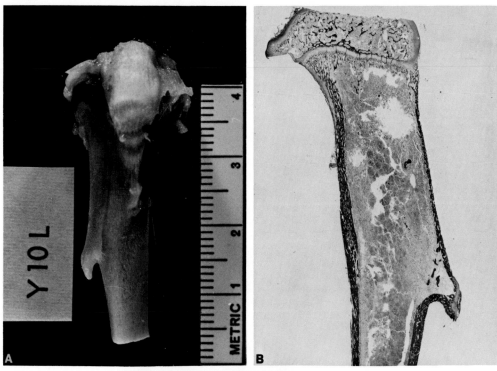

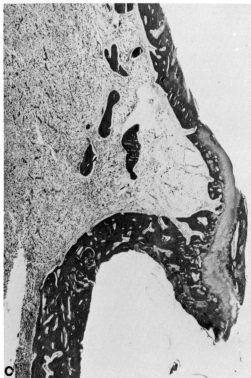

Figure 11.7. The laboratory creation of an osteochondroma in the rabbit by epiphyseal line transplant to the proximal metaphysis of the tibia. (*A*) The gross specimen reveals cartilage cap and widened metaphysis behind the osteochondroma. (*B*) The effect on the width of the medullary cavity and of the cortex proximal to the lesion is related to failure of modeling, a characteristic of chondrodysplasia. Remodeling is evident in those areas not affected by the growth of the cartilage cap. (*C*) Detail of the cartilage cap and demonstration of continuity of the medullary cavity into the lesion (8 weeks posttransplant).

	GROWTH PRODUCED				REMODELING
ZONE OF ENCHONDRAL OSSIFICATION	TOTAL RABBITS	NO GROWTH	OSTEOCHONDROMA	CARTILAGE ISLAND	REMODELING
TOWARD TIBIA	13	3	10	0	10
AWAY FROM TIBIA	13	4	0	9	0
CONTROL	8	8	0	0	0

Figure 11.8. Polarization of the transplant so that the metaphyseal side of the cartilage is toward the cortex is very important in achieving experimental osteochondroma formation. When polarity was reversed, only a cartilage island remained. The controls had a periosteal defect made but not carried to the point of inserting a cartilage transplant from the epiphyseal line.

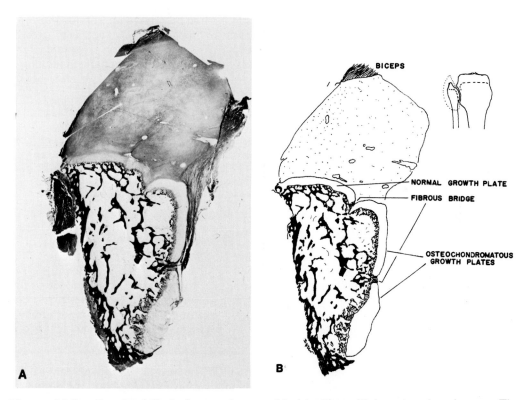

A   B

Figure 11.9. Proximal fibula from a 4-year-old girl with multiple osteochondromas. The osteochondromas are separated from each other and from the normal growth plate by fibrous bridges. The cell columns appear vacuolated, disarrayed, and are lightly stained. These osteochondromas were juxtaposed to a similar osteochondroma of the lateral proximal tibia. (*A*) Gross specimen with separation of osteochondromatous growth plates from the epiphyseal line. (*B*) Diagram of the photograph of the gross specimen (cut surface). The areas are labeled for easy identification in the photograph. (Courtesy of John Ogden, M.D.)

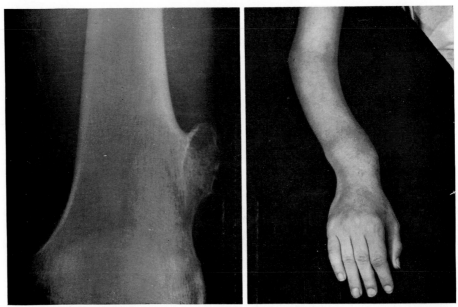

Figure 11.10 (*Left*). Osteochondroma of the distal femoral metaphysis. Note that the area supporting the cartilage cap is not subject to normal metaphyseal remodeling.

Figure 11.11 (*Right*). Multiple osteochondromas are frequently involved with growth abnormalities at the epiphyseal line. This is not so true of the solitary exostosis. Here deficient ulna growth has resulted in bowing of the radius and a resultant Madelung's deformity.

line. A portion of the cartilage of the epiphyseal line is not converted to bone. The area of bone beneath this peripheral anomaly is not subject to remodeling. Thus as the epiphyseal line grows away from the cartilage cap left behind, the normal remodeling of the metaphyseal bone takes place, leaving the osteochondroma jutting out as the metaphysis falls away. On top of the unremodeled bone lies a cartilage cap which has many of the characteristics of the epiphyseal line from which it came. Although initially the osteochondroma is not wider than the epiphyseal line, if further growth remains to the child, the cartilage cap may also grow, resulting in an increase in size of the bony mass as the cartilage is converted to apparently normal bone. This eccentric growth may result in pressure defects in an adjoining bone, bursae over the prominence, bowing deformity of a paired bone, snapping tendons as the muscle course must fall over the prominence and be displaced as motion occurs, or, finally, limited motion due to bony abutment.

The cartilage cap seems to be subject to the same influences as the epiphyseal line.

As the end of growth nears, the adventitious cartilage becomes less cellular and cell columns begin to disappear. Growth in an osteochondroma is not to be expected after general body growth has ceased.

Malignant change is heralded from the x-ray point of view by the development of increasing density in the tumor or by continued growth after the normal epiphyseal lines have closed. Malignant change as a possibility is rated from 17% down to 8% of the cases seen, but the real incidence is not really known inasmuch as most series have been preselected by referral of the more unusual cases to an authority. Malignant change is more likely in the case with multiple exostoses.

Solitary exostoses, although identical on microscopic examination, are not ordinarily accompanied by the profound disturbances of growth from the involved epiphyseal line. In the instance of single lesions, a case can readily be made to support the contention that they represent the end result of a traumatic peripheral detachment of a portion of an epiphyseal line which is otherwise normal.

Treatment

Excision of the osteochondroma may be done because it is producing deformity, interfering with growth or joint motion, or is cosmetically unappealing (Fig. 11.12). Rarely, pain due to overlying bursitis or tendinitis may occur.

It is possible to produce disability if the exostosis is not correctly removed. The base should be well beyond the cartilage cap area and should depress into the parent bone. It is very easy to take out too little.

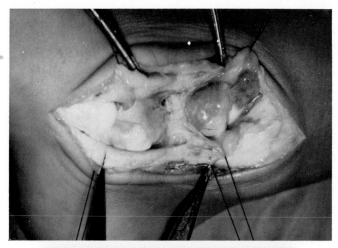

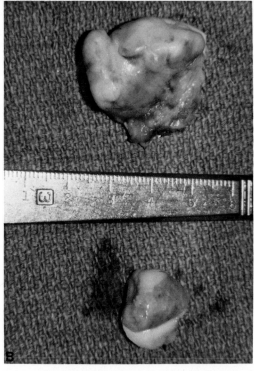

Figure 11.12. (*A*) Epiphyseal osteochondroma of talus and navicular. The approach is from the medial side of the foot the talus exhibits a cartilage capped irregular protuberance (*left*) followed next in line by a similar lesion projecting from the navicular. (*B*) The excised osteochondromas. This left the parent bones of normal size and shape. The astragalar lesion is on top.

The overlying soft tissue should be repaired across the defect of bare bone that is left. This is particularly important where a broad flat surface of muscle will lie against the defect and could adhere to it. The end result of this occurrence would be limited motion of the involved joint.

Cast immobilization aids postoperative comfort, prevents excessive hematoma formation, and allows healing of the repaired tissues without tearing apart and subsequent adherence. The cast should be on for at least 3 weeks.

Reference

1. D'Ambrosia, R., and Ferguson, A. B., Jr.: The formation of osteochondroma by epiphyseal cartilage transplantation, *Clin. Orthop. Res., 61:* 103, 1968.

SIMPLE BONE CYST

If we carry on the concept of origin from the epiphyseal line by failure of conversion to normal bone we find that the simple bone cyst fits readily into this picture. Very definite is the feature of these lesions which is evident roentgenographically—namely, that in the case of simple bone cysts the entire epiphyseal line is involved. The lesion, once fully formed, extends from cortex to cortex. It always is limited to the metaphysis. It never extends beyond the width of the epiphyseal line and accordingly has no evidence for the existence within it of autonomous growth.

As a form of chondrodysplasia the area involved by the cyst responds to the fundamental rule of areas so involved—that is, it does not respond to remodeling. Consequently the normal bone distal to it remodels to meet the diaphysis, and, proximally, once normal bone has again been laid down by the epiphyseal line, it too begins to remodel. This leaves the area occupied by the cyst apparently expansile—an optical illusion, for it never progresses beyond the maximum width of the metaphysis or the epiphyseal line (Fig. 11.13). The area of radiolucency extending the width of the bone has no evidence of independent density within it.

It is occupied by fluid and a thin membrane tending to be pale rather than reddish or brown, which would be its characteristic color with the hemosiderin deposits of recent trauma and fracture. It is one large cavity occasionally ridged but not divided by bone septa. The septa contain fibroblast macrophages with hemosiderin and occasional clusters of giant cells. The predominance of any cell is not such that one would consider the diagnosis of tumor.

It is often said that this is a lesion of the growing years—roughly from 3–16. One wonders why it is so rarely seen in adult life. The explanation is fairly obvious when one

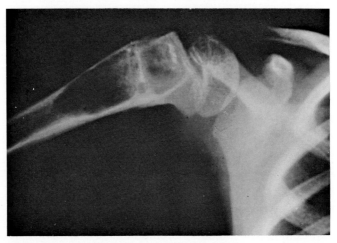

Figure 11.13.   The simple bone cyst involves the entire width of the metaphysis at its widest point. This should not be wider than the epiphyseal line. The cystic tissue narrows as the epiphyseal line begins once again to lay down normal bone, leading to a false appearance of expansion. The cyst area is not subject to remodeling—the bone proximal and distal to it is.

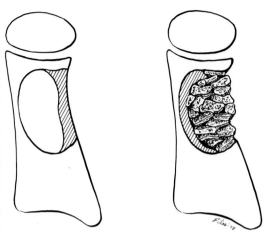

Figure 11.14. To make certain the cyst cavity is obliterated, the surgeon can reverse one cortex against the remaining intact wall. The membrane of the cyst is thoroughly removed. The cortex is then placed in reverse fashion against the far wall. Bone grafts fill in the remaining space.

Fracture through the cyst exerts a healing influence of callous formation for about ⅛ inch on either side of the fracture line and exerts a neglible effect on large cysts.

ANEURYSMAL BONE CYST

The name derives from the fact that this lesion breaks through the cortex of the parent bone and new bone is laid down about it. This gives rise to the appearance of "blow out" or "soap bubble"—terms that have been used to characterize the lesion. Because of its vascular nature, the term "aneurysmal bone cyst" has stuck.

On occasion, the location, combined with the expansile characteristic, has given rise to secondary complications. In vertebra, where the lesion occurs in the posterior elements and progresses forward, pressure on the spinal cord has given rise to paraplegia.

remembers that in older children bone usually begins to be laid down once again by the epiphyseal line. The cyst comes to lie more distally in the metaphysis. The bone continues to enlarge and new cortex is formed over the cyst area, obliterating it from x-ray view, as the cortex resumes normal thickness.

Treatment

Most series agree that the later in life that a cyst is operated upon the greater the chances of success. Some feel this is due to the removal of the cyst from direct contact with the epiphyseal line. It is also apparent that the further down the metaphysis toward the diaphysis the cyst occurs the easier it is for strong cortex to form in a bone now enlarging beyond the character of the cyst.

Some cysts in the proximal metaphysis have been extraordinarily troublesome to obliterate and Fahey has replaced most of the cyst with bone graft, on occasion, leaving only a thin strut of bone to maintain the normal anatomic outline.

The thoroughness with which bone grafts are packed into the defect obliterating unfilled space has played a part in healing the lesion.

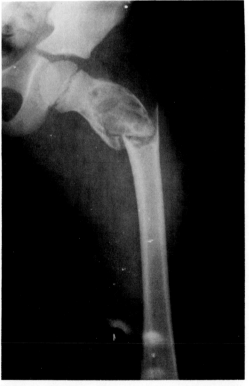

Figure 11.15. Bone cysts involving the femoral neck lead to varus deformity with repeated fractures and must be attacked early by grafting to prevent deformity.

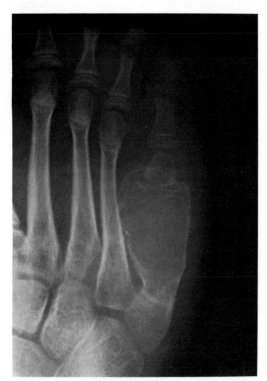

Figure 11.16. The aneurysmal bone cyst destroys the old cortex and lays down a thin shell of new bone about the lesion. In this fifth metatarsal it occupies the entire width of the bone, but in long bones it is more usual for it to be eccentric.

The lesion produces pain, low grade usually, but the patient has noted its painful nature when pressure has been accidentally applied. If superficial, a mass or swelling about it has been noted. It is a lesion of late childhood extending into early adult life. The youngest case reported, however, was 2 years and 3 months of age.

Roentgen Appearance

It is a cyst of bone, totally lucent in the area it occupies. It is distinguished in long bones from simple cysts by several characteristics. It is eccentric in its location in the metaphysis rather than extending completely across it. The fact that it has broken through the cortex rather than being enclosed by it is usually evident. A thin layer of new bone encloses it, but this layer extends beyond the original width of the epiphyseal line. The long axis parallels the long axis of the bone. It may extend well beyond a line dropped from the edge of the epiphyseal line parallel to the parent bone. This feature is never seen in simple bone cyst.

In vertebra its appearance is very characteristic. The spinous process is enlarged and a lacelike new bone envelops it. As the lesion extends through the posterior elements it may invade the body, but only from its posterior aspect, giving rise to a very diagnostic appearance. Only the posterior one-third or one-quarter of the vertebral body is involved.

Pathology

On cutting into the lesion blood wells up, tending to obscure sight of the lesion. It is not filled with dense tissue, but the abundant vascular spaces make the tissue appear fragmentary. It may be gritty to cut, as calcification of the tissue is occasionally present. Extraperiosteal dissection is simple as the lesion easily separates from surrounding tissue. Dissection from the bone is difficult as it invades the intraosseous area. There are fibrous septa. Spaced in these septa are small giant cells of the foreign body type (Fig. 11.18). The vascular spaces do not have well marked endothelial lining. The septa have a collagenous matrix with occasional areas of osteoid formation, some of which may be calcified.

Treatment

The lesion responds well to simple curettage. Apparently the surgical trauma and division of blood supply is sufficient to ablate most lesions. The bone then goes on to repair itself with normal bond. There have been recurrences after simple curettage, however, and it must be thoroughly ablative (Fig. 11.19). The lesion also responds to x-ray therapy, and, once the diagnosis is made, this form of therapy may be indicated in inaccessible locations.

Reference

1. Donaldson, W. F.: Aneurysmal bone cyst, *J. Bone Joint Surg*, 44A: 25, 1962.

CHONDROMYXOID FIBROMA

Chondromyxoid fibroma is a painful and rapidly progressive tumor of bone, a considerable number of which have occurred in children. This statement charcterizes the lesion. It is true that the peak of incidence is in the third decade. It is rather definitely a metaphyseal lesion giving rise to the suspicion that the parent cells may represent offshoots from the epiphyseal line which have failed to heed their genetic code.

Roentgen Appearance

The area of bone involvement is totally lucent—it appears to arise at the cortical edge, perhaps in the subperiosteal region, with a multipronged involvement of the metaphysis. There is considerable periosteal reaction. Nothing, however, suggests malignancy, the edge remaining smooth despite considerable sclerotic reaction. The lesion appears to have bone septa, as the bone extends into areas between lobular extensions; it definitely is eccentric rather than extending across the total width of the bone.

Pathology

There is a greyish yellow cast to the tissue. A lobulated appearance is confirmed as the whole lesion is viewed in cross section. The mass is stiffened by fibrous tissue septa, not bone. The cells lying in a homogenous ground substance are scarce and stellate or triangular in shape. The ground substance is

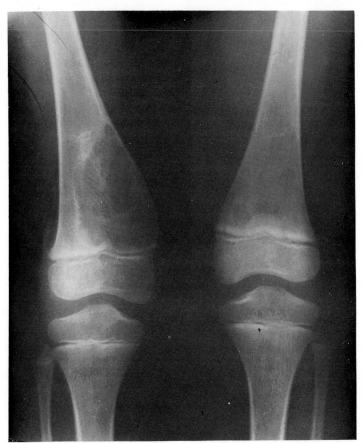

Figure 11.17. Aneurysmal bone cyst occupying the medial portion of the distal femoral metaphysis. Note the eccentric position, the destruction of the old cortex, and the laying down of a thin layer of new bone about the lesion which extends beyond the confines of the old bony outline.

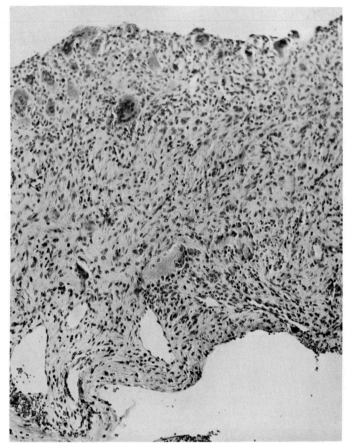

Figure 11.18.   Septa from aneurysmal bone cyst, primarily fibrous with some giant cell formation. Osteoid formation is not uncommon.

abundant and enclosed by the fibrous tissue septa, giving form to the lesion. Metachromasia of the ground substance has been noted by Scaglietti and Stringa.[2]

Treatment

Definite, complete local excision beyond the edges of the tumor is indicated. There have been recurrences after simple curettage. Because of the normal bone still remaining due to the eccentric location it is usually possible to easily graft the area of removal with reasonable expectations of filling in as the grafts are replaced by normal bone.

References

1. Dahlin, D. C., Wells, A. H., and Henderson, E.: Chondromyxoid fibroma of bone, *J. Bone Joint Surg,* 33A:831, 1953.

2. Scaglietti, O., and Stringa, G.: Myxoma of bone in childhood, *J. Bone Joint Surg, 43A:*67, 1961.

3. Stout, A. P.: Myxoma, the tumor of primitive mesenchyme, *Ann. Surg, 176:*706, 1948.

DESMOPLASTIC FIBROMA

This lesion looks so much like a simple bone cyst that it could escape recognition on first encounter (Fig. 11.20). There is one important difference: it can occupy the diaphysis as well as the metaphysis of the bone. This is a very important difference as it establishes the fact that it does not arise from the epiphyseal line but is a tumor arising from fibroblasts in a local area, and as experience with it grows one might expect that many bizarre locations would eventually be reported. Two cases have been reported that extended into the epiphysis.

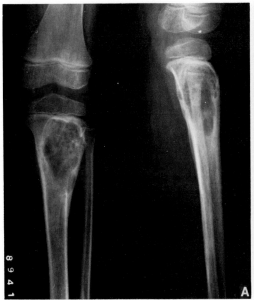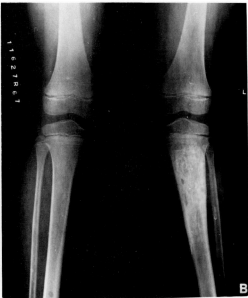

Figure 11.19. (A) The eccentric position of a recurrent aneurysmal bone cyst is a distractive feature when contrasted with a simple bone cyst which occupies the entire width of the metaphysis. Note the junction of the lesion with the distal cortex of the tibia. The old metaphyseal cortex has been destroyed, and the new bone laid down about the lesion abuts onto the exterior surface of the old cortex. It is not a direct continuation of the cortex as in a simple bone cyst. (B) After excision and grafting, the lesion is ablated, but growth of the lateral portion of the epiphyseal line appears deficient as some valgus of the tibia is apparent.

It occurs principally in children, although cases have been reported at age 40. Series of cases have run an age span from 8–21 years in one and 8–40 years in the other. The humerus, radius, femur, and tibia carry by far the majority of the cases, although scapula, illium, calcaneus, and lumbar vertebrae have been reported as involved. There is no sex predilection.

The clinical complaint that calls attention to the lesion is the presence of pain or pathologic fracture.

Roentgen Appearance

Like a simple bone cyst the lesion is totally lucent and tends to extend across the full width of the bone without exciting a marked bony reaction or periosteal proliferation. As one grows more sophisticated it is possible to appreciate that, as in giant cell tumor, there is a density to the lucent area all its own, giving a homogeneous appearance to the lucent area occupied by the tumor. The edge is smooth as it meets bone, not invasive.

Pathology

The defect in the bone is totally filled by the lesion. It does not consist of a few scrapings from the wall of a cyst. The material is greyish white and collagenous. The characteristic cell is the fibroblast, and careful study of the cells in necessary to differentiate the lesion from fibrosarcoma. The cells are small by comparison with those associated with fibrosarcoma, approximately half the size of those seen in the malignant lesion. The cells are sparse, spindle shaped, and with uniformly small, oval nuclei. Mitotic figures are not seen.

Treatment

Complete local extirpation of the lesion is indicated. This is better done by so-called segmental resection than by curetting, leaving the periosteum and hopefully a stub or two of uninvolved bone. Bone grafts are then used to maintain its skeletal outline. The

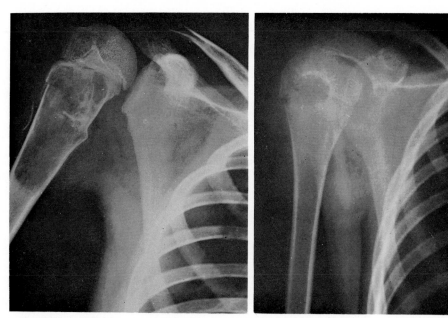

Figure 11.20 (*Left*). Desmoplastic fibroma giving a very similar appearance to simple bone cyst. There is a hazy density to the lesion as the result of being filled with fibrous tissue very difficult to differentiate on occasion from fibrosarcoma. (From P. Cohen and R. R. Goldenberg: Desmoplastic fibroma of bone, *Journal of Bone and Joint Surgery, 47A:* 1620, 1965.)

Figure 11.21 (*Right*). Chondroblastoma occupying an epiphyseal location of the humerus. Small flecks of calcification are occasionally seen.

results of surgical attack to date have been good.

References

1. Cohen, P., and Goldenberg, R. R.: Desmoplastic fibroma of bone, *J. Bone Joint Surg.,* 47A: 1620, 1625, 1965.
2. Sheer, G. R., and Kuhlman, R. E.: Vertebral involvement by desmoplastic fibroma, *J.A.M.A.,* 185: 669, 1963.
3. Whitesides, T. E., and Acherman, L. V.: Desmoplastic fibroma, *J. Bone Joint Surg.,* 42A: 1143, 1960.

CHONDROBLASTOMA

Ewing in 1928 referred to atypical giant cell tumors producing areas of punctate calcification in the humeral head as essentially benign. Codman[2] referred to these tumors as epiphyseal chondroblastomas, Their chondroblastic nature was still further delineated by Jaffe and Lichtenstein as they sharpened their delineation from giant cell tumors of bone.

A chondroblastoma is a lesion that occurs in adolescents and young adults. As the chondroblast fades as a type cell with the closure of the epiphyseal line, one would expect that the origin of these tumors must have taken place prior to epiphyseal line closure.

Recognition of the tumor may occur in adolescents and young adults, but it is often possible to trace the origin to an earlier date.

Pain occurs as the presenting symptom in some; for others, existence has been prolonged sufficiently and pain has been so low grade that a mass is the presenting symptom.

Roentgen Appearance

An epiphyseal location is characteristic, but extension from the original site may occur into the metaphysis. The tumor produces a radiolucent defect with a benign smooth edge often accompanied by a thin scalloping of bone. There is very little reaction in the adjacent bone, although, as the tumor progresses into lower reaches of the metaphysis, some periosteal reaction may occur. The presence of flecks of calcification within the tumor is very characteristic (Figs. 11.21 and 11.22).

Pathology

Because there is often considerable cartilage produced by the tumor, it tends to a pale grey or reddish grey color. The presence of calcified cartilage areas gives a gritty sensation as it is cut.

The lesion appears to be derived from proliferation of the chondroblast, a cell that disappears from the area the epiphyseal line closes. This accounts for its characteristic age group onset in adolescence. The rounded chondroblast may produce little cartilage, giving rise to highly cellular areas. There is considerable variation from section to section with myxomatous and collagenized fibrous tissue also present. The presence of giant cells accounts for its earlier inclusion in the giant cell variant group of tumors.

Treatment

The tumor is highly responsive to local excision, including incomplete removal, and one suspects the cartilaginous material produced within the lesion could be induced to convert to bone with the trauma of surgery. Radiation seems contraindicated and has been implicated in one case where this ordinarily benign tumor later developed into a chondrosarcoma.

References

1. Aegerter, E., and Kirkpatrick, J. A.: *Orthopaedic Diseases*, Ed. 2, pp. 574–580; Philadelphia: W. B. Saunders, 1963.
2. Codman, E. A.: Chondroblastoma, *Surg. Gynecol. Obstet.*, 52: 543, 1931.

EOSINOPHILIC GRANULOMA

This disease produces an area of radiolucency within bone without any particular habit so far as location is concerned (Fig. 11.23). It is inserted here under the category of "mentioned in passing." It does not conform well to the habits of true tumors and its cause is unknown. However it does produce a cyst lesion in bone which may lead to confusion.

The picture is still further complicated by the fact that Hand-Schüller-Christian disease produces lesions in bone which are indistinguishable from the standpoint of pathology. The clinical picture is vastly different, however, with one child (Hand-Schüller-Chris-

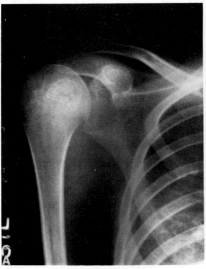
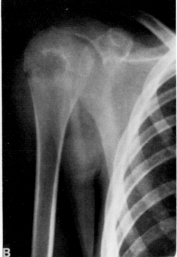

Figure 11.22. (*A*) Chondroblastoma involving the proximal humeral epiphysis. There are irregular flecks of calcification in the lesion. (*B*) After excision.

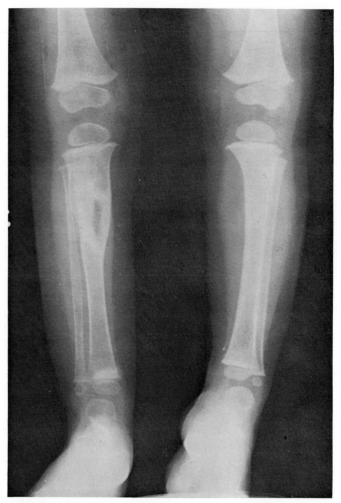

Figure 11.23. Eosinphilic granuloma of the tibia—considerable sclerosis about the lesion may occasionally be seen. This particular lesion has had roentgen therapy, resulting in considerable bony density. A thin area of sclerosis is more typical. The lesion is totally lytic.

tian disease) subject to a severe illness which involves liver and spleen enlargement and leading to anemia and a fatal termination. The child with eosinophilic granuloma as a solitary lesion exhibits no systemic manifestations whatever and is in exceedingly good general health. Despite this obvious difference many authors have attempted to link the two conditions together. It leads one to think that eosinophilic granuloma may be one of the ways that bone can react as visualized pathologically, and there easily may be no relation between the two conditions.

Most of the cases in our series have occurred about the pelvis and proximal femur.

Eosinophilic granuloma does represent an important consideration in the differential diagnosis of radiolucent lesions of bone in childhood. There is usually some bone reaction consisting of a very thin walling off of the lesion which does not extend for any distance into the general bone structure.

On the microscopic slide the appearance is exceedingly characteristic. Histiocytes, rather pale and large, reticulate with one another in a characteristic background. Over them flows a mass of eosinophilic leukocytes, occasionally exceedingly dense in concentration, varying to relatively thinly populated areas. Charcot-Leyden crystals have been reported in the cytoplasm, leading to a suspicion that the lesion represents an allergic reaction. Occasionally giant cells occur. Lipid-filled cells are not obvious except in very long standing lesions.

It should be mentioned that this lesion has been implicated as the cause of vertebral collapse which occurs in Calvé's disease or vertebral plana, a condition which runs a benign course.

The only real connection between patients with solitary eosinophilic granuloma and Hand-Schüller-Christian disease lies in the fact that initially the picture might momentarily be very similar if one considered only the microscopic findings. The differentiation into a systemic disease soon occurs in the latter, however, leading to a very sick child.

Treatment

Many lesions have been cured by the curettage which accompanied biopsy. It is very sensitive to low doses of x-ray therapy as well. It is important to biopsy the initial lesion if possible—one or two others may occur. If this occurs, the possibility of dealing with Hand-Schüller-Christian disease must be kept in mind.

References

1. Compere, E. L., Johnson, W. E., and Coventry, M. B.: Vertebra plana (Calvé's disease) due to eosinophilic granuloma, *J. Bone Joint Surg.*, 36A:969, 1954.
2. Green, W., Farber, S., and l-Dermott, L.: Eosinophilic granuloma, *J. Bone Joint Surg.*, 24:499, 1942.

GIANT CELL TUMOR

It is difficult to consider the giant cell tumor as anything but a malignant tumor which is locally invasive but rarely metastasizes. It characteristically occurs after closure of the epiphyseal line, but most series report a considerable percentage in the group from 10–20 years of age. This is partially explained by the high incidence in females in this younger age group. In one series, 8 of 11 patients under 20 were girls, but only 2 of these were under 15 years of age. The female sex predominates over all, almost 2 to 1. The highest age group incidence occurs between the ages of 20 and 30.

It was originally described in 1818 by Cooper and Travers, but it was clearly recognized as an entity distinct from other tumors containing giant cells by the delineation of Jaffe, Lichtenstein, and Portis[1] in 1940.

The area about the knee, either distal femur or proximal tibia, accounts for most cases, but two other sites deserve particular mention. The distal end of the radius is thought of as highly characteristic, but surprisingly high is the occurrence in the sacrum. This is true in most series. Other sites include the proximal humerus, distal ulna (Fig. 11.24), and proximal fibula. It can occur in vertebra and in small bones but is rare there.

Pain is a prominent presenting feature, although it may be sufficiently low grade that a number of months elapse before the patient comes to clinical attention. A mass or pathologic fracture may be the presenting complaint.

Roentgen Appearance

A giant cell tumor in a long bone has features that give it sufficient personality that the diagnosis should be readily made.

The epiphyseal origin is obvious, although the lesion readily extends into the metaphysis. It destroys bone, but leaves in its place the x-ray density of the soft-tissue mass which is homogenous and recognizable. No bone is formed except that which walls off the tumor at its periphery and appears definitely as a host reaction rather than tumor bone. Such bone as appears in the lesion has been left behind by the enveloping tumor. At the junction of the tumor with normal cortex of metaphysis, the lesion has clearly broken through, and new periosteal bone has been laid down over the cortex, which extends often as a thin layer of bone about the expanded tumor. This layer may not be complete but ceases shortly after it leaves the tumor-cortex junction.

In the vertebra or sacrum the lesion may start in the posterior element and has considerable tendency to fill the outline of the vertebrae before breaking out through the cortex.

Reaction of the host bone to the tumor is not marked.

Pathology

The tumor fills the area of destruction with a reddish gray mass with occasional hemorrhagic areas. The edge may cut with the gritty feel of a thin layer of bone. It is not unusual to find the tumor invading into the surrounding soft tissues. Some cyst formation may occur within the tumor secondary to necrosis.

The tumor is cellular with the stromal cells fairly uniform in size (Fig. 11.25). The supportive collagen framework is moderately abundant. Mitoses are extremely variable, a factor that led to grading the lesion, although there is little correlation with grading and subsequent course. Various parts of the lesion may exhibit variable giant cell concentration as well. These cells contain abundant nuclei.

Treatment

The results of treatment with irradiation, curettage, and partial excision are extremely poor with recurrence the rule. In one series of 9 patients treated by irradiation, 8 recurred. The course following the other two forms of treatment is similar and leads to clear definition of the most advantageous treatment.

The lesion should be thought of as invasive, locally recurrent, and malignant. Neither the term "benign giant cell tumor" or grading the tumor help the clinical approach.

En bloc excision is the treatment of choice, leaving the defect to be filled by surgical reconstructive measures. This en bloc excision usually means partial removal of a long bone or even amputation. Grafts and pros-

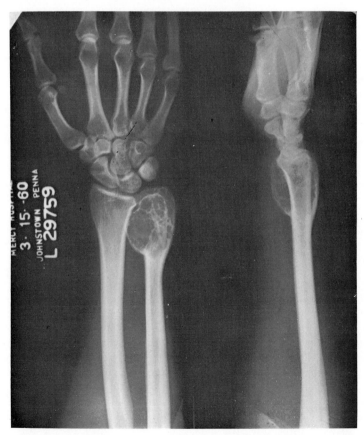

Figure 11.24. Giant cell tumor of the distal ulna. The bone has been totally destroyed and the tumor is now walled off by a thin layer of new bone. Note the typical junction of this new bone with the remaining old cortex. It is seen on the radial side most characteristically.

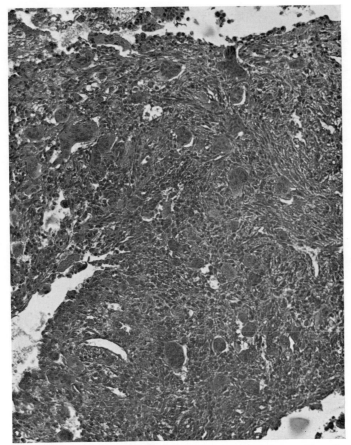

Figure 11.25.   The active stroma of giant cell tumor with tumor rather than foreign body giant cells.

theses may be used to fill the area of excision and maintain function.

Sacral tumors have a poor prognosis because of the difficulty of applying en bloc excision. There seems to be little justification for the use of the phrase "malignant transformation." Good results are obtained in anatomic locations where en bloc excision is easy. Poor results are obtained where it is difficult or impossible.

References

1. Jaffe, H., Lichtenstein, L., and Portis, R. B.: Giant cell tumor of bone, its pathological appearance, grading supposed variants and treatment, *Arch. Pathol,* 30: 993, 1940.
2. Johnson, E. W., Jr., and Dahlin, D. C.: Treatment of giant cell tumor of bone, *J. Bone Joint Surg,* 41A: 895, 1959.
3. Mhaymneh, W. A., Dudley, H. R., and Mhaymneh, L. G.: Giant cell tumor of bone, *J. Bone Joint Surg,* 46A: 63, 1964.
4. Schajowicz, F.: Giant cell tumor of bone (osteoclastoma); a pathological and histological study, *J. Bone Joint Surg,* 43A: 1, 1961.

CONGENITAL GENERALIZED FIBROMATOSIS

This rare condition has been noted at birth. It is characterized by multiple fibrous tumors available for clinical inspection in the subcutaneous tissues, but it is also found in such other tissues as the muscles, viscera, and bone.

Of the 16 cases found in the literature by Schaffzin et al.,[3] bone involvement occurred in only 4. Death in infancy is common, but regression can occur. The fata cases have all had visceral involvement. No cases of devel-

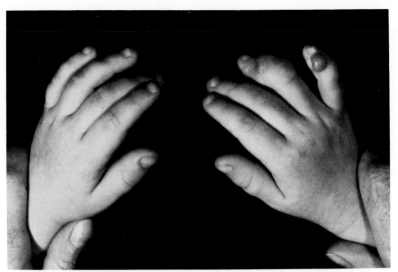

Figure 11.26. Multiple fibromas of the hand in a child.

opment of the lesion after the first few months of life have been described.

The lesions consist of fibroblastic tissue, with elongated spindle cells. The mass is not encapsulated, and there is a striking lack of atypical nuclei or mitoses. The histologic pattern of neurofibromatous tissue is absent. The fibrous tissue invades bone. Heiple et al.[1] described a case apparently limited to the skeleton with regression of the lesion in 9 months.

The cases may be confused with congenital fibrosarcoma or neurofibromatosis. The other possibilities are reticuloendotheliosis,

neuroblastoma, fibrous dysplasia, hemangioma, lymphangioma, and lipomatosis. The microscopic examination differentiates this condition from the others.

References

1. Heiple, K. G., Perrin, E., and Aikawa, M.: Congenital generalized fibromatosis, *J. Bone Joint Surg.,* *54A:* 663, 1972.
2. Kauffman, S. L., and Stout, A. P.: Congenital mesenchymal tumors, *Cancer,* *18:*460, 1965.
3. Schaffzin, E. A., Chung, S. M. K., and Kaye, R.: Congenital generalized fibromatosis with complete spontaneous regression, *J. Bone Joint Surg.,* *54:*657, 1972.

MALIGNANT TUMORS

BY JAMES H. McMASTER, M.D.

OSTEOGENIC SARCOMA

Osteogenic sarcoma is the most common primary malignancy of bone and is characterized by rapid growth, early metastasis, and a grave prognosis. Typically arising in the metaphysis of a long bone (Fig. 11.27), its distribution pattern in the body is directly related to the rate of bone growth. Thus, the distal femur, proximal tibia, and proximal humerus are the most frequently involved sites. Osteosarcoma in children is seen from

ages 3 through 20 with most cases concentrated in the pubertal years. A 2 to 1 male to female ratio has been reported by many authors. The etiology of childhood and adolescent osteosarcoma is unknown.

In adults this tumor is seen in association with Paget's disease, previous enchondromas, and bone infarcts. There are many differences between osteosarcoma in the adult and osteosarcoma in children. In children, the site predilection is for the lower extremity, distal to midfemur. In adults preexisting disease, such as Paget's disease of bone, or previous irradiation is a common antecedent. Also, it has been induced through the use of localized radiation therapy in excess of 1,500 R, radium implants, strontium-90 ingestion, beryllium ingestion and the use of Thoratrast. No convincing epidemiologic, virologic, or immunologic evidence exists implicating a virus as the etiologic agent. Although a history of trauma is frequently obtained from patients presenting with osteosarcoma, its role as an etiologic factor has not been demonstrated.

Symptoms

The insidious onset of extremity pain which becomes unrelenting, associated with a palpable mass in an adolescent is characteristic of osteosarcoma. The tumor is usually metaphyseal in location and produces minimal to severe functional impairment.

Physical Examination

The patient presenting with osteosarcoma usually appears to be in good health, although one occasionally is first seen with anorexia and distant metastasis. The tumor mass is palpable in the metaphysis of the long bone with variable tenderness on direct palpation. Highly vascular lesions are usually warm with distention of the overlying veins. Metastases are typically blood borne, although regional lymph node involvement has been reported. Because osteogenic sarcoma arises from intramedullary elements, x-ray examination reveals an alteration in the normal bony structure of the metaphysis (Fig. 11.28). A portion of the cortex is usually destroyed, and adjacent to it is subperiosteal new bone formed in response to periosteal elevation. The amount of extraosseous bone formation varies from tumor to tumor. The sclerosing osteosarcomas may form a large extraosseous mass. Other tumors are more nodular, and the lytic variety forms virtually no new bone at all. The intraosseous reaction beneath the cortical destruction causes areas of radiolucency due to dissolution of the trabeculae of cancellous bone by the tumor. Other areas demonstrate endosteal or tumor bone proliferation. The tumor is usually contained by the adjacent epiphyseal line, but there is no barrier to its diaphyseal extension. X-ray examination usually fails to reveal the true extent of the diaphyseal spread.

Computerized tomography is invaluable in helping to determine size and location of the tumor mass as well as its relationship to surrounding muscles, major vessels, nerves, and joints. It also permits accurate evaluation to establish the presence of calcium within the mass. With the advent of more sophisticated surgical approaches in the treatment of

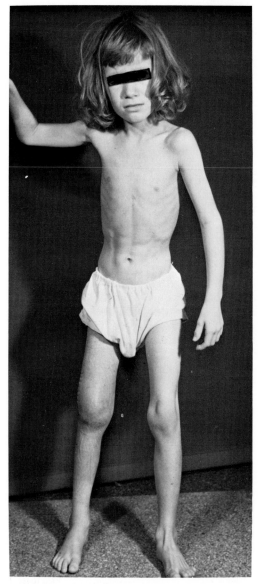

Figure 11.27. Clinical appearance of patient with osteogenic sarcoma. There is swelling of the metaphyseal area of the distal right femur.

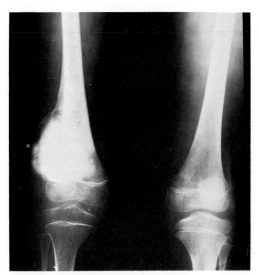

Figure 11.28. Roentgen features of osteogenic sarcoma: metaphyseal location, bone formation, globular shape, early destruction of the cortex, Codman's triangle of subperiosteal bone at the periphery, active destruction, sunburst appearance, and radial deposition of bone.

osteosarcoma, this tool will become increasingly valuable in helping with the selection of proper biopsy sites and the surgical approach. Computed tomographic studies of the pulmonary area should be performed routinely to rule out the presence of metastatic deposits that are undetectable by other roentgenographic techniques.

Laboratory Data

The usual clinical laboratory studies on patients suffering from osteogenic sarcoma add little to the diagnosis. In some cases, the serum alkaline phosphatase and erythrocyte sedimentation rate may be elevated, but these findings are variable and nonspecific. To make a definite diagnosis of osteogenic sarcoma, biopsy material must be obtained. It should be taken under tourniquet so that the best possible selection of gross material can be made. The biopsy should be adequate in size and taken from the radiolucent portion of the tumor, avoiding areas of necrotic or liquefied material. Accuracy of daignosis is of overriding importance in evaluating the biopsy material obtained, with care taken to avoid hasty, inaccurate interpretation. Per-

manent sections should be made and evaluated thoroughly by special, competent bone pathologists before definitive therapy is instituted.

Pathology

Osteogenic sarcoma most often arises from within the intramedullary canal of the metaphysis of the long bone. The tumor fills the intramedullary canal and perforates the cortex, forming a nodular, asymmetric mass about the shaft. Longitudinal sections of such a specimen usually demonstrate containment of the tumor by the epiphyseal line with variable diaphyseal extension through the intramedullary canal. The peripheral, actively growing portion of the tumor is usually fibrous or cartilaginous in nature and not as densely sclerotic and calcified as the more central regions. Most tumors remain metaphyseal in location; occasionally one is seen that extends throughout the length of the involved bone. Failure to amputate above the level of diaphyseal involvement is the cause of local recurrence of tumors when midshaft amputation is performed. For this reason some surgeons advocate routine disarticulation at the joint proximal to the long bone involved. The microscopic examination of an osteogenic sarcoma shows great variation from tumor to tumor and even within different areas of the same tumor. One constant feature is tumor bone or osteoid formation. This new osseous tissue may arise from a stroma predominantly of cartilaginous tissue. Other areas of sclerotic bone are so dense that the cellular details are obliterated. A supposedly typical field is that of very active pleomorphic osteoblasts forming irregular tumor bone with a vascular marrow and occasional malignant giant cells.

Classification

A great deal of energy has been expended on classifications of osteogenic sarcoma. In general, such classifications are based on the amount of bone produced by the tumor and on the type of stroma producing it. Thus, the tumor which destroys bone and produces little of its own would be called an "osteolytic osteogenic sarcoma." Other sarcomas cause much bone production and are called "scle-

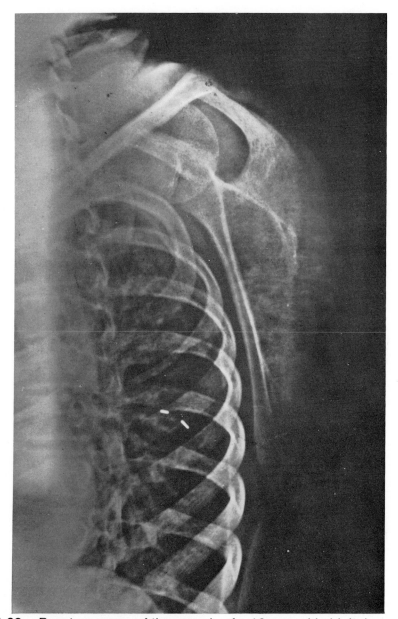

Figure 11.29. Roentgenogram of the scapula of a 13-year-old girl. It demonstrates an osteogenic sarcoma that was probably radiation induced. At age 2 years, this child had a hemangioma that was removed by x-radiation, and two randon seeds were implanted. The sarcoma quickly metastasized and caused her demise.

rosing osteogenic sarcomas." There are other classifications based on the predominant stroma of the tumor, and thus terms such as "telangiectatic," "chondroblastic," and "fibrous" osteogenic sarcoma may be used. The classification of osteogenic sarcomas is criti-cal to the proper interpretation of therapeutic results as assessed by 5-year survival rates. The typical osteosarcoma is an anaplastic malignant tumor which occurs in metaphyses of major tubular bones. Primary lesions of the skull and the trunk should not be grouped

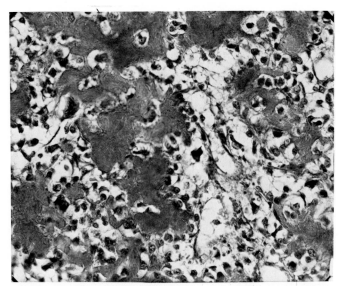

Figure 11.30.   Bone formation in osteogenic sarcoma.

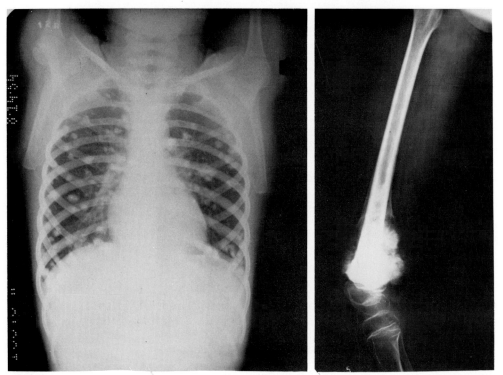

Figure 11.31.   Osteogenic sarcoma of the femoral metaphysis with osteoplastic metastases to the lungs.

with the typical tumors due to their obvious unresectability. The more distal the location of the primary tumor, the more favorable its prognosis. In evaluating therapeutic results it is important that patients with known metastatic deposits be segregated from those who are free of detectable metastases. As indicated earlier, computerized tomographic studies are invaluable in defining this distinction. Any series reported must have a sufficient number of cases to allow a valid sampling and statistical analysis. All biopsy material should be reviewed by at least one pathologist who is familiar with osseous disease to exclude benign lesions such as aneurysmal bone cyst and heterotopic ossifications, which not infrequently are misdiagnosed as osteosarcoma. Variants of osteosarcoma known to be biologically distinct from the typical tumor include the following: (1) osteosarcoma of the jawbone, (2) osteosarcoma in Paget's disease, (3) periosteal osteosarcoma, (4) multicentric osteosarcoma, (5) low grade central osteosarcoma (intramedullary), (6) parosteal osteosarcoma, (7) postradiation osteosarcoma, and (8) dedifferentiated chondrosarcoma.

Other rare variants of osteosarcoma that Dahlin suggests should be separated from ordinary tumors include: (1) telangiectatic osteosarcoma, (2) osteosarcoma resembling malignant fibrous histiocytoma, and (3) osteosarcoma known to arise in benign tumors or dysplasias.

Parosteal osteogenic sarcoma typically occurs between the ages of 10 and 40 years as an extraosseous lesion adjacent to the planum popliteum of the femur. It appears as 1–3 islands of dense new bone with a surrounding mass and causes a proliferation of the posterior cortex of the femur. As the tumor ages, the extraosseous new bone becomes confluent with the posterior cortical reaction and progresses to the entire shaft of the femur. It may assume a remarkable size with little systemic effect on the patient.

Parosteal osteogenic sarcoma can be successfully treated by local excision, if this is technically feasible. If the tumor is so large that it demands amputation, this can be done with an excellent chance of long survival in the majority of cases.

Grossly, the parosteal osteogenic sarcoma does not invade the intramedullary canal of the bone to any great extent. The tumor seems to arise from the periosteal region and to mushroom out into the soft tissue. The tumor is sclerotic toward the center and becomes less so peripherally.

Finally, it must be noted that the position of origin of osteogenic sarcoma influences the survival rate. Osteogenic sarcomas arising in the proximal metaphysis of the humerus or femur give practically no survival. Those tumors arising in the distal femoral metaphysis give a small percentage of 5-year survival. Those arising in the proximal tibial metaphysis give a still better prognosis.

Recent studies may provide a clue as to why this neoplasia is so well tolerated by its host. The host immune resonse has long been implicated as a vital component in the body's defense against neoplasia. Extensive investigation into the role of the immune response in patients with osteosarcoma has been performed. These studies clearly indicate that osteosarcoma patients are immunologically competent but their tumor is nonantigenic. This lack of antigenicity permits tumor growth to occur, unimpeded by the suppressive effect of the host immune system.

Clinical studies indicate the presence of abnormal carbohydrate metabolism in the majority of patients with osteosarcoma. In vitro experiments have demonstrated production of a peptide with marked hypoglycemic properties by cultured human osteosarcoma cells. The relationship of these biochemical observations to the etiology of the tumor is being investigated.

Treatment

Recent reports indicate significant improvement in the previously dismal prognosis associated with osteosarcoma. Classically 85% of patients with histologically proven osteosarcoma succumb to their disease within 24 months after diagnosis. Reports published by Taylor et al. indicate a 50% 5-year survival rate in patients with typical osteosarcoma treated with amputation alone. Confirmation of this observation by other institutions with a comparable group of patients would establish this as the current standard of care in treatment of this tumor. No case of spontaneous regression has been recorded, nor has cure attributable to the use of radiation therapy and/or chemotherapy without amputation been seen. These results support amputation as the best treatment available at this time and clearly indicate the need for basic investigation into the biology of this tumor.

The statistics regarding osteogenic sarcoma reveal that patients with late amputation (that

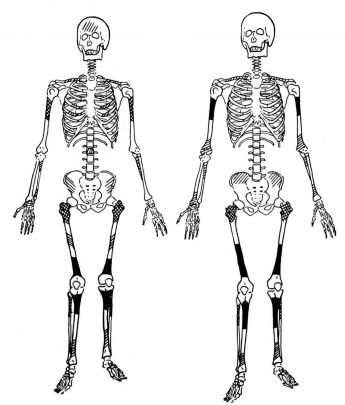

Figure 11.32. Distribution of sclerosing (*left*) and osteolytic (*right*) osteogenic sarcoma. The greatest incidence is in the metaphyseal areas above and below the knee (*shaded black*). (From C. T. Geschickter and M. M. Copeland: *Tumors of Bone*, Ed. 3; Philadelphia: J. B. Lippincott, 1949.)

is, amputation after a period of months in which the tumor was known to exist) have a higher survival rate than those with immediate amputation (Ferguson[5]). Whether this finding reflects only a lower degree of malignancy among the former group of patients or is a valid indication of correct treatment may still be argued. However, patients who have had a delayed amputation and preliminary x-ray treatment have had a better than expected course in our direct observation. These tumors are thought to be insensitive to x-ray therapy. There is however, a maturing influence, because the tumor tends to become more osteoplastic, denser by roentgenogram, and less painful after x-radiation.

The patient gains weight; fever, if it is present, subsides; and the sedimentation rate, if it has been elevated, declines. When the tumor is quiescent and has no new radiolucent areas, the limb is amputated. The level

of amputation is not necessarily that of disarticulation, but it is as far removed from the tumor as possible. Recurrence in the stump is rare.

Other modes of therapy currently under investigation include the following:

1. Routine postoperative administration of adjuvant chemotherapy using a variety of agents, varying routes of administration and duration of treatment.

2. Preoperative administration of chemotherapeutic agents followed either by amputation or prosthetic replacement of the involved bone.

3. Preoperative irradiation of the primary tumor coupled with preoperative irradiation of lung fields followed by amputation in cases in which metastases have failed to appear.

4. Section and allograft replacement of primary tumor in selected cases. This may or

may not be combined with postoperative adjuvant chemotherapy or radiation therapy.

5. Use of interferon to elicit a systemic immune response against both the primary tumor and its metastases.

6. The administration of high dose intra-arterial chemotherapeutic agents in conjunction with amputation.

It is imperative that the guidelines discussed earlier be kept in mind in evaluating the efficacy of each of these therapeutic methods. Current data indicate that a 50% 5-year survival rate is the standard of treatment in osteosarcoma.

References

1. Badgley, C. E., and Batts, M., Jr.: Osteogenic sarcoma, *Arch. Surg.* 43:541, 1941.
2. Colby, B. L.: *Neoplasms of Bone and Related Conditions,* New York: Paul B. Hoeber, 1949.
3. Coventry, M. B., and Dahlin, D. C.: Osteogenic sarcoma, *J. Bone Joint Surg.* 39A:741, 1957.
4. Dahlin, D. C.: Problems in the interpretation of results of treatment for osteosarcoma, *Mayo Clin. Proc.* 54:621, 1979.
5. Ferguson, A. B.: Treatment of osteogenic sarcoma, *J. Bone Joint Surg.* 22:916, 1940.
6. Goodman, M. A., McMaster, J. H., Drash, A. L., Diamond, P. E., Kappakas, G. S., and Scranton, P. E., Jr.: Metabolic and endocrine alterations in osteosarcoma patients, *Cancer,* 42:603, 1978.
7. Hatcher, C. H.: The development of sarcoma in bone subjected to roentgen or radium irradiation, *J. Bone Joint Surg.* 27:179, 1945.
8. Jenkil, R. D. T., Allt, W. E. C., and Fitzpatrick, P. J.: Osteosarcoma, *Cancer,* 30:393, 1972.
9. Marcove, R. C., Mike, V., Jajek, J. V., Levin, A. G., and Hutter, R. V. P.: Osteogenic sarcoma under the age of 21; a review of 145 operative cases, *J. Bone Joint Surg.* 52A:411, 1970.
10. McMaster, J. H., Ferguson, R. J., and Weinert, C.: The host-immune response in osteosarcoma, *Clin. Orthop.* No. III: 76, 1975.
11. Schumacher, T. M., Genant, H. K., Korobkin, M., and Bovill, E. G.: Computed tomography; its use in space-occupying lesions of the musculoskeletal system, *J. Bone Joint Surg.* 60A:600, 1978.
12. Sweetnam, R., Knoweldon, J., and Seddon, H.: Bone sarcoma; treatment by irradiation, amputation, or a combination of the two, *Br. Med. J.* 2:363, 1971.
13. Taylor, W. F., Ivins, J. C., Dahlin, D. C., Edmonson, J. H., and Pritchard, D. J.: Trends and variability in survival from osteosarcoma. *Mayo Clin. Proc.* 53:695, 1978.

EWING'S SARCOMA

Original Description

In 1921 Ewing[5] described a lesion he called diffuse endothelioma of bone. He reported a total of 7 cases and characterized the disease as a primarily lytic lesion of bone that is extremely radiosensitive and readily metastasizes to the lungs and to other bones. All of his patients apparently died of the disease. Histologically, the tumor was stated to be "composed of broad sheets of small polyhedral cells with pale cytoplasm, small hyperchromatic nuclei, well defined cell borders, and complete absence of extracellular material." He postulated the probable endothelial origin of this tumor. No postmortem examination was performed on any of these patients. The course was that of rather rapid development of metastases to the lung and skull and of exophthalmos.

Since this original report, the literature has contained an interesting running debate as to whether such a disease entity actually exists and, if it does, what its clinical and histologic picture really presents.

Clinical Picture

The most common period of onset of Ewing's sarcoma is the second decade of life. The average age is about 15 years, but the extremes are 3 and 40 years of age. Most reports suggest it is twice as common in boys as in girls.

SYMPTOMS

The first complaint is pain in the region of a bone. The pain may be intermittent for several weeks or months, but it then becomes constant. It is unrelated to activity, and it usually interferes with sleep. If the lesion is in the region of a rather superficial osseous structure, it may present a tender mass, but otherwise it causes a diffuse swelling of an extremity. The symptoms quickly become totally disabling. Fever may be noted soon after the onset of pain, and it is usually intermittent.

SIGNS

Physical examination early in the disease reveals tender enlargement of the shaft of a long bone. Should the lesion be near the metaphysis of a long bone, it causes some limitation of motion of a major joint. If the patient is seen when two or more bones are involved, he appears cachectic and may have fever.

X-ray Examination

Much has been written of the characteristic roentgenographic appearance of Ewing's sarcoma. It should be a lytic diaphyseal lesion of subperiosteal new bone that has an onion skin appearance. Such a typical lesion was seen in 65% of cases in a review of a series by Sherman. Coley et al.[4] found the typical roentgenographic picture in less than half of their cases.

Ewing's sarcoma causes rapid lysis in whatever bone it affects. It appears locally multifocal, as if arising from myeloid elements. Its rapid growth results in sudden elevation of the periosteum, and the roentgenogram reflects this by evidence of periosteal new bone beyond the limits of the lesion (Fig. 11.33). Directly over the area of destruction, the tumor cells may be growing so rapidly that subperiosteal new bone may not be seen. Within the medullary canal, the tumor grows so quickly that the host bone rarely responds by sclerosis. Only 10% of the lesions in Sherman's series showed sclerosis.

Laboratory Data

The most consistent change in the hemogram is a hypochromic, normocytic anemia. The erythrocyte sedimentation rate is elevated. In patients with fever, there may be a moderate leukocytosis.

Pathology

Grossly, Ewing's sarcoma causes a much more extensive involvement than the roentgenogram suggests. Nodules of tumor are found in the intramedullary canal beyond the areas of obvious bone destruction. These tumors appear as grayish white, glistening nodules.

Microscopically, the characteristic lesion differs from that which Ewing originally described. The tumor appears as sheets of closely packed, dark-staining, rather uniform cells (Fig. 11.34). There is very little cytoplasm and no clearly defined cell boundaries. The typical cell nucleus contains finely divided chromatin and is about twice the size of the nucleus of a lymphocyte. Vascularity is not the predominant picture. True rosettes are not seen in this lesion.

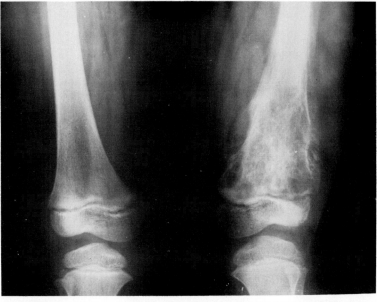

Figure 11.33.   Roentgenogram of Ewing's sarcoma exhibiting infiltrative type of destruction, tendency to run axially along the shaft, and multiple layers of subperiosteal ossification. A disphyseal location is more typical.

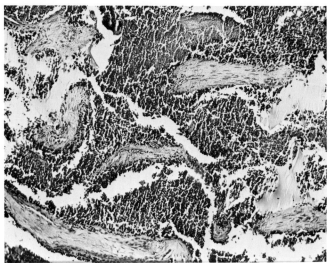

Figure 11.34.   Ewing's sarcoma with sheets of endothelial cells separated by fibrous tissue septa.

Differential Diagnosis

From the foregoing description, it is evident that the clinical picture may be confused with those of other more common diseases. Not infrequently, a patient with pain in an extremity, fever, leukocytosis, and a roentgenogram showing a destructive mottled lesion of bone may be considered to have osteomyelitis. Grossly at surgery, fluid-simulating pus may be seen surrounding a sequestrated portion of diaphysis. Microscopic examination may show tissue that suggests an abscess lining. Further research on the tissue may reveal the sheets of cells that are considered to characterize a Ewing's sarcoma. The prognosis in these cases that resemble osteomyelitis seems universally poor.

Eosinophilic granuloma may present with the same clinical and roentgenographic changes as Ewing's sarcoma and must be included in the differential diagnosis.

Treatment

One of the characteristics of this tumor that was originally noted by Ewing is its very gratifying disappearance after roentgen therapy. He also noted that the lesion soon reappeared, if not in its original site, as a "metastasis" to another bone or in the lungs (Fig. 11.36). Some report long term survivals following roentgen treatment of a single lesion, but these are exceptions. Surgical ablation, locally or by amputation, has not given any more satisfactory results. The combination of surgery and x-ray therapy has failed to increase the survival rate. At present the most universal treatment is roentgen therapy to the destructive lesion of the bone and to as much of the adjacent normal-appearing bone as possible.

Past experience amply documents the futility of radical amputation in this disease. Recently, the combination of supervoltage radiation in combination with vincristine and cyclophosphamide has greatly improved the patient's chances of surviving this tumor. The role of the orthopaedic surgeon should be strictly limited to obtaining adequate biopsy material to permit accurate histologic diagnosis. Radical surgical procedures are no longer indicated in patients suffering from Ewing's sarcoma.

Course

The patient presenting originally with a single lesion receives dramatic relief from 3,000–4,000 R of x-radiation. Usually, the symptoms of persistent pain return within 6–12 months, and a second course of treatment gives much less relief or none at all. It is not uncommon for the presenting lesion to re-

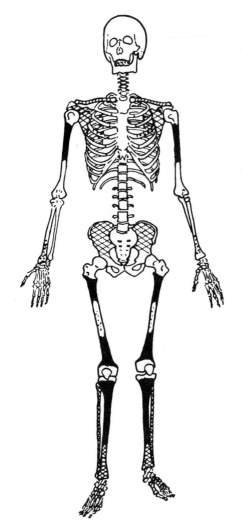

Figure 11.35. Distribution of Ewing's sarcoma. (From C. T. Geschickter and M. M. Copeland: *Tumors of Bone*, Ed. 3; Philadelphia: J. B. Lippincott, 1949.)

main quiescent, yet for the patient to expire from pulmonary metastases. Regardless of treatment, 95% of all patients with this disease succumb to it within 5 years.

References

1. Bardin, R. P.: Similarity of clinical and roentgen findings in children with Ewing's sarcoma and neuroblastoma, *Am. J. Roentgenol., 50:* 575, 1943.
2. Boyer, C. W., Jr., Barkner, T. J., and Perry, R. H.: Ewing's sarcoma; case against surgery, *Cancer, 20:* 1602, 1972.
3. Charpure, V. V.: Endothelial myeloma, *Am. J. Pathol., 17:* 503, 1941.
4. Coley, B. L., Higenbotham, N. L., and Bowden, L.: Endothelioma of bone, *Ann. Surg., 128:* 533, 1948.
5. Ewing, J.: Diffuse endothelioma of bone, *Proc. N. Y. Pathol. Soc., 21:* 17, 1921.
6. Foote, F. W., Jr., and Anderson, H. R.: Histogenesis of Ewing's tumor, *Am. J. Pathol., 17:* 497, 1941.
7. Histo, H. O., Pinkel, D., and Prah, C. B.: Treatment of clinically localized Ewing's sarcoma with radiotherapy and combination chemotherapy, *Cancer, 30:* 1522, 1972.
8. Stout, A. P.: A discussion of the pathogenesis and histogenesis of Ewing's tumor, *Am. J. Roentgenol., 50:* 334, 1943.
9. Wang, C. C., and Schultz, M. D.: Ewing's sarcoma, *N. Engl. J. Med., 248:* 571, 1953.
10. Willis, R. A.: Metastatic neuroblastoma in bone presenting the Ewing syndrome, *Am. J. Pathol., 16:* 317, 1940.

NEUROBLASTOMA

This tumor is derived from sympathetic formative cells. The primary tumor is, therefore, located wherever the sympathetic ganglia are found or in the suprarenal medulla. Neuroblastoma should be considered as an embryonal tumor in spite of the fact that it is seen in patients in the second decade of life. In children less than 2 years old, it is usually confined to the thorax or abdomen. Such tumors are usually amenable to surgical ablation and x-ray therapy, and they give an appreciable survival rate. Neuroblastoma of this clinical type does not frequently metastasize to bone.

The orthopaedist is concerned with those cases of neuroblastoma in which the initial complaint is due to an osseous metastasis. Such cases are unusual before the age of 2 years and are most commonly seen between 5 and 15 years of age. Because of the retroperitoneal origin of neuroblastoma, it may give rather unusual complaints and findings. Ten cases in the literature simulated appendicitis closely enough to force an abdominal exploration, which revealed a large retroperitoneal tumor in the right iliac fossa. Neuroblastoma arising anterior to the sacroiliac joint may cause pain in the femoral nerve distribution or femoral nerve paralysis. The most common complaint, however, is the spontaneous onset of constant deep pain in the extremity, which is usually accompanied by swelling and is ultimately disabling.

The patient not infrequently presents with weight loss and fever, as if he were suffering

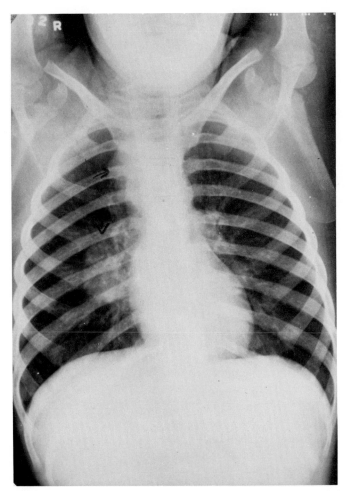

Figure 11.36.   Metastases to the lung from Ewing's sarcoma of the femur.

from an infectious process. Laboratory data may support this impression by showing anemia, leukocytosis, and an elevated sedimentation rate. Gaffney et al.[6] reported finding characteristic tumor cells in the bone marrow smears from 15 patients with neuroblastoma. In 13 of these 15 positive cases, the marrow smears contained tumor cells when the patients were first observed.

Roentgenographic examination of the osseous lesion reveals bone destruction and usually no bone reaction. The periosteum is soon elevated, and there is an adjacent soft-tissue mass. Some suggest that femoral lesions tend to be symmetric.

Microscopic examination of biopsy material shows a tumor composed of sheets of deep-staining cells of uniform size. These cells possess very little cytoplasm and no extracellular material. There are usually large areas of necrosis within the tumor. A supposedly characteristic microscopic finding is the presence of rosettes (Fig. 11.37). These are circular collections of tumor cells around a central collection of fibrils. They may not, however, be present in a metastasis of neuroblastoma or even in all of the primary lesion.

Treatment

Neuroblastoma of bone is a metastatic lesion that is usually sensitive to x-radiation. Because the osseous lesion is a metastasis, surgical ablation is not rewarding. After the administration of large doses of x-radiation (2,500–3,500 R) to the neuroblastoma, the tumor usually recedes, only to recur locally or as another metastasis.

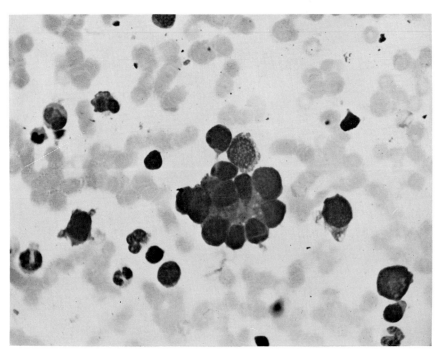

Figure 11.37. Marrow smear from a child with metastatic neuroblastoma. Illustration shows neuroblastoma cells assuming a rosette-like arrangement. (From P. C. Gaffney, C. F. Hansman, and G. H. Fetterman: Experience with smears of aspirates from bone marrow in diagnosis of neuroblastoma, *American Journal of Clinical Pathology, 31:* 213, 1959.).

This tumor tends to metastasize to the skull, orbit, and maxilla, as well as to the lungs. The course is usually very rapid and ends fatally 6 months to 1 year after diagnosis.

Neuroblastoma is unique in its high rate of spontaneous regression, particularly in young infants. This phenonemon is seen more frequently in neuroblastoma than in any other human cancer. Considerable investigative effort has been extended in attempting to define the role of the host immune system in this disease. The concept of host suppression of tumor through the immune mechanism is supported by the positive correlation of lymphocyte infiltration of tumor with enhanced survival. Also important in the prognosis is the age of the patient (younger patients having the more favorable prognosis) and the presence of the primary lesion in the chest. Bone marrow involvement does not preclude survival, but lytic bone disease usually has a fatal outcome. Although chemotherapy and radiation therapy are widely used in treatment of this disease, their role remains poorly defined.

Bodian[1] was enthusiastic about the arresting effect of vitamin B_{12} on the tumor. His enthusiasm has not been shared by others, for the most responsive cases occurred in the younger age group, in which the tumor has a good prognosis under surgical and radiation therapy also. A combination therapy of α-methopterin, actinomycin D, and Cytoxan is being used, and a new agent, Leuropristin, shows some promise. The nitrogen mustards have not been effective.

It should be evident from the foregoing description of Ewing's sarcoma and neuroblastoma—the onset, clinical and roentgenographic findings, pathologic description, and course—that these lesions are quite similar. Not infrequently it is impossible to distinguish between the two entities unless an autopsy is performed. The literature records that frequently a postmortem examination of a patient who dies of what seemed to be Ewing's sarcoma reveals a large retroperitoneal tumor that proves to be a neuroblastoma, and the original diagnosis is changed. At the Children's Hospital of Pittsburgh, there have been 45 diagnoses of neuroblastoma in the past 10 years. Twelve of these have been confirmed by autopsy. Ewing's sarcoma has been diagnosed in 15 patients, but none of these have been autopsied. For the arguments in favor of the opinion that these lesions differ, one should read Foote, Charpure, Lichtenstein, and Jaffe. Friedman and Hanaoka have pointed out the value of electron microscopy in differentiating Ewing's sarcoma from neuroblastoma. The presence of cytoplasmic glycogen deposits strongly suggests the diagnosis of Ewing's sarcoma. Conversely, the demonstration of neurofibril by the electron microscope establishes the diagnosis of neuroblastoma. It is imperative, therefore, that orthopaedic surgeons involved in biopsying these lesions anticipate the need to obtain specimens for electron microscopy and also have the necessary preservatives available to permit proper handling of the tissue. A recent review of 64 children with neuroblastoma was reported by Haas et al. The most common sites of involvement were the abdomen and thorax. Those patients under 1 year of age without evidence of bony metastasis have a highly favorable outcome (13 of 15). Those patients with bony lesions failed to attain long term disease-free survival despite the combined use of radiation therapy and chemotherapy (33 of 34). Histologic and biochemical characteristics were of no prognostic value. The urinary secretion of vanillylmandelic acid, however, was useful as an index of response to treatment. The sex of the patient played no role in determining the outcome of the disease process.

References

1. Bodian, M.: Neuroblastoma, *Pediatr. Clin. North Am.*, *6:* 449, 1959.
2. Charoche, H.: Neuroblastoma, *Am. J. Surg.*, *87:* 545, 1954.
3. Evans, A. E.: Treatment of neuroblastoma, *Cancer*, *30:* 1695, 1972.
4. Farber, S.: Neuroblastoma, *Am. J. Dis. Child.*, *66:* 749, 1940.
5. Friedman, B., and Hanaoka, H.: Round cell sarcomas of bone (a light and electron microscopic study), *J. Bone Joint Surg.*, *53A:* 1118, 1971.
6. Gaffney, P. C., Hansman, C. F., and Fetterman, G. H.: Experience with smears of aspirates from bone marrow in the diagnosis of neuroblastoma, *Am. J. Clin. Pathol.*, *31:* 213, 1959.
7. Hendren, W. H.: Pediatric surgery, *N. Engl. J. Med.*, *289:* 562, 1973.

RETICULUM CELL SARCOMA

Reticulum cell sarcoma was distinguished as an entity by Parker and Jackson[2] in 1939. It is believed to be derived from the reticulum cells of the bone marrow and offers a more hopeful outlook than Ewing's sarcoma. Typ-

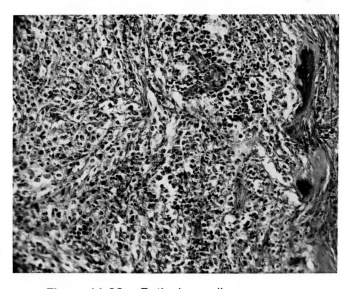

Figure 11.38. Reticulum cell sarcoma.

ically, the general condition of the patient is unaffected. The tumor has a tendency to remain localized to a single bone for a considerable time before it metastasizes to regional lymph nodes or distantly via the blood stream. The tumor ordinarily affects adults, but some cases have been seen in children.

The roentgenographic picture resembles that of Ewing's sarcoma somewhat, except that the reticulum cell sarcoma involves the metaphyseal area. It is osteolytic and tends to break out through the cortex on one side. There is little or no cortical or periosteal reaction. The tumor readily involves the epiphyseal region.

The tumor cell has a round or oval nucleus, approximately twice the size of a lymphocyte. It may be elongated or lobulated. There may be a fair amount of cytoplasm. Giant cells are not seen, but mitoses are present. A reticulum stain brings out strands running around areas of tumor cells (Fig. 11.38).

The prognosis, if appropriate treatment is given, is apparently much better than in cases of Ewing's tumor. Treatment includes amputation or radical resection followed by roentgen therapy.

References

1. Francis, K. C., Higenbotham, N. L., and Caley, B. L.: Primary reticulum cell sarcoma of bone, *Surg. Gynecol. Obstet.*, *99:* 142: 1954.
2. Parker, F. Jr., and Jackson, H., Jr.: Primary reticulum cell sarcoma of bone, *Surg. Gynecol. Obstet.*, *68:* 45, 1939.
3. Valls, J., Muscolo, D., and Schajowicz, F.: Reticulum cell sarcoma of bone, *J. Bone Joint Surg.*, *34B:* 588, 1952.

CHAPTER 12

The Neck and Shoulder

CONGENITAL DEFORMITIES

Spina Bifida

Spina bifida is the term applied to the hiatus or gap due to failure of fusion of the laminae of the neural arches, through which a sac may protrude. This sac may or may not contain nerve elements, and the degree of defect determines the type of resulting deformity.

ETIOLOGY

Spina bifida occulta occurs on occasion in the neck as a congenital skeletal defect without any protrusion of the dura. Occasionally a meningocele, perhaps containing spinal fluid but no neural elements, originates from the dura and protrudes through the laminal defect.

CLINICAL PICTURE

A spina bifida occulta is suspected if superficially on the neck there is a localized overgrowth of hair or a small dimple. Very rarely is there a lump or protrusion large enough to palpate. A dimple responsible for repeated attacks of meningeal irritation may be hidden by occipital hair.

TREATMENT

The dimple may be a clue to a congenital dural sinus, particularly if it has a midline location. The sinus may be responsible for meningeal irritation and even for meningitis if infection arises from it. Its removal is indicated. Great care in the excision and adequate closure of the dura are essential to a successful result. Removal of the frank occipital and cervical myelomeningocele falls in the province of neurosurgery.

Klippel-Feil Syndrome

The Klippel-Feil syndrome might better be termed a congenital fusion in which two or more vertebrae become anatomically fused to each other. Such spines appear quite disorganized by roentgenogram (Fig. 12.1).

ETIOLOGY

The origin of such deformities cannot be laid to the failure of ossification centers to develop because it antedates the period of their formation.

CLINICAL PICTURE

The cervical spine is limited in motion. The neck appears to be short, and, if sufficient involvement has occurred, the head may seem to be resting between the shoulders, and broad "webs" of skin and soft tissue extend out to the shoulders (Fig. 12.2). Some neurologic changes may accompany this deformity owing to involvement of the cord. X-rays reveal vertebral disorganization with multiple anomalies (Fig. 12.3). There is no characteristic distribution of the involved vertebrae.

TREATMENT

Severe though this disability may be, there is no treatment that will fully correct the deformity. Stretching by traction and passive exercises are used. Plastic improvement of the skin "webs" may be indicated.

There is a significant association of major anomalies with the Klippel-Feil syndrome. Of great significance are those involving the renal system. In our seriess of 20 patients, 16 were found to have absence of one kidney. Cardiac anomalies and other musculoskeletal anomalies, such as congenital absence of the thumb, also occur. An intravenous pyelogram is important as part of the work-up

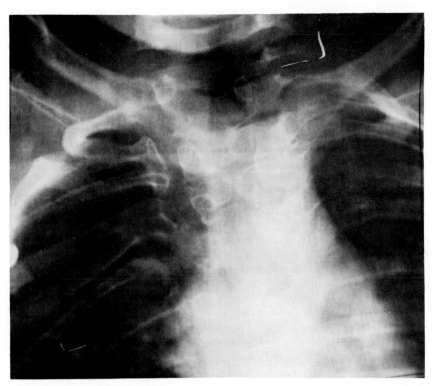

Figure 12.1. Multiple vertebral and rib anomalies in upper thoracic spine in patient with Klippel-Feil syndrome.

because ptosis of the other kidney and secondary involvement may also occur.

The excessive motion of those joints that are free above and below the fixed segments may lead to cord impingement in adult life.

Sprengel's Deformity

A cephalad position of the scapula, which lies above its normal position and between the spines of the second to seventh dorsal vertebrae, appears to be congenital (Fig. 12.4). This deformity has also been designated congenital elevation of the scapula, congenital high scapula, and undescended scapula. Sprengel made a preliminary report on the omovertebral connection in 1880 and reported 4 cases of the deformity in 1891.

Cavendish[2] has researched still earlier reports. The first description was that of Ealenberg in 1863. Willett and Walsham reported 2 cases in 1880 and 1883 and included excision of the omovertebral bone with improvement of function in their treatment.

Putti's operation entailed transplantation of the scapula to a lower level by excision of the protruding part of the scapula and its muscle attachment. Modification and various methods of holding the scapula down have been described by Delchef (1922), Schrock (1926), Green (1957),[4] and Allen (1964).[1] Woodward's[9] procedure in 1961 was a radical departure from these methods. Macfarland (1950)[6] made a case for massive scapula excision, particularly of the protruding elements, leaving only the glenoid and coracoid processes as a means of improving the appearance of the patient.

The anlage of the scapula can be differentiated at the fifth week in the embryo. At this point, it lies opposite the lower four cervical and upper two thoracic vertebrae. During the ninth week of embryonic development, the descent of the scapula begins. By the third month, its descent is complete. It is the rule rather than the exception to find associated anomalies of the cervical and thoracic spine as well as of the ribs. In one-third of the cases, an omovertebral bone is found. It may be osseous, fibrous, or cartilaginous. It arises from the proximal vertebral border and may be joined to processes of the lower cervical vertebrae.

ETIOLOGY

Various origins of the deformity have been suggested. Horwitz in 1908 mentioned a number of possibilities, including excessive intrauterine pressure related to an improper amount of amniotic fluid. Defective musculature or an abnormal articulation could in essence tie the scapula to its embryonic position and arrest its development.

The "bleb" theory was stated by Engel,[3] who, in 1943, postulated such an abnormal condition as failure to achieve midline union sufficiently early. Cerebral spinal fluid could, in such a case, escape from the fourth ventricle into the subcutis of the adjacent neck region. Such blebs, as they spread over the

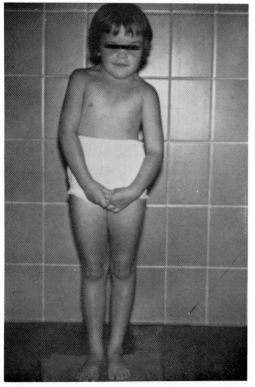

Figure 12.2. In Kleippel-Feil syndrome, the shortening of the cervical spine brings the head toward the chest. The deformed appearance is accentuated by a tendency toward webbing over either shoulder.

neck, would result in pressure and inflammation. A Klippel-Feil deformity could then occur in the neck and a Sprengel's deformity in the shoulder area. Engel believed that the escape of fluid from the fourth ventricle normally forms the subarachnoid space. If the bleb spreads over the upper limb, deformities of the humerus, radius, and ulna, and ultimately syndactylism and other anomalies of the fingers, could occur.

CLINICAL PICTURE

The condition is unilateral and results in an elevated shoulder and a neck that appears short. The youngster does not appear to be standing fully upright, and indeed some scoliosis of the upper dorsal and lower cervical region is usually present (Fig. 12.5). The palpable outline of the scapula, measured from its superior to its inferior border, reveals the fact that it is smaller than the scapula of the opposite side. On the other hand, roentgenogram confirms the fact that both the axillary and vertebral borders are increased. There is a rotary change that cocks the upper medial angle of the scapula toward the midline and the inferior angle consequently toward the axilla.

The omovertebral connection, by its union to the lower cervical area and by its being, in substance, a complete bony union, may limit motion of the scapula markedly.

As Greenville and Coventry[5] have remarked, surgical intervention is determined by three considerations: (1) the deforming appearance, (2) the loss of a function, such as abduction of the arm, and (3) pain.

Pain is not ordinarily a factor in the childhood period. The deforming appearance is the principal presenting complaint, and the child is usually seen at approximately age 7–10. It is important to recognize that the appearance may worsen because the deformity is of the type that progresses with growth. Function may become increasingly limited, and pain may eventually result.

TREATMENT

From a conservative viewpoint, voluntary elevation of the opposite shoulder markedly improves the appearance. Exercises for the opposite shoulder may be helpful in this regard. Although we have tried such a pro-

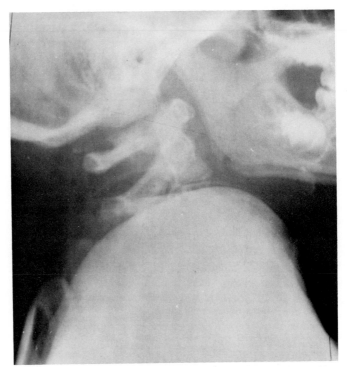

Figure 12.3. Short cervical spine in Klippel-Feil syndrome.

gram during several years with a number of children, we have not been able to procure persistent voluntary elevation of the scapula. The range of motion can occasionally be improved by stretching and by such exercises as chinning on a bar.

Operative procedures that have been developed include (1) removal of the omovertebral bone alone to improve motion, (2) extensive subperiosteal stripping of the scapula and removal of a large part of its upper portion, and (3) complete freeing of the scapula by subperiosteal dissection and anchoring of it as far as possible distally by attachment to a rib through fascia.

GREEN PROCEDURE

William T. Green has a long follow-up of the surgical correction of congenital elevation of the scapula by a method he originally applied in 1941. The procedure gets high marks, not only for the cosmetic appearance, but for the improvement in function. The incision is not as objectionable as the long spinal scar obtained with the Woodward procedure.

The child is prone and the incision follows the superior and medial border of the scapula. Using sharp dissection, the muscles connecting the scapula to the trunk are divided at their insertion into the scapula. Tight bands connecting the lower pole of the scapula to the chest wall are divided as well. Once freed, the scapula is pulled distally an obtainable amount. The muscles are then reattached at their new relationship to the scapula. The scapula is held by skeletal traction in its new position for 3 weeks.

To do the procedure well, the trapezius must be clearly removed from the spine of the scapula and retracted medially. If this is not done, the anatomy of the muscles inserting on the scapula will not be well visualized. The trapezius will be replaced after the reconstruction.

The levator scapulae muscle is divided from the scapula and the omovertebral bone visualized. This is removed extraperiosteally. The proximal portion may be difficult anatomically and requires great care.

An important cosmetic improvement is gained by removal of the superior portion of the scapula beneath the medial portion of the supraspinatus muscle. The muscle is later reattached to the spine of the scapula.

A heavy steel wire in the spine of the scapula is the instrument to pull the scapula distally. It exits to pull the scapula distally. It exits through the skin distal to the scapula. It is essential to avoid overpull which could put

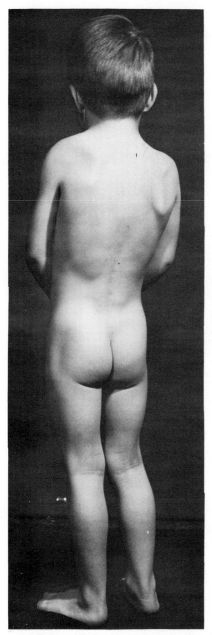

Figure 12.4. High scapula on the left constituting Sprengel's deformity.

traction on the brachial plexus. The wire is attached distally, and function of the patient is carefully observed in the postoperative course.

In any procedure, the danger of decreasing the traction of the scapula on the brachial plexus, which may result in paralysis of the arm, must be borne in mind. Such an eventuality shows up principally as deltoid and biceps weakness and must be carefully watched for. Here Robinson has added an important procedure. Its value lies in preventing this complication and thereby allowing a more radical descent of the scapula no matter which procedure is used. This increases the validity of the end results in terms of better cosmesis and function. Robinson's addition is essentially morcellation of the middle third of the clavicle. The middle third is excised subperiosteally. It is divided into small segments and replaced in a manner to hold the periosteal cuff open. The cuff and soft tissues are then resutured.

In Woodward's procedure (Figs. 12.10–12.12), a midline incision is made from the fourth cervical to the ninth dorsal spine. The skin and subcutaneous tissues are undermined to expose the vertebral border of the scapula. It is now possible to lower the scapula without moving the skin with it if the medial attachments (midline) holding it are cut.

The trapezius is identified in the lower reaches of the incision and is separated from the latissimus dorsi by blunt dissection. The origin of the trapezius is removed from the spinous processes by sharp dissection. The major and minor rhomboids are divided at their origin as dissection progresses. The rhomboids and the proximal trapezius are separated from the serratus and sacrospinalis. This continuous sheet of muscle is retracted to give access to the omovertebral bone or fibrous bands arising from the superior vertebral border. The spinal accessory nerve lying on the undersurface of the trapezius may easily be stretched and must be guarded during this phase of the operation. This is also true of the nerve to the rhomboids.

Any breaking of the supraspinatous portion of the scapula is removed by rongeurs at this stage. Subperiosteal stripping is avoided. The superior portion of the trapezius usually has to be sectioned at about the fourth cer-

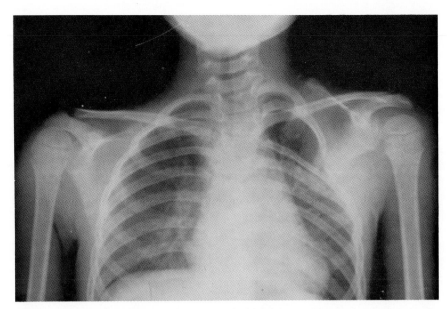

Figure 12.5. Roentgenogram with congenital high scapula and accompanying lower cervical-upper dorsal scoliosis.

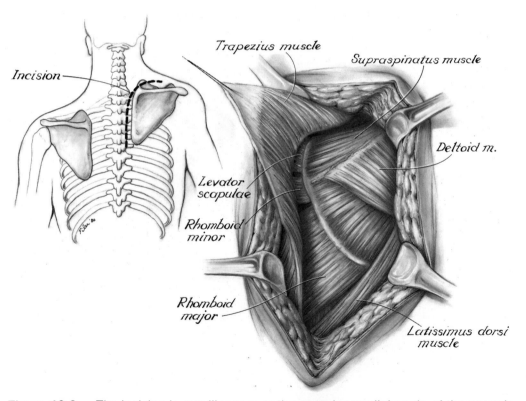

Figure 12.6. The incision is curvilinear over the superior-medial angle of the scapula. It should be proximal enough to permit excision of the superior angle of the scapula and its extension to the cervical spine as necessary. Identification of the trapezius muscle and its release and medial retraction permit visualization of the anatomy of the scapula. (Redrawn from W. T. Green: Sprengel's deformity. *American Academy of Orthopaedic Surgeons Instructional Course Lectures*, Vol. XXI, 1972.)

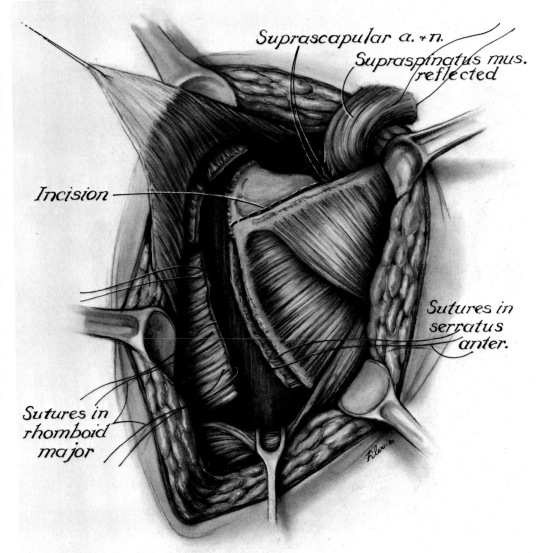

Suprascapular a. + n.

Supraspinatus mus. reflected

Incision

Sutures in serratus anter.

Sutures in rhomboid major

Figure 12.7. The posteromedial angle of the scapula is resected, and the medial muscle insertions of the medial edge of the scapula are released.

vical level. The levator scapulae muscle is released.

It is now possible to pull this muscle sheet distally until the spine of the scapula lies about opposite the one on the normal side. The inferior angle should not be used as a measure of correction because overpull might result.

As the aponeurosis of trapezium and rhomboids is held down, it is sewn into its new position at the midline. Because one works from above downward, a fold is created. It may be clipped off at the lower end, and the defect created may be sutured.

A Velpeau type dressing is worn for several weeks before active use of the shoulder is begun. In Woodward's series, 1 patient had demonstrable weakness and sensory loss which returned after a 6-month interval. Keloid formation in scars in this area is not unlikely.

DISCUSSION

Cavendish has classified congenital elevation of the scapula into the following grades: Grade I: very mild, the shoulder joints are level and deformity invisible when the pa-

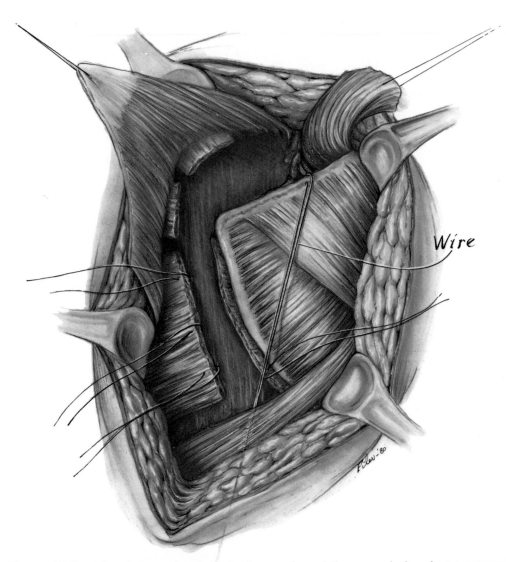

Figure 12.8. The deformed supraspinatus portion of the scapula has been removed. The rhomboids have been divided at their insertion and marked by sutures. A wire has been attached to the spine of the scapula in order to put traction on the scapula, drawing it distally.

tient is dressed; Grade 2: the shoulder joints are almost level, but there is a visible protuberance when the patient is dressed; Grade 3: moderate, the shoulder joint is elevated 2–5 cm, a very visible deformity; and Grade 4: severe, the shoulder is elevated so that the superior angle of the scapula is near the occiput with or without neck webbing.

Loss of ability to fully abduct the arm—a very definite loss of function—enters into the consideration for surgery, as does cosmetic appearance.

If surgery is to be considered for correction, then because of the tendency of this lesion to be progressive, it should be done in the young age group, roughly from 4–7 years. One can expect improvement in function and appearance, but absolute anatomic likeness to the opposite shoulder is frequently not obtained. However, the change is sufficient to justify the procedure.

An important addition to any procedure for an elevated scapula is morcellation of the middle third of the clavicle. This allows a

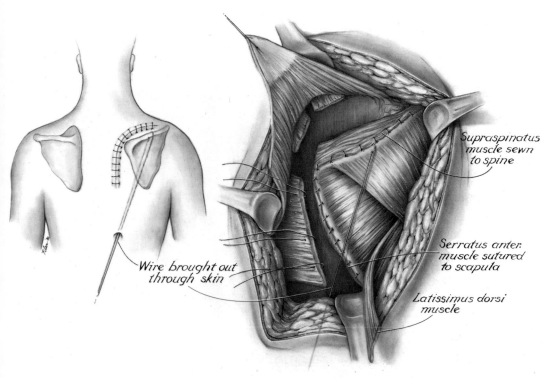

Figure 12.9. The supraspinatus is sutured back against the spine of the scapula. The serratus is reattached, and the rhomboids marked by sutures will be reattached to the scapula in its new position. The scapula is drawn distally into a pocket beneath the latissimus dorsi. Holding traction will be applied to wire brought out through the skin.

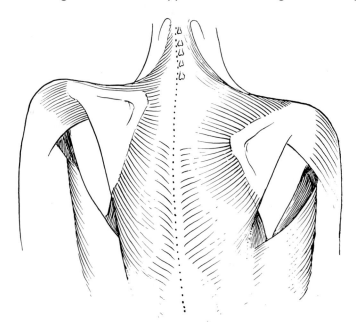

Figure 12.10. In the operation for Sprengel's deformity reported by Woodward, the incision is made in the midline from the fourth cervical to the ninth dorsal spine. The skin is undermined to the vertebral border of the scapula. (From J. W. Woodward: Congenital elevation of the scapula, *Journal of Bone and Joint Surgery, 43A:* 219, 1961.)

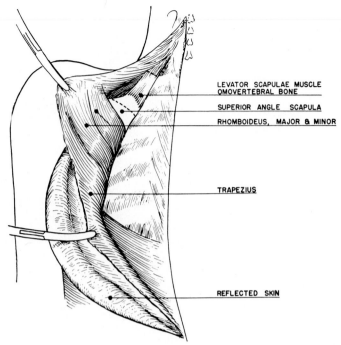

Figure 12.11.   Dissection of the muscle flap is begun inferiorly by detaching the origin from the spine. The omovertebral attachment is sectioned. (From J. W. Woodward: Congenital elevation of the scapula, *Journal of Bone and Joint Surgery, 43A:* 219, 1961.)

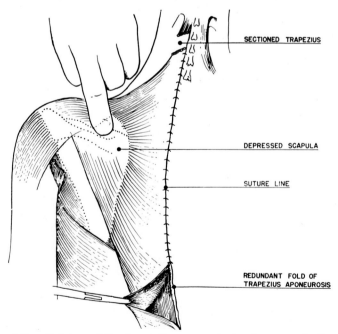

Figure 12.12.   After division of the trapezius superiorly, the muscle flap is drawn down until the scapula lies approximately opposite that of the normal side. Care must be taken to avoid overstretching the spinal accessory nerve and the brachial plexus. The muscle flap is sewn into its new attachment on the spine. (From J. W. Woodward: Congenital elevation of the scapula, *Journal of Bone and Joint Surgery, 43A:* 219, 1961.)

more radical descent of the scapula to be obtained by surgical correction without an accompanying loss of function of the cords of the brachial plexus.

References

1. Allen, F. G.: The surgical treatment of Sprengel's shoulder, *J. Bone Joint Surg. 46B:* 162, 1964.
2. Cavendish, M. E.: Congenital elevation of the scapula. *J. Bone Joint Surg. 54B:* 395, 1972.
3. Engel, D.: The etiology of the undescended scapula and related syndromes, *J. Bone Joint Surg. 25:* 613, 1943.
4. Green, W. T.: The surgical correction of congenital elevation of the scapula (Sprengel's deformity), *J. Bone Joint Surg., 39A:* 1439, 1957.
5. Greenville, W., and Conventry M.: Congenital high scapula (Sprengel's) deformity, *Proc. Mayo Clin., 31:* 465, 1956.
6. McFarland, B. L.: Congenital deformities of the spine and limbs, In *Modern Trends in Orthopaedics,* Chap. 6, p.. 107; London: Butterworth & Co., 1950.
7. Duthie, R., and Ferguson, A. B., Jr.: *Mercer's Orthopaedic Surgery,* Ed. 7, p. 148; Baltimore: Williams & Wilkins, 1973.
8. Pessolano, C.: Sprengel's deformity, *Pa. Med. J., 14:* 99, 1958.
9. Woodward, J. W.: Congenital elevation of the scapula, *J. Bone Joint Surg., 43A:* 219, 1961.

Absence of Muscles or Muscle Groups

Congenital absence of a muscle or muscle group may result in contracture if the function of the absent muscle is not substituted for by other muscles controlling the part. Bracing and exercises carrying the part through a full range of motion may be indicated until the function of the absent muscle can be substituted for by transplant if necessary. Not all absences of muscle groups lead to deformity, because the extent of the damage varies with the anatomic location. Thus, absence of the palmaris longus is not significant, but unilateral absence of the sternocleidal mastoid may lead to deformity.

The muscle group most frequently affected is the pectoral (Fig. 12.13), and the trapezius is next in order. Although any muscle may be affected, proximal or trunk muscles seem most liable to involvement. Absence of the sternocleidal mastoid is not infrequent (Fig. 12.14).

Familial Nuchal Rigidity

This condition is one of rigidity of the cervical spine. It is probably the direct antith-

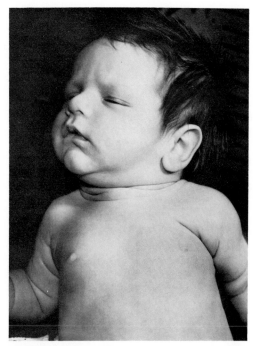

Figure 12.13. Congenital absence of the pectoralis major muscle with the creation of an abnormal skin fold across the area normally occupied by that muscle.

esis of Ehlers-Danlos syndrome, which is one of hypermobility of all joints of the body.

ETIOLOGY

Enler-Danlos syndrome, which is associated with hyperelasticity of the skin and fragility of the skin and blood vessels, has been proved to be an inherited, dominant constitutional dyscrasia. It is thought that familial nuchal rigidity is likewise inherited by dominant transmission.

CLINICAL PICTURE

This condition is characterized by an inability to flex the neck due to relatively short ligaments and soft tissues on the posterior or dorsal aspect of the vertebral column. It is sometimes confused with ankylosing arthritis.

TREATMENT

Treatment is unavailing.

ACQUIRED DEFORMITIES

Deformity Due to Position in Utero

Considrable interest has been aroused in recent years concerning the question of just how much fetal position determines the presence of deformities existing at birth. We do on occasion see a child born with what seem to be bilateral contractures of the sternocleidal mastoid muscles.

ETIOLOGY

Rarely this is due to a congenital loss or a stretching of the antagonistic posterior cervical muscles and ligaments. More often, however, it appears to be a positional contracture and is associated with a generalized rounded kyphosis of the entire spine similar to that of the fetal position.

CLINICAL PICTURE

There is a flexion deformity of the neck. Frequently the deformity is accompanied by an acute hip flexion deformity or by such severe flexion that the legs lie up along the abdominal wall. The head is flexed on the neck, and the whole of the spine presents a generalized, rounded dorsal and lumbar kyphosis.

TREATMENT

In such a case, gradual correction by traction, starting in the line of deformity with the child on a hard bed and with pads or pillows placed to conform to the deformities and then continuing with less and less padding until the spine and head are flat, brings about complete correction. If the legs are involved, the line of traction is gradually shifted. Correction is not sufficient and treatment should not cease until a normal lumbar curve has been obtained and the head can be easily hyperextended. Many minor contractures can be overcome merely by manual manipulation. Maintenance of the corrected position for a period may be necessary to allow overstretched muscles to become relatively shortened with growth of the skeleton.

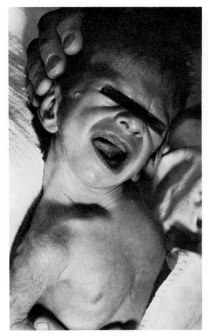 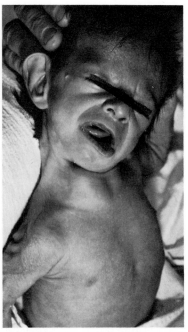

Figure 12.14. Congenital absence of the sternocleidomastoid muscle. The area normally occupied by the sternocleidmastoid muscle is retracted on inspiration and expanded on expiration.

Muscular Torticollis

Muscular torticollis does not seem to be a congenital anomaly but has a high association with breech births. There are many other possible reasons for a characteristic tilt and rotation of the head in childhood other than a contracture of the sternocleidomastoid muscle, but this causation is most common in childhood (Figs. 12.15 and 12.16). Osseous defects, neurogenic disturbances, ocular and middle ear pathology as well as underlying emotional disturbances have been suggested as possible causes of the deformity.

Frederick Taylor (1875) writing in London first described the pathology of the muscle as an "induration of the sterno-mastoid muscle or sterno-mastoid tumour." He found fibrous tissue displacing the muscle fibers and interspersed among them so that the muscle was enlarged. The changes were present throughout the muscle in his particular case, a 6-week-old infant. Isacius Minnius (1685), a Dutch surgeon, had reported tenotomy of the muscle for torticollis.

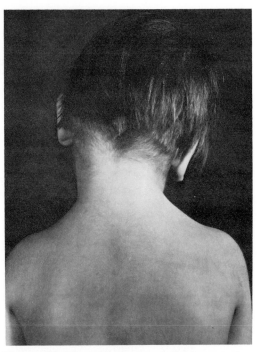

Figure 12.15. Posterior view of muscular torticollis in older child showing tilt and elevation of shoulder on affected side.

EMBRYOLOGY OF STERNOCLEIDOMASTOID MUSCLE

Lidge, Bechtol, and Lambert[18] reviewed the evolutionary development of the sternoclei—domastoid muscle. They pointed out that in a mammals both the trapezius and the sternocleidomastoid are innervated by the spinal part of the accessory nerve and by branches of the anterior rami of the cervical nerves, and this double innervation is unique. This muscle was apparently originally developed in the bronchial arch region. The visceral nerve supply shifted with its relocation. In lower forms this mass is supplied by the vagus nerve; in higher forms the main nerve supply is the spinal accessory nerve. (The nucleus of this nerve is closely related to the nucleus of the vagus nerve.) In higher forms of life, the nerve supply to both the sternocleidomastoid and trapezius may be related to the nerve supply to the muscles of the gastrointestinal tract.

The muscles are derived from the mesoderm and arise in the lateral portion of the occipital region as a common muscle mass. As they migrate to the shoulder girdle, the accessory nerve is carried along with the muscle mass. The muscle mass first appears in the 7-mm embryo as the caudel member of the bronchial arch series. In the 11-mm, embryo the trapezius portion is separate and extends to the sixth cervical nerve. The sternocleidomastoid extends virtually to the clavicle. At the 16-mm stage, the muscles are separate through their length. The sternocleidomastoid extends from the mastoid process to the clavicle by the 20-mm stage, the trapezius extends to the occipital cartilage.

The accessory nerve supply from the cervical region is secondary—not developed directly as if the muscle came from a myotome.

The vagus complex consists of both vagus and accessory nerves, the more caudal portion of the vagus becoming a motor nerve primarily known as the spinal accessory to innervate both the sternocleidomastoid and trapezius. Additional innervation to this nerve as it is carried down the neck is obtained from the roots of the spinal cord down as far as the fourth cervical segment.

The sternocleidomastoid arises from the anterior end of the superomedial line and at the mastoid process anteriorly. The two distal heads are divided into an attachment to the superior border of the medial third of the

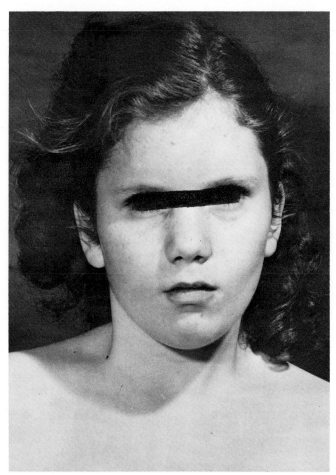

Figure 12.16.   Muscular torticollis becoming more evident with growth and involving primarily the clavicular portion of the sternocleidal mastoid.

clavicle—the other head crosses the sterno-clavicular joint and extends by fibrous bands to the sternum.

The proximal blood supply consists of a short but major supply to the upper end and is derived from the occipital artery. The sternal head is supplied by a branch of the superior thyroid artery. The clavicular head is supplied by an artery running upward as a branch of the thyrocervical trunk or from one of the branches of this trunk, the transverse scapular artery. The venous drainage is multiple, numerous, and overlapping to all the major veins of the neck.

ETIOLOGY

The process present in the sternocleidomastoid muscle is unique and is not completely understood, making theories of causation of muscular torticollis difficult. The breech presentation incidence in this condition may be brought on by a preexisting position of the head. As early as 1670 von Roonhysen attributed the condition to the abnormal pressure on or position of the head in utero. Stromeyer in 1838 thought that the sternocleidomastoid muscle was ruptured during birth. Unfortunately, evidence for the hemorrhage when a resected muscle is examined pathologically does not exist.

In 1883 experimental hematoma was produced by Witzel by tearing muscle. Not resemblance to the hyperplastic process present in this condition was found. Petersen[24] in 1886 felt that adhesions had formed between the amnion and the face of the embryo, bringing about a position of the head which interfered with development of the sternocleidomastoid muscle.

Volkman (1885) believed that the process was an infectious myositis. In 1980 Golding-Bard initiated a neurogenic theory—the deformity being secondary to a cerebral lesion occurring during intrauterine life. Anderson in 1893 believed that there was both an intrauterine type of torticollis and a birth injury type. In 1895 Mikulicz mentioned ischemia as a possible cause—a general anoxia and local trauma to the muscle. By 1906 Nove-Josserand and Viannaz developed a concept of each of the three segments of blood supply to the muscle being independent to a given segment of the muscle. In extreme rotation during labor the tensed sternocleidomastoid may compress blood vessels supplying the muscle as they pass beneath it.

The first recorded case of bilateral torticollis was reported by Morse in 1915. Bilaterally shortened muscles after a cesarean delivery were obviously not the product of birth trauma. Morse felt that it was due to a hyperextended position of the fetal head.

In 1923 Jones and Lovett felt that abnormal intrauterine pressure was the cause and called attention to the association of the disease with forefoot and equinovarus deformity.

Krogius (1924) called the condition a defect in the muscle blastoma itself—connective tissue formation at the expense of muscle fiber formation. And uniquely he called attention to the fact that this could be an active process continuing in the years after birth.

Middleton in 1930 stated that he was unable to demonstrate thrombosed veins in the sternocleidomastoid, and he found no evidence to support the hematoma theory. He pointed out that the mass palpable in the sternocleidomastoid is from the outset firm, hard, and cartilaginous in feel. He noted also the development of the tumor several weeks after birth as being inconsistent with a hematoma. Greenstein reported a case of congenital muscular torticollis in 1950. The delivery was a cesarean section performed before the onset of labor and 2 weeks prior to the expected date of delivery.

PATHOLOGY

Taylor's original description in 1875 brought out the histologic character of the lesion. Fibrous tissue had developed between bundles of muscle fibers destroying and displacing them. The middle portion of the muscle was most densely occupied by the process with fibrous tissue alone being seen.

Numerous observations have been made of the fact that no evidence for hematoma is found, including those by Whitman (1891) and Parker (1893). Witzel described the secondary changes in skull and face that occur with growth in this disease (1883). The affected side of the head and face becomes relatively atrophic.

In 1929 Von Lachun reported that in 3 cases that he examined the muscle was normal above and below the site of the fibrous hyperplasia. In 1 case, however, the process extended throughout the muscle rim into both clavicular and sternal heads. Muscle fibers were interspersed with the fibrous tissue.

At infancy on gross examination the tumor appears to be glistening fibrous tissue resembling a soft fibroma. Microscopically there is young and cellular fibrous tissue with remnants of the original muscle fibers. Some of these fibers are vacuolated and undergoing degeneration. In the older child the process has matured there is no degenerating muscle or young fibrous tissue. There are scattered collections of muscle fibers in the fibrous tissue. The author has found calcification in this fibrous tissue (Fig. 12.17).

The fibrous tissue has been observed to be continuous with the tendon at either end where it has extended that far.

Adams stated that giant cells have been sent and described them as masses of sarcolemmic nuclei possibly representing attempts at regeneration of muscle fibers.

CLINICAL PICTURE

The mass in the sternocleidomastoid muscle may be evident at birth, but most frequently it is not noticed until after approximately 10 days to 2 weeks, when it is seen as a hard, immobile, fusiform swelling in the muscle. Delivery has usually been difficult or a breech presentation. The swelling increases in size for 2–4 weeks and then gradually subsides over a 5 to 8 month period.

The deformity is produced by contracture of the involved muscle, the occiput being held constantly toward the involved side and the chin being rotated toward the opposite shoulder.

With persistence of the deformity, the

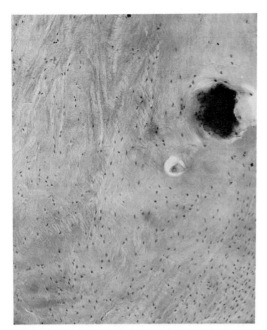

Figure 12.17. Fibroplastic process in congenital torticollis. The dark area in the upper right portion of the section represents calcium deposition (×140).

skull becomes foreshortened, the level of the eyes changes, the side of the face on the involved side becomes flattened, and the mastoid process becomes more prominent. The clavicle and shoulder become elevated as compared to the opposite normal side. With continued growth and no treatment, a lower cervical-upper dorsal scoliosis will develop.

TREATMENT

When recognized early after birth, deformity can be corrected by gentle, yet even and persistent, stretching to an overcorrected position; i.e., the head is stretched over toward the shoulder opposite to the side of involvement, and the chin is rotated toward the side of involvement. Many useful tricks and artifices may be used to stimulate the child to turn the head toward the involved side. The crib may be placed so that he must turn to the desired position of overcorrection in looking for window light or for a favorite rattle. A special skull cap with an arm attachment has been used so that weight and use of the arm pull the head over. Placing sandbags along the head has been found useful.

Removal of the tumor is not necessary and has the disadvantage of deforming the outline of the neck. In the rare case that is not fully corrected after exercises, the sternal portion of the muscle can be lengthened and divided from the mastoid process at its origin. Such a procedure preserves the neck outline.

In older patients, correction of deformity can usually be obtained by lengthening of the sternal portion and detachment of the clavicular head of the sternocleidal muscle. An upper pole myotomy can also be done, if it is necessary. The overcorrected position can be maintained by a special collar.

Rotary Subluxations

An inability to rotate the head may occur as an acute episode in children who undergo some injury, even a minor one, in the course of play. There is usually some history of trauma, mild or severe, after which the child suddenly develops an inability to rotate the neck to one side. A sore throat or upper respiratory infection may also precede the symptoms in some cases. The resulting "wryneck" or torticollis is characterized by spasm and tenderness on the long side of the torticollis instead of on the short side, where it is

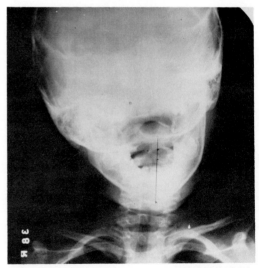

Figure 12.18. Open-mouth view of cervical spine in patient with muscular torticollis, revealing tilt but accurate alignment of chin, spine of C2, and base of odontoid; there is no evidence of cervical subluxation.

seen in such conditions as myositis. There is also limitation of motion toward the long or stretched side. Stimson and Swenson[30] stated that this acquired deformity is the result of a unilateral subluxation without associated fracture of the second or the third cervical vertebra. A. B. Ferguson, Sr., described a rotary subluxation that causes such a deformity between the atlas and axis. In a series of cases of our own, we were able to demonstrate that subluxation occurred in both places simultaneously in this deformity, there being a subluxation between C1 and C2, as well as between C2 and C3. It is the opinion of many that these subluxations occur in childhood because of the slope of the articular facets, which gradually change until the more stable adult situation is reached. The subluxation occurs in the upper three vertebrae, in which the more horizontal slope of the facets allows sufficient rotation (Fig. 12.19).

CLINICAL PICTURE

Following a respiratory infection or some injury at play, or in connection with muscle spasm as the result of a cervical gland infec-

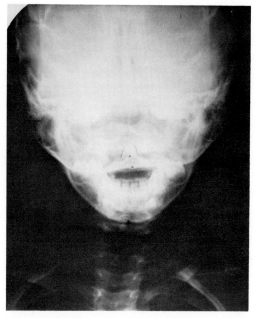

Figure 12.19.   Cervical subluxation at C1 and C2 evidenced by malalignment of axis of C2 (base of odontoid and spine of C2) in relation to chin (correlating with C1).

tion, the child complains of pain and inability to move the head. The head is tilted to one side and can be pushed further toward that side without pain. The rotation is limited to one side, and when the anomaly is acute, lateral tilt is also limited. Muscle spasms and tenderness are also evident on the long or stretched side. There may also be tenderness of the spine of the first and second cervical vertebrae.

PATHOLOGY

The pathology can be demonstrated by roentgenogram. An open-mouth anteroposterior view of the first and second cervical vertebrae is necessary for diagnosis. The symphysis of the mandible, the body of the second cervical, and the spine of the second cervical lie in a position of constant relationship, one to the other. If a true anteroposterior view is taken, they all lie on the same line. If the view is slightly oblique, they all are displaced in relative proportion to each other. If, however, a rotary subluxation has taken place, one of these points will be out of line in relation to the other two. The mandible is carried to one side since its position is associated with the first cervical vertebra. The body of the second cervical and its spine give a line indicating the plane of rotation, which deviated from that indicated by the mandible. In the lateral stereo view, the unilateral subluxation between the second and third cervical vertebrae can be seen, the facet of the second cervical riding upward and forward on its mate below without complete dislocation.

TREATMENT

Reduction may occur quite easily and quickly with the use of cervical traction, and often within 24–48 hr the neck is freely movable. A modified Thomas collar may be used for a period thereafter to prevent recurrence, usually until all tenderness and any respiratory infection have subsided.

References

1. Berkhizer, D. J., and Siedler, F.: Non-traumatic dislocations of the atlanto-axial joint, *J. A. M. A.,* *95:* 517, 1931.
2. Chandler, F. A.: Muscular torticollis, *J. Bone Joint Surg.,* 30A: 556, 1948.

3. Chandler, F. A., and Altenberg, A.: Congenital muscular torticollis, *J. A. M. A., 125:* 476, 1944.

4. Coakley, W. A., Teplitsky, D., and Diaz, A.: Infections of head and neck, *Am. J. Surg., 77:* 469, 1949.

5. Compere, E. L.: Excision of hemivertebrae for correction of congenital scoliosis, *J. Bone Joint Surg., 14:* 555, 1932.

6. Compere, E. L.: Neck, shoulder, and arm syndrome, *New Orleans Med. Sci. J., 104:* 473, 1952.

7. Coutts, M. D.: Atlanto-epiphyseal subluxation, *Arch. Surg., 29:* 297, 1934.

8. Hartley, J. B., and Burnett, C. W. F.: Spina bifida and its associated skull defects, *Arch. Dis. Child., 18:* 173, 1943.

9. Herz, E., and Hoefer, P. F. A.: Physiologic analysis of involuntary motor activity. *Arch. Neurol. Psychiatry, 61:* 129, 1949.

10. Horwitz, A. E.: Congenital elevation of scapula, *Am. J. Orthop. Surg., 6:* 260, 1908.

11. Howorth, M. B.: Spasmodic torticollis, In *Textbook of Orthopedics*, p. 1963; Philadelphia: W. B. Saunders, 1952.

12. Jacobson, G., and Alder, D. C.: Evaluation of lateral atlanto-axial displacement in injuries of the cervical spine, *Radiology, 61:* 355, 1953.

13. Jeanopolous, C. J.: Congenital elevation of the scapula, *J. Bone Joint Surg., 34A:* 883, 1952.

14. Jones, R. W.: Spontaneous hyperemic dislocations of the atlas, *Proc. R. Soc. Med., 25:* 1, 1931–32.

15. Kaplan, E. B.: Personal communication.

16. Keith, A.: *Human Embryology and Morphology,* Ed. 6; Baltimore: Williams & Wilkins, 1933.

17. Lewis, W. H.: The development of the arm in man, *Am. J. Anat., 1:* 145, 183, 1901–1902.

18. Lidge, R. T., Bechtol, R. C., and Lambert, R. C.: Congenital muscular torticollis, *J. Bone Joint Surg., 39A:* 1165, 1957.

19. Mercer, R. D.: Atlas-axis dislocation following cervical adenitis, *Cleve. Clin. Q. 11:* 161, 1952.

20. Nelson, W. E.: Skeletal defects, In *Textbook of Pediatrics,* Ed. 5, p. 1449; Philadelphia: W. B. Saunders, 1950.

21. Nicholson, J. T.: Spontaneous reduction of cervical spine dislocations, *J. A. M. A., 115:* 2063, 1940.

22. Patton, E. F.: Cervical subluxation, *Ann. West. Med. Surg., 3:* 258, 1949.

23. Peters, K., et al.: *Handbuch der Anatomie des Kindes,* Vol. 2, 1938.

24. Petersen, J.: Zur Frage des Kopfricher Hamatoms bei Nengeborenen, *Zbl. Lymak, 10:* 797, 1886.

25. Pick, D. M.: Spina bifida and its associated malformations, *Wis. Med. J., 50:* 659, 1951.

26. Schrock, R. D.: Congenital elevation of scapula, *J. Bone Joint Surg., 8:* 207, 1926.

27. Shands, A. R.: Affections of neck and shoulder, In *Handbook of Orthopedic Surgery,* Ed. 2, p. 434; St. Louis: C. V. Mosby, 1940.

28. Shoul, M. I., and Retro, M.: Manifestations of Klippel-Feil syndrome, *Am. J. Roentgenol., 68:* 369, 1952.

29. Smith, A. D.: Congenital elevation of scapula, *Arch. Surg., 42:* 529, 1941.

30. Stimson, A. B., and Swenson, P. C.: Unilateral subluxation of the cervical vertebrae without associated fracture, *J. A. M. A., 104:* 1578, 1935.

31. Sutra, C. J., and Mishkin, R. D.: Familial nuchal rigidity; form of hypomobility of vertebral column which clinically may be misdiagnosed as ankylosing arthritis (antithesis to Ehler-Danlos disease), *Bull. Hosp. Joint Dis., 13:* 155, 1952.

32. Taylor, J. C.: Breech presentation of hyperextension of the neck and intrauterine dislocation of cervical vertebrae, *Am. J. Obst., Gynec., 56:* 381, 1948.

33. Townsend, E. H., Jr., and Rowe, M. L.: Mobility of the upper cervical spine in health and disease, *J. Pediatr., 10:* 567, 1952.

34. Ward, J., and Learner, H. H.: A review of the subject of congenital hemihypertrophy and a complete case report, *J. Pediatr., 31:* 403, 1947.

35. Wycis, H. T., and Moore, J. R.: The surgical treatment of spasmodic torticollis, *J. Bone Joint Surg., 36A:* 119, 1954.

CHAPTER 13

Infections of the Bones and Joints

SEPTIC ARTHRITIS

BY HAROLD SWENSON, M.D

Thomas Smith's classic review in 1874[13] discussed 21 cases of septic arthritis in infants, 13 of whom died. Treatment through the years was restricted to surgery, which reduced both the death rate and complication rate. Sulfa drugs, introduced in the late 1930s changed the course very little, but the antibiotic era beginning in the 1940s resulted in significant changes. The greatest effect was a dramatic drop in mortality in bone and joint infections uncomplicated by major systemic illness. Death is no longer so possible, and prevention of permanent joint destruction and growth alteration are the goals. Anything less than a normal joint falls short of that goal.

Etiology

Joint infection is usually the result of hematogenous spread from a primary focus. In the majority of cases the site of entrance into the body is not of clinical importance. The most common portal of entry is the upper respiratory tree. Furunculosis, otitis media, pneumonia, meningitis, and urinary tract infections are all known to precede joint invasion. Direct penetration, either by trauma or iatrogenically, is also a cause.

Enough experience has now been amassed so that the etiologic agent is predictable in a high percentage of cases. This accomplishes two things. First, treatment can be initiated prior to complete bacteriologic identification, and second, treatment can be successfully accomplished when bacteriologic diagnosis cannot be made. An uncomfortably large number of cases occur in which no etiologic agent is isolated (Table 13.1).

The most common organism producing septic arthritis from birth to age 16 is still

Staphylococcus aureus. In all series reviewed this proved to be the case.

However, different organisms tend to predominate at different ages. In the first 6 months staphylococcal and streptococcal infections are encountered most frequently. Most of these tend to occur in the first 3 months. Recent reports seem to demonstrate a reduction in incidence of streptococcal bone and joint infections over what it was in preantibiotic and early antibiotic years.

Infections by pathogens of the colon-bacillus family of bacteria are also seen occasionally in infancy, but rarely later. These are aerobic, gram-negative nonsporogenous rods found typically in the excreta of man and animals. Relative immunity against these pathogens develops within 6 months in an otherwise healthy child.

The past 20 years has seen a significant increase in septic arthritis secondary to *Haemophilus influenzae.* This gram-negative pleomorphic bacillus generally strikes the child in the 6 to 36-month age range producing bronchitis, pneumonitis, otitis media, and meningitis, as well as arthritis.

After age 3 the most common infecting organism is the staphylococcus, with no particular age group evidencing a predilection. However, with the increase incidence of gonorrhea, there also has been an increase in gonococcal arthritis in children, most particularly in the teenage years.

Clinical Picture

The onset of septic arthritis may be preceded by a variety of infections, but in most cases the focus is the upper respiratory tract. In the newborn the umbilical stump is a potential invasive site. A history of trauma may be given in cases involving active, otherwise healthy children. Such systemic diseases as blood dyscrasias, dysgammaglobulinemia, and rheumatoid arthritis are also on occasion complicated by pyogenic arthritis.

Table 13.1
Reported proved etiology of septic arthritis

Series	Cases	Positive cultures	
		no.	%
Nelson and Koontz[8]	117	57	48.7
Borella et al.[3]	52	17	32.7
Almquist[1]	50	16	32.0
Children's Hospital of Pittsburgh	92	24	26.1

Fever, anorexia, and irritability usually herald the onset of septic arthritis anywhere from hours to several days prior to specific joint involvement. In the infant the initial symptoms may be subtle, with the baby failing to feed well and displaying a greater than usual amount of fussiness. Pseudoparalysis of the affected limb may also occur.

The child with septic arthritis usually appears acutely ill or "toxic." The temperature may be 39.5C or higher. Tachycardia and tachypnea are present. Those children on steroid therapy may have significant masking of symptoms.

Pain, loss of motion, and a local increase in heat then involve the joint. Refusal to walk or an antalgic gait are early signs when the lower extremities are involved. Erythema and articular swelling are evident in the more superficial joints. Swelling may even be seen around the hip and shoulder if the process is more advanced. The hip is typically held in a position of abduction, flexion, and external rotation to accommodate the effusion and an increased intra-articular pressure. Most other joints are rigidly splinted in flexion, and any attempt at passive motion produces pain.

Pathology

Bacterial invasion of the joint occurs by the hematogenous route with involvement of the synovium as the initial stage. Less frequently, infection results secondary to direct extension from an osteomyelitic focus. This is particularly true in the hip where the proximal femoral metaphysis is within the articular capsule.

Edema and hyperemia of the synovial tissue occur first. An effusion develops, which, if aspirated early, may appear turbid or cloudy and, within 24–48 hr, frankly purulent. Polymorphonuclear leukocytes predominate. The protein content of the fluid is high, and fibrin pannus may be evident as early as 3 days after invasion. If opened at this point, the joint appears to contain much debris, usually fibrinous, as well as pus.

Destruction of articular cartilage seems to result from loss of nutrition because of the local environment and more actively by proteolytic enzymes. Studies by Curtiss and Klein[4] demonstrated release of hexosamines from cartilage in the presence of lysosomes and streptococcal and leukocytic proteinases. They felt that the matrix was initially lost, and the subsequent breakdown of collagen might be secondary to pressure and use. This process of cartilage breakdown and loss seems to occur most rapidly in staphylococcal and streptococcal infections, although it is seen with all.

Extension of the infection from the joint may occur with the further passage of time. In the untreated case extension to the adjacent osseous structures generally does not occur in less than 5 days. Spread is probably along vascular channels because direct penetration through the articular cartilage and growth plate is rarely seen.

The hip, which is the most commonly infected joint, may also develop septic necrosis of the capitular femoral epiphysis. Increased pressure and/or thrombosis of the intra-articular vessels resulting in ischemia seems to be the cause. In addition, because the growth plate and metaphysis are within the capsule, bony destruction and growth arrest are more likely to occur. Growth arrest and avascular necrosis are rare in any other joint.

X-ray Appearance

Initially there is evidence of deep soft-tissue swelling with displacement or obliteration of fat pads particularly at the elbow and knee. Later, not much earlier than 1 week, there may be evidence of osteoporosis about the joint. Subluxation or dislocation of the hip joint can occur and may be evident within several days after onset of the septic process.

Evidence of bone destruction or new bone formation can be seen later, most particularly in the region of the hip. Actual loss of cartilage space is not usually seen radiologically, at least not until after there has been resumption of some degree of activity.

Diagnosis

Critical in the handling of any case of septic arthritis is the bacteriologic diagnosis. No child with an inflamed joint should receive antibiotics prior to aspiration of that joint and culture of the fluid obtained. In addition, nose and throat cultures and at least two blood cultures should be gotten. If the initial urinalysis demonstrates a pyuria, the urine should also be cultured.

Of all inflammatory conditions of joints, pyogenic arthritis is the most rapidly destructive and potentially one of the most treatable. If the suspension of septis is present, aspiration should be done. Anaerobic and some gram-negative infections produce a lesser effusion; consequently, it may be necessary to irrigate the joint with saline to obtain sufficient quantities for study. The aspirate may appear creamy yellow in the case of staphylococcal sepsis, gray and possibly bloody with streptococcal sepsis, and dirty, watery, gray-yellow in the presence of haemophilus infections.

Culture and Gram stain should be done immediately after arthrocentesis. Thioglycolate broth is inoculated and may be most productive in the isolation of microaerophilic and anaerobic organisms. Plating should be done on blood agar and chocolate agar specifically to culture haemophilus organisms. There are a number of commercially available enriched media which will satisfactorily accomplish specific bacterial growth.

Bacterial morphology and staining characteristics are then determined on the Gram stain. *Haemophilus influenzae* is pleomorphic and classed as a gram-negative coccobacillus. It is important that an expert review slides when *H. influenzae* is suspected because identification is sometimes difficult other than by a bacteriologist. White cell type and predominance can also be observed on the Gram stain. Granulocytes will be present in the greatest percentage, often with many immature forms in evidence.

Fluid should also be placed in a tube with heparin to determine the cell count. This should be diluted to the proper concentration with saline. In septic arthritis the count may be as low as 10,000 or as high as 100,000, but generally it is about 30,000–50,000 cells per cubic millimeter.

If a sufficient amount of fluid remains, a joint fluid glucose content is determined. Simultaneously a blood glucose level is done. In the presence of joint sepsis, the synovial fluid glucose level may be one-half or less than that of blood. If sufficient fluid remains, it may be checked for mucin content. In the presence of infection, the mucin clot may not form or it may be very friable. Peripheral blood will usually reveal an elevation in the white blood count with the predominance of polymorphonuclear leukocytes and a shift to the left. This count may be as high as 35,000 but, particularly in the case of infants, not notably elevated. Often the hemoglobin and hemotocrit are lower than expected, an indication of the preinfection status of the child or as the result of hemolysis. Almost invariably the sedimentation rate is elevated (Table 13.2).

Table 13.2
Synovial fluid analysis*

	Appearance	Viscosity	Mucin clot	Cell count	Cell type	Glucose	Bacteria
Normal	Clear	Normal	Good	<200		>80% of serum	None
Posttraumatic	Clear, bloody, or xanthochromatic	Normal	Good	Few to many < peripheral blood	Mononuclear to many RBCs	>80% serum	None
Rheumatic fever	Cloudy, yellow turbid	Decreased	Good to fair	18,000	50% polys, RBCs		None
Rheumatoid arthritis	Cloudy, yellow turbid	Decreased	Fair to poor	15,000	60% polys	>80% of serum	None
Septic arthritis	White, yellow-gray, turbid	Decreased	Poor	20,000–100,000	90% polys	50% of serum	Present

* From Ropes, M., and Bauer, W.: *Synovial Fluid Changes in Joint Disease;* Cambridge, Mass.: Harvard University Press, 1953.

Treatment

Antibiotic therapy is initated after all culture samples are obtained. The smallest needle used in aspiration of the joint should be 18 gauge. Note should be made of the amount of particulate matter aspirated and whether or not the needle clogs. Irrigation with saline can be accomplished after samples are obtained, if there is a free flow of fluid. A smaller syringe, such as a 5 or 10 cubic milliliter, facilitates aspiration because less suction is applied and synovium is not drawn into the needle tip. The synovial fluid is often under enough pressure so that one may not have to apply any force.

Enough is now known about septic arthritis so that different treatment modalities can be applied rationally without being excessively dogmatic. The goal is to restore a normal joint with no loss of growth potential (Figs. 13.1–13.5). Our predecessors have given us the tools to prevent death so that it is rarely, if ever, of great concern unless the septic joint is but one of multiple body sites infected by microorganisms. Early recognition followed by adequate therapy invariably ends in the desired results. Therefore, education of colleagues in general medicine and pediatrics will result in referral for early definitive treatment. If partially treated or untreated cases are being seen at pediatric treatment centers 1 week or longer after onset, those involved in definitive care have not been fulfilling their proper role in education of their colleagues. Cases seen 12 hr after onset may not present the so-called classical or full blown picture, but they do allow some latitude in treatment in terms of time.

If seen early, satisfactory drainage can be accomplished by means of arthrocentesis. This means within 48–72 hr of onset. Beyond that period it becomes difficult or impossible to satisfactorily remove pus and debris from most septic joints by repeat aspiration. An arthrotomy must then be done.

Decompression of hips is obviously a treatment necessity and this is accomplished only temporarily and partially by needle drainage. Therefore, arthrotomy by the posterior Ober muscle splitting approach should be done as soon as it is possible for the child to receive an anesthetic safely. Retrospectively, it seems evident that open drainage of the hip has reduced necrosis of the femoral head and damage to the femoral growth plate.

Numerous studies have demonstrated that antibiotics readily cross the synovial membrane barrier in sufficient concentrations to destroy sensitive bacteria. Consequently, it is unnecessary to instill antibiotics directly into the involved joint in acute cases. There is also evidence that high antibiotic concentrations injected directly into a joint may produce additional synovial irritation, an undesirable side effect of an unnecessary mode of therapy.

The antibiotic of choice prior to identification of the infecting organism is determined primarily by two factors. One is the result of the Gram stain where morphology and stain characteristics are decided, and the second is the patient's age. As mentioned before, gram-positive cocci are found most often in the septic joints of infants. Therefore, penicillin and penicillinase-resistant synthetic penicillins are used in this young age group until cultures and sensitivities are obtained. In the age group from 6–36 months, *Staphylococcus aureus* or *Haemophilus influenzae* are generally isolated. In this age group ampicillin is the therapy of choice when the organism cannot be differentiated on Gram stain. In a child beyond 3 years of age, the staphylococcus is far and away the most commonly isolated bacteria; therefore, penicillin and the penicillinase-resistant penicillins are the drugs of choice.

Repeat joint aspiration after initiation of antibiotic therapy will usually produce fluid in which no organism can be seen by staining or isolated by culture. In those cases where no organism can be retrieved because of prior antibiotic therapy, the safest choice seems to be to treat on the basis of the child's age and the usual infecting agent of that age group.

Intravenous administration provides the surest route by which satisfactory levels of antibiotic concentrations can be reached. Intramuscular injections also seem to give high enough serum levels, although this method of therapy may prove to be difficult, particularly in the infant where the subcutaneous tissue and muscle mass is not so great. Unpredictable levels are achieved by the oral pathway because absorption varies in different individuals and is also affected by the time relationship to feedings.

The satisfactory duration of antibiotic therapy is difficult to assess objectively. If therapy has been started early after the onset of joint involvement, it logically follows that

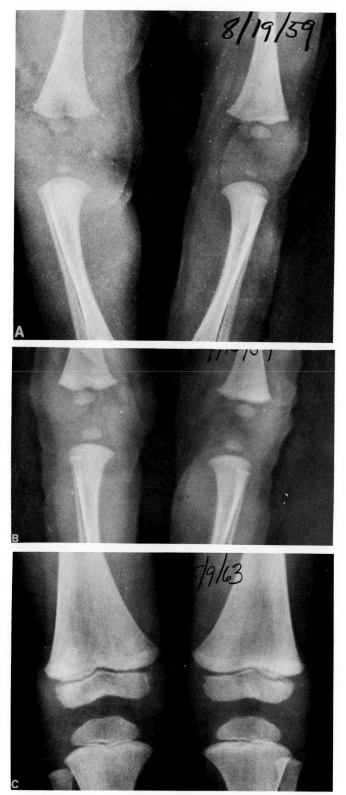

Figure 13.1. (*A*) Three-week-old infant. Two-day history of fever and swelling of right knee and distal thigh. Note lytic area in distal femoral metaphysis. Penumococcus was isolated from the knee. (*B*) Three weeks after incision, drainage, and immobilization. Note irregularity of epiphyseal line; the right knee is still swollen. (*C*) Four years later. No evidence of growth disturbance and right knee appears intact.

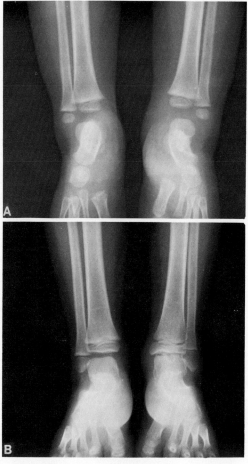

Figure 13.2. (*A*) Two-year-old girl, treated at home for 10 days for fever and hot, swollen left ankle. Had received penicillin and tretracycline. Culture of joint fluid was sterile. (*B* and *C*) Two and a half years later; now age 4 1/2. Film demonstrates loss of articular cartilage and flattening and irregularity of talus. (*D*) Four years after onset; advanced degenerative changes.

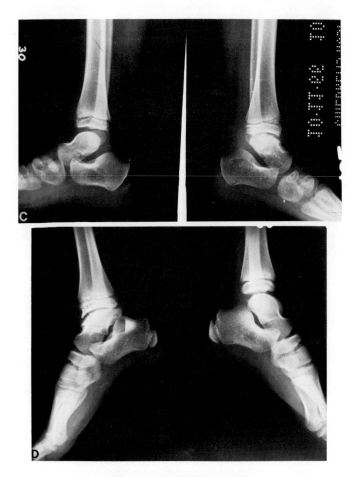

Figure 13.2 (*C* and *D*)

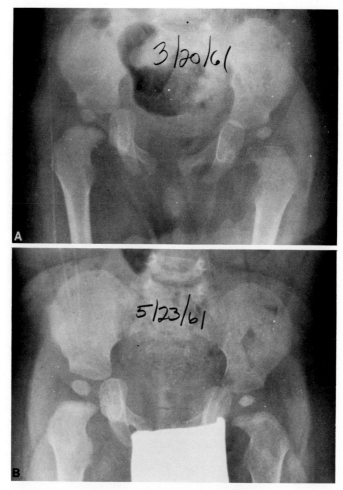

Figure 13.3. (*A*) Six-month-old boy treated with antibiotics at home for 3 weeks for fever, irritability, and failure to move the left lower extremity. Left hip is subluxed. (*B*) Two months after incision and drainage and spica immobilization. *Haemophilus influenzae* was isolated. Note dense left capital femoral epiphysis. (*C*) One year later there is absence of the osseous growth center and widening of the proximal femoral metaphysis. (*D*) Age 5. Coxa magna and plana. (*E*) Age 11. Femur is 1/2 inch shorter on left. Coxa magna and plana.

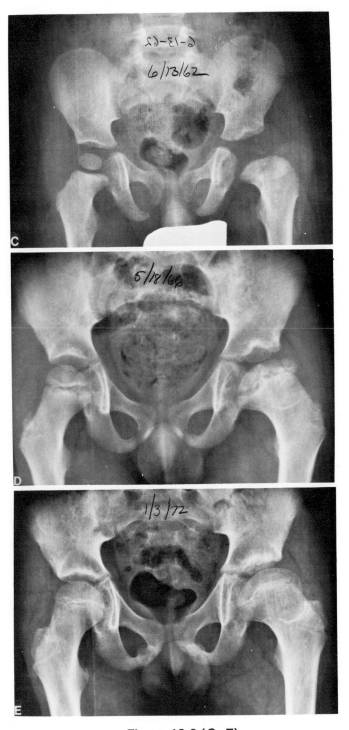

Figure 13.3 (C–E)

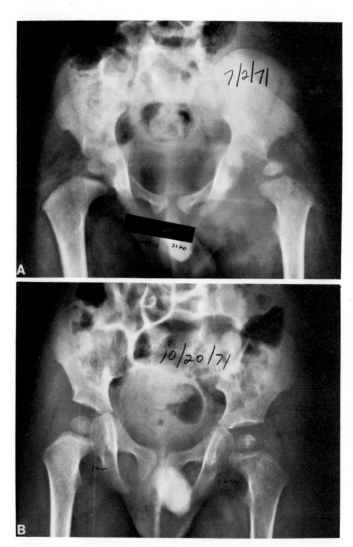

Figure 13.4. (A) Septic dislocation of left hip in 21-month-old boy. Had been treated with penicillin. *Staphylococcus aureus* was isolated from blood culture. (B) Three and a half months after incision, drainage, and cast immobilization. (C) Eleven months after onset. (D) Now age 3 1/2. Full range of motion and no limp. New bone formation at proximal femoral metaphysis.

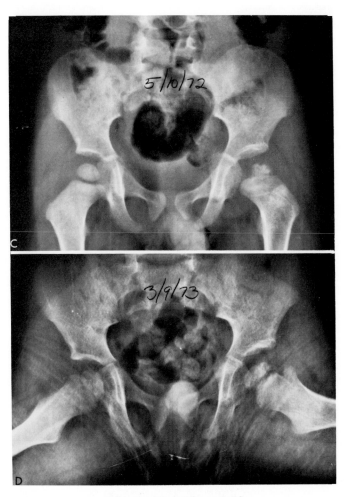

Figure 13.4 (*C* and *D*)

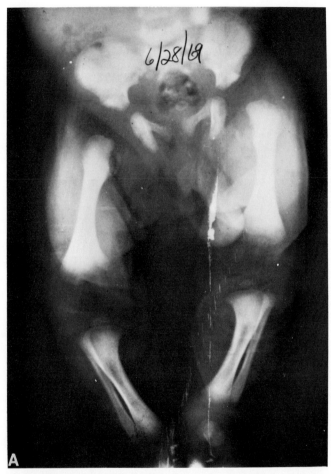

Figure 13.5.   (A) Four-day-old infant with fever and irritability for 1 day. Subluxation of both hips. Bilateral incision and drainage was done on the same day. *Staphylococcus aureus* was isolated from blood and hips. (B) One month later. Treatment by cast immobilization and methicillin for penicillin-resistant Staphylococcus. Note proximal femoral new bone formation. (C) Two years later. Clinically normal.

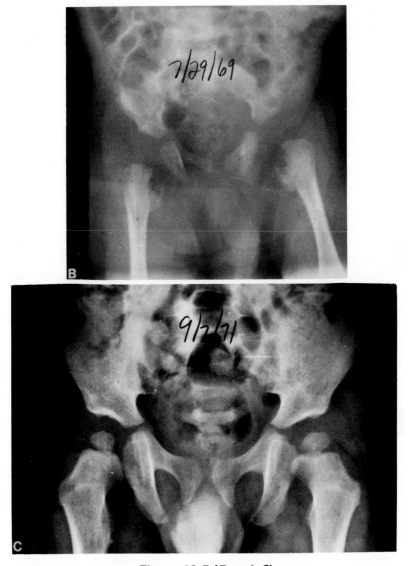

Figure 13.5 (B and C)

eradication of the organism will occur early if that particular bacteria is sensitive to the antibiotic being given. Successful reversal of the infectious process also occurs more rapidly in the infant and the younger child. Experience seems to indicate that the intravenous and intramuscular method must be used for at least 1 week in these cases. In those instances where prior antibiotics have been given and successful isolation has not occurred despite the persistence of signs and symptoms of joint infections, therapy must necessarily be continued by parenteral means for a longer period, usually for 2 weeks or more. On those occasions where septic arthritis is complicated by the presence or apparent presence of osteomyelitis, parenteral therapy should be continued for 3 weeks or more.

When arthrocentesis has been chosen as the means of joint drainage, repeat aspirations are necessary. How often this is done is dependent upon the reaccumulation of the effusion, the continued presence of bacteria in the synovial fluid, a persistently high while blood count, and a failure to improve systemically. As noted before, if local and systemic signs and symptoms persist for longer than 72 hr from the time of onset, arthrotomy should be performed. There does not seem to be any necessity for insertion of drains in acute cases.

In all cases the joint should be put at rest. This may satisfactorily be done in the case of the shoulder, hip, and knee by the use of cast immobilization or suspension. All other joints seem to respond best to splinting or whole cast immobilization.

Successful therapy transfers the joint to a sterile state very rapidly. An aseptic synovitis will usually persist to some degree for a number of days or even weeks. Immobilization or splinting should continue until all evidence of joint inflammation has cleared, even though antibiotic therapy may have been stopped (Table 13.3).

References

1. Almquist, E. E.: The changing epidemiology of septic arthritis in children, Clin. Orthop., 68: 96, 1970.
2. Badgely, C. E.: Study of the end-results in 113 cases of septic hips, J. Bone Joint Surg., 18: 1047, 1936.
3. Borella, L., Goobar, J. E., Summitt, R. L., and Clark, G. M.: Septic arthritis in childhood, J. Pediatr., 62: 742, 1963.
4. Curtiss, P. H., and Klein, L.: Destruction of articular cartilage in septic arthritis, J. Bone Joint Surg., 47A: 1595, 1965.
5. Eyre-Brook, A. L.: Septic arthritis of the hip and osteomyelitis of the upper end of the femur in infants, J. Bone Joint Surg., 42B: 11,1960.
6. Lloyd-Roberts, G. C.: Suppurative arthritis of infancy; some observations upon progress and management, J. Bone Joint Surg., 42B: 706, 1960.
7. Nelson, J. D.: Antibiotic concentrations in septic joint effusions, N. Engl. J. Med., 284: 349, 1971.
8. Nelson, J. D., and Koontz, W. C.: Septic arthritis in infants and children, Pediatrics, 38: 966, 1966.
9. Ober, R.: Posterior arthrotomy of the hip joint, J. A.M.A., 82: 1500, 1924.
10. Samilson, R. C., Bersani, F. A., and Watkins, M. B.: Acute suppurative arthritis in infants and children, Pediatrics, 21: 798, 1958.
11. Schmid, F. R., and Parker, R. H.: Treatment of infection forms of arthritis, Mod. Treat., 6: 1969.
12. Schmid, F. R., and Parker, R. H.: Ongoing assessment of therapy in septic arthritis, Arthritis Rheum., 11: 529, 1969.
13. Smith, T.: On the acute arthritis of infants, St. Bartholomew Hospital Rep., 10: 189, 1874.
14. Weissman, G., and Spilberg I.: Breakdown of cartilage protein polysaccharide by lysosomes, Arthritis Rheum, 11: 162, 1968.

Gonococcal Arthritis

The incidence of gonorrheal infections has climbed steadily since 1960. Along with the increase in genitourinary infections, there has been a concomitant rise in gonococcal arthritis. However, joint involvement has been reported to occur in less than 1% of cases of gonorrhea.

Systemic manifestations in addition to arthritis include tenosynovitis, meningitis, en-

Table 13.3
Remission of septic arthritis

Etiology	No. of cases	Time for complete remission in days	
		Range	Average
Staphylococcus	13	10–70	28
Streptococcus	9	10–30	21
Haemophilus influenzae	4	10–50	
Diplococcus pneumoniae	2	8–38	
Escherichia coli	2	37–45	
Pseudomonas	2	40–45	
Proteus	2	65–80	
Salmonella	1	27	

docarditis, maculopapular skin lesions, and septicemia. Arthritis and tenosynovitis are the most common complications in disseminated gonorrhea. Females are afflicted with joint sepsis 3 or 4 times as often as males, a reversal of statistics from the preantibiotic and early antibiotic eras. This is most likely because genitourinary symptoms in men are more apparent, and consequently successful treatment is received earlier. Symptoms of disseminated infection occur disproportionately more often during menses and pregnancies.

Gonorrheal arthritis, other than neonatal, has occurred as early as age 3. However, most cases are seen in the late teens and 20s. In the majority of instances, involvement is polyarticular. Wrists, knees, ankles, and the small joints of the hands and feet are the most frequent sites of involvement.

Two phases of gonococcal arthritis have been described. The first is the bacteremic phase, characterized by fever, chills, skin lesions, and tenosynovitis or polyarthritis. Little or no fluid is evident in the joints in this phase. The second or septic joint phase occurs later and is characterized by single joint infection with a large effusion. The gonococcus recovery rate is generally much higher from the joint aspirate in this phase.

Diagnosis requires, first, a high index of suspicion. Blood and cervical or urethral cultures could be obtained as well as those from joints. In addition to the usual plating, inoculation should be done on a Thayer-Martin medium. Gram staining will frequently reveal the gram-negative intracellular dipplococci. The peripheral white blood count is usually elevated. Synovial fluid cell count may exceed 50,000. The synovial fluid glucose level will be less than one-half that of the serum. A poor mucin clot is formed.

Most cases respond within several days to parenteral penicillin G therapy. This should be in a range of 10 million units per day in a mature patient. In the face of penicillin allergy, tetracycline is the alternative drug of choice. Arthrotomy and joint debridement are usually not necessary, but splinting or cast immobilization should be done to protect the inflamed joint.

The response to parenteral penicillin therapy is usually rapid, and reversal of the process occurs in several days. It is now relatively unusual to see a gonococcal arthritis which has produced any significant degree of damage in a joint, when treatment has been begun within 5 days of onset.

TUBERCULOSIS OF HIP

The onset of this disease is seen as a rule in young children. It accounts for 20% of the cases of bone and joint tuberculosis. The hip is more frequently involved with tuberculosis than any other single joint.

The infection is hematogenous and due to Koch's bacilli. The initial lesion may be synovial in the superior acetabulum or in the inferior neck adjacent to the epiphyseal line. Because it is impossible to excise the local site of involvement with hope of success, it is best to think of the disease as generally involving the joint.

Clinical Picture

The onset is insidious, and there is a history of chronic limp and hip or knee pain, usually encompassing many months, when the patient is first seen. Cries and sudden awakening in the night may mark the illness. There are systemic complaints that often include anorexia, loss of weight, and afternoon fever. The child limps, drops out of activities with his fellows, and avoids weight bearing.

On physical examination, the atrophy of the limb is often striking. The hip motion is limited, and a hip flexion contracture is evident when the uninvolved hip is flexed so that the lumbar spine is flattened. The patient may guard against pain on attempted motion in all planes, but early in the disease, most particularly in internal rotation and abduction as well as in extension.

The rate of progression of the disease may vary from individual to individual.

The limp is antalgic, and there is a short stance phase on the involved leg. Hip flexion contracture may result in marked lumbar lordosis on standing. Local tenderness of the joint may be evident over the femoral head, located beneath the femoral artery one finger's breadth below the inguinal ligament. Posterior joint tenderness may be present as well.

It is not common in these times to see a tuberculous hip accompanied by abscess formation when it is first diagnosed. Shortening of the limb from bone destruction is also a late finding. Relative shortening due to an adducted position may, however, be present in the early stages. Some cases late in the disease show extensive shortening—as much as 10 inches. Gill has shown that such shortening may be due in part to premature central closure of the distal femoral proximal tibial epiphysis.

Pathology

The disease can begin in the synovia, in the metaphysis adjacent to the proximal femoral epiphysis as in the acetabulum. The place of origin is not important.

Even if synovial, the tuberculous granulation tissue begins to invade the subchondral area very quickly. Metaphyseal foci spread to the same area, but usually not by going through the epiphyseal line. A primary epiphyseal foci is uncommon. The trabeculae of the articular cortex are absorbed, and there are granulations both over and under the joint cartilage. This cartilage may be free of its attachment to the parent bone. Areas of contact of joint cartilage constitute a barrier to the extension of the disease and cause destruction to take place first at the joint margins.

With the advancement of the disease, complete destruction of cartilage and subchonral bone occurs. Lymphocytes and plasma cells infiltrate the granulomatous tissue lying intermixed with fibroblasts and vascular tissues. The typically tuberculous arrangement of epipeloid and giant cells about a central area of caseation may be found. In children, healing may occur spontaneously, but when it does, a fibrous ankylosis usually results.

Roentgen Picture

Despite the relative resistance of cartilage to the infection, the most noticeable roentgen finding may be narrowing of the joint space (Fig. 13.6). Apparently no proteolytic enzyme that will digest cartilage, as in pyogenesis, is associated with tuberculous infection. Nonetheless, progression of the disease is so slow and chronic that narrowing of the joint space actually stands out.

There is active destruction of bone, which proceeds irregularly rather than in a rounded distribution as in a tumor; both sides of the joint are often affected. Later, marked bone atrophy occurs in the involved area (Fig. 13.7). There is distention of the capsular shadow and a hazy loss of distinctness of the trabeculae over a wide area. The disease may progress to gross destruction.

Treatment

The first objective is to make a diagnosis of this destructive lesion that is without doubt. While studies are proceeding, the child should be confined to bed, and traction should be applied at the line of his flexion deformity with the object of reducing the degree of contracture (Fig. 13.8), eliminating muscle guarding, and securing comfort for the patient.

There is a positive tuberculin test virtually without exception. A negative test in a patient suspected of having tuberculosis should cause the antigen to be checked and another source to be used. The laboratory work usually reveals an elevated sedimentation rate and may reveal a leukocytosis. The lymphocyte-monocyte ratio may be altered. Secondary anemia may be present.

The joint should be inspected, and a biopsy should be done. The degree of cartilage involvement in both sides is noted at the time of biopsy. With confirmation of the diagnosis, one proceeds with treatment.

An attempt should be made to save a joint that still has intact surfaces. This usually means immobilization in a hip spica which also covers the unaffected leg to the knee. The spica is bivalved, and the patient is allowed to carry the joint briefly through a range of motion twice daily. The spica is not applied until the joint flexion and adduction contracture has been corrected in traction.

The patient's systemic response should subside rapidly if the treatment is to be successful.

Chemotherapy with streptomycin, isoniazid, and p-aminosalicylic acid is used as outlined in the treatment of the knee with this disease.

Failure of the systemic symptoms to subside rapidly and progression of destruction seen by roentgenogram indicate a need for

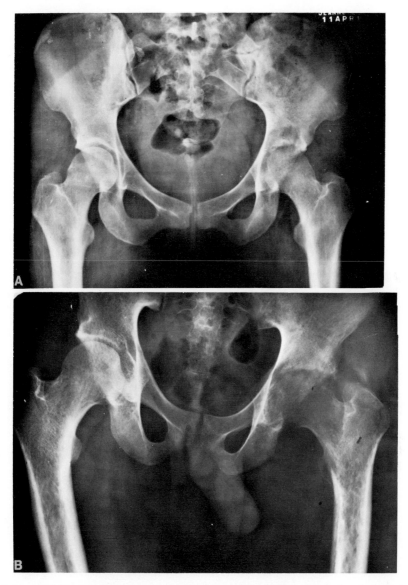

Figure 13.6. (*A*) Early tuberculosis of the hip. Note destruction of subchondral bone of the acetabulum with narrowing of the joint. (*B*) Later development of the disease reveals extensive bone atrophy on the affected side. In addition, destruction of bone on both sides of the joint has become marked.

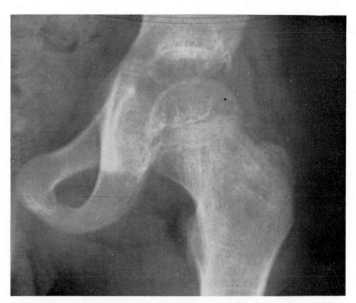

Figure 13.7.　Early tuberculosis of the hip with atrophy and bone involvement.

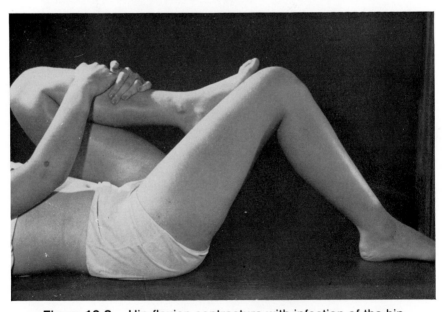

Figure 13.8.　Hip flexion contracture with infection of the hip.

complete immobilization with the hip in neutral position in relation to the pelvis.

Such treatment is also indicated if the patient first presents with a destroyed joint which cannot be functional. Abscesses of the hip are drained and closed primarily.

When the case is destined for fusion, the systemic symptoms are first brought under control. The younger the patient, the more difficult the fusion is to secure and, therefore, the longer the delay in attempting it. For patients younger than 10, fusion is frequently inadvisable.

Attempts at fusion directly through the area involved by disease do not do well and subject the grafts to the ravages of the tuberculous granulation tissue. Operations for hip fusion try in general to bypass the diseased area by proceeding either above or below the hip joint.

In Wilson's technique, a rectangular section of ilium is turned down into the trochanter. In Hibb's technique, the greater trochanter and a portion of the shaft are cut out and reversed, and the shaft end is sunk into a hole in the ilium, the cortex of which has been levered out. The cut surface of the graft faces the neck, which can be denuded where healthy. All fusions superiorly have one defect in common: the muscles guarding the hip tend to pull it into adduction, and thus to separate the graft from bony contact. Thus some forces tend to compress into the graft when it is inferior. Brittain's method runs the graft from the femoral to the ischial region. A tibial graft is run through a subtrochanteric osteotomy of the femur into an ischial bed. In the Trumbell operation the tibial graft runs from femoral shaft to ischium, but without a subtrochanteric osteotomy.

In all hip fusion operations the task is easier if hip motion is limited and the joint quite firmly fixed; the joint is unstable, difficulty in fusion may be encountered. The simultaneous use of a subtrochanteric osteotomy in order to obtain fusion has been found of great value by the author.

All of these operations require immobilization in a bilateral hip spica for at least 6 months. Thereafter, release from immobilization depends on the state of bone fusion. Bony union takes place last through the diseased area. The bypass graft acts as a stabilizing start to eliminate motion and to permit healing of the diseased area.

References

1. Bosworth, D. M.: Treatment of bone and joint tuberculosis in children. *J. Bone Joint Surg.*, 41A:1255, 1959.
2. Cleveland, M.: Surgical treatment of joint tuberculosis. *J. Bone Joint Surg.*, 21:607, 1939.
3. Girdlestone, G. R., and Somerville, E. W.: *Tuberculosis of Bone and Joint;* New York: Oxford University Press, 1952.
4. Key, J. A.: Pathology of tuberculosis of spine, *J. Bone Joint Surg.*, 22:799, 1940.
5. Luck, V.: *Bone and Joint Diseases;* Springfield, Ill.: Charles C Thomas, 1950.
6. Phemister, D. B.: Changes in articular surfaces in tuberculous arthritis, *J. Bone Joint Surg.*, 7: 835, 1925.
7. Phemister, D. B., and Hatcher, C. H.: Correlation of pathological and roentgenological findings in the diagnosis of tuberculous arthritis, *Am. J. Roentgenol.*, 29: 736, 1933.
8. Pimm, L. H., and Waugh, W.: Tuberculous tenosynovitis, *J. Bone Joint Surg.*, 39B: 91, 1957.
9. Pomeranz, M. M.: Roentgen diagnosis of bone and joint tuberculosis, *Am. J. Roentgenol.*, 29:753, 1933.

RETROPERITONEAL ABSCESS

In septic arthritis of the hip, the muscle spasm is marked and resistance occurs when rotation is attempted either way from a usual fixed externally rotated and abducted position.The internal rotation mode may be limited in retroperitoneal abscess, but further external rotation may be possible. Both septic hip and retroperitoneal abscess, of course, have a flexion contracture held so by the patient to maintain comfort. March et al. considered the possibility of the physical signs of septic hip being duplicated in children by retroperitoneal abscess. They stated that rectal examination is very helpful in differentiating the two, as a tender mass may be palpated by this route.

Any condition that could cause a hip flexion contracture can cause diagnostic confusion. Uncorrected inguinal hernia and the multitudinous causes giving rise to psoas and retroperitoneal abscess must be considered. This includes appendicitis with abscess formation. It includes spinal abscess descending via this route anteriorly.

PYOGENIC INFECTION OF HIP

The septic hip problem is still very much with us. The long term trend since the advent of antibiotics is an increased incidence, and in the early 1970s specifically an increased incidence due to *Haemophilus influenzae.*

Not only is the incidence increased, but the disease is often masked by early antibiotic therapy for undiagnosed illness. This leads to softening of the diagnostic signs, delay in arrival of the concept that a serious destructive process is going on in an infant's hip, and consequent important tissue destruction—never to be replaced.

A contrast of the picture of septic hip, prior to the advent of antibiotics and since, reveals that the mortality has virtually been eliminated by antibiotic therapy. The masking of symptoms and signs and the delay in diagnosis exhibit increased incidence and severity since antibiotics have arrived on the scene. The epiphyseal line is destroyed and the femoral head isolated from its blood supply and possibly destroyed as well during this delay.

Over age 2 *Staphylococcus aureus* becomes increasingly the etiologic agent, arriving fairly obviously via the blood stream from a skin lesion. In the early months of infancy. *Staphylococcus* and *H. influenzae* are the common organisms.

Infected hip joints are seen most frequently in infancy and may easily be overlooked in the early stages; yet early diagnosis is necessary to save the hip joint. Pyogenic infection occurs most often as a complication of a general septicemia. The initial lesion may be respiratory, dermal, or enteric, or it may be an umbilical vein infection. It is not unknown as a complication of femoral vein puncture in a septicemic infant.

The disease may begin as an osteomyelitis of the femoral neck metaphysis rather than as a primary synovial infection. The femoral neck, because it is contained within the joint, allows the infection to progress rather easily directly into the joint. Destruction of cartilage is particularly possible with staphylococcic infection owing to its proteolytic enzyme.

Clinical Picture

The patients fall into two groups: those who are acutely ill and appear so, and those who are acutely ill and do not appear so. In infants, fever and a high leukocyte count help to determine the diagnosis but are not necessary to it. The child's failure to move the limb may be the first clinical observation. Swelling in the hip and trochanteric area may be another. Some possible portal of entry for the organism is usually known. The most common agents are the streptococcus, staphylococcus, pneumococcus, or *Escherichia coli*.

Examination reveals limited motion of the hip. Neither internal nor external rotation is evident. Swelling obscures bony prominences and makes palpation of the femoral head beneath the femoral artery difficult or impossible. Tenderness is present both anteriorly and posteriorly over the hip joint.

Roentgen Picture

The early signs are those of distension of the capsular shadows of the hip joint and widening of the joint space (Fig. 13.9). Later, areas of destruction in the metaphysis of the femoral neck may be seen. If the infecting

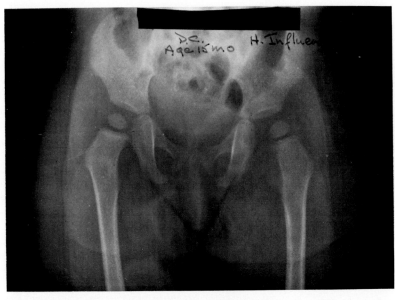

Figure 13.9. Fifteen-month-old infant with widened hip joint space and lateral displacement of the femur with extensive soft-tissue swelling.

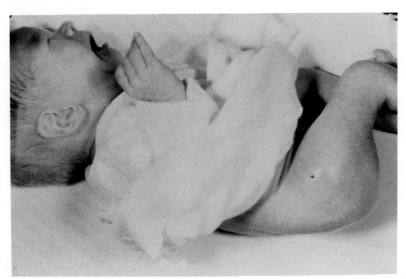

Figure 13.10.   Abscess of the thigh secondary to infection of the hip in a 3-week-old infant. Progression of the disease unrecognized to this point means virtually certain destruction of the femoral head and neck.

agent is the staphylococcus, bony proliferation may also be noted relatively early. In infants, because much of the femoral epiphysis and neck consists of cartilage, the amount of destruction may not be evident (Figs. 13.10 and 13.11).

In the untreated case, further distension of the joint with purulent material, plus the associated muscle spasm, leads to dislocation (Fig. 13.12). Subperiosteal new bone may be present well down the diaphysis in late cases.

Treatment

The disease is an emergency, because drainage and removal of purulent material in contact with the cartilage of the femoral epiphysis may be the only means of saving the epiphysis from destruction. The general condition of the patient may, if necessary, be reinforced by blood transfusion before proceeding.

On clinical suspicion, the joint is aspirated anteriorly with a No. 18 spinal needle. When the needle enters the distended hip joint, purulent material wells up into and out of it. Smears and cultures of this material are made. If pus is obtained, the patient is turned over and the buttock area is reprepared and redraped. Drainage of the hip is done through a linear Ober type incision. This incision is made in line with the femoral neck and over it. The landmarks are a point one-third of the distance along the iliac crest from the posterior superior spine and the trochanter of the femur. In infants, care should be taken to keep the incision well lateralward to avoid the sciatic nerve. The incision splits the fibers of the gluteus maximus, separates the quadratus femoris from the gemellus, and then incises the hip joint capsule. The joint is thoroughly irrigated so that all fibrin clots are removed. A suitable chemotherapeutic agent is instilled. The edges of the capsule are sewn open with a few catgut sutures. A catheter is led down to this opening, but not into the joint itself, and held in place by a skin silk. The wound falls together, and the skin is loosely approximated.

Postoperatively the patient is treated on a Bradford frame (Fig. 13.13). The posterior incision allows for gravity drainage and does not interfere with nursing care. The catheter is gradually removed whenever, during the next 5 days, the patient's clinical course suggests that it may be.

During therapy and from the time of recognition, the patient has both legs in traction in order to prevent dislocation and allow for the resumption of early motion. Immobilization in a hip spica during this period is contraindicated because it is too likely to lead to a limited hip motion.

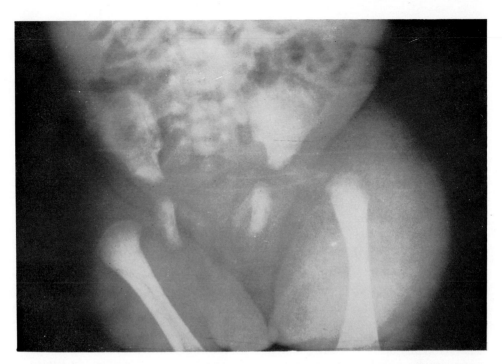

Figure 13.11. Soft-tissue inflammatory swelling, widening of the joint space, and displacement of the femoral shaft at the hip in acute pyogenic infection of the hip.

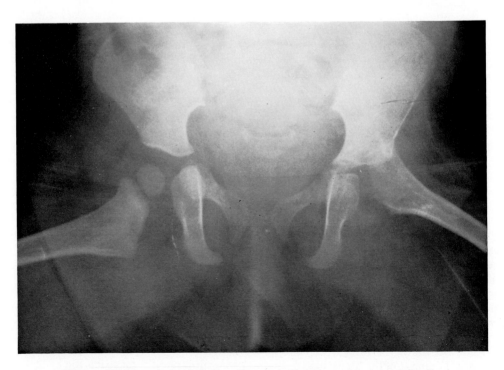

Figure 13.12.   Actual dislocation resulting from hip joint infection.

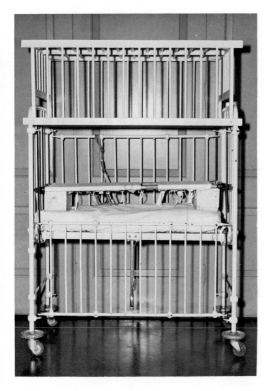

Figure 13.13. A Bradford frame for the care of infants in a hip spica. The pelvis is higher than the head on this frame, and plastic inserted into the plaster spica leads to the bed pan. The patient's cast is strapped to the frame to prevent an accident. The frame, made of pipe with canvas laced tightly around it for support, is sent home with the patient along with instructions for its use in order to prevent soiling of the cast. The frame on top of the crib is used for those youngsters who are standing and inquisitive to the point of leaving the crib, but it is not necessary with a Bradford frame patient who is strapped to the frame and in a plaster spica. Although there are youngsters who could surmount this handicap, they are rare.

Reconstruction of Old Septic Hip

The indications for the reconstruction are: (1) the loss of the normal anatomy with the head and neck frequently destroyed by the original septic process, (2) the unilaterality of the disease with the need for preventing a secondary deformity due to unequal growth of the limb, and (3) the need for stability to correct an unsightly limp (Figs. 13.14 and 13.15).

When the deformity is recognized in infancy, the femur is kept pulled down opposite the acetabulum and abducted until the age of 2. Weight bearing or other activity that will cause the femur to slide up the face of the ilium is not allowed on the basis that it complicates the eventual reconstruction.

The reconstruction procedure is borrowed in part from Colonna's arthroplasty. There are, however, no loose capsular tissues to enclose the trochanter. The object is to seat the trochanter in the newly carved acetabulum and have the trochanter convert to a femoral head substitute. To do this, all tendinous portions of muscles attaching to the greater trochanteric area—such as gluteus medius, gluteus minimus, the gemelli, piriformis, and so forth—are left on the trochanter in as great an abundance as possible. The procedure is done at a relatively young age in the hope of getting greater adaptation and conversion of these tissues. The trochanter is placed against the bare bone of the newly reamed acetabulum and the trochanteric musculature allowed to lie against the bare femoral shaft by widely abducting it. The youngster is kept in position in a spica for 6 weeks. Motion from the bivalved spica is then allowed for the next several months.

References

1. Dunham, E. C.: Septicemia in the newborn, *Am. J. Dis. Child,* 45:229, 1933.
2. Ferguson. A. B., Anderson, R. L., and Braude, A. I.: Bacteriostatic effect of tetracycline in bone, *Antibiot. Chemother,* 9:2, 1959.
3. Obletz, B. E.: Acute suppurative arthritis of the hip in the neonatal period, *J. Bone Joint Surg,* 42A:23, 1960.
4. Sieber, W. K., and Ferguson, A. B., Jr.: Surgical and orthopedic aspects of infections in newly born and young infants, *Pediatrics* 24:145, 1961.
5. Watkins, M. B., Samilson, R. L., and Winters, D. M.: Acute suppurative arthritis, *J. Bone Joint Surg,* 38A: 1313, 1956.

OSTEOMYELITIS

Although osteomyelitis occurs directly— for example, after compound fractures—we

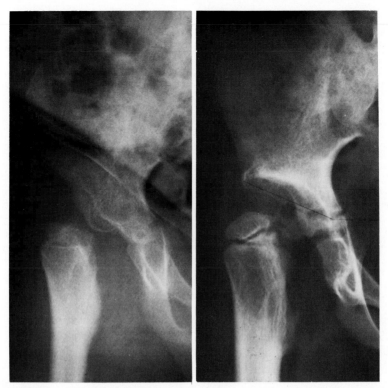

Figure 13.14 (*Left*).   Preoperative roentgenogram reveals destruction of head and neck due to sepsis of the hip joint. If the femur is left in this position, the gait is poor, and shortening of the limb with lack of normal stress becomes excessive.

Figure 13.15 (*Right*).   Postoperative follow-up roentgenogram of reconstructed hip joint. The trochanteric epiphysis and shaft have been transplanted into a reconstructed acetabulum.

are considering here principally the blood-borne, hematogenous infection of bone. This disease once occupied a most prominent position in texts as a difficult and dangerous entity requiring great skill in treatment. The incidence of bone infection has been greatly reduced, but unfortunate situations in which the disease has been underestimated or not recognized are still regularly seen, particularly in the first 3 years of life. It is primarily a disease of early childhood, and it is 4 times as frequent in boys as in girls.

Osteomyelitis is most commonly caused by one of the pyogenic organisms. Green and Shannon have noted the high incidence of streptococcal infections apparently secondary to respiratory involvement in the first 2 years of life. The *Staphylococcus aureus* rises in incidence, as skin lesions liable to cause a

bacteremia begin to occur in the ensuing decade.

Etiology

The disease is most frequently secondary to a blood-borne organism which tends to localize in the metaphysis of bones, owing apparently to a peculiarity of the vessels, and which, with its anatomic loops, tends to produce a relatively stagnant situation.

The tendency to localize in the metaphysis is so strong that it frequently is helpful in differential diagnosis. Although the staphylococcus and streptococcus lead the list, infections with gram-negative organisms occur and must be considered as diagnostic possibilities early in the disease when the organism may not yet be known. The pneumococcus, *E. coli,* and typhoid bacillus are occasional offending agents.

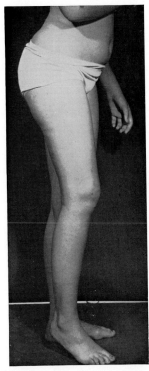

Figure 13.16. Hip flexion and adduction with fixed deformity following previous sepsis of the hip joint.

Clinical Picture

The most usual history in these times of antibiotic agents is a primary respiratory infection, skin abscess, abscess of the teeth, or intestinal infection which was treated apparently in adequate fashion. However, 1 or 2 weeks later, the child may have a recurrence of fever, lassitude, and usually pain in an extremity. The primary infection may not have required medical attention, however, and the child in this case is first seen because of the secondary infection.

In an infant, the tendency of the involved extremity to lie flaccidly may lead to confusion with diseases such as poliomyelitis. If a lower extremity is involved, a limp may lead to similar confusion.

The most helpful diagnostic sign is the anatomic position of the tenderness, which early in the disease is maximal in the metaphyseal area. Late in the disease, a spread of an abscess to the midshaft may result in more diffuse tenderness. There is often local heat and swelling, depending on the area involved. The child frequently experiences such agony upon motion of the limb that any attempt to move it is resisted. It is possible, if one is careful not to press on a tender area, to gain enough cooperation from the patient to carry the joints of the area through a range of motion and thus to rule out pathology in the joint itself.

The child may be seriously ill with a septicemia in addition to his local disease. The

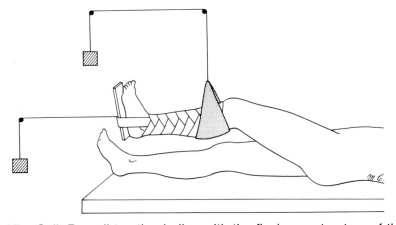

Figure 13.17. Split Russell traction in line with the flexion contracture of the irritated hip.

blood picture indicates an inflammatory response with a rise in polymorphonuclear leukocytes and an increase in young forms. Rarely the osteomyelitis in infants may be part of an overwhelming infection that does not elicit the usual systemic response.

The antibiotic regime to which the child has previously been subjected may make diagnosis quite difficult. The bone may be carrying an abscess with a low grade inflammatory response, development of physical signs may be slow, and only a stubborn failure of the fever to subside from a low grade elevation to normal following treatment may arouse suspicion.

In infants osteomyelitis is still occasionally seen late in its development. Such infections, if in the region of the shoulder or hip, may have broken through into the joint, and the proteolytic enzymes of the purulent material may have done irreparable damage to the cartilage of the epiphysis. Phemister is responsible for calling our attention to the existence of these enzymes and to the rapidity of the digestion of cartilage.

Advent of Antibiotics

Gilmour,[3] analyzing the Perth Children's Hospital figures, noted that penicillin treatment beginning in 1944 constituted a massive experiment. *Staphylococcus aureus,* always the predominant organism, was virtually wiped out. There was progressively a tendency to regard the disease as completely curable by administration of penicillin alone. The staphylococcus reacted by developing a resistant strain. This was evident by 1951. The disease began to increase in frequency. Sequestra reappeared. The disease appeared at a lower age and neonates became prominently involved. The mortality went from 25–30% prior to antibiotics to 1% or less, depending on the incidence of neglected cases. Papers appeared bent more on promoting a medical stance than the child's welfare. One proved that osteomyelitis was no longer a surgical disease by showing that 7 cases involving the distal femur failed to drain and subsided without recurrence. Four of these 7 children had their epiphyseal lines destroyed in the process. What was becoming evident was that the mortality due to septicemia was markedly improved. On the other hand, the disease could not be inadequately treated, the symptoms masked, and the morbidity due to tissue destruction increased.

A review of the statistics at Pittsburgh Children's Hospital revealed that the essential truths were there with the advent of penicillin. The mortality went down, but masking

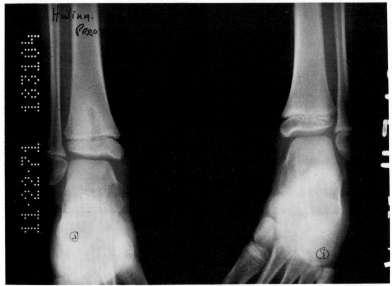

Figure 13.18. Swelling of the ankle joint in a 5-year-old child with evidence of metaphyseal destruction, pointing to origin of disease mistaken for rheumatoid arthritis (8-week duration).

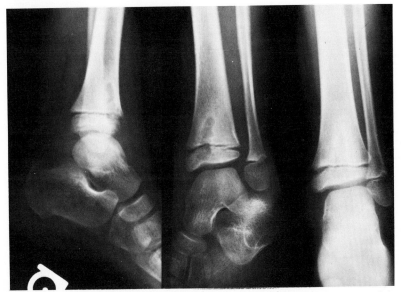

Figure 13.19. Six weeks after incision and drainage, the metaphyseal involvement extending into the epiphysis and then anteriorly to the ankle joint is clear as the ankle joint swelling subsides.

the disease with antibiotic therapy led to a rise in aseptic necrosis and total destruction of the infant's hip with late diagnosis of the condition.

Dennison, dividing the patients into preantibiotic, those treated with sulfathiazole, and those treated with penicillin, noted the progressive decrease in mortality. The incidence of complications did not subside, however. Twenty-seven of 75 patients died before any antibiotics. Even sulfathiazole reduced this to 12.7%. Pathologic fracture and limb overgrowth as well as arthritis by direct extension remained common problems. He found that aspiration was not enough.

As the staphylococcus learned to live with penicillin, the battle between new chemicals and the ability of the staphylococcus to adapt was joined. A review of the history of this battle reveals that, in moments of enthusiasm when surgical drainage has been neglected, later review has left us with destroyed tissue and complications for full function in the life of a growing child.

Paterson[7] in Adelaide, Australia, adopted an immediate arthrotomy program with installation of penicillin for septic hips in 1960. The improvement in results thereafter was dramatic. Fifty joints were clinically and radiographically normal on follow-up. Of 33 other joints treated by a variety of other methods, 15 were destroyed.

Pathology

Osteomyelitis tends to begin in the metaphysis because the circulation slows at the endarteries. Cells to combat the infection become less evident as these sinusoids abut against the epiphyseal line. Inflammation and exudate follow the initial lesion. The pressure forces the purulent material out beneath the periosteum, raising it up—it runs into the epiphyseal line and often through it and into the epiphysis and, in the case of the hip and shoulder, where the metaphysis is intracapsular, frequently into the joint.

The metaphyseal abscess may follow any one of many possible courses. It may subside with treatment and not extend. If a condensation of bone forms around it, the abscess may become chronic. This kind of abscess was more frequently seen before the introduction of antibiotics and was known as Brodie's abscess. The infection may spread through the cortex, elevate the periosteum, and form a subperiosteal abscess. A more massive development of the same trend causes the purulent material to extend up and down the diaphysis and circumferentially around the bone. The entire shaft, or a portion of it, may be cut off from its blood supply, and a sequestrum may form (Fig. 13.20). Such an avascular segment of bone complicates treatment. New bone of a coarse type may wall off the abscess by forming what is called an involucrum. Pathologic specimens have been obtained in which the original bone is encased in an involucrum of similar form.

A less common course for the metaphyseal abscess is that of rupturing into the joint and forming a pyogenic arthritis. Such a development is more common at the shoulder or the hip where, depending on the location of the infection, little or no periosteum or fibrous septa may separate it from the joint space.

Although the disease is most commonly localized in the metaphyseal areas of long bones such as the femur and the tibia, it should be remembered that other metaphyseal areas, such as that of the os calcis, have

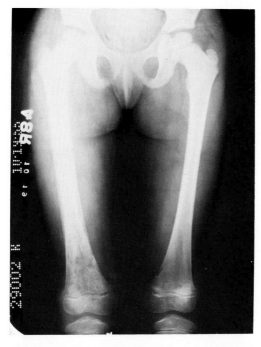

Figure 13.20. Osteomyelitis of proximal femoral metaphysis with involvement of the diaphysis, sequestration of the shaft, and wrapping of the diaphysis in reactive subperiosteal ossification (involucrum).

the same arterial configuration and are surprisingly common sites of involvement.

Roentgen Picture

The x-ray is very helpful and indeed most helpful early in the disease (during the first 11 days), when it is commonly thought to be valueless.

To diagnose osteomyelitis at this stage, when it is most helpful to do so, the examiner must be able to distinguish deep from superficial swelling (Figs. 13.21 and 13.22). Deep swelling involves the area spoken of as of muscle density and having the anatomic configuration of muscle. The area of the subcutaneous tissue is not involved. A superficial skin abscess, on the other hand, involved the subcutaneous tissue with increased vascular markings and the hazy loss of definition associated with inflammation. The deep shadows in superficial cellulitis are not thickened or swollen. It is also necessary to remember that, in the early stages, osteomyelitis is metaphyseal in location. Thus a deep swelling of the inflammatory type localized to the metaphysis is most helpful in recognizing osteomyelitis before changes of bone destruction have appeared.

Later bone destruction, inflammatory swelling, periosteal new bone (involucrum), and new bone distant from the lesion associated with stasis of the circulation make an obvious picture.

The radiolucent areas that appear track irregularly through the metaphysis. The destroyed areas may break out through the cortex. The destruction may progress into the epiphysis. Soft-tissue swelling appears down into the diaphyseal region. The original metaphyseal location can usually be seen, however.

In late disease solitary radiolucent areas with hazy outline may appear. These are often filled with granulomatous tissue. Periosteal ossification is often evident.

Certain specifics in the x-ray pictures enable the physician to gain an impression of the probable causative organism. The staphylococcus is rapid, acutely destructive, and early on provokes an ossifying reaction about the areas of involvement. Salmonella involving children with sickle cell anemia tends to run up and down the shaft in a chronic way, providing minimal reaction but extensive

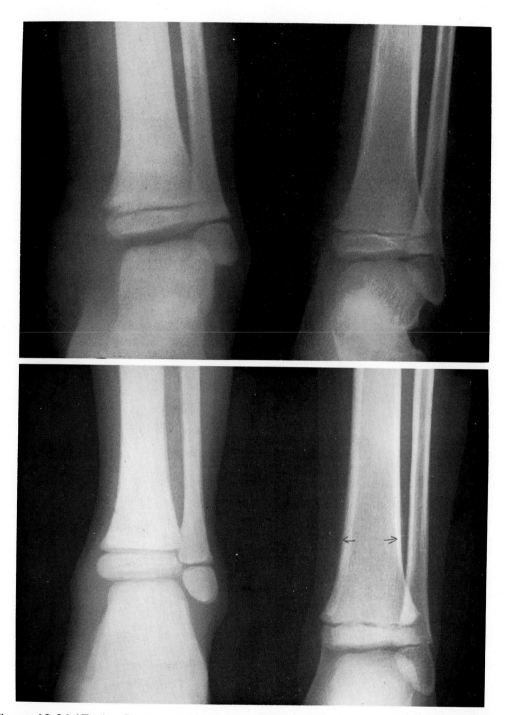

Figure 13.21 (*Top*).   Deep metaphyseal swelling in early osteomyelitis as compared to superficial cellulitis. On the left, the swelling involves superficial subcutaneous as well as deep tissues. On the right, the swelling involves the deep soft tissues only.
Figure 13.22 (*Bottom*).   On the left, the cellulitis area is seen 1 week later. On the right, subperiosteal reaction can be seen 11 days later.

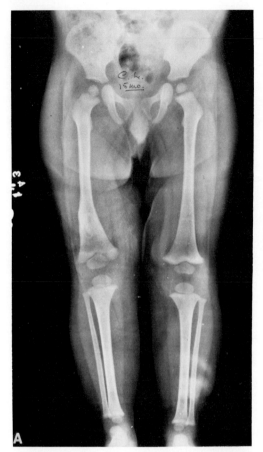

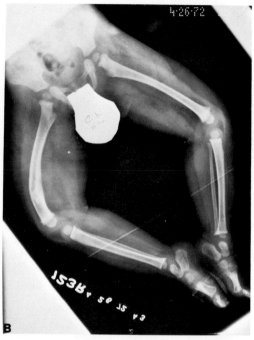

Figure 13.23. (*A*) Chronic osteomyelitis can occur in children as in this 15-month-old patient. There is sclerosis and proliferation of bone about a metaphyseal focus. (*B*) Lateral view of the femur with bone proliferation and deformity.

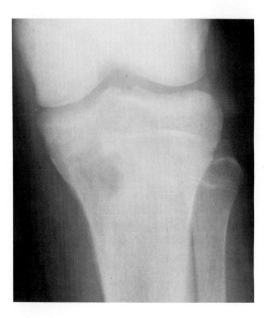

Figure 13.24. Osteomyelitis of proximal tibial metaphysis with bone abscess, destruction of adjacent cortex, and periosteal reaction.

prominent, such as atrophy of the bone and musculature. This evidence for chronicity is prominent, relative to the amount of active destruction and walling off by ossific reaction that may appear. Streptococcus excites little ossific reaction but much cellulitis as evidenced by soft-tissue swelling.

Treatment

If the disease involves only a metaphyseal focus, it may be treated and cured with the correct antibiotic, given a sufficiently long period of time to prevent recurrence and

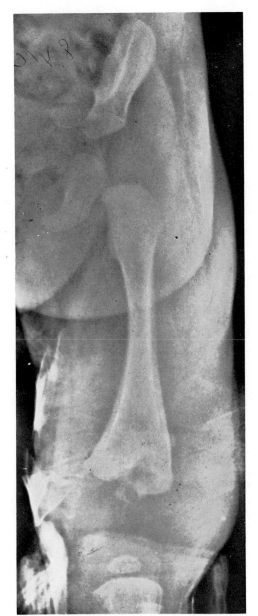

Figure 13.25. In this infant, the osteomyelitis that was originally centered in the metaphysis (where an area of destruction can be seen) has extended through the epiphyseal line into the epiphysis. New bone is laid by the periosteum, and deep soft-tissue swelling is apparent.

mottling of the bone over most of its length (Fig. 13.29).

Tuberculosis does everything the staphylococcus does in the x-ray but takes months to do it. This evidence of chronicity becomes

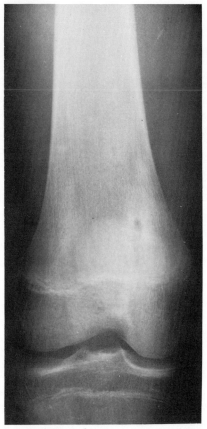

Figure 13.26. Chronic osteomyelitis in childhood. This 15-year-old boy had a 2-year history of pain, limp, and inability to use the extremity actively. Previous treatment included 1 year's use of antibiotics of various types without amelioration of symptoms. In this anteroposterior view of the distal femoral metaphysis, destruction and new bone proliferation about it can be seen.

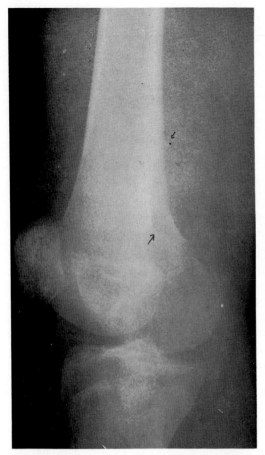

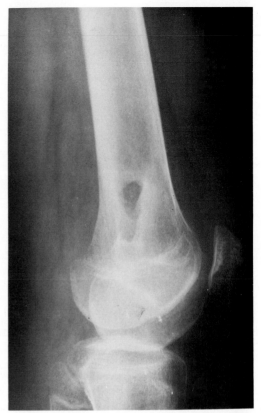

Figure 13.27. The lateral view of patient shown in Figure 13.26 shows the original nidus and a dimly seen tract toward the cortex proximally.

Figure 13.28. The postoperative view of patient shown in Figures 13.25 and 13.26 shows excision of the infected granuloma and primary closure of the wound. Full healing resulted, and activity was regained without further antibiotic therapy. The body tends to isolate the infected lesion from the systemic circulation and thus renders antibiotics useless.

provided that the limb is immobilized during that time.

Some of the cases in which there is a small subperiosteal abscess in addition may get by with antibiotics alone. Most, however, need aspiration or drainage to avoid unnecessary complication, such as interference with growth, the development of a sequestrum, or a prolonged course.

Cases which have already developed beyond this point may need surgical intervention to save the child, the limb, an epiphyseal line, or a joint or to secure a sequestrum and prevent the development of chronic osteomyelitis.

The judgment as to what procedure will secure the maximal benefit for the child must be based on bedside findings, not on a text-book; but, in general, unnecessary guttering and removal of bone are to be avoided. The healing powers of childhood are equal to restoring even a sequestration of the entire shaft. Cartilage of the epiphyseal line, if damaged, is damaged permanently, however.

The general antibiotic approach is through wide spectrum drugs, which are used until the organism is known and the most useful drug can be prescribed (Tables 13.4–13.7). Dosage is high; it is continued for a minimum of 3 weeks and at least 2 weeks beyond the subsidence of fever and preferably also of the sedimentation rate. A slight elevation of the sedimentation rate may persist for several

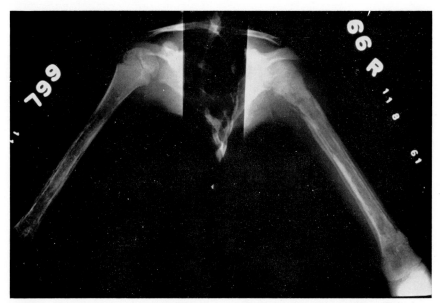

Figure 13.29. Extensive osteomyelitis due to Salmonella infestation. This low grade, widespread process is seen in blood dyscrasias (in this case, sickle cell anemia) in children.

Table 13.4
Antibacterial spectrum of antimicrobial agents

Mode of action	Gram positives	Broad spectrum	Gram negatives
Bactericidal	Penicillins Bacitracin	Kanamycin-Neomycin Cephalothin Ampicillin (Penicillin)*	Streptomycin Polymyxin B-Colistin Gentamycin
Bacteriostatic	Erythromycin Oleandomycin Lincomycin	Tetracyclines Methacycline Sulfonamides Chloramphenicol	Nalidixic acid

* In very large doses, penicillin may be bactericidal against a number of gram-negative organisms.

months, however, if there has been extensive tissue destruction.

Rest is still good treatment for infection, and, in the presence of resistant organisms. it gives the natural antibody processes the greatest help in overcoming the disease. Bed rest alone, however, has many times been found insufficient rest for the part. A comfortable splint or bivalved cast ensures real rest for the extremity involved.

A general principle and safe working rule is to incise and drain the subperiosteal abscess when it is clearly evident and fluctua-tion is apparent, or when there is any possibility of involvement of the epiphyseal line. Cellulitis alone is not drained in infants. To drain the bone, an incision is made and holes are drilled through the cortex without elevating the periosteum. It is important to maintain the blood supply to the bone and yet secure adequate decompression of the medullary cavity. In infants, this cavity has a tendency to decompress spontaneously due to the spongy nature of very young bones.

In older children with an established bone abscess, the abscess must be reached and

Table 13.5
Choice of anti-infective agents

Organism (and gram reaction)	Drugs	
	First choice	Second choice
Actinomyces (+)	Penicillin + tetracycline	Sulfonamide
Aerobacter aerogenes (−)*	Kanamycin, neomycin, cephalothin	Streptomycin + tetracycline, polymyxin, colistin, gentamycin
Bacillus anthracis (+)	Penicillin	Tetracycline, erythromycin
Bacteroides (−)*	Tetracyclines	Penicillin
Brucella (−)	Tetracycline + streptomycin	Kanamycin
Clostridium (+)	(Antitoxin) penicillin	Erythromycin, kanamycin
Corynebacterium diphtheriae (+)	(Antitoxin) penicillin	Erythromycin, lincomycin
Diplococcus pneumoniae (+)	Penicillin	Erythromycin, cephalothin, tetracyclines, lincomycin
Erysipelothrix (+)	Penicillin	Tetracyclines, erythromycin
Escherichia coli (−)*	Ampicillin	Kanamycin, streptomycin, tetracyclines, colistin, cephalothin, sulfonamides
Haemophilus influenzae (−), H. pertussis	Ampicillin	Chloramphenicol + streptomycin
Klebsiella pneumoniae (−)	Kanamycin, neomycin, cephalothin	Streptomycin + tetracyclines, polymyxin, colistin, gentamycin
Leptospira icterohaemorrhagiae	Tetracyclines	Penicillin
Listeria monocytogenes	Tetracyclines	Penicillin, bacitracin
Lymphogranuloma venereum, psittacosis, and trachoma agents	Tetracyclines	Chloramphenicol, sulfonamide
Mycobacterium leprae (+)	Sulfones	Sulphetrone, diphenylthiourea, sulfoxone
M. tuberculosis (+)	Isoniazid + streptomycin + p-aminosalicylic acid	Viomycin, cycloserine, ethionamide, pyrazinamide
Moniliasis (Candida albicans)	Amphotericin B	Nystatin
Mycoplasma (Eaton agent)	Tetracyclines	
Neisseria gonorrhoeae (−)	Penicillin	Ampicillin, tetracyclines Erythromycin, chloramphenicol
N. meningitidis (−)	Penicillin + sulfonamides	Ampicillin, cephalothin, erythromycin, tetracyclines
Nocardia (+)*	Sulfonamides + tetracyclines	Sulfonamides + agent chosen by sensitivity tests
Pasteurella pestis, P. tularensis (−)	Streptomycin + tetracyclines	
Proteus mirabilis (−)*	Ampicillin, penicillin	Cephalothin, neomycin
P. vulgaris, P. morganii,* P. rettgeri (−)*	Kanamycin, streptomycin	Cephalothin, chloramphenicol, gentamycin
Pseudomonas aeruginosa (−)*	Polymyxin B, colistin	Gentamycin, tetracyclines, kanamycin, neomycin
Rickettsia (−)	Chloramphenicol	Tetracyclines
Salmonella (−)	Ampicillin	Chloramphenicol, cephalothin, tetracyclines, kanamycin
S. typhosa (−)	Chloramphenicol	Ampicillin
Shigella (−)	Sulfonamides	Ampicillin, tetracyclines, cephalothin, chloramphenicol

Table 13.5—*Continued*

Organism (and gram reaction)	Drugs	
	First choice	Second choice
Spirrillum minus (−)	Penicillin	Tetracyclines
Staphylococcus (+)*, if sensitive	Penicillin	Erythromycin, lincomycin, oleandomycin
Staphylococcus (+), if resistant	Methicillin, oxacillin, nafcillin, cloxacillin	(See above)
Streptococcus (+)	Penicillin	(See above)
S. faecalis (+)*	Penicillin + streptomycin	Ampicillin
Treponema pallidum	Penicillin	Cephalothin, erythromycin, tetracycline

* Sensitivity tests usually indicated.

emptied completely. It will often contain granulation tissue requiring curettement. The abscess is left unroofed, and the soft tissues are closed primarily with catgut rather than with silk or cotton. The periosteum is not stripped to accomplish this surgery.

References

1. Altermeier, W. A. and Helmsworth, J. A.: Penicillin treatment in acute osteomyelitis, *Surg. Gynecol. Obstet,* 81:138, 1945.
2. Altermeier, W. A., and Helmsworth, J. A.: An evaluation of penicillin therapy in acute osteomyelitis, *J. Bone Joint Surg,* 30A:657, 1948.
3. Gilmour, W. N.: Acute hematogenous osteomyelitis, *J. Bone Joint Surg,* 44B:840, 1962.
4. Harris, N. H., and Kirkaldy-Willis, W. H.: Primary subacute pyogenic osteomyelitis, *J. Bone Joint Surg,* 47B:526, 1965.
5. Hook, E. W., Campbell, C. G., Weens, H. S., and Cooper, G. R.: Salmonella osteomyelitis in patients with sickle-cell anemia, *N. Engl. J. Med,* 257:403, 1957.
6. Morse, T. S., and Pryles, C. V.: Infections of the bones and joints in children, *N. Engl. J. Med,* 262:846, 1960.
7. Paterson, D. C.: Acute suppurative arthritis of infancy and childhood, *J. Bone Joint Surg,* 52B:474, 1960.
8. Trueta, J.: The three types of osteomyelitis, *J. Bone Joint Surg,* 41B:671, 1959.
9. White, M., and Dennison, W. M.: Acute hematogenous osteitis in childhood, *J. Bone Joint Surg,* 34B:608, 1952.

INFLAMMATION OF INTERVERTEBRAL DISC SPACE IN CHILDREN

Particularly in the child age 2–6, the clinical syndrome accompanying inflammation of the intervertebral disc can be a puzzling diagnostic problem. The child frequently refuses to walk.

The child will characteristically splint the entire spinal column rigidly. This results in a stiff gait with minimal flexion of the hips and difficulty with a sitting posture. On the floor the child tends to sit with the trunk thrown back and rising on the outstretched arms behind the body. (The old tripod sign of poliomyelitis and occasionally meningitis.) The child in imitable.

Palpation of the spine with the child prone when done carefully will elicit highly localized tenderness. The straight leg raising may reveal marked hamstring spasm. The lumbar lordosis is straightened.

The average age of the child is 4 years, but cases have been reported from 15 months to 15 years. The vast majority are under 6 years of age.

In addition to refusal to walk (the commonest complaint), back pain and thigh pain are common complaints. Loss of appetite and vomiting may occur.

The most common disc spaces involved are at the thoracolumbar junction or at L4-L5 or L5-S1 interspaces.

Laboratory Findings

The sedimentation rate usually shows a mild elevation but may be slow in developing. The white blood cell count tends to run in the high normal range, only occasionally getting over 10,000 per cubic millimeter.

Tuberculin, brucellergin, and febrile agglutinin tests are ordinarily negative, but we

Table 13.6
Sensitivity of common pathogens to major antibacterial agents: minimal inhibitory concentration, μg/ml

Pathogen	Sulfonamide (0.029)	Penicillin G (0.02–2)	Ampicillin (0.02–5)	Methicillin (0.15–2.6)	Cephalosporin (0.15–8)	Erythromycin (0.03–1)	Vancomycin (0.5–1)	Tetracycline (0.25–2)	Chloramphenicol (0.5–16)	Streptomycin (0.1–32)	Kanamycin (1–8)	Polymyxin (0.1–1)
Staphylococcus aureus (a)	PS	[0.03]	0.06	2	0.25	0.12	1	0.12	4–8	2	0.5	R
S. aureus (b)*	V	R	R	[2]	0.25	0.12	1	0.12	4–8	V	0.5	R
Streptomyces pyogenes	S	[0.015]	0.03	0.12	0.12	0.03	0.5	0.25	2	32	R	R
Streptococcus faecalis	R	[2]	2.0	32	>8	0.5	1	0.5	2	[64]	64–128	64–128
Pneumococcus	S	[0.015]	0.06	0.25	0.12	0.03	0.5	0.25	2	64	R	R
Mycobacterium tuberculosis	R	R				5–20		10	10	[0.1]	0.5	R
Gonococcus	[S]	[0.015]	0.12	0.06		0.06	R	1	1	4	8	R
Meningococcus	[S]*	[0.03]	0.06	0.25	0.12		R	1	1			R
Haemophilus influenzae	PS	0.25–2	[0.25]	2	8	1.0	R	1	[0.5]	2–4	2	0.1–1
Haemophilus pertussis	PS	0.5–2				0.2		0.2–2	0.2–2	2–64		0.2–1
*Escherichia coli**	[S]	16–R	[8]	R	16	R	R	1	2–8	4	[1–4]	0.25
*Klebsiella-Aerobacter**	PS	R	16–R	R	8–R	R	R	2–R	2–R	2–R	4–R	0.25
Proteus mirabilis (a)*	V	[16–32]	[4]	R	16	R	R	32–64	4–16	4–8	4–8	R
P. mirabilis (b)*	V	R	R	R	[16]	R	R	32–64	[4–16]	4–R	[4–8]	R
*Proteus vulgaris**	V	R	64	R	128–R	R	R	4–32	[4–8]	2–8	[1–4]	R
*Proteus morgagni**	V	R	128	R	R	R	R	4–64	[4–64]	4–R	[2–4]	R
Salmonella sp.	PS	[2–16]	[2]	R	4–8		R	1	2	8	2–4	0.12
Shigella sp.	[PS]	16	[4]	R	8–16		R	[0.5–2]	1–8	8	4	0.12
*Pseudomonas**	R	R	R	R	R	R	R	20–R	R	16–64	64–128	[0.12]

* Variable sensitivities—should always be tested. (a) = nonpenicillinase producers, (b) = penicillinase producers, □ = preferred antimicrobial(s) in clinical use. R = all resistant; S = all sensitive; PS = probably sensitive; V = variable.

Table 13.7
Incompatibilities of commonly used drugs for intravenous administration

Agent	Incompatible agents
Amphotericin B	Potassium penicillin G, tetracyclines
Cephalothin	Calcium chloride or gluconate, erythromycin, polymyxin B, tetracyclines
Chloramphenicol	B-Complex vitamin preparations, hydrocortisone, polymyxin B, tetracyclines, vancomycin
Methicillin	Tetracyclines
Nafcillin	B-Complex vitamin preparations
Potassium penicillin G	Amphotericin B, metaraminol, phenylephrine, tetracyclines, vancomycin, ascorbic acid
Polymyxin B	Cephalothin, chloramphenicol, heparin, tetracyclines
Tetracyclines	Amphotericin B, cephalothin, chloramphenicol, heparin, hydrocortisone, methicillin, potassium penicillin G, polymyxin B
Vancomycin	Chloramphenicol, heparin, hydrocortisone, potassium penicillin G

have had one patient with a very high brucellosis titer.

Blood cultures and cerebrospinal fluid determinations are ordinarily negative.

Cultures obtained by needle biopsy have generally been negative, with an occasional coagulase-positive *Staphylococcus aureus* entering the picture.

Roentgen Findings

Narrowing of the disc height is the earliest finding, usually present by the second to third week of symptoms. There follows invasion of the adjacent cortical bone of the vertebrae on either side of the disc space (Figs. 13.30 and 13.31). This is clearly defined active destruction. Smith and Taylor[3] pointed out that this destruction may progress to well defined cavities in the vertebrae, the vertebrae do not lose height, and there may be some reactive sclerosis, but it is minimal.

Treatment

The usual treatment is immobilization in a double hip spica for 3 months. Antibiotics are used for a period of 3 weeks at onset of treatment. This usually consists of methicillin, oxacillin, or penicillin in combination with broad spectrum agents. Even though positive cultures are not frequent and the value of the spica immobilization well established, there is still sufficient evidence of delayed response without antibiotics that their use continues to be justified.

Course

The clinical course is ordinarily benign and the patient is left without residual symptoms or vertebral deformity. The patient never appears to be in critical condition. Spontaneous interbody fusion is rare. Six months following onset, the child is usually back on full activity, with roentgen signs stable or possibly with some irregularity of the cortical surface of the vertebrae remaining, but no loss of height.

References

1. Bremmer, A. E., and Neligan, G. A.: Benign forms of acute osteitis of the spine in young children, *Br. Med. J*, 1:856, 1953.
2. Menelaus, M. B.: Discitis; an inflammation affecting the intervertebral discs in children, *J. Bone Joint Surg*, 46B:16, 1964.
3. Smith, R. F., and Taylor, T.: Inflammatory lesions of intervertebral discs in children, *J. Bone Joint Surg*, 49A:508, 1967.
4. Wiley, A. M., and Trueta, J.: The vascular anatomy of the spine and its relationship to pyogenic vertebral osteomyelitis, *J. Bone Joint Surg*, 41B:796, 1959.

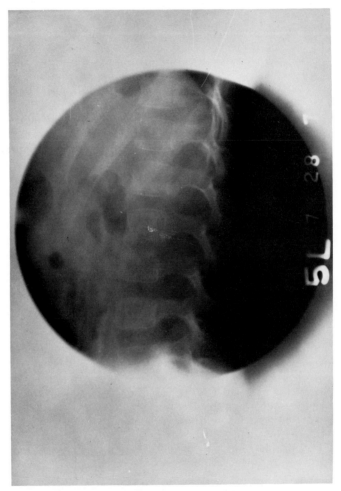

Figure 13.30. Narrowing of the intervertebral disc space with destruction of subchondral bone on either side of the disc space.

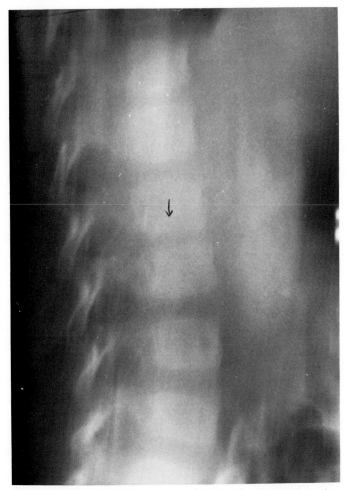

Figure 13.31. The tomogram further accentuates the irregular destruction of the subchondral bone on either side of the intervertebral disc space.

CHAPTER 14

Neurogenic Affections

POLIOMYELITIS

Although the diagnosis of poliomyelitis frequently falls on the shoulders of the medical pediatric practitioner, the treatment of its effects is the responsibility of orthopaedic surgery. A thorough knowledge of the disease, of the requisites for maximal recovery, of the prevention of deformity, and finally of the methods of reconstruction gives the orthopaedic surgeon tools of great use in understanding and treating other conditions in childhood.

The disease may produce an asymmetric, flaccid, irregular paralysis without sensory involvement. Such an effect is duplicated by very few conditions.

History

Ghormley[3] stated that the first monograph of poliomyelitis was published in 1840 by Jacob Heine of Connstatt. Heine put the age group affected by 6–36 months and noted that the children were enjoying unusually good health when stricken. Pain and paralysis of both lower extremities were forecast as the result.

Caverly may have been the first to describe the nonparalytic form of poliomyelitis when he reported an epidemic in Vermont in 1894. One hundred ten patients were noted to have had paralysis in some form, and at least 50 of these had fully recovered.

The first great epidemic appeared in 1905 in Norway and Sweden. Eighteen months after this epidemic broke out, 56% of the 550 patients originally reported paralyzed still had some residual paralysis, and 44% had recovered completely.

In a 1917 monograph on poliomyelitis, Rohrah and Mayer harked back to Badham, who in 1835 initiated the use of heat for comfort. They advocated wrapping the extremities in flannel and supplying heat in the form of hot water bottles.

Peabody, Draper, and Dochez in 1913 classified the forms of the disease as follows: (1) abortive cases, (2) cerebral cases (spastic paralysis evident), and (3) bulbospinal cases (flaccid paralysis). They remarked that, preceding paralysis, there is a period marked by prodromal symptoms, and they recommended quarantine during this stage.

Ghormley, in his article on the history of the treatment of poliomyelitis, showed that Peabody and his co-workers recommended the use of heat, passive motion, and rhythmic motion, along with active training of muscles, to prevent contractures and hasten recovery. Placing the children in a warm bath was considered an aid to the exercising of their limbs.

Draper emphasized that resistance to anterior flexion of the spine was typical of poliomyelitis and was greater in this disease then in either the stiff neck or Kernig's sign of meningeal irritation.

Vulpian, in the same era, remarked on the muscle contracture and deformity that followed the initial stage of the disease. In total paralysis, he noted the relaxation of the joint capsule and the tendency of the limb to adapt itself more to the demands of gravity than to those of function. The shortening of active muscle groups and the development of contracture were responsible for deformity in partial paralysis. The involved muscles undergo marked atrophy and decrease in size, and the atrophied fibers become yellowish white owing to fatty degeneration. Vulpian recommended wet or dry packs (1912).

Lovett,[9] who was a keen student of poliomyelitis, laid the groundwork (1916) for much of the understanding of the disease as it occurs today. To Lovett, poliomyelitis was a generalized disease that acted on viscera as well as on the central nervous system. Spinal cord pathology could produce a fatality via the nerve cells that control respiration, or spontaneous repair of it could allow complete recovery. He described the symptoms as follows:

The symptoms are in general those of an acute infection. In many instances, however, gastrointestinal symptoms predominate; while in others, those referable to the respiratory tract, are the most marked. Stiffness of the neck to flexion of the head, sweating, marked nervous irritability and general hyperesthesia are present in many instances before the onset of paralysis, but they are not all constant.

Lovett believed that "muscle training forms the basis of the modern treatment of poliomeylitis." In theory, this training attempts to make the patient send a voluntary impulse to contract a muscle and aids the muscle to contract by means of passive movement. The limb is placed in such a position that gravity aids the movement, and further assistance is given by the hand.

There is one very important point in this connection that is often lost sight of. In an affected limb, some muscles are as a rule paralyzed, some weakened, and some comparatively normal. The muscles that we wish to exercise are those that are paralyzed or weakened. If the exercises are not carefully controlled and located, the patient is sure to use strong muscles instead of the weak ones and thus to make the muscular imbalance still worse. Exercises loosely given by untrained persons and encouragement of the child to kick about and do anything he can are likely to do harm rather than good.

Lovett emphasized that splints to prevent deformity are an aid to treatment.

He also gave us a system of grading muscles which is in common use today for following the patient's progress.

Diagnosis

Despite widespread familiarity with the cardinal signs of poliomyelitis, the disease continues to be much misdiagnosed. During the summer and fall months, virtually every child with a limp, stiff neck, or pain in the extremities is suspected to having the disease. The problem is often to separate out the cases of multiple neuritis (Guillain-Barré), meningitis, cord tumor, disease of the hip, knee, and spine from the cases of Heine-Medin's disease or poliomyelitis. The stages of poliomyelitis are:

I. The acute stage
II. The convalescent stage
   A. With sensitivity
   B. Without sensitivity
III. The chronic stage

Acute Stage

ONSET

The onset of poliomyelitis is like that of many other acute illnesses. Fever and symptoms of malaise referable to the gastrointestinal tract—i.e., vomiting, headache, and signs of a mild coryza—may all be present. The early period of mild illness may be followed by a week in which the patient feels essentially well. But the fever returns (a chart of the fever produces a double-humped curve), and it is followed rapidly by signs of meningeal irritation. When the onset is more continuous, as it quite commonly is, the fewer does not subside, and the symptoms and signs gradually spread to include the central nervous system. The initial symptoms may have been overlooked because of their mildness.

In the second phase of the onset, muscle aches in the extremities are common. Stiffness of the back and neck are noted, and headaches become a frequent complaint. The irritability that is common to involvement of the central nervous system becomes prominent.

Paralysis begins usually in the second to fifth day of the febrile period. It may be maximal 2–4 days after recognition. Subsidence of the fever has been thought by many observers to signify the end of the development of paralysis. Sensitivity may, however, cause muscles to belie this characteristic of the disease. Marked persistence of the fever may occur in cases that eventually lead to death.

As Caverly noted, there may be no paralysis at all. Sensitivity precedes paralysis. In infants, the response may be one of flaccidity such that muscle spasm, and sensitivity are not appreciated by the examiner. The fever is usually approximately 101F and occasionally 103F, higher but it is rarely higher than this. An exceptionally high fever is associated ordinarily with the encephalitic type.

CLINICAL PICTURE

The patient is a very irritable child who resents attempts to handle or move the extremities. Unless the disease is encephalitic, the patient is alert and clear. Spasm of the back, neck, and hamstrings is usual. Forward flexion of the neck is painful (Brudzinski). There is a positive Kernig test. Lying on his side, the patient does not allow forward flexion of the spine. When he sits, he presents the so-called "tripod" sign of poliomyelitis (Fig. 14.1). With legs extended on the table, sitting is limited, and the patient supports himself in a partial sitting posture with his arms. Straight-leg raising is limited usually in a quite symmetric fashion; the leg which will later show most involvement is not necessarily more limited than the other.

Muscles may be sensitive to pressure. Muscle sensitivity should be distinguished from nerve sensitivity by palpation of the anatomic distribution of the large nerve trunks. Spasm of the trunk muscles may be acute anteriorly as well as posteriorly and may result in confusion with intra-abdominal conditions. Even in the so-called nonparalytic type of poliomyelitis, some mild weakness may be seen on careful examination.

DIFFERENTIAL DIAGNOSIS

As Britt, Christie, and Batson have shown, the problem in diagnosis in a medical community that is alert to the disease is not that of overlooking poliomyelitis, but that of misdiagnosing other entities as poliomyelitis. Entities to be considered as the same time as nonparalytic poliomyelitis are meningitis, encephalitis, brain tumor, gastroenteritis, bacillary dysentery, meningococcemia, tick typhus, fecal impaction, and intussusception.

In patients presenting paralysis or pseudoparalysis, poliomyelitis must be differentiated from the Guillain-Barré syndrome, brain and cord tumors, osteomyelitis, pyelonephritis, scurvy, and fractures.

TREATMENT

In the acute phase, the patient is on bed rest and is protected against deformity by general measures, including positioning. A bed board is used so that excessive lumbar lordosis is readily seen. The bed board should not be one piece, however, because treatment of the disease includes periodic positioning of the patient in gentle spinal flexion when mobilization is begun. A knee roll that allows slight flexion of the knee is a matter of great comfort to the patient. The foot board is separated from the end of the mattress, and

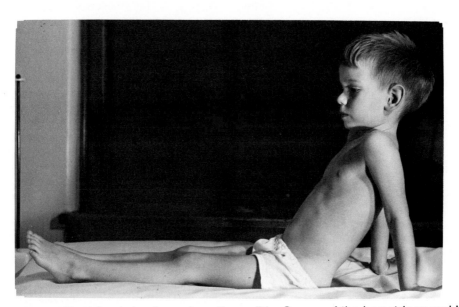

Figure 14.1. The tripod sign in acute poliomyelitis. Spasm of the hamstrings and back muscles limits the patient's ability to sit up.

the heels are allowed to drop into the interspace. A small neck roll may be comfortable. Hot packs are used to diminish sensitivity. They also aid the performance of stretching type exercises when they are used just prior to the stretching. If they produce discomfort, they have little value. Hot packs in general are wrapped around an extremity and laid on the trunk. Continuous use of packs can be debilitating to the patient.

There are many special therapeutic problems at this stage which cannot be covered here. They include measures to relieve difficulty in swallowing, respiration, and micturition. The respirator, rocking bed, and tracheotomy have special and definite indications.

While the patient is febrile, it is important that disturbances and handling be minimized and that supportive measures be gentle and adequate. Positioning in bed to avoid deformity results in a very sensitive patient if it overstretches irritable muscles.

Convalescent Stage

The convalescent stage begins with the subsidence of fever and continues for $1\frac{1}{2}$ years after the onset. It has been found that, during this period, the disease has a marked tendency to improve spontaneously insofar as paralytic involvement is concerned. With the appearance of paralysis and sensitivity there is a marked tendency toward deformity. The paralyzed muscles, when they are opposed by muscles in spasm, become overstretched. Spastic paralysis has been seen very rarely in encephalitic types of involvement. Flaccid paralysis is the general rule.

The bulbospinal respiratory type needs special emphasis because it may be fatal. Prompt and early recognition is essential to the treatment. Facial nerves may be involved in bulbar poliomyelitis.

Examination in the stage of sensitivity must be gentle. Much can be learned merely from observing the patient's characteristic position in bed. Tendencies such as external rotation of the lower extremity, drop foot, and adduction of the upper extremity are readily appreciated. Assessment of muscle weakness at this initial stage may be general rather than specific, but it should be thorough enough to reveal what measures are necessary to block the development of deformity.

Muscle spasm in poliomyelitis is largely due to an attempt on the part of the patient to protect sensitive muscles. Spasm of this type may seem to indicate more paralysis than actually exists because the opposing muscles may be inhibited by reflex. The duration of the paralysis varies with the degree of involvement. Mild involvement may result in transient weakness only. The degree of intial paralysis is of some help in prognosticating the time of eventual recovery. The subsidence of sensitivity greatly aids the patient's progress. The rate of recovery is greatest in the early phases of the disease and decreases as the final stages of the convalescent period are reached. The patient at the end of this period passes to the chronic or reconstructive stage of poliomyelitis.

PATHOLOGY

Areas other than the central nervous system are involved. Lymphoid tissue generally is hyperplastic. A myocarditis has been noted at autopsy, and it occurs in approximately 25% of cases that terminate in death. The nerve cells themselves are the seat of primary injury, however. The virus is located within the neurons, and degeneration of them leads to secondary tract and nerve degeneration. There is an inflammatory and hemorrhagic reaction, the subsidence of which in the presence of undamaged ganglion cells may account for the "recovery tendency" of the disease.

The ganglion cells undergo coagulative necrosis, chromatolysis, and neuronophagia. There is no evidence that damaged ganglion cells recover. The motor cells of the cord are apparently more susceptible than cells of the cerebral cortex. The effects of the disease are not limited to the cord, however, but have been noted in medulla, pons, midbrain, cortex, and cerebellum as well. A neurogliar proliferation tends to produce a scar in 3–4 weeks.

The lesions typically tend to be distributed in the anterior horn, i.e., predominantly dorsomedially. The distribution accounts for the tendency of the clinical picture to follow certain distributions of paralysis. The anterior horn involvement is most severe, and lateral columns and posterior horns are affected.

In the late stages of the disease, the axis cylinders of the peripheral nerves degenerate. The muscles undergo the changes associated with denervation atrophy. There is a loss of striations, reduction in sarcoplasm, and alteration in electrical response. This is followed by atrophy, fibrosis, and fat replacement. Bone atrophy is a late development that follows disuse of the limb.

The development of cold legs that have a tendency to appear mildly cyanotic may be due to palsy of parasympathetic nerves from damage to the bulbar cord; the sympathetic system is spared through the lateral columns of lumbar nerves 1 and 2. Damage of anterior horn cells affects the parasympathetic system more than the sympathetic and results in failure of bladder and rectum to contract; it thereby produces the clinical problems in these areas that are occasionally seen in poliomyelitis.

TREATMENT

Once the patient is afebrile, the paralytic involvement is estimated. The estimate may be inaccurate owing to muscle spasm and sensitivity; it may indicate more severe involvement than actually exist. Tendencies toward deformity are noted, and the patient is positioned against them periodically during the day. The bed may be used to aid in developing spinal flexion and hamstring stretching. No positioning should be considered static, but changes in position should be frequently made.

Splints are often necessary. With young children, they are used in place of the footboard because it is sometimes difficult to keep the youngster against the board. The splint holds the foot in a neutral position so far as dorsiflexion and inversion-eversion are concerned. An outrigger attached to the splint to prevent chronic hyperextension of the knee by holding it in slight flexion is occasionally used. Splints should not be misused by being left on the patient for excessively long periods.

All of the joints should be carried through a range of motion within the limits of pain regularly during the day. Stretching is begun early and is carried to, but not beyond, the point of producing pain. Limbs are held at bony prominences, not in areas of large muscle masses, in tender patients. The period of convalescence is greatly shortened by early stretching and mobilization. The spine should be stretched in rotation as well as in flexion.

The drop foot deformity is well known in poliomyelitis. When the patient is prone, the feet should be allowed to drop into the interval between the mattress and the footboard. Less well known but quite common is the development of a flexion abduction deformity at the hip. This deformity begins with spasm of the iliopsoas, sartorius, and tensor fascia lata muscles, which tilts the pelvis forward and produces excessive lumbar lordosis. When the spasm is unilateral, a curve in the spine is produced. Full spine roentgenograms made while the patient is recumbent are often helpful in picking up early tendencies toward spinal deformities.

By the end of the first month, the patient ordinarily has full straight leg raising and spine flexion, and an accurate estimation of the paralysis has been obtained. The following muscle-grading system is usually used:

Muscle Rating	Definition
Zero	No palpable contraction
Trace	Palpable contraction but no movement of the part
Poor	Part moves through its range but not against gravity
Fair	Part moves through its range against gravity, but not against resistance
Good	Part moves through its range against gravity and against resistance
Normal	Normal

In general, a muscle rated "zero" cannot be expected to progress beyond a "poor" rating. A muscle needs to be rated "fair" in the early stage of the disease in order to develop to "good" or "normal" in most instances. The degree, not the extent, of the involvement is of some help in prognosis. Certain muscles have a marked tendency to be involved together—e.g., biceps femoris and gastrocnemius—and the clinical problem can often be predicted when the involvement of one is known.

The basic exercise rule is to exercise the muscle according to its rated grade. Exercising the muscle beneath its capabilities does not produce improvement except in endurance. In order to increase in power, the muscle must perform maximal work at each contraction. An increase in power is more helpful to the poliomyelitis patient at this stage of his disease than an increase in endurance. Repetitive exercises to increase endurance may be used at a late date. When the limb can be moved against gravity, progressive resistance exercises are added.

In general, bed rest is continued as long as something is to be gained from it. Residual sensitivity or tightness should be overcome before the patient is allowed up. Asymmetric tightness in the trunk should not be allowed to persist. Weakness of the trunk often calls for continued bed rest. The development of an extremely important muscle, such as the gastrocnemius, gluteus medius, or gluteus maximus, may deserve further attention before ambulation is permitted.

Except in nonparalytic cases, crutches are almost routine when ambulation is begun. Even in abortive cases, the child may have difficulty in raising the body weight with the gastrocnemius, and crutches and heel lifts help to procure the return of full function of the gastrocnemius within 2 weeks after the patient is allowed up.

Bracing is a means of preventing deformity and allowing greater activity than would otherwise be possible (Fig. 14.2). Many of these children can walk without braces but with severe tendencies toward deformity in their gait. A brace aids in the prevention of overstretching a muscle, which may result in regression rather than in an increase in the power of a muscle. The gastrocnemius is so important a muscle in a child's gait that it must be protected at all costs. The young

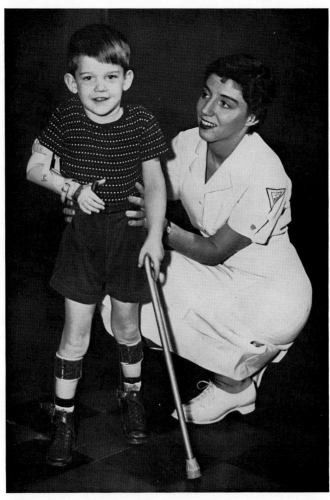

Figure 14.2. Bracing is a means of expanding the child's horizon, not of limiting it.

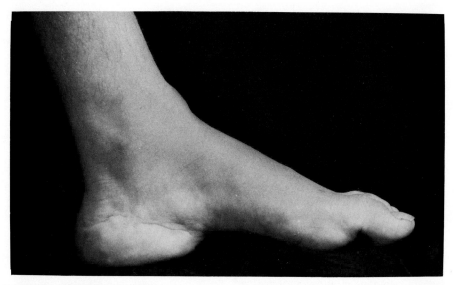

Figure 14.3. Calcaneous foot produced by attempting take off in the gait without gastrocnemius power.

child without the gastrocnemius walks with hyperextended knees and frequently needs a long leg brace. The older child can be taught to keep the knee flexed if sufficient muscle power is present.

A weak gastrocnemius must be prevented from allowing a calcaneus foot to develop (Fig. 14.3). The particular type of brace used varies from child to child according to the individual muscle picture.

Paralytic shoulders (weak deltoid), drop feet (weak anterior tibial), and knee weakness (weak quadriceps or hamstrings) are among other anomalies that must be improved by apparatus. A weak trunk must be braced according to the degree of involvement. Abdominals are particularly prone to being overstretched when the upright posture is resumed.

The pool is particularly useful in exercising patients with trunk and hip weakness, in handling large patients with extensive involvement, in stretching out resistant tightness, and in beginning ambulation in patients with minimal musculature.

So far as electrical stimulation is concerned, the present evidence indicates that in the initial phase of involvement, it temporarily slows the progress of atrophy. However, atrophy progresses nonetheless and eventually reaches the same degree in a stimulated muscle as in an unstimulated one that is similarly involved. Cessation of the stimula-

tion causes the atrophy to progress rapidly to the level expected. There seems to be no justification for its routine use, although it may be of some help in enabling the patient to find a muscle in cases of facial paralysis or virtually flail extremities, for example.

Chronic or Residual Poliomyelitis

At the end of the convalescent period of poliomyelitis, that is, 18 months after the onset, the patient enters a period that is dominated, for the physician, by three important aims: (1) to prevent deformity, (2) to increase muscle power, and (3) to reconstruct and substitute for paralysis.

Although no further recovery can be expected, the patient may improve in the performance of practical functional tasks.

CLINICAL DESCRIPTION

These patients have usually recovered from the initial mental depression of poliomyelitis. They enter the residual stage attempting to gain as much functional ability as possible. Except in the case of a completely flail extremity, they are left with muscle imbalance, which, alone and unprotected, is sufficient to cause deformity. To this imbalance may be added the tendencies toward deformity due to use and to gravity. Atrophy of the extremity is noted within 6 weeks of the onset. A markedly diminished circulation in childhood has an effect on growth. The patient up to this point has not been allowed to substitute muscles to gain function and has become well schooled in exercise routines. The economic factor, an important consideration in adults, is not important for children.

This stage may be attended by loss of function due to progressive deformity. Flaccid paralysis is sufficient disability, but its effects may be augmented by contracture. Gravity and function may stretch ligaments and joint capsules to the point that they no longer act as adequately functioning units.

BRACING

The brace is a means of allowing increased activity without increased deformity. It is not a means of limiting activity. Bracing should be as dynamic as possible. The following outline of its uses is greatly simplified.

Lower Extremities. The foot, if completely flail, must be supported on both sides, as well as anteriorly and posteriorly, by a double upright brace with stops to limit both dorsal and plantar flexion. Such a brace ordinarily allows 10 degrees of motion at the ankle as an aid in walking.

When the peroneal musculature alone is weak, a single upright brace placed on the medial side may be sufficient. An anterior T-strap is ordinarily added. This strap runs from the shoe to the lower tibia and upright. Lateral wedges may be used on the shoe. Stops are added when there is weakness anteroposteriorly. An anterior stop aids in preventing overstretching of the gastrocnemius. A posterior stop aids in preventing drop foot and overstretching of the anterior tibial.

Anterior or posterior tibial weakness is protected by a lateral single upright with an inner T-strap. Medial wedges on the shoe and a longitudinal arch pad are often necessary additions. Anterior or posterior stops or both may be necessary.

Different combinations of paralysis may demand double upright braces where, at first glance, a single upright may seem to be all that is necessary.

Knee. A "poor" or worse gastrocnemius may result in a tendency to hyperextend the knee despite good knee musculature. For children 6 years old and younger, a doubt in

regard to the necessity for a long leg brace should result in its use. Older children can be taught to protect their knees by walking in flexion.

Surprisingly, both strength of the quadriceps in the presence of weak hamstrings and weakness of the quadriceps may result in hyperextension at the knee. A brace to support the knee must of necessity be of double upright construction. The leather knee cap should not be so tight that it forces the knee into hyperextension. Knee braces have a number of ingenious locks designed to allow flexion when the child is sitting. The single so-called "drop lock" works well with children.

Hip. Gluteus medius and gluteus maximums limps are largely eliminated by the use

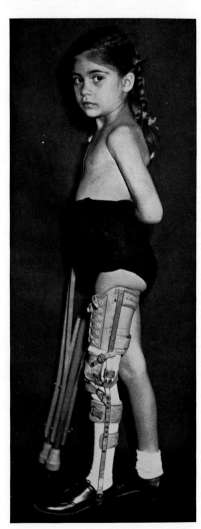

Figure 14.4. Long-leg brace for flail leg.

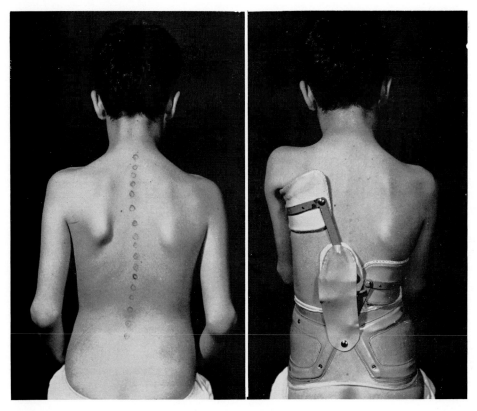

Figure 14.5. Barr-Buschenfeldt brace used to hold early paralytic scoliosis.

of crutches or canes. The hip weakness cannot be substituted for by a brace alone. When the hip is flail, it may be necessary to join a long leg brace to a trunk brace by means of a hinge.

Trunk. When abdominal weakness alone is present and is relatively symmetric, a corset may suffice. The corset should be laced from the bottom upward to support the abdominal contents properly. Lateral deviations of the spine may be held well by a brace of the Barr-Buschenfeldt type whose arms are appropriately placed to eliminate the deviation (Fig. 14.5). In general the lower arm supports the slump, and the upper arm corrects the curve. Check roentgenograms may be taken while the patient is held by supporting hands in the position of the arms of the brace. An x-ray film taken with the patient in the brace reveals a need for further adjustment, if there is one.

Neck. Asymmetric weakness of the sternocleidomastoids may call for holding braces of the Buchminster-Brown or collar type for a growing child. When the weakness is quite

general, braces built with chin cups and occipital supports and held by a pelvic band in the fashion of Blount's brace may be needed.

Upper Extremity. The shoulder joint is subject to gravity, and weakness of the deltoid may result in a tendency toward overstretching of the capsular structures. Support for the humerus may come from the trunk or from a sling anchored at the neck. Allowing a subluxation to develop renders a later reconstruction more difficult and eliminates all possibiity of improvement.

The flail elbow may be simply kept at a right angle by a sling or by a combination shoulder and elbow brace.

Hand bracing, which varies in method with each patient, attempts to encourage the position of function; it has been more fully described by Dr. Stelling in Chapter 17, "The Upper Extremity."

The child presents a different picture from that of the adult. In children, growth in length of bone relative to soft tissue is a factor in the production of severe contractures. A child may have to be supported for many years before the skeletal maturation of a joint is sufficient to permit an arthrodesis. Children wandering from supervision may, in a short time, develop more severe deformity than adults. The problems of rehabilitation, from the points of view of both surgery and vocation, are quite different.

PROGRESSIVE RESISTANCE EXERCISE

Exercises during the chronic stage of poliomyelitis may be aimed at development of hypertrophy. Progressive resistance exercises, as popularized by DeLorme and Watkins, are particularly valuable in this regard. The principle is that, to gain strength, the muscle must undergo a maximal contraction—that is, maximal in relation to the work load performed. Thus, if a muscle can life 5 lb against gravity, it should be exercised at this level until it can lift 6 lb. Repeated submaximal contractions may increase endurance, but not strength.

Because a heavy load increases the sensory response in a muscle, progressive resistance exercises aid also in isolating and strengthening transplanted muscle. DeLorme has advocated preoperative use of this type of exercise in order to isolate function. The problem of training the muscle in the new position is then greatly simplified. The first stage in educating a transplanted muscle is to achieve use of the muscle and to suppress the use of antagonists to it. The muscle must be repeatedly "set" until a powerful sustained contraction is reduced. The proprioceptive response aids in finding the muscle when some form of resistance is used. The motion of the part involved aids in suppressing the antagonist muscles. The synergists are then suppressed one by one until the transplanted muscle alone is left. Once it has been isolated in this manner, the muscle can progressively develop greater force with increasing resistance.

STRETCHING EXERCISES

These exercises are of greatest usefulness in combatting contractures which play an active role in the development of deformity. Many of these contractures are residual from the onset of the disease—when muscle spasm resulted in habitual positioning of joints. Myostatic contractures take place only in innervated muscle and are much more likely to be seen in partially involved than in completely flail extremities.

Fixed equinus of the foot due to anterior tibial weakness in the presence of a strong gastrocnemius is most common. Flexion contractures of the hip aided by a strong iliopsoas and a weak gluteus maximus are frequently unrecognized until they are well marked. This is particularly true of a flexion-abduction contracture in which the sartorius and tensor fascia lata enter as additional factors.

Contractures of the trunk that limit the lateral bend, forward flexion, or rotation may be factors in the development of trunk deformity.

Stretching type exercises must be performed in the correct position so that the joint proximal to that being moved is immobilized. The knee is extended when the Achilles tendon is stretched, for example. Correct use of stretching exercises requires a detailed knowledge of anatomy.

Stretching exercises accomplish their purpose when they are done to the maximum each day, rather than when they are repeated many times in a single day. Muscles like the hamstrings are particularly easy to stretch. Those about the pelvis with heavy fascia and short muscle bellies are particularly difficult.

FUNCTIONAL TRAINING

The simplest example of functional training is the teaching of a patient to negotiate stairs. It is obvious that the strong leg pulls the patient upstairs and steadies him as he advances downstairs. The difficulty of such a task is appreciated when the patient confronts it, however; and the bracing and muscle power that a patient has must be converted to use in the tasks of life. The simple act of getting out of a chair can be a very complicated thing when one is handicapped. The combining of crutches and the use of them as an aid rather than a hindrance can be quickly taught. Yet if he is left to his own devices, the patient may find it impossible to leave the chair with any facility. The necessity of arms, the use of the upper extremity to extend the trunk, and the locking of braces in turn become aids under guidance.

The practical problems that the patient has to face must be met and solved. These include eating, the use of the bathroom and stairs, entering and leaving public transportation,

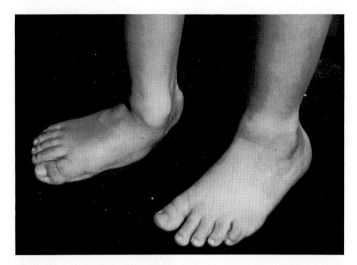

Figure 14.6. Peroneal strength and anterior and posterior tibial weakness leads to valgus deformity of the foot, as on the *left*.

and many others. One need not have expensive equipment to duplicate these tasks. Ingenuity and forethought bring the patient to the successful solution of these problems if they are met in some form in advance of activity.

RECONSTRUCTION OF PARALYTIC PATIENT

No operation of this type is justified unless it either (1) enables the patient to use less apparatus, (2) prevents progressive deformity, or (3) increases the patient's ability to perform. It is recognized that there are many alternative procedures to the one more or less standard procedure given here.

Unstable Foot. Various types of situations have to be met under this heading, because all possible ones cannot be covered specifically. In various borderline situations, individual judgment must determine treatment. Bone deformity must be corrected; the use of muscle transplant alone is of limited usefulness in the presence of deformity.

Peroneal strength, anterior and posterior tibial weakness, and good gastrocnemius— This situation results ordinarily in a valgus foot or a drop foot. Before the age of 10, the foot has been stabilized, from the skeletal point of view, by the subtalar bone block procedure of Grice.[5] A transplant alone in the presence of this deformity cannot pull the medial arch up against the body weight. In Grice's procedure, the subtalar joint is exposed. The os calcis is inverted beneath the astragalus, and a notched bed is made in the inferior surface of the astragalus and the superior surface of the os calcis, just distal to the posterior third of this joint.

The height of the bed is measured by compass. Two grafts from the proximal tibial cortex are then inserted exactly into this bed to block the ability of the os calcis to evert laterally. The grafts are wedge shaped and are of greatest height laterally.

A transplant of the peroneus longus is then performed. The peroneus longus tendon is divided just proximal to the os peronei. The peroneus brevis is detached from the base of the fifth metatarsal and sewn to the stump of the longus. A bed is then made for the insertion of the tendon in the base of the second metatarsal. (In some feet, a still more medial insertion may be indicated.) An insertion that has worked well is accomplished in the following manner. A drill hole sufficiently large to accept the tendon is created in the superior cortex, and two small drill holes are made just distal to it. A third incision is now made on the lateral calf. The peroneus longus is identified and then retracted into the proximal wound. A long incision is made into the anterior muscle compartment. A tendon passer is introduced into this compartment and is run beneath the deep fascia to the bed prepared in the base of the second metatarsal. Silk sewn into the peroneus longus is drawn

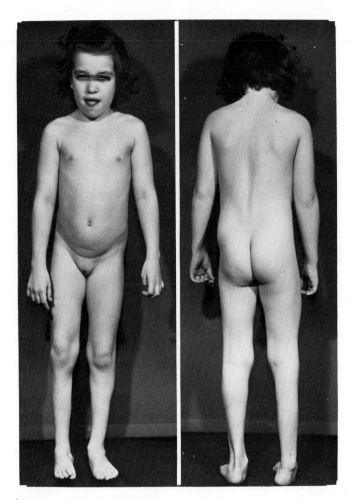

Figures 14.7 and 14.8. Inverted foot with poor gastrocnemius and good peroneal and anterior and posterior tibial power.

by the tendon passer down this route. If the procedure is done quickly and smoothly, the peroneus longus will lie flat without twisting.

With the use of a good tendon suture technique, the two ends of the thread (2-0) are individually passed out through the distal drill holes. The tendon is drawn down into the bone, and the thread is tied. The tendon should be taut when the foot is in maximal dorsiflexion and inversion. The patient is kept in a long leg plaster cast in the corrected position for 6 weeks and then in a bivalved cast in which the peroneal transplant can be exercised until it is working well. When bone union is demonstrated in the grafts, the patient begins weightbearing with crutches. When it can be established that the transplant is used in the gait (about 2 months later), the crutches are discarded.

For patients past the age of 10 whose feet have a fixed valgus deformity, a triple arthrodesis is indicated. In addition, however, the muscle balance of the foot must be restored by a peroneal transplant, or the deformity will probably recur.

A triple arthrodesis corrects bony deformity by the shape of the wedges removed and provides stability for the foot by fusing the midtarsal and subtalar joints.

A lateral incision over the sinus tarsi is made. The muscle belly of the short extensor to the toes is reflected from its origin on the os calcis. The long extensor tendons are retracted superiorly, and the peroneal tendons are retracted inferiorly. The fat filling the sinus tarsi is removed. The head of the astragalus, the astragalar surface of the navicular, and the cubocalcaneal and subtalar

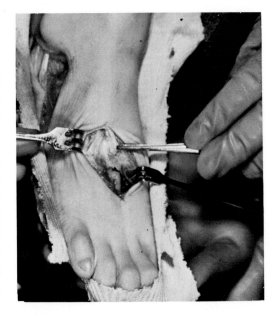

Figure 14.9. Peroneus longus muscle implanted into base of second metatarsal.

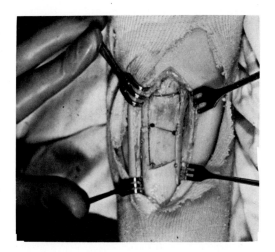

Figure 14.10. Subastragalar arthrodesis described by Grice. The tibial cortex is cut on a carefully measured triangle twice the height of block needed, and the center cut is angled so that grafts can be wedged into the subastragalar joint.

joints are exposed. The first osteotome cut is made in the astragalus in line with the coronal plane of the ankle joint without involving the bone further than is necessary to get in this plane. Navicular and cuboid joint surfaces are removed at right angles to the forefoot. The subtalar joint surfaces are removed, as-

tragalar surface parallel with the weight-bearing plane of the ankle joint, calcaneal surface with sufficient wedge to correct the hindfoot eversion. Inversion should not be produced as it will increase with weight bearing.

At the conclusion, joint surfaces should be flatly opposed. The tissues are repaired to eliminate dead space. The foot is held by the operator as a long leg plaster cast is applied. This cast is kept on for 6 weeks. When it is removed, roentgenograms are taken, and a short leg cast is applied if early fusion is apparent. The short leg cast is used for 2 weeks with crutches and a walking heel, then for 2 more weeks to stimulate maturation of the fusion. The cast is then removed, and partial weight bearing with crutches is begun.

When a transplant has been simultaneously done, the cast is bivalved at 6 weeks, and exercises for the transplant are done and continued, usually for a 4 to 6-week period, until maturation of the fusion is revealed by roentgenogram as well as by the action of the transplant. Partial weight bearing with crutches is then begun.

Anterior tibial absent, peroneals strong, posterior tibial strong, toe extensors strong— When the posterior tibial balances the everting pull of the peroneals, equinus of the forefoot may result in a cavus deformity. If it is done before fixed bony changes occur, a transplant of the extensor tendons into the metatarsal necks gives dorsiflexion.

Weak gastrocnemius, strong peroneal, and strong anterior and posterior tibial muscle

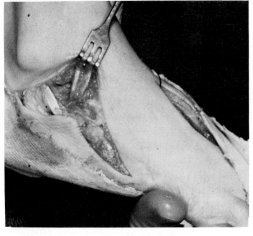

Figure 14.11. The tibial cortical grafts in place.

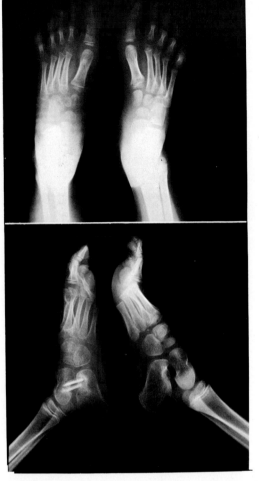

Figure 14.12. Postoperative roentgenogram of tibial cortical grafts blocking subastragalar joint into inversion.

power—Before the age of 14, the peroneal longus, posterior tibial, and long toe flexor may be moved and inserted into the posterior inferior angle of the os calcis. When there is no gastrocnemius power, such a transplant, although it does not give sufficient power to substitute for a brace, may prevent progression of a calcaneous deformity.

When there is some gastrocnemius power, such additions may be sufficient to substitute for a brace and to give a normal gait.

After the age of 14, an ankle fusion is preferable in the presence of a laterally stable foot.

An incision is made anteromedially and is carried down to the ankle joint between the long extensors of the toes and the anterior tibial tendons. A Hatt type of procedure is followed. The cartilage surfaces of the ankle joint are denuded and fitted together. A graft of tibial cortex is elevated from the anteromedial surface of the distal tibia. The most distal inch of tibial cortex is left intact as a bridge. A Hatt osteotome is inserted into the medullary cavity of the tibia and driven across the ankle joint and well into the astragalus. The bone graft is then driven down the track made by the osteotome. The foot is very carefully positioned as this is done so that the position determined as optimal preoperatively can be achieved and held by the graft. Ten degrees of equinus are usually necessary, but there may be some variety, depending on sex, type of heel worn, and other factors.

Knee. *Hyperextension deformity of knee* —This deformity quite frequently needs to be corrected. It results from the gait habit of locking the unstable knee by placing it in hyperextension. The procedure for correcting it is not done until growth is completed. A Steinmann pin or Kirschner wire is driven into the most proximal tibia. Force is applied to the pin as the tibia is divided distal to it. The proximal fragment is thus held in hyperextension as the distal fragment is lined up with the femur. This position is held as a plaster cast is applied.

Absent quadriceps; strong semimembranosus, semitendinosus, and biceps femoris—Not every patient who lacks a quadriceps needs muscle power anteriorly at the knee. Where a fundamental gain is possible, one or more of the hamstrings may be transplanted forward to the patella.

Hip. The most troublesome situation here is that of weak or absent gluteals with a strong hip flexor. The result is a tendency toward hip flexion contracture, which unleases a series of events that may result in a paralytic dislocation of the hip.

Barr found that anterior fasciotomy at the hip with reinforcement posteriorly did not prevent a recurrence of deformity. Such reinforcement is available in the erector spinae transplant of Ober.[10] It is insufficient to substitute for a gluteus maximus, but it can be used as a check to the development of a hip flexion contracture.

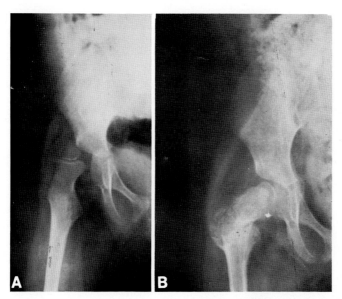

Figure 14.13. (A) The unstable hip in a patient with myelomengocele. (B) The same hip after a varus osteotomy to gain stability in the acetabulum.

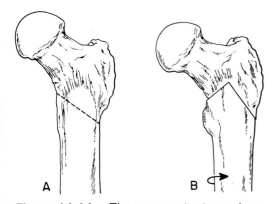

Figure 14.14. The varus osteotomy done in the intertrochanteric region with the hip internally rotated as in (A). In (B), as the distal fragment is rotated externally, the head and neck slide into varus.

In this procedure, after preliminary fasciotomy anteriorly, a second incision is made to detach the fascia lata at its insertion into the fibula. It is withdrawn and run from the insertion of the tensor fascia lata into it through a subperiosteal tunnel below the greater trochanter, posteriorly over the pelvis, through the substance of the gluteus maximus, to the erector spinae. The lower end of the erector spinae is fashioned into a cone in its lower segments, and the fascia lata is sewn around it while the hip is in an extended position.

Shoulder. Paralysis of the deltoid can be very well substituted for by fusion (Fig. 14.15). There are fundamental conditions to be met, however, before fusion can be considered. The muscles controlling the scapula must be rated "good" or better, and the hand and elbow must be functional. The situation of the other arm must be considered. The patient should be past age 12. The joint is usually denuded of cartilage, the surfaces are opposed, and the acromion is osteotomized and bent down to notch into the humerus.

The usual position is such that the hand reaches the mouth when the elbow is flexed. This usually means about 45 degrees of abduction, 15 degrees of forward flexion, and 15 degrees of internal rotation.

The postoperative shoulder spica is made preoperatively so that the position is accurate. The spica is removed and replaced after operation. The usual period of necessary immobilization is 4 months.

Elbow. Lack of elbow flexion must be overcome to restore useful function to the upper extremity. It is fairly common to have good forearm flexors with weak or absent biceps. If the hand has function, a Steindler transplant may be performed (Figs. 14.16–14.18).

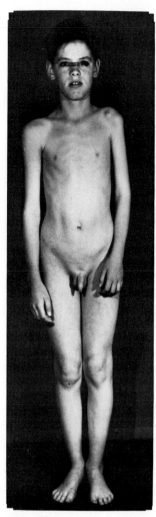

Here the common flexor tendon is isolated at its origin from the medial epicondyle and transplanted approximately 1½ inches proximally up the shaft of the humerus. This improves the lever action across the elbow joint so that the hand can be elevated against gravity and against some resistance.

References

1. Bouman, H. D., and Schwartz, R. P.: The degree, the extent and the mechanism of muscle spasm in infantile paralysis, *N. Y. J. Med,* 44:147, 1944.
2. Colonna, P.: Hamstring transplantation for quadriceps paralysis, *J. Bone Joint Surg,* 5:472, 1923.
3. Ghormley, R. K.: History of the treatment of poliomyelitis, *J. Iowa Med. Soc,* 37:343, 1947.
4. Green, W. T.: Diagnostic and therapeutic considerations in anterior poliomyelitis, *R. I. Med. J,* 28:89, 1945.
5. Grice, D. S.: Further experience with extra-articular arthrodesis of the subtalar joint, *J. Bone Joint Surg,* 37A:246, 1955.
6. Johnson, R. W.: Results of modern methods of treatment of poliomyelitis, *J. Bone Joint Surg,* 27:223, 1945.
7. Jones, R.: On arthrodesis and tendon transplantation, *Br. Med. J.,* March 28, 1908.
8. Legg, A. T., and Merrill, J. B.: *Physical Therapy in Infantile Paralysis,* Hagerstown, Md.: W. F. Prior, 1932.
9. Lovett, R. W.: *The Treatment of Infantile Paralysis;* Philadelphia: Blakiston, 1916.
10. Ober, F. R.: Tendon transplantation in the lower extremity, *N. Engl. J. Med,* 209:52, 1933.
11. Peabody, C. W.: Tendon transplantation—an end-result study, *J. Bone Joint Surg,* 20:193, 1938.
12. Sabin, A. B.: Pathology and pathogenesis in human poliomyelitis, *J.A.M.A,* 120:506, 1938.
13. Steindler, A.: *The Rehabilitation of the Paralyzed Patient;* New York: Appleton-Century-Crofts, 1925.
14. Yount, C. C.: The role of the tensor fascia femoris in certain deformities of the lower extremities, *J. Bone Joint Surg,* 8:171, 1926.

Figure 14.15. Functional hand and elbow with flail deltoid but good scapular muscles—a candidate for fusion.

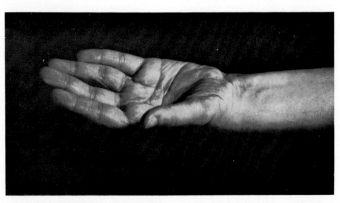

Figure 14.16. Muscle transplant—in this case, the fourth sublimus tendon to the metacarpal and first phalanx of the thumb.

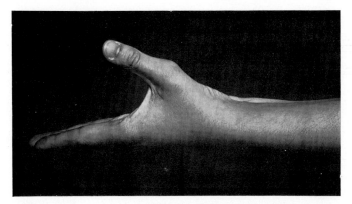

Figure 14.17. Muscle transplant provides motor power.

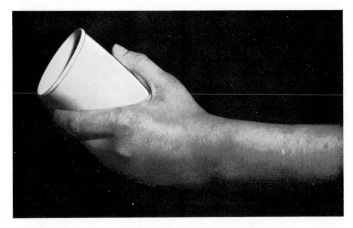

Figure 14.18. Muscle transplant increases function.

PROGRESSIVE MUSCULAR ATROPHY OF THE PERONEAL TYPE (PERONEAL ATROPHY, CHARCOT-MARIE-TOOTH DISEASE)

BY PIERCE E. SCRANTON, JR., M.D.

Charcot-Marie-Tooth disease, or peroneal muscle atrophy, was first described in 1886. The disease has been defined as a neurologic disorder, and it ultimately affects the muscles of the upper and lower extremities to varying degrees. Much of what is known about this heredofamilial disease has come from the classic descriptions by Charcot and Marie in France[4] and, independently but concurrently, by Tooth in England.

Since 1886, many authors have made considerable progress in defining the various features of this disease. Mixed pictures among neuromuscular disorders, both clinically and pathologically, have made this task quite difficult. Lucas and Forester concluded that "Charcot-Marie-Tooth disease, spinocerebellar ataxias, and possibly muscular dystrophy are variants of a common hereditary predisposition to neuromuscular degeneration." Thus, these disease entities have been classified under three broad categories. The primary myopathies fall under the heading "muscular dystrophies." There are also spinal-muscular atrophies, and peroneal muscular atrophy falls into the general classification of "neurogenic muscular atrophy."

Clinical Picture

The age of onset of clinical manifestations for patients with Charcot-Marie-Tooth disease may vary widely. Few cases have been diagnosed before the age of 2 years. When the disease occurs at such an early age, the diagnosis is most likely made on the pes equinovarus and claw toe deformities and further aided by the fact that a positive family history already exists.

Charcot-Marie-Tooth disease is essentially a neurologic process with secondary involvement of muscle through degeneration of peripheral nerves and their corresponding motor units. This ultimately leads to neurogenic (denervation) atrophy of skeletal muscles. The disease affects primarily the muscles of the extremities, with truncal sparing. The first physical sign is usually a mild equinovarus deformity of the feet, secondary to weak peroneals. There may also be early clawing of the toes. The ultimate appearance of the foot consists of a severe cavoequinovarus deformity (Fig. 14.19). However, because muscular involvement progresses insidiously, the patient is usually unaware of the initial findings. Involvement is symmetric, continuing in a centripetal direction, at times to include all muscles of the lower leg and most muscles of the thigh, occasionally in a radicular pattern. Especially involved are the muscles below the middle one-third of the thigh, producing the classic "stork leg" or "inverted champagne bottle." The involvement of the lower limbs usually precedes that of the upper limbs, but a similar progression will occur there as well. Upper extremity involvement is heralded by atrophy and weakness of the intrinsic hand muscles and later the forearm muscles. There is usually sparing of the shoulder muscles. As in the feet, a mild claw deformity may develop in the hands to produce the so-called "monkey fist."

The patient's first complaint may be the inability to keep up with peers in physical activities, or problems in the fitting of shoes. Physical findings may vary, depending upon the point in the disease's course when the physician is consulted. One may see fasciculations along involved muscles, and there may be paresthesia and pain in the limbs. Vibratory sensation has also been reported as being depressed or absent early in the dis-

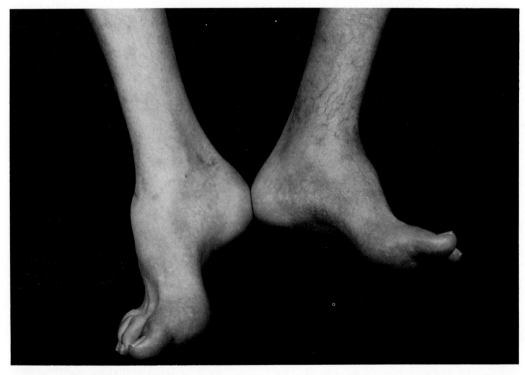

Figure 14.19. Cavus feet often develop in patients with Charcot-Marie-Tooth disease. Varus of the heel, forefoot equinus, and claw toes distinguish this deformity.

ease, although these findings are infrequent. More commonly, the sensory examination is normal. Muscle weakness is often found and usually coincides with the amount of atrophy in the muscle being tested. Considerable muscle wasting may be present before total debility supervenes.

Inheritance

Charcot-Marie-Tooth disease has heredofamilial inheritance and, according to some authors, has multiple patterns of transmission. Allan[1] proposed that the disease was due to unit traits that are transmitted by a single defective gene. He described a triple pattern of inheritance: (1) simple recessive, (2) sex-linked recessive, and (3) autosomal dominant. According to Allan, for those with the simple recessive inheritance, the disease becomes manifest in the first decade, and afflicted patients evidence severe involvement by the second decade. In this case, the patient has inherited double recessive genes of the disease trait; hence, there is no normal counterpart on the chromosome to ameliorate the disease effects. Those with a sex-linked recessive inheritance pattern begin to show the disease in the middle of the second decade. They, too, progress to the point of being severely handicapped. In this inheritance pattern, males receive one defective gene from the mother (X chromosome), who does not have clinical manifestations of the disease. Because there is no corresponding normal gene from the father, the disease is fairly severe. The third type of inheritance is a dominant pattern, in which the penetrance is variable, but disease effects generally become evident in the third decade. In this instance, the atrophy is moderate, and the patient can usually continue to work into old age.

Irrespective of the pattern of inheritance, these patients by and large have a normal life expectancy. Schwartz reported on a "mixed" family whose average age at death for those involved was 60 years, whereas the unaffected members had an average death age of 47. This finding could not be explained by the author, as the disease has certainly not been known to bestow longevity. More commonly, the age at the time of death does not seem to be significantly different between the afflicted and nonafflicted.

Neurophysiology

A fairly extensive study of nerve conduction velocity was carried out by Dyck, Lambert, and Mulder.[9] Conduction characteristics of the median, ulnar, and peroneal nerves of 103 patients with Charcot-Marie-Tooth disease were studied, measuring latency, amplitude, and duration of muscle action potential. Latency was defined as being less than 47 m/second in the ulnar nerve, 45 for the median, and 40 m/second for the peroneal nerve. According to their criteria, latency of response was abnormal if it exceeded 4 msec for the ulnar nerve, 4.7 msec for the median, and 7 msec for the peroneal nerve for patients over 5 years of age. In this study, all patients with a confirmed diagnosis of Charcot-Marie-Tooth disease had abnormal conduction time and exhibited latency of response. Another group with a diagnosis based purely on clinical grounds had low conduction velocities in all nerves tested. There were also several young children who had not manifested the disease clinically but had low conduction times. Therefore, conduction velocities can be a valuable adjunct to identifying the latent carrier.

Treatment

The management of patients with this disease is multidisciplinary. The geneticist, neurologist, neuropathologist, and orthopaedist may each be involved in some aspect of diagnosis and treatment. Genetic determination of the pattern of inheritance, and ultimately genetic counseling, is extremely important. We believe that all patients initially seen and diagnosed should be referred to determine the inheritance pattern. Thus, the more severe or progressive forms of Charcot-Marie-Tooth disease may be delineated and treatment based upon the predicted course of the disease.

For these patients, the operative management has been mainly addressed to the ankles and feet. Significant intrinsic atrophy in the hands has been observed in patients who presented with disabling feet, but this was not regarded by these patients as a significant problem. When evaluating a progressive foot deformity, the family history makes it possible to regard each patient's deformity in the light of the pattern of disease progression for that family. Thus, for those patients with recessive, sex-linked, or severe penetrance, autosomal dominant patterns of inheritance, it can be predicted that there will be a rapid progression of deformity. Therefore, a definitive triple arthrodesis should be performed at an appropriate age. In children from families with mild penetrance who present with early cavus deformity, but with other older family members without severe disability, a Dwyer calcaneal osteotomy with or without tendon transfers or plantar fascia release may be entirely satisfactory. However, most patients treated have been from families evidencing rapid progression of deformity, and here triple arthrodesis is the treatment of choice.

When considering a Dwyer calcaneal osteotomy, it is important to act before there is fixed forefoot deformity. Thus, this osteotomy is generally more successful as a definitive procedure only when hindfoot varus is the predominant deformity. If lateral displacement of the posterior calcaneus is resisted by the plantar fascia, this should also be released. Generally, a satisfactorily performed Dwyer will obviate the need for toe procedures such as flexors-into-extensors. As the years pass, there will be a recurrence of the hindfoot deformity, and a second Dwyer or triple arthrodesis may be necessary. Once there is satisfactory recovery from the Dwyer, the patient's gait should be carefully followed (biannually) to determine whether weakness is developing in the anterior tibialis and is noticeable during the swing phase of gait. Weakening of this muscle usually occurs before the posterior tibialis (as in muscular dystrophy), and this imbalance will predispose to the development of forefoot equinus and a drop foot gait. Early recognition of this problem and treatment by a posterior tibial tendon transfer will assist in the prevention of progressive deformity and the maintenance of normal gait.

There are those children who will present with both a varus hindfoot and a weak anterior tibialis. The Dwyer osteotomy and posterior tibial tendon transfer should be performed separately, in that order, with several months allowed for recovery from the initial Dwyer.

A Hoke type triple arthrodesis will be satisfactory in providing permanent correction for severe, fixed deformity. It should be performed after the age of 12, and the osteotomy cuts may be planned to correct the cavoequinovarus deformity in such a way that the drop foot is corrected as well (see Chapter 4).

References

1. Allan, W.: Relation of hereditary pattern to clinical severity as illustrated by peroneal atrophy, Arch. Intern. Med., 63: 1123, 1939.
2. Brodal, A., Boyesen, S., and Frovig, A.: Progressive neuropathic (peroneal) muscular atrophy (Charcot-Marie-Tooth disease): histological findings in muscle biopsy specimens in fourteen cases, with notes on clinical diagnosis and familial occurrence, Arch. Neurol. Psychiatry, 70: 1, 1953.
3. Brody, I., and Wilkins, R.: Charcot-Marie-Tooth disease, Arch. Neurol., 17: 552, 1967.
4. Charcot, J., and Marie, P.: Sur une forme particuliere d'atrophie musculaire progressive souvent familiale dubutant par les pieds et les jambes et atteignant plus tart les mains, Rev. Med., 6: 97, 1886.
5. Christie, B.: Electrodiagnostic features of Charcot-Marie-Tooth disease, Proc. R. Soc. Med., 54: 321, 1961.
6. Dawson, C., and Roberts, J.: Charcot-Marie-Tooth disease, J. A. M. A., 188: 659, 1964.
7. Drachman, D., Murphy, S., Nigam, M., and Hills, J.: Myopathic changes in chronically denervated muscle, Arch. Neurol., 16: 14, 1967.
8. Ducan, J., and Lovel, W.: Hoke triple arthrodesis, J. Bone Joint Surg., 60A: 795, 1978.
9. Dyck, P., Lambert, E., and Mulder, T.: Charcot-Marie-Tooth disease; nerve conduction and clinical studies of a large kinship, Neurology, 13: 1, 1963.
10. Dyck, P. J., Ellefson, R., Lois, A., Smith, R., Taylor, W., and Von Dyke, R.: Histologic and lipid studies of sural nerves in inherited hypertrophic neuropathy; preliminary report of a lipid abnormality in nerve and liver in Dejerine-Sottas disease, Mayo Clin. Proc., 45: 280, 1970.
11. Earl, W., and Johnson, E.: Motor nerve conduction velocity in Charcot-Marie-Tooth disease, Arch Phys. Med. Rehabil., 44: 247, 1963.
12. England, A., and Denny-Brown, D.: Severe sensory and trophic disorders in peroneal muscular atrophy, Arch. Neurol. Psychiatry, 67: 11, 1952.
13. Haase, G., and Shy, G.: Pathological changes in muscle biopsies from patients with peroneal muscular atrophy, Brain, 83: 631, 1960.
14. Herringham, W.: Muscular atrophy of the peroneal type affecting many members of a family, Brain, 11: 230, 1884.
15. Hoyt, W.: Charcot-Marie-Tooth disease with primary optic atrophy, Arch. Ophthalmol., 64: 145, 1960.
16. Jacobs, J., and Carr, C.: Progressive muscular atrophy of the peroneal type (Charcot-Marie-Tooth disease), J. Bone Joint Surg., 32A: 27, 1950.
17. Low, P., McLeod, J. C., and Prineas, J.: Hypertrophic Charcot-Marie-Tooth disease; light and electron microscopic studies of the sural nerve, J. Neurol. Sci., 35: 93, 1978.
18. Lucas, G., and Forester, F.: Charcot-Marie-Tooth

disease with associated myopathy, *Neurology, 12:* 629, 1962.

19. Washington, R., Scranton, P., and Martinez, J.: Charcot-Marie-Tooth disease; clinical presentation, histopathology, and treatment, *Orthop. Surv., 2:* 314, 1979.

PARAPLEGIA IN CHILDHOOD

The most frequent causes of paraplegia in childhood are congenital. But whether the paraplegia is congenital or acquired, severe deforming forces are at work and may be expected to cause progression until growth ceases. Excessive lumbar lordosis, kyphoscoliosis, and fixed pelvic obliquity all act to affect the deformities present in the lower extremities. Kilfoyle, Foley, and Norton[1] have studied the natural history of these spine and pelvic deformities. Patients with acquired paraplegia have their lesion principally at L1 level and above into the dorsal spine, usually with complete paralysis. In congenital lesions the principal site of involvement is the lumbar spine with patchy loss of sensation and motor power.

The spinal deformities may be divided into the following:

Lordosis. The development of increased lordosis occurs in almost all of these children. It may be low, ending at the third lumbar vertebra, or high, extending through the lumbar spine into the lower dorsal segments.

The development of lordosis is favored by the frequent finding of innervation of the iliopsoas and loss of the gluteus maximus due to its sacral innervation—a more distal level more likely to be involved is with congenital etiologies. In addition, the natural tendency of the child with paraplegia to stand with a forward inclination of the trunk when using crutches in order to maintain balance favors lordosis development. In order to become erect the lordosis must be increased, and, if the child is going to be balanced as defined by Kilfoyle et al.,[1] the kyphosis above it must bring the center of gravity of the trunk over the feet. Crutches are needed if off balance, and the deformity of one area of the spine may be so great when not compensated by an anteroposterior curve either above or below it that standing even with crutches is impossible.

Lateral curvature of the spine may be added to the lordosis or kypkosis; and, again,

if unbalanced, may progress to the point of inability to sit without external support.

Balance would mean level shoulder and pelvis with occiput centered over the first sacral body.

Lordosis primarily affects walking, and scoliosis affects the ability to sit.

Pelvic Obliquity. The accurate determination of pelvic obliquity in terms of the area causing it to be fixed is an exercise in physical diagnosis. A fixed abduction deformity at the hip can be appreciated by performing a Thomas test—stabilizing the opposite side by full flexion. Full abduction of the involved hip is then necessary to eliminate the tendency of the limb to go into flexion if an abduction contracture is present. The abduction or adduction component at the hip can be further evaluated by bringing both hips into a position in which the pelvis is at right angles to the spine; this may result in considerable displacement of the limbs to either side. Inability to get the pelvis to neutral by this maneuver speaks for a contracture above the pelvis. Further evaluation can be made by pulling the limb downward against the quadratus lumborum and erector spinae musculature above.

With poliomyelitis, infrequent fixed pelvic obliquity is principally caused by paralysis and chronic posture associated with spina bifida syndromes.

Collapsing Spine. The collapsing flaccid spine is principally seen in high thoracic levels of paralysis and has been designated as a "rope spine" by Kilfoyle et al.[1] It is a clear-cut indication for spine fixation before deformity that is fixed develops.

Kyphosis. Increasing kyphosis can involve the lumbar spine and culminate in a jackknifed position of the spine, making it impossible for the patient to stand without support. The sitting posture tends to be supported by the upper extremities as the center of gravity is thrown forward. In dorsal hemivertebra the vertebrae above and below may converge in front of the hemivertebra to form an extreme deformity for which there seems to be no treatment.

Treatment

Treatment is based on a careful assessment of the forces producing the deformity and a

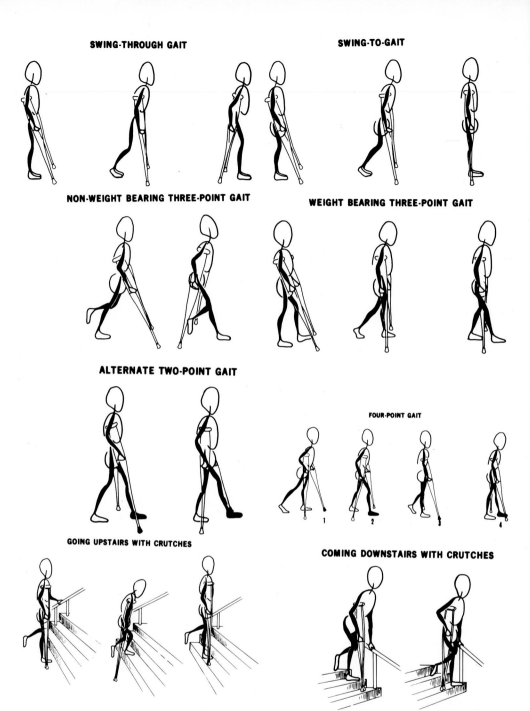

SWING-THROUGH GAIT

SWING-TO-GAIT

NON-WEIGHT BEARING THREE-POINT GAIT

WEIGHT BEARING THREE-POINT GAIT

ALTERNATE TWO-POINT GAIT

FOUR-POINT GAIT

1   2   3   4

GOING UPSTAIRS WITH CRUTCHES

COMING DOWNSTAIRS WITH CRUTCHES

Figure 14.20. Diagrammatic representation of the various crutch gaits. The swing-through gait is a rapid means of ambulation fondly used by children once the arms are built up to their use. The legs progress ahead of the crutches. The swing-to gait brings them even with the crutches. The non-weight-bearing, three-point gait requires a flexed knee of the involved leg and is difficult over distances. If the foot can touch down, the involved leg can go through the usual gait motions and requires less energy. In the alternate two-point gait, the crutch on the same side is brought forward with the leg and repeated on the alternate side. The four-point gait is a good stable gait, easier, but slower, and requiring a rhythmic cadence. On going upstairs with crutches the good leg leads to pull the patient upstairs; on going down the good leg remains on the step behind to let the patient down.

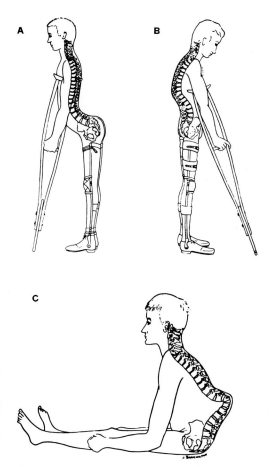

The attention is to the spine before the hips, because hip position cannot be maintained if the spine cannot be controlled. Spine fusion is used early in preventing excessive kyphosis, lordosis, and scoliosis.

Sectioning of adductors, transplant of the iliopsoas, and adductor tendon division are all necessary in controlling the pelvis if deforming contracture exists. When correcting hip flexion contractures, the opposite hip must be held in a flexed position in plaster to stabilize the pelvis while the correction is being obtained or the result will be disappointing.

The usual orthopaedic procedures are used as indicated to stabilize the lower extremity at the ankle, foot, and knee. Harrington instrumentation seems to have a place in the treatment of some of the severe lordotic deformities, but it is not fully established as yet. Spine fusion accompanying the correction frequently must include the sacrum.

Reference

1. Kilfoyle, R. M., Foley, J. J., and Norton, P. L.: Spine and pelvic deformity in childhood and adolescent paraplegia, *J. Bone Joint Surg.*, 47A: 659, 1965.

NEUROFIBROMATOSIS

Manifestations of neurofibromatosis are seen in childhood as the cause of some difficult and bizarre orthopaedic problems. Café au lait spots and skeletal and joint changes are an entity in a variety of conditions (Fig. 14.22).

Von Recklinghausen in 1882 originally described the relationship between peripheral nerves and the subcutaneous nodules which are typical of the disease in the adult. The advanced form of the disease he described has been supplemented by childhood manifestations in which tumors of the skin and subcutaneous tissue are seldom evident visually but may be palpable. The incidence has been variously calculated at between 1 in 2,500 and 1 in 3,300 of the general population.

Clinical Picture

The pigmentation and skin nodules of the adult are a serious cosmetic problem. In

Figure 14.21. (*A*) Strong iliopsoas and weak glutei result in increasing forward tilt of the pelvis and secondary lordosis. (*B*) Balance must be achieved by getting head and shoulders over the pelvis. To enable the patient to get the pelvis tilted back up to this position, surgery may be necessary. (*C*) Increasing kyphosis in the lumbar spine may result in "jack-knifing" of the spine and the necessity to support the sitting posture with the upper extremity. (From R. M. Kilfoyle, J. J. Foley, and P. L. Norton: Spine and pelvic deformity in childhood and adolescent paraplegia, *Journal of Bone and Joint Surgery*, 47A: 659, 1965.)

recognition of the inevitable further progression if active forces in a growing child cannot be held by bracing, training, and careful attention to sitting and crutch-walking posture. The child's whole day must be laid out with attention to the posture used in performing all functions.

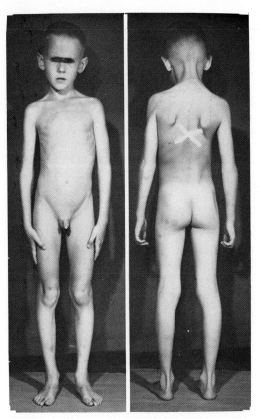

Figure 14.22. Patient with neurofibromatosis involving spine. There are a mild structural scoliosis of the dorsal spine and café au lait spots of skin pigmentation.

childhood the cutaneous manifestation consists of café au lait pigmentation and occurs in 80% of the cases. Still more threatening manifestations of the disease include a rapidly progressive scoliosis. Tumors extending from the spinal canal into the major body cavities may undergo sarcomatous change with a grave prognosis.

Soft-tissue involvement of an extremity is a cause of massive enlargement through lymphatic and vascular proliferation. It tends to be unilateral.

The skeletal changes include scoliosis and a very stubborn type nonunion in the tibia but that may also occur in such other bones as the clavicle and radius.

Recognition

The macules of neurofibromatosis are tan in color with smooth margins (coast of Cali-

fornia) as compared to the irregular (coast of Maine) configuration seen in Albright's disease. Although an occasional spot is seen in normal persons (20% of 100 student nurses), their presence in any number and their grouping in skeletally involved areas is significant. The café au lait spot immediately raises clinical suspicion. The development of tumors and pigmentation increases with puberty.

Tumors with central nervous system involvement tend to occur in 20% of the persons without the café au lait spots. Cranial nerves with optic glioma and widening of the optic formamen are found. Acoustic neuromas involving the eighth nerve occur. According to the study of Gardner and Frazier, 84% of bilateral nerve neuromas occurred in patients with neurofibromatosis.

The neurofibromas occur both centrally and peripherally and show malignant degeneration in 5–15% of recorded series.

There is an element of mental retardation. In Borberg's series of 71 patients, 85% had low normal or moron intelligence levels.

Peripherally the tumors are of three types: (1) those resulting in a "fibroma molluscum" subcutaneous lesion, (2) discrete lesions along the course of peripheral nerves, and (3) the plexiform neuroma associated with hamartomatous overgrowth resulting in local giantism. The plexiform neuroma may result in a large pedunculated mass, a "pachydermatocele."

Skeletal Lesions

About 50% of patients with this disease have at least some x-ray evidence of skeletal involvement. Erosions or scalloping along the ribs are the most common. When the neurofibroma is adjacent to the cortex of a long bone, a saucer-like depression will occur in the cortex. The thinning of the cortex in this area will give a cystlike impression when the x-ray is taken at right angles to it. Periosteal new bone may form about the lesion. The edges are smooth—metaphysis or diaphysis could be involved. When the lesion occurs at the point of exit of spinal or cranial nerves, the opening is smoothly eroded. The spinal nerve lesion thins the pedicles and enlarges the neural foramen.

SCOLIOSIS

The incidence of scoliosis has been reported as from 5–17%.

Scott[10] (1965) studied the scoliosis of neurofibromatosis and found no uniform length or direction of curves and no association with the number of café au lait spots or with tumors. Of 33 patients with scoliosis, 9 had gradual "C"-shaped curves, i.e., ≤30 degrees; the other 24 had curves ≥30 degrees, mostly thoracic and thoracolumbar. He noted the similarity of these acute curves with those of "progressive infantile idiopathic scoliosis."

The point to be made is that, although the severe angular curve with twisted ribbon ribs and erosions is pathognomonic of neurofibromatosis, often these findings are not present. Often the curve is indistinguishable from idiopathic scoliosis.

The x-rays of 18 patients seen here at Children's Hospital since 1957 confirm the findings of Scott. A third of these scoliosis lesions are not the "characteristic" type, with short, sharp, angular curves.

NONUNION

The nonunion of the tibia associated with neurofibromatosis is associated with bowing of the tibia and a thin, waving fibula. Congenital nonunion of the tibia can occur for several reasons, including fibrous dysplasia. The occurrence of nonunion in patients with neurofibromatosis is a real clinical fact, although actual demonstration of the neurofibroma has been rare. Green and Rudo[3] reported a case, and we have seen one adult with nonunion of the radius and gross clinical neurofibromatosis. The entity was described by Cucroquet in 1937. The nonunion is characteristic in that there is progressive narrowing and sclerosis of the tibia (pencilling) toward the nonunion site with obliteration of the marrow cavity. In Meszaros' 11 cases of pseudarthrosis, 9 had neurofibromatosis. The clavicle is a fairly common site in addition to the tibia.

Skeletal overgrowth occurs with gigantism and with marked involvement of the soft tissues of a limb.

ORBITAL DEFECTS

Orbital defects were first reported as part of the syndrome by LeWald in 1933. Hunt and Pugh found the defect in 7% of a series of 192 patients.

The defect involves the posterior wall of the orbit. It may be due to erosion, but more often no neurofibroma is found and dysplasia must be evoked. Usually the greater and lesser wings of the sphenoid and the orbital part of the frontal bone are absent. Pulsating exophthalmos results because of the direct contact of the temporal lobe with the orbital soft tissues.

OVERGROWTH

Asymmetric disorders of bone growth can be due to neurofibromatosis. Brooks and Lehman reported shortening of bones of the lower extremity secondary to invasion of the epiphyseal plate by neurofibroma. Several investigators, including Holt[4] (1948), found only increased bone length, presumably secondary to increased blood supply. According to Meszaros, the altered bone growth is found most often in association with plexiform neuroma and local gigantism.

In localized areas of hypertrophy, café au lait spots, palpable nodules, enlargement of the part, and erythema are all seen. If such a process involves an entire leg, it gives rise to a picture very much like that of elephantiasis. In a growing child it produces great inequality of leg length and overgrowth of the affected side.

Sarcoma

Sarcomas associated with the disease are often found contiguous with other neurofibromatous tissue. Such sarcomas are difficult to excise as they ramify through and around major nerve plexuses and appear usually as a neurofibrosarcoma under the microscope. Bone cysts in localized subperiosteal areas have been described. The treatment of these various lesions is highly individualized, and the general principles have been described elsewhere.

A large mass occurring in the chest or abdominal cavity identified as neurofibromasarcoma carries with it a dire prognosis in our experience. A fatal outcome may be expected due to the inability to excise the lesion.

References

1. Aegarter, E. E.: Possible relationship of neurofibromatosis, congenital psyeudarthrosis, and fibrous dysplasia, *J. Bone Joint Surg.*, 32A: 618, 1950.
2. Benedict, M.: Melanotic macules in Albrights and Von Recklinghausen, *J. A. M. A.*, 205: 618, 1968.
3. Green, W. T., and Rudo, N.: Pseudarthrosis and neurofibromatosis, *Arch. Surg.*, 46: 639, 1943.
4. Holt, R.: Radiologic features of neurofibromatosis, *Radiology*, 51: 647, 1948.
5. Hunt, E., and Pugh, D.: Skeletal lesions in neurofibromatosis, *Radiology*, 76: 1, 1961.
6. Laws, S.: Spinal deformities in neurofibromatosis, *J. Bone Joint Surg.*, 45B: 675, 1963.
7. Levin, M.: Neurofibromatosis—clinical and x-ray manifestation, *Radiology*, 71: 48, 1963.
8. McCarroll, H. R.: Clinical manifestations of congenital neurofibromatosis, *J. Bone Joint Surg.*, 32A: 601, 1950.
9. Moore, B. H.: Some orthopaedic relationships of neurofibromatosis, *J. Bone Joint Surg.*, 23: 109, 1941.
10. Scott, J.: Scoliosis and neurofibromatosis, *J. Bone Joint Surg.*, 47B: 240, 1965.

RADIAL NERVE PARALYSIS ASSOCIATED WITH FRACTURES OF HUMERUS

Approximately 20% of radial nerve paralyses following fractures of the humerus occur in children. In virtually all cases, the trauma has been severe. Virtually all fractures are located in the middle or lower third of the humerus, and the severe injury with marked displacement and angulation or comminution appears more important than whether it is spiral, oblique, or transverse. However, the medial angulation of the proximal portion of the distal fragment is significant. The outlook can be very optimistic when the paralysis is partial, and it is the usual rule for full recovery to occur in those patients whose paralysis occurred when the humerus was fractured. The onset of spontaneous recovery usually occurs by 2 weeks. The time required for full recovery varies from 3 days to 8 months, the average being 4 months. Two-thirds of the patients with complete paralysis will regain full nerve function spontaneously.

In all the patients with partial paralysis, recovery begins within 2 months, so that lack of spontaneous recovery or evidence of beginning spontaneous recovery at 2 months justifies exploration.

The findings at exploration may include divided nerves, large neuromas in continuity with partial involvement of the nerve, small neuromas, and contusions of the nerve. Neurolysis alone of the nerve is not associated with a good prognosis; and, although approximately 25–30% will evince some recovery, many will not. If the nerve is really crushed at the time of exploration and recovery not evident 7–8 weeks after operation, a resection of the neuroma and resuture should be performed. If the paralysis follows open reduction of the humeral fracture, prognosis is also excellent, the average time for full recovery being approximately 3 months for partial paralysis and 8 months for complete paralysis. In this instance, should recovery be delayed, neurolysis would be of some help.

CONGENITAL INDIFFERENCE TO PAIN

Children are seen in pediatric clinics who early on develop swelling about the epiphyses due to repeated trauma, but who are not subject to abuse. Underlying the problem is a neurologic deficit centering about a congenital indifference to pain. The condition is

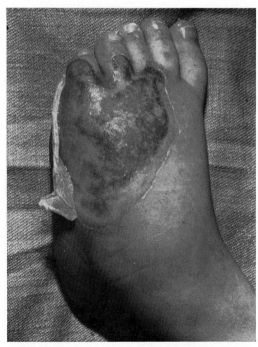

Figure 14.23. Thermal injury to foot with diminished sensation secondary to myelomeningocele.

rare and may be confused with rickets, as bowing of unrecognized fractures may take place along with the epiphyseal swelling evidence on clinical examination. The children are otherwise normal.

The complicating features that might be expected are burns (Fig. 14.23) and bruises, trauma to the eye, and biting of the fingers, tongue, or lips as the teeth appear. When subject to repeated trauma, the joints develop synovial thickening and laxity of the ligaments secondary to chronic hemarthroses. As in hemophilia, aseptic necrosis of the femoral head can occur.

As the age of the patient progresses the trauma to weight-bearing joints, particularly the ankle, may lead to dissolution and a picture of a Charcot neuropathic joint. The appearance of such a joint in a child without obvious neurologic deficit, such as that due to myelodysplasia, should arouse suspicion of congenital pain indifference.

The peripheral and central nervous system is otherwise intact except for the failure to respond to pain. The peripheral nerves should be demonstrated as being intact by electromyographic and nerve conduction studies.

There are other syndromes (all very rare) which may be thought of in connection with this syndrome, including the Riley-Day syndrome (familial dysautonomia). These children are of Jewish ancestry and tend to be mentally and emotionally operating at a below normal level. There is no lacrimation at birth. There is excessive sweating and temperature control abnormalities.

There is a lack of fungiform papillae on the tongue, and the normal reflex to histamines of the cornea and axion is absent.

In congenital sensory neuropathy all modalities of reaction to light touch, pain, and temperature change are affected. Conduction is absent over sensory cutaneous nerves, although the motor nerve conduction is normal. It may be inherited as a dominant trait.

Obviously recognition of the underlying defect in these children is of prime importance in saving them from marked disability secondary to unrecognized trauma. With recognition and maturity, the incidence of repeated difficulty diminishes. Bracing of the neuropathic joints is necessary.

References

1. Abell, J. M., Jr., and Hayes, J. T.: Charcot knee due to congenital insensitivity to pain, *J. Bone Joint Surg.*, *46A:* 1287, 1964.
2. Denny-Brown, D.: Hereditary sensory radicular neuropathy, *J. Neurol. Neurosurg. Psychiatry*, 14: 237, 1951.
3. Dimon, J. H., Funk, F. J., Jr., and Wells, R. E.: Congenital indifference to pain with associated orthopaedic abnormalities, *South. Med. J.*, *58:* 524, 1965.
4. Johnson, J. T. H.: Neuropathic fractures and joint injuries, *J. Bone Joint Surg.*, *49A:* 1, 1967.
5. Mooney, V., and Mankin, H.: A case of congenital insensitivity to pain with neuropathic arthropathy, *Arthritis Rheum.*, *9:* 820, 1966.
6. Riley, C. M., Day, R. L., Greely, D. M., and Lanceford, W. S.: Central autonomic dysfunction with defective lacrimation, *Pediatrics*, *3:* 468, 1949.

CHAPTER 15

Myelomeningocele

DAVID H. BAHNSON, M.D.

The actual birth of the child with myelomeningocele defect is a deceptively innocent event. Usually unheralded by any prenatal abnormalities, the labor and delivery may be quite normal. The face and upper torso of the child may be completely normal, and he may interact with his environment in a seemingly natural and typical manner. The parents have little reason to suspect the immensity of the problems that lie ahead, and they are usually overwhelmed enough with the culmination of the gestation period and the birth itself that realistic understanding of the magnitude of their problem is impossible.

The aftermath of such a birth is a disastrous problem. From the day of birth, the child born with myelomeningocele begins a course in life that will never be normal. Opportunities for the development of normal motor milestones will be hampered, social environment will be awkward and unnatural, and the child will draw into its future a seemingly endless association with a variety of doctors, nurses, therapists, social workers, orthotists, and many other care specialists. Even with the best of care and the most up-to-date facilities, the survivors of this condition will experience multisystem handicaps that seldom remain static, even though the neurologic deficit is not progressive.

In the past, many of these children died of complications relating to meningitis, ventriculitis, hydrocephalus, sepsis, renal failure, and other causes. Many others were institutionalized with massive hydrocephalus and crippling deformities. Today, with improved treatment techniques, the population of surviving patients has increased dramatically, and we are faced with an expanding dilemma of priorities. Ethical and financial considerations come to play a significant role in determining treatment plans, and as physicians we are caught in a balance between optimal care for the patient and optimal responsibility to society. Neither can be neglected.

TERMINOLOGY

The use of overlapping terms has caused considerable confusion of terminology in describing various spinal abnormalities. Common usage has assigned a somewhat different meaning to what initially were synonymous terms.

Spinal dysraphism is a broad term implying literally "defective seam" and, according to Lichtenstein,[34] includes a variety of embryonic ectodermal, mesodermal, and neuroectodermal defects, as well as neural dysplasia resulting from nonfusion of the dural layer. Some neurosurgeons prefer to exclude myelomeningocele and its variants from this terminology and reserve the term "spinal dysraphism" for congenital defects such as diastematomyelia, dermal sinus, intradural lipoma, tethered cord, and other closed lesions. It implies a lesion that is less obvious and results in insidious neurologic progression with growth.

Spina bifida is also a very broad term implying failure of fusion of the vertebral arches. It is further subdivided to spina bifida aperta (open) and spina bifida occulta (covered). *Spina bifida*, then, may be used to include myelomeningocele, simple meningocele, rachischisis, etc.

Meningocele is a form of spina bifida in which the lesion contains a herniated sac covered by meninges but does not contain neural elements. These are relatively rare, but are more common in the cervical spine than in the thoracic or lumbar region.

In *myelomingocele* the exposed meninges contain neural elements including distended nerve roots but, also, a portion of the spinal cord which is usually present as a neural plaque (Figs. 15.1 *A–C* and 15.2). Because of the distention of these neural elements, there is usually little or no function distal to the level of lesion.

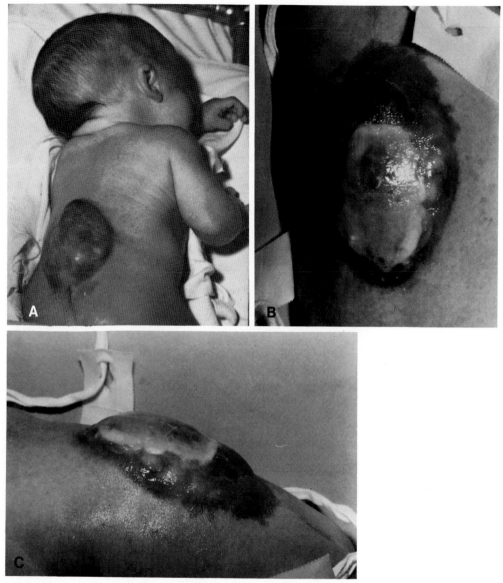

Figure 15.1. (*A*) Typical myelomeningocele involving the lumbar region. (*B* and *C*) Neural plaque covered with meninges.

Rachischisis, although technically synonymous with myelomeningocele, has come to imply a more extensively involved defect in which there is complete absence of the skin and sac so that uncovered neural and sometimes osseous elements are exposed.

Finally, *myelodysplasia* indicates disease associated with the spinal cord; although bony abnormalities may be present (such as in myelomeningocele), the overlying vertebral structures may be completely normal.

Clinical usage of this term places appropriate emphasis on the neurologic loss associated with a broad variety of pathology of the spinal cord.

EMBRYOLOGY

Mechanism of formation of the myelomeningocele defect is unknown but seems to be the result of two possible etiologies. This includes (1) failure of the neural tube closure or (2) rupture of the already formed neural tube.[5] The latter hypothesis is well supported and is useful in its application to such other related defects as diastematomyelia, syringomyelia, and spina bifida occulta.[5] The debate, however, is by no means resolved.

Further evidence exists that the condition arises quite early, perhaps before the fetus is 30 days old,[12] and that it may be influenced by a number of environmental as well as genetic factors, including geographic location, socioeconomic status, and others.[32, 49, 54, 69] Although a definite genetic influence has been established, more than 90% of all pregnancies with neural tube defects occur in families with no preceding affected members.[20]

In addition to the myelomeningocele defect itself, other abnormalities may be present. Important in this respect is the frequent occurrence of hydrocephalus (80% or higher) often associated with the Cleland-Arnold-Chiari malformation. Although some degree of hydrocephalus may be present at birth, brain atrophy is usually not present at this point.[12] Therefore, early ventriculoperitoneal shunting is essential in preventing progressive central nervous system deterioration due to hydrocephalus, and many children shunted early have normal intelligence.

Other congenital defects include congenital bony vertebral anomalies (hemivertebrae, diastematomyelia, unilateral unsegmented bars, etc.) and anomalies of the kidney and urinary collecting system. Severe congenital anomalies, such as limb deficiencies and car-

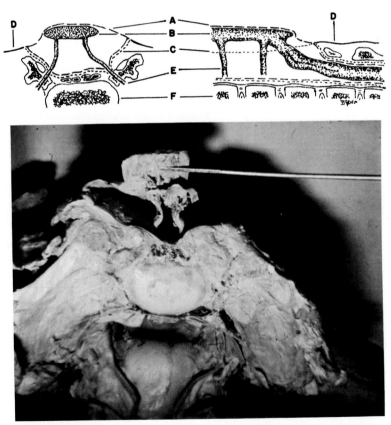

Figure 15.2. (*Top*) Schematic transverse and logitudinal views of myelomeningocele. (*A*) Arachnoid, (*B*) dysplastic cord, (*C*) dura, (*D*) skin, (*E*) peripheral roots, (*F*) vertebral body. (*Bottom*) Gross appearance of lumbosacral myelomeningocele in 2-month-old infant.

diac anomalies, might be considered as relative contraindications to initial treatment. Certainly the presence of spinal anomalies should alert one to look closely for other associated anomalies.

NATURAL HISTORY AND ETHICAL CONSIDERATIONS

The majority of patients with open spinal defects who are not treated at all will die within several months, with the more severe dying within hours of birth. Nontreatment may be defined as absence of *all* medicines (including topical or systemic antibiotics), withholding of any surgical procedure, and feeding orally by demand only. A representative series[41] suggests that 63% die by 1 month of age and 89% before 6 months. Other series[23, 29, 31, 32, 39, 42] support the contention that more than 90% and in some series 100% will not survive if untreated. The survivors in these groups of untreated individuals tend to be simple meningoceles or low level myelomeningoceles, and many are reported as being continent and without evidence of hydrocephalus, supporting the theory that untreated survival tends to be a function of lesser involvement.[30] In the few survivors who represent more severe involvement, it is highly speculative to assume that aggressive early intervention would have markedly improved the eventual functional outcome of the child.

In short, the likelihood of a severely involved patient surviving completely without treatment is small, whereas lesser involvement may be compatible with life even when completely neglected. In some cases "partial" treatment (e.g., intravenous antibiotics without closure and without shunting) has resulted in survivors with a multitude of problems compatible with life, but not compatible with a meaningful existence. Total neglect, with all its ethical considerations, may have been a more suitable alternative.

To put into perspective the outcome of untreated patients, we must compare and evaluate the outcome of the aggressively treated patients. An analysis of 524 unselected patients described by Lorber in 1971[41] sheds light on this issue. Based on evaluation of results of aggressive treatment available

during that time period (1959–1968), he concluded that:

1. Overall survival was 41%.
2. Only 7% of children treated were considered to have physical and mental capabilities consistent with self-respect, independent earning capacity, and eventual independence.
3. Of the survivors, 66% had an IQ less than 80.
4. Thirty-one per cent were confined to wheelchairs.
5. Selection criteria would be useful to determine maximal effective use of resources in treating this population.

It should be pointed out here that improved treatment techniques available today would probably modify survival rate and functional results, so that a direct application of his data to current treatment is not entirely valid. However, it should also be recognized that the oldest patient in his series was 12 years of age and complete understanding of results should include longer periods of follow-up. Recent investigators[3, 4, 24, 25] have noted a "peak" functional capacity attained in the childhood and early adolescent years that later diminishes toward adulthood. This will be discussed more fully later.

The work by Lorber, as well as subsequent studies by others, makes us question our own effectiveness in treating this condition, particularly when evaluating long term results. It also emphasizes the magnitude of the obstacles to be overcome.

An interesting insight with respect to selection criteria for treatment is provided by Freeston.[15] He interviewed parents of children treated for spina bifida and found that less than half of them had heard about spina bifida before the birth of their child, and of those who had heard of it, very few had any idea of how it would affect the child. Four years following the birth of the child, only one-fifth of these parents felt that severely handicapped people should be encouraged to live regardless of the condition. Those who advocated allowing the child to die felt that survival was unfair from the child's point of view, not with respect to burdening the parents.

If we are to improve upon the results of children treated for spina bifida, we must consider two important approaches. The first is improved methods of treatment, and the second is selection of patients as candidates for treatment. The first of these has been accomplished and is constantly being refined, but, as Lorber has pointed out, improved techniques did not lead to fewer, but to more, handicapped children because of the higher survival rate of the more severely affected infants. This led him to propose the following selection criteria for treatment: (1) Severe paraplegia (hip flexors and adductors, or less); (2) gross enlargement of the head (2 cm above the ninetieth percentile); (3) kyphosis; (4) associated gross congenital anomalies or major birth injuries.

These criteria were designed to apply to decision making at the time of birth or shortly thereafter but were also to be reconsidered at any time a life-threatening condition existed. Several other considerations have been suggested subsequently by other authors that need to be mentioned. These include lacunar skull defects,[65] professional and financial resources, infection, mental development, and social factors (e.g., illegitimacy).

Although not absolute in any sense, these factors should be kept in mind when formulating selection criteria as well as treatment protocols.

Perhaps the only satisfactory management of this disorder lies in prevention of its occurrence. Amniocentesis for alpha fetal protein during the second trimester, when positive, has an extremely high correlation with neural tube defects. This is useful in determining the condition in utero, but it is not a useful screening procedure. Recent techniques of obtaining *serum* alpha fetal protein determination during the sixteenth and seventeenth weeks could identify risk pregnancies in which amniocentesis would be indicated.[20] Therefore, this may be a useful clinical screening method of prenatal detection. This would provide some time for parental understanding of the conditions, but it still carries the ethical consideration with respect to termination of the pregnancy.

TREATMENT

General Principles

In many centers, the orthopaedist is seldom called upon to participate in the initial treatment geared toward survival of the infant. Nonetheless, he should have an understanding of the issues involved in the total treatment plan. He should be prepared to make decisions based on sound judgment and knowledge of facts and experience of others, because this will provide a means of formulating a practical and realistic set of objectives in treating what has been referred to by Bunch[5] as "the most complex treatable congenital anomaly of the central nervous system consistent with life."

Once the patient has been considered a candidate for treatment, using whatever criteria are appropriate for a particular treatment center, every effort should be made on the basis of available resources to establish a long range goal of independence for that child. This is not a simple task. Any objective evaluation of long term survivors of this condition will emphasize that to a large extent we are currently unsuccessful in this respect. Yet there are varying degrees of independence, and ultimate functional level is related to the child's ability to interact physically and socially with a minimal amount of assistance from others. Even though we do not often achieve the goal of total independence, we should continue to direct our efforts toward it. Abandonment of this goal at an early age is associated with the worst survivors of this condition.

Achieving independence has many facets from the multidisciplinary point of view, and treatment protocols must interfere with each other as little as possible. Several considerations should be briefly mentioned.

The pediatrician usually initiates the management in general and helps serve as a coordinator of the other disciplines in the total treatment plan. He frequently will be involved in the early decision of treatment versus nontreatment and may be called upon to participate in the difficult task of educating the parents as to what lies ahead. His role in establishing reasonable parental expectations and understanding is essential. Later this role may be taken over by a clinic coordinator (often a pediatrician as well) when the child's care is centered in a multidisciplinary clinic.

The neurosurgeon, in addition to providing a careful neurologic evaluation of function and anticipated level of involvement, may have an important role in the treatment decision. If treatment is "feasible," prompt closure of the spinal defect and coverage with muscle, fascia, and skin provides the best resistance against infection, although it probably does not improve neurologic function. Delayed closure (several days) of an unsterile sac results in a high incidence of meningitis. The neurosurgeon must also evaluate for the presence or absence of hydrocephalus, treat accordingly with shunting procedures when indicated, and observe closely after closure for the development of "delayed" hydrocephalus or shunt malfunction. The technique of closure using flank relaxing incisions[19] provides excellent immediate coverage over the spinal defect, having the advantage of providing durability in this region for future spine bracing, although it also may involve split-thickness coverage near the area of future pelvic band placement.

The urologist must manage neurogenic bladder dysfunction, with all efforts directed toward preservation of renal function while providing as sterile a urinary tract as possible plus a socially acceptable means of urine control. This latter involves Credé's maneuver (suprapubic massage), intermittent catheterization, or surgical urinary diversion techniques. The latter is being used much less commonly now because of a higher incidence of pyelonephritis in long term follow-up, and intermittent self-catheterization is used most often in our clinic. Renal failure as a cause of death in these individuals is a much less common occurrence with improved urologic management.

Perhaps equally as important as the physician speciality care mentioned above is the complex ancillary care provided by the nurse specialist, physical therapist, occupational therapist, orthotist, social worker, and many others. These personnel, in addition to providing much essential care directly, are often capable of providing to the physician information that is otherwise unavailable or difficult to extract. Their value in rehabilitation of the child cannot be overstated. Local assistance agencies, such as the Spina Bifida Association, can be extremely helpful as well. A team approach is mandatory.

At this point mention should be made of the parents of these children. Many physicians and others do not appreciate the intense emotional and psychological complex involvement that these parents may have with their children. Spawned by elements of guilt, misunderstanding, and uncertainty at the time of birth, they may respond to imminent helplessness of the child by taking tremendous burdens upon themselves at a time when rejection of the child and delegation of responsibility to others seem more intuitively "appropriate." This dependent relationship must be dealt with carefully. Obvious efforts on the part of the physician to interfere with this relationship will be met with distrust and anger. On the other hand, the goal of independence for the child must continuously be kept in mind. The only way to deal with the family is in a direct, honest fashion with realistic principles in mind and realistic expectations at hand.

ORTHOPAEDIC MANAGEMENT

The orthopaedist must attempt to minimize the myelomeningocele child's inability to meet normal motor milestones necessary to provide an environment consistent with intellectual, emotional, and social development. When possible he must provide mobility for the child, even though he realizes that ultimately, for some children, this mobility may be lost or substantially reduced.

For purposes of analyzing functional levels of ambulation, the classification provided by Hoffer et al.[24] is most often used. This provides four functional categories.

1. *Community ambulators*—Able to walk indoors or outdoors for most activities, wheelchairs used only for long trips out of the community.

2. *Household ambulators*—Able to walk indoors and transfer. Wheelchair use within the community and often for indoor activities.

3. *Nonfunctional ambulators*—Can walk as part of therapy sessions, but use their wheelchair for most transportation needs.

4. *Nonambulators*—Wheelchair bound.

Structural deficiencies, such as scoliosis, dislocated hips, contractures, etc., may interfere with the patient's ability to attain functional levels. The orthopaedist should correct the problems as they relate to each individual patient's needs or projected needs. This means that similar problems may have totally different methods of management in patients with different levels of involvement.

Although many factors (such as intelligence, motivation, home environment, etc.)

are involved, the most consistent and perhaps most significant factor in determining ultimate functional level is the level of neurologic lesion itself—that is, the root level or levels at which useful neurologic function is disrupted. Treatment methods, therefore, must account for difference in anticipated levels. For example, dislocated hips in the thoracic level paraplegic may be better left untreated. The same condition in the low lumbar level patient may have markedly adverse effects unless treated aggressively.

Therefore, long and short term goals must be considered with the level of involvement in formulating the practical approach to management of the many orthopaedic problems that are likely to arise. Treatment of the spine, hips, and feet is to be considered in light of their status and effects on walking, standing, sitting, and fitting in braces. Progressive spinal deformity may be a major determinant in deterioration of sitting and standing ability. In addition, some forms of spinal deformity may have marked effects on cardiopulmonary function. All anticipated problems must be considered in the treatment plan of these severely affected children.

Several general principles and concepts must be kept in mind at all times:

1. The neurologic level is usually determined by the lowest functioning motor root level. This delineation is not absolute by any means, and "spotty" innervation of lower levels is quite common. Also, the presence of activity at a motor level does not mean normal strength for that muscle group, so that lowest functioning motor levels should normally include only those muscles with good or normal voluntary strength, even though others *may* cause deformity.

2. Sensory levels do not seem to be reliable when predicting corresponding motor behavior, but they are extremely important in bracing considerations.

3. Neurologic "level" is seldom 100% symmetric, and variations of 1 or 2 root levels (or more) between left and right sides are not at all uncommon (Fig. 15.3).

4. Hydrocephalus, meningitis, neonatal hypoxia, spinal cord (versus root) compression of higher levels, and other upper motor neuronal conditions may introduce an element of spasticity, with corresponding propensity of particular muscle groups to exert a more substantial deforming force.

5. Neurogenic deformity predictably passes through three phases. They are: (1) Passively correctible deformity without contractures; (2) fixed deformity with soft-tissue contracture but no bony change; and (3) fixed deformity with secondary bony change. The implications of this are obvious. The earlier such deformity is corrected, or preferably *prevented*, the easier it is to maintain normal anatomic relationships with a minimal amount of surgery. This usually implies early surgical intervention in the presence of predictable progressive deformity.

6. *A joint deformity caused by a neurologic imbalance cannot be permanently corrected or prevented without altering the muscle imbalance in some way to achieve balance of power across the joint.* This basic concept cannot be overemphasized. Soft-tissue or bony procedures that attempt to correct neurogenic deformity without correcting or altering muscle forces are likely to fail. Serial casting, stretching exercises, and even surgical measures done in the face of neurologic imbalance should be viewed as a temporary form of treatment only.

SPECIFIC TREATMENT CONSIDERATIONS

The following discussion presents some of the many factors to be considered in planning a therapeutic approach to the myelomeningocele orthopaedic problems. The reader is referred to the literature for more detailed discussion of specific problems, as well as descriptions of surgical technique. Although the neurologic level may not be as precise as is often implied, it is useful to plan the treatment based on approximate motor level, with analysis of functioning motors for each particular child. Many options exist, many existing forms of treatment need more time for objective analysis of therapeutic results, and protocols for treatment are in constant revision. The following discussion will relate to levels of involvement; it is arbitrarily divided into thoracic (T12 and above), upper lumbar (L1-2-3), lower lumbar (L4-5), and sacral levels of involvement. Sharrard[59] has provided a table of muscle innervation corresponding to specific lower limb root levels (Fig. 15.5).

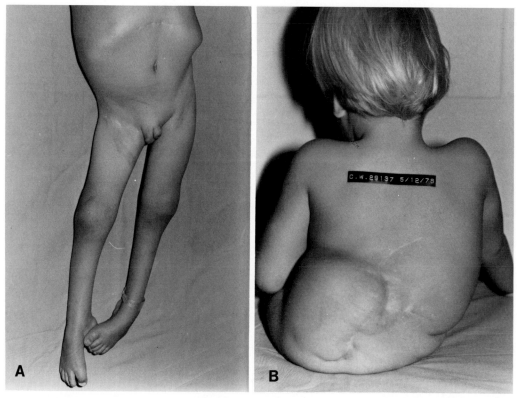

Figure 15.3. Asymmetric neurologic involvement of the lower extremities may result in "windswept" deformity (*A*), which may accentuate difficulty in sitting secondary to pelvic obliquity.

Thoracic Level

These children are severely involved and, as pointed out earlier, present with adverse criteria for selection as defined by Lorber. Complete paraplegia requires bracing to include pelvic support for standing and ambulation with swing-to gait. With present treatment, virtually all of these children ultimately will lose their ambulatory function—in their teens or sooner.

SPINE

At this level 100% of the patients will develop some degree of spinal deformity manifested by kyphosis, scoliosis, thoracic lordosis, and varying combinations of all of these. Compensatory *thoracic* lordosis above the fixed kyphus in the low thoracic level may become structural and progressive, and it is a significant factor in reducing cardiopulmonary function by narrowing the antero-

posterior diameter of the chest. Developmental spinal deformity may be markedly aggravated by a unilateral dislocated hip or other fixed infrapelvic obliquity. It should be kept in mind that when spinal fusion is required, it must be performed to the sacrum, thereby losing some flexion-extension mobility ordinarily used in sitting. This may influence consideration and treatment of the hips, when treatment may cause loss of hip mobility.

HIPS

At this level the hips are flaccid (Fig. 15.7), and gravity is the main deforming force, so that hips tend to assume a position of abduction, external rotation, and some degree of flexion. A hip maintained in the reduced position by splints or other methods is anticipated to remain stable as further development progresses, because there is no deforming force tending to dislocate the hip.

If unilateral dislocation is present, this should be treated early with splinting and other closed methods if possible.[43, 44] This may include abducting both hips in the first few weeks of life while the child is prone for care of the neurosurgical closure. The main consideration of a unilateral dislocated hip should be to prevent secondary spinal deformity relating to infrapelvic obliquity.

If bilateral dislocations are present and cannot be reduced early with minimal difficulty, strong consideration should be given to allowing them to remain dislocated. These hips tend to be pain free, have a range of motion consistent with both sitting and standing, and do not seem to influence pelvic obliquity to the degree a unilateral disloca-

tion does. The postoperative stiffness often associated with surgical procedures at this level is a significant disability for a minimal gain, that gain often being only a radiographically acceptable position. Pressure sores that develop in the presence of a stiff hip may be markedly aggravated by fusion of the spine to the sacrum at a later age.

Therefore, the goal of therapy is to maintain hip motion and a level pelvis, with a conscientious effort to avoid overtreatment.

KNEE

This joint is also flaccid, and deformity can usually be corrected by passive stretching with a goal toward maintenance of full exten-

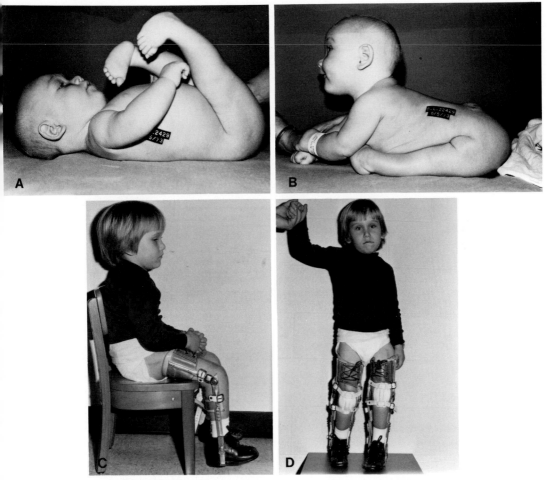

Figure 15.4.   Treatment of the infant should be directed toward realization of maximum ultimate potential. This patient with upper lumbar level of involvement is ambulatory in long leg braces and is able to sit comfortably.

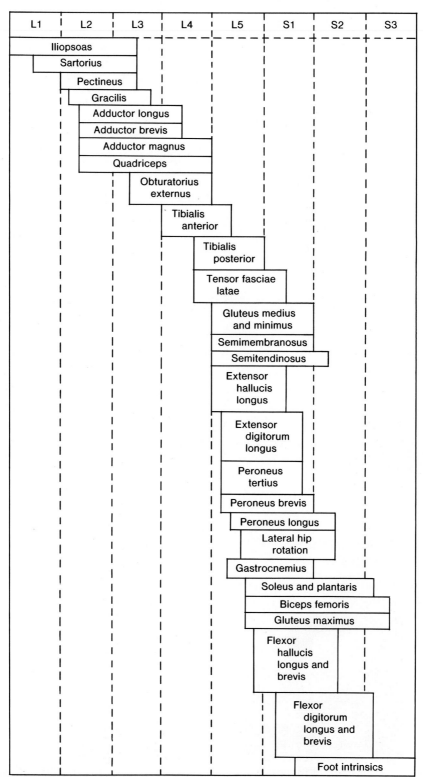

Figure 15.5. Root innervation of muscles of the lower limb. (From W. J. Sharrard: Posterior iliopsoas transplanting in the treatment of paralytic dislocation of the hip, *Journal of Bone and Joint Surgery, 46B:* 426, 1964.)

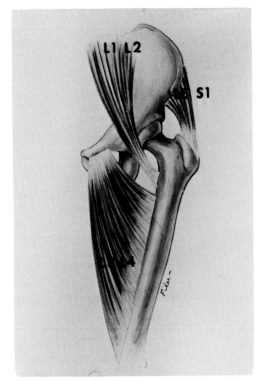

Figure 15.6. Innervation of muscles about the normal hip.

sion and 90 degrees of flexion to permit standing and sitting while in braces. Angular deformities of more than 20 degrees may present significant difficulties in fitting of braces. Femoral osteotomy can be performed if necessary, but stiffness and propensity to pathologic fractures secondary to immobilization must be anticipated. Early postoperative weight bearing in casts or braces and early mobilization of the extremities can minimize these adverse effects. With growth, valgus deformity may result secondary to static tightness of the iliotibial band and may be treated by a Yount[70] type fasciotomy.

FEET (Fig. 15.10)

The foot and ankle also will be flaccid with no protective sensation present. A plantigrade foot capable of bracing without breakdown of skin is the desirable result and the goal of treatment. Early cast correction with meticulous care to avoid damage to the insensate skin when deformities are present is the treatment of choice, and recurrent deformity based on neuromuscular imbalance

is not predicted. In the rigid and more severe deformities, soft-tissue release may be necessary, but frequently a talectomy[45] provides satisfactory long term correction. Recurrent deformity in flaccid feet should make one suspicious of neuromuscular imbalance, and not infrequently this will be of the reflex arc, nonvoluntary type of control. Also, one should be alert to the presence of paralytic vertical talus in the myelomeningocele population.[11]

Upper Lumbar Level

This neurologic level is characterized by the presence of strong hip flexors and in midlumbar levels by adductors and some knee extensors. When these latter muscle groups are strong, it is considered in the lower lumbar (L4 or lower) level. Ultimate ambulatory ability is quite variable and less predictable than in either thoracic or sacral level. The knees and feet must be braced, usually with pelvic attachment to achieve standing ability and control rotation.

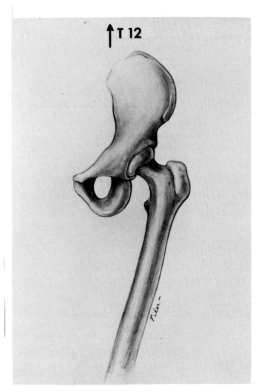

Figure 15.7. At level of T12, the hip is flail.

SPINE

There is a relatively high propensity for spinal deformity, although it may be more gradual or less severe than in the thoracic levels. The iliopsoas, in addition to producing a deforming force at the hip, has the effect of producing or exaggerating lumbar lordosis. As in the thoracic level, spine fusion to the sacrum may be required, reducing the mobility in flexion and extension at the pelvis necessary for sitting.

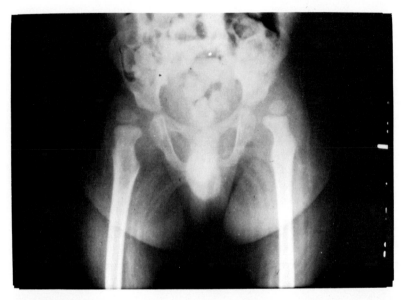

Figure 15.8. Anteroposterior roentgenogram of the pelvis showing irreducible neurogenic dislocated hips without skeletal adaptation. Note normal appearing acetabuli.

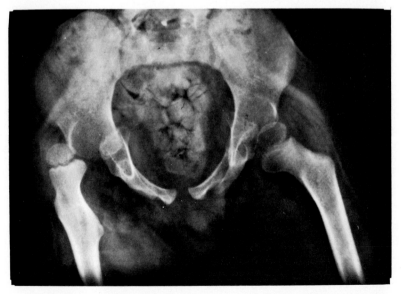

Figure 15.9. Anteroposterior roentgenogram of the pelvis showing neurogenic dislocated hips with skeletal adaptation. Note shallow acetabuli and formation of false acetabuli superiorly.

HIPS

At the high level lesion the iliopsoas and sartorius combine to provide flexion and external rotation (Fig. 15.11), but the tendency to dislocate is not nearly as great as in lower levels where adductors are strong. Pelvic obliquity may play a major role in dislocation, with the hip dislocating on the "high side" despite sometimes rather aggressive efforts to keep it located. Partial resection of the iliopsoas at its insertion or transfer to the anterior capsule is preferable to lateral transfer to the greater trochanter in this level of involvement. It should be remembered that isolated hip flexion in the absence of other hip motors is probably not a useful function.

Abduction splinting should be started early. Flexion and abduction contractures should be allowed to occur to some extent, with care taken to prevent adduction contracture of either hip. This should allow physiologic development of the acetabulum. Release of the hip flexors and adductors may be

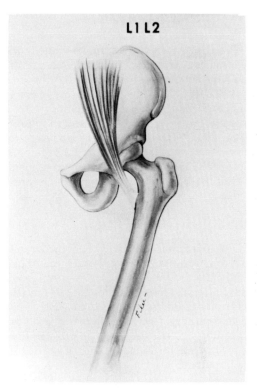

Figure 15.11. Innervation of muscles about the hip in the patient denervated below L1 or L2.

performed surgically before 12–18 months through a medial approach.[14] This regimen should provide located and mobile hips that permit standing in braces by age 18 months.

KNEE

Weak knee extension may be present but can be offset by functioning sartorius and gracilis unless the sartorius become a perverted extensor by displacement of the axis anterior to the femoral condyle. Passive stretching of the knee to achieve a 90-degree arc of motion usually allows for sufficient range to permit bracing. Surgical measures include sartorius release, quadriceps lengthening (V-Y plasty), femoral osteotomy, or iliotibial tract resection.

FEET

At this level there are still no functioning motors in the foot, and treatment is similar to that discussed for the thoracic level.

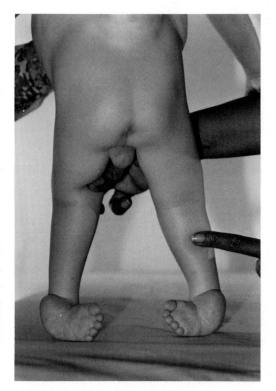

Figure 15.10. Severe equinovarus foot deformities in a thoracic level myelomeningocele.

Lower Lumbar Level

The presence of voluntary functional quadriceps "or better" defines this group, and a recent review has implicated the importance of quadriceps function for realistic long term independent ambulation.[25] Frequently short leg braces or thermoplastic AFOs (ankle, foot orthosis) are sufficient to provide full ambulatory potential. Neurologic hip instability is common, and its treatment is essential to provide maximum overall function.

SPINE

Developmental deformity is considerably less common than in the thoracic or upper lumbar levels, but it needs to be evaluated and followed closely, although no specific deformity is unique to this area. Fixed scoliosis resulting in pelvic obliquity should be prevented, because its effects on hip stability, as well as ability to stand and sit correctly, are important.

HIPS

The L4 lesion has the highest propensity to dislocate (Fig. 15.12). As further levels are innervated, hip abductors (parital L5) and hip extensors (S1) make dislocation less likely as the hip is more evenly balanced (Figs. 15.13 and 15.14). These hips are usually located at birth and develop neurogenic dislocation with time. When adductors and flexors are strong (this will usually be associated with active quadriceps and presence of anterior tibial muscle in the pure L4 lesion), the hip will likely dislocate despite any nonoperative method to reduce it or any operative method in which muscular imbalance is not corrected in some manner.

To permit standing and attempted ambulation before 18 months of age, the hips should be balanced and located by this age. After closed management with appropriate splinting before the age of 1 year, the neuromuscular imbalance must be specifically corrected. Lateral transfer of the iliopsoas[48, 59] (Fig. 15.15) is one means of accomplishing this. This procedure is controversial. Although it does not provide the active abduction desired, it does seem to relieve the deforming force and provide at least a tenodesis effect to help balance the hip structure. Lat-

eral transfer of the iliopsoas is, however, a balancing procedure only. The hip must be reduced for the transfer to be effective. The best means of accomplishing this is to reduce the hips manually at an early age, splinting them in a reduced position until the child is old enough for lateral transfer.[43, 46] When the hip is already dislocated, it should be reduced and stable at the time of transfer. This may require a combination of open reduction and varus derotation osteotomy, or occasionally pelvic osteotomy.

This procedure is associated with a high complication rate, especially postoperative fractures and redislocation.[13, 52] In addition, it is not likely to be effective in the presence of pelvic obliquity, as the hip on the high side is particularly prone to redislocate in the face of pelvic obliquity. Some authors[13, 25] recommend this procedure only in the presence of strong functioning quadriceps musculature, as soft-tissue releases alone will be equally effective with less morbidity in light of ambulatory potential in the children who do not have strong quadriceps.

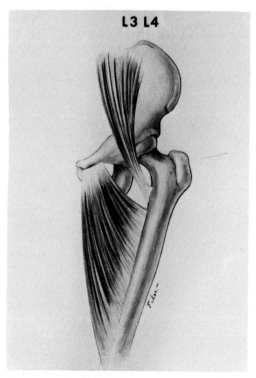

Figure 15.12. Innervation of muscles about the hip in the patient denervated below L3 or L4.

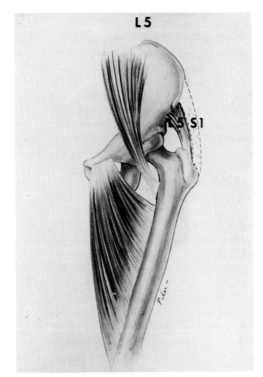

Figure 15.13. Innervation of muscles about the hip in the patient denervated below L5.

Another drawback to lateral transfer through the ilium is that it effectively destroys a large portion of the iliac donor site used for bone grafting in spinal fusions and may necessitate use of alternate bone graft donor techniques, such as bank bone or other graft sites, when spinal fusion is required.

At the L5 level, when abductors are present, the hip is less likely to dislocate and should be followed closely for development of flexion or adduction contractures. If contractures do develop, they should be released early to prevent dislocation. Psoas transfer at this level is not recommended.

When operative procedures are contemplated for the hips, careful assessment of the knees and feet should be made; if neurogenic deformity is predicted, then it is preferable to correct all of these at one sitting if possible. Menelaus[46] recommended performing bilateral hip procedures plus knee and foot procedures all at one sitting. Although this may seem a formidable undertaking, it is geared toward rapid achievement of correction of deformity with minimal long term immobilization.

KNEE

The presence of active quadriceps function with variable strength of knee flexors causes considerable variability of deformity at this level. Hyperextension deformity may be caused by overactive quadriceps. Every attempt should be made beginning in infancy to maintain at least a 90-degree range of motion of the knees. However, if hyperextension deformity persists in the presence of active quadriceps, then lengthening V-Y plasty with possible open reduction of the knee is appropriate.

Flexion contractures may be caused by overactive knee flexors or prolonged positioning in flexion. Flexion contracture represents a severe disability with respect to bracing and ambulation. As with other deformities, early maintenance of motion from infancy is essential. When apparent that this regimen will not be successful in preventing fixed deformity, then early surgical intervention is more likely to succeed than is waiting for more significant fixed deformity to de-

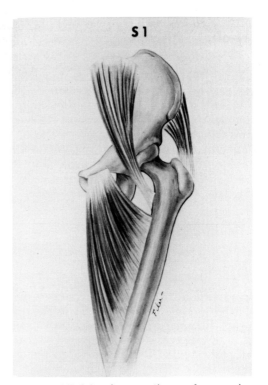

Figure 15.14. Innervation of muscles about the hip in the patient denervated below S1.

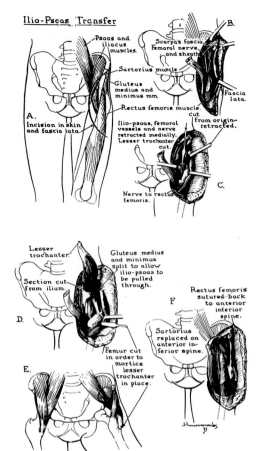

Figure 15.15. The iliopsoas transplant devised by Mustard to aid abduction. The iliopsoas is mobilized with the lesser trochanter, passed laterally through the ilium, and sutured to the femur by means of a trap door type of fixation. (From W. T. Mustard: A follow-up study of ilio-psoas transfer for hip instability, *Journal of Bone and Joint Surgery*, 41B: 289, 1959.)

velop and having to attempt correction of the more severe deformity.

A reasonable approach to the problem of knee flexion contracture is to perform percutaneous hamstring tenotomies in attempts to achieve reduction of the contracture to less than 20 degrees. If this is unsuccessful, the surgeon should be prepared to do femoral osteotomies under the same anesthetic to fully correct the deformity. Ideally, the arc of motion should remain greater than 90 degrees.

FEET

In the lower lumbar level, marked variation of both intrinsic and extrinsic foot musculature is responsible for a multitude of neurogenic deformities, sometimes influenced by intrauterine positioning factors. The skin problems associated with foot deformities in the low lumbar and sacral level myelomeningoceles may be further aggravated by a more active ambulatory status in the presence of insensate feet.

Carefully applied corrective plaster casts before 8–12 months of age may be successful in correcting deformity, but once corrected these feet should be watched closely for recurrence. In the event of recurrent deformity, muscular imbalance must be strongly suspected and treated appropriately by muscle transfer or release. The reader is referred to an excellent review by Drennan[10] for a discussion on a variety of specific foot deformities.

A common problem seen at this level is calcaneus deformity produced by functioning dorsiflexors (especially anterior tibial) in the absence of plantar flexors (especially gastrocnemius). A useful procedure to correct this problem and prevent deformity at an early age is transfer of the anterior tibial tendon through the interosseus membrane to os calcis.[53]

Sacral Level

These patients should be anticipated to maintain completely independent community ambulation and usually do not require lower extremity or spinal orthoses. The majority of their management revolves about urologic problems and care of the feet.

SPINE

Significant spinal deformity is uncommon in this region as compared to the more proximal levels of involvement. The absence of significant scoliosis or lordosis, however, should not divert one's attention beyond other bony spinal involvement, such as diastematomyelia, or other forms of spinal dysraphism distant to the presenting site of involvement. At this level, serial neurologic examination to detect possible progressive neurologic loss is essential.

HIPS

At the sacral neurologic level, the hips are nearly completely balanced, although there may be some weakness of hip extension (Fig. 15.16). Neurogenic tendency for dislocation, therefore, is quite low, and in most respects the hips behave in a manner similar to those that are normally innervated.

KNEE

The musculature about the knee in sacral level paraplegia also shows less tendency toward imbalance; therefore, the anticipation of paralytic deformity is low. Bracing of the knee to improve stability is seldom necessary.

FEET

At the sacral level of involvement, the care of the feet assumes prime importance. Particularly due to lack of more proximal deformities, or paralysis, the child may be considerably more active in terms of weight bearing

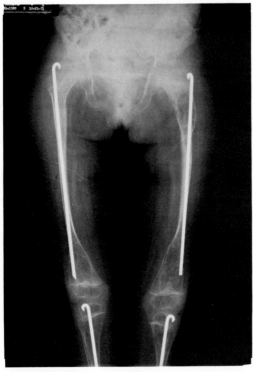

Figure 15.16. Anteroposterior roentgenogram of lower extremities treated by prophylactic rodding for multiple pathologic fractures.

and ambulation. In addition, these children may be expected to retain their ability to ambulate, so that surgical procedures affecting the resiliency of the foot should not be undertaken lightly. Perhaps the most important factor to consider is the sensory status of the sole of the foot. In the absence of the protective sensation, foot deformities affecting the weight bearing relationship of the forefoot and hindfoot are considerably more likely to cause skin ulcerations and secondary problems. Each foot deformity, of course, must be individually analyzed with respect to presence or absence of both intrinsic and extrinsic motor function. Every attempt should be made to provide a plantigrade foot that is flexible, able to withstand normal weight-bearing stresses, and balanced so as to obviate progressive deformity. Tendon transfer should be performed, when indicated, prior to progression to the point of fixed deformity. This is usually sometime in the age between 1 and 2 years. Similarly, soft-tissue releases may be helpful at an early age.

If deformity is allowed to persist to the point that it becomes fixed, then the surgeon may have to resort to more extensive bony procedures, such as arthrodesis of one or more joints. This significantly detracts from the resiliency of the foot, and thus reduces its ability to provide functional, evenly distributed weight bearing.

A common deformity seen in the low level myelodysplasia patient is that of a cavo varus foot with claw toes. Heel varus should be looked for carefully (Fig. 15.17). Various forms of surgical treatment are available for deformity, including soft-tissue releases of plantar structures or osteotomy of the calcaneus to correct varus heel deformity. A separate procedure is usually required for the claw toe deformity and may include transfer of flexors into extensors, extensor tendon recessions to the metatarsal necks, tenodesis of the great toe (as advocated by Sharrad[62]), or, when deformity is fixed, interphalangeal fusion.

FRACTURES

Lower extremity fractures are common in the myelomeningocele population and are

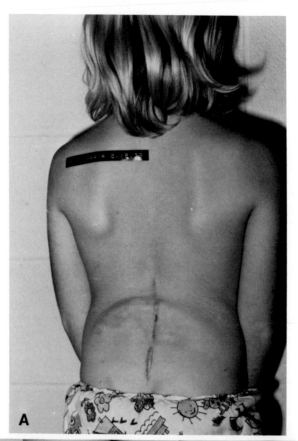

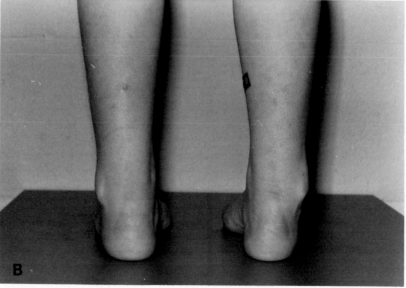

Figure 15.17. (*A*) In the sacral level myelodysplastic child, one should look closely for development of a varus heel (*B*). This is often associated with a cavus foot and clawing of the toes.

especially likely to result after immobilization following surgical procedures. Therefore, one of the effective forms of treatment of fractures is prevention, and this may be accomplished by careful planning of the surgical procedures to avoid excessive immobilization. In addition, weight bearing while in the postoperative cast has a substantial benefit on prevention of disuse osteoporosis that may accompany prolonged non-weight bearing and nonactivity. When fractures do occur, they may present only as swelling, redness, and warmth at the area of the fracture site without history of injury or significant degree of pain, and they may often be misdiagnosed as infection. Fever, swelling, erythema, and heat about a lower extremity in a myelodysplastic child should be considered to be a fracture until radiographically proven otherwise.

Stable and undisplaced fractures may be treated by immobilization in existing braces. When this regimen is utilized, the braces should be worn 24 hr per day (except to monitor skin care) with the joints locked until swelling has disappeared. Weight bearing should be resumed as early as possible.

Unstable fractures must be reduced and immobilized in plaster, again with attempt at early weight bearing when this is feasible. Fracture healing time is not prolonged in the myelodysplastic patient.

Finally, recurrent fractures in the same extremity frequently will represent a vicious cycle caused by repeated immobilization to treat fractures caused by immobilization initially. In this event consideration should be given to intramedullary rodding of the extremities to allow earlier functional weight bearing (Fig. 15.18).

The myelodysplastic child presents the orthopaedist, as well as other specialists, with a challenging complexity of problems that frequently tax our therapeutic resources. A

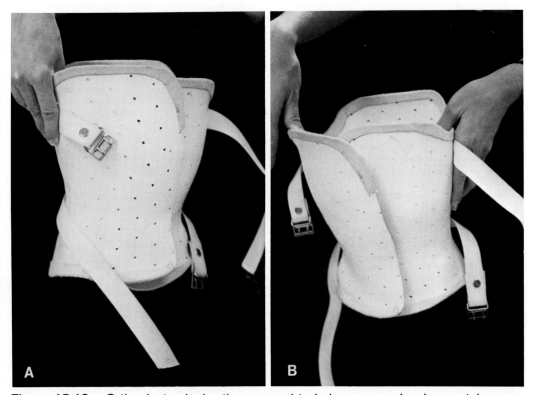

Figure 15.18. Orthoplast spinal orthoses used to help manage developmental curves or for postoperative immobilization. The univalved construction with opening in front fits well and is easily managed in those patients who do not have an ileal loop. In patients with higher curves, the anterior portion can be brought up higher for infraclavicular pressure. Minimal or no padding is necessary in these total-contact orthoses. A window in front can be added if desired.

team approach is essential, and yet each child's problems must be individualized. Realistic goals must be established. With appropriate care these children's lives may be substantially improved.

References

1. Abraham, E., Verinder, D., and Sharrard, W. J. W.: The treatment of flexion contracture of the knee in myelomeningocele, *J. Bone Joint Surg., 59B:* 433, 1977.
2. Asher, M., Olson, J., Weigel, J., Morantx, R., Harris, J., Lieberman, B., and Wallace, W.: The myelomeningocele patients, a multidisciplinary approach, *J. Kans. Med. Soc., 80:* 403, 1970.
3. Banta, J. V., Whiteman, S., Dyck, P. M., Hartleip, D., and Gilbert, D.: Fifteen year review of myelomeningocele, *J. Bone Joint Surg., 58A:* 726, 1976.
4. Barden, G. A., Mayer, L. C., and Stelling, F. H.: Myelodysplasias—fate of those followed for twenty years or more, *J. Bone Joint Surg., 57A:* 643, 1975.
5. Bunch, W. K.: Myelominingocele: general concepts, *A. A. O. S. Instruct. Course Lect., 25:* 61, 1976.
6. Carroll, N. C., and Sharrard, W. J. W.: Long-term follow-up of posterior iliopsoas transplantation of paralytic dislocation of the hip, *J. Bone Joint Surg., 54A:* 1364, 1970.
7. Cruess, R. L., and Turner, N. S.: Paralysis of the abductors in spina bifida; results of treatment by the Mustard procedure, *J. Bone Joint Surg., 52A:* 1364, 1970.
8. DeSouza, L. J., and Carroll, N.: Ambulation of the braced myelomeningocele patient, *J. Bone Joint Surg., 58A:* 1112, 1976.
9. Drennan, J. C.: Management of neonatal myelomeningocele, *A. A. O. S. Instruct. Course Lect., 25:* 65, 1976.
10. Drennan, J. C.: Management of myelomeningocele foot deformities in infancy and early childhood, *A. A. O. S. Instruct. Course Lect., 25:* 82, 1976.
11. Drennan, J. C., and Sharrard, W. J. W.: The pathological anatomy of convex pes valgus, *J. Bone Joint Surg., 53B:* 455, 1971.
12. Emery, J. L., and Lendon, R. G.: Neurospinal dysraphism syndrome, In *A. A. O. S. Symposium on Myelomeningocele;* St. Louis: C. V. Mosby, 1972.
13. Feiwell, E., Sakai, D., and Blott, T.: The effect of hip abduction on function in patients with myelomeningocele, *J. Bone Joint Surg., 60A:* 169, 1978.
14. Ferguson, A. B., Jr.: Primary open reduction of congenital dislocation of the hip using a medical adductor approach, *J. Bone Joint Surg., 55A:* 671, 1973
15. Freeston, B. M.: An inquiry into the effect of a spina bifida child upon family life, *Dev. Med. Child Neurol., 13:* 456, 1971.
16. Fried, A.: Recurrent congenital club foot: the role of m. tibialis posterior in etiology and treatment, *J. Bone Joint Surg., 41A:* 243, 1959.
17. Gordon, L. H., Shurtleff, D. B. and Fortz, E. L.: Myelomeningocele, *J. Bone Joint Surg., 47B:* 381, 1965.
18. Griffin, G. D., and Stark, G.: Correlation of neurological deficit and limb deformity in myelomeningocele, *J. Bone Joint Surg., 53A:* 386, 1971.
19. Habal, M. B., and Vries, J. K.: Tension free closure of large meningomyelocele defects, *Surg. Neurol., 8:* 177, 1977.
20. Haddow, J. E., and Macri, J. M.: Prenatal screening for neural tube defects, *J. A. M. A., 242:* 515, 1979.
21. Handelsman, J. E.: Spontaneous fractures in spina bifida, *J. Bone Joint Surg., 54B:* 381, 1972.
22. Hayes, J. T., Gross, H. P., and Dow, S.: Surgery for paralytic defects secondary to myelomeningocele and myelodysplasia, *J. Bone Joint Surg., 46A:* 1577, 1964.
23. Hide, D. W., Williams, H. P., and Ellis, H. L.: The outlook for the child with a myelomeningocele for whom early surgery was considered inadvisable, *Dev. Med. Child Neurol., 14:* 304, 1972.
24. Hoffer, M. M., Feiwell, E., Perry, R., Perry, J., and Bonnet, C. Functional ambulation in patients with myelomeningocele, *J. Bone Joint Surg., 55A:* 137, 1973.
25. Huff, C. W., and Ramsey, P. L.: Myelomeningocele: the influence of the quadriceps and hip abduction muscles on ambulatory function and stability of the hip, *J. Bone Joint Surg., 60A:* 432, 1978.
26. James, C. C. M., and Lassman, L. P.: Spinal dysraphism, the diagnosis and treatment of progressive lesion in spina bifida occulta, *J. Bone Joint Surg., 44B:* 828, 1962.
27. James, H. E., McLaurin, R. L., and Watkins, W. T.: Remission of pes cavus in surgically treated spinal dysraphism, *J. Bone Joint Surg., 61A:* 1096, 1979.
28. Kilfoyle, R. M., Foley, J. J., and Norton, P. L.: Spine and pelvic deformity in childhood and adolescent paraplegia, *J. Bone Joint Surg., 47A:* 659, 1965.
29. Knox, E. G.: Spina bifida-Birmingham, *Dev. Med. Child Neurol., 13:* 14, 1967.
30. Lawrence, K., and Tew, B. J.: Natural history of spina bifida cystica and cranium bifidum cysticum, *Arch. Dis. Child., 46:* 127, 1971.
31. Lawrence, K. M.: The survival of untreated spina bifida cystica, *Dev. Med. Child Neurol.* (Suppl. 11) 10, 1966.
32. Lawrence, K. M.: The recurrence risk in spina bifida cystica and anencephaly, *Dev. Med. Child Neurol.* (Suppl. 20) 23, 1969.
33. Letts, R. M., Fulford, R., and Hobson, D. A.: Mobility aids for the paraplegic child, *J. Bone Joint Surg., 58A:* 38, 1976.
34. Lichtenstein, B. W.: Spinal dysraphism, spina bifida and myelomeningocele, *Arch. Neurol., 44:* 726, 1940.
35. Lindseth, R. E.: Bilateral posterior iliac osteotomy for fixed pelvic obliquity, *J. Bone Joint Surg., 57A:* 1172, 1975.
36. Lindseth, R. E.: Treatment of the lower extremity in children paralyzed by myelomeningocele (birth to 8 months), *A. A. O. S. Instruct. Course Lect., 25:* 176, 1976.
37. Lindseth, R. E.: Posterior iliac osteotomy for fixed pelvic obliquity, *J. Bone Joint Surg., 60A:* 17, 1978.
38. Lindseth, R. E., and Glancy, J.: Polypropylene lower extremity braces for paraplegia due to myelomeningocele, *J. Bone Joint Surg., 56A:* 556, 1974.
39. Lorber, J.: Incidence and epidemiology of myelomeningocele, *Clin. Ortho., 45:* 81, 1966.
40. Lorber, J.: Spina bifida cystica, *Arch. Dis. Child., 13:* 279, 1971.
41. Lorber, J.: Results of treatment of myelomeningocele, *Dev. Med. Child Neurol., 13:* 279, 1971.

42. Lorber, J.: Selective treatment of myelomeningocele: to treat or not to treat, *Pediatrics, 53:* 307, 1974.

43. McKibbin, B.: Conservative management of paralytic dislocations of the hip in myelomeningocele, *J. Bone Joint Surg., 53B:* 758, 1971.

44. McKibbin, B.: The use of splintage in the paralytic dislocation of the hip in spina bifida cystica, *J. Bone Joint Surg., 55B:* 163, 1973.

45. Menelaus, M. B.: Talectomy for equinovarus deformity in arthrogryposis and spina bifida, *J. Bone Joint Surg., 53B:* 468, 1971.

46. Menelaus, M. B.: The hip in myelomeningocele: management directed toward a minimum number of operations and a minimum period of immobilization, *J. Bone Joint Surg., 58B:* 448, 1976.

47. Mustard, W. T.: Iliopsoas transfer for weakness of the hip abductors; a preliminary report, *J. Bone Joint Surg., 34A:* 647, 1952.

48. Mustard, W. T.: A follow-up study of iliopsoas transfer for hip instability, *J. Bone Joint Surg., 41B:* 289, 1959.

49. Naggan, L., and MacMahon, B.: Ethnic differences in the prevalence of anencephaly and spina bifida, *N. Engl. J. Med., 227:* 1119, 1967.

50. Ober, F. R.: An operation for the relief of paralysis of the gluteus maximus muscles, *J. A. M. A., 88:* 1062, 1927.

51. Padget, D. H.: Spina bifida and embryonic neuroschisis—a causal relationship, *Johns Hopkins Med. J., 123:* 233, 1968.

52. Parker, B., and Walker, D.: Posterior psoas transfer and hip instability in lumbar myelomeningocele, *J. Bone Joint Surg., 57B:* 53, 1975.

53. Peabody, C. W.: Tendon transposition: an end result study, *J. Bone Joint Surg., 20:* 193, 1938.

54. Renwick, J. H.: Potato babies, *Lancet, 2:* 336, 1972.

55. Rueda, J., and Carroll, N. C.: Hip instability in patients with myelomeningocele, *J. Bone Joint Surg., 54B:* 422, 1972.

56. Sharrard, W. J. W.: Congenital dislocation of the hip in children with myelomeningocele, *J. Bone Joint Surg., 41B:* 622, 1959.

57. Sharrard, W. J. W.: Immediate closure of myelomeningocele and management of paralytic deformities in myelomeningocele, *J. Bone Joint Surg., 45B:* 43, 1963.

58. Sharrard, W. J. W.: Paralytic deformity in meningomyelocele, *J. Bone Joint Surg., 45B:* 616, 1963.

59. Sharrard, W. J. W.: Posterior iliopsoas transplantation in the treatment of paralytic dislocation of the hip, *J. Bone Joint Surg., 46B:* 426, 1964.

60. Sharrard, W. J. W.: Paralytic deformity in the lower limb, *J. Bone Joint Surg., 49B:* 731, 1967.

61. Sharrard, W. J. W.: The management of deformity and paralysis of the foot in myelomeningocele, *J. Bone Joint Surg., 50B:* 456, 1968.

62. Sharrard, W. J. W., and Smith, T. W. D.: Tenodesis of flexor hallucis for paralytic clawing of the hallux in childhood, *J. Bone Joint Surg., 58B:* 224, 1976.

63. Smyth, B. T., Piggot, J., Forsythe, W. I., and Merritt, J. D.: A controlled trial of immediate and delayed closure of myelomeningocele, *J. Bone Joint Surg., 56B:* 297, 1974.

64. Sriram, K., Bobechko, P., and Hall, J. E.: Surgical management of spinal deformities in spina bifida, *J. Bone Joint Surg., 54B:* 666, 1972.

65. Stein, S. C., Schultz, L., and Ames, M. D.: Selection for early treatment in myelomeningocele: a retrospective analysis of various selection procedures, *Pediatrics, 54:* 553, 1974.

66. Thomas, L. I., Thompson, T. C., and Straub, L. R.: Transposition of the external oblique muscle for abductor paralysis, *J. Bone Joint Surg., 32A:* 202, 1950.

67. Walker, G.: The early management of varus feet in myelomeningocele, *J. Bone Joint Surg., 53B:* 462, 1971.

68. Winter, R. B.: Myelomeningocele, In *Scoliosis and Other Spinal Deformities,* Moe, J. H., Winter, R. B., Bradford, D. S., and Lonstein, J. E. (eds.), p. 239; Philadelphia: W. B. Saunders, 1978.

69. Yen, S., and MacMahon, B.: Genetics of anencephaly and spina bifida, *Lancet, 2:* 623, 1968.

70. Yount, C. C.: The role of tensor fascia femoris in certain deformities of the lower extremities, *J. Bone Joint Surg., 8:* 171, 1926.

SPINAL DEFORMITIES IN MYELODYSPLASIA

BY CARL D. FACKLER, M.D.

The management of spinal deformities in patients with myelodysplasia is one of the most difficult problems in orthopaedics today. In the past, most patients died with renal, neurologic, or septic problems before their spinal deformity became a significant factor. However, with recent urologic and neurosurgical advances, these patients' life span is markedly increased, their intelligence is often normal, and the management of their spinal deformity has emerged as the major problem affecting their length and quality of life.

More than 60% of all patients with myelodysplasia either have or develop significant spinal deformity by the age of 10.[6] The results of orthopaedic management of these problems in the past have not been satisfactory. Bracing was not successful, and with surgery success rates of 50% or less were reported.[2-4, 8] The surgical complications included unacceptably high infection, pseudarthrosis, and mortality rates. The problems encountered are major and different from other spinal deformities due to anesthetic skin, urinary tract infection, osteopenic bone, deficient posterior vertebral elements, previous surgery, and poor donor bone. Unfortunately, because of the magnitude of these problems,

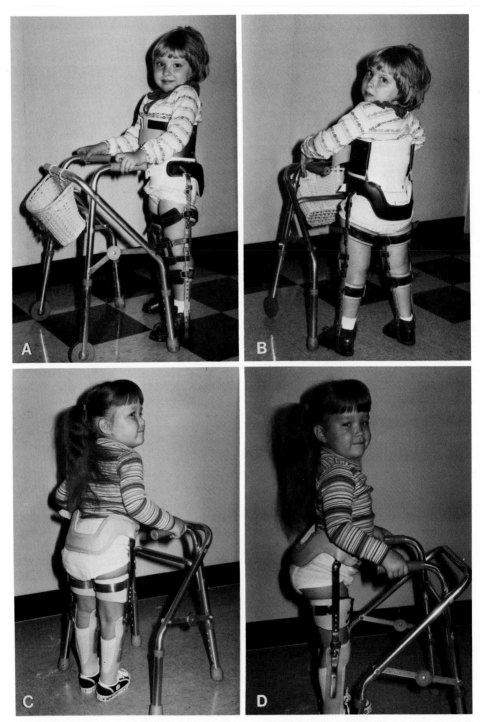

Figure 15.19. (*A* and *B*) Pelvic band with long leg braces that has been properly fitted around orthoplast body jacket. (*C* and *D*) Poorly fitting pelvic band that is too high in back and does not control the patient's increased lumbar lordosis.

many spinal deformities have gone untreated or have been ignored.

Thankfully, there have been many major advances in the past 10 years in both the understanding of the natural history of these deformities and in bracing and surgical techniques. Earlier, aggressive management utilizing these methods has led to a much higher success rate.

Natural History and Classification

Raycroft and Curtis described a method of classification of these individuals that is quite useful and is based on their natural history.[6] They divided them into two distinct groups—congenital and developmental.

Congenital curves are those present at birth and are due to vertebral anomalies other than the spina bifida. These occur in approximately 20% of all patients with myelodysplasia.[6] These can be further subdivided into the type of vertebral anomaly and the type of deformity—scoliosis, lordosis, or kyphosis. These curves are similar in behavior to congenital curves in patients without spina bifida. These deformities are stiffer, almost always progress early in life, and often develop significant compensatory curves. Lumbar kyphosis is generally included in this group.

Developmental curves are similar to paralytic curves and are the most common. These occur in patients who have been born with a normal spine without deformity except for the spina bifida. The curve subsequently slowly "develops" due to muscular or structural imbalance. In the series of 103 patients reviewed by Raycroft and Curtis, 79% of the patients had a normal spine except for the spina bifida, and 50% of these had a developmental scoliosis by the age of 10.[6] The higher the neurologic lesion, the more likely this type of deformity is to develop. After reviewing the literature and his own experience, Winter reported that a spinal deformity will develop in all patients with a T12 level or above, 90% at L1, 80% at L2, 70% at L3, 60% at L4, 25% at L5, and 5% at S1.[10] These curves initially progress slowly, but there is a rapid increase in the curve during the adolescent growth spurt. The most common deformity in this group is scoliosis with lordosis and pelvic obliquity. If untreated, these curves become quite severe.

Clinical Management

OBSERVATION

The key to successful management is early recognition of the problem. Each patient must be carefully evaluated and followed, starting early in life. Yearly upright spine films allow early detection so that treatment can be started at the proper time. Management of the hip and other lower limb problems to keep the pelvis level and the spine in balance in sitting and standing may prevent or delay the onset of progression of developmental scoliosis. A hip flexion contracture will increase lumbar lordosis in standing, and hip extension contractures will increase lumbar kyphosis in the sitting position. Each of these hip contractures should be treated surgically if it causes or significantly increases spinal deformity.

In patients who require lower extremity bracing to walk, one should strive for the "extension posturing" as described by Menelaus to prevent excessive lumbar lordosis.[5] This often can be achieved by modifying the posterior portion of the pelvic band to push in on the buttocks. A thoracic extension is sometimes also needed. The balance of the spine must always be kept in mind when ordering braces for the lower extremities.

Bracing

Early bracing of developmental scoliosis is an effective method of slowing down or delaying progression of the curve, thereby allowing further growth before surgical fusion is needed. Brace treatment of congenital deformities is ineffective, but it can be used to manage compensatory curves.

A light-weight, total-contact, underarm plastic body jacket is made from a cast of the patient's torso taken in the corrected position. Cutouts can be made for accommodation of stomas that may be present, and the jackets are bivalved or univalved. A univalved jacket that opens in the front fits better and is better tolerated, but a bivalved jacket may on occasion be necessary because it is easier for parents to apply and easier to remove for skin care.

Bracing for developmental scoliosis should generally be started when the curve is between 10 and 20 degrees as measured on upright spine x-rays. Bracing is started early and maintained until just before the adolescent growth spurt, when the brace will no longer hold the curve and surgery is indicated. If the scoliosis is 40 degrees or more, a brace will probably not be effective, and surgery should be considered at that time. Likewise, if the curve progresses to 40 degrees or more in the brace, then surgery is indicated at that time. If the scoliosis extends to the upper thoracic area or is associated with increased thoracic kyphosis, then a Milwaukee brace is indicated. The pelvic girdle for the Milwaukee brace is made in the same fashion as the underarm body jacket described above.

The patient should be encouraged to wear the brace full time, but if this is not possible he should wear it when standing or sitting. The brace can be worn over anesthetic skin providing the skin is checked frequently for pressure areas and meticulous skin care is given. If skin problems do develop, the brace must be discontinued or modified until these clear up and proper adjustments made to prevent recurrence.

Surgical Management

Spinal fusion is the only definitive treatment of significant spinal deformities in patients with myelodysplasia. Early aggressive surgical management before these deformities become severe yields the best long term result.

Patients with congenital spinal deformities other than lumbar kyphosis should be fused at the first sign of progression, no matter what the patient's age. In very young patients, the fusion should be no longer than necessary to control the congenital curve; bracing can be used to control the compensatory curve until the patient is older.

Patients with developmental scoliosis should be fused when the patient's curve exceeds 40 degrees, which, if the patient has responded well to brace treatment, is generally just before the adolescent growth spurt. Developmental curves should be fused from the high thoracic area to the sacrum. Because of the deficient posterior elements and poor results with anterior fusion alone or posterior fusion alone, both anterior and posterior fusion are indicated. The maximum use of internal fixation both anterior and posterior is essential. If abundant bone graft is not available from the iliac crests, it should be supplemented with tibial graft or bank bone.

A careful preoperative evaluation is essential. The patient should be admitted to the hospital at least 3–4 days before surgery to allow orientation of the patient to the hospital and for evaluation, including the patient's urologic and neurologic systems and status of the skin. If the patient has a ventricular shunt, it must be working prior to surgery. Skin care and treatment of urinary tract infections prior to surgery decrease the chance of postoperative infection. Preoperative myelography is indicated if there has been a change in the patient's neurologic status that cannot be explained by shunt malfunction and cord tethering is suspected. If a patient has concurrent hip or other lower extremity problems, it is recommended that the spinal deformity be approached first and maximally corrected before the other problems are treated.

The goal of surgery should be to correct the deformity as much as possible, to balance the spine, and to fuse the spine in the balanced position. One should strive for maximum correction and balance. Careful planning and staging of the operation is necessary preoperatively, and each patient must be considered on an individual basis. To achieve greater correction, the surgeon must be prepared to release soft tissues and resect vertebral elements as needed. Preoperative traction prolongs the period of hospitalization and immobilization. It is not recommended because the patient's bone becomes more osteopenic in this process, making internal fixation more difficult and less secure, and little additional correction is gained by the traction. The maximum use of internal fixation is essential to obtain and maintain correction.

Blood loss at surgery can be high and needs to be carefully monitored. The surgeon should be prepared to stop the operation if blood loss becomes excessive and return the patient to the operating theater at a later date to complete the surgery if necessary.

Postoperative care has dramatically changed in the past 5 years. Plaster body casts and pantaloon spicas are no longer used in many centers.[10] A plastic body jacket is

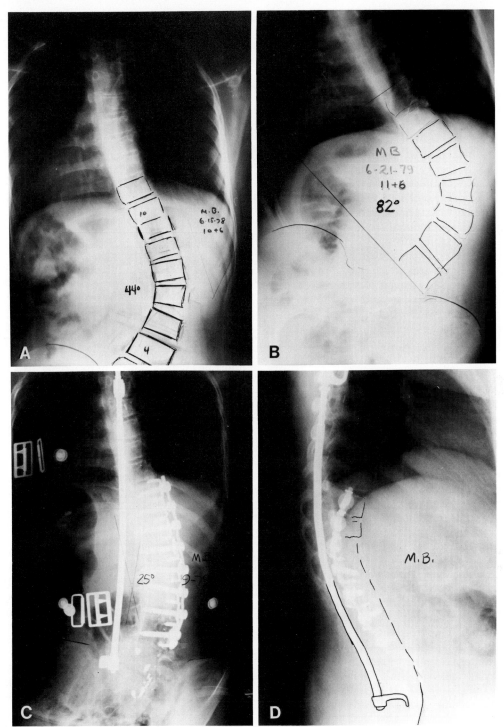

Figure 15.20. (*A*) Upright anteroposterior spine film of 10-year-old patient with upper lumbar level and scoliosis measuring 44 degrees. There was also an increased lumbar lordosis on the lateral x-ray. This curve will rapidly progress unless spinal fusion is performed as outlined in the text. (*B*) The patient was untreated and 1 year later the curve has increased to 82 degrees. The parents then agreed to proceed with surgery. (*C*) Postoperative x-rays following anterior spinal fusion with Dwyer instrumentation and a long posterior fusion from high thoracic spine to sacrum. (*D*) Postoperative lateral x-ray. Notice the Harrington rod has been bent to conform to the contour of the spine.

fabricated postoperatively from a plaster mold and applied within the first 2 weeks after surgery. The patients are generally able to resume their preoperative level of ambulation with these jackets on within 2 weeks of spinal surgery even if the fusion extends to the sacrum. This approach has decreased the incidence of pseudarthrosis and decreased the complications associated with prolonged immobilization. It also decreases the overall cost of treatment and makes postoperative management much easier. The use of maximum internal fixation and balance at surgery enables this approach to be successful. These body jackets can be removed when the patient is supine for skin care if needed. Univalved body jackets usually fit better than the bivalved jackets and are only slightly harder to remove, but bivalved jackets are still occasionally needed to facilitate skin and stoma care. These body jackets are worn for 1 year or until mature graft is present on x-ray. The fusion mass is not reexplored unless there is clinical or x-ray evidence of pseudarthrosis.

If postoperative infection develops after spinal fusion, the wound is opened, debrided, thoroughly irrigated, and left open, leaving the internal fixation in place even if it is exposed. Appropriate antibiotics are given parenterally and frequent wet-to-dry dressing changes are performed until infection has cleared; then secondary closure is performed.

LUMBAR KYPHOSIS

Lumbar kyphosis is specific to myelodysplasia. It is present at birth and always progresses. A compensatory thoracic lordosis develops that severely compromises pulmonary function. These patients almost always have a high complete neurologic lesion. Bracing does not prevent progression. Definitive surgery of the kyphosis is usually not possible until the patient is at least 4 years of age. If surgery is necessary prior to that because of nursing care problems, then a kyphectomy should be performed, realizing that a definitive surgical procedure will be needed at a later date. At age 4 or when the kyphosis reaches 50 degrees or more, the single stage operation with excision of vertebra just above the apex as described by Hall is indicated.[1] Enough vertebrae must be excised to achieve

reversal of the kyphosis. Anterior fusion is achieved by resecting the intervertebral discs above and below the resected area and laying in abundant graft anteriorly. Resection of the nonfunctioning cord is often necessary to facilitate exposure and closure. If the cord is resected, the cord itself should not be surgically closed but only the distal dural sac.[9] Harrington compression hooks can be successfully placed in the intervertebral foramen, and the uppermost hooks are usually placed in lamina.

SCOLIOSIS WITH LORDOSIS

This is approached surgically in two stages. First, an anterior fusion with Dwyer or Zielke instrumentation is performed, striving for a maximum correction. This is followed in 2 weeks by a posterior spinal fusion from high thoracic to the sacrum utilizing 2 or more Harrington rods and a sacral alar hook. Care must be taken at this point to achieve balance of the spine over the pelvis. Generally not much corrective force can be put through these rods because of osteopenic bone. The use of 2 or more rods distributes the corrective stress over more lamina and improves security of the fixation. These rods are bent as needed to fit the contour of the spine.

SCOLIOSIS WITH THORACIC KYPHOSIS

The kyphosis is often due to a posterior hemivertebra with the apex of the kyphosis at the level of functioning spinal cord. Myelography with lateral tomagrams is indicated if spinal cord compression is suspected. Surgical treatment of this deformity is done in 2 stages. First, an anterior release and fusion is performed with anterior decompression added if needed. Halo traction is then used postoperatively to help decrease the kyphosis, and in 2 weeks a long posterior fusion with Harrington compression and distraction instrumentation is performed. If additional strut grafts are needed, they must be large and placed over the full extent of the kyphosis in a third stage.

INCREASED LUMBAR LORDOSIS

This is rarely seen and is generally the result of a lumboperitoneal shunt.[7] Anterior

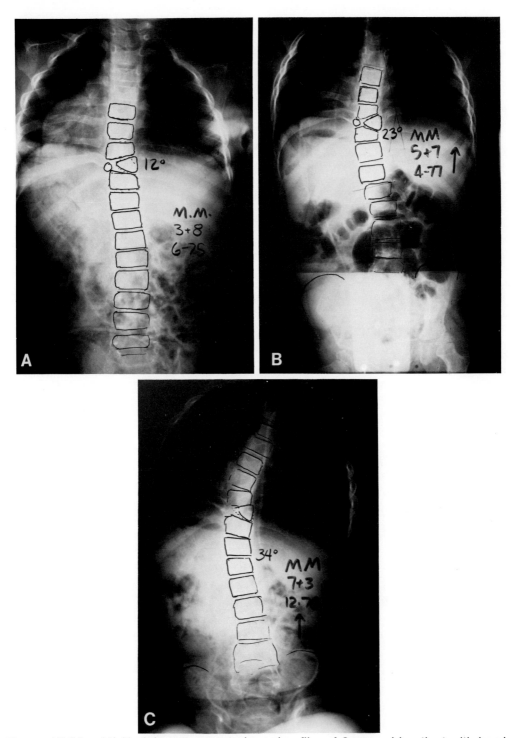

Figure 15.21. (*A*) Upright anteroposterior spine film of 3-year-old patient with hemivertebra in mid-thoracic spine. The scoliosis measures 12 degrees. (*B*) Two years later the curve has progressed to 23 degrees. Posterior spinal fusion, as described in the text, is indicated at this time. (*C*) Surgery was not done and 20 months later the scoliosis has increased to 34 degrees. It will continue to progress until posterior fusion is performed.

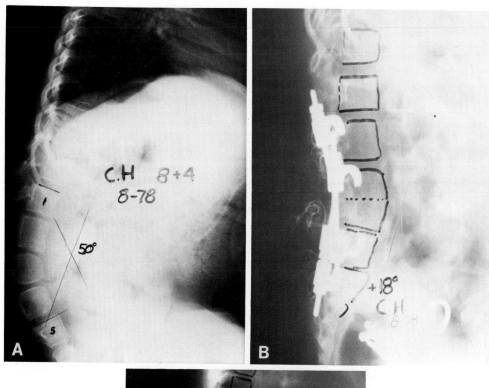

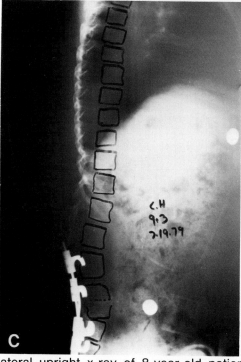

Figure 15.22. (*A*) Lateral upright x-ray of 8-year-old patient with lumbar kyphosis measuring 50 degrees. This was treated with single stage anterior and posterior fusion as described in the text. Minimal vertebral excision was necessary. (*B*) Intraoperative x-ray demonstrating reversal of the lumbar kyphosis. A better result could have been achieved if the apex of the resection was one level higher. (*C*) Upright lateral x-ray taken 1 year postoperatively, after brace removal, demonstrating maintenance of correction.

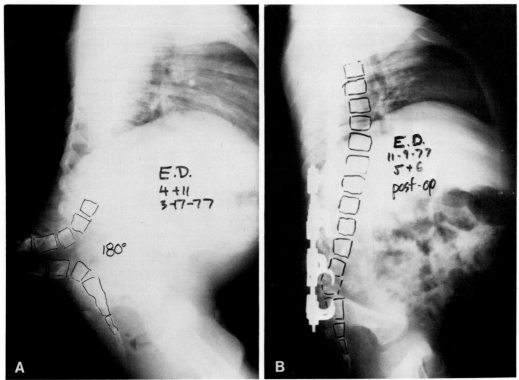

Figure 15.23. (*A*) Upright lateral spine x-ray of 4-year-old patient with severe lumbar kyphosis measuring 180 degrees. A one stage resection with anterior and posterior fusion was performed as described in the text. (*B*) Postoperative x-ray demonstrating correction of the kyphosis.

approach to resect the apical vertebral body and intervertebral discs as needed is performed followed by 90–90 traction to decrease the lordosis. The second stage is a posterior spinal fusion with Harrington distraction instrumentation over the full extent of the deformity.

SPINAL DEFORMITY WITH DIASTEMATOMYELIA

Diastematomyelia is found in approximately 5% of all patients with congenital scoliosis,[11] and its incidence in spina bifida patients with congenital scoliosis is probably higher than that. If a patient is growing and a diastematomyelia is diagnosed, the child must be carefully followed. Excision is recommended at the first sign of increased neurologic deficit. Unfortunately, such deficits are not reversible. If corrective spinal surgery is contemplated, the diastematomyelia must be removed before any significant correction

of the deformity can be performed safely. This need not be performed as a separate procedure but is best combined with the spinal fusion provided it is released and freed from its attachments before any corrective forces are placed through the spine.

References

1. Hall, J. E., and Poitras, B.: The management of kyphosis in patients with myelomeningocele, *Clin. Orthop.*, *128:* 33, 1977.
2. Hull, W. J., Moe, J. H., Lai, C., and Winter, R. B.: The surgical treatment of spinal deformities in myelomeningocele, *J. Bone Joint Surg.*, *56A:* 1767, 1974.
3. Kilfoyle, R. M., Foley, J. J., and Norton, P. L.: Spine and pelvic deformity in childhood and adolescent paraplegia; a study in 104 cases, *J. Bone Joint Surg.*, *47A:* 659, 1965.
4. Lindberg, C., Brown, J. C., and Bonnett, C. A.: The surgical treatment of spine deformity in myelodysplasia, Paper presented at the Scoliosis Research Society, Louisville, September, 1975.
5. Memelaus, M.: Myelomeningocele, principles, Paper presented at Pediatric Orthopaedic International Seminar, May, 1978.

6. Raycroft, J. F., and Curtis, B. H.: Spinal curvature in myelomeningocele, *A. A. O. S. Symposium on Myelomeningocele*; St. Louis: C. V. Mosby, 1972.

7. Sharrard, W. J. W.: The kyphotic and lordotic spine in myelomeningocele, *A. A. O. S. Symposium on Myelomeningocele*; St. Louis: C. V. Mosby, 1972.

8. Sriram, K., Bobechko, W. P., and Hall, J. E.: Surgical management of spinal deformities in spina bifida, *J. Bone Joint Surg., 54B:* 666, 1972.

9. Winston, J., Hall, J. E., Johnson, D., and Micheli, C.: Acute elevation of intracranial pressure following transsection of non-functioning spinal cord, *Clin. Orthop., 128:* 41, 1977.

10. Winter, R. B.: Myelomeningocele, In *Scoliosis and Other Spinal Deformities*, Moe, J. H., Winter, R. B., Bradford, D. S., and Lonstein, J. E. (eds.), pp. 239–287; Philadelphia: W. B. Saunders, 1978.

11. Winter, R. B., Haven, J., Moe, J. H., and Lagaard, S.: Diastematomyelia and congenital spine deformities, *J. Bone Joint Surg., 56A:* 27, 1974.

CHAPTER 16

Cerebral Palsy

CARL L. STANITSKI, M.D.

The act of birth did occasionally imprint on the nervous and muscular systems of the nascent organism very serious and peculiar evils—

W. J. Little, 1843[77]

For more than 200 years orthopaedists have been instrumental in the management of patients with cerebral palsy. In 1741 in his classic textbook, *Orthopaedia*,[1] Nicholas Andrey noted "cerebral diplegia" that developed spontaneously or after an acute illness in the young who had appeared normal at birth. William J. Little (whose foot deformity was treated by tendo achillis tenotomy) had a long standing interest in deformities of the musculoskeletal system.[76] In 1853 he published "Lectures on the Nature and Treatment of Deformities of the Human Frame."[77] In these he included a discussion on "infantile spastic paralysis," which later became referred to as "Little's disease." As he saw more patients with spasticity and deformity, his interest turned to the possible etiology of these conditions. In 1862[78] he delivered a lecture to the Obstetrical Society of London, "On the Influence of Abnormal Parturition, Difficult Labours, Premature Birth and Asphyxia Neonatorum on the Mental and Physical Condition of the Child, Especially in Relation to Deformities" (Fig. 16.1). Although his concepts were initially met with hostility and resistance by the obstetrical community, this paper became a classic monograph whose title stimulated many practitioners to correlate perinatal events and subsequent neuromuscular dysfunction.

Nonorthopaedists have been involved as well. Sir William Osler popularized the term "cerebral palsy" and, in a series of lectures in 1888 at the Philadelphia Infirmary for Nervous Diseases,[93] he emphasized the cortical nature of the lesion with its resultant peripheral effects. It began to be recognized that all cases were not equivalent to Little's "spastic paralysis" and that many forms of involvement existed depending on the site of the neurologic lesion. Prior to his involvement in dreams and psychic phenomena, Freud provided the first working classification of seven types of cerebral palsy by combining the region involved with the most dominant neurologic feature in an 1897 monograph on "Infantile Cerebral Paralysis."[47]

Interest in cerebral palsy management waxed and waned until the 1930s when Dr. Winthrop Phelps stimulated the study of this condition and helped to further popularize the term "cerebral palsy."[101] In 1949 he helped organize the American Academy of Cerebral Palsy, a group that provides an interdisciplinary forum among physicians and allied health personnel who utilize the "team concept" of management of patients with chronic neurologic dysfunction.

DEFINITION

Cerebral palsy is a disorder of motor function secondary to a nonprogressive lesion occurring above the foramen magnum in a developing nervous system. Associated deficits involving intellectual, sensory (visual, tactile, auditory, etc.), speech and perceptual areas occur as well as personality lability and hyperactivity. The definition emphasizes the point that there is no active central nervous system disease and that the insult to the central nervous system occurs early. The exact upper limit for this "early age of involvement" is unknown, but ranges from 2–5 years have been noted, the higher figure being the one chosen by the American Academy of Cerebral Palsy. The most commonly associated neurologic dysfunction is a seizure disorder, particularly in the group of spastic patients, with approximately one-third of the patients having childhood seizures and 10% continuing to have significant seizures during adult life.[105]

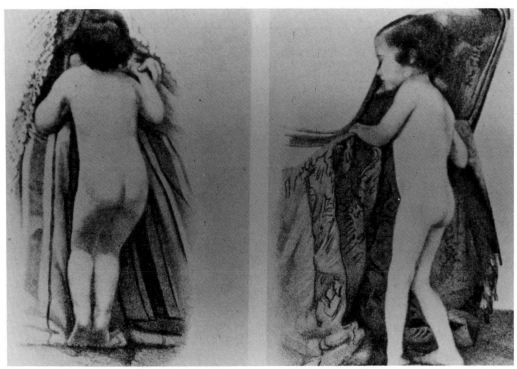

Figure 16.1. Illustrations of diplegic children from Little's paper, 1862.[78]

Cerebral palsy may be considered a static encephalopathy, i.e., the basic lesion does not change. For example, a patient with a right hemiplegia does not spontaneously become a left hemiplegic. Deformities when untreated may progress, but any change of the basic pattern of involvement should alert one to the improper diagnosis and suggest the possibility of a progressive lesion, usually a neoplasm of the neuraxis.

Cerebral palsy must not be considered a diagnosis but really a peripheral manifestation due to a constellation of the etiologic circumstances. Cerebral palsy refers to a heterogenous group of patients and is a useful organization term for a motor disorder with the motor involvement being but one of many problems.

United States, approximately 700,000 patients have the diagnosis "cerebral palsy."[140] In approximately three-fourths of the patients, involvement has been secondary to birth circumstances, with the remaining 25% being secondary to head injuries or other cranial insults in early life. The past decade has seen a dramatic decrease from 20,000 to 10,000 new cases annually. This diminution has been attributed to improved prenatal and perinatal care. Early recognition of maternal and fetal risks, therapeutic abortions, increased frequency of elective cesarean sections for infants at risk, phototherapy and immunologic management of Rh and ABO incompatibility, establishment of neonatal intensive care units, and improved care of the premature infant are all examples of such improvements.[131]

PREVALENCE

The prevalence of patients involved with cerebral palsy varies from 0.06–5.9 per 1,000 births in reported series.[89, 101, 140] In the

CLASSIFICATION

A multitude of classifications have been made since Freud's, including those by Minear,[85] Perlstein and Hood,[95] and Phelps.[101] Disagreements on terminology, definition, and classification have led to decreased communication among workers in the field. As with any classification, there tend to be "lumpers and splitters," and arriving at the correct conclusion may be as difficult a task as that faced by the blind men of Hindustan who attempted to describe an elephant.

Essentially the two basic types are: (1) the neurophysiologic, i.e., spastic (pyramidal) or ataxic, dyskinetic, or mixed (extrapyramidal) in an effort to localize the main neurologic lesion; and (2) the topographic classification that specifies the extremities involved such as hemiplegia, diplegia, or tetraplegia. Most classifications are modifications of Phelps',[101] whose clinical categories were a function of muscle tone, amount of involvement, and topographic distribution.

Hoffer[59] has distilled the classification to provide an assessment of functional goals and considered the neurologic types as spastic, motion disorder (ataxic, athetoid, dyskinetic, rigid, dystonic), or mixed and topographically as hemiplegia, diplegia, or total body involvement. I feel that total body involvement may also be considered a pentaplegia with the head-neck segment acting as a fifth extremity.

Hemiplegic patients have ipsilateral involvement of the upper and lower extremities with such involvement being more manifest in the upper than the lower extremity and involvement distal more so than proximal (Fig. 16.2). Cranial nerves may be involved with an associated hemianopsia, which may impede use of the upper limb. In general there is good intelligence and overall function, but often seizures and an aggressive temper-tantrum type behavior cause delay in functional gains. Prognosis for ambulation is excellent with motor milestones being delayed only 6–8 months. Almost all hemiplegic children walk between the ages of 2 and 3 years in the face of no fixed deformities.[31, 89] No difference has been noted in walking capabilities in right versus left hemiplegic patients. Upper extremity handicaps[115, 137, 139] (astereognosis, impaired two-point discrimination and position senses) and limb length inequality of the lowers greater than the uppers may also exist, parts of the so-called "parietal lobe syndrome."[65] The length dif-

ferential is usually small, rarely exceeding 2 cm.

Diplegia refers to those patients with spasticity of the lower extremities but with mild upper extremity involvement that may be asymmetric. This is the "classical" cerebral palsy described by Little and often referred to as the type where both the thighs and eyes are crossed. It is the most frequent pattern of involvement seen in most clinics and accounts for one-third of the patients followed in our clinic. This pattern is seen in low birth weight single children or children who are products of multiple births, with prematurity (by weight and age) accounting for from one-fourth to one-third of the cases of diplegia. Proximal involvement is more so than distal, with common lower extremity patterns demonstrating excessive hip flexion with internal rotation and adduction. Increased knee flexion with an equinovalgus or varus foot deformity and a crouched gait are also predom-

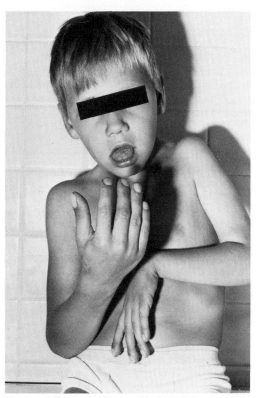

Figure 16.2. Left spastic hemiplegia from embolus due to cyanotic septal cardiac disease. Note marked finger clubbing.

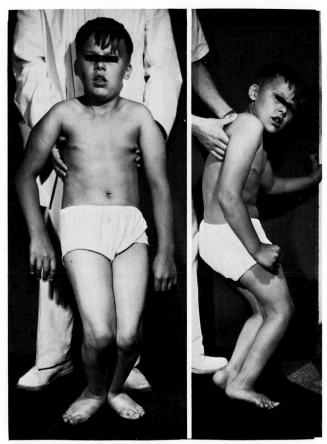

Figure 16.3. Crouched stance and poor balance in diplegic child.

inant features (Fig. 16.3). If upper extremity involvement is not manifest, as in an occasional rare form of spastic paraplegia, spinal lesions must be ruled out as a cause for the lower extremity spasticity. Diplegics all have deficient equilibrium reactions and poor balance. Locomotion and not upper extremity function is their main problem. However, most of these children will walk by the age of 3–4 years if significant deformities do not exist.[8, 15, 31] Twenty per cent will require ambulatory assist devices (canes, crutches, walker), usually because of poor balance.[89] The quadriplegic (tetraplegic) group, if examined closely, will usually be found to be diplegic patients, i.e., lower extremity involvement greater than upper extremity but with variable upper extremity handicaps. Many tetraplegic patients have mixed involvement that is a combination of spasticity and motion disorder, particularly athetosis.

In pentaplegic patients the lower extremities are involved more than the upper extremities, head control is absent, and marked dysfunction of swallowing and phonation and loss of bowel and bladder control are noted. An increase in mental retardation and seizure disorders is found among this group, who may initially present as hypotonic babies, even up to the age of 2 years. Most patients in this category will require total care and have limited if any ambulatory potential.[15]

The incidence of the type of patient seen in an outpatient cerebral palsy clinic setting will vary markedly as a function of patient age, functional capability, therapeutic needs, and source of referral, i.e., home versus custodial care facility. The most common type of patients are the spastics, who account for approximately 60%, with 25% being motion disorder or mixed patients.

ASSESSMENT

All too often in modern medicine the most valuable test is overlooked, i.e., the history and physical examination. Osler cautioned, "Listen to the patient, he is telling you his disease." The diagnosis of cerebral palsy is usually based on a history of failure to meet normal developmental milestones accompanied by physical signs of neurologic impairment. A single examination often does not establish with certainty either the diagnosis or the classification of the individual patient's disease. Usually the patient's family reports events to aid in the diagnosis. A mother's concern that this child is different from her other children or a neighbor's children is often the first clue and a valuable historical point. Such narrative often refers to children in the 6- to 12-month age range.

Possible etiologic circumstances must be considered in terms of prenatal, natal, and postnatal events (Fig. 16.4). Prenatal influences include toxic exposures to heavy metals, medications, radiation, or infections, including the "TORCH" syndromes (toxoplas-mosis, rubella, cytomegalic inclusion body disease, and herpes). Also, intrauterine dysmaturity syndrome, a history of bleeding during various parts of pregnancy, decreased fetal motion, toxemia of pregnancy, or trauma to the mother or fetus are important perinatal events.

Natal problems include fetal anoxia secondary to a variety of circumstances, including umbilical cord compromise and placenta previa (often reflected in the Apgar I and II scores), respiratory distress syndrome (RDS), cranial trauma, and prematurity, the most common single factor.[27]

Postnatal difficulties include seizures, jaundice secondary to blood type or group incompatibility, transfusions, the need for respiratory support, and a history of the child being unable to return home at the usual postdelivery interval. Postnatal factors also include head injuries, cerebral infarctions or hemorrhage, anoxic episodes, such as following drowning or seizures, and meningitis in the first 2–3 years of life. No significant history of possible pathologic episode(s) is obtained in 20–30% of cases presented in the clinics with a complaint of delayed motor milestones and significant motor involvement.

The clinical pattern of involvement that is noted may be related to the source and site of the encephalopathy. Anoxia is the common factor to cortical damage. Trauma, hemorrhage, infections, and vascular occlusions also can cause changes, but the anoxia that these processes produce is the major source of pathology. The lesions subsequent to such anoxic episodes tend to be diffuse and lack specificity.[27] However, in premature infants, the periventricular infarcts or hemorrhages adjacent to the lateral ventricles affect the pyramidal tracts with resultant spastic diplegia with lower greater than upper extremity involvement.

Kernicterus causes basal ganglia damage with resultant athetosis, and cerebellar involvement will produce ataxia. A mixed pattern is seen when both cortical and basal ganglia are affected.

Developmental history is critical to the evaluation of the maturity of the central nervous system.[68] When a child holds its head up, sits up, is able to pull to stand, cruises, and achieves independent ambulation are major motor milestones. Creeping or crawl-

PRENATAL	MEDICATIONS
	RADIATION
	HEAVY METALS
	INFECTIONS
	(TORCH)
	BLEEDING
	TOXEMIA
	TRAUMA
	NUTRITION
NATAL	CORD COMPROMISE
	PLACENTA PREVIA
	RDS
	PREMATURITY
	CRANIAL TRAUMA
	MULTIPLE BIRTHS
POSTNATAL	SEIZURES
	ANOXIA
	JAUNDICE
	MENINGITIS
	INFARCTION
	HEMORRHAGE
	CRANIO-CEREBRAL
	TRAUMA

Figure 16.4. Possible etiologic factors of delayed motor ability at various times during development.

ing patterns are extremely variable in onset and type and usually of little diagnostic help.

A constant "fisted" position of the hand over the age of 3 months may be the intial manifestation of spasticity. Also, if the child has a preference for only one extremity to the exclusion of the other, one must suspect a lesion causing this discrepancy. Normal children usually do not demonstrate a preference for handedness before 20–24 months of age.

Bladder and bowel training patterns are also important to note, particularly if the child had been toilet trained and then loses such control. The onset of communication between child and parent is another notable achievement.

The abnormal physical findings in the child with motor handicap are often subtle. The best platform from which to assess such aberrant behavior is a solid understanding of the broad spectrum of "normal" in the infant and toddler.[22, 29, 49, 119] When one is faced with a crying, writhing, uncooperative child, physical examination seems a formidable task. However, if this examination is carried out in a sequential manner, the necessary information will easily be obtained. The child is observed for evidence of spontaneous motion

and symmetry of that activity. Head and chest diameter should be measured, because direct correlation (up to 1 cm) is present to about 3 years of age. This may be used in assessing macrocephaly or microcephaly. In children who are not capable of standing or sitting, primitive neonatal reflexes should be assessed, for they provide information regarding the state of maturity of the central nervous system as well as prognostic signs of ambulation potential.[45] Asymmetric tonic neck (Fig. 16.5), symmetric tonic neck, Moro and parachute reflexes (Fig. 16.6), as well as step-and-place response (Fig. 16.7), should be checked. As noted by Bleck,[15] the obligatory persistence of any one of the first 3 reflexes after the age of 6 months and the absence of step-and-place response and parachute reflex after the age of 1 year bode poorly for later ambulating capability (Fig. 16.8).

Many patients with spasticity often are initially hypotonic, particularly in the first 6–12 months of life, the so-called "prespastic phase" noted by Beals.[8] Although many patients with cerebral palsy go through this "floppy infant" stage, most hypotonic babies do not later manifest signs of spasticity.[37] As a general rule, if the child is able to maintain a limb against gravity, there is probably not

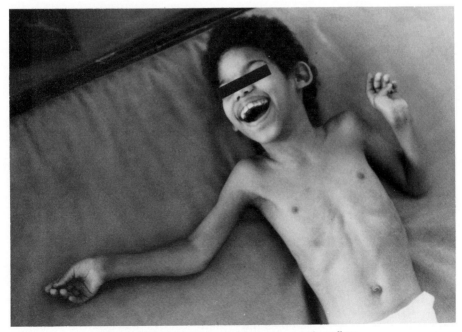

Figure 16.5. Asymmetric tonic neck reflex.

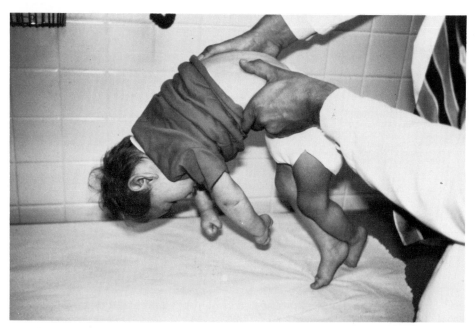

Figure 16.6. Negative parachute response. Note clenched fists in nonprotective position and head in flexion.

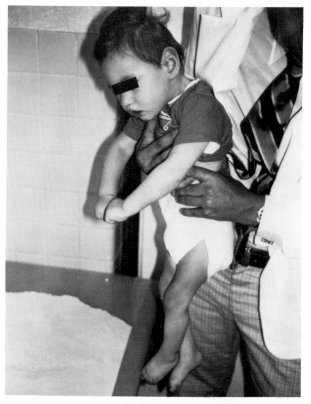

Figure 16.7. Negative step-and-place response and positive crossed-extensor reflex.

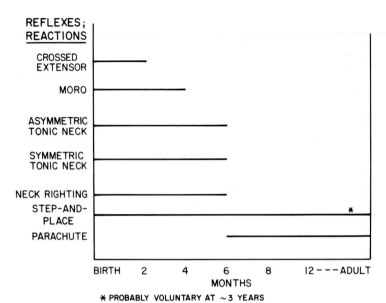

Figure 16.8. Onset and disappearance of primitive reflexes and postural responses.

excessive weakness. If weakness is present, then such conditions as infantile spinal muscular atrophy (Werding-Hoffman disease), central core disease, or nemaline myopathy must be ruled out. Also, such conditions as myasthenia gravis, poliomyelitis, or various muscular dystrophies must be considered in older patients.

Head control and head lag should be assessed by having the child rise from the supine to a sitting position either independently or assisted. Having a child rise from the sitting to standing position aids in ruling out evidence of proximal muscle weakness as would be evident by a positive Gower's test. Sitting capability is examined, because it, too, may serve as a motor ability prognositc test.[89] Standing, walking, and running are done to provide gait analysis.

Children with mild hemiplegia may not manifest any distinct upper or lower extremity abnormality while standing or walking slowly. However, while running, overt "posturing" of the upper extremity in adduction (elbow and wrist), finger flexion, and forearm pronation occur. The lower extremity will usually also show an equinovarus attitude. These changes are due to the compromised central nervous system being bombarded by the increased sensory input and the motor cortex not responding quickly enough to the challenge of the more complex motor act of running.

Normal gait is often considered a series of "controlled" falls. More formally defined by Perry,[96] it is a "sequence of standing postures which advances the body while retaining balance and security." It requires the ability to have a stable standing posture and to accomplish an effective stride. Because the problem in cerebral palsy is usually not one of strength but of proportional muscle control, the gait in such a petient is nonsynchronous, with subsequent increased energy demands because of inefficient patterns. In general, spastic children will have a decreased stance phase with a variable cadence. It must be recognized that a child with cerebral palsy does not have a normal gait and will never have a normal gait despite all the currently available therapeutic modalities, including surgery. It is essential that parents understand that surgical procedures will not produce a normal gait but may provide a more efficient gait. Gait analysis per se is beyond the scope of this chapter, and the reader is referred to various articles on this topic.[22, 32, 99, 117]

Ambulatory aides (crutches, canes, walkers) are noted, and any type of orthosis (including "corrective shoes") should be assessed for appropriate fit and function. One should ascertain whether the child does indeed still require the use of such devices.[11]

Neurological examination of the cranial and peripheral nervous systems is carried out. Many children with spastic diplegia have strabismus, but nystagmus is an uncommon finding and when noted requires further investigation into the possibility of cerebellar lesions. Arrested hydrocephalus may cause associated ataxia, especially with associated spasticity.

The range of motion of the upper extremities, spine, and lower extremities is assessed for fixed versus nonfixed deformities. Rapid stretch of joints must be avoided, because this will only cause increased muscle tone with a false impression of the arc of motion of the particular joint. The type of increased tone is noted, i.e., lead pipe, clasped knife, or rigid. Slow, steady assessment of the joint's range of motion will allow a much more accurate measure. Local blocks with either intramuscular alcohol or xylocaine into peripheral nerves (external obturator, posterior tibial, or median) are helpful to determine the status of myostatic contractures. Muscle grading of spastic muscles is a futile exercise because of the marked variance in muscle tone depending upon emotions, joint positions, or stress reactions in spastic patients, especially in those muscle groups not under voluntary control.

Physical and occupational therapists test functional capacities of these children, and their objective recordings provide an ongoing

CHILDREN'S HOSPITAL

NAME		BIRTHDATE	

DIAGNOSIS

FUNCTIONAL TASK	Age (mos.) Test Date Score		
1. Prone: Lifts & Controls Head 5/0			
2. Rolling: Either supine to prone or vice versa 5/0			
3. Sits unsupported 5/0			
4. Assumes Sitting 5/3/0			
5. Transfers Chair to Standing 5/3/0			
6. Walks 50 feet 5/4/3/0			
7. Crawls 15 feet 5/0			
8. Cruises 5/0			
9. Timed 50 foot walk			
10. Timed 15 foot crawl			

5=without help
0=unable to perform task
3=with assistance
4=ambulatory aide(s)

Figure 16.9.   Childrens Hospital, Pittsburgh, Cerebral Palsy Clinic, Physical Therapy Assessment Form.

record of the child's progress (Fig. 16.9). Such data allow a more critical assessment of the child's performance than the usual " . . . seems to be doing better" noted anecdotally by the parent and/or physician. In new patients, roentgenograms of the skull are done to rule out deformity as well as intracerebral calcification. Such roentgenograms are used to assess deformity and interpedicular distances, and roentgenograms of the pelvis provide information on the status of the hip joints. Serum thyroid, calcium, sodium, potassium, and phosphorus levels are obtained in new cases where the history is not clear regarding possible etiology of the neurologic condition. Muscle enzyme assessment and chromosome studies may also be required to aid in diagnosis. Computerized axial tomography can further assess spinal or skull lesions, particularly in patients with seizure disorders or acquired cerebral spasticity. If a full term neonate has seizures without an obvious metabolic or infectious cause, a computerized axial tomography scan should be done to rule out intracranial hemorrhage.

Gait analysis may be recorded on movies or videotape to provide a study that may be reviewed in a more leisurely and detailed manner. Films with ambulatory electromyograms and computerized force plate data integration are a current research tool (Fig. 16.10) that should find widespread application after sufficient numbers of preoperative and postoperative profiles are obtained for specific groups of patients.[32, 97-99, 126, 135]

PROGNOSIS

The adult brain possesses from 10^{10}–10^{11} neurons. Peak synaptic density occurs between 12 and 24 months of age, which may account for the ability of children to recover following injury.[35, 50, 57] As early as the time of Cajal, it was recognized that the brain is a highly structured system and not as randomly organized as might appear on initial examination. Unfortunately, much information is still needed to understand how the central nervous system develops, specializes, and repairs itself following insult. The high oxygen requirement for cerebral tissue was well emphasized by Little in his original paper.[78] At rest, the brain receives one-fifth of

the cardiac output and accounts for one-fifth of the body's oxygen consumption.

In general, in the normal child, neuromaturation is a function of the emergence of cortical dominance from spinal to brainstem to mid-brain control in an orderly, building sequence of events. Independent sitting, standing, and walking are not pinpoint episodes for all, but occur at a wide variety of intervals in normal children. The most primitive spinal level is characterized by mass flexor and extensor responses and is compatible with prone and supine lying of the type normally seen in children about the age of 2 months. With brainstem level maturation, asymmetric and symmetric tonic neck reflexes predominate and are present to the age of 4–6 months in normal children. The emergence of mid-brain control allows righting reflexes to occur and, therefore, quadripedal gait is possible. With cortical control, equilibrium responses are not present, and bipedal ambulation may occur. Children with cerebral palsy lack varying degrees of development of the normal postural reflex mechanism (righting, equilibrium, etc.) and have inability to inhibit the primitive neonatal reflexes and responses, the combination of which produces motor disability (Fig. 16.11).

To help parents understand the nervous system, a useful model is one of a telephone and switchboard to explain the effects of cortical control and peripheral response. The telephone (periphery) is normal but the switchboard (CNS) provides it with an inappropriate number.

Sherrington coined the concept of the "final common pathway" to emphasize the link between the brain and the motor neurons that affect muscle action. His concept of "proprioception" recognized the sensory inputs that arise during the course of motion. Hence, the stimuli to the receptors were delivered by the organism itself and provided a feedback based on the individual's own motion. Muscles both provide and resist motion and require the calibration of force, velocity, and displacement. Muscle length receptors trigger contraction to oppose elongation, whereas the tension receptors sense force and cause inhibition of associated motor neurons. "Ordinary" alpha motor neurons provide muscle contraction, with fine tuning of the motor system being done by the gamma neurons that act on muscle spindles to regulate sen-

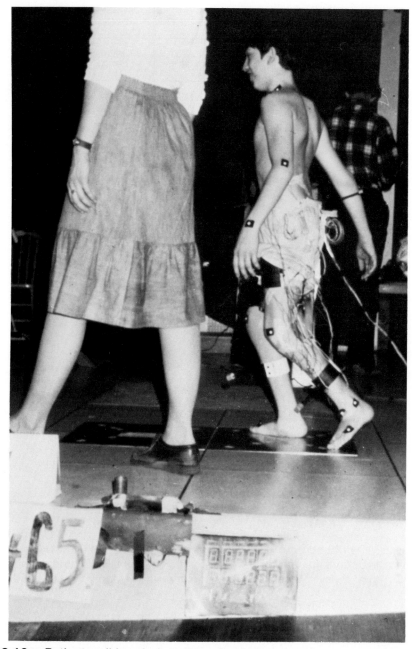

Figure 16.10. Patient walking during dynamic electromyogram gait assessment. Note force plate for vector analysis. (Courtesy of Children's Hospital Medical Center, Boston, Massachusetts.)

sitivity of the length receptors. Spasticity is noted via increased muscle tone and an exaggerated response to the stretch reflex. The spasticity is thought to result from gamma system release from control by higher centers. Aberrant patterns of firing with prolon-

gation of phasic activity are noted as consistent findings during functional electromyogram analysis in spastic patients.[32]

Volitional movements are considered those with a goal or purpose. Select motor control is that which allows sophisticated motion,

STATUS	REFLEXES; REACTIONS	MOTOR ABILITY
APEDAL	PRIMATIVE SPINAL AND BRAIN-STEM REFLEXES	PRONE-SUPINE POSITIONS
QUADRIPEDAL	MID-BRAIN; RIGHTING REACTIONS	TURN-OVER, SITTING, CRAWLING
BIPEDAL	CORTICAL CONTROL, EQUILIBRIUM REACTIONS	UPRIGHT STANDING AND WALKING

Figure 16.11. Progressive central nervous system maturation and functional ability.

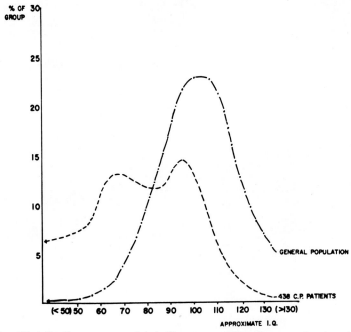

Figure 16.12. Distribution curve of intelligence rating for cerebral palsy patients as compared to the curve for the general population. (From B. Crothers and R. Paine: *History of Cerebral Palsy*; Cambridge, Mass.: Harvard University Press, 1959.)

such as a single joint moving while other associated joints maintain a fixed posture to permit that individual motion. Such selective control is often missing in patients with neurologic impairment, as in those with cerebral palsy.

Histochemical evaluations of muscle biopsies in spastic patients do not demonstrate any consistently abnormal pattern. In general, both types I and II muscle fiber atrophy due to central and peripheral nerve dysfunction are noted. In severely involved patients, atrophy of disuse is also seen.

Intelligence in patients with cerebral palsy varies from extremely low to rather high IQ scores.[31, 94, 140] However, approximately 50-70% of patients with the diagnosis of cerebral palsy fall in the category of the mentally retarded range of IQ testing (Fig. 16.12). Often, such testing is difficult because of limited communication capability of such patients. However, one must constantly be on guard not to assume that all patients with cerebral palsy are mentally deficient (Fig. 16.13).

Severely handicapped cerebral palsy patients had been noted by Schlesinger et al. in

1959[118] to have a 13–17 times increased death rate compared with normal children up to the age of 14, with a 4–5-fold increase among those mildly involved. Because modalities of newborn care have changed dramatically since that time, particularly in the salvage of the premature infant, these statistics may no longer be valid.

Bleck[15] found a 90+% accuracy when presence or absence of postural responses were used as predictors of later ambulatory ability in 1-year-olds. Persistence of obligatory Moro and obligatory tonic neck reflexes and extensor thrust with absence of step-and-place and parachute responses provided an accurate prognostic scheme for later ambulation. Beals[8] described a motor quotient equivalent to the motor age over the chronologic age. Results of motor tests done at 2 years were markedly uniform. He noted that the prespastic phase lasted 6–24 months and was then followed by a period of rapid linear improvement from ages 2–6 years, with the rate of improvement being inversely proportional to the severity of involvement. After the age of 7 years, a plateau of motor development was noted, and it was believed by Beals to represent the approximate end of

any spontaneous motor improvement (Fig. 16.14). A direct correlation with Beals' ambulatory prognosis was a decreased walking capability in patients with seizures. It must be recalled, however, that seizures are much more common in severely involved patients with limited original ambulation potential. As did other authors, Beals noted an inverse relationship between the severity of involvement and the quality of surgical result. Independent sitting by 2 years of age shows a good correlation with later independent ambulating ability, whereas inability to sit independently at 4 years of age is an ominous prognostic motor sign for later ambulation.[89]

Minear[85] advocated the classification of cerebral palsy patients according to functional classes I–IV and therapeutic classes A–D. Functional class I was essentially those with no limitation of activity, functional class IV was those incapable of any meaningful function activity, and classes II and III fell in between. Therapeutic class A consisted of those who needed no treatment, and class D was those requiring long term institutionalized total care.

The final function status achieved by patients is usually due to factors other than

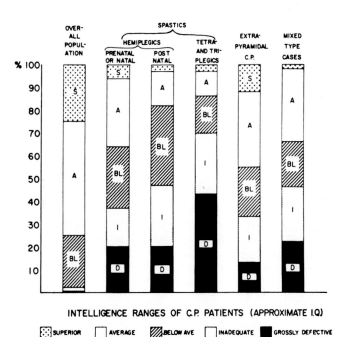

INTELLIGENCE RANGES OF C.P. PATIENTS (APPROXIMATE I.Q.)

SUPERIOR   AVERAGE   BELOW AVE   INADEQUATE   GROSSLY DEFECTIVE

Figure 16.13. The intelligence ranges of victims of cerebral palsy of various types is compared to that of the general population. (From B. Crothers and R. Paine: *History of Cerebral Palsy*; Cambridge, Mass.: Harvard University Press, 1959.)

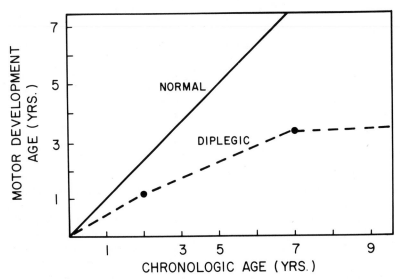

Figure 16.14. Motor development in normal versus diplegic children. Note plateau after 7 years. (According to Beals.)

physical ones, particularly personality and behavorial components. In general, the severity of motor and mental handicaps is proportional to the physical handicaps that are present. Speech handicaps, visual deficits (hemianopsia, strabismus), mental retardation, and seizure disorders are the common limiting factors to ultimate functional capabilities.[105] Optimally, about 35–50% of adult patients with cerebral palsy with the help of vocational training and rehabilitation will become self-supporting, particularly those with hemiplegia or athetosis.[28, 72, 88, 92, 105, 147]

GOALS

The data from the Department of Health, Education, and Welfare[140] estimate that the annual cost for patient care with "cerebral palsy" is $3.75 billion. Cerebral palsy must be considered a chronic disease, that is, one not cured but managed. Often this concept is difficult for orthopaedists to keep in focus because they are accustomed to treating conditions where cure is affected, such as following excision of a torn meniscus. Realistic goals must be set to avoid a chronic feeling of dependency by the parents as well as not providing false hope for them. If no potential exists, then limited goals must be empha-

sized. Efforts are directed to obtain the maximum function from whatever potential exists. It must be constantly kept in mind that a handicapped patient means a handicapped family. Counseling of the family, including siblings, is vital to provide needed understanding and to help alleviate the guilt, anger, and depression of the parents and to assuage anxiety regarding prognosis and treatment.[143]

The most commonly asked question of the orthopaedist by the parents of children with developmental delay, is "When will my child walk?" Although orthopaedists are enthusiastic to provide ambulation for patients, patient priorities place ambulation at the lowest portion of the scale (Fig. 16.15). Communication, independence of activities of daily living (dressing, feeding, and hygiene), and mobility rank far ahead of the patient's feeling of a need for ambulation. Ambulation per se must be considered at three levels:[80] (1) community, one who uses walking for routine outdoor activities; (2) household, one who uses walking as a means of room-to-room transportation; and (3) performance, one whose ambulation is limited to a physical therapy setting. The ambulatory category may change from community to household with advancing age and weight and subsequent increased cardiopulmonary demands with limited cardiac reserve. Such patients then realistically use a wheelchair for mobility.

Sitting should be considered in three categories: (1) independent, i.e., without any support; (2) propped, with head control; and (3) propped, without head control. Goals for each sitting and ambulatory category must be different, especially in terms of activites of daily living (Fig. 16.16).

MANAGEMENT

The team approach is an often misused term and concept. For it to function properly, communication between all members of the team must occur at frequent intervals. If not, the patient feels like a therapeutic football

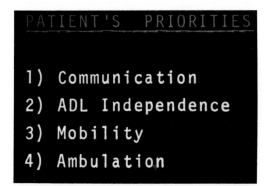

PATIENT'S PRIORITIES

1) Communication
2) ADL Independence
3) Mobility
4) Ambulation

Figure 16.15. Ambulation is lowest (by far) on the list of functional desires by the patient.

being passed from one evaluator to another. For a chronic disease such as cerebral palsy, the input of the social worker, speech pathologist, and developmental pediatric specialist is often much more important than that of the orthopaedist in terms of achieving the long range goals of these patients.[141] Treatment programs are a function of the patient's age, diagnosis, and available facilities. The aim of such programs is the treatment of the child and not the eradication of the disease.

An infant stimulation program is appropriate to provide techniques for improving balance, reflex inhibition, and reinforcement. It must be kept in mind that one must stand before one can walk; therefore, unless someone has standing capabilities, walking potential does not exist.

In general, two types of physical therapy programs exist. In the traditional mode, stretching, passive, and active resisted motion with specific muscle groups or joints are used to increase the range of motion. In the neuromuscular facilitation concept,[18] efforts are not directed at specific joints or muscles but attempts are made to alter posture and tone aberrations to elicit desired responses.

Occasionally, patients are placed in short leg casts in an attempt to provide a more stable base for ambulation and allow the therapist to work more toward proximal control, i.e., hips and trunk.

Any therapy program should not require the patient and his parents to become its

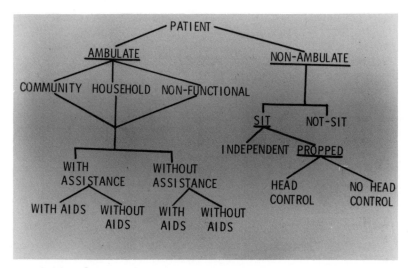

Figure 16.16. Scheme for assessment of patient's functional capabilities.

slaves, but rather should be realistically structured, because much effort must be expended at home and not in a single therapy setting. "Therapy" once weekly or less is essentially useless unless an appropriate home program is developed and understood by the parents. Despite enthusiastic and well meaning efforts on the part of many therapists, no program has yet proven its value in providing an increased rate of achieving ambulatory capability for children as compared with the "normal" progression of maturation of the central nervous system.[15, 94, 128, 145] An impossible set of variables exists among patients, therapists, and therapeutic modalities. The socially stimulating contribution of the patient-therapist interaction to the adjustment of the child, although impossible to quantitate, may be the most important factor.

It has been well recognized since the polio era that neurogenic deformity passes through several stages (Fig. 16.17): (1) a passively correctable one; (2) one with soft-tissue fixed deformity without bony change; (3) a fixed deformity with bony change. It must be emphasized that fixed deformity cannot be corrected by exercise.[30] Therefore, it is essential that the physician and therapist determine the progression or regression of deformity and take active steps to correct unchecked deformity progression. Persistent excessive stretching of spastic muscles somehow seems rather unphysiologic, especially in muscles that are hyperresponsive to stress.

Various medications, including L-dopa, sodium dantroline, and diazepam, have been tried in an attempt to reduce spasticity, but none have demonstrated any significantly consistent results.[33, 46] Diazepam seems to work primarily as a tranquilizer without an-

tispastic effect. Sodium dantroline causes nonspecific, inconsistent subjective feelings of decreased tightness, but no positive correlation was noted when assessment was done by objective task testing.

Neurosurgical manipulations of the central nervous system, including implantable stimulators, have not produced predictable success and must be considered experimental procedures at this time[52, 53]

Orthotic management requires the capability of an orthotist to provide orthoses to correct deformity and maintain its correction, not just to have such devices built in line of deformity. Serial assessment of correction maintenance is required, and adjustments must be correlated with any improvements. Orthotic principles applicable to the polio era are not appropriate for cerebral palsy patients where control and not power is the main deficit.[17, 96] Current fabrication techniques with thermoplastics allow the construction of orthoses that are lightweight and adjustable. These materials have revolutionized orthotic capabilities and have supplanted for the most part the cumbersome leather and metal devices that cause excessive burdens for children already handicapped by imprisonment within their neuromuscular system (Fig. 16.18).

Lower extremity orthotics are primarily for dynamic equinus deformities, and current lightweight plastics allow for ankle-foot orthotic fabrication that may be worn inside a shoe (Fig. 16.19). The high-top shoes with metal upright type orthosis usually do nothing more than hide persistent equinus deformity or, worse, rocker-bottom deformity of the mid-foot (Fig. (Fig. 16.20).

Upper extremity splinting to prevent deformity in spastic patients has met with limited success. Hemiplegic patients tend to remove the splint because of its interference with activity. In young patients, opponens and wrist extension splints are extremely difficult to fit.

Assist devices—e.g., long or large handled utensils, rocker knife, button hooks, etc.— often allow dramatic gains toward activites of daily living independence.

Mobility aides are required for severely handicapped children to allow transport about the home as well as in family or public conveyances. Correctly made, such custom-made devices can prevent spinal deformities in patients who require prolonged, propped

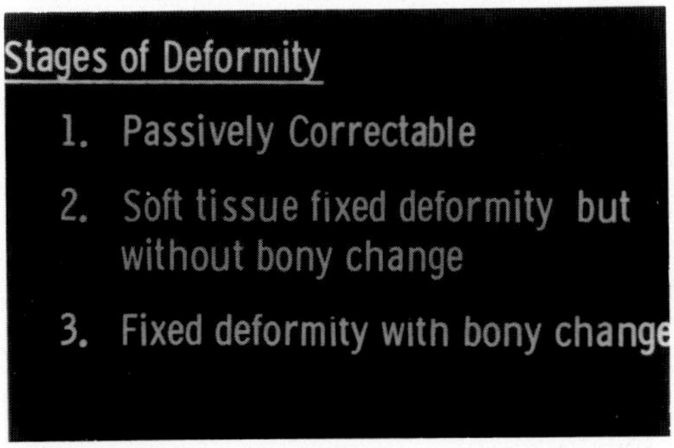

Stages of Deformity

1. Passively Correctable

2. Soft tissue fixed deformity but without bony change

3. Fixed deformity with bony change

Figure 16.17. Progressive stages of deformity.

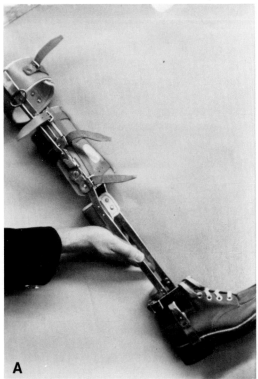
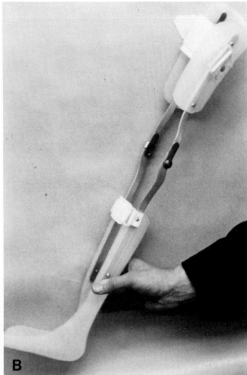

A   B

Figure 16.18. Cumbersome, heavy knee, ankle-foot orthosis of leather and metal contrasted with similar one made of polymers and metal.

sitting.[24, 48, 74, 91, 144] Balance and head control may be improved to the point where upper extremities can be used for basic functional tasks (Fig. 16.21).

With the miniaturization of electronic components, communication aides of a print-out type are becoming more readily available and allow the transfer of information for even basic needs among these patients to their attendants.[58]

SURGICAL TREATMENT

The role and benefits of surgery for the child with cerebral palsy have been disputed for some time, with enthusiasm for surgical modalities waxing and waning. With better preoperative assessment techniques,[32, 62, 97, 127] improved surgical procedures, and more enlightened postoperative management programs, surgery plays a significant role in the care of the involved child. Surgery is not meant to be a cure all—it is not.

This chapter is not designed as a text of surgical technique, and the reader is referred to the standard works on the topics regarding the surgical procedures as mentioned in the bibliography.

In the presence of limb or spine deformity, maximal function cannot be gained (Fig. 16.22). Thus, the primary goal of surgery for cerebral palsy patients is to provide maximal function, with a secondary goal being form or cosmesis. Most surgery is done for the spastic patient group, although the presence of a motion disorder, particularly athetosis, is not a contraindication per se to surgery. Surgery is designed to help the child obtain maximum potential, but it will not influence function where no potential exists.

The initial approach of surgery is usually with the soft tissues and then bone or combined bone and soft-tissue procedures. Judicious soft-tissue procedures may obviate the need for later bony surgery, particularly about the hip, wrist, and elbow.

The age at surgery varies, but it is usually done for children 4–6 years of age who can provide some measure of cooperation in a postoperative regimen. However, it must be

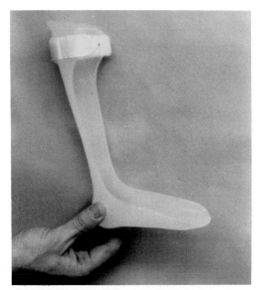

Figure 16.19. Plastic ankle-foot orthosis. It easily fits into a shoe and is lightweight; note the cosmetic appearance.

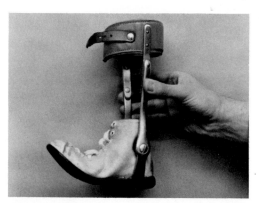

Figure 16.20. Ankle-foot orthosis with 90 degree stop without foot plate and rocker-bottom deformity.

recognized that surgery is necessary to overcome fixed, structural deformities at any age. We agree with Bleck[16] that a surgeon's goal should be a functional person and not a permanent patient. Therefore, staged surgical procedures may not be necessary when appropriate surgery can be carried out at one sitting. There has been much debate in the past regarding the sequence of surgery i.e., hips, knees, or foot/ankle procedures. No "recipe" is known, inasmuch as each patient's neurologic deficit and functional loss are

unique. With advances in dynamic electromyographic analysis, appropriate patient and procedure selection may be improved. Attempts to change radically the existing pattern of activity levels of a cerebral palsy patient will usually lead to a functional disaster for that patient. In the less severely involved patients, particularly the hemiplegics, much surgery is designed toward "fine tuning" and not correction of gross motor dysfunction.

Hips

It must be kept in mind that the hip is but one segment of an articulated, integrated,

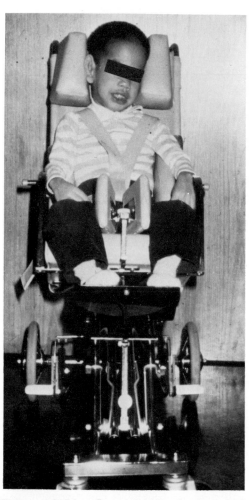

Figure 16.21. Specialized adaptive chair for patient requiring propped sitting, i.e., poor head control.

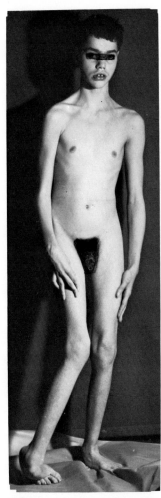

Figure 16.22. Motor system defect in cerebral palsy increased by deformity.

linkage system with a complex interaction between the lumbar spine, knee, foot, and ankle. The main problems in the hips of cerebral palsy patients are flexion, internal rotation, and adduction deformities, particularly in diplegic and pentaplegic patients. Rarely do these deformities occur in isolated fashion. Subluxation and dislocation of the hips are also commonly noted in the more severely involved patient. In nonambulatory patients, supple hips and a straight spine are basic requirements for sitting capability.

Excessive femoral antetorsion is noted in the spastic patient with diplegia or pentaplegia but, interestingly, not in hemiplegics. True coxa valga is rare and is an often misinterpreted finding on a routine anteropos-

terior roentgenogram of the hip.[9, 75] Instead of the usual regression of the infantile anteversion angle of 3–30 degrees to the 15–20 degrees seen in the adult,[42, 81, 112, 121] anteversion in spastics persists to an average of 55 degrees.[16] The exact reason for this increase is unknown, but several authors attribute it to muscle imbalance about the hip.[2, 9, 12, 108]

The cause of hip flexion contracture and deformity is not completely understood, and its management is a significant source of controversy.[2, 13, 103, 108, 116] The hip flexors include the sartorius, tensor fasia femoris, pectineus, rectus femoris, adductors, and primarily the iliopsoas.[84] Compensation for hip flexion deformity is by anterior pelvic tilt, with increased lordosis in the lumbar spine and increased flexion at the knees.

On physical examination, patients will often have a markedly positive Thomas test (Fig. 16.23) as well as a positive prone rectus (Ely) test. Rotation should be checked both with the hip at 90 degrees of flexion and in full extension to assess clinically the amount of antetorsion noted by the differential between the amount of external and internal rotation available in flexion and extension.

During gait, three patterns have been recognized in spastic patients:[12] (1) flexed, internally rotated hips with flexed knees secondary to spastic hamstrings; (2) flexed, internally rotated hips with extended knees due to spastic quadriceps; and (3) flexed, internally rotated hips with balanced knees because neither the quadriceps nor the hamstring predominate.

Roentgenographic assessment of the pelvis and hips should be done on all new patients to check containment of the femoral head within the acetabulum. This should be repeated at serial intervals of 6 months to 1 year to rule out progressive subluxation or dislocation (Fig. 16.24). Bleck[14] has advocated analysis of the sacrofemoral angle as measured on a standing lateral roentgenogram of the lumbar spine and pelvis where the angle created by the mid-shaft of the femur and the top of the sacrum is determined. This measurement is to provide an accurate assessment of the relationship between the hip and spine. In normals, the angle is between 50 and 60 degrees, whereas in patients with hip flexion contractures (and knee flexion contractures) this angle will be reduced to less than 50 degrees.

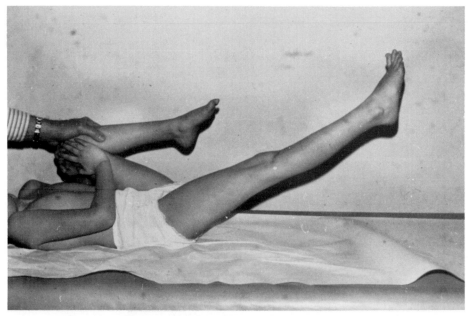

Figure 16.23. Positive Thomas test.

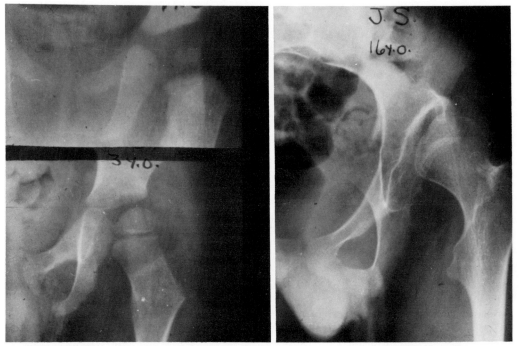

Figure 16.24. Progressive dislocation of a spastic hip from ages 1–16 years.

Surgical treatment for hip disorders includes soft-tissue, bony, or a combination of soft-tissue and bony procedures. A commonly performed procedure for adduction deformity and scissoring during gait is an adductor myotomy. In nonambulatory patients, adductor myotomy is most commonly performed to permit perineal hygiene care.

However, myotomy is not indicated in such patients unless fewer than a total of 90 degrees of abduction is present. The indication for complete adductor myotomy is rare. Overvigorous adductor release can cause excessive abduction, resulting in abduction contractures that are very difficult to correct[123] (Fig. 16.25).

Obturator neurectomy of the external branch is often done in association with adductor releases,[5, 114] particularly in total bed care patients (Fig. 16.26). In such patients, intrapelvic obturator neurectomy is easily performed and will usually produce long standing results to allow for hygiene care. In ambulatory patients, caution must be taken not to provide excessive release of the adductors with secondary loss of their usual function of stabilizing the hip in preparation for stance phase. In ambulatory patients, the adductor longus is usually the only one released because it is most commonly the prime offender. Muscular blocks with alcohol or blocks of the external obturator nerve with xylocaine will aid in patient selection and the need for neurectomy at the time of adductor release surgery.

Rectus femoris release is indicated in patients with combined hip flexion and knee extension deformity.[32, 38, 134] Rectus release should not be performed in patients with combined hip and knee flexion contractures because of already compromised quadriceps power.

Judicious soft-tissue surgery about the hip, including psoas recession, may allow improved muscle balance and prevent later subluxation or dislocation.[13, 70, 98, 100, 116, 132] The release of the psoas tendon from the lesser trochanter is performed in patients with persistent hip flexion deformity (Fig. 16.27). In ambulatory patients, as advocated by Bleck,[13] it is wise to transfer the tendon laterally and superiorly on the hip capsule following tendon lengthening in order to maintain some hip flexion power. If this power is markedly diminished (as noted following complete release), tasks such as climbing stairs or entering buses become formidable.

Progressive hip subluxation with secondary acetabular changes is due to combined psoas and adductor action with diminished abductor function, particularly in patients utilizing walking aids that unload the hip joint. Subluxation is commonly noted as stage one on the way to dislocation in a nonambulatory patient. In Samilson et al.'s[116] series, the average age of dislocation in non-

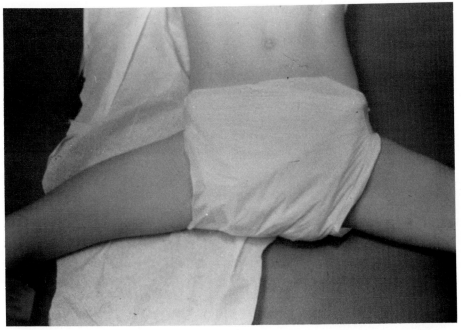

Figure 16.25. Excessive hip abduction following complete adductor releases and obturator neurectomies.

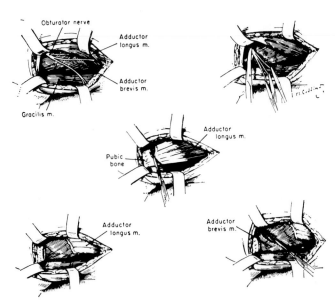

Figure 16.26. Drawing of adductor lengthening as done through a medial thigh incision over the adductor origins. (From H. H. Banks and W. T. Green: Adductor myotomy and obturator neurectomy for correction of adduction contracture of hip in cerebral palsy, *Journal of Bone and Joint Surgery, 42A:* 111, 1960.)

ambulatory patients was 7 years. Persistently subluxed or dislocated hips can cause pain as well as loss of sitting balance and pelvic obliquity, especially when unilateral (Fig. 16.28). Significant pain in the hip does not usually occur until the late teens or early 20s with the onset of degenerative joint disease and seems to be noted more often in patients with more neurologic maturity, i.e., those with decreased involvement.[90] Surgery for subluxated and dislocated hips is performed to prevent a progressively painful degenerative hip, to prevent or correct pelvic obliquity and improve sitting balance, to provide improved hygienic care in the perineum, and to eliminate greater trochanteric pressure areas secondary to pelvic obliquity.

Intertrochanteric derotational varus femoral osteotomy is the most common bony procedure performed with the neck shaft angle adjusted to between 100 and 110 degrees. Samilson et al.[116] advocated correction to 90 degrees in nonambulatory patients. Such an osteotomy may accompany a femoral shortening[73] with resection of a centimeter of bone at the level of the lesser trochanter with complete proximal release of the psoas.[43] This procedure is particularly helpful in attempting to correct combined severe hip and knee flexion deformities (Fig. 16.29). Using

the medial approach as advocated by Ferguson[44] and Keats and Margese,[70] I have been able to do combined bony and soft-tissue procedures (Fig. 16.30). Through such entre', adductor release, external obturator neurectomy and psoas recession or open reduction may all be carried out in addition to an intertrochanteric derotational varus femoral osteotomy using lateral percutaneous pins and casting or an external fixator for stabilization[129] (Figs. 16.31 and 16.32).

After the age of 9 or 10 years with evidence of subluxation or dislocation, marked acetabular dysplasia is commonly noted. In addition to a femoral osteotomy (possibly with shortening), a pelvic osteotomy is required of the innominate type.[26] With dislocated hips, the hip must be able to be centered at the acetabular level prior to the iliac osteotomy.

To manage the long standing, painful, dislocated hip in a total-care patient, the interposition resection technique described by Castle and Schneider[25] seems to be a rational way to solve this perplexing problem.[60] Care must be taken to resect an adequate amount of bone and release the psoas as well, prior to capsular interposition.

The spastic subluxed or dislocated hip is a significant challenge to the orthopaedist and requires judgment for the timing of surgery

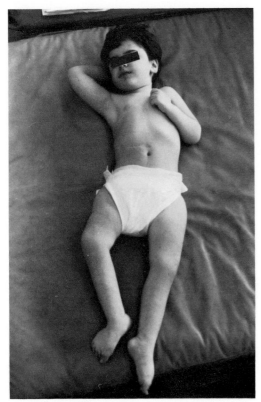

Figure 16.27. Spastic pentaplegic child with a right dislocated hip. The left hip had early soft-tissue surgery and has remained located. The patient had not returned for surgery on the opposite side.

and the correct choice of procedures to provide a stable but flexible hip that permits sitting without pelvic obliquity.

Knee

The knee is a key to gait adjustment capabilities in normal as well as spastic patients. The main knee deformities are flexion or recurvatum attitudes; they may be due to muscle imbalance between the quadriceps and hamstrings or be secondary to abnormal hip or foot-ankle postures. Knee flexion up to 15 degrees will still permit a functionally normal gait pattern on level ground.

Many diplegic patients require a crouched gait because it provides adequate stability for those patients with poor balance reactions. If such a patient is pushed backward and reacts

quickly and maintains his croched posture, he may very well require a certain amount of knee flexion to maintain balance. If he topples directly over when pushed from the front, knee flexion is usually not part of his compensatory balance mechanism.

With marked knee flexion contractures and fixation of the patella,[79] patellofemoral reaction force is significantly increased and will lead to degenerative joint disease. Forces across the knee may be great enough to cause patellar fragmentation.[110]

Prior to hamstring lengthening, excessive quadriceps spasticity should be determined because hyperextension may occur following such a release and markedly compromise sitting ability. Lengthening or release of the gracilis and semitendinosis only may be required for correction. Sectioning of the hamstring tendon sheath(s) should also be done because they are part of the structural changes that cause perpetuation of the deformity.

Posterior capsulotomy is occasionally required to permit further correction of a long standing knee flexion deformity. Care must be taken to prevent excessive manipulation following hamstring release, because fracture of the tibia or femur can occur in bone porotic from prolonged disuse (Figs. 16.33 and 16.34).

With dynamic internal rotation gait with increased knee flexion, a transfer of the semitendinosis laterally may act as a dynamic balancing force or tenodesis that will reduce the internal rotation and knee flexion position.[104] Caution must be taken not to compromise the posterior neurovascular structures with overaggressive correction of the knee flexion deformity.

Proximal release procedures of the hamstrings were reviewed by Drummond et al.,[36] and an increased lumbar lordosis with genu recurvatum was noted postoperatively in a significant number of patients. This lordosis was secondary to loss of posterior stabilization of the pelvis by the hamstrings with secondary anterior pelvic tilt and increased lordosis with further increase in hip flexion deformity. The Eggers procedure[41] (hamstring release and transfer to the femoral condyles) provides no significant advantage and may actually increase hip flexion deformity because of the loss of function of the hamstrings as secondary hip extensors (Fig. 16.35).

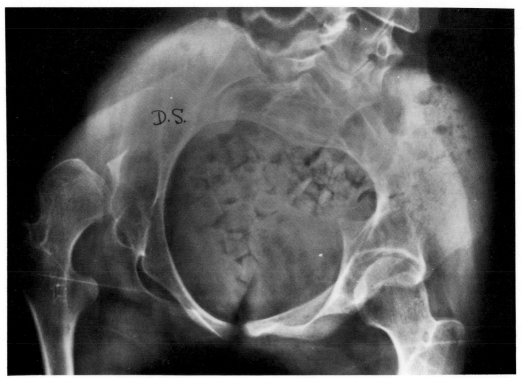

Figure 16.28. Spastic dislocated hip, pelvic obliquity, and scoliosis in 15-year-old with "wind-swept" lower extremities.

Dynamic genu recurvatum may be due to uncorrected ankle dynamic equinus deformity and may be treated with the ankle-foot orthosis advocated by Rosenthal.[109]

Foot and Ankle

Equinus is the most common deformity at the foot and ankle in spastic patients. In hemiplegic and diplegic patients, this usually begins as a dynamic deformity. Care should be taken in observing a toe-walking patient who has only recently begun to gain motor milestones. Many normal children will pass through a period of toe walking between 6 and 8 months following the onset of independent ambulation. In a child with delayed motor milestones, such a toe-walking phase may be transitory and part of their "normal" development.[22]

Excessive tibial torsion may be noted as a compensatory mechanism associated with excessive femoral antetorsion and internal rotation. The role of the lateral hamstrings in providing persistent external rotation deformity following medial hamstring release has been suggested[7] (Fig. 16.36).

During gait, the main role of the triceps surae is the deceleration of the tibia at stance phase to aid in roll off. Various procedures have been advocated to decrease triceps surae force (Fig. 16.37), including neurectomies of the gastrocnemius and soleus, gastrocnemius proximal recession, and open or percutaneous Achilles tendon lengthening.[4, 122, 133, 138] The Silfverskjold test has been used to differentiate gastrocnemius versus soleus function by flexing or extending the knee. Electromyographic data, however, have shown the test to be unreliable, because both muscles tend to be active with the ankle dorsiflexed beyond neutral, regardless of knee position.[99]

Tendo achillis lengthening is the most pernicious procedure in surgery of cerebral palsy patients (Fig. 16.38). Overlengthening either at time of surgery or casting following surgery may cause a calcaneus gait and marked disability, including progressive knee flexion,

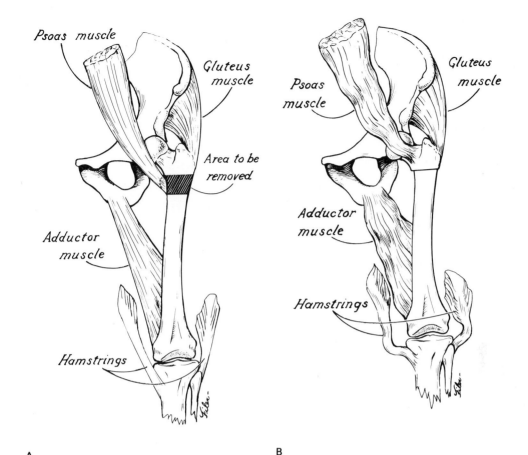

A   B

Figure 16.29. (A) Diagram of area for removal of bone segment from proximal femur. (B) Removing segment allows relative increase in length of iliopsoas (because lesser trochanter is removed), hamstrings, and adductors. (From A. B. Ferguson, Jr.: The effect of femoral shortening on severe spastic paraplegia, *Archives of Surgery*, 99: 349, 1969.)

increased hip flexion, and secondary increased lumbar lordosis. A lateral roentgenogram of the ankle is routinely obtained following tendo achillis surgery to make certain the tibiotalar joint is in neutral or 5 degrees of plantar flexion and not in dorsiflexion (Fig. 16.39).

Because the triceps surae is a triarticular muscle (knee, tibiotalar, subtalar), it may produce varus or valgus deformity at the heel. If a valgus heel is present, a percutaneous tenotomy is done of the tendo achillis in a hemisection fashion using the distal cut on the lateral side and then proceeding with proximal-medial and proximal-lateral section prior to sliding the tendon. If a varus deformity is present at the heel, the procedure is to go from distal to proximal in a medial-lateral-

medial sequence. In patients who have had previous open tendo achillis lengthening or in those with long standing fixed deformities without bony change, open tendo achillis lengthening is done in preference to the percutaneous type (Fig. 16.40). With equinus deformities of some duration, posterior capsular release may be required in addition to elongation of the flexor digitorum communis, flexor hallucis longus, and plantar fascia. Increased amounts of dorsiflexion at the tibiotalar joint following tendo achillis lengthening and capsulotomy will often unmask tightness in these plantar structures.

Pes varus deformity may be dynamic—i.e., in swing phase secondary to excessive anterior tibial function—or be present in stance phase secondary to excessive posterior tibial

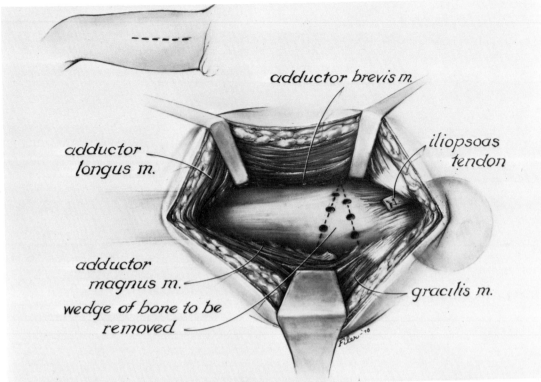

Figure 16.30. Exposure via medial approach. Psoas is recessed and osteotomy wedge outlined at lesser trochanter.

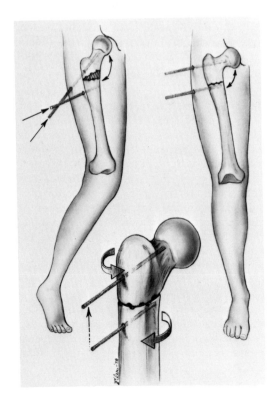

Figure 16.31. Percutaneous pins inserted with hip in abduction, internal rotation. Following osteotomy, pins are aligned in parallel manner to allow varus and derotation.

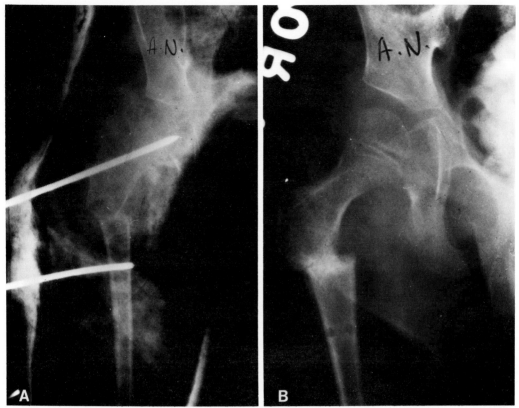

Figure 16.32.   Postoperative varus derotational femoral osteotomy.

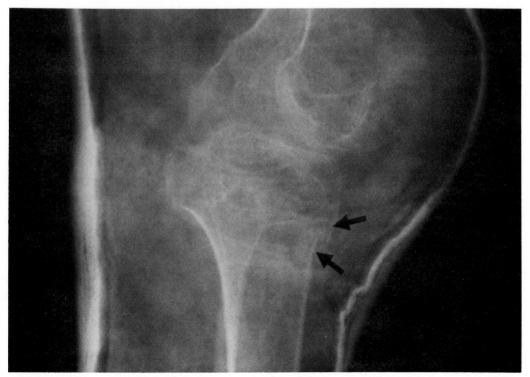

Figure 16.33.   Fracture of the proximal tibia following manipulation post-hamstring release.

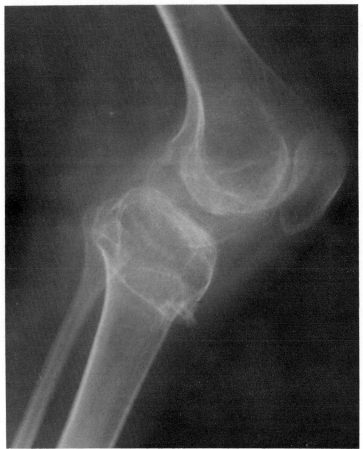

Figure 16.34. Healed fracture (see Fig. 16.33) with persistent subluxation of tibia and fixed patella.

function.[6, 63] Merely releasing the posterior tibial tendon may cause collapse of the longitudinal arch at the talonavicular joint with marked midfoot valgus. The role of posterior tibial transfer anteriorly is still questionable in spastic patients because of the excessive amount of force being transferred anteriorly.[10] For dynamic midfood varus deformities, i.e., without fixed deformity, the split anterior tibial transfer advocated by Hoffer et al. is a helpful procedure, especially in a hemiplegic patient.[63]

With a fixed hindfoot varus, a laterally based calcaneal wedge[125] with associated lengthening of the posterior tibial and Achilles tendon and plantar fascial release provides a plantigrade foot and eliminates the "razor-edge" deformity. With persistent, fixed midfoot and hindfoot deformity, a triple arthrodesis will provide a stable stance platform (Fig. 16.41). This procedure should not be reserved for only those older than age 13 but should be done when other techniques are not capable of correcting the fixed deformity.

Fixed pes valgus deformity with combined calcaneal eversion and equinus and associated forefoot abduction may best be treated with a calcaneal wedge osteotomy[40, 125] and associated peroneal tendon lengthenings. Extra-articular subtalar arthrodeses[54, 69] in spastics have not met with consistent success, the graft often dissolving and not providing the appropriate buttress affect (Fig. 16.42). Talo-calcaneal fusions have been advocated by some to provide stability at the subtalar joint in the optimal weight-bearing line.[34]

Metatarsus adductus is most commonly secondary to a spastic abductor hallucis and will respond to releasing the offending muscle. Hallux valgus is a common foot deformity in severely involved diplegic patients and

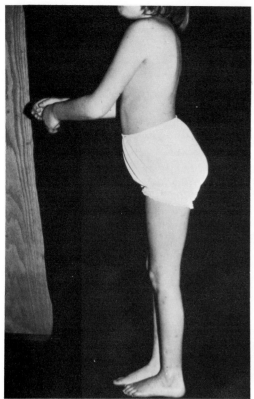

Figure 16.35. Increased lumbar lordosis, hip flexion deformity, and straight knees post-hamstring transfer to femoral condyles.

is best treated with adductor release and either proximal or distal first metatarsal osteotomy. At the same surgery, derotation of the proximal phalanx may also be required, depending on the severity of the disorder. With fixed hyperflexed toes, simple interphalangeal joint fusions will provide stability and prevent excessive wear both dorsally and plantarly.

Cavus deformities in spastic children are probably secondary to spasticity of the intrinsic musculature of the foot, and, in the presence of fixed deformity with bony change, triple arthrodesis is required. Occasionally, release of the plantar fascia alone in young children will allow for temporizing in their management.

With total body involvement in a nonambulatory patient, surgery around the foot and ankle is indicated to improve foot position while sitting (thus preventing pressure areas) or to improve stance stability to permit assisted transfers.

Spine

The deformities of the spine produced by muscular imbalance in cerebral palsy are usually progressive and often severe. Little has been written regarding the incidence of scoliosis associated with cerebral palsy.[3, 106, 111, 113] Various series report the incidence to range between 6 and 64%,[19, 80, 87] with the higher figure reflecting an institutionalized and for the most part bedridden population requiring total care. This contrasts with the incidence of scoliosis in the general population of approximately 1.9%.[107, 120, 146]

Because of the immature central nervous system with persistence of neonatal reflexes and sustained unbalanced muscle activity, significant dynamic forces are present on the spine (Fig. 16.43). Abnormal prolonged sitting or lying postures often aggravate appropriate spinal alignment.[48] Associated intrapelvic or infrapelvic obliquity will increase the severity of the spinal deformity, particularly with an unbalanced dislocated hip and "wind-blown" lower extremities[83] (Fig. 16.44).

The scoliotic type of curve may be either a "C-type" single curve or multiple curves,

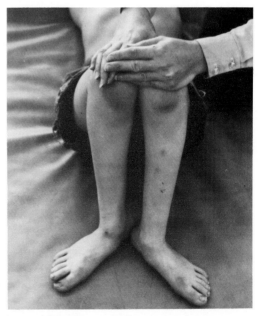

Figure 16.36. Excessive tibial torsion associated with marked femoral antetorsion. Patient had also had bilateral medial hamstring releases.

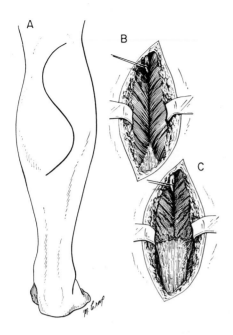

Figure 16.37. The gastrocnemius recession described by Strayer. The incision exposes the gastrocnemius muscle. The sural nerve is identified. The gastrocnemius muscle bellies are isolated and dissected from above downward to the attachment of the gastrocnemius and soleus. The tendon is then severed to make certain that all fibrous bonds between the soleus and gastrocnemius have been divided. The bellies then retract upward to their new location as the foot is dorsiflexed.

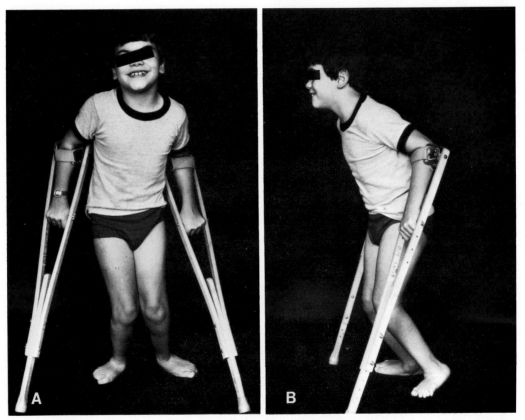

Figure 16.38. Diplegic patient post-tendo achillis lengthening with calcaneus gait and increased crouch with loss of balance requiring crutches for support.

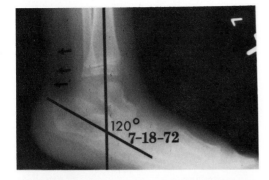

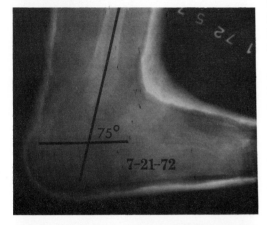

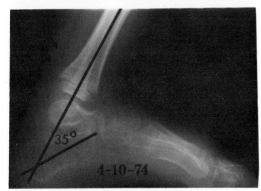

Figure 16.39. Progressive calcaneus deformity after tendo achillis lengthening and casting in dorsiflexion. Note loss of substance of Achilles tendon.

particularly the thoracolumbar type. Increased thoracic kyphosis has been noted, the kyphoses averaging over 70 degrees[71] (Fig. 16.45). Cervical spine degenerative joint disease with neural canal compromise may be seen in patients with motion disorders, particularly of the athetoid type.

Spinal orthotic devices may be helpful in sitting patients to control minor curves (less than 20 degrees) and perhaps to prevent their progression[21] (Fig. 16.46). However, the use of the Milwaukee brace in spastic patients has met with limited success. A plastic thoracolumbar jacket can provide improved sitting balance for less severely affected patients. Long term use of such devices has been implicated in a decrease in anterior-posterior thoracic cage diameter, with subsequent reduction in cardiopulmonary function.[87] Current orthotic techniques can allow for proper management of curves of smaller magnitude or as temporizing devices prior to surgery for the young child.

Until recently, surgical correction of spinal deformities in cerebral palsy was uncommon.[19, 87, 130] In the past decade, the use of the anterior approach and fusion with Dwyer-Sherwood instrumentation has become a powerful tool for correction of spinal deformity (Fig. 16.47). In addition, posterior fusion with instrumentation is also advised in spastic patients because of the pseudarthrosis rate following anterior fusion alone.[19] Such combined fusions provide excellent early rigidity postoperatively and permit mobilization of the patient with reduction of common bed-bound problems such as urinary calculi, infection, pneumonitis, and pressure areas. Postoperatively, cast application must be meticulous with fastidious attention to relieving pressure areas, particularly over bony prominences.

The exact degree and location of the curve to be fused in the cerebral palsy patient has not been precisely defined. Surgical stabilization is recommended for scoliotic curves of more than 40 degrees or for curves that show evidence of rapid progression.[130] The criteria for correction of lordotic or kyphotic deformities have not been delineated to date. Anterior longitudinal ligament release and in situ fusion can prevent progression of the kyphotic deformity.

In certain patients a staged procedure that includes muscle release and halo wheelchair traction followed by anterior and then posterior instrumentation and fusions may be required to provide appropriate correction. If an associated pelvic obliquity exists, it should be corrected prior to spinal surgery; if any residual obliquity is present, the fusion

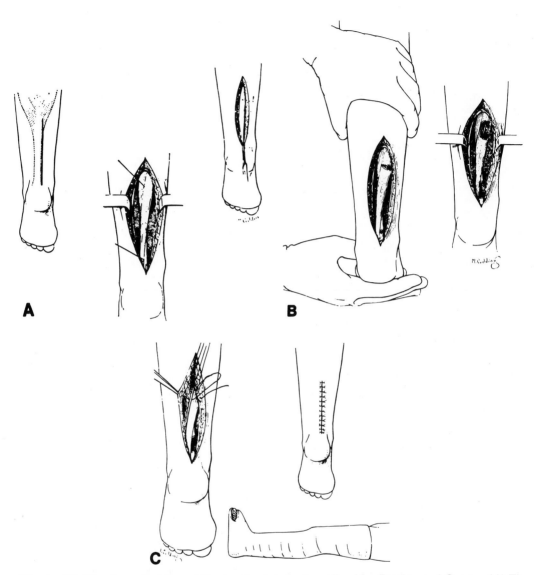

Figure 16.40. Lengthening of the heel cord as described by Banks and Green. (*A*) The incision is medial. (*B*) The rotation of the fibers of the tendon is studied, both cuts being made laterally. Those fibers inserting medially are divided superiorly; those inserting laterally are divided inferiorly. (*C*) The sheath is repaired after the tendon has been slid in order to avoid skin adherence. A long leg plaster is applied. (From H. H. Banks and W. T. Green: Correction of equinus deformity in cerebral palsy, *Journal of Bone and Joint Surgery, 40A:* 1359, 1958.)

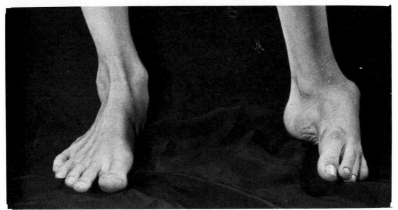

Figure 16.41. Foot deformity in patient with hemiplegia.

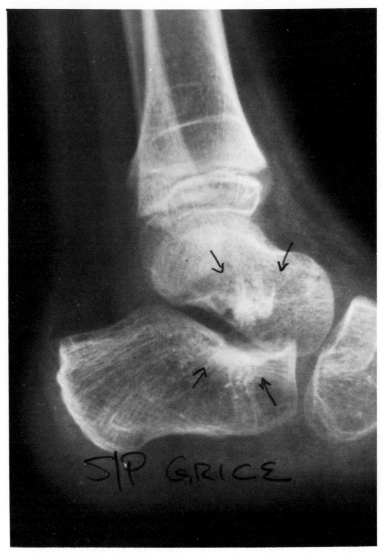

Figure 16.42. Dissolution of extra-articular subtalar graft for valgus deformity, 8 months postsurgery.

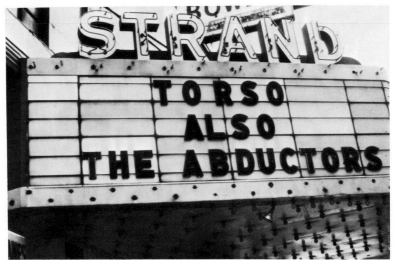

Figure 16.43. Movie marquee announcing importance of interrelationships of the trunk and pelvis.

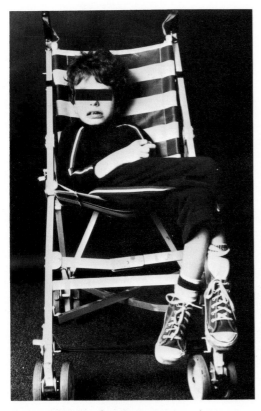

Figure 16.44. Seating allowing deformity. Note wind-swept lower extremities.

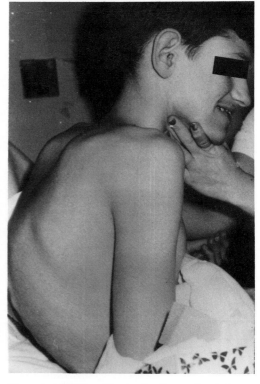

Figure 16.45. Kyphotic thoracic deformity.

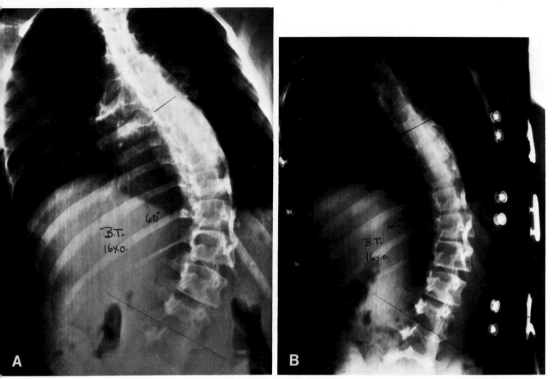

Figure 16.46. Progressive scoliosis in tetraplegic patient who was unable to sit because of imbalance. Thoracolumbar orthosis did not contain progression.

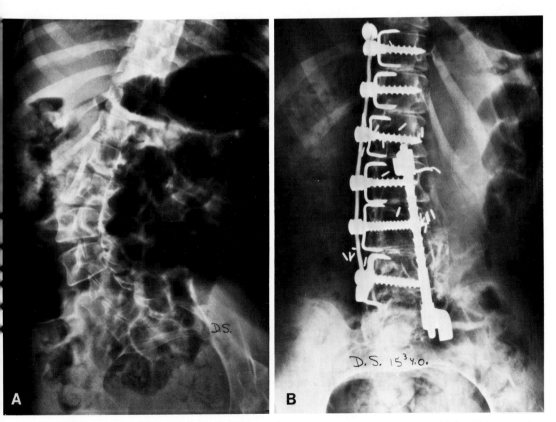

Figure 16.47. Progressive scoliosis with imbalance and pelvic obliquity. Note dislocated hip. Scoliosis corrected and pelvic obliquity improved following anterior and posterior instrumentation and fusions.

should extend to the sacrum to prevent further curve progression. Surgery is indicated to permit relief of back pain in these patients, many of whom have difficulty pinpointing the site of their pain because of communicative dysfunction. Surgery will also permit patients confined to a wheelchair to maintain adequate trunk posture that will permit maximum upper extremity function.

Upper Extremity

Involvement of the upper extremity in the cerebral palsy patient results in complex interrelated deformities along with significant sensory deficits.[51, 64, 115, 137] The main sensory deficits include marked proprioceptive and stereognostic losses that have been estimated to occur in 40–70% of hemiplegic patients. The lack of use of the upper extremity in the young child is often the initial manifestation of hemiplegia. This continued sensory deprivation may result in the patient completely ignoring the presence of this extremity, with resultant limited functional use as a "helper hand" (Fig. 16.48).

The primary goal of orthopaedic treatment is to improve gross function of the handicapped upper extremity, with a secondary goal of cosmesis. That proximal control must precede distal function is extremely well demonstrated in the upper extremity. Surgical intervention in the upper extremity in cerebral palsy is usually limited to the spastic patient and only rarely done for patients with motion disorders, specifically the athetoid type.

Upper extremity function needs to be tested in a proprioceptive realm by asking the patient to move the extremity to appropriately positioned targets. If the patient is unable to accomplish this basic task of positioning the hand, then functional goals must be extremely limited. A functional classification has been proposed by Green and Banks[55] and modified by Samilson and Morris[115]; it consists of four classes: *excellent*, good dressing and eating habits, effectual grasp and release and control; *good*, use of hand as a helper with dressing, eating, and effectual grasp and release and control; *fair*, use of the helper but without effectual eating or dressing function and only fair control; *poor*, use of the hand only as a paperweight

with poor or absent grasp and release and poor control.

Stereognostic deficits by themselves are not a contraindication to surgery in a cooperative patient who is able to obtain excellent visual clues. During assessment it is vital to check the basic functions of the hand in terms of not only grasp and pinch but release as well, because many patients require palmar flexion to permit release to occur. To improve dorsiflexion and grasp in these patients may be detrimental if they cannot then provide palmar flexion for subsequent release. As noted by Hoffer et al.,[62] the problem is usually with weak release and not with weak grasp.

The main deformities in the upper extremity consist of wrist and finger volar flexion, thumb-in-palm, forearm pronation, and elbow flexion. The thumb-in-palm deformity may progress from a simple dynamic one to a fixed contracture of the web space as well as the adductor pollicis. With fixed thumb-in-palm deformity, in addition to the de-

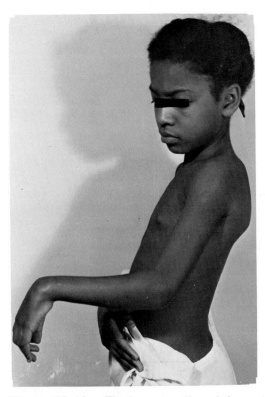

Figure 16.48. Flexion-pronation deformity with wrist extensor compromise.

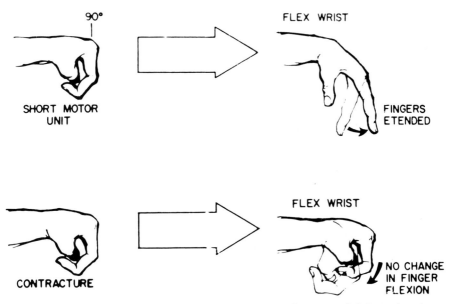

Figure 16.49.   Differentiation of short motor unit versus joint contracture.

crease of hand function from lost thumb capability, the thumb also becomes an obstacle to other fingers functioning appropriately.

Usually a Z-plasty of the web space is combined with an adductor pollicis and first dorsal interosseus release.[51, 82, 115, 124] Most thumb-in-palm deformities are also associated with metacarpal phalangeal or interphalangeal joint instability and weak thumb extensors and abductors secondary to flexor-extensor imbalance. To correct this instability, arthrodesis of the metacarpal phalangeal and interphalangeal joints may be carried out, or volar capsulorrhapy of the distal joint may be done if excessive flexion is not present.[136] Flexor pollicis longus lengthening is necessary with a fixed deformity. Augmentation of weak thumb extensors and abductors is performed by reinforcement with the brachioradialis, flexor carpi radialis, or flexor digitorum superficialis. Inglis et al.[67] presented an approach to the surgical correction of thumb-in-palm deformity by stepwise corrections of deformities that are unmasked at the time of surgery.

Bone block procedures between the first and second metacarpal are contraindicated in most patients except for those with persistent severe thumb-in-palm deformity where hygiene is impossible despite previous soft-tissue procedures. When faced with a patient with a wrist and finger flexion deformity, the source of the deformity must be ascertained and differentiation done between a myostatic contracture of wrist or finger flexors or a fixed capsular or joint contracture (Fig. 16.49). Testing is done by placing the wrist in volar flexion and demonstrating whether further passive extension may be gained at the finger joints. If this is not possible, a block at the median and ulnar nerves using xylocaine will often decrease muscle spasticity and permit passive examination of the range of motion in extension of the fingers (Fig. 16.50). Likewise, prior to flexor carpi ulnaris transfer[55] to improve supination and dorsiflexion at the wrist, assessment of the passively available range of motion and active extension of the fingers must be determined in order not to worsen the finger flexion deformity with the wrist in increased amounts of dorsiflexion.

Wrist flexion deformity is associated with weakness of the wrist extensors. The flexor carpi ulnaris may require a lengthening if adequate wrist dorsiflexors are present for balance. More commonly, the flexor carpi ulnaris transfer as recommended by Green and Banks[55] provides reinforcement of wrist dorsiflexion as well and serves to remove the powerful flexor deforming force at the wrist. Hoffer and associates,[62] using dynamic electromyography for preoperative and postoperative assessment, have recently recom-

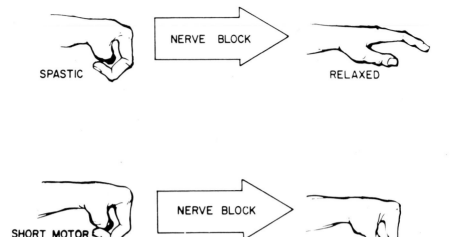

Figure 16.50. Effect of nerve block to aid in determination of spasticity versus short motor unit.

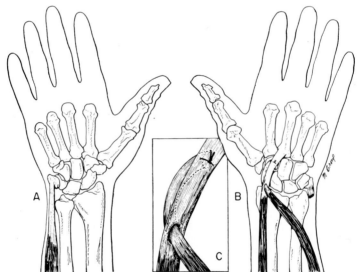

Figure 16.51. Transplantation of the flexor carpi ulnaris (*A*) to the long radial extensor (*B*). (*C*) Detail of insertion of tendon into tendon.

mended the use of the flexor carpi ulnaris transfer to augment finger extension and not just wrist extensor function because a combined weakness is usually present. They feel that, because spastic muscles are phase dependent and will not change phase, if the muscles are active throughout grasp and release of if a fixed finger flexion contracture is present, tendon lengthening rather than transfer should be done.

Radiocarpal-metacarpal arthrodesis is rarely indicated but is helpful to restore wrist

and hand alignment in severely involved patients following appropriate resection of the carpal row to provide correction.

Finger flexion deformities rarely occur independently and are almost always associated with significant wrist flexion deformity. Selective lengthening of both the superficial and profundus finger flexors at the wrist may be done to increase finger extension with the wrist in neutral position. Such lengthening provides a more anatomically appropriate result than proximal flexor muscle origin

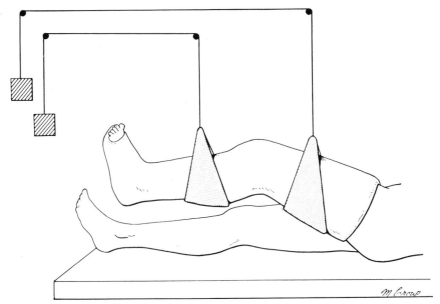

Figure 16.52.   Elevation of the limb in plaster helps control postoperative edema.

"slide."[66, 142] Decompression of the carpal canal at the time of finger flexor lengthening is also advocated to increase volume following increased dorsiflexion and to prevent median nerve compression. In the nonfunctional hand, sublimus to profundus transfer as advocated by Braun, Vise, and Roper[20] is a useful technique to eliminate chronic hygienic difficulties. With a forearm pronation deformity, pronator teres release is usually done in conjunction with flexor carpi ulnaris transfer to increase the range of supination. Persistent elbow flexion deformities that provide significant cosmetic loss during gait in hemiplegic patients may be managed with anterior elbow release as advocated by Mital.[86] For success to be achieved with this procedure, early assisted motion is required to maintain the elbow extension obtained at surgery.

The statement of Green and McDermott[56] in 1942 is still pertinent: "Surgical procedures, by reducing deformity, establishing better balance of motor power, decreasing spasticity of muscles and simplifying the problems of control are often an indispensable part of the process of habilitation." A vigorous postoperative program of appropriate physical therapy measures, orthotic use, and follow-up is as vital as any technique performed in the operating theater.

The principles of management of the patient with cerebral palsy have not changed markedly since the time of Little who in 1843 noted[77]: "I have had many of these cases under observation from one to twenty years and may mention as an encouragement to other practitioners that treatment based upon physiology and rational therapeutics affects an amelioration surprising to those who have not watched such cases."

Appreciation is expressed to Miss Sally Schneider, Mrs. Elizabeth Schaeffer, and Mr. Norman Rabinowitz for their assistance.

References

1. Andry, N: Orthopaedia 1741.
2. Baker, L. D., Dodelin, N. D., and Bassett, F. H.: Pathological changes in the hip in cerebral palsy: incidence, pathogenesis, and treatment, J. Bone Joint Surg., 44A:1131, 1962.
3. Balmar, G. A., and MacEwen, G. D.: The incidence of scoliosis in cerebral palsy, J. Bone Joint Surg., 52B:134, 1970.
4. Banks, H. H., and Green, W. T.: Correction of equinus deformity in cerebral palsy, J. Bone Joint Surg., 40A:1359, 1958.
5. Banks, H. H., and Green, W. T.: Adductor myotomy and obturator neurectomy for correction of adduction contracture of hips in cerebral palsy, J. Bone Joint Surg., 42:111, 1960.
6. Banks, H. H., et al.: The varus foot in cerebral palsy, J. Bone Joint Surg., 58A:729, 1976.
7. Bassett, F. H., et al.: Hamstring procedures in cerebral palsy: a sequence after long follow-up. B. Recommendations for current practice, J. Bone Joint Surg., 58A:725, 1976.
8. Beals, R. K.: Spastic paraplegia and diplegia: an

evaluation of non-surgical and surgical factors influencing the prognosis for ambulation, *J. Bone Joint Surg., 48A:* 827, 1966.

9. Beals, R. K.: Developmental changes in the femur and acetabulum in spastic paraplegia and diplegia, *Dev. Med. Child Neurol., 11:* 303, 1969.

10. Bisla, R. S., Lovis, H. J., and Albano, P. S.: Transfer of the tibialis posterior tendon in cerebral palsy, *J. Bone Joint Surg., 58A:* 297, 1976.

11. Bleck, E. E.: The shoeing of children: sham or science? *Dev. Med. Child Neurol., 13:* 188, 1971.

12. Bleck, E. E.: The hip in cerebral palsy, In *Instructional Course Lectures, American Academy of Orthopaedic Surgeons;* St. Louis: C. V. Mosby, 1971.

13. Bleck, E. E.: Surgical management of spastic flexion deformities of the hip with special reference to iliopsoas recession, *J. Bone Joint Surg., 53A:* 1468, 1971.

14. Bleck, E. E.: Deformities of the spine and pelvis in cerebral palsy, In *Orthopaedic Aspects of Cerebral Palsy,* Samilson, R. L. (ed); Philadelphia: J. B. Lippincott, 1975.

15. Bleck, E. E.: Locomotor prognosis in cerebral palsy, *Dev. Med. Child Neurol., 17:* 18, 1975.

16. Bleck, E. E.: *Orthopaedic Management of Cerebral Palsy;* Philadelphia: W. B. Saunders, 1979.

17. Bleck, E. E., and Berzins, U. J.: Conservative management of pes valgus with plantar flexed talus, flexible, *Clin. Orthop., 122:* 85, 1977.

18. Bobath, K. *The Motor Deficit in Patients with Cerebral Palsy,* Clinics in Developmental Medicine No. 23; London: Heineman Medical Books, 1966.

19. Bonnett, C., Brown, J. C., and Grow, T.: Thoracolumbar scoliosis in cerebral palsy, *J. Bone Joint Surg., 58A:* 328, 1976.

20. Braun, R. M., Vise, G. T., and Roper, B.: Preliminary experience with superficialis-to-profundus tendon transfer in the hemiplegic upper extremity, *J. Bone Joint Surg., 56A:* 466, 1974.

21. Bunnell, W. P., and MacEwen, G. D.: Non-operative treatment of scoliosis in cerebral palsy: preliminary report on the use of a plastic jacket, *Dev. Med. Child Neurol., 19:* 45, 1977.

22. Burnett, C. N., and Johnson, E. W.: Development of gait in childhood—parts I and II, *Dev. Med. Child Neurol., 13:* 196, 207, 1971.

23. Cajal, R. S.: *Degeneration and Regeneration of the Nervous System;* London: Oxford University Press, 1928.

24. Carlson, J. M., and Winter, R.: *The "Gillette" sitting support orthosis, Orthot. Prosthet., 32:* 35, 1978.

25. Castle, M. E., and Schneider, C.: Proximal femoral resection—interposition arthroplasty, *J. Bone Joint Surg., 60A:* 1051, 1978.

26. Chiari, K.: Medical displacement osteotomy of the pelvis, *Clin. Orthop., 98:* 55, 1974.

27. Churchill, J. A.: On the etiology of cerebral palsy in premature infants, *Neurology, 20:* 305, 1970.

28. Cohen, P., and Koh, J. G.: Follow-up study of patients with cerebral palsy. *West. J. Med., 130:* 6, 1979.

29. Coon, V., Donato, G., Houser, C., and Bleck, E. E.: Normal ranges of hip motion in infants six weeks, three months and six months of age, *Clin. Orthop., 110:* 256, 1975.

30. Cooper, R. R.: Alterations during immobilization and degeneration of skeletal muscle in cats, *J. Bone Joint Surg., 54A:* 919, 1972.

31. Crothers, B., and Paine, R. S.: *Natural History of Cerebral Palsy;* Cambridge: Harvard University Press, 1959.

32. Csongradi, J., Bleck, E. E., and Ford, W. F.: Gait electromyography in normal and spastic children with special reference to quadriceps femoris and hamstring muscles, *Dev. Med. Child Neurol., 21:* 738, 1979.

33. Denhoff, E., Feldman, S., Smith, M. G., Litchman, H., and Holden, W.: Treatment of spastic cerebral palsied children with sodium dantrolene, *Dev. Med. Child Neurol., 17:* 736, 1975.

34. Dennyson, W. G., and Fulford, R.: Subtalar arthrodesis by cancellous grafts and metallic fixation, *J. Bone Joint Surg., 58B:* 507, 1976.

35. Dobbing, J., and Sands, J.: Quantitative growth and development of the human brain, *Arch. Dis. Child., 48:* 757, 1973.

36. Drummond, D. S., Rogala, E., Templeton, J., and Cruess, R.: Proximal hamstring release for knee flexion and crouched posture in cerebral palsy, *J. Bone Joint Surg., 56A:* 1598, 1974.

37. Dubowitz, V.: *The Floppy Infnat,* Clinics in Developmental Medicine, No. 31; London: Spastics Society with Heineman, 1969.

38. Duncan, W. R.: Release of rectus femoris in spastic children, *J. Bone Joint Surg., 37A:* 634, 1955.

39. Duncan, W. R.: Tonic reflexes of the foot, *J. Bone Joint Surg., 42A:* 859, 1960.

40. Dwyer, F. C.: Osteotomy of the calcaneum in the treatment of grossly everted feet with special reference to cerebral palsy, In *Proceedings of the 8th Congress of Orthopedic Surgeons and Trauma,* New York, September 1960; Brussels: Imprimerie Medicale of Scientifique, 1960.

41. Eggers, G. W. N.: Transplantation of hamstring tendons to femoral condyles in order to improve hip extension and to decrease knee flexion in cerebral spastic paralysis, *J. Bone Joint Surg., 34A:* 827, 1952.

42. Fabry, G., MacEwen, G. P., and Shands, A. R.: Torsion of the femur, *J. Bone Joint Surg., 55A:* 1726, 1973.

43. Ferguson, A. B., Jr.: The effect of femoral shortening on severe spastic paraplegia, *Arch. Surg., 99:* 349, 1969.

44. Ferguson, A. B., Jr.: Primary open reduction of congenital dislocation of the hip using a median adductor approach, *J. Bone Joint Surg., 55A:* 671, 1973.

45. Fiorentino, M. R.: Reflex testing methods for evaluation, In *C.N.S. Development;* Springfield, Ill.: Charles C Thomas, 1973.

46. Ford, L. F., Bleck, E. E., Collins, F. J., and Stevick, D.: Efficacy of dantrolene sodium in the treatment of spastic cerebral palsy, *Dev. Med. Child Neurol., 18:* 770, 1976.

47. Freud, S. *Infantile Cerebral Paralysis* (1897); Miami: University of Miami Press, 1962.

48. Fulford, G. E., and Brown, J. K.: Position as a cause of deformity in children with cerebral palsy, *Dev. Med. Child Neurol., 18:* 305, 1976.

49. Gesell, A., and Amatruda, C. S.: *Developmental Diagnosis,* 2nd Ed.; New York: Hoeber Medical Division of Harper and Row, 1947.

50. Goldman, P. S.: An alternative to developmental plasticity: heterology of central nervous system structures in infants and adults, In *Plasticity and*

Recovery of Function in the Central Nervous System, Stein, P. G., Rosen, J. J., and Butters, N. (eds.); New York: Academic Press, 1974.

51. Goldner, J. L.: The upper extremity in cerebral palsy, In *Orthopaedic Aspects of Cerebral Palsy*, Samilson, R. L. (ed.); Philadelphia: J. B. Lippincott, 1976.
52. Gornall, P., Hitchcock, E., and Kirkland, I. S.: Stereotaxic neurosurgery in the management of cerebral palsy, *Dev. Med. Child Neurol.*, 17: 279, 1975.
53. Grabow, J. D.: Cerebellar stimulation for the control of seizures, *Mayo Clin. Proc.*, 49: 759, 1974.
54. Grice, D. S.: Extra-articular arthrodesis of the subtalar joint for correction of paralytic flat feet in children, *J. Bone Joint Surg.*, 34A: 927, 1952.
55. Green, W. T., and Banks, H. H.: The flexor carpi ulnaris transplant and its use in cerebral palsy, *J. Bone Joint Surg.*, 44A: 1343, 1962.
56. Green, W. T., and McDermott, L. J.: Operative treatment of cerebral palsy of the spastic type, *J. A. M. A.*, 118: 434, 1942.
57. Guth, L.: History of central nervous system regeneration research, *Exp. Neurol.*, 48: 3, 1975.
58. Hagen, C., Porter, W., and Brink, J. D.: Non-verbal communication: an alternative mode of communication for the child with severe cerebral palsy, *J. Speech Hear. Disord.*, 38: 445, 1973.
59. Hoffer, M. M.: Basic considerations and classification of cerebral palsy, In *American Academy of Orthopaedic Surgeons Instructional Course Lectures*, vol. 25, p. 106; St. Louis: C. V. Mosby, 1976.
60. Hoffer, M. M., Abraham, E., and Nickel, V.: Salvage surgery at the hip to improve sitting posture of mentally retarded, severely disabled children with cerebral palsy, *Dev. Med. Child Neurol.*, 14: 51, 1972.
61. Hoffer, M. M., Feiwell, E., Perry, R., Perry, J., and Bonnett, C.: Functional ambulation in patients with myelomenigocele, *J. Bone Joint Surg.*, 55A: 137, 1973.
62. Hoffer, M. M., Perry, J., and Melkonian, G. J.: Dynamic electromyography and decision-making for surgery in the upper extremities of patients with cerebral palsy, *J. Hand Surg.*, 45: 424, 1979.
63. Hoffer, M. M., Reswig, J. A., Garrett, A. M., and Perry, J.: The split anterior tibial tendon transfer in treatment of spastic varus of the hindfoot in childhood, *Orthop. Clin. North Am.*, 5: 31, 1974.
64. Hohman, L. B., Baker, L., and Reed, R.: Sensory disturbances in children with infantile hemiplegia, triplegia and quadriplegia, *Am. J. Phys. Med.*, 37: 1, 1958.
65. Holt, K. S. *Growth Disturbances*, Clinics in Developmental Medicine, vol. 4, p. 39; London: Spastics Society, 1961.
66. Inglis, A. E., and Cooper, W.: Release of flexor-pronator origin for flexion deformities of the hand and wrist in spastic paralysis: a study of eighteen cases, *J. Bone Joint Surg.*, 48A: 847, 1966.
67. Inglis, A. E., Cooper, W., and Bruton, W.: Surgical correction of thumb deformities in spastic paralysis, *J. Bone Joint Surg.*, 52A: 253, 1970.
68. Jones, M.: Differential diagnosis and natural history of the cerebral palsied child, In *Orthopaedic Aspects of Cerebral Palsy*, Samilson, R. L. (ed.); Philadelphia: J. B. Lippincott, 1976.
69. Keats, S.: Warning: serious complications caused by the routine re-routing of the peroneus longus and brevis tendons in performing the Grice procedure in cerebral palsy (abstract), *J. Bone Joint Surg.*, 56A: 1304, 1974.
70. Keats, S., and Margese, A. N.: A simple anteromedial approach to the lesser trochanter of the femur for the release of the iliopsoas tendon, *J. Bone Joint Surg.*, 49A: 632, 1967.
71. Keller, R. B.: Spine deformity in the retarded, Paper presented at the Scoliosis Research Society Meeting, September 1978.
72. Klapper, Z. S., and Birch, H. G.: The relationship of childhood characteristics to outcome in young adults with cerebral palsy, *Dev. Med. Child Neurol.*, 8: 645, 1966.
73. Klisic, P., and Jankovic, L.: Combined procedure of open reduction and shortening of the femur in treatment of congenital dislocation of the hips in older children, *Clin. Orthop.*, 119: 60, 1976.
74. Letts, R. M., Fulford, R., and Hobson, D. A.: Mobility aids for the paraplegic child, *J. Bone Joint Surg.*, 58A: 38, 1976.
75. Lewis, F. R., Samilson, R. L., and Lucas, D. B.: Femoral torsion and coxa valga in cerebral palsy—a preliminary report, *Dev. Med. Child Neurol.*, 6: 591, 1964.
76. Little, W. J.: *A Treatise on the Nature of Club Feet and Analogous Distortions*; London: W. Jeffs, 1839.
77. Little, W. J.: Lectures on the nature and treatment of the deformities of the human frame, *Lancet*, 1: 350, 1843.
78. Little, W. J.: On the influence of abnormal parturition, difficult labours, premature birth and asphyxia neonatorum on the mental and physical condition of the child, especially in relation to deformities, *Trans. Obstet. Soc. Lond.*, 3: 293, 1862.
79. Lotman, D. B.: Knee flexion deformity and patella alta in spastic cerebral palsy, *Dev. Med. Child Neurol.*, 18: 315, 1976.
80. Madigan, P. R., and Wallace, S. L.: Scoliosis in the institutionalized cerebral palsy population, Paper presented at the Scoliosis Research Society Meeting, September 1979.
81. Magilligan, D. J.: Calculations of the angle of anteversion by means of horizontal lacteral roentgenography, *J. Bone Joint Surg.*, 38A: 1231, 1956.
82. Matev, I.: Surgical treatment of spastic "thumb-in-palm" deformity, *J. Bone Joint Surg.*, 45B: 703, 1963.
83. Mayer, L.: Fixed paralytic obliquity of the pelvis, *J. Bone Joint Surg.*, 13: 1, 1931.
84. Michele, A. A.: *Iliopsoas*; Springfield, Ill.: Charles C Thomas, 1962.
85. Minear, W. L.: A classification of cerebral palsy, *Pediatrics*, 18: 841, 1956.
86. Mital, M. A.: Lengthening of the elbow flexors in cerebral palsy, *J. Bone Joint Surg.*, 61A: 515, 1979.
87. Moe, J. H., Winter, R. B., Bradford, D. S., and Lonstein, J. E.: *Scoliosis and other Spinal Deformities*; W. B. Saunders, Philadelphia, 1978.
88. Moed, M., and Litwin, D.: The employability of the cerebral palsied; summary of two related studies, *Rehabil. Lit.*, 24: 266, 1963.
89. Molnar, G. E., and Taft, H.: Pediatric rehabilitation. Part I. Cerebral palsy and spinal cord injury, *Curr. Probl. Pediatr.*, 7: No. 3, 1977.
90. Moreau, M., Drummond, D. S., Rogala, E., Ashworth, A., and Porter, T.: Natural history of the dislocated hip in spastic cerebral palsy, *Dev. Med.*

Child Neurol., *21*: 749, 1979.

91. Motloch, W. M.: Seating and positioning for the physically impaired, *Orthot. Prosthet.*, *31*: 11, 1977.

92. O'Reilly, D. E.: Care of the cerebral palsied: outcome of the past and needs of the future, *Dev. Med. Child Neurol.*, *17*: 141, 1975.

93. Osler, W.: *The Cerebral Palsies of Children.* A clinical study from the Infirmary for Nervous Diseases, Philadelphia, 1889.

94. Paine, R. S.: On the treatment of cerebral palsy: the outcome of 177 patients, 74 totally untreated, *Pediatrics*, *29*: 605, 1962.

95. Perlstein, M. A., and Hood, P. M.: Infantile spastic hemiplegia, intelligence, oral language and motor development, *Courrier*, *6*: 567, 1956.

96. Perry, J.: Pathomechanis, In *Atlas of Orthotics—Biomechanical Principles and Applications*, American Academy of Orthopaedic Surgeons; St. Louis: C. V. Mosby, 1975.

97. Perry, J., and Hoffer, M. M.: Preoperative and postoperative dynamic electromyography as an aid in planning tendon transfers in children with cerebral palsy, *J. Bone Joint Surg.*, 531, 1977.

98. Perry, J., Hoffer, M., Antonelli, D., Plut, J., Lewis, G., and Greenberg, R.: Electromyography before and after surgery for hip deformity in children with cerebral palsy, *J. Bone Joint Surg.*, *58A*: 201, 1976.

99. Perry, J., Hoffer, M., Giovan, P., Antonelli, D., and Greenberg, R.: Gait analysis of the triceps surae in cerebral palsy, *J. Bone Joint Surg.*, *56A*: 511, 1974.

100. Peterson, L. T.: Tenotomy in the treatment of spastic paraplegia with special reference to the iliopsoas, *J. Bone Joint Surg.*, *32A*: 875, 1950.

101. Phelps, W. M.: *Cerebral Birth Injuries, Their Orthopaedic Classification and Subsequent Treatment*; New York: New York Academy of Medicine, January 15, 1932.

102. Phelps, W. M.: Long-term results of orthopedic surgery in cerebral palsy, *J. Bone Joint Surg.*, *39A*: 53, 1957.

103. Phelps, W. M.: Prevention of acquired dislocation of the hip in cerebral palsy, *J. Bone Joint Surg.*, *41A*: 440, 1959.

104. Ray, R. L., and Ehrlich, M. G.: Lateral hamstring transfer and gait improvement in the cerebral patient, *J. Bone Joint Surg.*, *61A*: 719, 1979.

105. Robinson, R. O.: The frequency of other handicaps in children with cerebral palsy, *Dev. Med. Child Neurol.*, *15*: 305, 1973.

106. Robson, P.: The prevalence of scoliosis in adolescents and young adults with cerebral palsy, *Dev. Med. Child Neurol.*, *10*: 447, 1968.

107. Rogala, E. J., Drummond, D. S., and Durr, J.: Scoliosis: incidence and natural history, *J. Bone Joint Surg.*, *60A*: 1973, 1978.

108. Roosth, H. P.: Flexion deformity of the hip and knee in spastic cerebral palsy: treatment by early release of spastic hip-flexor muscles, *J. Bone Joint Surg.*, *53A*: 1489, 1971.

109. Rosenthal, R. K.: A fixed ankle below-the-knee orthosis for the management of genu recurvatum in spastic cerebral palsy, *J. Bone Joint Surg.*, *57A*: 545, 1975.

110. Rosenthal, R. K., and Levine, D. B.: Fragmentation of the distal pole of the patella in spastic cerebral palsy, *J. Bone Joint Surg.*, *59A*: 934, 1977.

111. Rosenthal, R. K., Levine, D. B., and McCarver, C. L.: The occurrence of scoliosis in cerebral palsy, *Dev. Med. Child Neurol.*, *16*: 664, 1974.

112. Ryder, C. T., and Crane, L.: Measuring femoral anteversion: the problem and a method, *J. Bone Joint Surg.*, *35A*: 321, 1953.

113. Samilson, R. L., and Bechard, R.: Scoliosis in cerebral palsy, In *Current Practice in Orthopaedic Surgery*, Adams, J. P. (ed.); St. Louis: C. V. Mosby, 1973.

114. Samilson, R. L., Carson, J., James, P., and Raney, F.: Results and complications of adductor tenotomy and obturator neurectomy in cerebral palsy, *Clin. Orthop.*, *54*: 61, 1967.

115. Samilson, R. L., and Morris, J. M.: Surgical improvement of the cerebral palsied upper limb: electromyographic studies and results in 128 operations, *J. Bone Joint Surg.*, *46A*: 1203, 1964.

116. Samilson, R. L., Tsou, P., Aamoth, G., and Green, W. T.: Dislocation and subluxation of the hip in cerebral palsy; pathogenesis, natural history and management, *J. Bone Joint Surg.*, *54A*: 863, 1972.

117. Saunders, J. B., Dee, M., Inman, V. T., and Eberhart, H. D.: The major determinants in normal and pathological gait, *J. Bone Joint Surg.*, *35A*: 543, 1953.

118. Schlesinger, E. R., Allaway, N. D., and Pelton, S.: Survivorship in cerebral palsy, *Am. J. Public Health*, *49*: 343 1959.

119. Scrutton, D. R.: Foot sequences of normal children under five years old, *Dev. Med. Child Neurol.*, *11*: 44, 1969.

120. Shands, A. R., Jr., and Eisberg, H. B.: The incidence of scoliosis in the State of Delaware; a study of 50,000 minifilms of the chest made during a survey for tuberculosis, *J. Bone Joint Surg.*, *37A*: 1243, 1955.

121. Shands, A. R., and Stelle, M. K.: Torsion of the femur, *J. Bone Joint Surg.*, *40A*: 803, 1958.

122. Silver, C. M., and Simon, S. D.: Gastrocnemius muscle recession (Silfverskiold operation) for spastic equinus deformity in cerebral palsy, *J. Bone and Joint Surg.*, *41A*: 1021, 1959.

123. Silver, C. M., Simon, S. D., and Lichtman, H. M.: The use and abuse of the obturator neurectomy, *Dev. Med. Child Neurol.*, *8*: 203, 1966.

124. Silver, C. M., Simon, S. D., Lichtman, H. M., and Motamed, M.: Surgical correction of spastic thumb-in-palm deformity, *Dev. Med. Child Neurol.*, *18*: 632, 1976.

125. Silver, C. M., Simon, S. D., Spindell, E., Lichtman, H. M., and Scala, M.: Calcaneal osteotomy for valgus and varus deformities of the foot in cerebral palsy, *J. Bone Joint Surg.*, *49A*: 232, 1967.

126. Simon, S. R., Mann, R. A., Hagy, J. L., and Larson, L. J.: Role of the posterior calf muscles in normal gait, *J. Bone Joint Surg.*, *60A*: 465, 1978.

127. Simon, S. R., et al.: Genu recurvatum in spastic cerebral palsy, *J. Bone Joint Surg.*, *60*: 882, 1978.

128. Sparrow, S., and Zigler, E.: Evaluation of a patterning treatment for retarded children, *Pediatrics*, *62*: 137, 1978.

129. Stanitski, C.: Medial approach to the hip for combined bony and soft tissue procedures for cerebral palsy deformities, Paper presented at the Eastern Orthopaedic Association Meeting, Acapulco,

Mexico 1978.

130. Stanitski, C., Micheli, L., Hall, J., and Rosenthal, R.: Surgical treatment of spinal deformity in cerebral palsy, Submitted for publication.

131. Stanley, F. J.: An epidemiological study of cerebral palsy in Western Australia, 1956–1975. I. Changes in total incidence of cerebral palsy and associated factors, *Dev. Med. Child Neurol., 21:* 701, 1979.

132. Stephenson, C. T., and Donavan, M. M.: Transfer of hip adductor origins to the ischium in spastic cerebral palsy, *Dev. Med. Child Neurol., 13:* 247, 1971.

133. Strayer, L. M.: Recession of the gastrocnemius, *J. Bone Joint Surg., 32A:* 671, 1950.

134. Sutherland, D. H., Larsen, L. I., and Mann, R.: Rectus femoris release in selected patients with cerebral palsy: a preliminary report, *Dev. Med. Child Neurol., 17:* 26, 1975.

135. Sutherland, D. H., Schottstaedt, E. R., and Larsen, L. I.: Clinical and electromyographic study of seven spastic children with internal rotation gait, *J. Bone Joint Surg., 51A:* 1070, 1969.

136. Swanson, A. B.: Surgery of the hand in cerebral palsy in the swan-neck deformity, *J. Bone Joint Surg., 42A:* 951, 1960.

137. Tachdjian, M. O., and Minear, W. L.: Sensory disturbances in the hands of children with cerebral palsy, *J. Bone Joint Surg., 40A:* 85, 1958.

138. Throop, F. B., DeRosa, G. P., Reech, C., and Waterman, J.: Correction of equinus in cerebral palsy by the Murphy procedure of tendo-calcaneus advancement—a preliminary communication, *Dev.*

Med. Child Neurol., 17: 182, 1975.

139. Tizard, J. P. M., Paine, R. S., and Crothers, B.: Disturbances of sensation in children with hemiplegia, *J. A. M. A., 155:* 628, 1955.

140. United States, Bureau of Educational Handicaps, Department of Health, Education and Welfare: Estimated population of non-verbal individuals in the United States Conference on Communication Aids for the Non-vocal Severely Physically Handicapped Person, Alexandria, Va., 1977.

141. Vining, E. P. G., Accardo, P. J., Rubenstein, J. E., Farrell, S. E., and Roizen, N. J.: Cerebral palsy—a pediatric developmentalist's overview, *Am. J. Dis. Child., 130:* 643, 1976.

142. White, W. R.: Flexor muscle slide in the spastic hand, *J. Bone Joint Surg., 54B:* 453, 1972.

143. Williams, I.: The consequences of orthopaedic surgery to the adolescent cerebral palsied; medical, educational and parental attitudes, Paper presented at the Study Group on Integrating the Care of Multiply Handicapped Children, St. Mary's College, Durham, England; London: The Spastics Medical Education and Information Unit, 1977.

144. Winter, R. B., and Carlson, J. M.: Modern orthotics for spinal deformities, *Clin. Orthop., 126:* 74, 1977.

145. Wright, T., and Nicholson, J.: Physiotherapy for the spastic child: an evaluation, *Dev. Med. Child Neurol., 15:* 146, 1973.

146. Wynne-Davies, R.: Familial (idiopathic) scoliosis; a family survey, *J. Bone Joint Surg., 50B:* 24, 1968.

147. Yule, W.: Issues and problems in remedial education, *Dev. Med. Child Neurol., 18:* 674, 1976.

CHAPTER 17

The Upper Extremity

FRANK STELLING, M.D.

The hand of the child is fundamentally no different from the hand of the adult in its response to injury, in its healing characteristics, and in the therapeutic principles pertaining to it. Yet there are certain important differences that should be pointed out. In the adult, the major cause of disability is trauma due predominantly to industrial accidents. In the child, the major disabilities are caused by paralytic conditions and congenital abnormalities; trauma is a less frequent but a no less important cause. The same surgical principles apply to the child as to the adult; however, techniques must be varied to fit the individual problem. Some conditions, such as the spastic hand and congenital abnormalities, should be approached differently in the child than in the adult. With some problems encountered in childhood, the therapy must be a conservative one directed toward prevention of deformity until the patient has reached maturity, when definitive procedures can be performed. Occasionally, time-consuming reconstructive procedures that would not be attempted in adults because of the economic problem they would engender may be carried out in children.

There are many important differences between the hand of the child and that of the adult that affect the timing of surgical procedure; the type of suture material, dressings, skin graft, bracing, and immobilization used; the length of treatment; and the type of surgical procedure performed. These differences pertain to the size and maturity of the hand; the maturity, cooperation, and adjustment of the patient; the thickness of skin and the types of scar and contracture of skin; the maturity of bone and the reaction of bone to surgery; the mobilization and immobilization of joints and the reaction of joints to injury; the maturity of tendons and the attachment of tendons to growing bones; the maturity of the nervous system and the relationship of sensory impairments to reconstructive procedures.

This chapter deals mainly with conditions common to children and with the application of sound therapeutic principles. No attempt will be made to deal with functional anatomy or the many basic fundamentals of hand surgery, all of which are most important and absolutely necessary in any attempt to carry out the procedures to be described.

CONGENITAL ANOMALIES

Congenital anomalies of all types account for about 25–30% of all the admissions to children's hospital services throughout the United States. Deformities of the hand comprise 20–30% of this group. Of the total number of patients admitted to the Shriners' Hospitals as of April 1962, the records of 100,894 cases have been reviewed. Of this number of admissions, there were 52,203 congenital anomalies of all types. Approximately 2% of this total were congenital anomalies involving the upper extremity. No single deformity can be considered common, and some are extremely rare and need not be mentioned in this section. Most of the deformities are mixed in nature, and in nearly every instance treatment must be individualized. In spite of this, certain general principles of treatment for the more common groups of anomalies will be considered here.

The etiology of congenital anomalies of the hand has not been definitely established. The theories which have been advanced will not be discussed here, but it would seem that the most acceptable theory is that of mutations which are subsequently inherited.

Radial Meromelia (Hemimelia), Complete or Incomplete

Radial meromelia, hemimelia, congenital absence of the radius, congenital clubhand, clinarthrosis, and aplasia or hypoplasia of the radius are all terms used in the literature to denote a deformity of the hand manifested by radial deviation resulting from a defect in the radius (Fig. 17.1). Clubhand is a descriptive term denoting some type of deformity of the hand, but actually it means very little. Clinarthrosis, absence of the radius, and hypoplasia or aplasia of the radius are all medical terms relating to deformities of joint or

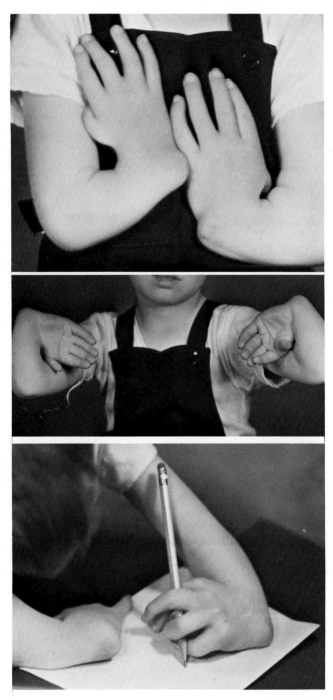

Figure 17.1. Typical bilateral clubhand with poor development of the thumbs.

of bone alone. In 1961 Frantz and O'Rahilly[3] pointed out that these deformities involve a great deal more than bone or joint and, therefore, suggested that everyone use the term, "radial hemimelia," which would describe the entire deformity. Recently, because of an argument based on the fact that hemimelia means half and that in many instances half is not particularly correct and that partial would be more explanatory, it has been suggested by the Committee on Prosthetics Research and Development that the term "hemimelia" be changed to "meromelia." Radial meromelia, therefore, can be further differentiated by describing it as "longitudinal, paraxial" when these are associated anomalies in the radial part of the hand or as "intercalary" when there is only an absence of the radius, etc., just as already written.

This condition is a manifestation of a defect in the radial elements of the limb bud. Similarly, an ulnar clubhand may occur in association with an ulnar defect. It has been found that the dividing line between radial and ulnar meromelias lies along the index finger. Quite often the thumb is absent in radial clubhands associated with a defect in the radius (Fig. 17.2), whereas often the last three fingers are absent in the defects in the ulna.

ASSOCIATED ANOMALIES

The skeletal changes which occur in the upper extremity usually involve most of the bones. The scapula is commonly reduced in size, and the clavicle may be short. The humerus is usually shorter than normal, and either end may present some deformity. The carpal bones are rarely complete in number. Most frequently absent is the navicular, which is followed by the greater multangular. Quite frequently, the first metacarpal is absent. Varying combinations occur with regard to the relationship of the first metacarpal and the thumb. If the first metacarpal is missing, the thumb usually has no function and very often is a soft-tissue appendage.

MUSCULAR DEFECTS

Numerous defects in the muscles accompany the condition. If the thumb and first metacarpal are present, the extensor pollicis longus and brevis and the abductor brevis are also present, and the muscles of the thenar eminence are usually normal. If the first metacarpal is absent, however, these muscles are commonly missing. The pronator teres may be missing if the radius is completely absent, or it may be underdeveloped if there is a partial defect in the radius. The flexor pollicis longus is apt to be absent unless the entire thumb and first metacarpal are present, in which case it is likely to be normal. The muscles about the shoulder and arm are frequently involved. The pectoralis major may have an abnormal insertion, or its clavicular or costal portions may be absent. The pectoralis minor and the deltoid are usu-

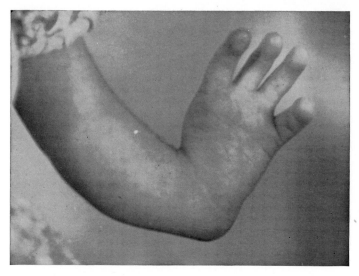

Figure 17.2. Clubhand with absence of thumb.

ally present, although the latter muscle may have an abnormal insertion or it may fuse with the triceps or the brachialis. The biceps is frequently missing; however, if it is present in a patient with complete absence of the radius, it inserts into the lacertus fibrosus. The brachialis varies but is usually present, and the triceps is usually normal. The brachioradialis is found to be missing when the radius is completely absent; however, occasionally it will be present and inserted into the ulna. The extensor carpi radialis longus and brevis may be absent, or they may be fused with the extensor digitorum communis, which is usually present and normal. The supinator is commonly absent unless the proximal radius is present.

VASCULAR DEFECTS

The arterial system shows numerous abnormalities. The brachial artery may be normal, or it may divide into two branches high in the arm. The ulnar artery is usually normal, but the radial artery is frequently small or absent. The median nerve is not infrequently the most superficial structure found on the radial aspect of the forearm. For the most part, the ulnar nerve is normal and supplies the usual intrinsic muscles in the hand.

TREATMENT

Many different methods have been devised through the years to improve these hands. Most of the operative procedures devised for the condition have varied from producing fair improvement to being of questionable value. The general methods of treatment of this condition at the present time are: (1) conservative stretching and splinting (Fig. 17.3) and the development of the use of the hand without a surgical procedure; (2) stretching and splinting followed by tenotomy and soft-tissue surgery to get the hand over the ulna, followed by fusion of the wrist or of the ulna into the carpus; and (3) conservative or surgical procedures to get the hand over the wrist, followed by some bony procedure in order to keep the hand in the new position without a definite stabilization. In general, the operative procedures that have been described in the literature have been confined to tenotomy of the contracted muscles, osteotomy of the curved ulna and addition of a

stabilizing bone graft to replace the absent radius, and splitting of the ulna into radial and ulnar portions (Figs. 17.4 and 17.5). Most of these procedures result in a fusion of the wrist joint; if such is the result, the appearance of the hand is certainly more pleasing, but sometimes it is questionable whether the functional value of the hand has been increased or not.

CONSERVATIVE TREATMENT

Conservative treatment should be started in all cases as early as possible. In the correction of the deformity, plaster casts, splints, or braces should be used until the soft tissues have been stretched to the greatest degree that the bony deformity will allow. As soon as possible, the deformity is corrected by plaster casts. Following this, small correction braces or splints may be used on a part-time basis while stretching is carried out as a daily routine by the parents. Some authorities believe that this is the only treatment that should be used. Quite often if treatment is continued during the entire growth period, the hand remains deformed, but the child adapts to the deformity. Stretching and the movement of the parts keep the hand functionally sound, and it is amazing to see how well these children can use the hand at the termination of the growth period. The appearance of the hand is not particularly pleasing, but quite often its function is very satisfactory, and perhaps better than that of a hand with a wrist fusion alone.

SURGICAL TREATMENT

In 1955, in the *Journal of Bone and Joint Surgery*, Riordan[6] reported a modification of the surgical method of Starr which he felt to be a more promising surgical procedure for the treatment of the radial meromelia or congenital absence of the radius, and quite a number of us undertook these surgical procedures with varying results. In actuality, the procedure functioned well for a number of years after the procedure had been performed, and, at first, it was the thought by Riordan and quite a number of us that this transplanted fibula into the ulna would grow. In a very few instances this actually occurred, but the number of cases of increasing growth was so small as to not make this the procedure of choice that we at one time hoped it

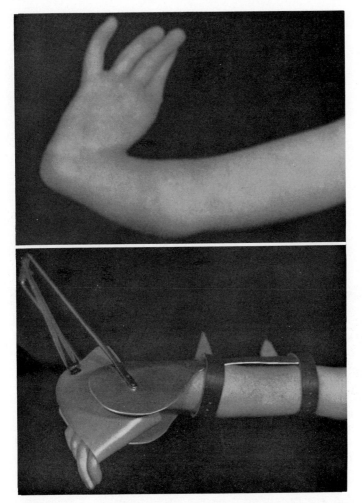

Figure 17.3.   Typical clubhand showing the use of a clubhand splint. The splint is used on a part time basis to give active stretch in order to lessen the deformity.

would be. In previous editions of this book, this has been written up as a surgical technique of value in the treatment of this condition. However, in 1963, at the meeting of the American Orthopaedic Association at Hot Springs, Virginia, Dr. Riordan reviewed all of his cases to that time and suggested a better method of treatment because the fibula transplant had failed to grow in most instances and, therefore, there was a recurrence of the deformity of the hand. At that time and since, he has advocated that the hand and wrist be surgically transposed over the distal end of the ulna, leaving the ulnar epiphysis intact. He found that if this were done at a very early age, the ulnar epiphysis would expand in breadth if the wrist were held over

it long enough. The expanded ulna epiphysis would act as a buttress and hold the hand over the distal ulna giving a good alignment between the forearm and the hand and also a mobile joint. So far, he has been pleased with this procedure. We have done these since 1960 and have been pleased with our results also. We have reviewed all of our cases that were performed according to Riordan's first method and we, too, have had the same problems that he experienced, as have others. We have been able to correct some of the difficulties of those cases that have been performed according to his first method by performing an osteotomy of the ulna just at the junction of the bifurcation between the fibular graft and the ulna, in other words at

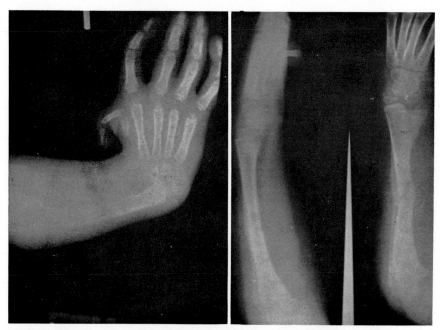

Figure 17.4 (*Left*).　X-ray of radial clubhand before surgery.
Figure 17.5 (*Right*).　X-ray of same case after correction, which involved a fibular graft to the ulna and an osteotomy of the ulna.

a low point and adjusting the osteotomy so that the hand is again in proper alignment with the forearm. In some instances some of the tendons must be lengthened in order to hold this, but this has allowed us to correct the radially deviated hand and still maintain good function. In performing the new procedure of Riordan, the carpus must be exposed through a radial incision and, as in his first procedure, one must be quite careful of the median nerve, which quite often is exposed directly under the skin with many small branches, particularly sensory branches, running out both to the dorsal and volar aspects of the radial side of the hand. The tendons are usually not lengthened, but fascial bands are resected and the carpus is exposed. Sometimes an incision must be made over the ulnar side to expose the ulnar epiphysis, and, in certain instances, the entire procedure has been performed through just a transverse ulnar incision. Care is of utmost importance as far as the distal ulnar epiphysis is concerned in that it be allowed to grow. Therefore, nothing is done as far as the ulnar epiphysis is concerned other than its exposure. If the soft tissues are too tight, several of the carpal bones may be removed so that the hand can be placed directly over the ulnar epiphysis. Sometimes the entire proximal

carpal row is removed, and, if this is not enough, some of the midcarpus in the distal row may be removed to allow the hand to be positioned over the ulna. All we need here is a joint with the ulna opposing the central part of the hand. This is then locked in place by the use of a longitudinal Kirschner wire and sometimes by a transverse Kirschner wire through the metacarpals, and a cast is applied with the hand in corrected position. Once this has been performed, the wounds are closed. There is usually redundancy on the ulnar side, and, if there is any tension on the longitudinal incision on the radial side, this should be closed by Z-plasty to relieve the tension on the scar. A long arm cast is applied with the wrist held in the neutral position and the elbow in flexion. The cast is maintained in this position and changed at intervals over a long period of time, sometimes as long as 1 year or more. Sometimes a brace is used instead of a cast. Many types of braces are used. In our experience they are not quite as useful as a well molded cast, except that the cast must be changed frequently and there is always the problem of water. It is of utmost importance, however, that the hand be maintained over the ulnar epiphysis until the ulnar epiphysis has grown and expanded so as to form a buttress to keep the hand from rotating back into a radially deviated position. Once stability has occurred by x-ray and by clinical observation, then, and only then, can all immobilization be discontinued. The procedure in our experience should not be performed after the child has attained the age of 5 years because the ulnar epiphysis will not grow enough to allow the proper expansion and buttressing effect. Riordan[6] has indicated that this is best done in children who are quite small and has actually performed this procedure during the first month of life. The cases in which we have performed this newer Riordan procedure have been followed long enough to be certain that we will be able to maintain in most instances a flexible part that is motored well for functional use. Riordan has indicated that in some instances this did not occur, but he was able to go ahead with wrist fusion and have still a more satisfactory extremity than if this had been left alone to develop as a clubhand.

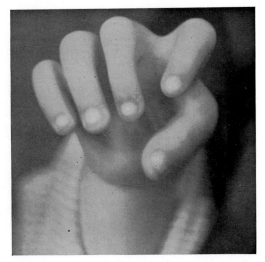

Figure 17.6. Thumb-clutched hand with finger deformities.

References

1. Albee, F. H.: Formation of radius congenitally absent; condition 7 years after implantation of bone graft, *Ann. Surg.*, 87:105, 1928.
2. Bunnell, S.: *Surgery of the Hand,* Philadelphia: J. B. Lippincott, 1944.
3. Frantz, C. H., and O'Rahilly, R.: Congenital skeletal limb deficiencies, *J. Bone Joint Surg.*, 43A: 1202, 1961.
4. Hiekel, H. V. A.: Aplasia and hypoplasia of the radius, *Acta Orthop Scand.*, Suppl. 39, 1959.
5. Kato, K.: Congenital absence of the radius, *J. Bone Joint Surg.*, 6:589, 1924.
6. Riordan, D. C.: Congenital absence of the radius, *J. Bone Joint Surg.*, 37A:1129, 1955.
7. Riordan, D. C.: Congenital absence of the radius; a 15 year follow-up, *J. Bone Joint Surg.*, 45A: 1783, 1963.
8. Starr, D. E.: Congenital absence of the radius, a method of surgical correction, *J. Bone Joint Surg.*, 27:261, 1943.
9. Stelling, F. H.: Surgery of the hand in the child, *Instruct. Lect. Am. Acad. Orthop. Surg.*, 15: 172, 1958.

Congenital Flexion and Adduction Deformity of Thumb (Pollex Varus, Thumb-clutched Hand, Congenital Clasped Hand)

This anomaly is a rare deformity that tends to be an inherited trait. The thumb is characteristically held adducted into the hand, and there is marked flexion of the metacar-pophalangeal joint. Quite frequently there are coexistent flexion deformities of the proximal interphalangeal joints of the fingers; such deformities give rise to the term "thumb-clutched hand" (Fig. 17.6). The skin of the flexor surface of the fingers and thumb is usually contracted. This contraction is thought to be secondary to the true pathology. The flexion deformity of the proximal interphalangeal joints of the fingers may exist without the thumb deformity, but this is considered to be a rare occurrence. In most instances, it has been found that there is a hypoplasia or absence of the extensor pollicis brevis and a secondary adduction flexion contracture of the thumb. In the finger deformities, it is believed that there is a hypoplasia or absence of the intrinsic musculature (Fig. 17.7).

TREATMENT

The results of treatment depend upon the stage in which therapy is started. Many of these cases have been noted in adults with persistent disabling finger and thumb deformities. If the deformity is seen early, conservative measures should be instituted. The thumb should be mobilized out of the palm into extension and abduction and should be held in this position by some type of splint. White and Jensen[2] use a special elastic abduction splint which can be easily removed for cleaning. Wechesser[1] uses a plaster case for several months and changes the cast at 4-

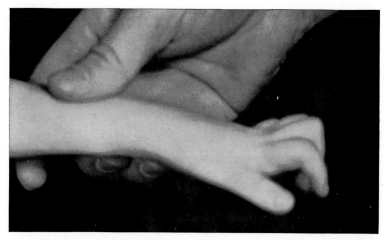

Figure 17.7.   Congenital absence of the intrinsic muscles without clutched thumb.

to 6-week intervals to allow for growth. Most of his cases develop good function with this conservative care. If the deformity returns following the release of the part after conservative immobilization, then it is to be expected that the tendon is either absent or nonfunctional, and tendon transplants should be done. White transplants the common extensor tendon of the index finger into the extensor surface of the metaphysis of the base of the proximal phalanx of the thumb and has shown excellent results in these cases. Sometimes the skin is tight on the flexor surface, and a Z-plasty or releasing incision with a full thickness graft should be utilized. The contracture has been limited to the skin and does not usually involve fascia and deeper structures in the small child. In the adult, contracture of all elements of the thumb web is to be expected.

References

1. Wechesser, E. C.: Congenital flexion-adduction deformity of the thumb (congenital "clasped thumb"), *J. Bone Joint Surg.*, 37A:977, 1955.
2. White, J. W., and Jensen, W. E.: The infant's persistent thumb clutched hand, *J. Bone Joint Surg.*, 34A:680, 1952.
3. Zadek, I.: Congenital absence of extensor pollicis longus of both thumbs: operation and cure, *J. Bone Joint Surg.*, 16:432, 1934.
4. Zumoff, B.: Congenital symmetrical finger contractures, *J.A.M.A.*, 155:437, 1954.

Stenosing Tenovaginitis of Thumb— "Trigger Thumb"

This condition is characterized by a flexion deformity of the interphalangeal joint of the thumb, and it occurs in adults as well as in children. In the adult, it is irritative in origin and due to repeated trauma, and in the child it is congenital. Snapping is usual in adults and rare in children. It is generally thought that the lesion is of congenital origin in infants, even though in some instances it is not present until weeks or months after birth. Zadek[6] cited a case that developed in an infant with a history of minor trauma of one thumb and that was thought to have been a result of the injury; however, a few months later, the other thumb developed the same deformity with no history of trauma. The pathology was found to be the same in both thumbs.

PATHOLOGY

The gross pathologic appearance of this lesion is that of an encircling constricting fibrocartilaginous band of the sheath of the flexor pollicis longus at the level of the metacarpophalangeal joint. Usually as this constriction is released, an indentation or groove in the tendon and thickening on either side of this identation are seen. Sometimes the tendon bulges to double its normal size on either side of the groove.

CLINICAL PICTURE

The interphalangeal joint of the thumb is held in a position of fixed flexion. There is inability to extend the joint actively. Usually the thumb can be flexed actively a few degrees. In some instances the distal joint can be forcibly extended, but it locks in flexion

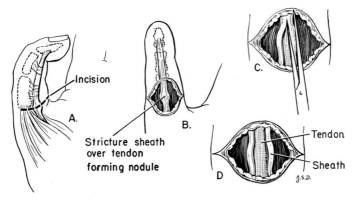

Figure 17.8. Operation for "trigger thumb." The incision in the skin is transverse, and the incision in the tendon sheath is longitudinal.

as soon as flexion is again initiated. The joint cannot be passively extended, and any attempt to do so causes pain. As extension of the joint is attempted, the tendon becomes taut distal to the metacarpophalangeal joint, and the skin of the flexor surface of the thumb at the level of the metacarpophalangeal joint. This area may at times be sensitive.

TREATMENT

If the interphalangeal joint can be passively extended and splinted in this position for 3 weeks, the thumb sometimes resumes normal function and is permanently rid of the deformity. In most instances, however, this treatment is unsuccessful, and the deformity recurs. The treatment of choice is incision of the flexor tendon sheath, preferably by means of two incisions through each side of the annular constricting band and removal of a small section of the sheath. The incision in the skin should be made transversely in a line with the crease at the metacarpophalangeal joint (Fig. 17.8). A longitudinal incision crossing the skin crease produces a serious, painful scar that can produce a flexion deformity. Care must be taken not to injure the digital nerves. The results of this therapy are usually excellent.

References

1. Fahey, J. J., and Bollinger, J. A.: "Trigger thumb" in adults and children, *J. Bone Joint Surg.*, 36A: 1200, 1954.
2. Jahss, S. A.: Trigger finger in children, *J.A.M.A.*, 107: 1463, 1936.
3. Miller, J. W.: Pollex varus, a report of 2 cases, *Univ. Mich. Med. Bull.*, 10: 1, 1944.
4. Sprecher, E. E.: "Trigger thumb" in infants, *J. Bone Joint Surg.*, 31A: 672, 1949.
5. White, J. W., and Jensen, W. E.: "Trigger thumb" in infants, *Am. J. Dis. Child.*, 85: 141, 1953.
6. Zadek, I.: Stenosing tendovaginitis of the thumb in infants, *J. Bone Surg.*, 24: 326, 1942.

Syndactylism

Syndactylism is the most frequent anomaly of the hand, and it occurs in all degrees of severity. The simplest involvement is an incomplete web formation between two fingers with no bone or joint deformity (Figs. 17.9 and 17.10). Extreme involvement may take the form of severe webbing of all the fingers accompanied by incomplete segmentation of the bony parts and multiple joint deformities. Syndactylism is frequently bilateral and is sometimes seen in conjunction with webbing of the toes or other deformities of the foot. The deformity is thought most frequently to be inherited. Of the series of cases reviewed at the Shriners' Hospital in Greenville, South Carolina, almost all of the patients have been found to originate from a single family.

In many instances syndactylism is complicated by associated deformities such as symphalangism, brachydactyly, and polydactyly. In our experience, one is more likely to find these complicating factors than not. They alter the prognosis considerably. The final prognosis in many instances of multiple congenital anomalies naturally depends upon what we have to work with. By means of a combination of basic procedures, including removal of proper parts, separation of syndactyly, and sometimes transposition of fingers, the best functional result is attained. The resulting hand is not going to be pretty or even normal in appearance, but function

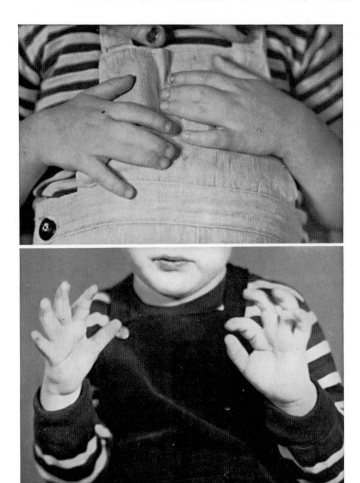

Figure 17.9 (*Top*).   Bilateral syndactylism involving two fingers. There is no bone, joint, or nail deformity. This child is only 2 years of age, and a good operative result should be expected.
Figure 17.10 (*Bottom*).   The functional and cosmetic results following surgery are good.

is always the first consideration. In these instances, the appearance should be the best that can be attained under the circumstances. Each case must be considered individually, and the surgeon himself must decide exactly what the total plan of treatment is to be and what function may finally be attained. The latter must be clearly stated, both to himself and to the family of the child.

TREATMENT

The results of therapy vary according to the degree of deformity, the number of fingers involved, and the amount of bony fusion. Partial webbing of the skin without bone or nail involvement can be totally cor-

rected. The presence of bone or joint deformities invariably causes some permanent deformity, in spite of the best operative procedures. Syndactyly is so varied in its manifestations and complications that it is impossible to prescribe one method of treatment. The basic principles are the same, but the timing of the procedure, the type of immobilization, and the follow-up are all affected by the severity of the condition and the complicating factors present.

Webbing without Concurrent Discrepancy in Length. In such instances, because the discrepancy of finger lengths present is not sufficient to cause increasing joint deformities, it is thought best to defer surgery until the child is almost school age. The primary reason for this is that the skin grafts are more easily held in place by rigid immobilization at this age and that neater primary healing, less scar, and better definitive results are obtained. Secondary operative procedures are rarely necessary, even when there is some bony attachment between the distal phalanges; however, better functional and cosmetic results can always be expected if there are separate nails, no bony attachment, and only intervening soft-tissue involvement. In such cases, the prognosis is excellent.

The surgical procedure for the separation of these fingers is always performed under a tourniquet. The incision is begun by constructing pedicles in the form of V-shaped flaps on both sides of the web at the level of the metacarpholangeal joint. The points of the Vs are toward the fingers, and the flaps extend out approximately ½ inch. The flaps are then dissected from the finger in a manner that permits some subcutaneous tissue to remain attached to the skin. The web is then separated from both fingers, care being taken to cut in an irregular line, either waving or angulating, to prevent longitudinal scarring when the graft is attached. The soft tissues are separated by blunt dissection after the skin incisions have been completed. The neurovascular bundles are carefully protected. If the phalanges are fused, they are separated with a bone cutter and trimmed back smoothly. In instances of a single nail for two fingers, the nail is split and a portion of it and of its matrix on the cut side is then removed so that the skin graft may be brought around the margin of the nail. The resulting defect produced on the opposing sides of the two fingers should then be covered by a skin graft.

Two different types of skin graft may be used. In very small children, because it is almost impossible to decide what thickness a split thickness graft would be, it may be best to use a full thickness skin graft. In older children, we like a thick split thickness skin graft, which can be removed from the volar aspect of the forearm on the same side as the hand to which it is to be grafted. This skin is taken with a dermatome and fashioned to cover the area so that its edges meet the wavy or angulated edges previously constructed (Fig. 17.11). The two V flaps are crossed and sutured across the existing web at the palm. It is not necessary to bring the points completely across; however, if this can be done

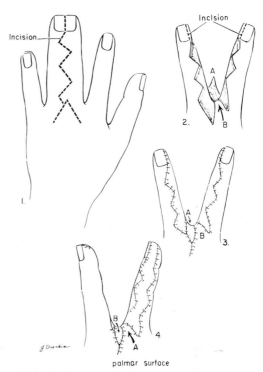

Figure 17.11. Method of surgical treatment for syndactylism. The sides of the finger are covered with split thickness grafts; the base, by two-triangular flaps that cross.

without producing tension and with discomfort to the child, it is performed. A small amount of overlap is also perfectly acceptable because the skin graft can be made to cover the defect. The sutures used are 4-0 or 5-0 interrupted catgut. These sutures do not cause any increased reaction, and they fall out at the proper time; therefore, there is no necessity to struggle with the child to remove sutures and no danger of pulling the new skin graft off, nor is there any reason to anesthetize the child to remove the sutures. The tourniquet is always released prior to skin closure, and a dry field is attained before any part of the wound is closed. The donor site is covered with scarlet red gauze, which is allowed to remain in place until the skin underneath has reepithelized. The recipient site is covered, preferably with paraffin gauze, and the hand is placed in a skeleton splint of steel or aluminum at the end of which small holes are drilled at the level of the end of the finger. The splint is padded to protect the back of the hand, and stainless

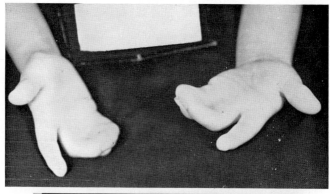

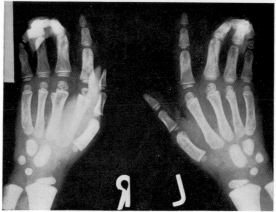

Figure 17.12. Syndactylism involving three fingers. Note the deformity of the nails and of the longer fingers. There is also lack of segmentation of the distal phalanges. A good result can be expected here, but there will probably be some fixed joint contracture of the middle finger. The patient should have been treated surgically at a younger age for a better result.

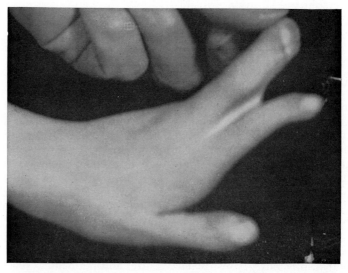

Figure 17.13. Brachydactylia, syndactylism, and symphalangism. The hand can be improved by separating the index and adjacent finger, but the middle finger joints will still be restricted in motion.

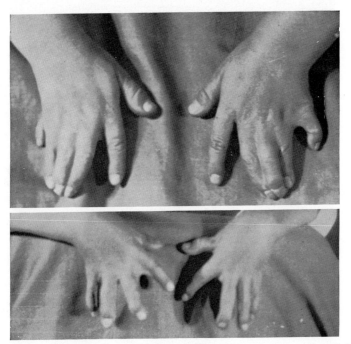

Figure 17.14 (*Top*).   Bilateral syndactylism of three fingers plus extra digits on the lunar side.
Figure 17.15 (*Bottom*).   Appearance after surgical release of the syndactylism and removal of the entire ray on the left and digit on the right.

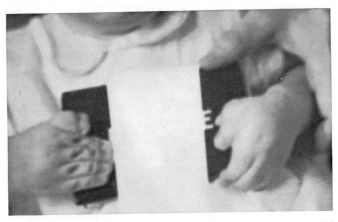

Figure 17.16.   Bilateral syndactylism of all four fingers and bifid thumbs.

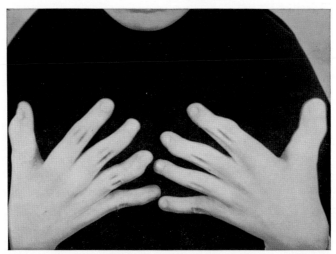

Figure 17.17. Same case as in Figure 17.16 after correction of the syndactylism and removal of the radial thumbs. There is some residual scarring of the flexor surface, but functional ability is excellent.

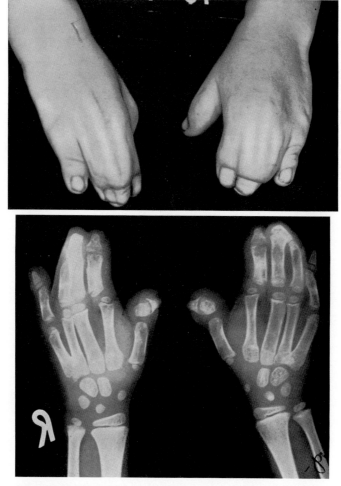

Figure 17.18. Severe syndactylism with deformity of only the middle and ring fingers. There is a wedged phalanx in the thumb. The result here will not be excellent, but the fingers will be greatly improved.

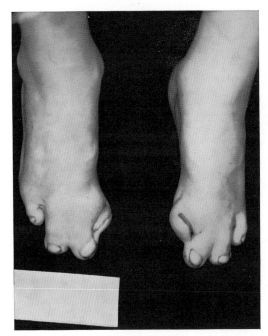

Figure 17.19. Same case as in Figure 17.18. Deformities of the feet.

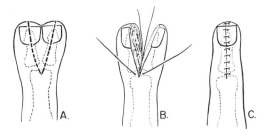

Figure 17.20. Surgical correction of bifid distal phalanx. This type of surgical correction of a bifid distal phalanx should not be performed in the growing child because of the probability that increased deformity will result from the growing epiphyses.

steel wire sutures are placed through the fingernail and then through the splint so that the fingers are held in full extension and also in abduction. The proximal end of the splint is then incorporated in a plaster cast extending beyond the elbow, which is at 90 degrees in the older age group. In very young children 1 or 2 years old, this cast is extended over the shoulder and chest to give more secure immobilization. The cast is left in place for a period of about 2 weeks, and then the dressing is removed. Most of the sutures come out

at that time. The wounds are redressed, and splints are left in place for a another week. At the end of that time, the stenuous immobilization is removed, and small splints are applied to keep the fingers in extension and abduction for at least 3 more weeks. During this period of time, it has been found, even in older children, that the joints do not stiffen, and there is no permanent joint damage due to the immobilization. In no instance should work be done on both sides of any one finger. This may jeopardize circulation and cause loss of the finger.

Syndactyly with Discrepancy in Length of Adjacent Parts. When the little finger is attached to the ring finger or the thumb to the index finger (which is rare), or when the entire group of fingers is involved in a mitten of skin, surgery should be performed much earlier. It should be done sometime after 1 year of age and before 2 years; otherwise increasing joint deformities in the longer finger will occur. In these cases, surgery is performed with the full knowledge that immobilization is difficult and almost impossible. If immobilization is not perfectly secure, motion occurs and causes many degrees of scarring and subsequent "scarring in" because of partial or total loss of the graft. This produces skin contracture usually of the flexion type, which is not as severe as lateral or rotary deformity. Later, Z-plasty or skin graft inlays after section of the cicatrix are necessary. Skin contracture need not always result. We should try our best to achieve perfect immobilization to avoid secondary scarring and secondary surgical procedures, but the parents should be told that these procedures may be necessary. The surgical procedure in

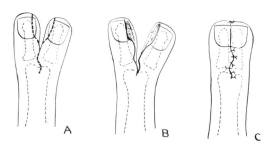

Figure 17.21. This procedure, which leaves the bone and joint untouched, would be used in the case of bifid distal phalanx. If further definitive surgery should be necessary, it should be done after the patient has reached maturity.

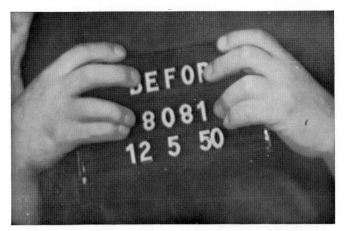

Figure 17.22. Bilateral syndactylism of two fingers with no bone or nail deformity. The child is young, and excellent cosmetic and functional results should be anticipated with proper surgery.

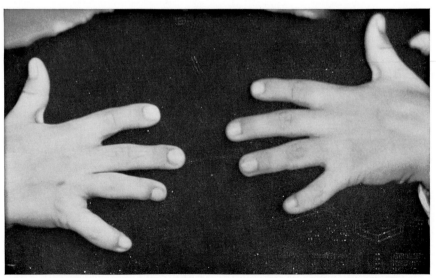

Figure 17.23. Same case as seen in Figure 17.22. Postoperative appearance shows a good functional result.

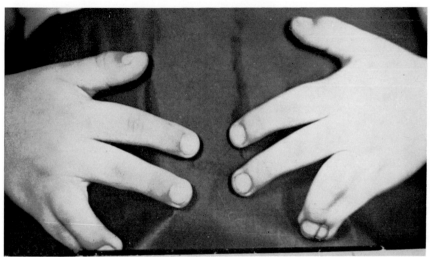

Figure 17.24. Bilateral syndactylism of two fingers. There is some nail and joint deformity.

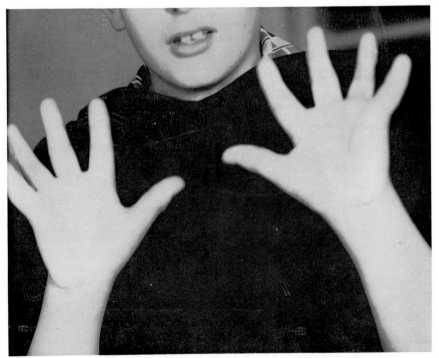

Figure 17.25. Same case as seen in Figure 17.24. Surgery was performed early enough to correct the joint deformity.

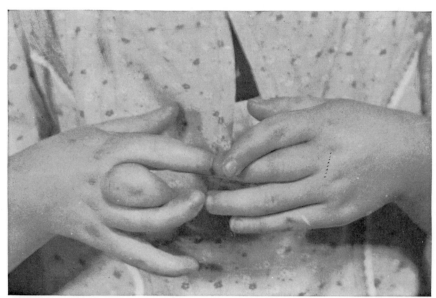

Figure 17.26. Congenital anomalous development of a joint in the fingers. There is a large double first metacarpal of the middle finger and marked joint contracture.

very young children is the same as that described above, except that immobilization may be obtained, if the finger is perfectly straight, by means of a small Kirschner wire inserted centrally through the phalanges. The wire may be left in place for a period of 3 weeks and then exchanged for a plastic or metal splint. Care must be taken that the wire be centrally located. The procedure of immobilization described above is then added to this, the plaster being extended above the shoulder in all instances. If there is doubt in these very young children as to the thickness of skin, it is best to use a full thickness skin graft taken from the flexor crease of the elbow of the same side.

Polydactylism

Polydactylism is inherited and often accompanies syndactylism, brachydactylism, and other congenital anomalies. It is probably the most common congenital anomaly, but because some of the small finger appendages attached by a fine skin pedicle are tied off with a suture in the nursery by the obstetrician or pediatrician, they are lost in statistical analyses.

The anomaly occurs in three main types: (1) an extra soft-tissue mass not adherent to the skeleton and frequently without bone joints or tendons; (2) a duplicate digit containing all elements and attached to a large metacarpal head or to a bifurcated metacarpal; and (3) a complete extra digit with a full metacarpal.

TREATMENT

Cases of the first type that show very small pedicle at birth can be easily treated by tying off the pedicle with a piece of silk. The result is usually a normal-appearing hand without deformity. Sometimes the soft-tissue attachment is too thick for this type of treatment, and, in such cases, it is best to wait until the child is older (4–5 years) before carrying out a surgical resection. Extra digits do not cause functional difficulty in the early years of life. In some instances, it is difficult to decide which digit should be sacrificed, and careful study and observation for a considerable period of time become necessary before the decision to operate can be made. If there is any doubt whatsoever in cases of polydactyly as to which finger should be sacrificed, it is best to wait until one can be definitely certain of the function of the various parts before deciding which part should be retained and which deleted. Structures should also have developed enough to be identified with certainty. In many cases of polydactyly, there are split tendons or a central tendon with a

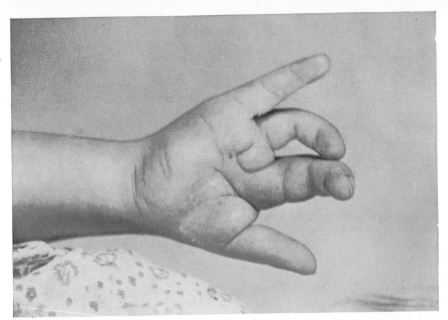

Figure 17.27. Same case as seen in Figure 17.26 after complete ray excision and narrowing of the hand. The child has very good function.

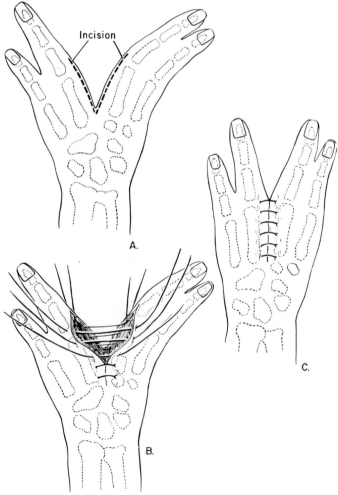

Incision

A.

B.

C.

Figure 17.28. Narrowing of the hand to improve its cosmetic appearance. Function should always be the main consideration, however.

Y-split to the two segments. Such variations should be checked at the time of surgery, and the functional structures should be left in the remaining part. In cases of double thumb in which there is one metacarpal or a partially segmented metacarpal, the dissection must be very careful. Too often when the radial thumb is removed, the abductor attachment should be searched out anatomically and reattached in proper relationship to the part remaining. When a part is removed, one must be sure that the part remaining can function properly. Occasionally, the tendons of an accessory digit may be transferred to provide function in the remaining digit.

Injury of the epiphysis, either traumatic or surgical, may produce deformities. For this reason certain surgical procedures that are of a definitive nature and involve the bone structure itself often must be delayed. In the treatment of a congenital duplication of the distal phalanx of the thumb, it has been suggested that central segments of the bone be removed, the remaining parts fitted together to form one bone, and the soft tissues closed over to form one distal thumb segment. If this procedure is performed in a growing child, it is nearly certain that deformity will occur from the damage to the epiphysis. It is believed far better in the young child to produce a syndactylism surgically, to leave the bone alone except for pulling the two bone segments toward each other, and to leave a broad distal thumb with two bones and nails covered with one envelope of skin. A split nail will be produced, but this should cause little difficulty, and if definitive reconstruction is necessary, it can be performed at or after maturity.

Cleft Hand

This is a rare deformity with many variations and often concomitant with other types of congenital malformations, such as syndactylism, brachydactylism, and symphalangism. The usual deformity is a central cleft dividing the hand in two parts (Fig. 17.32). The digits in each part may be webbed partially or completely, or they may be free. Most frequently, one or more rays are missing. In some cases, there may be a radial and ulnar ray with no digits between them. In others, the hand may be normal except that it lacks a central digit. In nearly all instances, the patient uses the hand almost like a claw, opposing one part to the other for grasping.

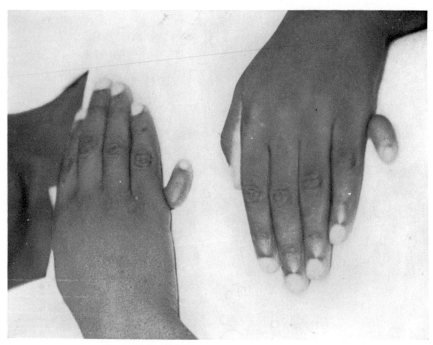

Figure 17.29.   Extra ulnar digits.

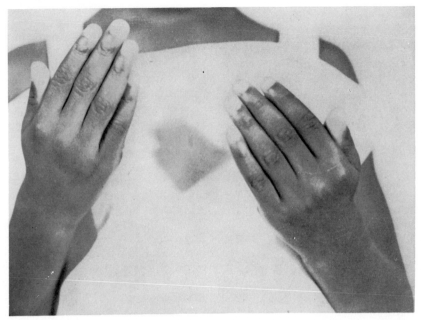

Figure 17.30.   Same case as seen in Figure 17.29, showing the final result after surgical excision.

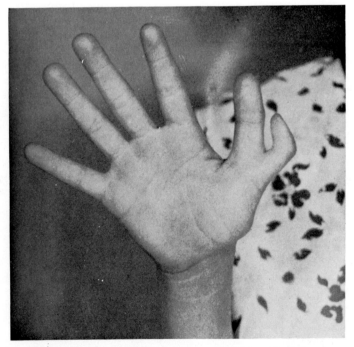

Figure 17.31.   Bifid thumb. Excision of the radial digit will give an excellent result.

TREATMENT

The treatment must be individualized to the type of deformity present. In instances in which only two functioning units are present and there is no webbing, the hand is best left untreated.

Webbing should be released as described in the section of syndactylism, and the cleft should be eliminated by closure of the palm and hand defect. If a central digit or digits are missing but there metacarpals are present, the metacarpal should be excised and the two parts of the hand closed.

Megalodactylism

Hypertrophy of one or more digits or of the entire hand is a rare anomaly (Figs. 17.33 and 17.34). These hypertrophies may be the result of true anomalies of development, but there is definite evidence that a large number of them have neurofibromatosis as the underlying pathology. McCarroll,[11] Moore,[13] and Brooks[3] have shown cases of increase in length as well as breadth or of soft tissues and bone due to neurofibromatous changes in the digit. The neurofibroma itself is usually unobstrusive, and the associated hypertrophy is the most notable condition.

TREATMENT

A good deal of the enlargement may consist entirely of soft-tissue hypertrophy in which large tortuous nerves and nodular tumor masses are located. When this is the case, resection of the soft-tissue masses, the grossly enlarged tortuous nerves, and the redundant skin may produce a nearly normal finger, although sensation may be somewhat diminished. It is advisable to perform this procedure in stages to avoid circulatory damage to the entire part. If the digital nerve is uninvolved, it should be preserved, and excess tissues should be removed from its periphery. In some instances, the length of the finger and of the associated bony deformity is too great, and parts of the finger may have to be sacrificed. If the finger is severely deformed and enlarged so that it is a poorly functioning unit in an otherwise normally functioning hand, it is probably best to sacrifice it. A ray amputation in these cases produces a result that is excellent functionally and cosmetically.

Annular Grooves and Congenital Amputations

These ringlike bands appear circumferentially about the arm, forearm, leg, fingers,

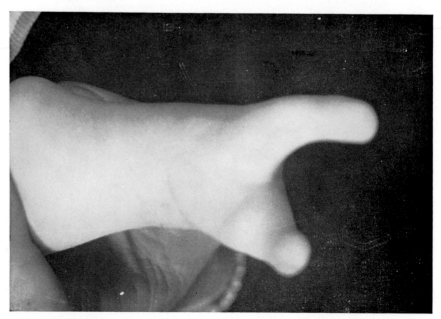

Figure 17.32. Lobster claw hand. No treatment is prescribed for this type of case.

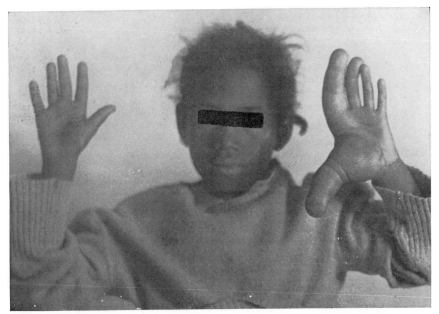

Figure 17.33.   Congenital hypertrophy or megalodactylia.

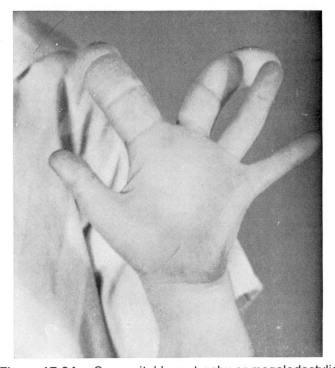

Figure 17.34.   Congenital hypertrophy or megalodactylia.

and toes. The exact etiology is unknown; however, they are not due to amniotic bands. The grooves may be shallow, involving only skin and subcutaneous tissue, or they may extend through the fascia to any depth. The deeper ones often interfere with lymphatic and venous return and cause distal edema. At times, the portion of the extremity that is distal to the groove is lost. This definitely occurs in utero, and amputations are then present in the newborn. Single or multiple amputations of fingers or of the hand frequently accompany these annular grooves (Figs. 17.35 and 17.36).

TREATMENT

When the grooving is superficial, no treatment is necessary and the groove should be left alone. Deep grooves, particularly those interfering with lymphatic drainage, should

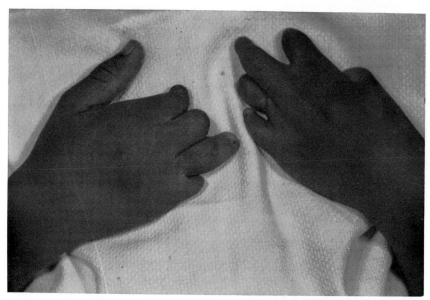

Figure 17.35. Congenital grooves and bands with amputations associated with partial syndactylism. Some improvement cosmetically and functionally can be obtained by deepening the webs.

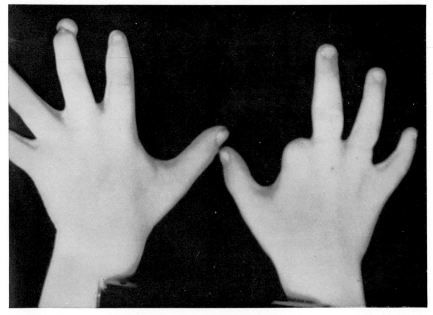

Figure 17.36. Typical Streeter's dysplasia (congenital amputation and annular grooves).

be corrected. The groove is excised by means of incisions that go beneath it until normal structures are encountered and that zigzag in a manner approximating the subcutaneous tissue and skin so that a constricting scar is avoided (Fig. 17.37). The excision should not be accomplished in one procedure, but rather in stages, one-half to one-third of the groove being released at a sitting, to avoid circulatory embarrassment.

Brachydactylism

Interference with embryonic development may cause shortening of one or more digits. The phalanges may be decreased in number of length, or the metacarpal may be shortened. Various combinations may occur simultaneously. It is not uncommon for this condition to occur concomitantly with syndactylism or polydactylism (Fig. 17.38).

TREATMENT

There is really no treatment for brachydactylia. The fingers may be almost normally formed, and they may function quite satis-factorily. The accompanying deformities of syndactylism or polydactylism should be corrected as described above.

Agenesis and Incomplete Development

Absence or incomplete development of parts may involve an entire extremity or parts of one (Fig. 17.39). This section deals with such deformities as amelia, or complete absence of an upper limb; hemimelia, or absence of the hand; adactylia, or absence, complete or incomplete, of the digits, including the metacarpals and phalanges; aphalangia, or absence of phalanges, complete or incomplete; and phocomelia, including complete phocomelia—or absence of an entire arm except the hand and fingers, proximal phocomelia—or complete absence of only the proximal segment of an arm, and distal phocomelia—or complete absence of only the forearm. In some instances, the involvement may be quite extensive, even to the point of producing a quadruple amputee. It may be so mild, however, as to produce a perfectly normal skeleton except for the absence of a phalanx or even a part of one phalanx. Some-

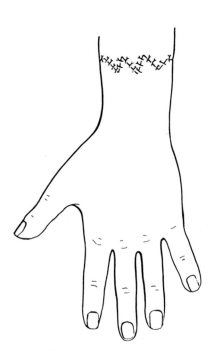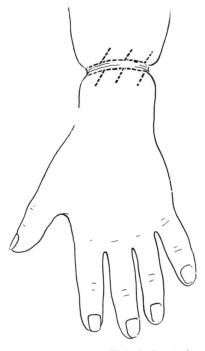

Figure 17.37. Correction of annular groove by surgical excision. This is best done in stages, with one-third to one-half of the circumference being released at one sitting.

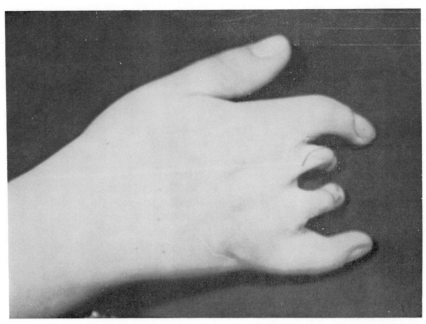

Figure 17.38. Severe partial brachydactylia and syndactylism. The child was very much upset by the deformity. Excision of the middle and ring fingers and moving the middle ray ulnarward would render the deformity much less noticeable.

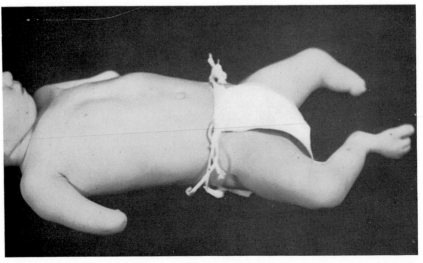

Figure 17.39. Congenital absence of both forearms and of left lower leg with flexion contracture of both knees. The flexion contractures were corrected by posterior surgical release and skeletal traction. The right leg was then braced, and a prosthesis was fitted on the left. The patient walked with crutches at the age of 3 years.

times the stump of a part is smooth and has no external evidence of a part distal to it; however, by x-ray there are at times evidences of incomplete development of the distal limb bud. In other instances, there is a fairly well developed arm but a poorly developed forearm and a limb bud for the hand. Usually these small processes are valueless

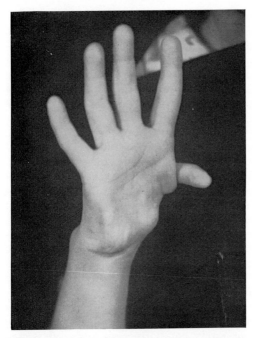

Figure 17.40. Congenital absence of the first metacarpal with poorly developed phalanges. There is some function in the long flexor and the extensor (adactylia, partial, intercalary) (floating thumb).

from a functional standpoint and are in the way as far as the fitting of prostheses is concerned.

A deformity of the fingers may be manifested in many ways (Figs. 17.40 and 17.41). There may be complete absence of a finger or an entire ray, or of the entire radial or ulnar side of the hand. The fingers may be present but incompletely developed, and there may be other associated anomalies such as partial or complete syndactylism, symphalangism, or any group of such associated deformities.

TREATMENT

Unfortunately, when a part is absent, there is no way to add or replace it. Usually one must accept deformity, particularly if there is incomplete loss of a part such as a forearm, arm, or hand. In cases of amelia, and of hemimelia and phocomelia in which no definite procedures can be accomplished to give satisfactory terminal usefulness to the part, prostheses should be used. Numerous factors have been shown to determine whether the prosthesis will be functionally useful or a failure. Two of the most important are (1) the

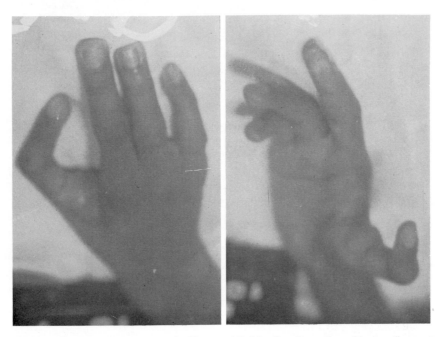

Figure 17.41. Same case as seen in Figure 17.40 after transfer of index finger to thumb position.

age at which the prosthesis is fitted and (2) the attitude of the family. Aitken and Frantz[1] have pointed out that when the child with an amputation is presented for care, it is imperative first to establish enough rapport with the family to convince them that the prosthesis is desirable and necessary. The family must exercise its authority to promote acceptance of the prosthesis, repetitive wearing, and practice until functional gain makes wearing the prosthesis seem desirable. This will not be done unless the family is first convinced that prosthetic restoration is a sound principle.

For years it was thought unnecessary to fit children who had limb deficiencies until they were old enough to decide for themselves whether they needed a prosthesis or not. In recent years, fitting was begun just before school age at about 4–4½ years (Figs. 17.42 and 17.43), but now most authorities who work constantly with this problem believe that the best final results are obtained in children only 6 months of age. As soon as the child can sit well and balance, it is well to fit these congenital limb deficiencies with a passive type of mitten that offers some cosmetic restoration and also permits palmar prehension. At the age of approximately 2½ years, the two-pronged, voluntary-opening, terminal device should be fitted. When these protheses are fitted early, the children are found to adapt to them quite nicely; the prosthesis actually becomes a part of the child.

Small, useless appendages, if present, should be sacrificed in order to gain an accurate fitting of the prosthesis (Fig. 17.44). When there is an abnormal appendage that may have some functional use in stabilizing a prosthesis or in helping to control some of the movable parts, it should be left intact, regardless of how small or unsightly it may be, and the prosthesis itself should be altered to fit and utilize this valuable part.

Children do well with quite short arm and forearm stumps. It is amazing to watch the function of a multiplying action joint with a short stump. People usually count stumps but rarely count fingers. Any useless part should be sacrificed. The appearance is always improved by such procedures, and quite often function is also improved. When children have been born without certain

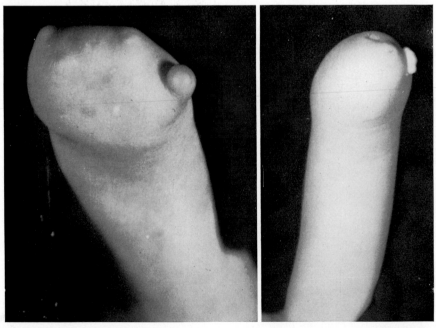

Figure 17.42 (*Left*). Congenital absence of the hand. A prosthesis should be fitted at an early age (about 4 years).
Figure 17.43 (*Right*). Congenital absence of the forearm and hand. This patient should have a prosthesis with an elbow joint at the age of about 4 years.

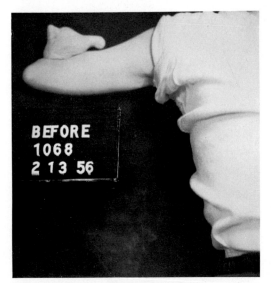

Figure 17.44. Rudimentary bud of forearm and hand. Improved function and appearance may be attained by sacrificing the bud and fitting the remaining arm stump with a prosthesis.

functions, they tend to adapt to the deficiency without great difficulty, to become quite agile, and to substitute very nicely for the missing parts. Such substitution should certainly be encouraged. If phalanges are absent but metacarpals are present, the webs may be deepened so that the metacarpals may be used for grasping. The first metacarpal is particularly valuable for such an adaptation.

Absence of Thumb. If the entire thumb ray is absent bilaterally, a pollicization may be performed on one side. It is better to perform this type of surgery in late childhood when the structures have some maturity and are relatively easy to work with and when the child is at an age of cooperativeness and understanding. The procedures we have been most pleased with have been done between the ages of 7 and 10.

We have been very happy in recent years with the results of the one-stage procedure of transfer of the index finger to the thumb position on a neurovascular pedicle, as described by Littler and Cooley,[10] for both congenital and traumatic absence of the thumb. It is generally thought that, if there is a unilateral absence of the thumb, the procedure is not necessary, but if the absence is bilateral, the mobile thumb ought to be developed.

Many procedures for dealing with the so-called floating thumb have been described. These procedures attempt to utilize the existing hypoplastic thumb as a post and, in some instances, to obtain a post plus a little mobility if any tendon structures are present in the hypoplastic thumb. Some of the procedures have been successful, but they always leave the thumb in a poor position. It is always a post, and its appearance and function are never as good as one desires. It is not nearly as functional as an index finger that has been properly moved to the thumb position.

Depending upon what structures are present, many modifications of the procedure may be necessary. In some instances, an existing first metacarpal allows a relatively simple procedure. In other instances, there may be no thumb tendons, either extrinsic or intrinsic, and no carpal bones. In such cases, the procedure is somewhat more difficult but certainly possible, and it gives, in our experience, excellent results. Usually when the entire digit, including all musculature, has been removed, we have found that a sublimis type of opponens transfer gives better stability and even more function of the moved finger. The procedure, which has been well described by Littler, involves making a flap on the radial side of the hand. A racket type of incision is made about the base of the index finger; it comes down radialward and dorsalward and then swings back from the dorsal surface of the hand to the level of the "take-off" position of the thumb. The entire wound, which circumscribes the index finger, is opened up; then, the surgeon working from the dorsal surface, the dorsal aponeurosis is sectioned between the second and third metacarpal ligament and any interdigitating fibers between the extensor tendons of the index and middle fingers. The vessels are demonstrated at this point, and the artery and vein to the radial side of the middle finger are identified, ligated, and severed in order that the vessels to the index finger may remain intact and that the entire finger may be mobilized. The nerve is usually separate at this level. If it is not, it can be mobilized by sharp dissection about as far back as one desires so that the nerve fibers are left running out to the middle finger and index finger separately. If the entire finger is moved, the interossei are detached and the metacarpal is exposed. The metacarpal may then be sec-

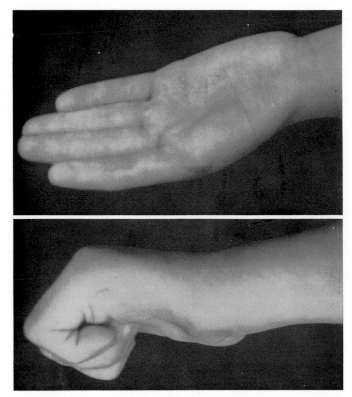

Figure 17.45. Congenital absence of the thumb with excellent function of fingers.

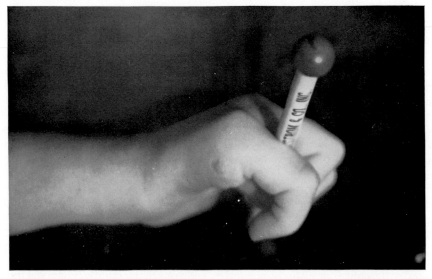

Figure 17.46. Same case as seen in Figure 17.45. Use of pencil showing substitution pattern. Surgery should not be considered unless the deformity is bilateral, in which case the index finger might be transposed for the thumb on one side.

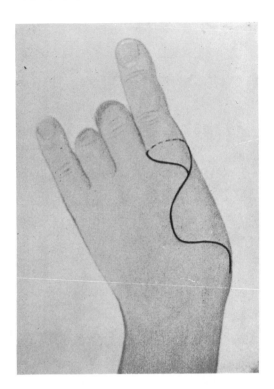

Figure 17.47. Plan of incision used in first stage of transfer of index finger to thumb position.

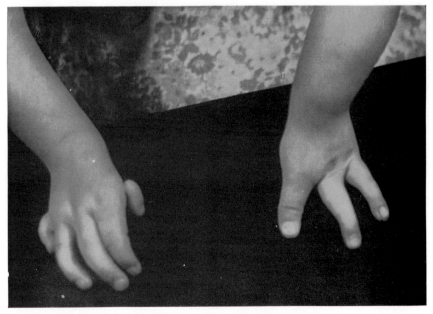

Figure 17.48. Congenital maldevelopment. The right hand can be improved cosmetically by removal of the poorly developed radial and ulnar digits.

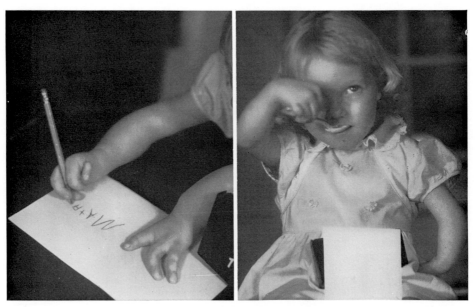

Figure 17.49. Same case as seen in Figure 17.48 showing adaptability at an early age. Function will improve in this patient with use and time.

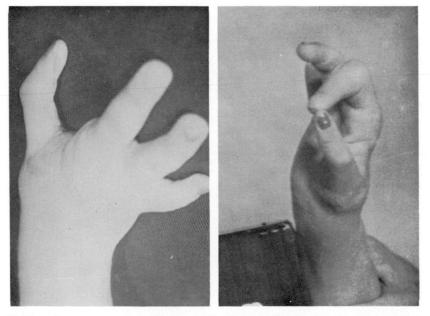

Figure 17.50. Same as seen in Figures 17.48 and 17.49 after transfer of index finger to thumb position.

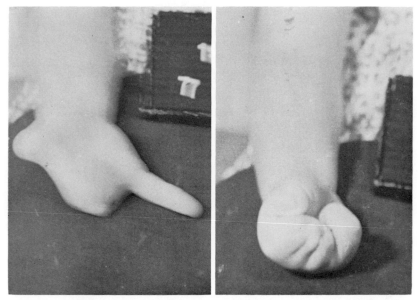

Figure 17.51.   Hand of child with multiple congenital anomalies.

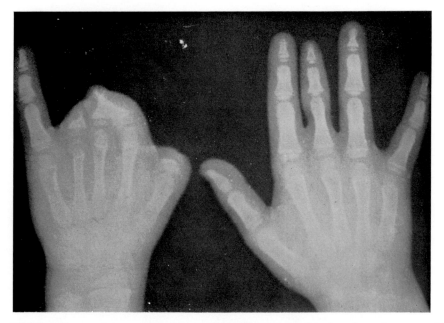

Figure 17.52.   X-ray of same hand as seen in Figure 17.51 showing absence of thumb phalanges, partial absence of finger phalanges, and syndactyly.

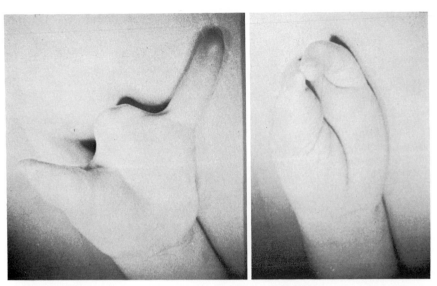

Figure 17.53. Hand shown in Figure 17.51 after syndactyly separation of index finger and transfer of entire index ray to first metacarpal. A usable thumb with good sensation has been constructed.

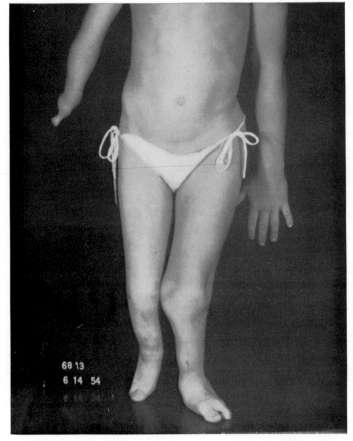

Figure 17.54. Multiple congenital skeletal anomalies. The child has adapted well to the use of one finger on the right. He can lace shoes and tie bows as quickly as anyone.

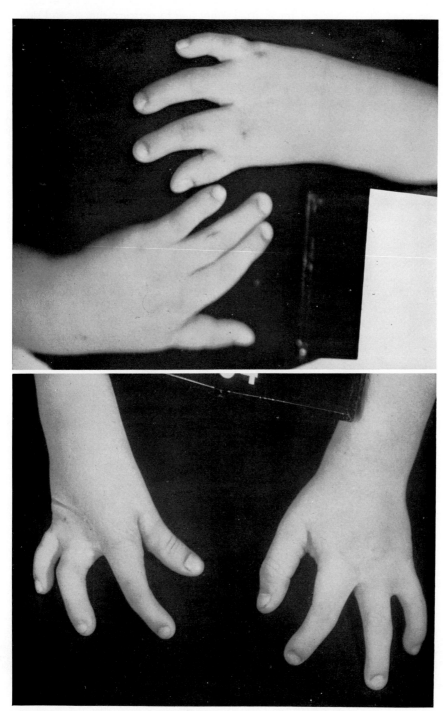

Figure 17.55 (*Top*).   Congenital absence of digit with webbing of the first metacarpal space. The child has congenital deafness and congenital anomalies of the ears in addition.
Figure 17.56 (*Bottom*).   The result after Z-plasty deepening of the thumb web.

tioned at the base and also at the neck so that its shaft is completely removed. We have utilized the head of the second metacarpal more or less as a carpal bone. In one instance, we attached this bone to its own base at an angle of almost 90 degrees. It united and, in spite of our wishes to the contrary, has continued to grow and to add length to the finger. In 2 other cases since that one, we left the head of the metacarpal in the position of the carpus and attached it to the base of the second metacarpal bone very insecurely so that bony union would not occur; in both instances, the head has remained as we desired it, so that it has been used as a carpal bone, and has not increased in length, the metaphysis being constantly absorbed. Therefore, we have a fibrous union at this level, and the proximal phalanx is utilized as the first metacarpal. The flexor and extensor tendons motivate the finger, and if after a year of use there is not enough take-up in these tendons, they can be shortened above the wrist. In our experience to data, we have not had to perform this second procedure.

A transfer of the index finger should be done any time after the child has reached a cooperative age. We have not thought it necessary to do this very early but like to get it done about the age of 5 or 6 years. After the procedure has been performed, the skin is sutured with interrupted 4-0 sutures or 51-0 chromic catgut, and a pressure dressing and a cast that holds the thumb in a position of opposition are applied. To date we have had no difficulties with arterial insufficiency. Venous stasis has at times presented a small problem, but not yet enough difficulty to warrant treatment other than observation. We have been very careful to observe Littler's original suggestion that as many venous structures as possible be saved in the skin so that there is little interference with venous return. This is very important.

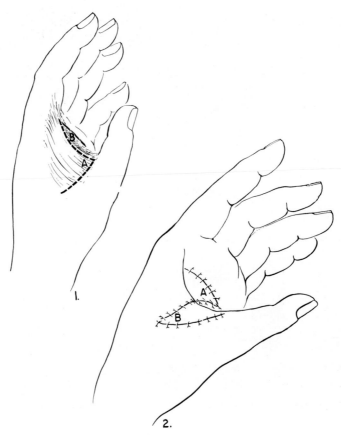

Figure 17.57. Widening the adductor web by Z-plasty to procure additional function of thumb.

Symphalangism

This condition results in failure of the interphalangeal joints to develop and occurs most frequently as a loss of the distal interphalangeal joint. The condition is frequently hereditary (Fig. 17.58). There is no treatment, and, as a rule, the patient does not realize the presence of the deformity and usually adapts well from a functional standpoint.

Triphalangeal Thumb

Sometimes a thumb develops the appearance of a finger. This may occur with failure of development of the thenar muscles and lack of a wide intermetacarpal space between the first and second metacarpals, along with the existence of three phalanges in the ray. Another variation is a more or less normally developed thumb with three full phalanges. This thumb is more satisfactory in that the function is more normal and treatment is usually unnecessary. On occasion, one of the three phalanges may be deformed or wedge shaped. In such instances, the deformed phalanx, which is fortunately most often the middle one, can be removed surgically so that the two normal phalanges will approximate each other (Figs. 17.59 and 17.60). They will form a good joint. The ligaments should be sutured, and most often the thumb will have very good function and appearance.

References

1. Aitken, G. T., and Frantz, C. H.: The juvenile amputee, *J. Bone Joint Surg., 46A:* 1376, 1964.
2. Barsky, A. J.: Congenital anomalies of the hand, *J. Bone Joint Surg., 33A:* 35, 1951.
3. Brooks, B., and Lehman, E. P.: The bone changes in Recklinghausen's neurofibromatosis, *Surg. Gynecol. Obstet., 38:* 587, 1924.
4. Bunnell, S.: Contractures of the hand from infections and injuries, *J. Bone Joint Surg., 14:* 27, 1932.
5. Bunnell, S.: *Surgery of the Hand*, Philadelphia: J. B. Lippincott, 1944.
6. Colonna, P. C.: Some common congenital deformities and their orthopedic treatment, *N. Y. J. Med., 28:* 713, 1928.
7. Frantz, C. H., and O'Rahilly, R.: Congenital skeletal limb deficiencies, *J. Bone Joint Surg., 43A:* 1202, 1961.
8. Johnson, H. M.: Congenital cicatrizing bands, report of a case with etiologic observations, *Am. J. Surg., 52:* 498, 1941.
9. Kanavel, A. B.: Congenital malformations of the hand, *Arch. Surg., 25:* 1932.
10. Littler, J. W., and Cooley, S. G. E.: Congenital dysplasia of the thumb, *J. Bone Joint Surg., 46A:* 912, 1964.
11. McCarroll, H. R.: Clinical manifestations of congenital neurofibromatosis, *J. Bone Joint Surg., 32A:* 601, 1950.
12. MacCollum, D. W.: Webbed fingers, *Surg. Gynecol. Obstet., 71:* 782, 1940.
13. Moore, B. H.: Some orthopedic relationships of neurofibromatosis, *J. Bone Joint Surg., 23:* 109, 1941.
14. Sachs, M. D.: Familial brachyphalangiae, *Radiology, 35:* 622, 1940.
15. Stelling, F. H.: Surgery of the hand in the child, *J. Bone Joint Surg., 45A:* 623, 1963.

CEREBRAL PALSY

Reconstruction of the hand disabled by cerebral palsy is one of the most difficult tasks confronting the surgeon who treats hand conditions. The results are frequently disheartening, and, in general, treatment should be conservative. There are very few cases in which surgical intervention is advisable or beneficial (Fig. 17.61). Many factors serve to complicate the treatment of these hands. One of the first and most important steps is the careful classification of these cases into one of the basic types, i.e., true spastics, athetoids, tension athetoids, ataxias, or rigidites. Therapy that may prove valuable in one of these groups can well be completely ineffective or contraindicated in another. Because the classification may at times be difficult, careful observation and repeated examinations are necessary before a definite therapeutic plan can be developed.

A second major factor that plays an important part in determining treatment is the mentality of the child. Many of these children are retarded and lack the cooperativeness necessary to hand surgery. Another factor that contributes greatly to the difficulties of treatment is that even in specific groups there are great variations in the severity of involvement. In certain cases, spasticity and poor coordination may seem to play the greatest part in dysfunction; however, there may also be a definite weakness of the opposing muscle. In the very young cerebral palsied child, major emphasis should be placed on preventing a fixed position. The fingers, thumb, wrist, and forearm should be stretched passively several times daily (Figs. 17.62 and 17.63). Frequently, children affected unilaterally do not recognize the effective hand as

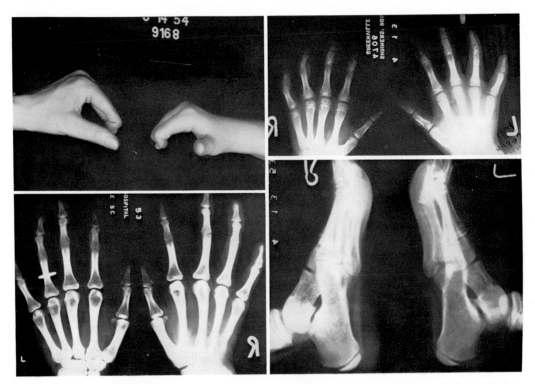

Figure 17.58. Symphalangism in mother and daughter. X-rays of the child's feet show incomplete segmentation of calcis, cuboid, talus, and navicular.

such and make no attempt to use it as a hand. Early recognition of the hand should be taught by means of toys, colored beads, and blocks to stimulate interest. Occasionally, the doctor or parent attempts to restrict the good hand to force the child to use the affected one. This procedure is condemned, as it has been definitely shown that restricting a dominant hand may lead to such serious psychologic difficulties as stuttering, loss or lack of speech, and behavior problems. Occasionally, after the child has discovered the dominant hand, restriction of the other may cure a psychologic complex.

Splinting and Physical Therapy

Following a period of observation, some of these children may be helped by the use of a small cock-up splint, or a splint with an outrigger to hold the thumb in extension may be necessary. Occasionally, rigid splints or plaster bivalves may be used at night or on a part-time basis during the day to hold the forearm in a supinated position and to aid in passive stretching exercises (Fig. 17.64). Later, as the child begins to develop and becomes more cooperative, active exercises can be added to the treatment program. Physical therapists are helpful in teaching the child and parents specific exercises outlined by the doctor. Major functions to be stressed are those of reaching, releasing the fingers, stabilizing the wrist in extension, grasping and releasing the fingers (Figs. 17.65 and 17.66). Patients with true spasticity usually tend to flex the wrist as the fingers are extended incoordinately. They also have difficulty extending the thumb out of the palm. As grasp is attempted, varying degrees of wrist flexion hinder active grasping function of the fingers (Fig. 17.67). Frequently, the thumb is in a position of adduction prior to finger flexion, and this position interferes severely with pick-up and attempted pinch. In most of these cases, if one extends the wrist to aid the strength of grasp, the patient may be unable to extend the fingers effectively for function. Treatment must be carried out many times daily, and parental cooperation and understanding are essential.

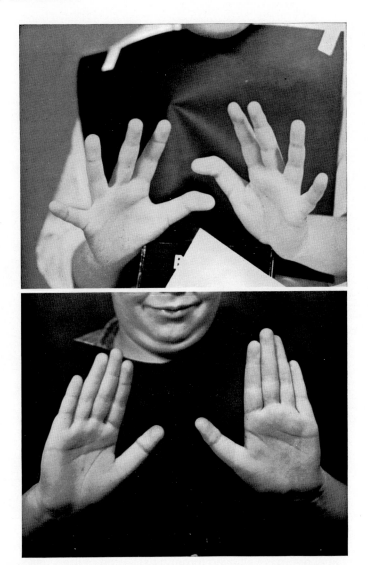

Figure 17.59 (*Top*).   Triphalangeal thumb bilateral; the middle phalanx is wedge shaped.
Figure 17.60 (*Bottom*).   Hands are shown after removal of middle phalanx. Excellent functional and cosmetic results.

The preceding conservative program is used in all types of cases and should be the only type of treatment for ataxias, athetoids, and tension athetoids. With athetoids, one of the prime initial efforts should be to teach the patient active relaxation. Time is a great factor here, but again understanding on the part of the family and helpfulness of those charged with the care of the patient may make a great difference. It is amazing to see one of these patients attempt to write or to use a typewritter while fighting the marked overflow. Surgery in some of these cases produces much poorer function, and in very few instances does it produce the desired effect.

Surgical Treatment

Occasionally surgical intervention definitely improves the function in these hands. At the North Carolina Cerebral Palsy Hospital, Goldner,[3] taking into consideration physical status and mental condition, found only 12 patients acceptable for hand surgery

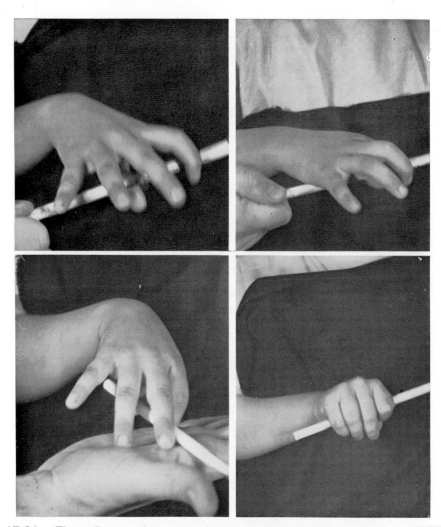

Figure 17.61. These figures show typical attempt of the spastic to grasp. Active flexion of the wrist is performed to release the spastic finger flexion. The fingers are incoordinately flexed, and final grasp is achieved through extension of the wrist, which enhances the use of the spastic finger flexors. The child with this pattern can be trained, and surgery can often be avoided.

out of 300 selected as eligible for general treatment.

Prior to selecting a case for surgery, it is advisable that the surgeon follow the patient for a long period to make sure that the proposed procedure has at least a reasonable chance of improving function. The use of casts or splints may be extremely helpful in making a decision. The brace or cast may be placed on the extremity so as to hold it in the position that might be attained by surgery. The use of the hand in the cast or splint is observed over a period of time before a decision is made. Before a definitive surgical procedure is attempted, a detailed examination of the muscles must be made. Phelps[8] has emphasized that, in addition to the charting and evaluation of spastic muscles, the power of other associated muscles must be evaluated and their degree of control noted. The importance of evaluating the power of nonspastic muscles is emphasized because certain antagonistic muscles may show a great weakness and at times may be com-

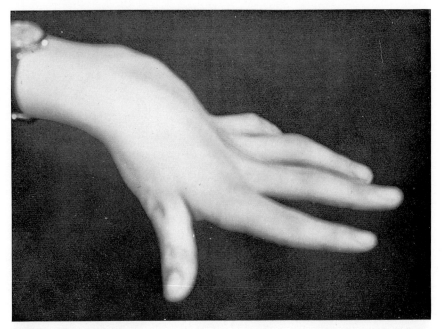

Figure 17.62. Cerebral palsy, spastic type, showing reach and poor ability to get the thumb away from the palm.

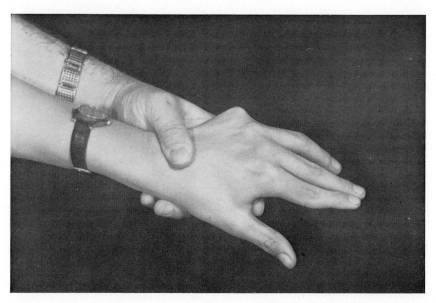

Figure 17.63. Same case as seen in Figure 17.62. Patient with wrist immobilized passively in extension and ulnar deviation, showing active ability now to get the thumb away from the palm for better function. Ability to extend the fingers is not quite as good, but it would still be quite effective for reach. This patient would profit from a wrist fusion.

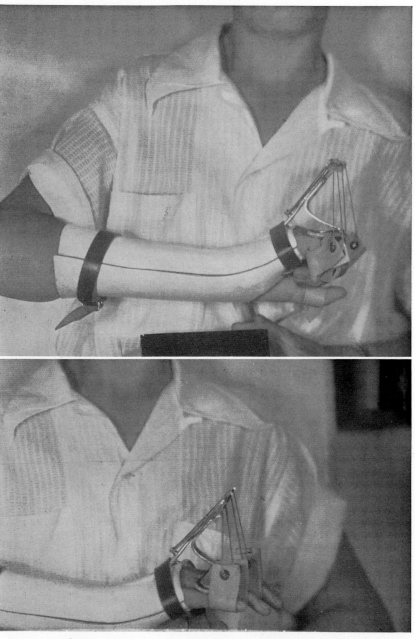

Figure 17.64. Removal plastic splint with active rubber band traction outriggers tor finger and thumb extension. The bar prevents hyperextension of the metacarpophalangeal joint. This splint is used on a part time basis in an attempt to teach proper patterns.

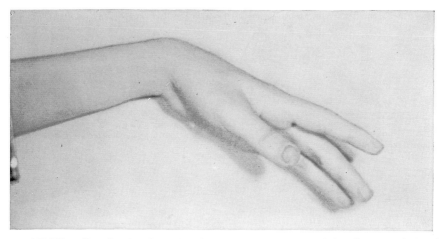

Figure 17.65. Cerebral palsy showing attempt to extend the fingers and wrist.

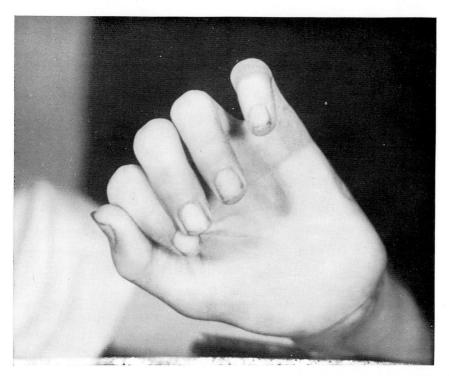

Figure 17.66. Same case as seen in Figure 17.65 after transplantation of the flexor ulnaris to the common extensors and the flexor radialis to the extensor pollicis brevis. The patient has a good grip but now hyperextends the wrist and is unable to extend the fingers away from the palm. The condition would be improved now by a wrist fusion in a neutral position. This pattern sometimes occurs after transplantation of wrist flexors into finger extensors owing to a resulting active insufficiency of wrist flexion.

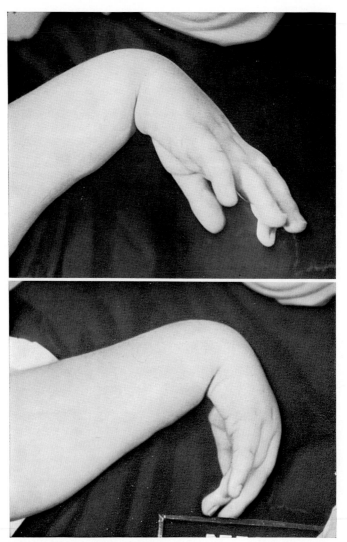

Figure 17.67. True spastic cerebral palsy showing patient's attempt to extend the fingers and wrist (*top*) and to grasp (*bottom*).

pletely flaccid. This is particularly true in the muscles controlling the wrist and fingers. If there is a flaccid paralysis in the antagonistic muscles, relieving the spasticity will not solve the problem.

Surgery should be used only as an adjunct to the general treatment of the hand in cerebral palsy. Many of the operative procedures have been devised for other types of neurologic involvement, and it should be emphasized that, when these procedures are used on the cerebral palsied child, the final results are never as satifactory. The procedures used in cerebral palsy for improvement of the

spastic hand should be those which stabilize the wrist to permit better finger function, get the thumb away from the palm to allow the hand to be opened and closed effectively, and improve supination. Certain minor procedures may be helpful, and occasionally, an excellent result may be obtained. Intricate procedures, which are often used for polio, should be left to the surgeon who is well versed in hand surgery.

Arthrodesis of the wrist is performed to improve the function of the digits and correct deformity of the wrist. The flexor carpi ulnaris is often a strong spastic muscle capable of producing considerable deformity. Steindler described a procedure in that the spastic flexor carpi ulnaris was released from its insertion, brought subcutaneously through a channel from the ulnar side across the dorsal aspect of the forearm, and transferred into an osseous opening in the distal radius in the radial styloid. This removed the deforming force of the ulnaris as a strong ulnar deviator and flexor, and aided in active supination of the forearm. Green[4] later modified this procedure by transferring the flexor carpi ulnaris into the extensor carpi radialis longus. This actually is a better procedure because it adds a powerful active dorsiflexion that improves wrist and finger control; also, because of the

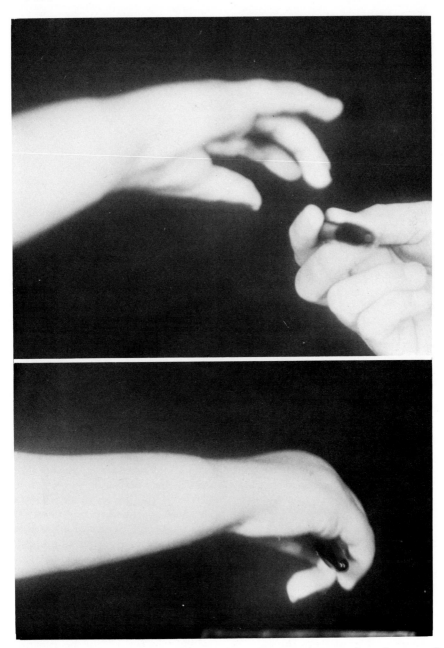

Figure 17.68. Same case as seen in Figure 17.67, showing reach and grasp after wrist fusion in a neutral position.

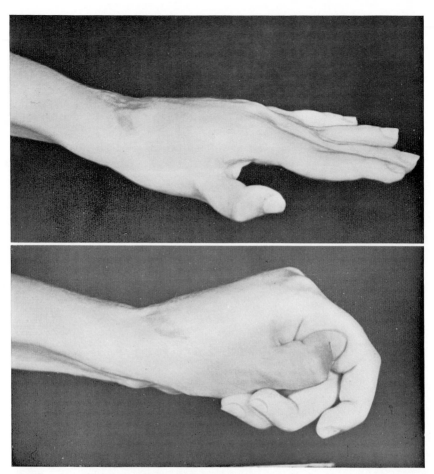

Figure 17.69. Reach and grasp following transplantation of the flexor ulnaris to the common extensors and the flexor radialis to the extensor pollicis brevis. Prior to surgery, the thumb was held flexed, the fingers were clenched, and the wrist was markedly flexed. Now the patient has better reach and grasp, but the thumb hyperextends. This has since been improved by an arthrodesis of the metacarpophalangeal joint.

position of the transfer, it will add some supinatory effect. It is less desirable than the Green transfer, which removes the deforming force of ulnar deviation and flexion and provides the active force of promoting dorsiflexion of the wrist in supination, however. In 1962 Green and Banks[5] reported an end result study of 39 cases and rated 24 in the excellent to good group, 15 in the fair group, and only 2 as poor results. They felt that surgical procedure was the single best way to improve function of the hand and fingers in cerebral palsy. They also noted that they had not had to perform a wrist arthrodesis in the past 20 years. They emphasized the importance of proper evaluation of cases before utilizing

this procedure. In every instance the transfer should not be performed until the soft tissues causing fixed deformity were corrected, such as release of flexion of the wrist or fixed pronation of the forearm. They felt it was very important to utilize proper follow-up care in the use of proper splinting and utilization of physical therapy in the form of active assistive exercises until the patients were able to function actively to the best possible ability before discontinuing all protection and functional training. In his discussion of the paper by Drs. Green and Banks, Goldner[3] indicated that he did not believe that arthrodesis should be abandoned. There are definitely some patients in whom previous procedures have failed or others in whom stability can only be obtained by arthrodesis. Hands requiring stability of the wrist are helped considerably by arthrodesis just past the neutral position in extension. This position allows more effective and efficient use of the fingers. Not infrequently this positioning of the wrist causes the fingers to be tightly clenched in the palm and unable to extend. This condition should be known prior to surgery, and a first procedure would be to transplant one of the strong wrist flexors into the finger extensors. Occasionally, this procedure is all that is necessary; however, a wrist fusion is usually needed to provide for adequate stability.

The thumb-in-palm deformity is one of the most disabling encountered in the spastic hand. If the deformity is mild, ulnar deviation of the hand at the wrist increases the tension of the extensor and abductor mechanism of the thumb and thus pulls the thumb phalanges and the first metacarpal toward the radial side. This was first emphasized by Cooper,[2] and it is wise, in arthrodeses of the wrist, to place the hand in moderate ulnar deviation in order that this mechanism may become effective in pulling the thumb up out of the palm. It should be remembered that if the flexor pollicis longus is spastic or contracted and the thumb web is tight, no amount of ulnar deviation of the hand produces an ef-

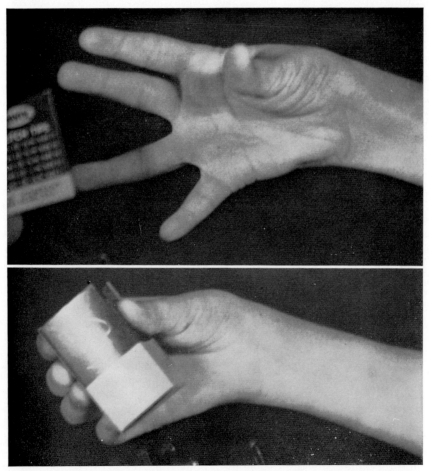

Figure 17.70. These figures show a hand of a child with cerebral palsy, true spastic type, following a wrist fusion in ulnar deviation with the wrist in a neutral position regarding flexion and extension. The patient is able to extend the fingers and to get the thumb away from the palm for grasping. Prior to surgery, the patient clenched the fingers and thumb into the palm and had difficulty attempting to get them away from the palm.

fective result in getting the thumb out of the palm. A hypermobile metacarpophalangeal joint often results in the deformity that pulls the thumb into the palm, and weakness of the intrinsic musculature of the thumb may lead to the thumb-in-palm position.

Spasticity or contracture of the thumb web may be treated by sectioning the web fascia and stripping the dorsal interosseous muscle from the first metacarpal, as well as tenotomizing the adductor pollicis. These procedures are often done in conjunction with fusion of the metacarpophalangeal joint. If the extensor mechanism is inactive or weak, transplantation of an active wrist or finger flexor to the extensor pollicis longus should be carried out. Sometimes this leads to an imbalance with hyperextension of the metacarpophalangeal joint and, when it does, a fusion of this joint should be added.

References

1. Burman, M. S.: The spastic hand, *J. Bone Joint Surg.*, 20: 133, 1938.
2. Cooper, W.: Surgery of the upper extremity in spastic paralysis, *Q. Rev. Pediatr.*, 7: 64, 1951.
3. Goldner, J. L.: Reconstructive surgery of the hand in cerebral palsy and spastic paralysis resulting from injury to the spinal cord, *J. Bone Joint Surg.*, 37A: 1141, 1955.
4. Green, W. T.: Transplantation of flexor carpi ulnaris for pronation-flexion deformity of the wrist, *Surg. Gynecol. Obstet.*, 75: 337, 1942.
5. Green, W. T., and Banks, H.: Flexor carpi ulnaris transplant and its use in cerebral palsy, *J. Bone Joint Surg.*, 44A: 1343, 1962.
6. Green, W. T., and McDermott, L. J.: Operative treatment of cerebral palsy of spastic type, *J. A. M. A.*, 118: 434, 1942.
7. McCarroll, H. R.: Surgical treatment of spastic paralysis, *Instruct. Lect. Am. Acad. Orthrop. Surg.*, 6: 134, 1949.
8. Phelps, W.: Prevention of acquired dislocation of the hip in cerebral palsy, *J. Bone Joint Surg.*, 41A: 440, 1959.

POLIOMYELITIS

Poliomyelitis frequently involves the upper extremity and results in residual weakness and a poorly functioning hand. In some instances, the hand is so severely involved that very little functional value is maintained; however, by certain operative procedures, the value can be increased. The aim of these procedures is to reroute tendons to prevent or correct deformities caused by strong musculature and to increase the efficiency of poorly functioning muscle. Occasionally, a completely paralyzed muscle can be replaced by tendon transplantation. In other instances, substitution patterns are developed, or can be developed with help, so that a fairly vulnerable hand is obtained. Occasionally these substitution patterns may be strengthened or enhanced by surgical procedures.

From the very onset of the acute disease, function should be the final goal of the care and treatment of the hand. The joints should be kept mobile, and secondary contractures and deformities should be prevented by proper utilization of active and passive exercises and by splinting the hand in the position of function. During the sensitive stages of the disease, passive splints may be used to rest the parts and thus to prevent stretching of painful, weakened muscles. Later, as sensitivity and muscle spasm disappear and muscle power begins to return, certain active splints are used. These splints are devised to afford helpful stabilization of the wrist action in some 10 of 15 degrees of dorsiflexion. They are made of spring type metal to afford support and yet maintain flexibility. Outriggers are used to help finger extension or flexion, or both, with spring metal or elastic bands. Opponens splints are usually rigid or semirigid to keep the thumb in the opposed, functioning position. They may be made of plastic or metal.

In the younger age groups (up to 10 years) it is best to utilize functional splinting for a period of years even though certain operative procedures might be available to improve function and thus to replace the splint. There are several reasons for this recommendation: (1) operative procedures are technically more difficult in the young child; (2) the refined hand movements that are necessary for taking over tendon transplants are lacking because of incomplete development of the nervous system; (3) the best results are attained with full cooperation, which is often lacking in the younger age group; and (4) bone growth should be complete, or nearly complete, to prevent disproportion between the bony framework and the tendon transplantation.

In some exceptional cases, waiting should definitely be avoided. These cases are mainly those in which the tendon to be transplanted is producing bone or joint deformity in spite of splinting and exercises.

Certain conditions that are present in polio are not always present in traumatic hands and are favorable to both the patient and the surgeon. On the other hand, other conditions exist which make rehabilitation more difficult and uncertain.

Unfavorable conditions:
1. Disseminated muscle weakness
2. Substitution patterns
3. Involvement of the trunk and other extremities

Favorable conditions:
1. Good skin and subcutaneous tissue
2. Normal sensation
3. Good mobility of joints

The procedures devised to improve hand function surgically may be divided into three groups: (1) arthrodeses, (2) tendon transfers, and (3) tenodeses. Of these three groups, the tendon transfers are the most valuable and produce a better functioning hand.

Arthrodeses

Arthrodeses should be used only as a last resort. Occasionally, an arthrodesis is indicated to free tendons for other usage, but, in polio, the loss of joint motion in the upper extremity may be disabling. All other methods of improving function should be carefully considered before such a procedure as fusing the wrist is undertaken. This procedure should be regarded as a last resort, and the relationship of a stiff wrist to the total function of the patient's extremity must be determined. Occasionally, it may be seen that the finger and thumb function could undoubtedly be improved by utilizing the wrist tendons following stabilization; however, after careful consideration, it may be found that wrist motion will be much more useful than an improved finger and thumb function. Fusion of the wrist in the wheelchair patient may cause loss of ability to use the chair, and may thus disable him completely if the chair is his only means of locomotion. Other patients need a flexible wrist in order to shift the body weight. A fusion of the wrist here might well prevent the patient from moving about. It is important in all instances to consider the affected hand in relation to body function as a whole before permanently stabilizing a joint. Arthrodesis of the metacarpophalangeal joint is certainly of value and sometimes necessary to correct deformity

and to increase the usefulness of the fingers; however, it should not be done if it can possibly be avoided. The avoidance of this procedure is especially necessary in a severely handicapped person who requires a flat hand to push himself about. It has also been found that arthrodesis weakens the grasp and thus makes the use of crutches extremely difficult. It is wise, when arthrodesis is considered, to defer the procedure as long as possible, preferably until maturity. The reason for this is that the person should be allowed to try a vocation first. The relationship of the hand to his vocation is extremely important, and he may be greatly handicapped by such a permanent procedure as an arthrodesis.

The bone block procedure may be helpful in improving the function of the hand, but it should be remembered that it is a poor procedure if the patient is a crutch walker.

Arthrodesis of the interphalangeal joint of the thumb is valuable if other means of stabilization are found impossible.

Tendon Transplantation

It has been found that tendon transplants are by far the best procedures for increasing the function of the hand. Occasionally, active motors are not available, and it has been found best to perform passive or active tenodeses, which will be discussed later. A tendon must never be moved without careful consideration and an accurate muscle evaluation. It is frequently necessary to retest the muscles several times to get an accurate picture of the muscle power, and it is often difficult in the young child to obtain an accurate muscle test. It is to be remembered that occasionally two muscles acting together may produce a functioning unit, even though each muscle has only 50% of normal power. A muscle used for transplantation should have at least 85% of normal power.

It should be remembered that transplanting a tendon should not excessively weaken the portion of the hand from which it is taken. For example, a strong wrist extensor should not be transplanted to gain finger flexion or opposition when the remaining wrist flexors are weak (Figs. 17.71 and 17.72). The procedure would result in loss of the stablizing function of wrist extension and would thereby defeat the purpose of the orig-

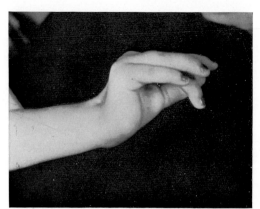

Figure 17.71. A hand in which all wrist flexors have been transplanted into finger and thumb extensors. The stabilizing effect of the wrist flexors has been lost; the wrist cocks back, and the fingers do not extend in the metacarpophalangeal joints.

inal transplant, which was to strengthen the grip. If there is any doubt regarding the power of a muscle, an incision should be made over the belly, and the color and texture of the muscle should be inspected.

In adults, it has been found advisable to wait for a period of 2 years before attempting a tendon transplantation. In children up to the age of 12, it is best to wait for even longer periods. With proper splinting, substitution patterns which will make surgery entirely unnecessary may evolve. In children, it is better to err on the side of waiting too long than to perform surgical procedures without careful consideration.

OPPOSITION

Paralysis of opposition is major disability. The transplant of choice for restoring opponens function is based on use of the sublimis tendon of the ring finger as a motor (Figs. 17.73 and 17.74). The prerequisites for this procedure are: (1) a profoundus of the ring finger that is adequate for flexion of the digit without the sublimis; (2) a strong flexor pollicis longus; (3) a strong extensor pollicis longus and abductor pollicis longus; (4) a good or normal flexor digitorum sublimis; (5) absence of bone, joint, or soft tissue deformity of the thumb; (6) a strong flexor carpi ulnaris; and (7) functional strength of the fingers and the palmar arch.

If these conditions do not exist, the profundus of the ring finger may be reinforced with an adjacent profundus or sublimis. The flexor longus, the abductor, or the extensor of the thumb may be strengthened by another transplant. The most suitable tendon for such strengthening is the long extensor of the wrist. The indicis propirus can often be used to great advantage for strengthening the extensor pollicis longus. The flexor carpi ulnaris may be reinforced by the extensor carpi ulnaris. These procedures will be described in detail later. If there is deformity or contraction of the thumb, it should be corrected prior to any attempts at tendon reconstruction. Sometimes a tenotomy of the adductor of the thumb is necessary to release soft-tissue contracture of the web space. Permanent tightness of the joints may be relieved by a rotation osteotomy of the first metacarpal. Occasionally, in a thumb with a strong flexor pollicis brevis and no disability other than a weakened or absent opponens, an osteotomy of the first metacarpal may produce a satisfactorily functioning result that obviates the necessity of an opponens transplant.

The opponens transfer should pull from the region of the pisiform for best mechanical efficiency. When the sublimis is used, this is accomplished best by bringing the tendon beneath and around the ulnar side of the

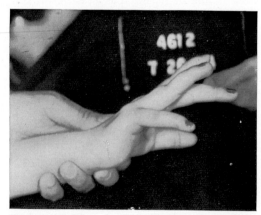

Figure 17.72. Same case as seen in Figure 17.71. If the wrist is stabilized toward flexion, the fingers then extend beautifully. It is always best to leave at least one wrist flexor intact when transferring a tendon, whether it be for cerebral palsy, polio, or brachial palsy.

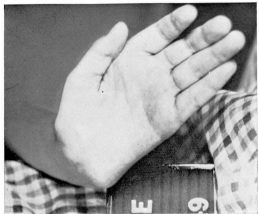

Figure 17.73. Loss of opponens and atrophy of thenar eminence.

flexor carpi ulnaris at its insertion as a pulley. The tendon should be attached to the thumb on the ulnar side of the proximal phalanx. The transplanted tendon should pass across the base of the palm subcutaneously from the pisiform to the metacarpophalangeal joint of the thumb. Proper tension is of utmost importance and is gained only by experience with the procedure. If the tendon is inserted too loosely, it will lack sufficient strength to oppose properly. If it is inserted too tightly, it may migrate over the metacarpophalangeal joint and cause a hyperextension contracture. Following transfer, the hand should be immobilized in a plaster splint that holds the wrist in approximately 30 degrees of flexion and 15 degrees of ulnar deviation. Immobilization should be continued for a period of 3 weeks. Active exercises should follow, but an opponens splint should be used for protection between exercise periods. If the sublimis of the ring finger is not sufficiently strong, the sublimis of the middle finger may be used satisfactorily. Occasionally, it may be necessary to reinforce a transplanted weaker sublimis. This can be done by suturing an additional tendon into the musculotendinous junction of the sublimis tendon. In the absence of sublimi, the extensor carpis ulnaris may be used, if its length is prolonged with a free tendon graft. It is passed around the ulnar border of the wrist proximal to the dorsal carpal ligament so that no pulleys are required.

Rerouting of Extensor Pollicis Longus. Frequently, the thumb drifts into ulnar deviation at the metacarpophalangeal joint. This position often cannot be corrected by opponens transfer. The condition may be alleviated and the opponens transfer made more effective, however, by rerouting the extensor policis longus tendon.

In this procedure, the dorsal carpal ligament is sectioned, and the extensor pollicis longus is removed from its groove and brought volarward in the subcutaneous tissue. Its position is maintained by a subcutaneous suture that holds the tendon in direct line with the thumb ray. The dorsal carpal ligament is then resutured.

Reinforcement of Pulley for Opponens Transfers. At times the opponens transfer migrates toward the radial border of the wrist, and thus reduces the power and effectiveness of the transplant. The usual reason for this migration is weakness of the flexor carpi ulnaris. It can be corrected by suturing the extensor carpi ulnaris into the tendon of the flexor carpi ulnaris, according to the following procedure.

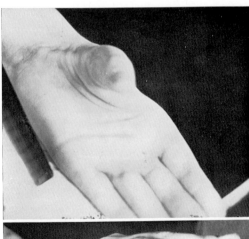

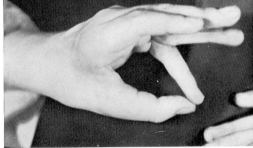

Figure 17.74. Same case as seen in Figure 17.73 after opponens transplantation of the sublimis of the ring finger to the base of the proximal phalanx of the thumb, with the flexor carpi ulnaris used as a pulley.

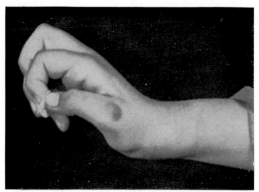

Figure 17.75. Typical pinch of opponens loss plus a weak first interosseous.

A hockey stick incision is made over the volar ulnar border of the wrist. The flexor carpi ulnaris is then freed, and the forearm is pronated. The extensor carpi ulnaris is isolated and sutured through a slit in the flexor carpi ulnaris. Fixation is maintained by interrupted silk sutures. The anastomosis is performed just proximal to the route of the opponens transfer around the flexor carpi ulnaris tendon.

The index finger stands next to the thumb in functional importance. Loss of intrinsic power of this finger along with weak or absent opposition of the thumb is more commonly seen than weakness in all the remaining extrinsic muscles of the hand in poliomyelitis. Absence of the intrinsic power of the index finger prevents extension of the distal two phalanges and abduction of the finger into a position opposite the opposed thumb in the formation of the pinching mechanism. Strong extrinsic flexors and extensors of the index finger do not replace the dorsal and volar interossei add lumbricale muscles in the pinching mechanism. The clinical picture is usually that of cocking or hyperextension of the metacarpophalangeal joint when pinching is attempted. It is due to a loss of stability in flexion of the metacarpophalangeal joint.

If restoration of the intrinsic factor, particularly with regard to stability in flexion of the metacarpophalangeal joint, is attempted, transfers must insert into the lateral band, and function is better mechanically when the insertion is from the volar aspect of the hand. Many procedures for the restitution of this function have been described. Probably the most popular is that of sublimis transfer into the lateral band, as described by Bunnell.[1] Even in the absence of actively functioning musculature, tenodeses according to the methods of Fowler and Riordan[12] are sometimes performed to stabilize these joints. These procedures will be discussed to some extent below. Frequently, the indicis proprius is transferred into the lateral band tendon to afford good abduction of the index finger. This transplant restores abduction and extension but does not stabilize the metacarpophalangeal joint in flexion. Irwin and Eyler[10] have described a procedure which is excellent for the restoration of the abduction element in flexion and extension and also the stabilizing effects of intrinsic power on the metacarpophalangeal joint. This is the split sublimis procedure.

In this procedure, a long finger sublimis is severed at the proximal joint of the finger and withdrawn at the musculotendinous junction. The tendon is split into two tails. One tail is introduced through the lumbricale canal and inserted into the lateral band past the lubricale insertion. The other is inserted into the volar and dorsal interosseous tendons of the first dorsal interosseous. The wrist is kept in neutral position, the metacarpophalangeal joints are flexed 80 degrees, add the interphalangeal joints are fully extended. The hand is immobilized for a period of 3 weeks, after which active exercises are begun.

Finger Flexion. Irwin[9] stated that weakened profundi may be successfully reinforced by being placed in continuity with other strong profundi or sublimi. When this pro-

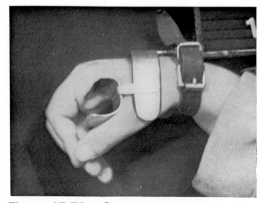

Figure 17.76. Same case as seen in Figure 17.75, showing the support given by an opponens splint.

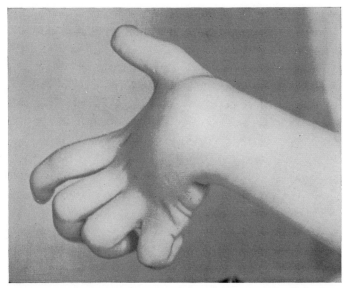

Figure 17.77. Effect of imbalance of the long flexors, intrinsics, and long extensors due to weak wrist extensors. Thenar muscles are absent, except for the long thumb flexor and extensor and the long abductor.

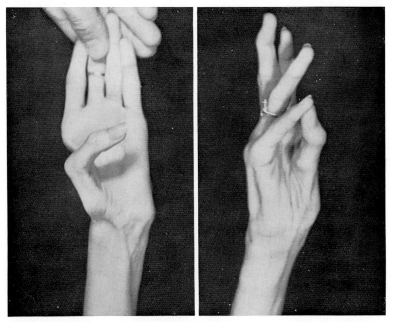

Figure 17.78. This opponens transplant functions well, but there is practically no abductor brevis or flexor pollicus longus to give stability.

cedure is performed properly, excellent results are obtained. It is accomplished by splicing the strong tendons into the weakened ones proximal to the volar carpal ligament. The wrist extensors work more or less synergistically with the long flexors of the fingers, and it has been found that wrist extensors work well in restoring finger flexion. The extensor carpi radialis longus has a good excursion and works well when it is woven

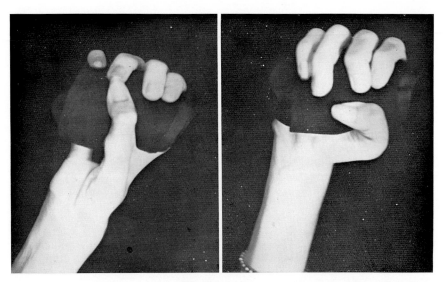

Figure 17.79. As strength is added, the grip is lost and the thumb flexes. This functional anomaly can be avoided by inserting one slip of the sublimis into the metacarpal and one into the phalanx so that the metacarpal is brought into opposition equally with the rest of the thumb.

into the profundus tendons at the musculo-tendinous junction. The anastomosis should be made under considerable tension; the little finger should be under the greatest tension, and each adjacent finger under progressively less tension. It should be made with the fingers in a position of relaxed flexion. A plaster splint is applied for about 3 weeks, and active motion follows its removal. Prior to utilization of an extensor of the wrist as a transplant, particularly to the flexor side, the ability to extend the wrist in the absence of this tendon must be assured. The remaining wrist extensor muscles should be inspected directly. If a strong extensor carpi radialis tendon is not available, transfer of the extensor carpi ulnaris into the flexor digitorum profundus tendons may give good restoration of finger flexion. The excursion of the flexor carpi ulnaris is not great enough to give satisfactory finger function. The brachioradialis works moderately well, but its excursion is less than that of the longer extensor of the wrist. Restoration of common extensor action restores the ability to extend the metacarpophalangeal joints and stabilizes these joints, but it does not extend the intraphalangeal joints in the absence of good intrinsics. The extensor carpi radialis also works very well in a restoration of common extensor function. It is transferred to the finger extensors more

easily and with less concern than to the flexors, inasmuch as it can work as a stabilizer of the wrist when it is anastomosed into the extensors.

In this procedure, the extensor of the wrist is sectioned at its insertion into the base of the metacarpal, freed up in a retrograde fashion from under the carpal ligament, and then redirected along the dorsal surface of the forearm subcutaneously and anastomosed into the extensor tendons at their musculotendinous junctions. The anastomosis must be made with the extensors in considerable tension and with the metacarpophalangeal joints in extension. Relative differences in tension are accomplished by suturing the little finger tighter than the adjacent ring finger, the ring finger slightly tighter than the middle finger, and so on. The extensor carpi radialis brevis can also be used to replace extensor communis function. The extensor carpi ulnaris is of fair usefulness, and the brachioradialis has been found to be an excellent motor for this purpose. The wrist flexors, being synergistic with finger extension, may be used quite satisfactorily as replacements for common extensor function. The flexor carpi radialis and ulnaris can be used succesfully; however, they are not as satisfactory as the radial extensors of the wrist.

Restoration of Finger Function by Tenodesis

As has been previously established, an arthrodesis, in the hand paralyzed by polio is rarely indicated. The procedure might be considered to free valuable tendons for transplantation to weakened fingers and thumb; however, in evaluating the activity of the patient, one might find loss of flexibility of the wrist to be a great handicap. Irwin[9] and his associates at Warm Springs have found instances of patients who could be aided considerably by a tenodesis. Wrist motion can be retained, and, in instances in which conventional transfers cannot be performed because of insufficient musculature, the tenodesis action can be utilized with quite effective results.

Grasp with the wrist extended is the result of two types of muscle action, namely, a primary flexion of the fingers caused by contraction of the flexor muscle mass and a secondary flexion of the fingers due to the increased distance, with the wrist extended, between the origin and the insertion of the long flexors. Conversely, flexion of the wrist may extend the fingers as a result of increasing the distance from the origin to the insertion of the long extensors. In the presence of weakness or loss of the long extensors or flexors of the fingers, grasp may be enhanced greatly by tenodesis of the afflicted motors. The fixation can be accomplished by implanting the common tendon mass into bone, which creates a tenodesis, or by transferring an actively contracting muscle into the tendon mass to form a dynamic tenodesis. Irwin emphasized that the distinction between a dynamic tenodesis and a standard transfer is a difficult one. A dynamic tenodesis is a transfer which, when the tendon is inserted into a common tendon group, such as the flexors of the fingers, relies mainly on wrist action for its function and only secondarily on the transplanted active muscle. Tenodeses should be reserved for patients who lack sufficient motors for conventional transfers. The patient must possess a mobile wrist that he can manipulate into flexion and extension, mobile fingers, and a functional elbow. An active wrist extensor greatly enhances the value of a flexor tenodesis; however, in the absence of active wrist extension, the wrist may be made to fall into the extended position by gravity when the forearm is supinated and the elbow flexed. The grasp that results is necessarily very slight, but an effective hook that the patient may utilize to considerable advantage is created. Active wrist flexion is less important than wrist extension to the grasp. In the absence of active motors, the wrist normally falls into a position of pronation and flexion when the elbow is flexed. The status of the intrinsics of the fingers plays an important role in the final result. Extensor tenodesis will not fully extend the fingers unless active intrinsics are present. Interestingly enough, finger extension may improve with flexor tenodesis if the lumbricales are functional. Lumbricale efficiency is increased when the profundi are stabilized.

According to the technique described by Irwin, flexor tenodesis is performed through a semilunar incision overlying the volar surface of the wrist. The median nerve is identified and carefully retracted from the field. The profundus tendons are identified by applying manual traction to each tendon and observing for flexion of the distal phalanges. The position of the fingers is adjacent to correspond to that assumed by the normal hand lying at rest on a flat surface with the wrist supinated. If the tenodesis is to be of the passive type, a small window is made in the distal end of the radius, and the profundus tendons are inserted into the bone with the aid of single wire suture. Should a dynamic tenodesis be indicated, the position of the fingers is fixed by anastomosing any available transfer into the common tendon mass. Anastomosis is secured with the aid of twisted steel wire sutures. The technique for insertion of the extensor tenodesis is the same. The common extensors are isolated through a semilunar incision from the dorsum of the wrist to the ulnar side of the tubercle of Lister. Anastomosis is accomplished while the hand is in a position of rest. Active transfers are inserted under moderate tension. Immediate postoperative immobilization is secured with dorsal and volar plaster splints. Flexor tenodeses are immobilized with the wrist in full flexion and the fingers extended, and extensor tenodeses with the wrist in full extension and the fingers extended. Three weeks postoperatively, the splints are removed and mobilization of the hand and wrist is initiated.

References

1. Bunnell, S.: Surgery of the intrinsic muscles of the hand other than those producing opposition of the thumb, *J Bone Joint Surg., 24:* 1942.
2. Bunnell, S.: Active splinting of the hand *J. Bone Joint Surg., 28:* 732, 1946.
3. Bunnell, S., and Howard, L. D.: Additional elastic hand splints, *J. Bone Joint Surg., 32A:* 226, 1950.
4. Coonrad, R., Eyler, D., and Irwin, C. E.: Splint sublimis transfer for paralysis of the intrinsic muscles of the index finger; Correspondence Club Letter, Duke Training Program, 1951.
5. Eyler, D. L., and Markee, J. E.: The anatomy and function of the intrinsic musculature of the finger, *J. Bone Joint Surg., 36A:* 1, 1954.
6. Foerster, O.: Fusion of metacarpals of thumb and index finger, *Acta Chir. Scand. 67:* 350, 1931.
7. Goldner, J. L., and Irwin, C. E.: An analysis of paralytic thumb deformities, *J. Bone Joint Surg., 32A:* 627, 1950.
8. Irwin, C. E.: Apparatus for the upper extremity disabled by poliomyelitis, *Instruct. Lect. Am. Acad. Orthop. Surg., 9:* 208, 1952.
9. Irwin, C. E.: Dynamic tenodesis, paper presented at the American Academy of Orthopaedic Surgeons, January 1956.
10. Irwin, C. E., and Eyler, D. L.: Surgical rehabilitation of the hand and forearm disabled by poliomyelitis, *J. Bone Joint Surg., 33A:* 825, 1951.
11. Kirklin, J. W., and Thomas, C. G.: Opponens transplant; an analysis of methods employed and results obtained, *Surg. Gynecol. Obstet., 86:* 213, 1948.
12. Riordan, D. C.: Tendon transplantation in median nerve and ulnar nerve paralysis, *J. Bone Joint Surg., 35A:* 312, 1953.
13. Royle, N. D.: An operation for paralysis of the intrinsic muscles of the thumb, *J. A. M. A., 111:* 612, 1938.
14. Thompson, C. F.: Fusion of metacarpals of thumb and index finger to maintain functional position of the thumb, *J. Bone Joint Surg., 24:* 907, 1942.

RHEUMATOID ARTHRITIS

Rheumatoid arthritis is a generalized systemic disease affecting both children and adults. In children, the disease may vary considerably in its mode of onset. Frequently, it begins in one joint and subsequently spreads to involve all joints. When it remains localized to one or two joints, as it occasionally does, it becomes a problem in diagnosis. It may be manifested by generalized joint involvement with marked toxicity, anemia, weight loss, splenomegaly, and fever.

When the hands are involved, marked deformity causing severe permanent dysfunction and disability frequently results (Fig. 17.80). Primary joint involvement is not the only deforming factor. Secondary muscle spasm and eventual myostatic contracture contribute to the hand deformity. The muscles are in spasm and eventual myostatic contracture contribute to the hand deformity. The muscles are in spasm because of irritation of the synovial reaction, but later they become fibrosed and permanently shortened. Microscopically, the muscles, tendons, and ligaments show multiple foci of inflammation and later fibrotic contracture. Some ligaments actually degenerate and thus permit subluxation of the joints. Some of the tendons may degenerate and rupture at focal spots of granulation. The joint changes and the ligamentous and tendinous involvement all play a part in the deformity, but the position of the deformity is largely due to a muscle imbalance among the long flexors, the long extensors, and the intrinsics. Because of this disturbance of the normal equilibrium in these three groups of muscles, all of the clinical forms of arthritis involving the hands and fingers result in two types of deformity, namely, the clawhand and the pillroller hand. In the clawhand, the metacarpophalangeal joints are pulled into hyperextension by the long extensors and thus overcome the resistance of the intrinsic mucles. The fingers flex in the middle joints and extend in the distal joints. The more usual of the two deformities is the pillroller hand, in which there is flexion of the metacarpophalangeal joints due to the intrinsic contracture. The middle and distal joints are thus pulled straight by the lateral bands, or at times the middle joint may be hyperextended and the distal joints may flex. The position of the wrist seems to play a great part in the effect of the deformity on the hands and fingers in both of these conditions. In the clawhand, the wrist is in flexion; therefore, the passive tension on the extensors leads to hyperextension in the metacarpophalangeal joints. In the pillroller hand, the wrist remains in extension and the finger extensors are relaxed. The spastic contracture of the intrinsic muscles, which are not being opposed by the relaxed finger extensors, causes the metacarpophalangeal joints to become markedly flexed. The interphalangeal articulations assume a position of hyperextension because of the contracture and tightness of the intrinsic musculature. The thumb is usually drawn into flexion and adduction. The imbalance between the short flexors and adductors and the abductor group

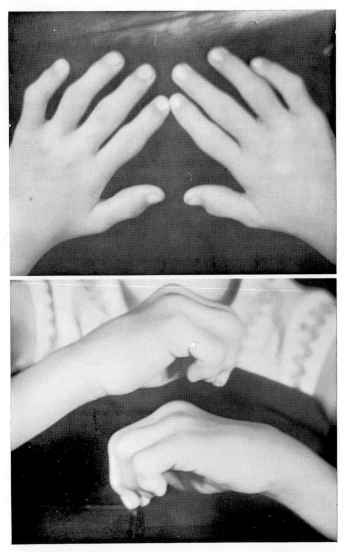

Figure 17.80.   Rheumatoid arthritis prior to therapy showing the range of extension and flexion.

usually results in adduction and flexion of the carpometacarpal joint. The metacarpophalangeal joint is overflexed and thus causes hyperextension of the distal joint because of the pull of the long extensor. Deformity of the thumb is more often noted in the pillroller type of hand.

Treatment

Because of the systemic nature of rheumatoid arthritis, treatment of it must first be generalized; however, great attention should also be given to the local involvement and the prevention or correction of deformity. It is rare to see a patient who has in any way been neglected from a general standpoint. It is not unusual, however, to find that the general treatment has been carried out but that there has been very little effort locally to prevent crippling contractures. With the advent of newer remedies for rheumatoid arthritis and the improvement in general care and treatment, conservative local measures should become much more efficient and promising in the prevention and correction of deformities such as those that occur in the hand. In cases that are seen early—prior to the development of contracture—the treatment to prevent the deformity should start early and proceed actively under careful observation. The development of deformity is insidious, and frequently the doctor and family procrastinate until a serious deformity results. The family physician or pediatrician should handle the general medical care of the patient, but the orthopaedist should see the child early during the stage of irritation and painful swelling, before the occurrence of permanent contracture and deformity. If the development of deformity due to the imbalance of musculature is anticipated, proper splinting may be instituted, and the occurrence of serious disability may be completely avoided. Bunnell[1] and Steindler[5] have emphasized that the muscles are contracted from irritation and are in a state of spasm. It is only later that they become structurally changed by progressive fibrosis. Steindler stated that a spastic muscle is an extensible one which has retained its elasticity, whereas a fibrosed muscles has lost its elasticity. The arthritic muscle remains in a reflex spastic state for a considerable period. The correction of this reversible condition by mechanical means and the restoration of balance by muscle reeducation offer a wide therapeutic opportunity for the acute and subacute case of rheumatoid arthritis. These factors greatly

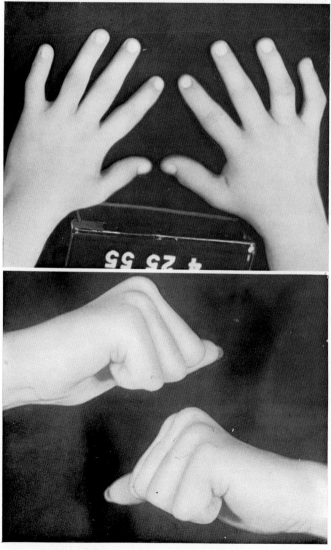

Figure 17.81. Same child as seen in Figure 17.80, 10 months later, after use of paraffin baths, whirlpool and active exercises, and active splinting.

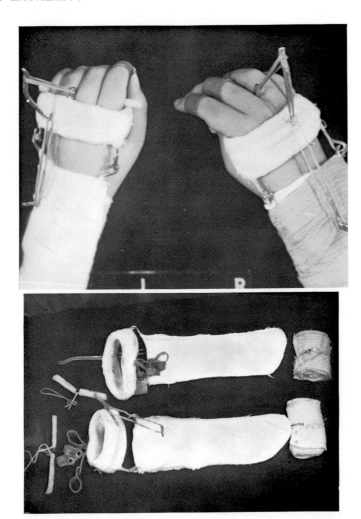

Figure 17.82. Active splints made of plaster with rubber band traction; they can be removed for use of the limb and for physical therapy.

improve the prognosis for the arthritic hand in children who are seen prior to the development of fixed contracture and bone deformity. Even when a definite contracture has developed, it is usually still in the stage of reflex spasm rather than of fixed myostatic contracture. Physical therapy in the form of heat, splinting, paraffin baths, and active exercises should be utilized to the fullest (Fig. 17.81). Surgery is rarely indicated. In the early stages of swelling, pain, and muscle spasm, paraffin and whirlpool baths are more effective. Early development of flexion contracture of the wrist can be prevented by passive splinting with a cock-up splint. Active use of the hand should be encouraged, and fixed immobilization is to be avoided. Splints should be retention ones, which are designed only to maintain position, and should not be applied for corrective effect.

Active splinting is quite effective (Figs. 17.82–17.84). The active splint should perform one purpose only; however, several splints, each exerting a different type of effect, may be used in the same patient at different periods. Active splints using mild elastic traction or spring effect may be made by the bracemaker. If there are none available, simple plaster splints using spring wire or elastic traction can be fashioned inexpensively. By utilizing the active splints part time to help overcome muscle spasm and imbalance, fixed deformities can be prevented.

Active exercises for the fingers, wrist, and forearm are essential in the treatment and should be combined and properly balanced

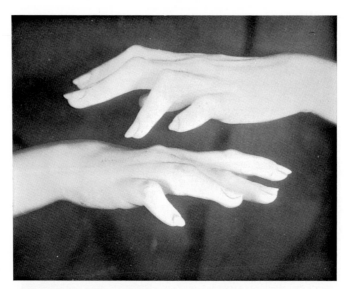

Figure 17.83. Hands with rheumatoid arthritis showing advanced stage of deformity: flexed wrist, hyperextended proximal finger joints, flexed middle joints, and extended distal joints.

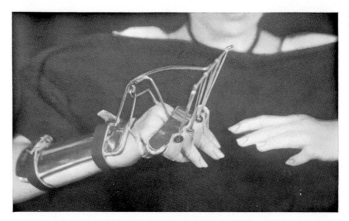

Figure 17.84. Metal active splint to hold wrist in dorsiflexion and bar to prevent metacarpophalangeal extension during active stretch on the proximal interphalangeal joints. This splint is worn part time while gentle passive stretching and active exercises are used and, at other times, during active use of the hand in general daily activity.

with gentle passive stretching of tight joints. Emphasis is placed on gentle stretching and manipulative treatment, which must be undertaken with great care never to approach the point of tearing capsular tissues. The treatment program is attended by some increase in pain, which may be allayed by the adminstration of salicylates. Children usually tolerate treatment better than adults and are quite cooperative.

Utilization of the foregoing measures, accompanied by proper education of the family regarding the chronicity of the treatment, usually produces gratifying results. Only after a period of from 2–10 years usually does the disease become completely burned out, and some residual deformities may be expected at the end of this period. However, major crippling can usually be minimized, and in many instances it can be completely prevented.

References

1. Bunnell, S.: Surgery of the rheumatic hand, *J. Bone Joint Surg.* 37A: 759, 1956.

2. Bunnell, S., and Howard, L. D.: Additional elastic hand splints, *J. Bone Joint Surg.*, 32A: 226, 1950.
3. Bunnell, S.: Active splinting of the hand, *J. Bone Joint Surg.*, 28: 732, 1947.
4. Peacock, E., Jr.: Dynamic splinting for prevention of deformities and correction of hand deformities, *J. Bone Joint Surg.*, 34A: 789, 1952.
5. Steindler, A.: Arthritic deformities of the wrist and fingers, *J. Bone Joint Surg.*, 33A: 849, 1951.

TRAUMA

Trauma in its many varieties, and particularly that due to the increased mechanization of the modern age, accounts for a vast number of hand disabilities and deformities. Children are susceptible to many of the same types of trauma as adults, and their reaction to injury, in spite of minor variations, is practically the same. Most of the variations have to do with skin thickness, growth and healing ability of bone, and joint mobility. Some of these variations from the adult tend to be helpful in treatment, but others make the treatment more difficult. Children have surprising powers of adaptation and are able to accommodate well to the loss of a part. They are able to substitute functions and to accept their disabilities and deformities better than one might at first suppose. Sometimes it is best to defer large reconstructive procedures until the child is older. Delay may result in sufficient accommodation to the difficulty to make treatment unnecessary. It is advisable also because young children do not cooperate well, and, because their small extremities are hard to immobilize, the postoperative care is difficult and sometiees unsuccessful.

The basic principles of treatment of traumatic deformities in children are the same as those in adults; therefore, the entire field is not covered here. Certain injuries which are common in children are discussed in detail, and variations in basic treatment of other types of trauma are given.

Volkmann's Ischemic Contracture

Volkman's ischemic contracture is one of the most serious deformities of the hand and forearm, and the most dreaded complication of injuries about the elbow and forearm, particularly in children. Steindler[33] stated that, from a purely pathologic viewpoint, ischemic contracture is a fibrous reaction of the muscles of the forearm, particularly those of the flexor group. The contracture may involve the muscles in toto or in part, and cases have been reported in which muscles of the hand alone were involved. In one instance, all of the muscles, except one sublimis muscle, escaped involvement.

The fully developed ischemic contracture actually is a combination of deformities. The characteristic picture is that of pronation of the forearm, flexion of the wrist and interphalangeal joints, and hyperextension of the metacarpophalangeal joints (Fiig. 17.85). The hyperextension of the metacarpophalangeal joints is largely a result of passive insufficiency of the extensors and is not necessarily indicative of intrinsic loss. Although this picture is the one most frequently seen, variations of it may be encountered. Common variations are the absence of hyperextension of the metacarpophalangeal joints and a flexion contracture of the wrist similar to that seen in radial nerve palsy. The thumb is frequently involved; an adduction contracture and the inability to oppose may place it in a plane with the involved fingers.

ETIOLOGY

Since Volkmann et al.'s original description,[34] numerous investigators have tried to solve the problem of pathogenesis of this lesion, and excellent papers, from both clinical and experimental standpoints, have been written on the subject. Each of these papers conveys the impression that the investigator has proved his premise to be the correct one. Bardenheuer[1] originated the venous obstruction theory, and his work has been adequately substantiated by other authorities in the field. Brooks and his associates[3] have done some excellent experimental studies that prove quite conclusively that the lesion can be produced experimentally by complete venous obstruction. Volkmann's original arterial deficit theory has been substantiated by numerous investigators and by much experimentation.

Griffiths[11,12] has produced an excellent work giving convincing proof that the lesion is due to arterial occlusion and muscle infarction. Others hold that the lesion is merely an unusual variety of contracture due to nerve injury. In many instances, it is undoubtedly true that there is peripheral nerve

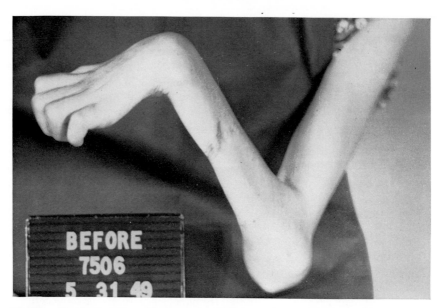

Figure 17.85. Typical deformity seen in Volkmann's contracture. There is atrophy of the forearm, acutely flexed wrist and interphalangeal joints, and hyperextended metacarpophalangeal joints.

damage in addition to the contractures, but there has been no definite proof that direct injury to the nerve is the primary cause of ischemic contracture. There can be little doubt, however, that constriction lasting for a long enough period of time to close large vessels does exert pressure over the median and ulnar nerves and leads to neuritis and degeneration. Leriche and his workers attributed great significance to irritation of the sympathetic nerve supply that results in peripheral vasoconstriction.

In view of these conflicting clinical and experimental impressions, the etiology of Volkmann's contracture could be either arterial or venous obstruction. It is also not illogical to assume that in certain cases all of the previously postulated factors might well play a part.

Because of the popularity of circulatory obstruction as the etiology of Volkmann's ischemic contracture, constricting casts, bandages, and dressings have long been associated with the condition. There are cases on record, however, in which no dressing or cast was used, and yet the condition developed. In spite of this, casts or bandages can be very definite contributing causes, and for this reason, careful supervision and vigilance are essential features in the treatment of all injuries about the elbow and forearm.

PATHOLOGY

In the initial stages, the subcutaneous tissues become cyanotic and infiltrated with blood. The superficial veins engorge, and there is swelling of the extremity. Deep fascia and muscle envelopes are tight, and, when cut, they tend to gap and retract markedly and to show a very pale, yellowish-gray musculature. In later stages, the muscles may become gray and may have shortened muscle fibers and evident fibrous cords. Within 48 hr after the onset, polymorphonuclear leukocytes accumulating about the fibers produce a typical inflammatory appearance. Organization of the exudate begins within 4 or 5 days and is usually well established within 10 days. Destruction of muscle fibers varies directly with the severity of the case. All gradations of involvement can occur. In mild cases almost all of the muscle fibers function normally, whereas in severe cases all of the muscle substance may be replaced by connective tissue.

Histologically, the connective tissue forms in bundles which ramify throughout the muscle bellies and replace necrotic muscle fibers. The fibrous tissue has a fibrillar aspect and forms a meshwork in which isolated areas are of viable muscle tissue.

CLINICAL PICTURE

Following the treatment of an acute injury such as a fracture or dislocation, there is usually a period of relative comfort to the patient. The earliest signs and symptoms of Volkmann's contracture usually appear within 4–6 hr, but they may develop as late as 48 hr after treatment. Cases are recorded in which the symptoms have developed as late as a week after the initial injury. Following the period of initial comfort, there is usually a sudden onset of severe pain in the arm and in the volar aspect of the forearm. The fingers become cold, cyanotic, and swollen. The pain increases in intensity and is often incompletely relieved by narcotics. Paresthesias develop, and even though the fingers may feel numb, they are often hypersensitive to touch. As the condition progresses, voluntary motion is lost, and the fingers assume a flexed position. Passive extension of the fingers causes severe pain. The radial pulse is usually absent. The pain disappears after about 48 hr, contracture of the flexor group of muscles occurs, add a clawhand subsequently develops. Clinically, the presence of coldness, swelling of the fingers, cyanosis, and absence of the radial pulse are most important early signs; however, it must be noted that pallor, rather than cyanosis, is sometimes present and is equally important. Pain in the forearm accompanied by fixed flexion of the fingers and increased pain in the forearm on passive extension of the fingers are serious signs; if preventive treatment is to be attempted with any hope of success, earlier signs must be sought.

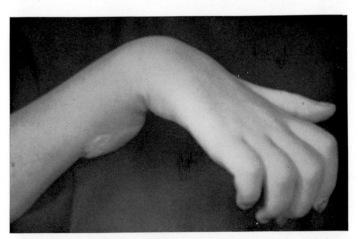

Figure 17.86. Severe Volkmann's contracture upon attempted flexion in an 8-year-old girl. Pedicle graft over the volar aspect of the lower forearm has been performed at the site of a skin slough.

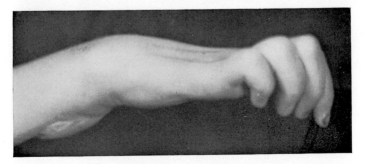

Figure 17.87. Attempted extension in patient seen in Figure 17.86. Below the elbow, only the wrist extensors, common extensors, and thumb extensors are functioning. These muscles are greatly inhibited due to the flexion contractures.

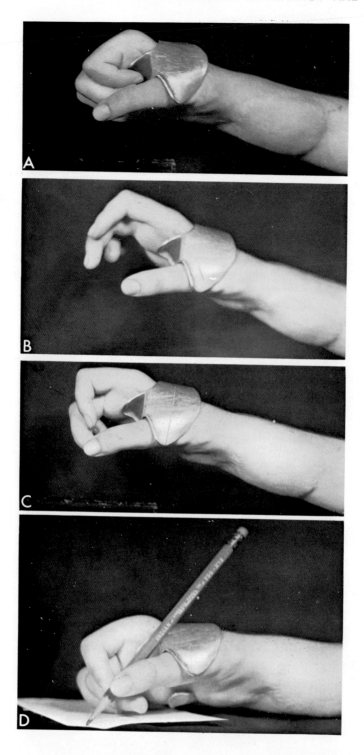

Figure 17.88. Same case as seen in Figure 17.86 after multiple tendon transfers. The figures show the function of the hand on active flexion (*A*) and extension (*B*) of fingers, opposition (*C*), writing (*D*), and grasping a glass (*E*). The procedures were the following: (1) the extensor radialis longus and brevis were transplanted to the profundus and

TREATMENT

The treatment of Volkmann's contracture is prophylaxis. The condition is easily missed in its earliest stages, and recognition is essential if successful preventive measures are to be initiated. As a result of the injury the patient is expected to have some pain and some swelling and tenderness of the fingers. Procrastination during this important stage is an easy matter, and differentiation between normal discomfort and an impending Volkmann's contracture may be difficult. It should be remembered that, following proper therapy of injuries such as fractures and dislocations the pain should rapidly subside. Cases of undue and prolonged pain should be watched with suspicion. All injuries about the elbow and forearm in children must be meticulously watched and preventive measures vigilantly initiated as soon as increased swelling, cyanosis, coldness, and pain appear. The time to treat Volkmann's contracture is at its very beginning. Once there has been degeneration and fibrosis with contracture of the muscle, no power can restore the muscle to normal. From then on, we must think in terms of improvement but never of cure.

Early Phase. As soon as the signs and symptoms of impending Volkmann's contracture appear, one must first remove all dressings, bandages, and splints and relieve the acute flexion of the elbow. One of the best methods of maintaining immobilization of the supracondylar fracture without acute flexion and without bandages or external splints is traction by means of a Kirschner wire in the olecranon. The use of repeated stellate ganglion blocks frequently improves circulation. Should notable improvement—evidenced by pink, warm fingers and the return of a radial pulse—appear with these measures, the case may be watched. If this happy state does not appear within 3 or 4 hr, surgical intervention is mandatory. Surgery is performed with the intent of relieving obstruction. The incision is made lengthwise over the flexor surface of the forearm, and it jogs across the antecubital space to avoid crossing the flexion crease of the elbow. The skin usually gaps as it is cut, and the deep fascia is found to be very tight as it is incised. The brachial, radial, and ulnar arteries are freed, and the muscle groups of the forearm are separated. In making incisions through the deep fascia, one must remember that the

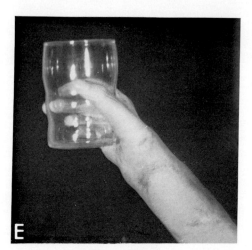

Fig. 17.88 (*E*)

sublimis tendons after all of the flexor tendons had been released, (2) the brachioradialis was transplanted into the flexor pollicis longus, (3) the extensor carpi ulnaris was elongated by means of grafts from the long toe extensors and was then transplanted through the intermetacarpal spaces to the lateral bands, and (4) the extensor pollicis brevis was elongated by means of the palmaris longus tendon and was rerouted around the ulna to replace the opponens function. (The last procedure gave only a fair result and is not a good procedure owing to the weakness of the extensor pollicis brevis. Function is enhanced by use of an opponens splint.)

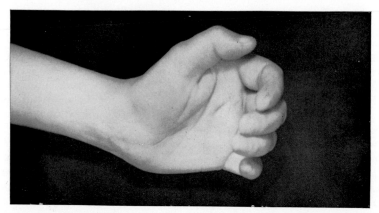

Figure 17.89. Volkmann's contracture of less severity. This patient had some function of the flexor profundus and sublimis, but these muscles were weak and had contractures. Wrist flexors were strong, but the extensors were poor.

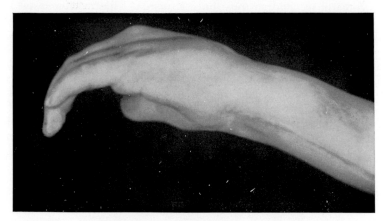

Figure 17.90. Same case as seen in Figure 17.89 showing extension.

forearm consists of a series of deep fascia compartments. The release of one compartment when another is involved is not the solution to the problem. It is important to relieve the tension in each compartment. Closure is confined to the skin, and if it cannot be accomplished without tension, a split thickness skin graft should be utilized.

Neurolysis of the ulnar and median nerves has been advocated and should be considered when primary involvement of the nerve seems to be present. At surgery, a few constricting bands or dense adhesions causing complete strangulation of the nerve may be discovered. The nerve, in this case, should be carefully freed by sharp dissection and saline neurolysis.

Late Phase. Treatment of the established contracture is as varied as the theories of pathogenesis. The reason for this is that the

established contracture is not always the same. Various combinations and degrees of muscle involvement with or without nerve damage present many types of contractures. Initial treatment during this stage should be conservative. In early cases, gradual stretching according to the method of Sir Robert Jones[18] is excellent treatment. By means of a rigid splint hinged at the wrist, first the interphalangeal joints are gradually extended, then the metacarpophalangeal joints are extended, and finally the wrist is brought into extension. The splint should be removed several times daily so that the hand may be actively and passively exercised and treated with heat and massage. Rapid or forceful correction of the deformity produces overstretching, laceration, and hemorrhage and invites recurrence. There are many other methods of gaining gradual correction of the

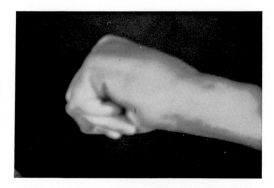

Figure 17.91. Same case as seen in Figures 17.89 and 17.90, showing flexion following mobilization by physical therapy and transfer of the flexor carpi ulnaris to the base of the third metacarpal. The result of these procedures was a dynamic tenodesis function whereby extending the wrist with the transfer allowed the tight finger flexors to grasp more or less passively.

deformity by the use of bivalve casts, semirigid splints, elastic traction splints, glove traction splints, and other pieces of apparatus. The general principle of gentle but persistent stretching of the deformity remains applicable to every method.

In patients in whom there is sufficient viable muscle to provide for practical function and muscle balance of the hand, passive stretching exercises and splinting may be the only treatment necessary. In some instances, it may be found that certain structures are not stretching and are more deforming than valuable. These structures should be sacrificed. Steindler[33] stated that the contracture resistance of muscle varies with the number of joints the muscle motivates. The short fibered, uniarticular muscles of the wrist joint are very much more resistant in contracture than are the muscles of the fingers, which have a wider contractile range because of the greater length of their muscle fibers. The flexor carpi ulnaris offers the most resistance, and lengthening or even sectioning of this tendon should be performed when necessary. The same principle holds true for the flexor carpi radialis and the flexor pollicis longus.

RECONSTRUCTION

A thorough knowledge of the mechanics and function of the hand and an ability to asssess the deformity with utmost care are prerequisites to attempting surgical reconstruction of the deformity caused by Volkmann's ischemic contracture. Surgical procedures must be meticulously designed to salvage as much as possible from a serious deformity. Excellent results are rarely obtained because of extensive damage to the functional mechanism of the hand. These hands have a poor appearance; however, some function which will greatly decrease the handicap of the patient can frequently be obtained. Occasionally, nothing can be done to improve function, and the surgeon must be satisfied to accept this fact and to improve the hand cosmetically if possible. The end results are innumerable, and because each case presents an entirely different problem, many operative procedures have been advocated for a single condition. A procedure which is suitable for one problem may be quite unsatisfactory for another. The general groups of procedures which are at present in common usage are: (1) sliding of the flexor muscle origin distalward; (2) lengthening of tendons; (3) shortening of static structures, including carpectomy and shortening of the radius and ulna; and (4) tendon transposition with or without carpal arthrodesis.

The first procedure releases flexion contractures of the wrist, but detachment is possible for only a short distance because of the restriction of the median nerve branches. Lengthening of the wrist flexors, combined with stretching and other operative procedures, is often helpful. Lengthening of the finger flexors is rarely of benefit. This procedure may allow the finger to be extended, but usually, when the length is increased, the active contractive power of flexion is diminished or lost in the functional range. Shortening of the long bones has decreased in popularity, and it is now thought that, if actual shortening of the static parts will aid function, carpectomy is the procedure of choice (Fig. 17.92). In well selected cases, this procedure provides good functional results and frequently improves the appearance of the hand. Tendon transplantations following a careful muscle evaluation frequently aid the functional improvement of the hand. This is especially true of the transplantations following a careful muscle evaluation frequently aid the functional improvement of the hand. This is especially true of the transplantation of extensors to the flexor muscles. Capsulectomies of the metacarpophalangeal joints are often

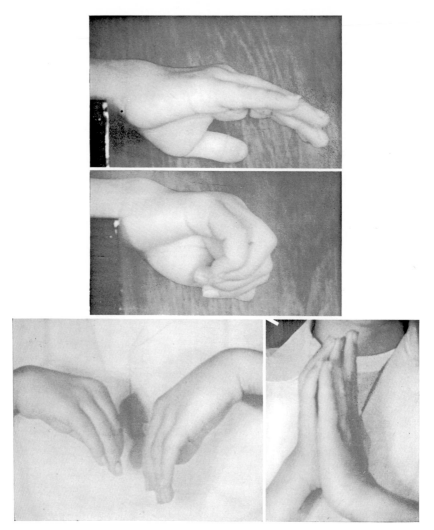

Figure 17.92. Function attained in a case of moderately severe Volkmann's contracture after carpectomy.

indicated; but, not infrequently, the contracture is so severe that the resection of the metacarpal heads or metacarpophalangeal arthroplasty is necessary.

The end results of treating established cases of Volkmann's ischemic contracture are by no means excellent in anyone's hands. The recovery of some degree of function in these cases is often more appreciated by the patient than a brilliant correction of a mild deformity in another condition. The rehabilitation of these hands presents a great challenge and offers great possibilities if a meticulous therapeutic plan is carried out.

References

1. Bardenheuer, E.: *Dtsch. Z. Chir., 108:* 44, 1911.
2. Brooks, B.:Experimental study of Volkmann's paralysis, *Arch. Surg., 5:* 188, 1922.
3. Brooks, B., Johnson, G. S., and Kirtley, J. A., Jr.: Simultaneous vein ligation, *Surg. Gynecol. Obstet. 59:* 496, 1934.
4. Bruce, J. R.: Localized Volkmann contracture, *J. Bone Joint Surg., 22:* 738, 1940.
5. Burman, M. S., and Suturo, C. J.: Brief communications; experimental ischemic contracture, *Ann. Surg., 100:* 559, 1934.
6. Cohen, H. H.: Adjustable volar-flexion splint for Volkmann's contracture, *J. Bone Joint Surg., 24:* 189, 1942.

7. Fleming, C. W.: Case of impending Volkmann's ischemic contracture treated by incision of deep fascia, *Lancet*, 2: 293, 1931.
8. Foisie, P. S.: Volkmann's ischemic contracture, *N. Engl. J. Med.*, 226: 671, 1942.
9. Garber, J. N.: Volkmann's contracture as complication of fractures of forearm and elbow, *J. Bone Joint Surg.*, 21: 154, 1939.
10. Glen, F. W.: Vascular injuries complicating supracondylar fractures of humerus in children, with case report, *Bull. Jackson Mem. Hosp.*, 3: 29, 1941.
11. Griffiths, D. L.: Volkmann's ischemic contracture, *Lancet* 2: 1339, 1938.
12. Griffiths, D. L. Volkmann's ischemic contracture, *Br. J. Surg.* 28: 239, 1940.
13. d'Harcourt, J., and d'Harcourt, M.: A contribution to the study of Volkmann's ischemic contracture, *Madrid Med.*, 6: 237, 1935.
14. Harris, C., and Riordan, D. C.: Intrinsic contracture in the hand and its surgical treatment, *J. Bone Joint Surg.*, 36A: 10, 1954.
15. Horwitz, T.: Significance of venous circulation about elbow in patho-mechanics of Volkmann's contracture, *Surg. Gynecol. Obstet.*, 74: 871, 1942.
16. Jepson, P. N.: Ischemic contracture, *Ann. Surg.*, 84: 785, 1926.
17. Jones, E. B.: Volkmann's ischemia; observations at open operation, *Br. Med. J.*, 1: 1053, 1940.
18. Jones, R.: Address on Volkmann's ischemic contracture with special reference to treatment, *Br. Med. J.*, 2: 639, 1928.
19. Jones, S. G.: Volkmann's contracture, *Am. J. Surg.*, 43: 325, 1939.
20. Laigle, L.: Evolution of ideas concerning Volkmann's syndrome, *Medicine*, 19: 893, 1938.
21. Massart, R.: Volkmann's disease, ischemic contraction of the flexor muscles of the fingers: pathogenesis and treatment, *Presse Med.*, 43: 1695, 1935.
22. Meyerding, H. W.: Volkmann's ischemic contracture, *J. A. M. A.*, 94: 394, 8, 1930.
23. Meyerding, H. W.: Volkmann's ischemic contracture, *Surg. Clin. North. Am.*, 10: 49, 1930.
24. Meyerding, H. W.: Fracture of elbow and Volkmann's ischemic contracture, *Minn. Med.* 22: 100, 1939.
25. Meyerding, H. W., and Krusen, F. H.: Treatment of Volkmann's ischemic contracture, *Ann. Surg.*, 100: 417, 1939.
26. Middleton, D. S.: Discussion of Volkmann's ischemic contracture, *Lancet*, 2: 299, 1928.
27. Murphy, J. B.: Myositis, *J. A. M. A.*, 63: 1949, 1914.
28. de Nuce: Ischemic contracture, *Rev. Orthop. 20*: 97, 1909.
29. Plewes, L. W.: Occlusion of brachial artery and Volkmann's ischemic contracture, *Br. Med. J*, 1: 1054, 1940.
30. Powers, C. A.: The ischemic paralysis and contracture of Volkmann, *J. A. M. A.*, 48: 759, 1907.
31. Pusitz, M. E.: Abortive treatment of Volkmann's ischemia, *J. Kans. Med. Soc.*, 35: 448, 1934.
32. Rowlands: *Lancet* 2: 1168, 1904.
33. Steindler, A.: Ischemic contracture, *Surg. Gynecol. Obstet.* 62: 358, 1936.
34. Volkmann, Pithia, and Bilrath: *Handbuch der Chirurgie*, 2: 846, 1882.
35. White, J. W., and Stubbins, S. G.: Carpectomy for intractable flexion deformities of the wrist, *J. Bone Joint Surg.*, 29: 131, 1944.

Wringer Arm

"Wringer arm" is a descriptive term applied to an upper extremity that has been caught between two rollers (Fig. 17.93). The injury occurs most frequently in childhood and is usually caused by a power-driven washing machine. Hardin and Robinson[3] reported 35 cases of which 30 were children under the age of 6 years.

PATHOGENESIS AND PATHOLOGY

The compressive force and friction produced by the rollers cause damage primarily to the skin and soft tissues of the hand, the forearm, and the elbow region. The severity of the damage depends upon the length of time the extremity has been between the rollers, the rapidity of revolution, the width of approximation, and the tension of the rollers. The prognosis is much better in the younger age groups because of the elasticity and flexibility of the bones, joints, and ligaments.

In these injuries, the hand usually enters the roller first with the fingers in the extended position. The rollers are usually elastic enough to allow the hand and the distal portion of the forearm to pass through them without great damage. As the forearm proceeds through the roller, however, tension usually builds up because of the increasing width of the upper arm and elbow, and the elbow usually bears the brunt of the avulsing action of the rollers.

Bones are rarely damaged, but muscles, tendons, and nerves may be crushed, torn, or avulsed without a break in the skin. The most common damage is that of separation of the skin from its subcutaneous attachments by the mechanical action of the moving rollers. A collection of blood and serum beneath such a full thickness skin area delays the reestablishment of good blood supply. If this condition goes unrecognized and untreated, the overlying skin remains separated and sloughs. Venous thrombosis and lymphatic obstruction occur frequently. The arteries in the affected zone are less easily injured than the veins; they continue to circulate blood

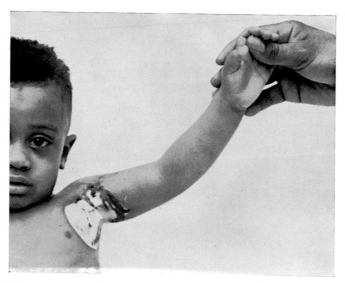

Figure 17.93. Wringer injury. Besides deep slough shown here, the child has paralysis of the radial, ulnar, and median nerves.

into the damaged area and thus cause engorgement and subsequent necrosis. Occasionally, flaps of skin are completely separated and expose contused or macerated muscle. At times, tendon ends are completely stripped from their muscle attachments.

CLINICAL EXAMINATION

Immediate evaluation should include the determination of nerve and tendon function distal to the site of the injury and roentgenographic examination for possible bone or joint damage. In cases seen immediately after injury, the swelling and echymosis may be mild to moderate and may mislead the physician who is inexperienced in treating these conditions. Occasionally, the damage may be limited to abrasion, contusion, and edema of the skin. In many instances, however, extravasation of blood and serum separate the skin as a flap from the forearm or arm, and severe sloughs occur. The extent of damage cannot always be determined early, and the prognosis should always be guarded.

TREATMENT

Regardless of the initial appearance of the injury, the patient should be hospitalized and observed for at least 48 hr. Conservative treatment, making use of viable skin to cover the damaged area, should be employed. Pres-

sure dressings and elevation of the extremity minimize the edema of the damaged limb. The area should be cleansed with soap, preferably Phisoderm with hexachlorophene, and water and dressed with sterile dressings. The use of pressure dressings applied as one dresses a new skin graft often prevents separation of the skin from the underlying tissues. The dressing should be changed after 48 hr and, if a hematoma has lifted the skin, aspiration should be performed and the pressure dressing reapplied. In late cases with severe extravasation, the collection of blood should be aspirated or released by multiple small incisions, and the wound should then be dressed with pressure dressings and subsequently ele-.ated and observed.

Definitive reconstructive surgery should be deferred until all inflammatory induration has subsided and the degree of soft-tissue destruction can be ascertained. The surface should be well covered in all cases before tendon and bone reconstruction is attempted. If the injury has produced a flap, resuture will usually be unsuccessful. Farmer[2] has successfully excised the fat and subcutaneous tissues to convert the flap into a full thickness graft. The depth of injury limits this type of treatment, which requires a suitable underlying bed. A split thickness graft should be used in cases of permanent loss of skin, but because this graft usually results in shrinkage, secondary coverage should be carried out. If bone, tendon, joint, or nerve is exposed, an immediate pedicle graft is imperative. Rotation or sliding flaps are usually unsuccessful because of tissue damage and circulatory impairment to the immediately surrounding tissues.

The thoracicoabdominal area is a convenient source of skin for covering these severely damaged areas according to the method of Hardin and Robinson.[3] The flaps are developed conventionally; they have a superior base and should be one-third larger than the defect to allow for shrinkage. The length should not exceed the base by more than two times. The flap is carried to the external oblique fascia and is transferred without any removal of fat. The abdominal defect may be closed by undermining, or, if it is too large for undermining, coverage may be completed with a split thickness graft. The graft is dressed with moderate pressure, and the joint is immobilized to relieve any motion or tension on the graft base. Detachment and revision are carried out in approximately 3 weeks. If tendon repairs or grafts are necessary, all joints should be thoroughly mobilized passively prior to surgery. The skin should be well healed and induration should have subsided before definitive work is attempted; otherwise summation of scarring is likely.

References

1. Dupertius, S. M.: An evaluation of skin grafts for hand coverage, *J. Bone Joint Surg., 34A*: 811, 1952.
2. Farmer, A. W.: Treatment of avulsed skin flaps, *Ann. Surg., 110*: 951, 1939.
3. Hardin, C. A., and Robinson, D. W.: Coverage problems in treatment of wringer injuries, *J. Bone Joint Surg., 36A*: 392, 1954.
4. MacCollum, D. W.: Wringer arm, a report of twenty-six cases, *N. Engl. J. Med., 218*: 549, 1938.
5. MacCollum, D. W., Berhard, W. F., and Banner, R. L.: The treatment of wringer arm injuries, *N. Engl. J. Med., 247*: 750, 1952.
6. Posch, J. L., and Weller, C. N.: Mangle and severe wringer injuries of the hand in children, *J. Bone Joint Surg., 36A*: 57, 1954.

Lacerations of Hand and Fingers

Damaged tendons may occur as a result of lacerations, burns, crushing injuries, friction wounds, or combinations of traumata such as those seen in wringer or mangle injuries, which are discussed above. Most lacerations are of the fingers and are due to grasping sharp cutting surfaces. The treatment of these wounds in children varies in no way from the treatment in adults. Boyes[3] has grafted tendons in 2-year-old children with excellent results. The tendons grow in length and continue to function well with growth. Because of the smallness of the parts, the difficulty of immobilization, and the poor cooperation of the very young, it is thought best to wait until the child is at least 2 years of age before performing tendon grafts. Joints should be kept mobile by passive exercise until surgery can be performed. No tendon surgery should be done until good skin coverage has been attained and all scars have been released. The bony parts should be intact, and all joints of the involved digits should be passively mobilized before tendon surgery.

If the profundus tendon has been cut distal to the sublimis attachment, the distal end of the cut profundus can be advanced to a bony attachment at the base of the distal phalanx (Figs. 17.94 and 17.95). The distal piece of the cut tendon is then removed. The suture is made by means of a stainless steel, pullout write suture attached into the bone at the base of the distal phalanx. The tendon soon accommodates to its new length, and a satisfactory functional result is obtained. If one or both tendons are cut in the area on the volar surface between the sublimis insertion and the distal palmar crease, both tendons should be removed. A graft should be placed from the profundus tendon in the palm out through the finger to a bony attachment into the proximal end of the distal phalanx. This is done according to the method of Bunnel[8, 10, 11] with No. 34 stainless steel wire sutures (Figs. 17.100 and 17.101). If pulleys have been destroyed, they are replaced by means of tendons wrapped about the phalanges or metacarpal necks and passing subcutaneously on the dorsal surface outside the extensor apparatus. The suture line in the pulley should be fixed in an area not in contact with the tendon graft. The hands are immobilized routinely in plaster splints to relieve tension on the graft for a period of 3 weeks. Following removal of the cast, active exercises and physical therapy are begun. If a tendon seems to be tied down, a tendolysis may be necessary, but such a procedure should not be premature in a child, inasmuch as adhesions, if they occur, often stretch out

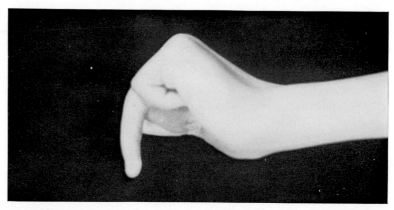

Figure 17.94. Attempted flexion after severance of the flexor sublimis and profundus in an 11-year-old boy.

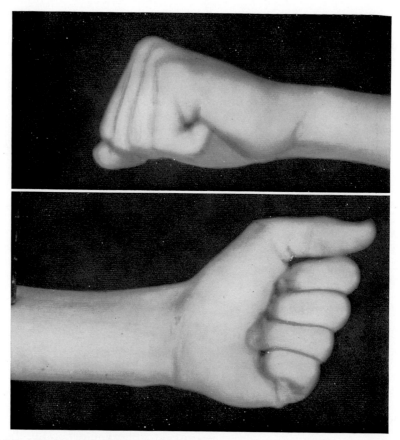

Figure 17.95. Same case as seen in Figure 17.94. Range of flexion after removal of the sublimis and profundus tendons and graft of the palmaris longus to the profundus in the palm. The graft was extended to the base of the distal phalanx.

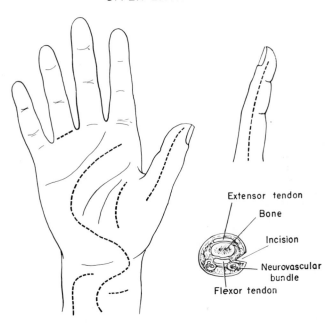

Extensor tendon
Bone
Incision
Neurovascular bundle
Flexor tendon

Figure 17.96. Incisions useful in hand operations.

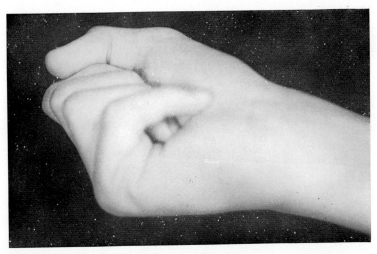

Figure 17.97. Severed profundus tendon in the right little finger between the proximal and middle creases of the finger. One slip of the sublimis had also been severed, and there was deep scarring and destruction of this pulley.

after several months of active and passive exercises. In the majority of instances, the tendon begins to function well within the first weeks after removal of the casts or splints.

Lacerations of the flexor aspects of the fingers are best treated by debridement, cleansing, and skin suture; the graft should be an elective procedure and should be de-ferred to a later time. In lacerations involving the extensor aspects of the hand and fingers, the extensor tendons should be sutured primarily.

Children are not infrequently seen with deformities of the hand and fingers that are due to unrecognized lacerations of the peripheral nerves higher in the arm or forearm. Many of these lacerations have been treated

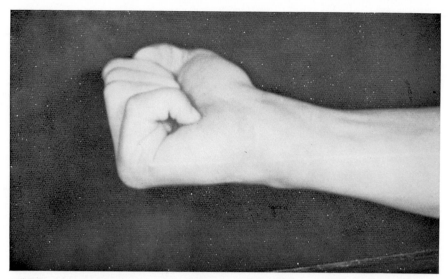

Figure 17.98. Same case as seen in Figure 17.97, showing flexion and extension after a tendon graft. The sublimis and profundus tendons were removed. The palmaris longus was grafted from the profundus in the palm through the finger to the base of the distal phalanx. The proximal pulley was reconstructed from a part of the removed sublimis tendon.

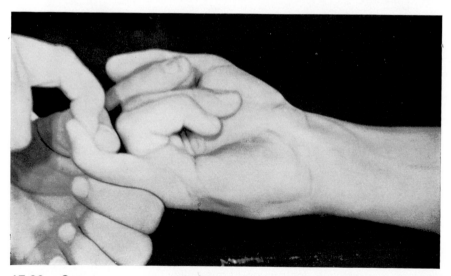

Figure 17.99. Same case as seen in Figures 17.97 and 17.98, showing the definite function of the profundus and its strength after the profundus graft.

as simple, small cuts, without due recognition of the nerve damage. Fixed contractures that have occurred should be corrected if the injuries are seen late, and the nerves should then be explored just as in the adult patient, the ends being sutured carefully with No. 6-0 silk on an atraumatic needle. If this proce-

dure is carefully performed, a great number of these children regain full function. Satisfactory results may be expected as late as 2 years after the injury for return of motor function and even later for the return of sensation. Digital nerves damaged in the hand and fingers should be sutured, accord-

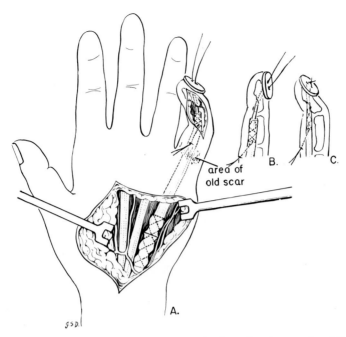

area of
old scar

B.

C.

A.

Figure 17.100. Free tendon graft after removal of profundus and sublimis and attachment of graft to distal phalanx according to the Bunnell technique.

ing to a meticulous technique, with No. 6-0 silk on an atraumatic needle at the time of debridement.

If motor function does not return, any of various reconstructive transplants can be performed with good results. In the case of a radial nerve loss (Fig. 17.102), good results are usually obtained by transplanting the wrist flexors into the finger and thumb extensors. The most common procedure is to move the flexor ulnaris into the common extensors, the palmaris longus into the abductor and extensor brevis of the thumb, and the flexor carpi radialis into the extensor policis longus. There are other methods of utilizing these same muscles just as effectively, but their use depends upon individual variations.

In ulnar and median paralyses, the main loss is that of intrinsics, and the consequent loss of finger extension and thumb opposition is quite disabling. The many different kinds of transplants that may be used to restore these functions will not be enumerated. Deformities can be overcome completely or partially by appropriate tendon transfers and arthrodeses designed to restore muscle balance and to bring the thumb and fingers to functional positions (Figs. 17.103–

17.105). Often there is a dearth of transferable tendons, so that only the most important intrinsic function can be restored. In children, it is best to avoid arthrodeses if possible. Irwin's dynamic tenodesis may give adequate function by utilizing a few tendons and retaining joint motions. Occasionally, injury makes it necessary to sacrifice digits or a portion of the hand. Such a loss is always disabling; however, the axiom that the thumb should be preserved or restored at all costs should always be kept in mind by the surgeon.

Sometimes parts of fingers or entire fingers must be sacrificed. The loss of a finger is disabling, but not nearly as disabling as the loss of a thumb. In instances of loss of the terminal part of the thumb, the simple procedure of deepening the web space by a Z-plasty may greatly improve the function. Sometimes when both phalanges are lost and the first metacarpal, along with its musculature, is retained, certain procedures may increase the length and usefulness of the thumb. Lewin[21] has described an advancement procedure that uses a bone graft into the metacarpal and a skin graft onto a non-opposing surface, lifts the intact skin up over

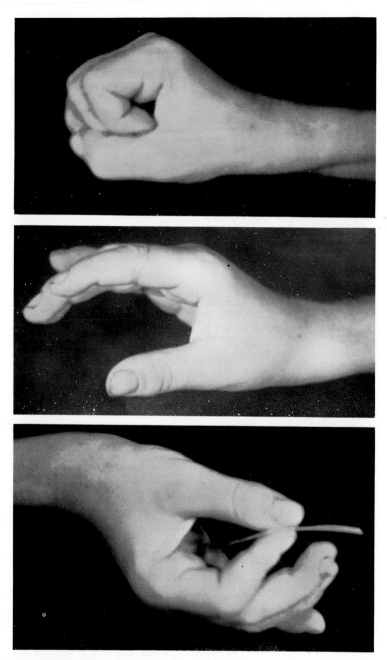

Figure 17.101. Application of Bunnell technique (Figure 17.100), showing function of hand following transplantation of flexor carpi radialis to extensor pollicis brevis and abductor pollicis longus, palmaris longus to extensor pollicis longus, and flexor carpi lunaris to common finger extensors.

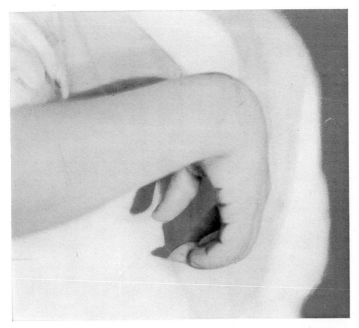

Figure 17.102.   Radial nerve palsy due to trauma.

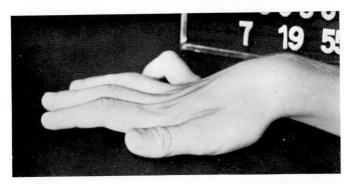

Figure 17.103.   Ulnar nerve palsy due to laceration over the flexor surface of the ulnar side of the elbow. This palsy is only 5 months old, and the wound is well healed. No finger contractures are present. The nerve should be explored and sutured at this time.

the bone graft, and inlays the skin below the surface. This procedure may add to the length and give sensation on the opposing surface to serve greatly for the previous loss. Littler,[24] who has gone even further, uses almost the same principle, except that when the thumb is retained and all of the fingers, including the metacarpals, have been lost, he elevates the skin flap and inserts a bone graft from the ilium uunderneath it, opposes normal skin from hand, with its sensation, against the thumb, and then fills the part that is not to be opposed with a skin flap from the abdomen. This procedure improves the function of the hand by providing an effective post for the intact thumb to work against; this post has good sensation in the part that opposes the thumb (Fig. 17.106).

A tube pedicle may be constructed and a bone equal to the length of the missing thumb may be moved into the pedicle and grafted into the first metacarpal. The motor function of such a reconstructed part is usually excellent, but, because its sensation is poor, its

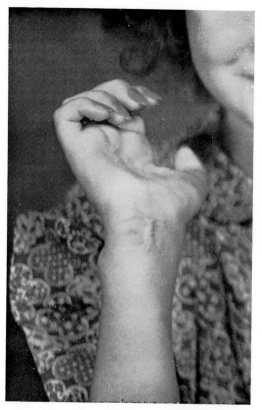

Figure 17.104. Attempt to extend fingers after laceration at the ulnar surface of the wrist. The ulnar nerve was severed at that level, and the intrinsic function was consequently lost.

usefulness is inadequate. This inadequacy may now be circumvented, however, by transferring skin from a less valuable finger, such as the little or ring finger. The skin is taken from the flexor surface at the tip and, with its neurovascular bundle, is transferred according to the method of Littler to the opposing end of the thumb. This addition should make for much better functional results, but great care is necessary in performing this type of surgery.

References

1. Abbott, L. C., Saunders, J. B., and Bost, F. C.: Arthrodesis of the wrist with the use of grafts of cancellous bone, *J. Bone Joint Surg., 24:* 883, 1942.
2. Boyd, H. B., and Stone, M. M.: Resection of the distal end of the ulna, *J. Bone Joint Surg., 26:* 313, 1944.
3. Boyes, J. H.: Flexor tendon grafts in fingers and thumb, *J. Bone Joint Surg., 32A:* 489, 1950.
4. Boyes, J. H.: Repair of motor branch of the ulnar nerve in the palm., *J. Bone Joint Surg., 37A:* 920, 1955.
5. Bruner, J. M.: Problems of postoperative position and motion in surgery of the hand, *J. Bone Joint Surg., 35A:* 355, 1953.
6. Bunnell, S.: Repair of tendons in the fingers and description of two new instruments, *Surg. Gynecol. Obstet., 26:* 103, 1918.
7. Bunnell, S.: Physiological reconstruction of the thumb after total loss, *Surg. Gynecol. Obstet., 52:* 245, 1931.
8. Bunnell, S.: Treatment of tendons of the hand, *J. Bone Joint Surg., 23:* 240, 1941.
9. Bunnell, S.: Surgery of the intrinsic muscles of the hand other than those producing opposition of the thumb, *J Bone Joint Surg., 24:* 1, 1942.
10. Bunnell, S.: Suturing tendons, *Instruct. Lect. Am. Acad. Orthop. Surg.,* Lect. 1–5, 1943.
11. Bunnell, S.: *Surgery of the Hand;* Philadelphia: J. B. Lippincott, 1944.
12. Bunnell, S.: Active splinting of the hand, *J. Bone Joint Surg., 28:* 732, 1946.
13. Bunnell, S.: Digit transfer by neurovascular pedicle, *J. Bone Joint Surg., 34:* 772, 1952.
14. Bunnell, S.: Primary and secondary repair of flexor tendons of hand, *Plast. Reconstructr. Surg., 12:* 65, 1953.
15. Dial, D.: Reconstruction of the thumb after traumatic amputation, *J. Bone Joint Surg., 21:* 98, 1939.
16. Dunlop, J.: The use of the index finger for the thumb: some interesting points hand surgery, *J. Bone Joint Surg., 5:* 99, 1923.
17. Goldner, J. L.: Deformities of hand incidental to pathological changes of the extensor and intrinsic muscle mechanisms, *J. Bone Joint Surg., 35A:* 115, 1953.
18. Graham, W. C.: Flexor tendon grafts to the fingers and thumb, *J. Bone Joint Surg., 29:* 553, 1947.
19. Joyce, J. L.: Results of new operation for substitution of the thumb, *Br. J. Surg., 16:* 362, 1929.
20. Koch, S. L., and Kanavel, A. B.: Purposeful splinting following injuries of the hand, *Surg Gynecol. Obstet., 68:* 1, 1939.
21. Lewin, M.: Partial reconstruction of the thumb in a one stage operation, *J. Bone Joint Surg., 35A:* 573, 1953.
22. Littler, J. W.: Free tendon grafts in secondary flexor tendon repair, *Am. J. Surg., 74:* 315, 1947.
23. Littler, J. W.: Tendon transfers and arthrodeses in combined median and ulnar nerve paralysis, *J. Bone Joint Surg., 31A:* 225, 1949.
24. Littler, J. W.: Architectural principles of reconstructive hand surgery, *Surg. Clin. North Am., 31:* 463, 1951.
25. Littler, J. W.: The neurovascular pedicle method of digital transposition for reconstruction of the thumb, *Plast. Reconstructr. Surg., 12:* 303, 1953.
26. Littler, J. W.: Transfer of free skin graft with neurovascular pedicle, paper presented at the American Society of Surgery of the Hand, 1956.
27. Riordan, D. C.: Tendon transplantation in median nerve and ulnar nerve paralysis, *J. Bone Joint Surg., 35A:* 312, 1953.
28. Siler, V. E.: Primary tenorrhaphy of the flexor tendons in the hand, *J. Bone Joint Surg., 32A:* 218, 1950.

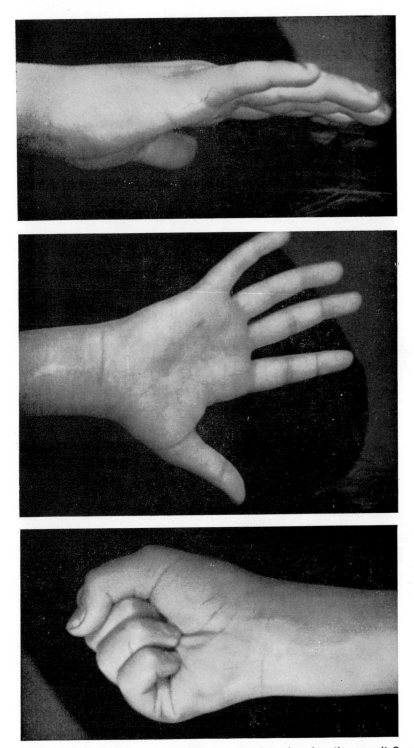

Figure 17.105. Same case as seen in Figure 17.104, showing the result 2 years after ulnar nerve suture. The patient has completely recovered intrinsic function and sensation in the hand.

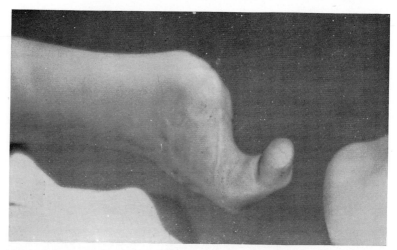

Figure 17.106. Loss of hand except for the thumb due to trauma. This patient would benefit greatly by Littler's procedure, which gives a post for the thumb to work against.

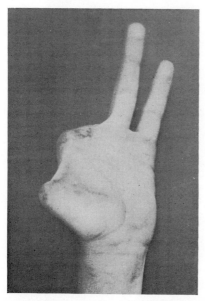

Figure 17.107. Loss of phalanges of the thumb and of the index and middle fingers due to trauma.

Burns

Burns involving the hands are unfortunately common injuries in children. Involvement of other parts of the body, which is very frequent, greatly complicates the overall treatment program. The burn usually involves only the skin and spares the tendons, bones, and joints; however, if it is treated improperly in the early stages, secondary involvement of these structures may cause severe crippling disability of the hand. The deformity produced may take almost any form and is often quite grotesque. The most common deformity is that of flexion of the wrist and hyperextension of the metacarpophalangeal joints combined with flexion of the interphalangeal joints or with flexion of the proximal interphalangeal joints and extension of the distal joints. This type of deformity tends to be most frequent since pain and muscle spasm cause overpull of the wrist flexors and stretching of the common extensors. This causes a hyperextension of the proximal finger joints, which often results in lateral slipping of the lateral bands to produce severe finger deformities. These burns are sometimes severe enough to cause loss of major deep structures, particularly of ligaments and tendons. Occasionally, fingers, parts of fingers, or practically the entire hand are lost. If the wounds are allowed to become septic or if there is an accumulation of necrosis after poor debridement, joints and tendons become fixed rapidly and often permanently. Because the skin of children and infants is relatively thin, deeper involvement may occur initially than would have been the case in an adult with a similar burn. Fortunately, the joints of a child do not stiffen quite as rapidly as those of an adult. On the other hand, children do not tolerate burns in general very well during the initial phases.

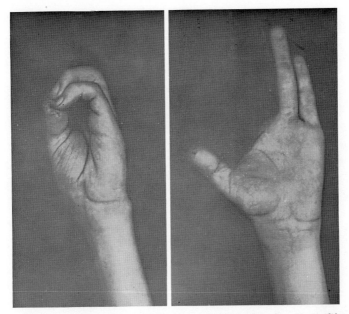

Figure 17.108. Same hand as seen in Figure 17.107 after bone grafting of the second metacarpal into the first metacarpal through a pedicle graft, release of the pedicle, and closure. Good functional and cosmetic improvement.

TREATMENT

The systemic treatment of burns in children does not differ from the therapy indicated in adults. The general care of toxemia, shock, and sepsis, all of which are of great importance, will not be discussed here. An attempt will be made to outline and cover only the more important aspect of the local care of the hand. It is essential that all efforts should be made to allay pain, prevent sepsis, debride early, and cover as soon as possible with skin grafts. Splinting in the position of function is extremely important to prevent deformity.

Early. Methods of early treatment are controversial, but the majority of authorities are of the opinion that open surgical drainage is the treatment of choice. Hand burns seen in the first 12 hr, or even those seen after sepsis has occurred, should be treated in the following manner with the general idea of gaining skin coverage as soon as possible. This goal can be attained by early debridement, daily cleansing, and use of wet dressings. As soon as the general condition permits, the entire hand should be cleansed gently and thoroughly by means of large gauze sponges with hexachlorophene and Phisoderm in water. The blisters should be opened and necro-

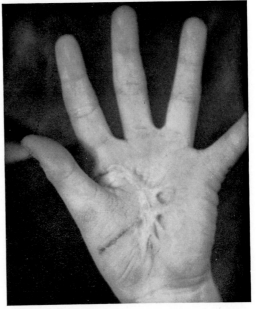

Figure 17.109. Burn healed by granulating in without any skin coverage. There is a severe cicatrix contracture.

tized, and charred tissue should be removed. This procedure should be exacting and meticulous. Several layers of fine mesh gauze should be wrapped around the part. Each

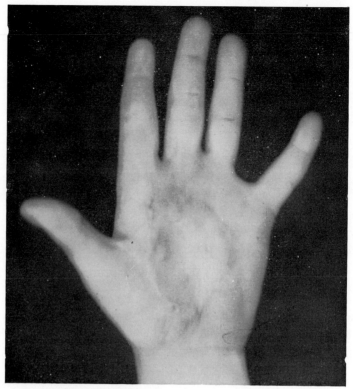

Figure 17.110. Same case as seen in Figure 17.109, after excision of scar and replacement of full thickness skin graft from the abdomen.

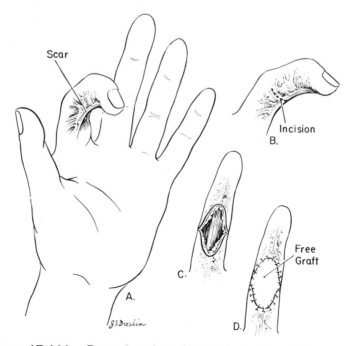

Figure 17.111. Procedure for release of cicatrix with free graft.

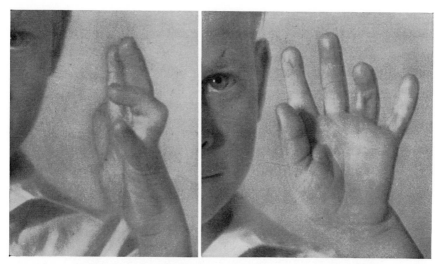

Figure 17.112. Longitudinal cicatrization after burn. The contracture may be released by a Z-plastic procedure with an excellent result.

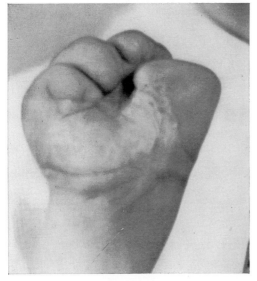

Figure 17.113. Severe scarring following a burn.

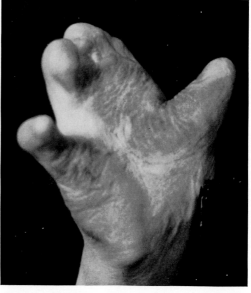

Figure 17.114. Same case as seen in Figure 17.113 after freeing of scar and application of a full thickness graft to release the thumb alone and the fingers en masse from the palm.

finger should be dressed separately and placed in the position of function. The wrist should be dorsiflexed, the fingers in semi-flexion, and the thumb slightly flexed and in opposition. Sterile mechanic's waste may then be applied to hold these positions, and the entire bulky dressing should be kept wet with normal saline solution. Metal or plastic splints may also be included, if they are necessary, but usually the bulky mechanic's waste dressing holds the position satisfactorily. The dressings are changed under water, and the patient is encouraged to move his fingers actively as much as possible. Necrotic tissue is trimmed away as it is encountered. Most burned hands can be prepared in this manner for split thickness coverage within 2–4 weeks. In most instances involving the dorsal aspect of the hand and fingers, split thick-

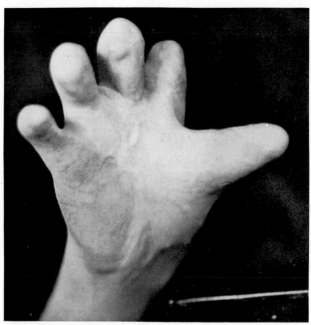

Figure 17.115. Same case as seen in Figures 17.113 and 17.114 after the webs between the fingers had been released as in syndactylism.

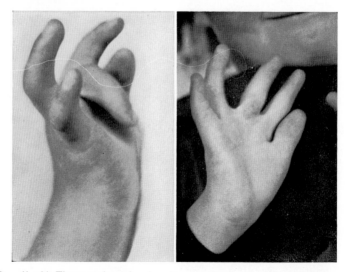

Figure 17.116. (*Left*) Flexor cicatrix due to an old burn. (*Right*) After release of scar and coverage by diamond inlay of free, full thickness skin from the abdomen.

ness skin will serve permanently. On the palmer aspect of the hand and fingers, the split graft is used only for temporary coverage. It is later replaced with full thickness skin grafts.

Late. Unfortunately, many burned hands are seen only after severe scarring and contractures have occurred. No burn wound should be allowed to "granulate and heal in (Figs. 17.109 and 17.110). Every burn should be covered as soon as possible.

When scarring of the dorsal surface of the fingers occurs (Fig. 17.11), athe scar can be dissected completely free, and the fingers flexed and immobilized on an aluminum splint. The area can be covered with a split

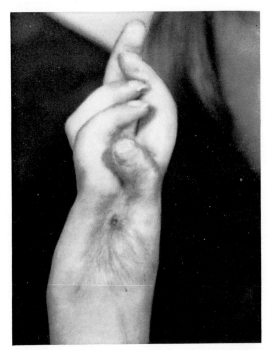

Figure 17.117. The result of poor early handling of a burn. There was no splinting. Healing has occurred by granulating in, which has produced heavy cicatrization and inexcusable deformity due to contracture.

thickness skin graft. The aluminum splint can be prepared and cut to the proper shape prior to surgery and then sterilized and molded into the position desired in the operating room. Pressure dressings are applied over the graft, and the entire part is dressed with bulky pressure dressings that incorporate the splint. The dressings are changed in about 10 days, and immobilization is continued for approximately 1 month; then mobilization is begun by means of physical therapy in the form of active exercises and whirlpool treatment. The splint is used on a part time basis until the end of the sixth week. Scars involving the palm should be removed, and the hand should be splinted with the fingers in extension after a full thickness graft has been applied. The grat is obtained from an area on the abdomen containing as little hair as possible.

The graft is outlined according to a pattern, and the dissection, which is carried out with the graft under tension, follows a plane in the fine white fibers that attach the skin to the subcutaneous tissue. No fat is removed with the skin. The graft is cut slightly larger than the wound to allow for shrinkage. It is sutured accurately into the bed, which should be perfectly dry to prevent formation of hematomas. A central holding stitch or two is often used to prevent slippage.

The donor site can usually be closed by excising the subcutaneous fat undermining the defect and closing. If the defect is very large, a split thickness graft may be needed to cover it without tension. In most instances, it is necessary to immobilize the elbow in flexion and to attach the part of the cast that covers the elbow to the splint to keep it from slipping. Longitudinal scars involving the flexor surfaces of the finger and web spaces are not uncommon in burns of the hand. They may be released by Z-plasty or multiple Z-plasties or but cutting the longitudinal scar transversely to allow the finger to extend and then inserting a diamond-shaped full thickness graft (Fig. 17.112). The release of tension by these methods results in the gradual disappearance of the scar and the contracture.

Dry fields are essential. Immobilization as decribed above is mandatory. When final coverage for hands and fingers has been secured and mobilization has been attained, fixed deformities due to tendon, bone, or joint damage may remain. If the middle extensor slip of the extensor apparatus scars

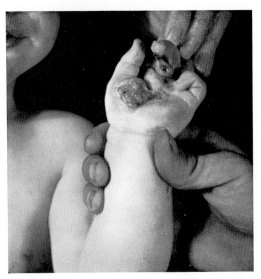

Figure 17.118. Soon after burn due to friction. This child grasped a belt of a rapidly rotating motor.

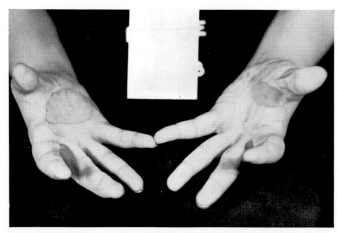

Figure 17.119.   Free full thickness grafts used in the palm to replace cicatrices.

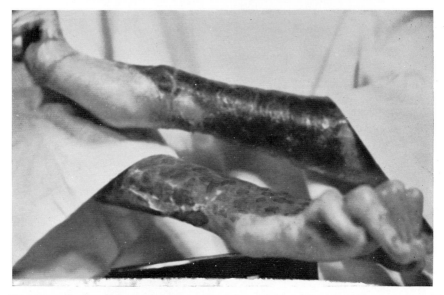

Figure 17.120.   Severe burn of hand and wrists mainly on the dorsal surfaces with fixed hypertension contractures of the metacarpophalangeal joints, flexion contracture of the proximal interphalangeal joints, and hyperextension of most of the distal interphalangeal joints.

down, the lateral bands slip laterally, causing flexion of the middle joint and extension of the distal joints. The middle slip should be freed and the lateral bands sectioned. This procedure allows the distal phalanx to flex into the mallet finger position but allows for better function in the proximal and middle joints. In several cases the joint surfaces may be extensively damaged and the tendons and ligaments scarred beyond repair. Arthrodesis in a functional position may be the treatment of choice. Occasionally, an amputation may be most desirable. The decision depends upon the individual case. If flexor tendons have been lost, they may be replaced by grafting as in other traumatic flexor tendon injuries (see "Lacerations of Hand and Fingers"). Frequently the results are rather discouraging because of other involvement, such as joint tightness and trauma to the capsule, caused by the burn itself. Tendon grafts should not be undertaken until good skin coverage has been secured in the area of transplantation. It is also imperative that a range of passive motion of maximal function be attained in the involved joint before the

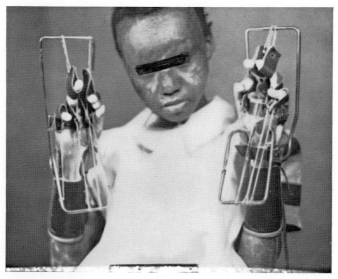

Figure 17.121. Same case as seen in Figure 17.120. Active splinting is used to help relieve some of the contractures.

tendon work is started. In many instances, only partial restoration is possible; however, because of the serious disability which occurs as a result of severe burns to the hand, reconstruction should always be attempted in order to gain at least some functional, and possibly cosmetic, improvement.

References

1. Barsky, A. J.: Surgical repair of unusual dermatological conditions, *Surg. Clin. North Am., 19:* 459, 1939.
2. Blair, V. P., and Brown, J. B.: Use and uses of large split grafts of intermediate thickness, *Surg. Gynecol. Obstet., 49:* 82, 1929.
3. Brown, J. B.: Surface defects of the hand, *Am. J. Surg., 46:* 690, 1939.
4. Brown, J. B., and McDowell, F.: Persistence of function of thin grafts through long periods of growth, *Surg. Gynecol. Obstet., 72:* 849, 1941.
5. Brown, J. B., and McDowell, F.: *Skin Grafting of Burns;* Philadelphia: J. B. Lippincott, 1943.
6. Bunnell, S.: Contractures of the hand from infection and injuries, *J. Bone Joint Surg., 14:* 27, 1932.
7. Bunnell, S., and Howard, L. D.: Additional elastic hand splints, *J. Bone Joint Surg., 32A:* 226, 1950.
8. Cohen, H. H.: An adjustable volar flexion splint, *J. Bone Joint Surg 24:* 189, 1942.
9. Conway, H.: Whole thickness grafts in correction of contractures due to burn scar, *Ann. Surg., 109:* 286, 1939.
10. Davis, J. S.: Use of small deep grafts in repair of surface defects, *Am. J. Surg., 47:* 280, 1940.
11. Dupertius, S. M.: An evaluation of skin grafts for hand coverage, *J. Bone Joint Surg., 34A:* 811, 1952.
12. Gillies, H.: Experience with tubed pedicle flaps, *Surg. Gynecol Obstet., 60:* 291, 1935.
13. Goldner, J. L.: Deformities of the hand incidental to pathological changes of the extensor and intrinsic muscle mechanism, *J. Bone Joint Surg., 35A:* 115, 1952.
14. Harris, C., and Riordan, D. C.: Intrinsic contracture of the hand and its surgical treatment, *J. Bone Joint Surg., 36A:* 10, 1954.
15. Hovens, F. Z.: Preoperative and postoperative care in skin grafting, *Surg. Clin. North Am., 20:* 1087, 1940.
16. Howard, L. D., Jr.: Contracture of the thumb web, *J. Bone Joint Surg., 32A:* 267, 1950.
17. Jones, R., Jr.: Management of old contractures of upper extremity resulting from third degree burns, *South. Med. J., 4:* 789, 1941.
18. Koch, S. L.: Complicated contractures of the hand, *Ann. Surg., 98:* 546, 1933.
19. Koch, S. L., and Kanavel, A. B.: Purposeful splinting following injuries of the hand, *Surg. Gynecol. Obstet., 68:* 1939.
20. Mason, M. L.: Plastic surgery of hands, *Surg. Clin. North Am., 19:* 227, 1939.
21. Padgett, E. C.: Free full thickness skin graft in correction of soft tissue deformities, *J. A. M. A., 98:* 18, 1932.
22. Padgett, E. C.: Skin grafting in severe burns, *Am. J. Surg., 43:* 626, 1939.
23. Padgett, E. C.: Skin grafting and three-quarter thickness skin graft for prevention and correction of cicatricial formation, *Ann. Surg., 113:* 1034, 1941.
24. Padgett, E. C.: *Skin Grafting;* Springfield, Ill.: Charles C Thomas, 1942.
25. Sheehan, J. E.: Use of free full thickness skin grafts, *J. A. M. A., 112:* 27, 1939.
26. Tanzer, R. C.: Prevention of postoperative hematoma in surgery of the hand: use of compression suture, *J. Bone Joint Surg., 34A:* 797, 1952.

BRACHIAL PALSY—BIRTH TYPE

A paralysis due to injury of the roots of the brachial plexus at birth became a more

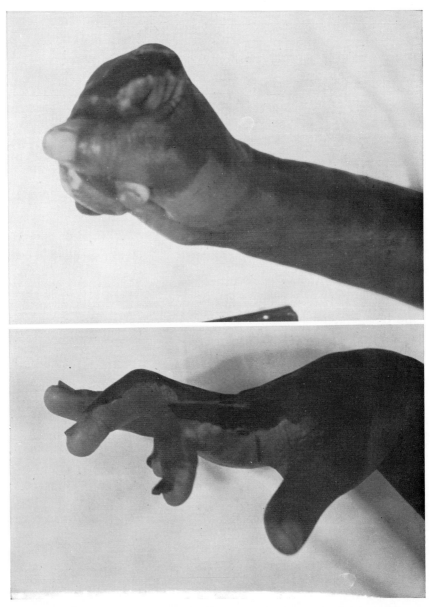

Figures 17.122. Same case as seen in Figures 17.120 and 17.121, after removal of the dorsal scar of the wrist, hand, and fingers to the proximal interphalangeal joints and coverage with split thickness grafts. Release of the distal extensors of the lateral bands may improve the fingers by releasing the extension contracture of the distal joint and the flexion of the proximal interphalangeal joint, which have occurred through buttonholing of the lateral hands.

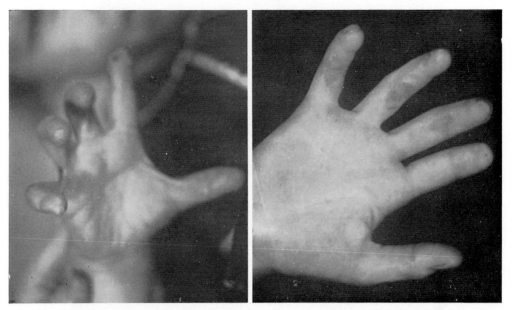

Figure 17.123. (*Left*) Flexion contractures in volar skin of all fingers. (*Right*) After a diamond-shaped, free, full thickness graft.

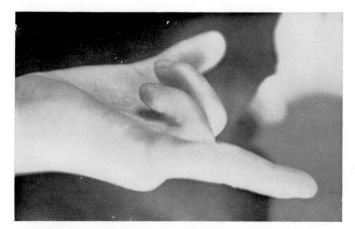

Figure 17.124. Flexion contracture of the ring and middle fingers is due to a burn. The skin only was involved on the ring finger. The tendons and the proximal interphalangeal joint were scarred in the middle finger. Both fingers were released and covered with a free, full thickness skin graft. Later, the middle finger was covered by a pedicle flap from the abdomen, and a free tendon graft was inserted. The tendon used was the palmaris longus tendon from the profundus tendon in the palm, and it was attached to bone at the base of the distal phalanx.

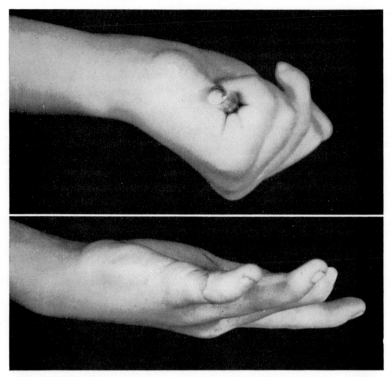

Figure 17.125. Same case as seen in Figure 17.124. Result 4 years after treatment. (In an adult, amputation of the middle finger would have been the procedure of choice.)

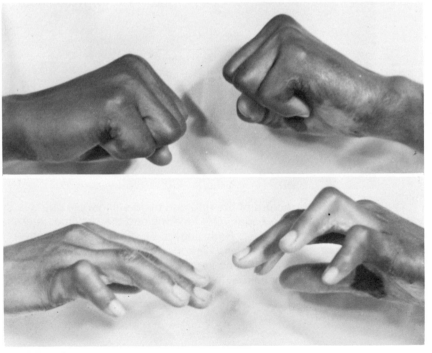

Figure 17.126. Result after release of a severe cicatrix in the palm due to burns. There is still flexion tightness of the skin in the fingers. The fingers will be released and the defect filled by a free, full thickness graft, just as in the palm.

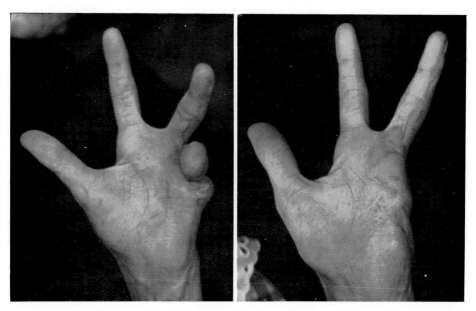

Figure 17.127. (*Left*) Severe burn with contracture of the middle finger and loss of the ring and little fingers in a 7-year-old girl. (*Right*) Release of the scar and removal of the fourth and fifth rays; some of the skin from the fillet was used to cover the scarred areas.

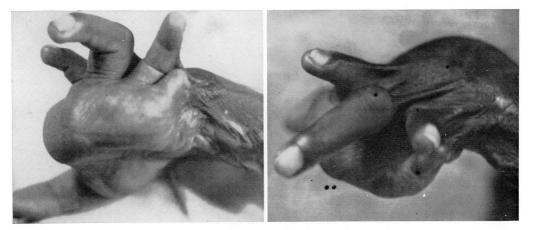

Figure 17.128. Severe deformity of the hand due to cicatrix of the skin involving mainly the dorsal aspect.

common clinical entity as fetal and maternal mortality associated with difficult deliveries was reduced. Still further refinement of obstetric technique has reduced the incidence in recent times.

Smellie mentioned this complication of delivery in 1764. The mechanism of the paralysis was described by Duchenne in 1872 and by Erb in 1874. The predominant upper arm lesion bears their names. Klumpke described the lower arm type in 1885.

Etiology

Fixation of the shoulder or head followed by traction and lateral flexion of the neck by means of either the trunk, an arm, or the

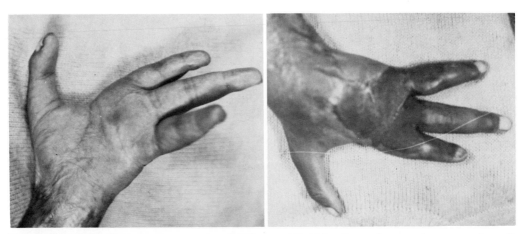

Figure 17.129. Same case as seen in Figure 17.128 after release of scar and application of free, full thickness grafts from the abdomen.

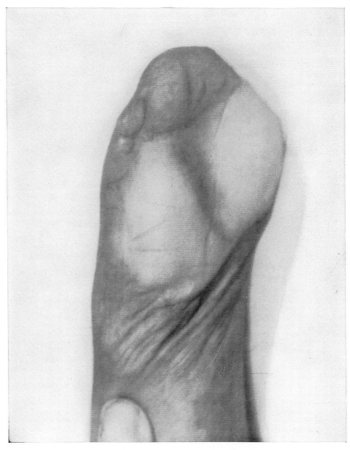

Figure 17.130. Severe burn with loss of all fingers. The first metacarpal remained, and its intrinsic muscle attachment is intact.

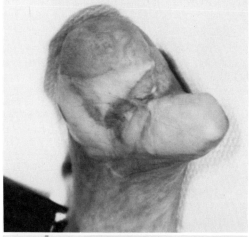

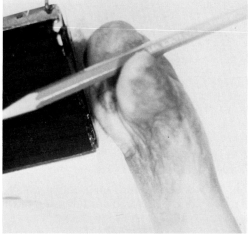

Figure 17.131. Same hand as seen in Figure 17.130, after a Z-plastic procedure and deepening of the web between the first and second metacarpals. The function of the hand is now much improved.

head, acting as a lever, has been thought to be the mechanism of injury.

Pathology

In 36 of 54 patients reviewed by Wickstrom et al.,[8] the involvement centered about the fifth and sixth cervical roots. In these cases of principally upper arm involvement, damage was most commonly minimal. It was represented at the root by edema and mild intraneural hemorrhage and by some tearing of fibers, although the root remained intact. Recovery sometimes occurred in only a few days, but more commonly complete return was evidenced in 3–6 months.

There were 14 patients in whom all roots were involved and 4 in whom paralysis was evidenced as involving primarily the eighth cervical and first thoracic roots.

In these there was disruption of the nerve fibers, including avulsion of the roots from the spinal cord, at multiple points. Complete laceration of the roots, multiple neuromata, and gross lesions of the cord have been observed on exploration.

There were three cases of Horner's syndrome and four of sensory as well as motor loss in Wickstrom's series.

Clinical Picture

EARLY

Although no signs may be noted other than the loss of the Moro reflex when the infant is startled, more frequently the stricken limb is observed to remain lifeless at the side with the elbow extended. In some infants, a traumatic neuritis persists, and the infant cries when the arm is moved. Pronation of the forearm and wrist, placing the limb in the attitude of receiving a "hidden tip," is a typical finding. There may be swelling in the supraclavicular fossa due to hemorrhage or inflammation. Occasionally a fractured clavicle or humerus is seen in concert with the paralysis. Signs consistent with Horner's syndrome may be found if the thoracic root has been injured.

The upper arm, or Erb-Duchenne, type of paralysis is most frequent; it is at least four times as common as other types. Here, damage to the fifth and sixth cervical roots results in paralysis of the deltoid supraspinatus, infraspinatus biceps, coraco brachialis, and supinator brevis.

In Klumpke's type, which involves the lower arm and the eighth cervical and first thoracic nerve roots, there is loss of the intrinsic musculature of the hand, the flexors of the wrist, and the long flexors of the fingers. Along with involvement of the sympathetic fibers, there is dropped eyelid (ptosis), narrowing of the palpebral fissure, and constriction of the pupil in the involved side.

Sensation is ordinarily intact.

In Sever's series,[6] the right side was involved in 64% of cases. In 63 of the 1,100

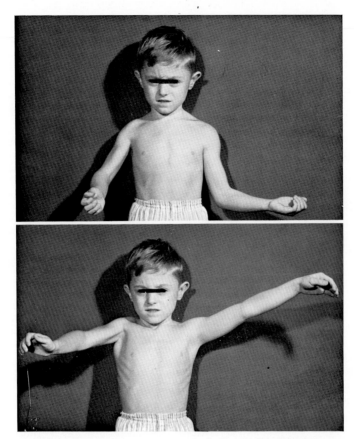

Figure 17.132. (*Top*) Limited external rotation due to contracture in brachial palsy. (*Bottom*) Limitation of abduction and elevation despite good deltoid power following birth type of brachial palsy.

cases analyzed by Sever, the involvement was bilateral.

The paralysis characteristically leads to internal rotation at the shoulder, pronation of the forearm, and flexion of the wrist.

LATE

The signs of this injury in the older child are those of residual deformity. The most marked imbalance of musculature involves the shoulder, in which the internal rotators are strong and the external rotators are paralyzed (Figs. 17.132–17.134).

The internal rotation contracture causes the child to hold the elbow away from the side in partial abduction in order to clear the arm from the trunk. The resulting deformity enables one to diagnose this condition on the street. Humeral scapular rhythm is lost, and there is limited abduction, most of which is really scapular elevation.

The humerus is frequently shortened out of all proportion to the muscular atrophy. The acromion may be hooked downward and elongated on x-ray examination. Posterior subluxation or dislocation of the humeral head may occasionally be present.

Pronation or supination deformities, depending on the kind of muscle imbalance, may be present in the forearm.

The most common muscle weakness by far is that of the deltoid, biceps, and external rotators at the shoulder. However, it is not unusual on examining a late case to find that the muscle power is good but inhibited from maximal function by contracture.

Treatment

Treatment cannot be based on the use of a position to prevent deformity 24 hr a day. Such therapy results in contracture in abduc-

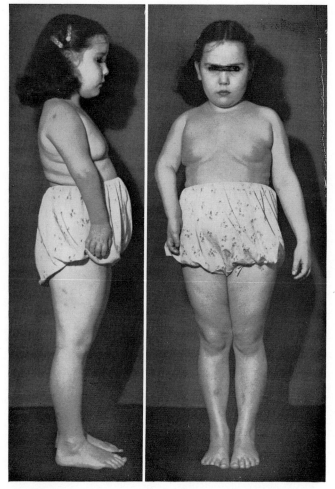

Figure 17.133. Involvement of the whole arm in brachial palsy. There are forearm, hand, and wrist contractures.

tion and internal rotation. Periodic change into the corrective position is the guiding principle of treatment. Neurologic exploration and repair of the injury have not been justified, the proximal nature of the lesion and the lack of suitable nerve sheath in young infants being major handicaps.

The arm may be pinned in abduction and external rotation by means of a diaper while the infant is recumbent. This position should be maintained for periods of 2–3 hr only, and there should be alternate periods during which the arm is free. In addition, at each diaper change the arm is passively abducted, the elbow flexed, the forearm supinated, and the wrist dorsiflexed so that a full range of motion of all joints, including those of the fingers, is gently carried out.

More efficient corrective immobilization is carried out by a so-called "Statue of Liberty" splint, with maintains abduction and external rotation and in addition controls the forearm and hand in a manner that mere splinting cannot equal. The splint is not worn continuously. It is alternated with periods during which the arm is entirely free and with periods of active and passive exercise. The splint is usually needed for the first 6 months intermittently through day and night and perhaps for an additional 6 months at night only. The child must be followed frequently enough so that the earliest opportunity to reestablish scapulohumeral rhythm through active use of the area is not missed. About one-half of the upper arm paralyses respond to this regimen with satisfactory shoulder

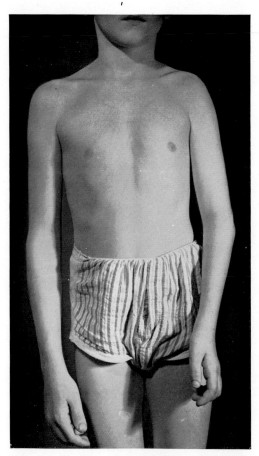

Figure 17.134. Involvement of the upper arm in brachial palsy. Note shortening, tendency to hold elbow away from trunk because of internal rotation contracture, flexed elbow but good hand.

function, but function is completely normal in only 10%.

In late deformity the splint does not solve the clinical problem.

The usual problem in late cases is to increase the range of external rotation and abduction. If there is no bony deformity, this may be accomplished in part by tenotomy of the subcapularis and pectoralis major muscles, as described by Sever. If active external rotation power is not present, it may be established by the muscle transplant described by L'Episcopo.[4] In this procedure, the teres major and often the latissimus dorsi are removed from their insertions and sutured under an osteoperiosteal flap on the posterior aspect of the humerus at the same level. They are thereby converted from internal to external rotators. Abduction is also frequently improved by this procedure.

In the presence of functioning musculature but fixed contracture, osteotomy of the humerus above the insertion of the deltoid and rotation of the distal fragment externally inside the periosteum may be indicated.

Improvement in appearance as well as in function can be expected from a correctly done operation that has been carefully selected for the particular case.

References

1. Clark, L. P., Taylor, A. S., and Prout, T.: A study of brachial birth palsy, *Am. J. Med. Sci., 130:* 670, 1905.
2. Fairbank, H. A. T.: Birth palsy: subluxation of the shoulder joint in infants and young children, *Lancet, 1:* 1217, 1913.
3. L'Episcopo, J. B.: Tendon transplantation in obstetrical paralysis, *Am. J. Surg., 25:* 122, 1934.
4. L'Episcopo, J. B.: Restoration of muscle balance in the treatment of obstetrical paralysis, *N. Y. J. Med., 39:* 357, 1939.
5. Sever, J. W.: Obstetrics paralysis; its etiology, pathology, clinical aspects and treatment with a report of four hundred and seventy cases, *Am. J. Dis. Child., 12:* 541, 1916.
6. Sever, J. W.: The results of a new operation for obstetrical paralysis, *Am. J. Orthop. Surg., 16:* 248, 1918.
7. Taylor, E. S.: Brachial birth palsy and injuries of similar type in adults, *Surg. Gynecol. Obstet., 30:* 494, 1920.
8. Wickstrom, J., Haslam, E. T., and Hutchison, R.: The surgical management of residual deformities of the shoulder following birth injuries of the brachial plexus, *J. Bone Joint Surg., 37A:* 27, 1955.

CHAPTER 18

The Spine

POSTURE IN EARLY ADOLESCENTS

Posture becomes a common clinical problem with girls between the ages of 10 and 15 years who have no abnormalities. This age group and sex is usually seen purely because of the parent's complaint that "I don't like the way she stands."

It should be recognized that much more than the way the child stands is embodied in the parental concern. The child is beginning to become a young woman of the age of social competition for the female. The mother, impatient that she put her best foot forward, wants the awkwardness of 12 to pass quickly to the poise of 18. The mother is motivated by the desire to obtain the best in life for her child.

The child, on the other hand, is motivated by a desire to conceal the developing lumps on her chest, which have reached the stage of being embarrassing. Very baggy sweaters and blouses become the rule. In addition, she really does stand poorly. The shoulders slope down and inward, the head protrudes forward, the abdomen is protuberant, and the buttocks are prominent. This posture, in part, is a reflection of an attitude toward life rather than a structural abnormality. The necessity for making oneself as inconspicuous as possible until some measure of understanding or mastery of the adolescent situation is gained is reflected in the stance.

Treatment

It is helpful first to explain to the mother why she is concerned about her daughter in terms of social competition and to assure her that, in any event, the child's stance at 12 will not be her posture at 18, when the motivations become quite different. It is obvious that if she constantly criticizes her daughter's posture, the only result will be the strained mother-daughter relationship that is so common among girls of 13. No amount of nagging correction will make a child stop concealing something about which she is embarrassed. Inasmuch as constant admonition to stand straight accomplishes nothing, it is better omitted.

It is possible to accomplish something with posture in this age group by exercises that tilt the pelvis. Exercises are a definite assigned task, like washing the dishes or doing homework, that hurts no one's psyche to have and to accomplish regularly. There are two commonly used forms of pelvic tilt exercises. One is the flexed knee sit-up in which the patient lies on the back on a table and flexes the knees on the chest. The head and shoulders are then lifted from the table by the use of the abdominal muscles, and the trunk is held off the table for a moment and slowly dropped back again.

Another form of pelvic tilt exercise consists of flattening the lumbar lordosis against the wall by the use of the abdominal musculature, holding the posture, and then releasing it.

A well tucked-in pelvis is the key to good posture.

BACK PAIN IN CHILDREN— DIFFERENTIAL DIAGNOSIS

The complaint of back pain in a child must always be taken seriously. In our own experience, the underlying cause has always been found to be a serious one, albeit occasionally of psychologic origin. The complaint has sometimes revealed a serious disturbance in the family situation, which, when brought to light early, has offered some hope of solution.

Every orthopaedist should be aware of the fact that leukemia not infrequently presents itself first as back pain. The pain is often fleeting and evanescent in character and gives

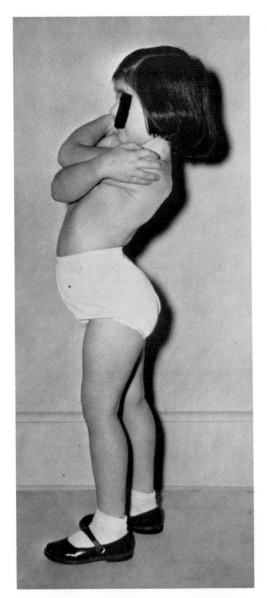

Figure 18.1. Posture can be affected as illustrated by hip flexion contractures with excessive lumbar lordosis and protuberant abdomen.

has become relatively rare, but it is still seen approximately 3–4 times a year in a children's hospital in a metropolitan area. Perhaps still more common is so-called osteomyelitis of the spine. The affected child presents with localized tenderness at a specific spinal level and a rigid spine due to muscle spasm. Roentgenograms reveal a narrowed interspace between two vertebrae and irregular destruction of the vertebral plate on either side. The presence of a well marked soft-tissue abscess shadow in addition would incline the observer toward a diagnosis of tuberculosis. Tuberculosis would, of course, tend to have a more insidious onset and a more prolonged history than osteomyelitis.

Osteomyelitis of the vertebrae occurs as a definite septic process, secondary to generalized sepsis or to the localized introduction of a needle, as in spinal puncture. There is also a type that has no predetermined etiology. The existence of an organism has not been proved in these cases. The disease tends to run a benign course, subsiding after a period of 4–6 months when the patient is immobilized in a cast and put on bed rest. Systemic signs are absent.

Tumor of the spinal cord may be extremely insidious, so much so that considerable time may elapse before sensory symptoms appear. Alertness to this lesion as a possible cause of low back pain when no other cause is evident requires making a lumbar puncture and an examination of spinal fluid, at the very least. It is frequently necessary to make a myelogram to rule out definitively the possibility of a spinal cord lesion.

Spondylolisthesis is common enough to receive eminent consideration as a diagnostic possibility. Tight hamstrings that limit straight leg raising are a frequent clinical sign. Localized tenderness at the spine of the fifth lumbar vertebra, or occasionally the fourth, is usually quite marked.

In early childhood, a severe slip of the fifth lumbar or the first sacral is unusual, and many of the so-called classic signs in the examination of the spine are not present.

Back pain due to so-called epiphysitis or Scheuermann's disease arises in the adolescent. Increased dorsal kyphosis is readily evident on physical examination and is confirmed by tenderness in the affected area. Roentgenograms reveal irregularity of the vertebral epiphyseal plates and wedging.

rise to a generalized complaint referable to the back rather than to one specific area. In difficult diagnostic problems, a sternal puncture and smear should always be included in the work-up.

There are a number of relatively common possibilities, including spinal cord tumor (often associated with paralytic bladder and urine retention). Tuberculosis of the spine

Eosinophilic granuloma may also produce wedging of the vertebra or a wafer-like appearance, as in Calvé's disease. Osteoid osteoma of the posterior element of the vertebra is not infrequently seen in childhood.

Rarely, malignant tumors of the vertebra, such as Ewing's sarcoma, are seen. Postural low back pain is not ordinarily seen in children. Underlying problems of the parent-child relationship may be suspected when both physical and laboratory examinations are negative.

CONGENITAL KYPHOSIS

An important childhood orthopaedic problem is kyphosis of the spine based on either a widespread disturbance of the ossification of the spine or a localized vertebral anomaly.

The patient is seen because of an increased anteroposterior curvature resulting in a rather sharp prominence that usually centers about the twelfth dorsal vertebra.

Etiology

There are at least three conditions in which this lesion is frequently seen. Widespread disturbance of the ossification of the spine is often seen in chondrodystrophy. In spines affected by this anomaly, the individual vertebrae frequently have a typical shape caused by lack of ossification of the anterosuperior and inferior angle (Fig. 18.2). Gargoylism and cretinism frequently have associated with

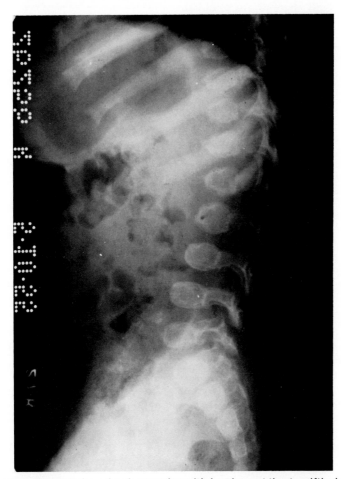

Figure 18.2. The spine in chondrodystrophy with kyphos at the twelfth dorsal vertebrae. The anteroposterior diameter of the vertebral body is increased, and ossification is deficient at the anteriorsuperior and inferior angles of some vertebrae.

them a hypermobility at the twelfth dorsal-first lumbar area (Fig. 18.3). The twelfth dorsal is often wedge shaped and irregular.

Individual vertebral anomalies of the type producing kyphosis are most often centered at the junction of the dorsal and lumbar spines. Such anomalies consist of partial absence of the vertebra involved; the posterior portion is present, the anterior absent.

Clinical Picture

MORQUIO'S SYNDROME

Morquio's syndrome is the form of chondrodystrophy in which changes are most prominent in the spine. It often is not recognized until the child is walking. The trunk is short beyond proportion to the shortening of the extremities. Skull changes are minimal.

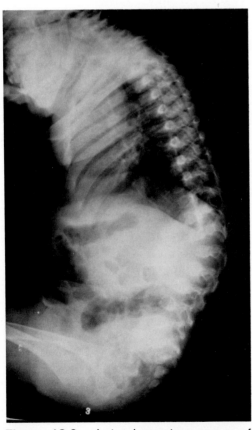

Figure 18.3. Lateral roentgenogram of the spine in a cretin, revealing hypermobility between the twelfth dorsal and first lumbar vertebrae.

The kyphosis is diffuse; there is wedging of the vertebrae in addition to localized changes at the twelfth dorsal. The extremities reveal widened epiphyses and bizarre bone shapes. Bone that is laid down has normal texture, however. There may be associated deformities, such as knock-knees. There is an epiphyseal disturbance of the vertebrae, as well as of the extremities. The epiphyseal line reveals a lack of cartilage column formation and, as a corollary, a lack of a provisional zone of calcification. There is no disturbance of membranous ossification.

The hand in chondrodystrophy is broad, and the fingers are short and have a tendency, when outstretched, to diverge, not at the metacarpophalangeal junction, but at the proximal interphalangeal joints.

HURLER'S SYNDROME

Hurler's syndrome, also known as gargoylism and dysostosis multiplex, resembles Morquio's syndrome closely. Many of the features of chondrodystrophy are found in this condition. Hurler's syndrome is associated with mental deficiency and clouding of the cornea. The hands sometimes exhibit an inability to extend the distal phalanges, resulting in a clawlike deformity.

The stored substance in gargoylism is not a lipid but a glycoprotein. At least three types of Hurler's syndrome have been delineated, as judged by various types of mucopolysaccharide found in large amounts in the urine and tissues. Greenback and Meyer found that chondroitin sulfate B predominated in 7 of 9 patients. Heparitin sulfate was found in varying lesser percentages. Neither of these compounds has been found in the urine of normal persons, although they are normal constituents of connective tissue.

In 2 of these 9 patients heparitin sulfate predominated, and in 1 it was the sole constituent. In this patient the intelligence quotient was normal.

In a third category of Hurler's syndrome, chondroitin sulfate B is found without heparitin sulfate.

KYPHOSIS ASSOCIATED WITH SINGLE AREAS OF BONY ANOMALY

When kyphosis is associated with single areas of bony anomaly, it is usually sharper and mentality is normal. It results in slight diminution in trunk height. Neurologic involvement has been reported in one-quarter of the published cases, according to Bingold.[1]

The most common site of involvement is the area between the tenth thoracic and the second lumbar vertebrae. The anomalous condition varies from complete absence of the posterior elements or body to a state in which some portion of these elements is present.

Treatment

In many orthopaedic clinics, considerable time and effort have been spent trying to maintain the patient's spine in a corrected position. Plaster shells, turnbuckle antero-posterior wedging jackets, and simple body casts and braces are all used.

In cases in which a considerable change takes place in the kyphos in flexion and extension in the upright posture, holding the spine in a corrected position has some merit. Such a condition frequently exists in various forms of chondrodystrophy. Where there is a single anomaly and the occiput is well centered over the pelvis, the follow-up films indicate that, although the condition enlarges with growth, the angle of the deformity remains the same.

Cosmetic attempts to reduce the deformity by excising the spine are usually misguided. The spines of the involved vertebrae are often rudimentary and have flat laminae enclosing the dural sac.

The consideration of spinal fusion as a means of maintaining the spine in a position of maximal extension through the kyphotic area is serious. Growth anteriorly in the presence of fused posterior elements may result in further correction. The posterior elements may be congenitally fused in localized anomalies of the spine. The type of congenital kyphosis most likely to benefit from fusion is that associated with excessive mobility at the area of kyphosis. The outlook in syndromes such as Hurler's, with its associated mental deficiency, must be considered in making a decision for surgery.

References

1. Bingold, A. C.: Congenital kyphosis, *J. Bone Joint Surg.*, 35B: 579, 1953.
2. Lombard, P., and LeGenissel, H.: Kyphosis congenitales, *Rev. Orthop.*, 25: 532, 1938.

VERTEBRAL PLANA (CALVÉ'S DISEASE)

Vertebral plana, characterized by a flattening of the vertebral body which gives a striking x-ray picture, was first reported by Calvé in 1925.[1] It occurs most frequently between the ages of 4 and 10 years but is occasionally seen in the early teens. The original etiology postulated by Calvé was aseptic necrosis—a process similar to coxa plana. Compere et al.[2] presented 4 cases which were diagnosed as eosinophilic granuloma. Similar deformities have been noted in patients who have widespread areas of involvement with eosinophilic granuloma.

Clinical Picture

The usual complaint is back pain. There is no radiation ordinarily. The symptoms are of short duration. If progression has taken place, there may be a gibbus, muscle spasm, and limited spine motion.

X-ray Picture

When seen early, the process may be osteolytic and may be gradually producing the thin, collapsed, "wafer-like" body which has been thought characteristic of this disease (Fig. 18.4). The picture is quite different from that of tuberculosis.

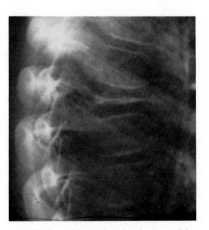

Figure 18.4. Vertebral plana with preservation of the disc spaces, but reduction of the single involved vertebra to wafer-like thinness.

Calvé noted that the discs adjacent to the involved vertebrae were intact, that ordinarily only one vertebra was involved, and that the flattened vertebra remained as a dense cortical disc.

Treatment

Rest in recumbency during the acute stage of symptoms followed by the wearing of a spine brace until the lesion is well healed and recalcified is the usual program. The brace is gradually discarded. The usual course varies between 1 and 3 years. Fripp[3] reported several cases for intervals as long as 22 years. He noted considerable reconstitution of the vertebra. A line of sclerosis was frequently left centrally as a ghost of the old collapse.

References

1. Calvé, J.: A localized affection of the spine suggestive of osteochondritis of the vertebral body with the clinical aspect of Pott's disease, J. Bone Joint Surg., 7: 41, 1925.
2. Compere, E. W., Johnson, W. E., and Coventry, M. B.: Vertebral plana (Calvé's disease) due to eosinophilic granuloma, J. Bone Joint Surg., 36A: 969, 1954.
3. Fripp, A. J.: Vertebra plana, J. Bone Joint Surg., 40B: 378, 1958.

SPONDYLOLISTHESIS

Spondylolisthesis, a low back condition, although most frequently noted as symptomatic in the age group from 30–40 years (Fig. 18.6), is also often seen in childhood.

The essential part of this lesion is a defect in the pars interarticularis of the involved vertebra at the junction of pedicle and lamina (spondylolysis). When the condition is bilateral, the body, pedicles, and superior articular processes are separated from the laminae, spine, and inferior articular processes (spondyloschisis). This situation may allow a forward slip of the body (spondylolisthesis).

The most commonly involved vertebra is the fifth lumbar (Figs. 18.7 and 18.8), but rarely the fourth lumbar may be involved.

Etiology

Ossification of the vertebra springs from three centers—one for the body and one for each half of the neural arch. Ossification starts in the pars interarticularis where the vessels originally penetrate the cartilage anlage.

Willis noted the "spondylolisthesis defect" in 6% of dissecting room subjects; 25% of these cases were unilateral. In no reported instance, not even in the unilateral type, has any evidence of bone repair been found. Hitchcock[5] noted that, despite a 5% incidence in the population at large, none has been found in fetal material. He found, in stillborn and infant cadavers, that hyperflexion of the spine fractured the neural arch in the lower lumbar region and tended to support fracture as the basic etiology. The hypothesis that the anomaly is a congenital defect is supported by a high incidence of associated defects, such as spina bifida, in the presence of the lesion. The argument as to whether the defect is a fracture or is of congenital origin is still open.

A third possibility exists, however, in that absorption may exceed accretion at the pars interarticularis. Such a situation would account for the failure of the lesion to be found in newborns, as congenital defects are, and for the lack of bone repair, which occurs in a fracture. It would also account for the high incidence in a group whose occupational habits include prolonged flexion of the spine, but the theory is as yet unproven.

Clinical Picture

The patients presenting in childhood are usually first seen in early adolescence. The male and female population seem to be equally involved. Low back pain with occasional radiation to both thighs posteriorly is the principal complaint. Unilateral leg pain, which is seen in one-third of the cases in adults, is rare in children. The low back pain is made worse by activity and is relieved by recumbency.

Hamstring spasm that limits straight leg raising is often present and symmetric. Forward flexion of the spine is limited and painful if the child is having symptoms. Excessive forward flexion has been found by us only in children who are asymptomatic and in whom spondylolisthesis was only an incidental finding. Tenderness over the spine of the involved vertebra is almost invariably present

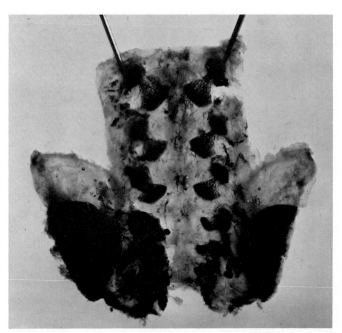

Figure 18.5.   Cleared specimen of lumbosacral spine from the newborn. The dark ossification centers of the posterior elements of the lower three lumbar vertebrae are seen coming down to the sacral spine and a portion of each ilium. The isthmus is the point of entrance of the vessels at the junction of pedicle and lamina. There is only one center on each side for the posterior elements, but the isthmus is the thinnest part of it.

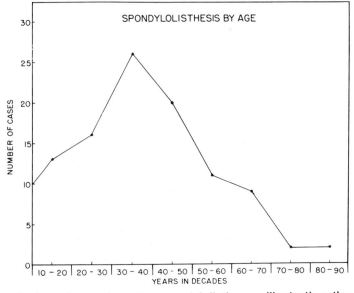

Figure 18.6.   Series of symptomatic spondylolistheses illustrating the age at which symptoms bring the patient to medical attention.

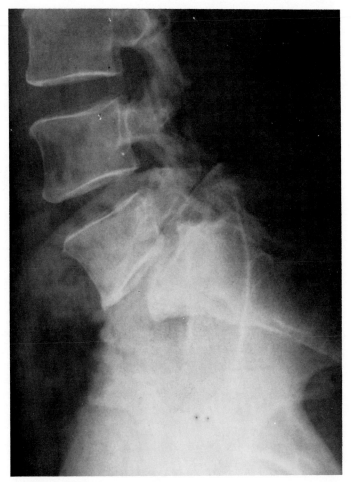

Figure 18.7. Spondylolisthesis with defect posterior to pedicle. The fifth lumbar vertebra has slipped forward, and there is cupping of the sacrum around the posterioinferior angle of this vertebra.

and localized. The trunk, when the patient is examined from the lateral view, appears to be displaced forward in relation to the pelvis.

Roentgen Findings

Forward displacement of the fifth lumbar on the sacrum can be recognized in minimal cases by drawing a line between the inferior angle of the first sacral and the superior angle of the fifth lumbar. A second line is drawn between the superior angle of the first sacral and the inferior angle of the fifth lumbar. These two lines should normally be parallel.

Forward slip is indicated by a deviation of these lines.

The defect in the pars interarticularis may be seen in either the lateral or the anteroposterior views of the lumbosacral joint. When it is not visualized, oblique views or a 45-degree anteroposterior view of the lumbosacral joint will flatten out the lamina so that it may be visualized, if present.

In long standing spondylolisthesis, the anteroposterior view is often diagnostic, because there tends to be considerable atrophy of the laminae involved (Fig. 18.9). A concavity in the inferior surface of the fifth lumbar vertebra, apparently due to excessive lumbosacral motion, may exist. The disc space may be narrowed more than is normal. Spina bifida of the neural arch is frequently seen.

Treatment

Gill et al.[4] recommended excision of an overgrowth of fibrocartilaginous tissue present beneath the defect and intruding on the fifth lumbar root. They demonstrated this in their cases, but we have found fusion necessary to relieve both symptoms and root pressure from whatever cause.

In general and depending on the individual patient, the attitude has been taken that the basic cause of the symptoms is lumbosacral instability and motion of the detached fragment directly over the roots.

A lumbosacral joint weak enough to give symptoms in the presence of the healthy musculature of childhood will almost certainly cause adult disability.

Excision of the spine and laminae and fusion of the first sacral to the fifth lumbar vertebrae, as recommended by Barr, have been carried out in our cases (Fig. 18.10). The result has been relief of pain, elimination of hamstring spasm, and good spine motion. The area between the fourth lumbar and first sacral is bridged by a continuous iliac graft on which bone chips are laid so that there is no danger of a reparative reaction involving the roots. Patients so treated are ordinarily kept in a double hip spica for 4 months.

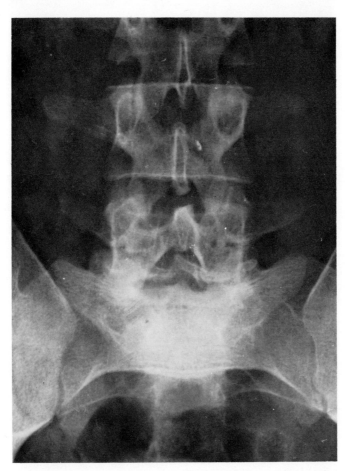

Figure 18.8. Marked atrophy of the laminae of the fifth lumbar vertebra in spondylolisthesis. The apparent laminae of the fifth lumbar vertebra are actually of the fourth. The fifth vertebra is represented by the vestiges of posterior elements below it.

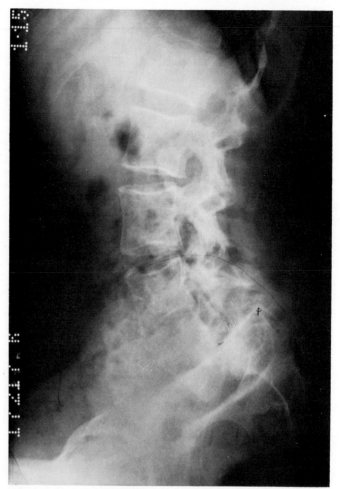

Figure 18.9. Severe spondylolisthesis slipping forward the entire width of the sacrum.

Asymptomatic patients are followed, but not operated on unless they become symptomatic. Strangely enough, mild degrees of slip seem more productive of symptoms than extensive slips involving the total vertebral surface.

References

1. Batts, M.: The etiology of spondylolisthesis, *J. Bone Joint Surg., 21:* 879, 1939.
2. Caldwell, G. A.: Spondylolisthesis, analysis of 59 cases, *Ann. Surg., 119: 485,* 1944.
3. *Friberg, S.: Studies on spondylolisthesis, Acta Chir. Scand. 82:* Suppl. 55, 1939.
4. Gill, G. G., Manning, J. S., and White, H. L.: Surgical treatment of spondylolisthesis without spine fusion; excision of the loose lamina with decompression of the nerve roots, *J. Bone Joint Surg., 37A: 493,* 1955.
5. Hitchcock, H. H.: Spondylolisthesis; observations on its development, progression, and genesis, *J. Bone Joint Surg., 22:* 1, 1940.
6. Roche, M. B., and Bryan, E. S.: Spondylolisthesis; additional variations in anomalies in the pars interarticularis, *Arch. Surg., 53:* 675, 1946.
7. Shore, L. R.: Report on a specimen of spondylolisthesis found in the skeleton of a Bantu native of South Africa, with further specimens illustrating an anomalous mode of development of the lower lumbar vertebrae, *Br. J. Surg., 16:* 431, 1929.

TUBERCULOSIS OF SPINE

Tuberculosis of the spine, although its incidence has decreased, is still frequently found on orthopaedic children's wards. It continues to account for a formidable percentage of all bone and joint lesions.

In former times, patients ordinarily were not seen until the lesions were well advanced.

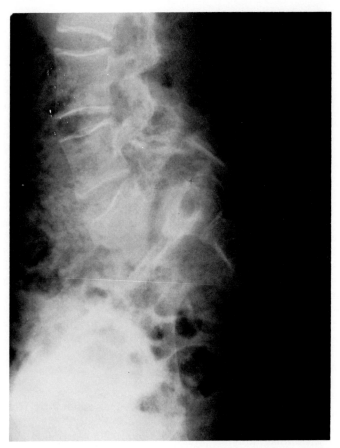

Figure 18.10. Postoperative view of the case seen in Figure 18.9, showing partial reduction of the slip, removal of the posterior element, and fusion posteriorly.

The fact that they are now seen in earlier stages demands a clinical awareness on the part of the examining physician of the nature of the disease. Tuberculosis does not affect only one localized area, but must be, at least potentially, a generalized infection. Even when the lesions are at first confined to the spine, the involvement there is often multiple. The causal organism, in order to have infected the spine, has been blood borne at some stage.

Potts first described the disease in 1779. After examining patients with well advanced cases and marked deformity, he noted that, in the histories, symptoms in the spine preceded the development of the deformity.

Etiology

Now that the incidence of bovine tuberculosis has been much reduced, the great majority of tubercular infections of bone seem to be caused by the human form of Koch's bacillus. The disease spreads by means of respiratory rather than alimentary infection, and it is most usual to find that the patient has had a close family association with an infectious individual. Although the possibility that infection spreads via the thoracic duct to the dorsal spine has been suggested, a blood-borne infection seems more likely and is supported by the initial localization in the vertebra. A primary lung complex is commonly found on a roentgenogram of the lungs in children.

Pathology

The involvement is most often in the center of the area supplied by the posterior spinal artery. From there the lesion spreads to the disc edge and then to the disc itself. Its progress encompasses the anterior and posterior ligaments but tends to spare the posterior elements, including transverse processes, spines, and facets.

Doub and Badgley note three types of lesions: intervertebral, central, and anterior. The rare anterior localization apparently reaches its destination via branches of the intercostal arteries; it involves a large number of vertebrae but often causes little deformity.

There may be several or many discrete lesions in the vertebra rather than mere direct extension. The initial lesion, after causing acute inflammation and lymphocytic infiltration, brings about central degeneration, caseation, and calcification. The bone is increasingly destroyed, and there is further debris and caseation and eventually the formation of an abscess. Dorsal abscesses tend to run along the ribs, lumbar abscesses to run down the psoas sheath and to point either posteriorward in the lumbar triangle or anteriorward beneath and distal to the inguinal ligament. In cervical lesions, the abscess usually gravitates into the mediastinum.

Cave[3] reported on a series of 162 cases, of which 7 were in the cervical spine and 115 in the dorsal spine. The dorsal spine is by far the commonest site. In this area, the normal dorsal round back accentuates anterior stress and, as contrasted to the cervical and lumbar areas, is more easily deformed.

The majority of initial infections of the spine occur between the ages of 3 and 10, although they also occur in adults.

Clinical Picture

Pain and stiffness in the back are the first symptoms. The parents note wasting, loss of appetite, night cries, withdrawal from activity, and easy fatigue. A low grade temperature elevation frequently accompanies the disease. A chronic, slowly developing course is typical.

The sign which immediately arouses suspicion of a tuberculous infection of the spine is a gibbus (Fig. 18.11). This localized prominence in the back is tender to pressure and may only be minimal to observation. There is accompanying muscle spasm and limitation of motion of the spine in all planes. Patients seen before the development of a gibbus exhibit dislike of jarring activity such as jumping, and some limitation of motion may usually be elicited. Further progression of the disease results in kyphos in the dorsal spine, shortening of trunk height, and descent of the ribs into the pelvis.

Abscesses radiating from the lumbar spine down the course of the iliopsoas may be palpable by abdominal examination posteriorly in the iliolumbar area, anteriorly in the thigh, or anteriorly. Abscesses and infections of the rib may be noted. Abscesses may be accompanied by flexion contracture of the hip.

Laboratory Findings

The sedimentation rate is elevated and becomes of value in following the patient's course rather than in diagnosis. The tuberculin test is positive and should first be used in dilution of 1:100,000. Those at 1:10,000 are virtually always positive. Failure to obtain a positive test in a suspicious case should result in reevaluation of the tuberculin used. The blood count may be unremarkable, but some authors have drawn attention to the lymphocyte-monocyte ratio. A rise in monocytes relative to lymphocytes above a ratio of 1:3 correlates well with activity of the disease and is one additional guidepost to the appropriate time for surgery, if it is indicated.

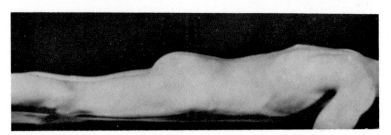

Figure 18.11.   Gibbus in dorsal spine marking the early development of deformity.

Roentgen Findings

In the stage at which the patient is most often seen today, narrowing of the intervertebral disc area is an outstanding sign (Fig. 18.12). Active destruction in the vertebrae, both above and below the narrowed interval between them, may often be found (Fig. 18.13). When these findings are coupled with the visualization of a soft-tissue mass adjacent to the involved area, the diagnosis of tuberculosis becomes most likely (Fig. 18.14). Such a mass should show a gravity effect; that is, it should be largest in its most distal portion and should gradually narrow in a cephalad direction. Obviously granulomatous masses show this effect less than masses composed of encased fluid pus.

In relation to its chronicity, a tubercular lesion, as compared to a pyogenic spondylitis, exhibits very little calcifying reaction. Infec-tions caused by organisms such as brucella may mimic the picture very well, however.

In late stages of the disease, there may be such complete destruction of vertebral bodies that deformity, particularly dorsal kyphos, is marked and a clear recognition of structure in the involved area is unobtainable. Abscess shadows may become especially prominent. In the lumbar area, the iliopsoas shadow may be obliterated by the developing abscess. The entire spine should be x-rayed, as unsuspected silent lesions may be found.

Treatment

One must be quite certain of the diagnosis, and those cases which are thought possibly to have another etiology should be constantly reappraised.

Needle biopsy is not thought to be indicated. Johnson et al.,[7] however, noted that

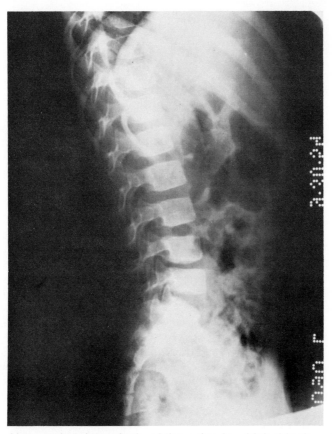

Figure 18.12. Very early tuberculosis of the spine in which thinning of the disc space at the fourth lumbar vertebra is the most striking feature. There is also involvement of the vertebral plates abutting the disc.

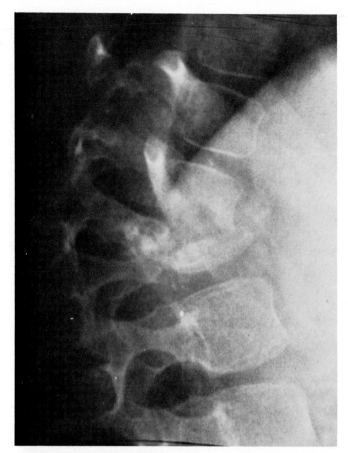

Figure 18.13.   Tuberculosis of the spine at the dorsolumbar junction with destruction in opposing vertebrae, collapse, and deformity, but without marked calcific reaction.

direct surgical biopsy should be done wherever possible as a considerable percentage of cases may be misdiagnosed without it.

The patient is suffering from a systemic as well as a local disease. The ideal treatment includes institutionalization so that bed rest can be enforced and the patient's progress readily reevaluated. Immobilization in hyperextension is not advocated because it unnecessarily prolongs the healing process of a disease which is attempting to heal by bony union. Various types of frames that hold the patient in a more normal position, but one which does not aggravate the deformity, have been used; the simplest type is an anterior and posterior plaster shell, which permits nursing care but aids immobilization. The patient may be turned from front to back in these shells.

A high calorie, high vitamin diet is instituted. Good nursing care is an important adjunct. Sunshine and fresh air, though aids to good health, do not occupy the center of the stage of treatment as they formerly did.

Chemotherapy has now become an important adjunct. The use of streptomycin, *p*-aminosalicylic acid, and isonicotinic acid hydrazide is discussed in Chapter 5, under "Tuberculosis of Knee." Other antibiotics helpful in tuberculosis are already on the scene. It has not been possible to supplant surgical measures with them, but under their cover the approach has become bolder.

A safe program to pursue includes observation of the child on a regime until definite progress in the direction of healing is obtained. This progress includes elimination of fever, weight gain, declination of the sedimentation rate, and a normal lymphocyte-monocyte ratio. When these signs are manifest, it is thought that the course can be influenced by fusion of the involved vertebra (Fig. 18.15).

Since it has been shown that the disease frequently involves adjacent vertebrae that exhibit no pathology by roentgenogram, a safe rule is to add two vertebrae above and two below the lesion to the fusion. Such a rule can be varied according to anatomic location, deformity, and activity of the disease. Fusion posteriorly is usually followed by fusion anteriorly and eventual cure of the disease. After the fusion the patient must remain on the general measures instituted until the disease is cured. Fusion by itself does not substitute for the general treatment of tuberculosis.

Fusion of the spine as a treatment for tuberculosis was instituted by Hibbs[6] in 1911. By Hibbs' method, multiple small chips were raised from the laminae, the articulations were curetted and denuded, and the spinous processes were split and bent over the interspinous area. Albee[1] also reported a spinal fusion operation the same year in which an autogenous cortical tibial graft was inserted between the split spinous processes. Many variations have subsequently been described, but fusion based on Hibbs' original concept has proved most successful (Fig. 18.16).

To a Hibbs'-type fusion, an osteoperiosteal shaving which is continuous has been added with benefit, particularly when the area of attempted fusion involves a deformity with an apex that, to be fused, needs much support.

Sinus formation, particularly when there is a secondary infection in addition to the tuberculosis, has proved responsive to chemotherapy. In general, abscesses are watched conservatively. However, large abscesses, pointing so that fluctuation is readily elicited, may be drained and an attempt to collapse the walls by compression may be made. Streptomycin is introduced into the cavity at the time of drainage. Abscesses requiring drainage are usually from lumbar, rather than dorsal, tuberculosis of the spine.

Paraplegia

This distressing complication of tuberculosis of the spine appears to originate in

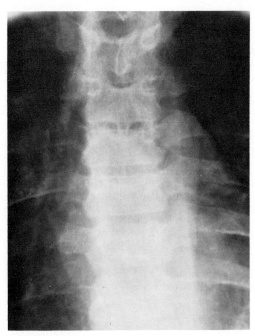

Figure 18.14.   Soft-tissue shadow of abscess on left with minimal evidence of vertebral involvement.

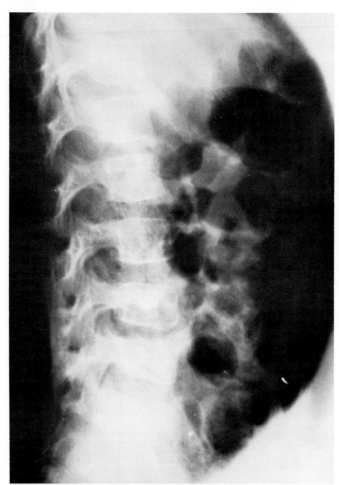

Figure 18.15.   Spine fusion for tuberculosis of the third and fourth lumbar vertebrae.

extradural pressure due to abscess formation (Fig. 18.17). Lesions are most likely to be mid-dorsal. Bony deformity, although undoubtedly contributing to the mechanics of the complication, has not been implicated to the degree that granulation tissue, debris, and purulent material have. Purulent material pressing on the cord in the form of a tight abscess sac has resulted in the slow development of paraplegia in 23.9% of cases in a series reported by Bosworth et al.[2] These authors noted that small abscesses tightly bound down by ligaments were of greater danger than large unconfined sacs.

Sustained clonus is a most reliable sign in the presence of a known tuberculous spinal lesion. It may be accompanied by sensory changes, muscular weakness, spasticity, and a positive Babinski sign.

Most authors are agreed that little improvement follows a posterior decompression by laminectomy. Conservative treatment alone results in improvement in many cases. Spine fusion is sometimes helpful. The operative approach of costotransversectomy with drainage of the abscess appears most likely to result in prompt improvement of the paraplegia. The ability of the cord to recover from pressure of this type with dramatic improvement or complete cure is remarkable in recorded cases of paraplegia of more than 2 years standing.

References

1. Albee, F. H.: Transplantation of a portion of the tibia into the spine for Pott's disease, *J.A.M.A.*, *57*: 885, 1911.

2. Bosworth, D. M., Dell Pietra, A., and Rahilly, G.: Paraplegia resulting from tuberculosis of the spine, *J. Bone Joint Surg.*, 35A: 735, 1953.
3. Cave, E. F.: Tuberculosis of the spine in children. *Instruct. Lect. Am. Acad. Orthop. Surg.*, 5: 114, 1948.
4. Garceau, C. J., and Brady, T. A.: Pott's paraplegia, *J. Bone Joint Surg.*, 32A: 87, 1950.
5. Girdlestone, S. R.: The operative treatment of Pott's paraplegia, *Br. J. Surg.*, 19: 121, 1931.
6. Hibbs, R. A.: An operation for progressive spinal deformities, *N. Y. State J. Med.*, 93: 1013, 1911.
7. Johnson, R. W., Hillman, J. W., and Southwick, W. O.: The importance of direct surgical attack upon lesions of the vertebral bodies, particularly in Pott's disease, *J. Bone Joint Surg.*, 35A: 17, 1953.
8. Ordell, S., and Blacklund, V.: Diagnosis and exact location of lesions by planigraphy in surgical treatment of tuberculosis, spondylitis under cover of streptomycin, *Acta Chir. Scand.*, 106: 61, 1953.

PREADOLESCENT AND ADOLESCENT KYPHOSIS

Preadolescent and adolescent kyphosis leads to the deforming and functional disability due to dorsal wedging round back (Fig. 18.18) that arises in the adult. The underlying condition exists in childhood, however. Ky-phosis juvenilis, Scheuermann's disease, and vertebral epiphysitis are other names for the condition.

Severe end stages of the condition are recognized in adolescence when wedging of the vertebra, irregular ossification of the vertebral epiphyses, and irregularity of the superior and inferior cortical plates of the vertebra may be striking x-ray features.

Youngsters below the age of 12 who are developing round back deformity should be treated with preventive measures in order to deter further deformity. Persistent anterior vascular grooves, recognizable by roentgenogram, leave the patient susceptible to further wedging.

Etiology

A number of factors have been implicated in the past. These include osteochondritis of the epiphyseal plates with deficient and irregular growth.

Schmorl's nodes have been implicated by some. These nodes appear as cartilage herniations into the vertebra. Associated with

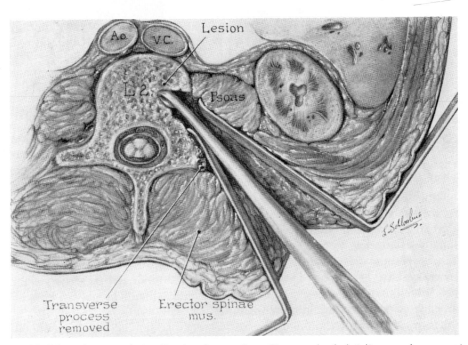

Figure 18.16. Approach to the lumbar spine. Removal of detritus and sequestra as part of the surgical approach to tuberculosis of the spine is becoming increasingly important. (From W. Southwich and R. Robinson: Surgical approaches to the cervical and lumbar regions, *Journal of Bone and Joint Surgery*, 39A: 631, 1957.)

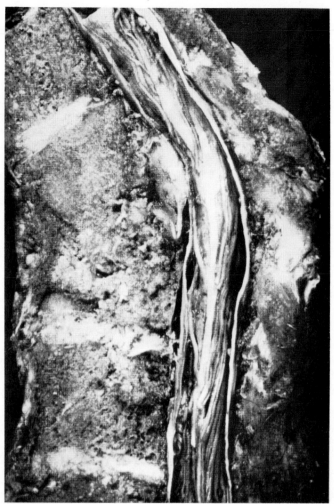

Figure 18.17. Soft-tissue abscess causing a paraplegia. Note that the pressure is anterior. (From S. J. Garceau and T. A. Brady: Pott's paraplegia, *Journal of Bone and Joint Surgery, 32A:* 87, 1950.)

deficient growth of the vertebra, they may actually represent a form of chondrodysplasia. In this area, bone formation has failed to take place. The edges are vertical and the base flat. Wedging of the vertebra may accompany their presence.

A third implicated factor is the anterior vascular groove (Fig. 18.19). This groove has been observed to close with anterior wedging (Fig. 18.20) and appears to be associated with the development of round back in preadolescents.

Whatever the underlying cause, stress appears to bring about the wedging in the defective vertebra. The upright posture forms stress enough. The mechanics that enter into upright posture, such as tight hamstrings (Fig. 18.21), put further stress on the dorsal spine in forward bend.

Normal Spine Development

In reviewing unselected normal lateral chest films in the age group from 6 to 11 years, certain observations were apparent. There is a normal dorsal kyphos, the curvature of which takes place in the area of the fifth, sixth, and seventh dorsal vertebrae. The time of development of this kyphos varies considerably, some youngsters still having a straight dorsal spine at age 10.

The anterior vascular groove, which is originally present in lumbar as well as dorsal vertebrae, is closed in more than 60% of the children reading 6 years of age. The wedging that develops in the fifth, sixth, and seventh dorsal vertebrae to form a so-called normal kyphos results in closure of the grooves in the upper dorsal area (Fig. 18.22).

By the time the age of 10 is reached, only 17% have some vestige of a groove remaining (Fig. 18.23). Seventy-one percent have developed a round back in the area of the fifth, sixth, and seventh dorsal vertebrae. The vestigial grooves are below this area in the dorsal spine. The lumbar spine grooves have long since been closed.

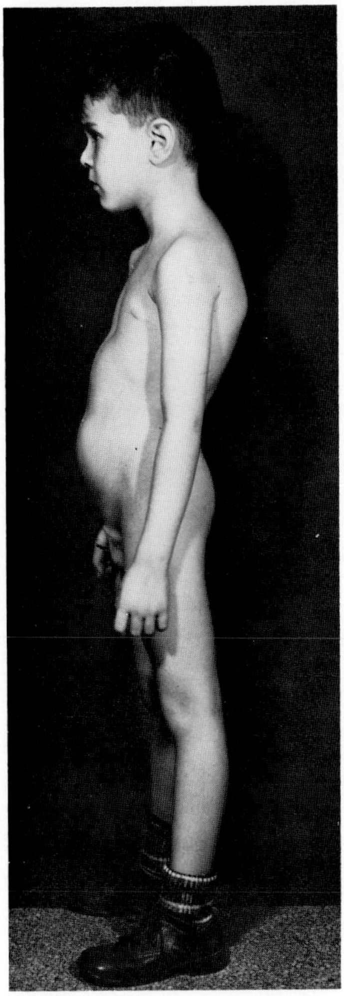

Figure 18.18. Developing dorsal wedging round back.

The indentation in the anterior border of the vertebra seen by the roentgenogram has been found by dissection to be occupied by a large endothelium-lined vascular lake formed by the confluence of veins at this point. Some cartilage is also present in the younger children. If the soft tissues are removed from the vertebral body, the groove depth varies, depending on the degree of closure.

Clinical Picture

The patient is often first seen as a posture problem. There may be a tired, aching sensation in the region of the dorsal spine. The round back due to accentuated dorsal kyphos is noted. There may be tenderness of the spine in this area. Accentuated forward bend may be painful. Tenderness may be localized to the region of the interspinous ligaments. The hamstrings may be tight and may limit straight leg raising.

The use of plaster body jackets and even spinal fusion is necessary in some cases to relieve the symptoms.

Roentgen Picture

Before the age of 10 and before the appearance of the epiphyses of the vertebrae, there may be wedging of vertebrae below the fifth, sixth, and seventh dorsal vertebrae. Such wedging added to the wedging above produces the accentuated round back. The anterior vascular grooves may persist or they may have closed, leaving a linear area of increased density in their wake. After the age of 10, the superior and inferior plates of the involved vertebrae may appear irregular. The epiphyseal plates tend to ossify irregularly in the affected area of wedging.

Treatment

The child who appears to be developing an excessive lumbar lordosis and an accentuated dorsal round back posture and who is then found, by lateral film of the dorsal spine, to have wide, open anterior vascular grooves becomes the object of special consideration.

There are preventive measures to relieve dorsal spine stress. Sleeping posture is im-

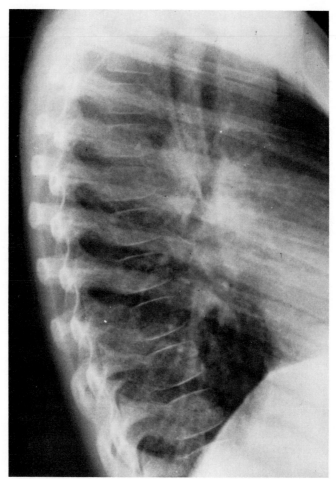

Figure 18.19.   Persistent anterior vascular grooves in the dorsal spine.

portant; any positions which flex the dorsal spine should be avoided. Sleeping on bed boards and without a pillow helps to maintain a flat surface. Relaxation flat on the back on the floor for 20-min periods relieves dorsal spine stress when the child is tired. Exercises to tilt the pelvis, to obliterate lumbar lordosis, and to stretch tight hamstrings are helpful.

As a constant means of relieving stress in the upright posture, we have used a low back brace which flattens the lumbar spine and thus causes a tendency to extend the dorsal spine on looking forward. In the case of the preadolescent, this is used until the anterior vascular grooves are closed. In the adolescent, it is used until the epiphyses are joined to the parent vertebra and the symptoms relieved.

"CAST SYNDROME"

In 1950, Doeph used the term "cast syndrome" to describe acute gastric dilatation after application of a body cast. When unrecognized severe hypokalemic alkalosis, hypovolemia, and death may result.

Evarts points out that the term is a misnomer since the traction causing the syndrome may be exerted without a cast. The traction exerted by distraction rods, halo-femoral apparatus, correction jackets, and the Milwaukee brace in some patients can result in vascular compression of the duodenum. The horizontal or third portion of the duodenum passes between the aorta and vertebral body posteriorly and the root of the superior mesenteric arterial trunk anteriorly. This anatomic situation gives rise to the possibility of the third portion of the duodenum being caught and partial or complete obstruction thereby resulting. Minimal pressure is needed to flatten the duodenum in this area. Persistent nausea and vomiting is the most common symptoms. Tenderness in the epigastrium occurs early. Severe metabolic alkalosis and dehydration result. Oliguresis, ruptured stomach, and death can ensue.

CONGENITAL SPINAL DEFORMITIES

BY CHARLES S. STONE, M.D.

Malformation of vertebrae originating during the 4th to 6th week of embryonic development can produce malignant progressive deformity leading to paralysis and to death if not properly evaluated and treated. This has been conclusively shown by Winter et al.[38,39] It is, therefore, imperative that congenital spinal anomalies be evaluated properly and not assumed to be benign entities. The fallacies that congenital curves do not progress and that little improvement can result from treatment must be put to rest. Every orthopaedist must be aware of the potential danger in congenital scoliosis and kyphosis.

Embryology

Failure of segmentation and/or failure of formation of vertebrae results in the abnormalities of congenital absences, congenital scoliosis, congenital kyphosis, and spina bifida syndrome. An understanding of the embryologic development of the spine may give helpful clues to understanding spinal deformities. The development of the neural axis precedes that of the surrounding mesodermal structures but is closely related to that of the bony spine. It is, therefore, not surprising that with congenital spinal deformities there coexists anomalies of the neural elements both grossly and microscopically. These congenital anomalies make the patient's cord more susceptible to either mechanical or vas-

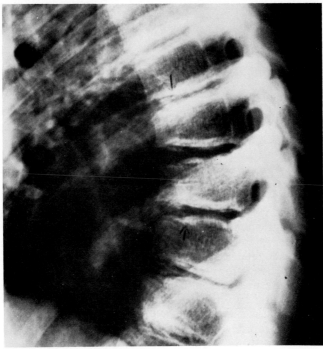

Figure 18.20. The central vertebra in this dorsal round back is wedged and has evidence of persistent anterior vascular groove.

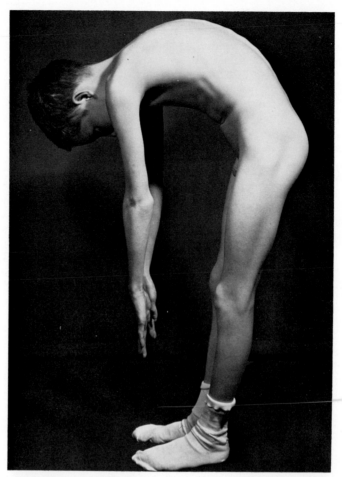

Figure 18.21. Dorsal spine flexion on forward bend with tight hamstrings. (Reprinted with permission from *Pediatric Clinics of North America*, W. B. Saunders Co., Philadelphia, 1955.)

cular injury during natural progression of deformity or during treatment.

There are three stages in vertebral development—membranous, cartilaginous, and osseous (Fig. 18.24). First, a neural plate forms from the dorsal ectoderm and a group of endodermal cells form the notochord. The neural plate then invaginates toward the notochord, becoming a solid cylinder called the neural tube at 21 days following fertilization. During the later period of invagination, the first pair of primitive somites appear as segmental accumulations of mesenchyme in the mesoderm beside the notochord. A group of cells, sclerotomes, derived from the ventromesial portion of each somite, migrates to each side of the notochord as the primordium of the ventral body. Each sclerotome pair, aligned beside the notochord, divides into a denser cephalic and a less dense caudal half. The cephalic portion of each sclerotome combines with the caudal portion of its neighbor causing the intersegmental artery to become situated in the middle of the vertebral body. By the sixth week, the caudal to cephalic combined quarters fuse side to side across the midline, undergo chondrification, and form the vertebral body. The cephalic-caudal cleavage creates the disc space, the center being occupied by the notochord which becomes the nucleus pulposus. Further maturation occurs, ribs grow out from the somites and, by the twelfth week, ossification centers appear in the ribs and vertebral bodies.

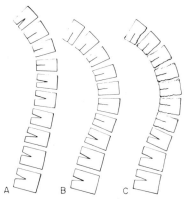

Figure 18.22. The effect of wedging due to persistent anterior vascular grooves when added to that normally expected in the upper dorsal spine. (*A*) The normal situation of wedging in the proximal dorsal spine to produce the normal dorsal kyphosis. (*B*) Persistent vascular grooves allowing wedging in the distal dorsal spine and creating a round back deformity. Such grooves should be closed by the age of 7 and certainly by age 10. (*C*) The effect of wedging and round back deformity is to produce irregularity in the epiphyseal plate ossification consistent with the diagnosis of Scheuermann's disease in the 13- to 16-year-olds.

Failure of vertebral formation probably results from lack of original sclerotome migration. Failures of segmentation can be related to lack of cephalic-caudal cleavage. Rib anomalies are closely related to vertebral development and frequently coexist.

After each vertebral centrum takes shape at the fifth week, paired mesenchymal cell concentrations extend dorsally and laterally to form the posterior elements. If normal neural tube formation has not taken place, it will negate dorsal closure of the posterior elements and, thus, create spina bifida syndrome.

All congenital vertebral anomalies probably occur by the sixth week of embryonic life. Experimental deformities of the spine of the congenital type have been produced in chicks by injecting insulin into the yolk sac of the fertile egg. Hypervitaminosis E in pregnant rats and hypoxia or injection of 6-aminonicotinamide to pregnant mice produce scoliosis of the congenital type.

Classification

A classification of congenital spine deformities is given in Table 18.1.

Congenital Scoliosis

Congenital scoliosis is a lateral curvature of the spine due to anomalous vertebral development. Any child with scoliosis requires adequate and complete x-rays to determine the vertebrae involved and to identify vertebral anomalies (Fig. 18.25).

Scoliosis is a physical finding. Establishing the correct diagnosis of this physical abnormality is required of any physician who will undertake its treatment. Treatment in its broadest sense includes as little as giving advice concerning prognosis and need for further follow-up. Correct and accurate diagnosis is particularly necessary in the area of congenital scoliosis. X-ray evaluation of the scoliotic vertebrae is difficult because ossification may not be complete, vertebral rotation may be present, and high quality radiologic technique may not be available. A full history and physical examination must be carried out looking particularly for indications of associated neurologic abnormalities such as small, club, or cavus feet, short extremities, calf atrophy, or skin lesions in the dorsal midline of the trunk. X-rays must be of high quality to show bony detail and, at a minimum, should include anteroposte-

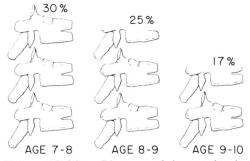

Figure 18.23. Diagram of decreasing incidence of persistent anterior vascular grooves in the dorsal spine (From A. B. Ferguson, Jr.: The etiology of preadolescent kyphosis. Dorsal wedging round back in preadolescents, *Journal of Bone and Joint Surgery*, 38A: 149, 1956.)

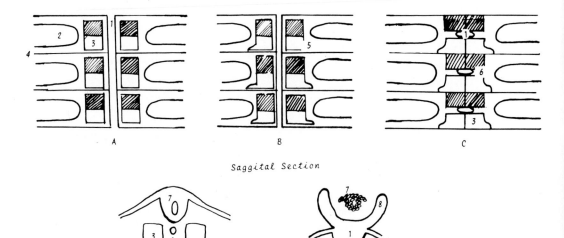

Figure 18.24. Vertebral embryology. (*A*) 3 weeks, (*B*) 4 weeks, (*C*) 6 weeks, (*a*) 3 weeks, (*b*) 5 weeks, (*1*) notochord, (*2*) myotome, (*3*) sclerotome, (*4*) segmental artery, (*5*) costal process, (*6*) disc space, (*7*) neural tube, (*8*) posterior elements.

Table 18.1
Classification of Congenital Spine Deformities

I. Congenital Scoliosis
  A. Failure of formation
    1. Wedge vertebrae
    2. Hemivertebrae
  B. Failure of segmentation
    1. Unilateral bar
    2. Bilateral (fusion)
  C. Mixed
II. Congenital Kyphosis
  A. Failure of formation
  B. Failure of segmentation
  C. Mixed
III. Congenital Lordosis
IV. Associated with Neural Tissue Defect
  A. Myelomeningocele
    1. Vertebral body anomalies
    2. Neuropathic type
    3. Kyphosis
    4. Lordosis
  B. Meningocele
  C. Spinal dysraphism
    1. Diastematomyelia
    2. Other

rior and lateral standing and supine views of the entire spine. Spot films and laminagrams may be required to determine the exact anatomy of the scoliotic vertebrae and, thus, a correct diagnostic classification. At the initial visit, bone age should be determined from hand x-rays that are compared with the standard Greulich and Pyle[11] *Atlas.* Other causes of vertebral body abnormalities should be ruled out such as osteochondrodystrophy, postirradiation changes, metabolic diseases, infection, tumor, and trauma. Only by correct diagnosis can the natural history of the patient's curve be known and adequate advice given.

NATURAL HISTORY

Anomalies with a unilateral unsegmented bar (Fig. 18.26) between two or more vertebrae are associated with severe progression. This unilateral failure of segmentation may be between the bodies alone, between the posterior elements alone, or between bodies, pedicles, and posterior elements. The next most severe group are those with multiple hemivertebrae one after the other on the

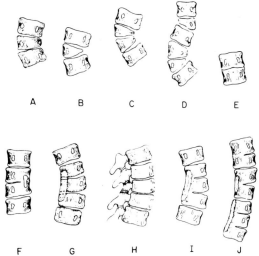

A   B   C   D   E

F   G   H   I   J

Figure 18.25. Classification of congenital scoliosis: (*A–D*) failure of formation: (*E*) failure of segmentation, bilateral; (*F–J*) failure of segmentation, unilateral. (From R. B. Winter, J. H. Moe, and V. E. Eilers: A study of 234 scoliosis patients treated and untreated, *Journal of Bone and Joint Surgery, 50A:* 3, 1968.)

same side of the spine. Common sense would lead us to analyze the balance of growth potentials in each anomalous spine. An absolute prediction of progression cannot be made except in the cases of unilateral tethering of bone (unsegmented bar). Thoracic and thoracolumbar curves in general have progressed to the most severe deformities. Any spine with congenital scoliosis can progress anytime during the growth period. Seventy-five percent of congenital curves are progressive. The average progression is 5 degrees a year. Except in those cases with associated neurologic deficit, no progression has been noted after closure of the vertebral ring apophyses.

TREATMENT PLAN

Ideally, any child with spinal deformity will be seen early and a diagnosis made by complete history, physical examination, and radiographic study. Unless the child has a unilateral unsegmented bar and/or neurologic deficit, he should be reexamined and x-rays taken every 6 months.

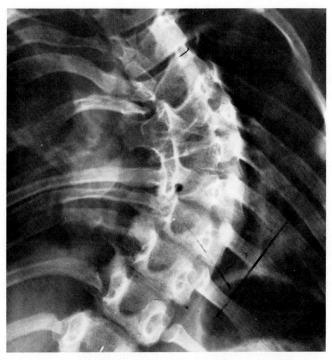

Figure 18.26. Unilateral unsegmented bar— a dangerous sign.

Initial work-up should include anteroposterior and lateral sitting, standing, and supine x-rays of the entire spine, spot films, and laminagrams, if needed. Repeat anteroposterior standing and sitting films should be obtained at 6-month intervals. The limits of each curve should be determined, the curve measured in degrees by the Cobb method, and each measurement recorded on a chronologic chart. In this way, the degree of original curve can be seen at a glance and compared with all subsequent measurements. The so-called eyeball technique will fail to note the 2- to 4-degree progression at each visit. In the 234 cases reported by Winter et al.,[38] failure to appreciate subtle but relentless progression was the most common error. Failure to act on this information was the second most common error. Congenital curves tend to progress and tend to be rigid. The lack of flexibility negating easy correction leads to the recommendation for early fusion. Any patient who is being followed either in a Milwaukee brace or by observation whose curve is nonprogressive must be checked until the vertebral ring apophyses fuse. If progression occurs during growth, arthrodesis is indicated regardless of age.

Classical arguments for not proceeding with early fusion of congenitally deformed spines have been retardation of growth and causation of lordosis. Certainly, in congenital scoliosis the growth potential of the concave side is already diminished or absent. Further growth of the spine will only result in more deformity and not contribute to vertical height. Lordosis has not been shown to increase in those patients who did not have a lordotic component prior to arthrodesis. Early spine fusion with massive bone is the only way to prevent deformity. Once deformity is established, it may be irretrievable. For those patients who have not consulted a physician knowledgable in the field of spinal deformities until their curves are severe, treatment is more involved, more dangerous, and less satisfactory. However, if these patients are abandoned, many will develop cardiopulmonary and neurologic complications leading to death. Operative treatment is the only choice.

When the patient with congenital scoliosis is seen in infancy and a correct diagnosis is made, the following plan is recommended. If the child has an unsegmented bar and the curve is under 35 degrees, a spinal fusion should be performed from at least one segment above to one vertebra below the area of segmentation failure. The child must be kept recumbent in a localizer for 10 months. We now ambulate the patient in a Milwaukee brace and continue biannual follow-up. If the curve increases, the fusion should be reinforced with bone graft and extended to the vertebrae which have been added to the curve pattern.

The patient with the unilateral posterior bar and a curve over 35 degrees should have an osteotomy of the bar, then localizer or traction correction followed by posterior fusion. The unilateral failure of segmentation may involve the vertebral bodies. Anterior osteotomy for correction is considered only with curves over 70 degrees because of the high risk of neurologic complications. Prior to surgical treatment, a myelogram is performed on all patients with congenital scoliosis. If anterior resection is necessary, preoperative selective spinal angiography could be helpful.

The remainder of infants with diagnosed congenital scoliosis are followed biannually with serial x-rays, careful measurements, and good records so that initial and present curve measurements can be noted. It is also important that the same level be measured each time. With any change in levels, the entire series of x-rays should be remeasured. If progression is noted in situ, spinal fusion is performed over the major portion of the curve. The patient is maintained in a Milwaukee brace until after the teen-age growth spurt when fusion may be extended to include a parallel vertebra at the top of the curve to a parallel vertebra at the bottom of the curve.

Frequently, the child with scoliosis is not referred to an interested orthopaedist until the deformity is quite severe. The goal is for all patients with congenital scoliosis to be seen, a diagnosis made, and treatment instituted before even cosmetically unattractive deformities occur. However, enlightened treatment is not yet available to all people, and some children will be seen with rather severe congenital scoliosis. Curves over 70 degrees and decompensated curves in which T1 is no longer over the gluteal crease in the erect position should be corrected. Their treatment may involve osteotomy of unsegmented bars posteriorly or anteriorly, vertebral resection, halo-femoral traction, and spinal arthrodesis.

MILWAUKEE BRACE

The Milwaukee brace has a place in the total treatment plan for congenital scoliosis. Mainly, it is useful following a short fusion in the young child to prevent progression of the curve above and below the fusion area. The brace also can be used for the rare mildly progressive but flexible scoliosis and for more severe flexible curves in children with congenital heart disease of the type rendering operative risk too great. The Milwaukee brace should not be used prior to spine fusion in unilateral unsegmented bars, nonflexible curves, and when the iliac crest skin is anesthetic. Serial x-ray examination and measurement must be carried out when a patient is undergoing nonoperative treatment. Nonoperative treatment should be abandoned in all cases in which satisfactory correction cannot be maintained or progression occurs. At this point spine fusion is indicated at any age.

SURGICAL TREATMENT

Posterior in Situ Fusion. Preoperatively, the routine admission work-up should include pulmonary function studies with blood gases. Myelography is done on all patients with congenital scoliosis prior to surgery. The embryologic development of the bony spine and neural elements are so closely related that associated unsuspected intraspinal anomalies such as diastematomyelia, developmental tumors, and tethered cord must be discovered and treated prior to fusion. Intravenous myelography is needed to rule out genitourinary anomalies. Preoperative marker films are obtained by taping a segment of paper clip transversely across the spine at the level of intradermal methylene blue skin markers on appropriate spinous processes. At surgery, the skin incision is outlined between the markers using a Steinmann pin as a guide for a straight line incision. Local pressure and self-retaining retractors are used to control hemorrhage during the skin incision and subcutaneous dissection. Subperiosteal stripping of the paraspinal musculature is facilitated by packing gauze sponges along the spinous processes and out onto the laminae with Cobb elevators. Meticulous soft-tissue removal is carried out prior to decortication. The cortex is removed out to the tips of the transverse processes in both the thoracic and lumbar areas. Strip grafts obtained from one iliac crest are placed across the prepared bed. Supplemental homologous bone may be used if the patient's crests do not yield enough volume. In patients below the age of 3, definite provision for bone-bank bone must be made. Postoperatively, the patients are kept at complete bed rest for 10 months. The first 6 months are spent in a well fitting localizer cast and the last 4 months in a body cast. If postoperative films at 6 months show evidence of pseudoarthrosis, exploration of the fusion mass is performed, and pseudoarthrosis is repaired with iliac crest bone.

When plaster is removed and the short fusion is solid, it is helpful to fit the patient with a Milwaukee brace in an attempt to prevent the addition of vertebral segments to the curve and to prevent bending of the solid spinal fusion in the plastic bone of a young child. Fusions that were solid at exploration 6 months postoperatively can undergo gradual loss of correction as the patient grows, indicating plasticity in the fusion mass. At the time of corrective osteotomy of the fusion mass, no pseudoarthroses have been identified.

Extension of the fusion may be required after the adolescent growth spurt to maintain a cosmetically and functionally good spine. However, severe rigid deformity will be prevented by the early fusion in all patients with an unsegmented bar and other categories of congenital scoliosis in which progression has been documented.

Fusion in situ is reserved for those patients whose deformity can be accepted and is too rigid for localizer correction. In children, Harrington distraction rods may be used as internal fixation devices, if the instrument size and bone size are compatible. Harrington rods are not to be used for intraoperative correction in these patients because the risk of neurologic damage is great even if a preoperative myelogram is normal.

Cast Correction and Posterior Fusion. Localizer cast correction and fusion with Harrington rods is the mainstay of operative treatment in scoliosis today. If the major curve can be corrected to 30 degrees or less on forced lateral bending films, this method is used. Under adequate sedation, a preoperative localizer cast is applied and cut out posteriorly as well as anteriorly for tracheal and abdominal windows. Spine fusion is carried out over the major curve extending to the neutrally rotated vertebrae above and below the curve. Meticulous fusion technique is used, taking care to adequately remove the soft tissue from transverse process to transverse process and decortication over the same area. Harrington rods are inserted in a careful manner. Ten days postoperatively, a new localizer is applied and the patient is ambulated. At 6 months, the localizer is removed and anteroposterior, lateral, and oblique x-rays are obtained of the fusion area. If there are any signs of pseudoarthrosis (loss of correction over 10 degrees or radiolucent defects), the fusion mass is explored and all areas of motion decorticated and packed with iliac crest bone. When no defects are found, a body jacket is worn for an additional 5 months. These patients are then followed clinically and by x-ray until after skeletal maturity.

Selected patients whose curves do not correct to 30 degrees or less on forced bending films are placed in Risser turnbuckle jackets for preoperative correction. Arthrodesis is done in this jacket. Postoperatively, a localizer jacket is applied and the patient is ambulated if Harrington rods have been used.

Halo-Femoral Traction and Posterior Fusion. When forced bending films give poor correction, halo-femoral traction is the method of choice. However, the pelvic-halo distraction method may be substituted. The halo and femoral pins are applied in the operating room under neuraleptic anesthesia. After 24 hr, correction is begun with the patient awake. Four pounds of weight are added initially, 2 lb at the head and 1 lb on each femoral pin. When the patient tolerates this weight, daily additions of 2 lb are made. The added weight should not exceed 50% of body weight. Twice daily, neurologic examinations must be carried out. Paralysis of the sixth cranial nerve with loss of lateral rectus muscle function is the most common neurologic complication. This can be quickly reversed by removing the traction weights. Anterior thigh pain is a common prodrome of paraplegia and should alert the physician to decrease the traction force. Inability to void is an early sign of cord dysfunction. In short,

any sudden onset of pain, weakness, numbness, or bladder or bowel disturbance is the indication for removing all weights and waiting for complete recovery before again applying traction. Weekly x-rays of the spine are obtained and measured. As long as correction is occurring and twice daily neurologic examination is normal, traction may be continued. Three weeks is the usual time but traction may be continued until maximum correction is achieved. The patient is taken to the operating room in traction. General anesthesia is induced and the patient intubated. One-half to two-thirds of the weights are removed and the patient placed in the prone position. The usual careful posterior fusion is carried out. Harrington rods are used if possible. Never attempt to achieve correction beyond that obtained in traction. Ten days postoperatively, a localizer cast is applied and the patient ambulated. If rods cannot be used the patient is continued in traction until skin healing has taken place and a cast is applied incorporating the halo frame and femoral pins. Bicycle hoop suspension is supplied for large children to facilitate nursing care (Fig. 18.27). At 6 months the fusion is evaluated by x-ray and a body jacket is applied. Ambulation is begun at 10 months.

Spinal Osteotomy. There are some patients in whom halo-femoral or halo-pelvic traction will fail to gain acceptable correction. Many of these patients will have hemivertebrae producing an intolerable pelvic obliquity. The ideal level for hemivertebrae excision is below L3. Technically, vertebral wedge resection or osteotomy can be done at higher levels. Leatherman[21] has reported 24 cases of vertebral resection without serious complications. Most neurologic complications of scoliosis are due to mechanical injury to the spinal cord or interference with its blood supply. At any level, the anterior spinal artery supplies two-thirds of the cross sectional area of the cord. The remainder comes from the bilateral posterolateral arteries. The blood supply to the cervical, upper thoracic, and lumbar cord including the cauda equina is abundant. The so-called watershed area of the midthoracic spine is the most precarious. Adamkiewicz in 1882 described the arteria radiculomedullaris magna. This vessel supplies the midthoracic cord and appears on the left side from T6 to L3 in 66% of cases. It originates from an intercostal or lumbar ves-

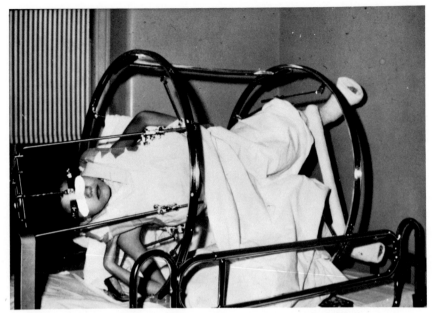

Figure 18.27.   Bicycle hoop suspension for easier nursing care.

sel near the intervertebral foramen and ascends along the anterior surface of the cord
as high as the fifth thoracic vertebra where it
makes a hairpin turn and descends as the
anterior spinal artery. Doppman et al.[6] have
described the technique of selective spinal
angiography using a femoral artery catheter
passed into the origin of each intercostal and
lumbar artery to be visualized (Fig. 18.28).
The radiographic technique of subtraction
allows the artery of Adamkiewicz to be visualized from its origin.

Paraplegia has been rare in anterior surgery
using Dwyer's instrumentation[8] even with
the division of 6–10 segmental arteries including the watershed area. Hall and King[12]
have shown arterial bleeding from both ends
of the segmental artery if it is divided well
away from the intervertebral foramen. This
suggests arterial collateral circulation outside
the spinal canal.

Selective spinal angiography to determine
the location of these arteriae radiculomedullaris magna and strict attention to technique
in sparing the arterial supply should reduce
neurologic sequelae of vertebral body resection (Fig. 18.29).

Leatherman[21] has described hemivertebrae
excision and his technique is applicable to
vertebral wedge resection. Following the appropriate transthoracic or retroperitoneal approach, the vertebral body is removed along
with the anterior half of the pedicle. Removal
of the disc above and below the vertebra to
be excised facilitates this resection. For correction to occur, the body resection must be
complete side-to-side. It is safer to resect
from the concavity but easier from the convexity of the curve. Care must be taken to
follow the neurovascular structures into the
intervertebral foramen and protect them during resection. When the anterolateral wound
is healed, the posterior spine is exposed
through a conventional midline dorsal incision. The posterior part of the hemivertebra
and the remaining portion of the pedicle are
removed. The wedge may then be closed
under direct vision using Harrington compression or distraction rods. Posterior fusion
is performed with abundant iliac crest graft.

An alternative method is proceeding with
the posterior resection first. Two weeks later
the anterior resection is undertaken, the vertebral end plates are removed, and the osteotomy is closed under direct vision by flexing
the operating table. The patient is placed in
a cast for 3 months, until anterior fusion is
solid. Posterior fusion is usually necessary
but in the young child the correction can be
maintained in a Milwaukee brace proceeding
with posterior fusion closer to skeletal maturity.

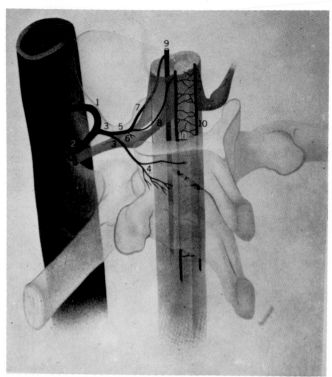

Figure 18.28.   Transverse section of spinal canal and contents with typical segmental artery pattern. Radiculomedullary originates from posterior branch of intercostal artery, supplies small vessel to dorsal root ganglion, and ascends to reach cord above level of entrance. Pattern is similar for posterior radiculomedullary arteries. (*1*) Intercostal artery, (*2*) anterior branch, (*3*) posterior branch, (*4*) muscular branches, (*5*) radiculomedullary artery, (*6*) ganglionic branch, (*7*) anterior radiculomedulary artery, (*8*) posterior radiculomedullary artery, (*9*) anterior spinal artery, (*10*) posterior spinal arteries. (Reprinted by permission from J. L. Doppmen, G. Dichiro, and A. K. Ommaya: *Selective Arteriography of the Spinal Cord*. St. Louis: Warren H. Green, 1969.)

It is necessary that knowledgable and adequate treatment of congenital scoliosis be carried out. If a unilateral unsegmented bar is present or, if the curve shows progression, spinal fusion is indicated regardless of age. The earliest successful fusion has been reported in a child 6 months of age. There should be no hesitation in performing an indicated spinal arthrodesis in the 1- to 5-year age group.

Congenital Kyphosis

Congenital kyphosis is an abnormal dorsal angulation of the spine due to anomalous vertebral development. Von Rokitansky[34] gave the first description of this condition in 1844. Van Schrick[33] described two groups: Type I—failure of segmentation, and Type II—absence of the vertebral body. In 1973 Winter et al.[40] studied 130 patients with congenital kyphosis and described the natural history and treatment of this deformity.

CLASSIFICATION AND NATURAL HISTORY

In Type I, failure of formation, nearly all of one or more vertebral bodies fail to form. The posterior elements, spinous processes, and pedicles are present but may be attenuated. Scoliosis frequently coexists in Type I kyphosis because of asymmetric failure of body formation. Type I occurs most frequently and is generally in the upper thoracic

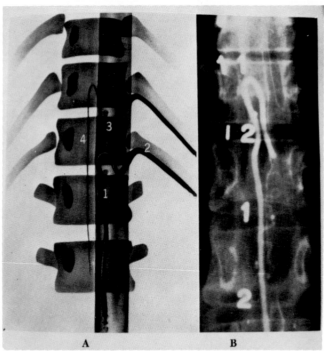

Figure 18.29. (*A*) Diagram of arteria radiculomedullaris magna and anterior spinal artery as opacified by selective intercostal arteriography: (*1*) catheter; (*2*) left twelfth intercostal artery; (*3*) arteria radiculomedullaris (*B*) arteriogram closely corresponding to sketch (*A*) (Reprinted by permission from J. L. Doppman, G. Dichiro, and A. K. Ommaya: *Selective Arteriography of the Spinal Cord.* St. Louis: Warren H. Green, 1969.)

area. It is associated with instability during infancy but becomes more rigid and fixed as it progresses past the age of 3. This type has sharp angular deformity, progresses more rapidly than the other two types, and is the only type with associated paraplegia in the Winters et al.[40] series (Fig. 18.30). Progression averages 7 degrees per year.

In Type II, failure of segmentation, the growth plates are absent anteriorly along with one or more disc spaces. The kyphosis of this type is symmetrical with the segmentation failure acting as an anterior bar. The curves are more gradual, less severe, and occur within the upper lumbar and thoracolumbar regions. Progression does, however, occur and treatment is necessary.

In a third category, Type III—mixed, there is a combination of Types I and II or the anomalies may be unclassifiable. Mixed kyphosis occurs in the thoracolumbar area, progresses more rapidly, and becomes more severe than occurs in Type II.

All types of congenital kyphosis do progress. Cardiopulmonary, neurologic, and mechanical pain complications occur. Early operative treatment gives the best results. Late operative treatment is better than none at all.

DIAGNOSIS AND PREOPERATIVE EVALUATION

The initial treatment is correct diagnosis. This requires a good history and physical examination with special attention to subtle signs of disturbed neurologic function such as a difference in thigh and calf girth or difference in foot size, early toe clawing and high arch or heel varus, tight hamstrings, and stretch reflexes. A full neurologic examination should be recorded. Radiologic evaluation should include an anteroposterior and lateral standing, sitting, and supine films of the entire spine, spot films from various angles, and laminagrams of the involved area. Lateral x-rays with maximum flexion and

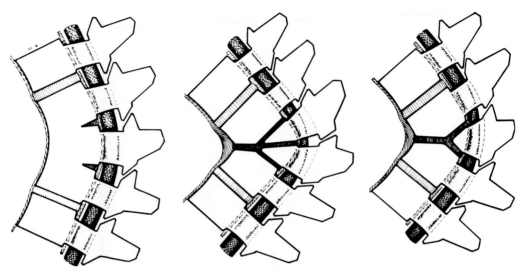

Figure 18.30. Congenital kyphosis—failure of formation (Type I) and failure of segmentation (Type II). (Reprinted by permission from R. B. Winter, J. H. Moe, and J. F. Wang: Congenital kyphosis, *Journal of Bone and Joint Surgery, 55A:* 255, 1973.)

extension should be obtained to determine flexibility. If scoliosis accompanies the kyphosis, maximum side bending films are needed. The construction of a perpendicular from the line drawn along the end plate of the maximally tilted vertebra cephalad to the apex of the kyphosis will intersect with a perpendicular line drawn from the end plate of the maximally tilted vertebra caudal to the kyphotic apex. Kyphosis is quantitated by measuring the angle formed by the intersection of these two perpendiculars. All lateral films are measured and compared. Flexibility and/or progression can be determined. Since progression is the rule and bracing of any type is not effective, operative treatment is indicated. Preoperative work-up should include routine preoperative laboratory work, the initial evaluation presented above, pulmonary function studies including blood gases, electrocardiogram, intravenous pyelogram, and complete myelography. A more useful myelogram will be obtained by removing the spinal needle, using a high volume technique, and positioning the patient with the kyphotic and scoliotic deformities in dependent positions. Carelessly done or inadequate myelograms are of no value and cannot be tolerated in patients with this severe deformity.

EARLY POSTERIOR FUSION

The most successful treatment is posterior spinal fusion in the child under 3 years of age with a kyphosis less than 50 degrees. No rods are used. A postoperative hyperextension type of localizer cast is applied and the patient is kept recumbent for 6 months. Fusion exploration is carried out at 6 months postoperatively and bone graft added even if a pseudoarthrosis is not present. Casting in a horizontal position is continued for an additional 6 months. Clinical and radiographic follow-up are recommended every 3 months, the second year postoperatively, and then biannually as unit bone growth proceeds. Type I deformities are unstable in children under 3, and correction may be noted on preoperative bending films. Successful posterior fusion is adequate treatment for most cases of congenital kyphosis regardless of age if bending films measure 50 degrees or less.

In the older child, Harrington compression rods may be used. If pseudoarthrosis is present at 6 months, anterior arthrodesis should be done by the technique described in the following sections.

Halo-femoral traction should not be used unless the curve is flexible as demonstrated by hyperextension films. A few patients will require halo-femoral traction and its incorporation into the postoperative cast to hold this correction.

LATER FUSION IN MODERATE DEFORMITY

Posterior fusion alone in the more severe curve is nearly always unsuccessful. This is most likely due to distraction forces on the posterior fusion mass. Any child over 3 years of age and any curve over 50 degrees are best treated by anterior strut grafting arthrodesis followed in 2–3 weeks by posterior fusion. Harrington compression rods are used posteriorly if the patient is large enough. Postoperatively, care and follow-up is the same as described for early posterior fusion in the preceding section. Routine exploration is carried out if the anterior and posterior fusions appear solid on x-rays taken at 6 months. Pseudoarthrosis can occur in spite of both anterior and posterior arthrodesis and should be repaired or the deformity will continue to progress. Postoperatively, Milwaukee bracing has been recommended to prevent loss of correction especially with associated scoliosis.

SEVERE KYPHOTIC DEFORMITY WITHOUT PARAPLEGIA

If hyperextension x-rays show no correction, halo-femoral traction is absolutely contraindicated. Such traction would further stretch the cord over the anterior gibbus leading to cord damage. Anterior spinal decompression and osteotomy with strut graft arthrodesis followed in 2–3 weeks by posterior fusion with Harrington compression rods is the only method to gain correction. The risk of paralysis from anterior resection surgery must be considered. The decision for correction should be based on the experienced surgeon's judgment that in situ anterior and posterior fusion would not prevent the later onset of anterior cord compression and paraplegia.

PARAPLEGIA

Ideally, fusion should be done early in the congenital kyphotic patient to prevent severe deformity and, thus, obviate the cardiopulmonary and neurologic complications. Some patients are not brought for adequate care until spasticity, paresis, or even complete paraplegia have developed. Most have Type I deformity. Posterior decompression by laminectomy alone is useless and contraindicated. Successful decompression requires removal of the anterior gibbus (the posterior portion of the apical vertebral bodies). Lateral rachiotomy and radical posterior decompression with transposition of the cord have been successful. These methods, however, do not effectively treat the entire problem of congenital kyphosis with paraplegia. Recurrence of the neurologic loss can occur. In any salvagable patient with complete or incomplete paraplegia secondary to congenital kyphosis, anterior decompression is indicated coupled with anterior strut grafting to be followed by a second stage posterior fusion with Harrington compression rods (Figs. 18.31, 18.32). Winter et al.[40] report nearly complete recovery in 5 patients undergoing this procedure. Their method is modified from that proposed by Hodgson et al.[16] for treatment of Pott's paraplegia and is applicable to any kyphosis-induced cord compression.

ANTERIOR DECOMPRESSION AND STRUT GRAFT ARTHRODESIS

The spine is exposed through a transthoracic or transthoracic-retroperitoneal approach. The rib chosen for removal should be the one above the most cephalad vertebra to be reached. Upon reaching the spine, the segmental vessels will be seen crossing the center of each vertebral body to enter the intervertebral foramina. A number of segmental vessels sufficient to reach all necessary vertebrae should be doubly ligated well away from the foramen and divided between ligatures. An incision is made along the anterior lateral side of each vertebra and disc space. A flap is raised by sharp and blunt dissection to the intervertebral foramen. A second flap is raised anteriorly and around the opposite side. The annulus fibrosus, adherent to each disc space and to the bone, must be raised sharply. The disc material from each space is removed completely back to the posterior longitudinal ligament so that the entire vertebral end plate may be visualized.

The apex of the kyphosis should be re-

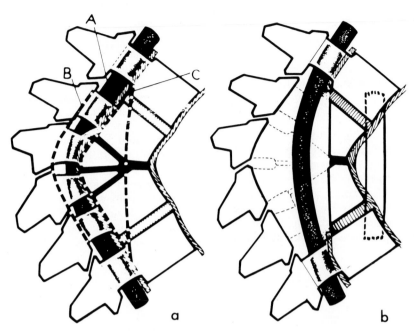

Figure 18.31. Anterior decompression of cord (*a*) *Broken lines* outline the bone removed for decompression of the spinal cord. *C* is the plane of anterior removal, and *A*, the posterior margin of the bone removed back to the bases of the pedicles. If a scoliosis is present the spine should be approached on the side of the concavity of the scoliosis and the pedicles should be removed (*broken line B*) to allow the spinal cord to move forward toward the operator. After removal of an adequate amount of bone, the cord may not move forward until the posterior longitudinal ligament is excised. The posterior longitudinal ligament, however may not be present in some cases. (*b*) Forward movement of the spinal cord after removal of the posterior longitudinal ligament. The appropriate location for insertion of the strut graft is shown. In this location, the graft cannot impinge against the cord even if dislodged. Usually, more than one graft is needed. The discs must also be excised and replaced with autogenous bone. (Reprinted by permission from R. B. Winter, J. H. Moe, and J. F. Wang: Congenital kyphosis, *Journal of Bone and Joint Surgery, 55A:* 254, 1973.)

moved for decompression and to facilitate a planned corrective osteotomy. Anterior fusion alone does not require decompression. The posterior longitudinal ligament has been identified through the disc space and through the intervertebral foramen. Its absence has been reported in some patients with congenital kyphosis. Begin to hollow out the center of the apical vertebra with a gouge and rongeur. Marked bleeding will occur from the cancellous bone. This is best controlled by bone wax which is preferentially removed prior to strut grafting. Curets and pituitary rongeurs are used to remove the bone posteriorly to the cortex across the entire width of the vertebral body. One or two other bodies are similarly prepared. The spinal canal must be entered either through the disc

space most distant from the apex or through a carefully made window in the posterior cortex of a distal vertebra. With removal of the posterior ligament, the dura may be seen. At this point, extensive epidural bleeding may occur and it is best controlled by pressure and the use of Gelfoam, topical thrombin, and Surgicel. Once the spinal canal is entered, the dura is identified and a small kerasin rongeur may complete the removal of the posterior aspect of each vertebral body, allowing the cord to move anteriorly into this newly acquired space. With true thoracic kyphoscoliosis, this procedure is most safely done from the concavity of the scoliosis to avoid any stretching of the cord.

After removal of the posterior bodies, a corrective osteotomy may be completed by

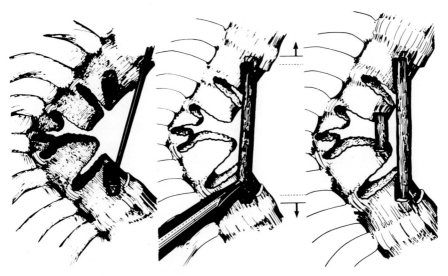

Figure 18.32. Technique of anterior strut grafting. (Reprinted by permission from R. B. Winter, J. H. Moe, and J. F. Wang: Congenital kyphosis, *Journal of Bone and Joint Surgery, 55A:* 252, 1973.)

cutting the remaining anterior vertebral body with an osteotome. In order to obtain correction, the cut must be complete from side to side. Care must be taken to protect the great vessels and segmental vessels entering the intervertebral foramen. Corrective osteotomy is never done without prior anterior decompression.

Anterior strut grafting is always done after osteotomy with decompression as well as after decompression alone. Slots are made in each end vertebra and hollowed out to the vertebral end plate with a curet. A second pair of slots is made in the next adjacent bodies in the kyphotic curve. Autogenous struts are prepared from ribs, fibula, or bicortical iliac crest bone. Each strut is first inserted into superior slots and, with the aid of manual distraction, slipped into the distal slot. The entire exposed cancellous vertebral bone is then cleared of bone wax and packed with autogenous cancellous iliac crest bone. If possible the periosteal flaps and the parietal pleura are closed. Chest tubes are inserted and the chest wound approximated in layers. Postoperatively, the patient is nursed in the horizontal position with frequent turning from side to side. If possible, the complete team of thoracic surgeon, neurosurgeon, orthopaedist, and anesthesiologist should work together in surgery of this magnitude. Blood loss is great. The patient's blood may be

recaptured in an auto-transfuser. The blood is heparinized and sent to be washed in a computerized centrifuge. The red cells suspended in saline can be returned to the patient during surgery and in the recovery room.

Several weeks later, a posterior spinal fusion is carried out using Harrington compression rods if possible. A postoperative hyperextension localizer cast is applied. The patient is sent home to bed rest. At 6 months, x-rays are evaluated and, if satisfactory, the patient remains in recumbency with a plaster body jacket for an additional 6 months.

Congenital kyphosis can be successfully managed. Early surgical treatment is best. If the patient's curve is advanced, anterior surgery is necessary. When doing transthoracic and retroperitoneal approaches to the spine, the orthopaedic surgeon must be prepared to treat associated operative and postoperative complications that differ from usual orthopaedic practice.

Myelomeningocele Spinal Deformity

Early in the care of the child with myelomeningocele, attention is directed to control of hydrocephalus, genitourinary infection, and lower extremity deformity. Frequently, the patient has pelvic obliquity associated with hip contracture and dislocation. When the obliquity persists after correction of its infrapelvic cause, attention is directed to the spine. X-rays will show a scoliosis extending into the pelvis causing the fixed pelvic obliquity. Again, a diagnostic classification of the scoliosis must be made. Seventy-five percent of children with myelomeningocele are born with straight spines and their only vertebral anomaly is that of the open posterior elements. At least 50% of these patients will develop a lateral spine curvature, many with associated lordosis. The onset of the curve is usually before the age of 5. The scoliosis is always progressive but at a variable rate. Five percent of children with myelomeningocele are born with scoliosis secondary to associated vertebral anomalies. These lateral curves have a natural history like those with congenital scoliosis alone. Spinal deformities occurring with myelomeningocele are consistently progressive. Early and adequate treatment is necessary to prevent severe deformities from deterring satisfactory levels of achievement. The spinal deformities associated with myelomeningocele are kyphosis, congenital scoliosis, developmental scoliosis, and developmental lordosis. All of these are associated with, and contribute to, fixed pelvic obliquity which is a dominant factor preventing adequate bracing and adequate sitting.

PELVIC OBLIQUITY

Pelvic obliquity in the coronal plane is present when the transverse plane of the pelvis is not parallel to the floor in the standing position (Fig. 18.33). It may be functional or fixed. Functional pelvic obliquity disappears when the patient is recumbent and may be due to a short extremity or lumbar muscle spasm. Fixed pelvic obliquity persists in all positions. The cause may be infrapelvic due to hip contractures as abduction contractures of the left hip and adduction contractures of the right hip. In order for the patient to stand, a functional type of scoliosis develops to balance the head over the pelvis. This cause may be suprapelvic due to structural scoliosis in which the sacrum is the last vertebra of the structural curve. In order to stand erect, a compensatory scoliosis develops above the major curve. Obliquity of the pelvis is only a physical finding. The cause may be infrapelvic (hips) or suprapelvic (spine). Fre-

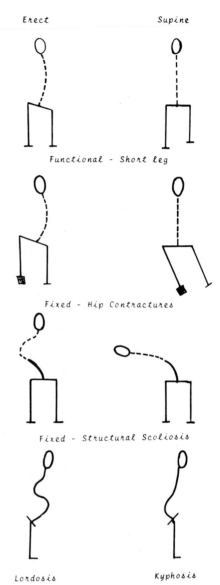

Figure 18.33. Pelvic obliquity.

quently, the patient with myelomeningocele will have both spine and hip type pelvic obliquity. Fixed pelvic obliquity occurs when the transverse axis of the pelvis is no longer at a right angle to the long axis of the patient and cannot be passively corrected. This describes pelvic obliquity in only the anteroposterior plane.

Saggital plane pelvic obliquity can be fixed or functional. Excessive posterior pelvic tilt is due to fixed lordosis and can produce secondary hamstring tightness and limited hip flexion. Excessive anterior pelvic tilting occurs with fixed lumbar kyphosis.

The third-dimension rotation must be considered when the scoliotic curve extends into the pelvis. The pelvis then behaves as a scoliotic vertebra. It may be like a true scoliotic vertebra taking part in the curve and having rotation. It may be like a neutral vertebral body below the curve having obliquity but neutral rotation. This added dimension causes difficulty in getting true anteroposterior x-rays of the hips and lumbar spine, thus confusing the true spatial relationships.

Most patients with myelomeningocele who have motor levels at L3 and above will function best as adults in the sitting position. Their spines must have nearly normal configuration and stability. The pelvis must be level in order to sit with the hands free (independent sitting). In addition, the head must be over the pelvis and the shoulders level for good sitting balance. In spite of special fabrication of seats, breakdown of sensory deprived skin will occur when weight distribution is unequal due to pelvic obliquity. The only successful treatment of spinal deformity and pelvic obliquity in the myelomeningocele patient is operative.

LUMBAR KYPHOSIS

Lumbar kyphosis commonly complicates a lumbar myelomeningocele with a motor level of T10 to L3. The posterior prominent spine presents as a subcutaneous mass across two-thirds of the width of the back with a neural plaque stretched over its apex (Fig. 18.34). Lateral x-rays show a kyphotic deformity of the entire lumbar spine with wedged-shaped apical vertebrae. Kyphosis most likely develops from a flexion pull of the paraspinal muscles which lie adjacent to the ventrally everted laminae. The untreated kyphosis is progressive. Kyphectomy is needed to facilitate posterior skin closure, to prevent skin breakdown, and to permit successful bracing. If possible, this procedure should be coupled with myelomeningocele closure during the first day of life.

KYPHECTOMY

The dura is freed from the skin edges and mobilized anteriorly and laterally in preparation for closure over the neural plaque. The functioning nerve roots are identified and traced to the intervertebral foramina. The lateral tips of the everted posterior elements are identified and the fascial attachments incised. The nerve roots are now identified passing ventrally through the foramina. They can be protected while the posterior elements are removed and blunt dissection is carried to the lateral aspect of the vertebral bodies and a tape passed across the anterior surface of the apical vertebrae. This allows the paraspinous psoas muscles to fall anteriorly and protect the retroperitoneal great vessels and ureters. With careful dissection, successive vertebral bodies can be exposed. Two vertebral bodies are usually removed through the disc spaces (Fig. 18.35). The end plates are then removed from the remaining vertebrae exposing bleeding bone. The pelvis is extended until vertebral apposition is accomplished preferably end to end. A portion of the resected bone is placed at the lateral aspect of the vertebral bodies as bone graft and the remainder is saved in the bone bank. The cord is now relaxed and the dura easily closed. The vertebra can be fixed by passing silk sutures through the vertebral bodies us-

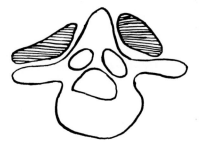 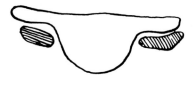

Figure 18.34. Congenital kyphosis. (*Left*) Normal vertebra with paraspinous muscle posterior; (*right*) kyphotic vertebra with paraspinous muscle anterior. (Reprinted by permission from J. F. Raycroft, and B. H. Curtis: Spinal Curvature in Myelomeningocele: Natural History and Etiology: *Symposium on Myelomeningocele, American Academy of Orthopaedic Surgeons.* St. Louis: C. V. Mosby Co., 1971.[23])

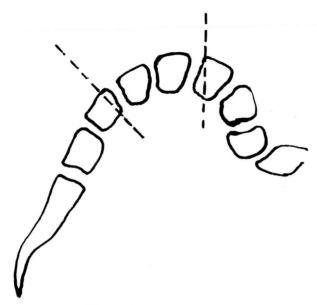

Figure 18.35.   Kyphectomy.

ing a heavy cutting needle. Sharrard[28,29] uses cross-threaded pins. However, the bone is quite soft and metallic fixation devices frequently cut out. The skin can be closed without tension. Care must be taken not to place the pelvis in an excessive lordotic position. Lordotic pelvic obliquity may stop hip flexion short of 90 degrees and, thus, interfere with sitting. The patient is nursed in a plaster shell until the skin is healed and then a double hip spica is applied extending above the nipple line. Plaster immobilization is required for 3–6 months until arthrodesis occurs. Extensive retroperitoneal bleeding accompanies this procedure and leads to fibrosis making later urinary diversion procedures technically more difficult, but not impossible.

If there is no neurologic function in the kyphosis resection area, the dura is oversewn and transected at the upper end of the proposed vertebral resection and removed distally. The spine may then be dissected free and transected without concern for the neural elements. Operating time is greatly shortened and hemorrhage reduced when dissection and preservation of the nerve roots is not necessary. Posterior interbody bone grafting aids in obtaining solid fusion.

Kyphectomy can be carried out in the older child (Figs. 18.36, 18.37). Usually there is posterior ulceration over the spine which must first be converted to clean granulation

tissue by good nursing care in the hospital. The granulating skin defect is excised when kyphos resection is performed. Skin can be easily closed when the bony ends are approximated. Plaster immobilization must be maintained in the older child for at least 6 months. The cast must extend to the toes to prevent unwanted incidental supracondylar fractures of the femora.

CONGENITAL SCOLIOSIS

If the patient with myelomeningocele has fixed scoliosis secondary to congenital bony abnormalities (Fig. 18.38), early correction should be attempted with halo-femoral traction followed by spine fusion. A myelogram should be done first to rule out diastematomyelia. Traction is frequently unsuccessful and vertebral resection becomes the method of choice. The pelvic halo has not been found useful in these children because iliac wings are small and flat preventing the seating of iliac transfixion pins. If vertebral resection is carried out above the level of neurologic deficit, the technique described in the section on congenital scoliosis is used. If the major deformity is at the level of the spina bifida and neurologic function is not present, hemivertebra resection or vertebral wedge osteotomy can be carried out from the posterior approach in the manner described for kyphectomy. Without the kyphotic deformity, however, greater care must be exercised in protecting the anterior great vessels.

Developmental Lordoscoliosis

These children are born with straight spines. Some have good motor function in the lower extremities. Scoliosis and lordosis begin insidiously around the age of 5 and are relentlessly progressive. Initially, both deformities are supple and correct almost completely with the child supine or suspended. These deformities become clinically important when they interfere with good bracing. Operative treatment is more easily carried out when the deformity is still flexible. The tendency is to delay until after the prepubertal growth spurt. However, we do not hesitate to proceed with correction and fusion at any

age if necessary to prevent fixed pelvic obliquity and loss of sitting balance.

At the discovery of scoliosis, anteroposterior and lateral recumbent and erect x-rays of the entire spine including the pelvis are made and measured. Serial examinations are done every 6 months and progression recorded. Correction and fusion are done when the curve is still supple and before the standard myelomeningocele bracing will not accommodate the associated pelvic obliquity.

TREATMENT

In the child whose scoliosis and lordosis is supple, a posterior approach for spine fusion may be carried out. Special care should be taken to begin the subperiosteal stripping of the paraspinous musculature at the level where normal spinous processes are palpable. Dissection is then carried distally to identify

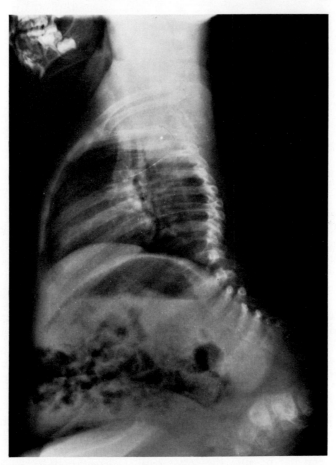

Figure 18.36.   Preoperative kyphos.

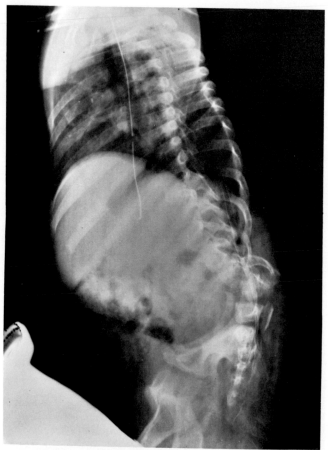

Figure 18.37.   Postoperative kyphectomy.

the lateral aspects of the everted posterior elements and stripping is carried out to the posteriolateral vertebral foramen. The open spinal canal is identified and dura protected. Wide decortication is performed and mass bone graft inserted. If no neurologic function is present in the area of wide open spina bifida, the dura may be oversewn, the nonfunctioning neural elements excised, and a posterior interbody decortication carried out. With a flexible spine, preoperative correction is not required. Posterior fusion to the sacrum can be carried out with wide decortication. Graft of iliac crest bone is supplemented with bone bank bone.

A Harrington rod is inserted from the ala of the sacrum to the first neutral thoracic vertebra. The modified deep-seated Moe hook placed on the ala of the sacrum is preferable to a sacral bar because the soft tissue can be more easily closed over the Harrington rod set closer to the vertebra.

Postoperative immobilization is maintained in a carefully fitted localizer jacket including the lower extremities for 1 year. The child may stand in the cast to facilitate urinary drainage. On ambulation, the patient is examined and x-rayed every 6 months. Breakage of the Harrington rod indicates pseudoarthrosis and repair must be undertaken. With meticulous technique, successful posterior fusion can be achieved. Pseudoarthrosis rate as high as 40% is not unusual, but pseudoarthrosis repair is successful.

Anterior Dwyer instrumentation[8] with interbody fusion has been advocated when posterior elements are absent. The technique is especially useful in the child with myelomeningocele (Fig. 18.39 A, B, and C), both for correction of supple lordoscoliosis and as a good technique for arthrodesis after preoperative correction. It has been our experience that the paralytic curve in the myelomeningocele must have arthrodesis to the sacrum

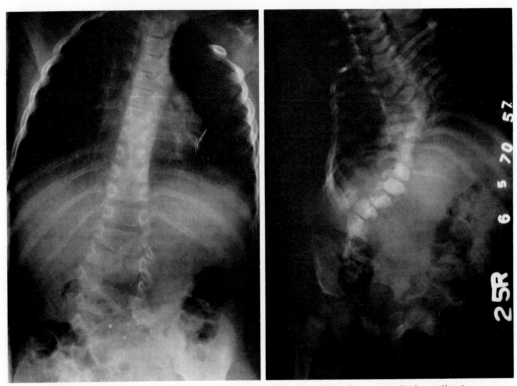

Figure 18.38.   Myelomeningocele with associated congenital scoliosis.

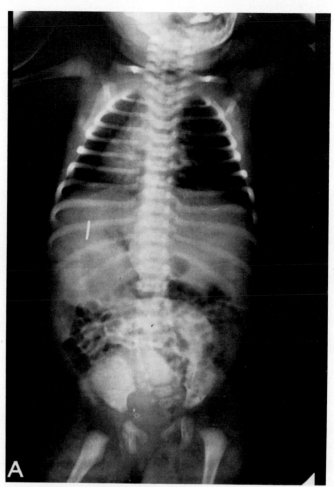

Figure 18.39.   Myelomeningocele developing scoliosis. (*A*) Birth, (*B*) age 5, (*C*) age 10.

in order to maintain adequate sitting stability and correction of pelvic obliquity. At the present time, the Dwyer instruments cannot be applied across the L5-S1 joint and the screws and staples are too large for the younger child. Dwyer instruments can be used over the major portion of the curve if either routine anterior interbody fusion is performed from L5 to the sacrum or complete posterior fusion with Harrington rod fixation is carried out as a second procedure. Combined anterior and posterior arthrodesis will reduce pseudoarthrosis in these neurogenic curves and is frequently indicated with thoracic level paralysis.

If the child's deformity in either or both planes has become rigid and does not significantly correct on forced bending films,

operative correction of scoliosis and lordosis is necessary. It is possible to obtain some correction of the rigid scoliosis and good correction of lordosis with one operative procedure using the anterior Dwyer technique. Again, however, the L5-S1 joint cannot be crossed with the Dwyer instrumentation. An alternate method is, therefore, described. Anterior lumbar osteotomy at the apex of the curve is carried out through a midline transperitoneal approach (Fig. 18.40). The abdominal contents are palpated and packed off with the patient in the Trendelenburg position. When lordosis develops, the bifurcation of the aorta and the common iliac veins ascend to lie over the body of L2-L3. The posterior peritoneum is opened and dissection carried down bluntly to the anterior

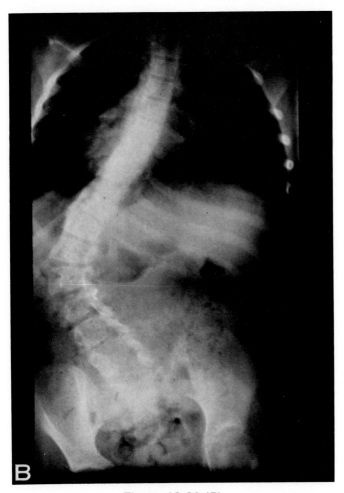

Figure 18.39 (B)

aspect of the body of L4. The great vessels are identified and, if necessary, mobilized and retracted with tapes for access to the bodies of L4-L5. The osteotomy should be carried out at the apex of the lordosis. Generally, the apex is at the L4-L5 disc space. The disc is excised. The posterior longitudinal ligament is identified and a rongeur is used to resect the posterior lip of the vertebral bodies of L4 and L5. A 35-degree wedge is cut from the body of L5 and the body of L4. The patient is placed in femoral traction with the hips maintained at 90 degrees for 2 weeks. When the lordosis is corrected, the patient is maintained in a hip spica with the hips and knees flexed at 90 degrees for 3 months until anterior arthrodesis is complete. If the osteotomy does not close, the L4 inferior articular facets and L5 superior articular facets are resected bilaterally via the intervertebral foramina through a posterior laminotomy approach and the patient is returned to traction. When the patient's lordosis is controlled, localizer cast correction and posterior fusion is carried out. Harrington rods are used when possible. Excessive fixed lordosis will not allow the skin to be closed without tension over Harrington rods. Therefore, anterior surgery for fixed lordosis is required prior to rod insertion. If the scoliosis is especially severe, a biplane anterior osteotomy may be done to obtain some degree of concurrent scoliosis correction. When the major fixed deformity is scoliosis, halo-femoral traction is useful for correction prior to fusion.

Developmental lordosis and scoliosis usually coexists in the patient with myelomeningocele, causing fixed pelvic obliquity in

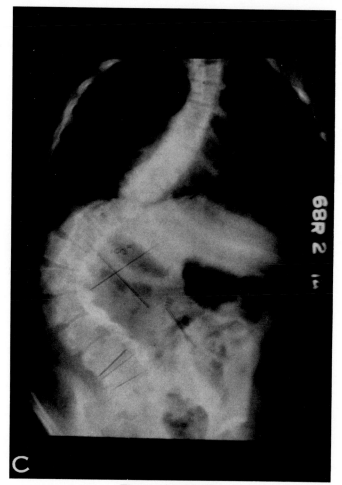

Figure 18.39 (*C*)

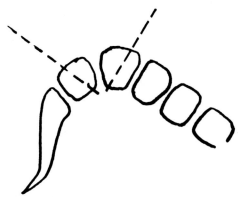

Figure 18.40. Anterior lumbar osteotomy.

both the saggital and coronal planes. Rotational deformity has not been corrected. Successful spinal arthrodesis from the neutral thoracic vertebra above the curve to the sacrum is absolutely essential if these children are to function in society. Enough correction of the deformities must be achieved so that stable unsupported sitting is possible. Any solid fusion that does not fulfill these criteria is a treatment failure and corrective osteotomy may be needed.

References

1. Bailey, H. J., Sister Mary Gabriel, Hodgson, A. R., and Shin, J. S.: Tuberculosis of the spine in children, operative findings and results in 100 conservative patients treated by removal of the lesion and anterior grafting. *J. Bone Joint Surg., 54A:* 1633, 1972.
2. Blount, W. P.: Congenital scoliosis, In *Transactions, 8th Congress, International Societe de chirurgie orthopedique et traumatolie,* New York, pp. 748–762, 1960.
3. Carlioz, H., Dubousset, J., and Guillaumat, M.: Therapeutic problems of scoliosis with pelvic obliquity, Reunion Commune, "Scoliosis Research Society,"

Groupe D'etude de la scoliose. Lyon, France, September, 1973.

4. Compere, E. L.: Excision of hemivertebrae for correction of congenital scoliosis; report of 2 cases, *J. Bone Joint Surg., 14:* 552, 1932.

5. Dewald, R. L., and Ray, R. D.: Skeletal traction for the treatment of severe scoliosis, *J. Bone Joint Surg., 52A:* 233, 1970.

6. Doppman, J. L., Di Chiro, G., and Ommaya, A. K.: *Selective Arteriography of the Spinal Cord;* St. Louis: Warren H. Green, 1969.

7. Duraiswami, P. K.: Experimental causation of congenital skeletal defects and its significance in orthopedic surgery, *J. Bone Joint Surg., 34B:* 646, 1952.

8. Dwyer, A. F., Newton, N. C., and Sherwood, A. A.: Anterior approach to scoliosis, *Clin. Orthop., 62:* 192, 1969.

9. Ehrehaft, J. L.: Development of the vertebral column as related to certain congenital and pathological changes, *Surg. Gynecol. Obstet., 76:* 282, 1943.

10. Gold, L. H., Leach, C. G., Kiefer, S. A., Chous, S. N., and Peterson, H. O.: Large volume myelography; an aid in the evaluation of curvature of the spine, *Radiology, 97:* 531, 1970.

11. Greulich, W. W., and Pyle, S. J.: *Radiographic Atlas of Skeletal Development of the Hand and Wrist,* Ed. 2; Stanford, Calif.: Stanford University Press, 1959.

12. Hall, J. E.: The anterior approach for spinal deformities, *J. Bone Joint Surg., 54B:* 765, 1972.

13. Hall, J. E., and King, J. D.: Hyperlordosis following lumbar peritoneal shunts for hydrocephalus, *J. Bone Joint Surg., 53A:* 198, 1971.

14. Hodgson, A. R.: Correction of fixed spinal curves, *J. Bone Joint Surg., 47A:* 1221, 1965.

15. Hodgson, A. R., and Stock, L.: Anterior spinal fusion, *Br. J. Surg., 44:* 266, 1957.

16. Hodgson, A. R., Stock, F. E., Fang, J. S. Y., and Ong, G. B.: Anterior spine fusion; the operative approach and pathological findings in 412 patients with Pott's disease of the spine, *Br. J. Surg., 48:* 172, 1960.

17. Hyndman, O. P.: Transplantation of the spinal cord; the problem of kyphoscoliosis with cord (Signs), *Surg. Gynecol. Obstet., 84:* 460, 1947.

18. Ingalls, T. H., and Curley, F. J.: Principles governing the genesis of congenital malformations induced in mice by Hypozia. *N. Engl. J. Med., 257:* 1121, 1957.

19. Klebanoff, G.: Early clinical experience with disposable unit for the intraoperative salvage and reinfusion of blood loss (intraoperative autotransfusion), *Am. J. Surg., 120:* 718, 1970.

20. Kuhn, J. G., and Hormell, R. S.: Management of congenital scoliosis; review of 170 cases, *Arch. Surg. 65:* 250, 1952.

21. Leatherman, K. D.: Resection of vertebral bodies, *J. Bone Joint Surg., 51A:* 206, 1969.

22. Macewen, G. D., Conway, J. J., and Miller, W. T.: Congenital scoliosis with unilateral bar, *Radiology, 90:* 711, 1968.

23. Raycroft, J. F., and Curtis, B. H.: Spinal curvature in myelomeningocele; natural history and etiology, In *Symposium on Myelomeningocele;* American Academy of Orthopaedic Surgeons, pp. 186-201; St. Louis: C. V. Mosby, 1970.

24. Riseborough, F. J.: The anterior approach to the spine for the correction of deformities of axial skeleton. *Clin. Orthop., 93:* 207, 1973.

25. Roaf, R.: Wedge resection for scoliosis, *J. Bone Joint Surg., 37B:* 97, 1955.

26. Schneider, R. C.: Transposition of the compressed spinal cord in kyphoscoliotic patients with neurological deficit, with special reference to the vascular supply of the cord, *J. Bone Joint Surg., 42A:* 1027, 1960.

27. Shands, A. R., Jr., and Bundens, W. D.: Congenital deformities of the spine; an analysis of the roentgenograms of 700 children, *Bull. Hosp. Joint Dis., 17:* 110, 1956.

28. Sharrard, W. J. W.: Spinal osteotomy for congenital kyphosis in myelomeningocele, *J. Bone Joint Surg., 50B:* 466, 1968.

29. Sharrard, W. J. W.: Osteotomy excision of the spine for lumbar kyphosis in older children with myelomeningocele, *J. Bone Joint Surg., 54B:* 50, 1972.

30. Simmons, E. H.: Observation on the technique and indication for wedge resection of the spine, *J. Bone Joint Surg., 50A:* 847, 1968.

31. Stiram, K., Bobechko, W. P., and Hall, J. E.: Surgical management of spinal deformities in spina bifida, *J. Bone Joint Surg., 54B:* 666, 1972.

32. Thomas, B. H., and Cheng, D. W.: Congenital abnormalities associated with vitamin E malnutrition, *Proc. Iowa Sci., 59:* 218, 1952.

33. Van Schrick, F. G.: Die angelorene Kyphose, *Z. Orthop., 56:* 259, 1932.

34. Von Rokitansky, K.F.: *Hanbuch der pathologiscen. Antomie,* Vol. II, Weir Braumuller, 1844.

35. Wiles, P.: Resection of dorsal vertebrae in congenital scoliosis, *J. Bone Joint Surg., 33A:* 151, 1951.

36. Williams, J. M., and Stevens, K.: Recognition of surgically treatable neurologic disorders of childhood, *J.A.M.A., 151:* 455, 1953.

37. Winter, R. B., and Moe, J. F.: Anterior fusion of the spine for difficult curvature problems, *J. Bone Joint Surg., 52A:* 833, 1970.

38. Winter, R. B., Moe, J. H., and Eiler, V. E.: Congenital scoliosis; a study of 234 patients treated and untreated. I. Natural history, *J. Bone Joint Surg., 50A:,* 1, 1968.

39. Winter, R. B., Moe, J. H., and Eiler, V. E.: Congenital scoliosis; a study of 234 patients treated and untreated. II. Treatment, *J. Bone Joint Surg., 50A:* 15, 1968.

40. Winter, R. B., Moe, J. H., and Wang, J. F.: Congenital kyphosis; its natural history and treatment as observed in a study of 130 patients, *J. Bone Joint Surg., 55A:* 223, 1973.

NONOPERATIVE TREATMENT OF KYPHOSCOLIOSIS

BY WILLIAM T. GREEN, JR., M.D.

Careful clinical and roentgenologic examination of the child permits early recognition of structural scoliosis before severe progressive spinal deformity occurs with growth. Until an effective nonoperative treatment was developed, most children were watched until the deformity became severe enough to warrant major surgery.

In 1958, a spinal distraction brace was introduced by Blount and Schmidt[4] of Milwaukee, Wisconsin. Experience has shown that this Milwaukee brace, complimented by an appropriate exercise program, can halt or even reverse the progression of scoliosis in the growing child when used judiciously.

Milwaukee Brace

In addition to a distractive force, the Milwaukee brace is designed to apply a bending and derotational force for the correction of the scoliotic curve (Fig. 18.41). The distractive force is applied between the pelvic girdle, which rests above the iliac crests, and the occipital rest. The head is held against the occipital rest by a chin piece or, more recently, by a throat mold. Use of this throat mold has eliminated the bite deformity often complicating use of the chin piece. The bending and derotational force is applied by the use of appropriate pads applied to the convexity of the curves, through the ribs in the thoracic spine or through the transverse processes in the lumbar spine. The brace is constructed in balanced alignment and by the application of these forces gradually brings the wearer into balance also.

The pelvic girdle, fabricated of leather and Monel Metal or thermoplastic, is connected to the neck ring by an anterior upright of aluminum and two posterior uprights of stainless steel. These uprights can be bent or lengthened as correction and growth occur, and they provide attachment for the corrective pads. Hinged laterally at the neck ring and anteriorly at the pelvic girdle, the brace is entered and secured at the back.

Best results are achieved when the Milwaukee brace and the corrective exercise program are supervised by a skilled team of orthotist, physical therapist, and orthopaedist. Under these conditions in children with juvenile or adolescent thoracic kyphosis (Scheuermann's disease), with idiopathic scoliosis measuring less than 40–50 degrees by the Cobb technique, or with congenital scoliosis, brace treatment is often indicated. This is particularly true when the curve is flexible, the child is young, and he is enthusiastic to participate in his own care. Treatment with this brace can be used to supplement surgical fusion. An early short fusion followed by control

with a brace is often indicated in progressive congenital scoliosis (Fig. 18.42).

Prescription for a Milwaukee brace should indicate to the orthotist the types of corrective pads desired and their initial placement: shoulder ring or axillary sling for high thoracic and cervicothoracic curves, "L"-shaped thoracic pad for lower thoracic and thoracolumbar curves, and an oval or upright-backed lumbar pad for lumbar curves. Also, it is good to note whether there is a pelvic obliquity or other special problems that will be encountered. The selection of the material for fabrication of the pelvic girdle is usually best left to the orthotist, allowing him to work with the material with which he is most comfortable. However, there is a strong preference for thermoplastic in the child who is not toilet-trained.

Prescription to the physical therapist should include general exercises to improve posture; pelvic tilt, spine extension and push-up exercises; also specific exercises to correct spinal deformity: shift of the torso away from the pad controlling the primary curve to restore spinal balance and thoracic flexion into the thoracic pad to derotate the spine and thereby to correct thoracic asymmetry.

Fit is a continuing problem. First the pelvic girdle must be fitted correctly. A common problem is failure to tighten the girdle adequately, allowing it to descend and painfully pinch the iliac crests laterally. This can be prevented by having the child grasp the girdle at the sides and hold it up while it is being tightened so it pinches inward above the crests. Once the pelvic girdle is in proper position the height of the occipital rest and throat mold can be adjusted so the former is just below the occiput and the latter is flush against the upper throat (Fig. 18.41 B). The trim line of the pelvic girdle should be just above the pubic symphysis anteriorly, the greater trochanter laterally, and the chair surface when seated posteriorly. It should allow enough room for hip flexion so the brace does not ride upward when seated. The anterior upright and the posterior upright on the side contralateral to the thoracic convexity should be adequately away from the thorax so that they make insignificant contact with deep inspiration or with thoracic flexion exercises. In contrast, the posterior upright on the side of the thoracic convexity backs the pad against the thoracic prominence.

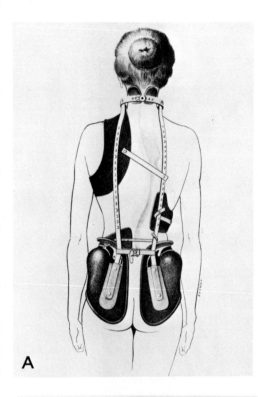

A

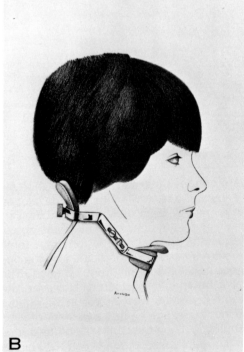

B

When appropriately placed, the wearer ought to be able to shift away from any pad ½ inch. A long-cassette standing roentgenogram (Fig. 18.42C) in the brace is very helpful in adjusting the position of the pads so their force is applied to the convexities of the curves, just inferior to their apices.

Initially it is usual for the child to wear the Milwaukee brace at all times, including sleep, except for twice daily. At these times, a total period less than 1 hr, he can come out of the brace for bathing and skin care with alcohol and powdered talc. The brace is best worn over one layer of underclothing. All activities including noncontact sports are encouraged since, when performed in the brace, corrective forces are applied to the spine with movement.

During the first 3–6 months of brace wear, the initial correction is usually achieved. Often it is preferable to apply the primary corrective pad initially alone until spinal balance from C-7 is corrected or slightly overcorrected, then to add the secondary pads.

The Milwaukee brace, correctly applied in a favorable case, can convert a child who is out of balance with a deforming curve to a child who is in balance with multiple smaller curves, a better physiologic and cosmetic situation (Fig. 18.43). The child's progress can be followed by long-cassette roentgenograms taken standing in the brace at decreasing intervals once correction has been achieved so radiation is minimized. It should be emphasized that if the brace does not adequately correct the scoliosis due to inappropriate selection, brace fabrication or application, then surgical correction should be done promptly. It is wise to advise the child and his parents before use of the Milwaukee brace is agreed upon that surgery may be required if adequate correction is not achieved and maintained.

If satisfactory correction is achieved and maintained by the Milwaukee brace when can it be discontinued? It is generally accepted that most scoliotic curves under 50 degrees do not progress after spinal growth is completed. Risser suggested that the ces-

Figure 18.41. (*A*) Young girl wearing a Milwaukee brace prescribed with a shoulder ring to control an elevated left shoulder and high left thoracic curve, an L-shaped thoracic pad to control a right thoracic curve, and a triangular shaped lumbar pad to control a left lumbar curve. (*B*) Position of the occipital rest and throat mold.

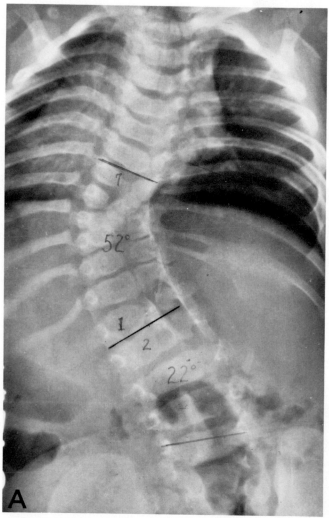

Figure 18.42.   This boy was born with a severe congenital scoliosis and low thoracic meningocele. The meningocele was closed at 5 days of age. At 7 months he developed a mild asymmetric spasticity in his legs. Spinal roentgenogram demonstrated hemivertebrae at T8 and T9, loss of definition of the pedicles on the concave side of the curve, failure of fusion of the primary ossification centers of the body of T11, fusion of the tenth and eleventh rib on the right, and a boney diastema at L1 and L2 (indicated by the *line* in *A*). This curve was convex to the left and measured 52 degrees from T7 to L1. The boney diastema was resected and, interestingly, the spasticity cleared. However, the infant was so badly out of spinal balance to the left that he was unable to sit without support until a localizer cast was applied. At 15 months of age he had a posterior fusion from T7 to L1 utilizing the posterior elements remaining along the convexity of the curve. Five months after the operation he was fitted with a Milwaukee brace which held him in balance (*B*). In a few months, he was up walking and playing normally (*C*). This scoliosis will need to be watched carefully, and will probably require further surgery and a Milwaukee brace until spinal growth is complete.

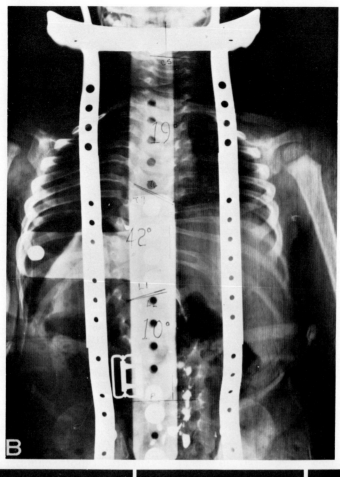

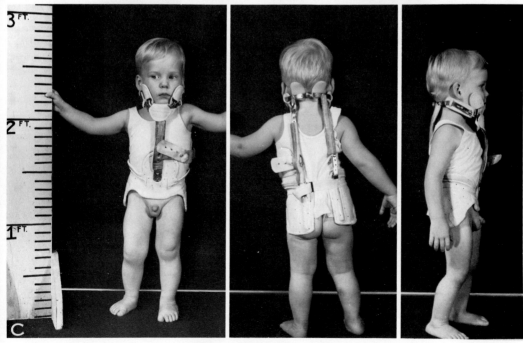

Figure 18.42 (*B* and *C*)

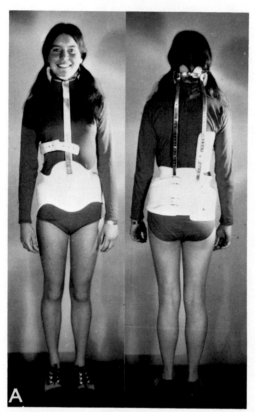
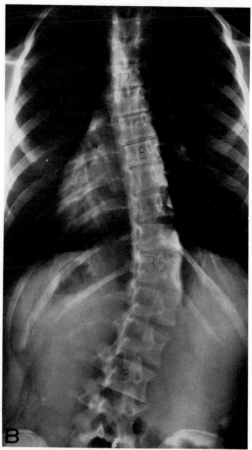

Figure 18.43.   This 15-year-old girl was seen with a right thoracolumbar curve from T8 to L3 out of spinal balance to the right. A Milwaukee brace with right L-shaped pad was prescribed (*A*). One year later standing in her brace, a roentgenogram (*C*) shows balance has been achieved into multiple small curves and the T8 to L3 thoracolumbar curve corrected from 35 degrees to 12 degrees as compared with her prebraced roentgenogram (*B*). Importantly, she is an athletic girl who did her exercises enthusiastically and has obtained a good correction despite her relatively advanced bone age as demonstrated by the maturity of her iliac apophyses (*B*).

sation of spinal growth occurs when the iliac apophyses have finished their ossification toward the sacroiliac joints; however, more recently the criterion of the fusion of these apophyses to the ilia or the ring apophyses to the vertebral bodies has been used. Both these events take place at a later age, of 17 to 20 years. Fortunately, in the adequately corrected, more mature, spine, part-time wear often holds this correction. Standing roentgenograms after the brace has been removed for increasing periods of time will determine whether the correction will be maintained when the brace is worn part time. Frequently it is possible to gradually discontinue brace wear until it is worn only during sleep until spinal growth has been completed. It is usually necessary to make several pelvic girdles during this period so the fit remains adequate as the child's pelvis changes. Thus the cost with this method of treatment is grossly comparable with surgical methods; however, in the correctly chosen case under favorable conditions the result can be very gratifying.

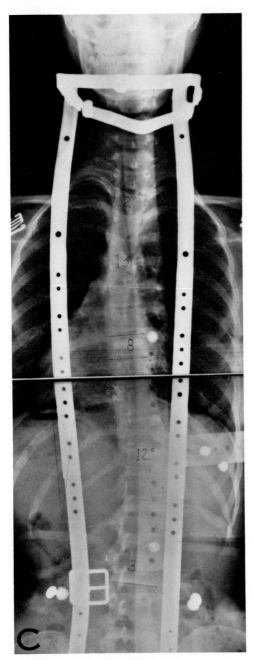

Figure 18.43 (C)

References

1. Blount, W. P.: Scoliosis and the Milwaukee brace, *Bull. Hosp. Joint Dis., 19: 152,* 1958.
2. Blount, W. P., and Bolinske, J.: Physical therapy in the nonoperative treatment of scoliosis, *Phys. Ther. 47: 919,* 1967.
3. Blount, W. P., and Moe, J. H.: *The Milwaukee Brace;* Baltimore: Williams & Wilkins, 1972.
4. Blount, W. P., Schmidt, A. C., and Bidwell, R. G.: Making the Milwaukee brace, *J. Bone Joint Surg., 40A: 526,* 1958.
5. Blount, W. P., Schmidt, A. C., Keever, E. D., and Leonard, E. T.: The Milwaukee brace in the operative treatment of scoliosis, *J. Bone Joint Surg., 40A: 511,* 1958.
6. Galante, J., Schultz, A., Dewald, R. L., and Ray, R. D.: Forces acting in the Milwaukee brace on patients undergoing treatment for idiopathic scoliosis. *J. Bone Joint Surg., 52A: 498,* 1970.
7. Moe, J. H.: The Milwaukee brace in the treatment of scoliosis, *Clin. Orthop., 77: 18,* 1971.
8. Moe, J. H., and Kettleson, D. N.: Idiopathic scoliosis; analysis of curve patterns and the preliminary results of Milwaukee-brace treatment in 169 patients. *J. Bone Joint Surg., 52A: 1509,* 1970.

SCOLIOSIS

BY WILLIAM F. DONALDSON, JR., M.D.

During the past 20 years, many workers have made significant contributions to our knowledge concerning the problems of patients with scoliosis. Its many diverse aspects are being given better definition. Certain strides have been made toward understanding the etiology of scoliosis, but there are still many gaps and much work must still be done to solve such questions as: Why does a scoliosis develop? What determines the curve pattern and its progression? Advances in treatment have been more concrete and dramatic. Even so, those involved in the management of these patients realize, all too well, the limitations of treatment currently available. We are still trying to control the effect, not the cause. Although much credit must be given to individual workers for the progress that has been made, the establishment of the Scoliosis Research Society in 1966 was of particular importance. This produced a much needed forum for the presentation and discussion of new and often preliminary ideas. The stimulus from this resulted in a reevaluation of old ideas, in the development of the new, in cooperative studies, etc. Thus, the care of these patients has become based less on empiric thought[83] and tradition.[89] As a result of the efforts of those involved in the Scoliosis Research Society, there is now a single acceptable method of measuring a curve (George and Reppstein[38], Cobb[10−14]) (Figs 18.44, 18.45). There is a standard way of recording rotation and vertebral

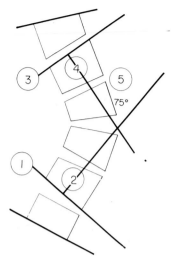

Figure 18.44. Scoliosis, measurement of a curve (Cobb.[10-14] *1.* Bottom vertebra: lowest one whose bottom tilts to concavity of curve. *2.* Erect perpendicular from bottom of bottom vertebra. *3.* Top vertebra: highest one whose top tilts to concavity of curve. *4,* Drop perpendicular from top of top vertebra. *5,* Measure intersecting angle. This is the accepted method of measurement of a curve according to the Scoliosis Research Society.

wedging.[97, 135] A standard nomenclature has been accepted. All of these advances provide a format within which more accurate comparison of patient studies can occur and truly scientific information can be exchanged.

Although numerous methods of conservative therapy have their advocates, the use of the Milwaukee brace has become widespread and is the most widely accepted method of nonoperative treatment for scoliosis. The technique of the construction and use of this brace is described earlier in this chapter. The necessary accompanying exercise program as described by Blount and Moe[8] is an indispensable part of this program. The current modification of the brace, as developed by Schmidt and Blount, are important. Anyone using this method must be conversant with all facets of the treatment program. An appropriate course of nonoperative treatment demands close cooperation between the patient and the patient's family, the orthopaedist, orthotist, and physical therapist.

In the surgical treatment of these patients, we owe a debt to such men as Albee,[1]

Hibbs et al.,[56] Cobb,[10-14] Moe,[85-89] and Goldstein[39-40, 42] for their contributions to the development of the surgical technique of spinal fusion for scoliosis. An exciting development has been the introduction and use of a method of posterior spinal instrumentation by Harrington.[49, 53-55, 75, 121] For many patients, this has resulted in a more satisfactory correction of their scolosis with less morbidity. A more recent innovation, anterior instrumentation as described by Dwyer,[27-29, 48, 51, 116] shows promise but its more exact role in our armamentarium is yet to be determined.

Preoperative surgical correction has undergone many improvements. Although the turnbuckle jacket (Fig. 18.46), as developed and modified by Ferguson,[32-34, 117, 124, 125]

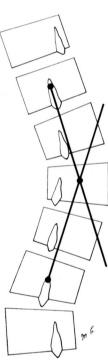

Figure 18.45. Scoliosis, measurement of a curve (Fergusen[32-34]). The central points of each end vertebra and of the apical vertebra are marked. The end vertebra are defined as the first nonrotated vertebra identified by the position of the spinous processes. The lines from the central point of the apical vertebra to those of each end vertebra form an angle. The deviation of these lines from 180 degrees is the angle of the curve.

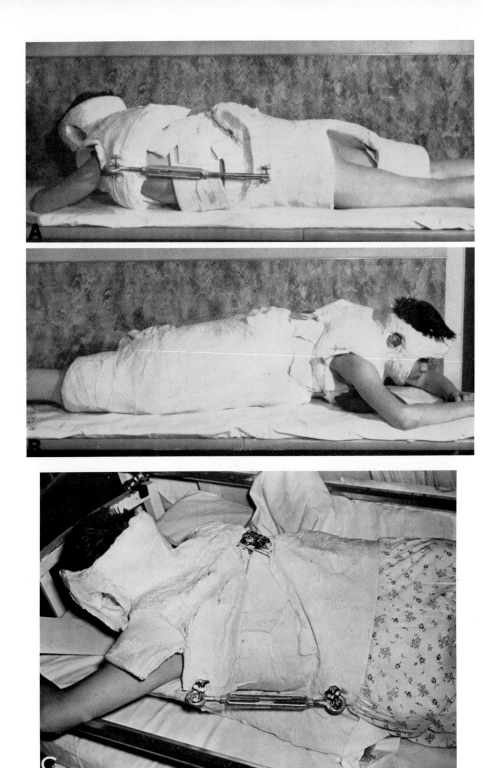

Figure 18.46. (*A*) Modified Risser turnbuckle jacket with full head piece and thigh extension of the side of the convexity of the major curve. The anterior and posterior hinges and the position of the turnbuckle can be seen. (*B*) A modified Risser turnbuckle jacket viewed from the side of the convexity of the major curve. Note the eccentric position of the anterior and posterior hinges. These hinges are made of aluminum and are, therefore, relatively radiolucent. (*C*) An overhead view demonstrating the position of the posterior hinge eccentric to and above the apex of the curve to be corrected. The

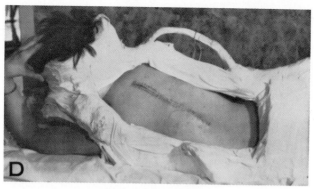

Figure 18.46 (D)

anterior hinge is directly opposite (D)—M.K. Patient is immobilized in her turnbuckle jacket. The portion over the sacrum is removable so that the posterior window is large enough to permit the taking of bone grafts from the posterior iliac crest.

Hibbs,[56] Risser,[107-112] and Cobb,[10-14] still remains one of the most efficient ways of correcting an angular deformity, other methods of preoperative treatment may be used in particular circumstances to improve the results obtained. These include the localizer cast of Risser, halo-femoral traction, halo-pelvic distraction, and Cotrell's cervical-pelvic traction.

We are learning more concerning the natural course of the patient with scoliosis, but most of these advances are concerned with those patients who have a specific etiologic basis for the development of their scoliosis such as congenital scoliosis with an unsegmented bar (Winter and Moe[130-132]), neurofibromatosis, etc. Cobb's work concerning untreated idiopathic scoliosis[14, 98] has not been followed up, and this leaves a great deficit in our understanding of the natural course of the disease.

Scoliosis has been defined as any lateral curve, tilt, or angular deviation of one or more vertebral segments of the spine from the normal straight position. Scoliosis may be divided into two major and distinct groups: functional and structural scoliosis.

A functional curve is one that the patient can voluntarily correct and that correction can be maintained in the erect position. In this type of scoliosis, there is no intrinsic involvement of the mechanics of the spine. There is no structural abnormality of the bone, nerve, or muscle elements of the spine. Conversely, in structural scoliosis, there is involvement of the intrinsic structure of the spine. This may be bone, neural, muscular, or a combination of any or all of these elements. In a structural scoliosis, complete correction cannot be obtained and maintained by the patient in the erect position.

Functional Scoliosis

Functional scoliosis may be seen in a variety of conditions. It may be due to poor posture alone, or it may represent a compensatory adjustment for an organic angular deformity such as a short leg, a pelvic tilt secondary to either an abduction or an adduction or a flexion contracture of the hip, "sciatic scoliosis," etc. (Fig. 18.47). These functional curves are not precursors of structural curves. Their nature must be understood and their significance appreciated if one is to evaluate appropriately and properly treat the patient with scoliosis.

By x-ray a functional scoliosis has different characteristics from those of a structural scoliosis. For example, in a functional curve, no evidence of wedging or other structural changes in the vertebrae are seen. No treatment is indicated for the functional scoliosis itself. The basic curve pattern, a C-curve, is such that it never crosses the midline in two directions. Therefore, it is a single curve and there are no minor or compensatory curves either above or below it.

Structural Scoliosis

While Cobb's classification (Table 18.2) of structural scoliosis has worked well for us in the past, with the newer knowledge available, it became clear that a more detailed and definitive segregation of patients according to etiology was necessary if we are going to be able to compare like groups of patients. Therefore, the current Scoliosis Research Society classification of patients with scoliosis is preferred (Table 18.3).

The importance of discovering the correct etiologic diagnosis cannot be overemphasized. It must be remembered that scoliosis is only a physical finding and is not, in itself, a diagnosis.

The etiology of the scoliosis has much to do with its characteristics and prognosis. The fact that the largest segment of the group must still be labeled idiopathic[66] does not detract from the value of determining the etiology, but rather emphasizes the importance of recognizing the other categories. This classification is based upon the systems and various disease processes that may be involved etiologically in the development of scoliosis.

Idiopathic scoliosis is divided into three separate groups, depending upon the age of

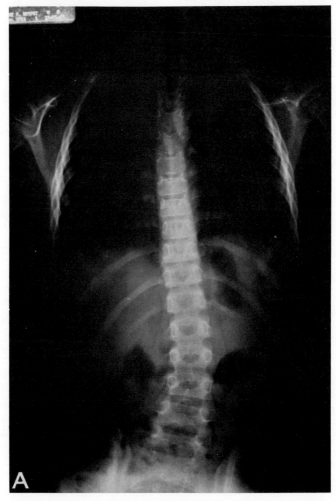

Figure 18.47. (A) Functional scoliosis, patient has 2-cm shortening of the left leg resulting in a pelvic tilt and functional scoliosis in the lumbar area. (B) With shortening corrected by a wooded block of appropriate height, the patient can maintain a straight spine in the erect position.

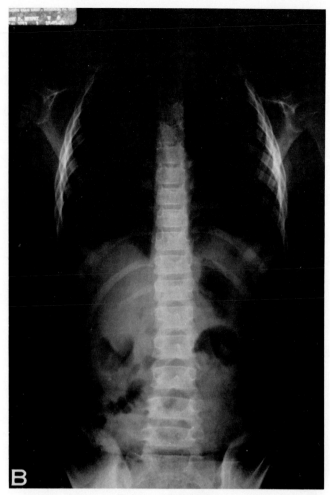

Figure 18.47 (B)

Table 18.2
Structural Scoliosis (Cobb's Classification)

I. Osteopathic
  A. Congenital
  B. Thoracogenic (postempyema, post-thoracoplasty)
  C. Postirradiation
  D. Other osteopathic
II. Neuropathic
  A. Congenital
  B. Postpoliomyelitis
  C. Neurofibromatosis, syringomyelia, etc.
III. Myopathic
  A. Congenital
  B. Muscular dystrophy
  C. Other myopathic
IV. Idiopathic

onset or recognition.[61] The infantile[35, 64, 65] age, 3 years and under, while quite uncommon in the United States, composes a significant group of patients in Great Britain. No specific explanation is currently available for the marked statistical difference. There are two subgroups of patients in this category: (1) the resolving type is found in patients who manifest a significant curve (20 degrees or more) that subsequently disappears without specific treatment; and (2) the progressive form is exceedingly difficult to manage because it has a great propensity for increase in the degrees of angular deformity regardless of the nonoperative treatment program used.

The juvenile patients (Figs. 18.48 and 18.49), ages 4–9, are a relatively small but important segment of patients for whom nonoperative treatment should be considered and

Table 18.3
Classification of Spinal Deformity

I. Idiopathic
  A. Infantile (3 years of age or younger)
    1. Resolving
    2. Progressive
  B. Juvenile (4–9 years of age)
  C. Adolescent (10 years of age or older)
II. Neuromuscular
  A. Neuropathic
    1. Upper motor neuron lesion
      a. Cerebral palsy
      b. Spinocerebellar disease
        (1) Friedriech's
        (2) Charcot-Marie-Tooth
        (3) Roussy-Lévy
      c. Syringomyelia
      d. Spinal cord tumor
      e. Spinal cord trauma
      f. Other
    2. Lower motor neuron lesion
      a. Poliomyelitis
      b. Other viral myelitis
      c. Traumatic
      d. Spinal muscular atrophy
        (1) Werdnig-Hoffmann
        (2) Kugelberg-Welander
      e. Myelomeningocele (paralytic)
    3. Dysautonomia (Riley-Day)
    4. Other
  B. Myopathic
    1. Arthrogryposis
    2. Muscular dystrophy
      a. Duchenne (pseudohypertrophic)
      b. Limb-girdle
      c. Facioscapulohumeral
    3. Fiber type disproportion
    4. Congenital hypotonia
    5. Myotonia dystrophica
    6. Other
III. Congenital
  A. Congenital scoliosis
    1. Failure of formation
      a. Wedge
      b. Hemivertebra
    2. Failure of segmentation
      a. Unilateral bar
      b. Bilateral ("fusion")
    3. Mixed
  B. Congenital kyphosis
    1. Failure of formation
    2. Failure of segmentation
    3. Mixed
  C. Congenital lordosis
  D. Associated with neural tissue defect
    1. Myelomeningocele
    2. Meningocele

    3. Spinal dysraphism
      a. Diastematomyelia
      b. Other
IV. Neurofibromatosis
V. Mesenchymal
  A. Marfan's syndrome
  B. Homocystinuria
  C. Ehlers-Danlos syndrome
VI. Traumatic
  A. Fracture of dislocation (nonparalytic)
  B. Postirradiation
  C. Postlaminectomy
  D. Other
VII. Soft-tissue contractures
  A. Burn
  B. Other
VIII. Osteochondrodystrophies
  A. Achondroplasia
  B. Spondyloepiphyseal dysplasia
  C. Diastrophic dwarfism
  D. Mucopolysaccharidosis
IX. Scheuermann's disease
X. Infection
  A. Tuberculosis
  B. Bacterial
  C. Fungal
  D. Parasitic
  E. Other
XI. Tumor
  A. Benign
  B. Malignant
XII. Rheumatoid disease
  A. Juvenile rheumatoid
  B. Adult rheumatoid
  C. Marie-Strümpell
XIII. Metabolic
  A. Rickets
  B. Juvenile osteoporosis
  C. Osteogenesis imperfecta
XIV. Related to lumbosacral area
  A. Spondylolisthesis
  B. Spondylolysis
  C. Other congenital anomaly
  D. Other
XV. Thoracogenic
  A. Postempyema
  B. Post-thoracoplasty
  C. Post-thoracotomy
  D. Other
XVI. Hysterical
XVII. Functional
  A. Postural
  B. Secondary to short leg
  C. Other

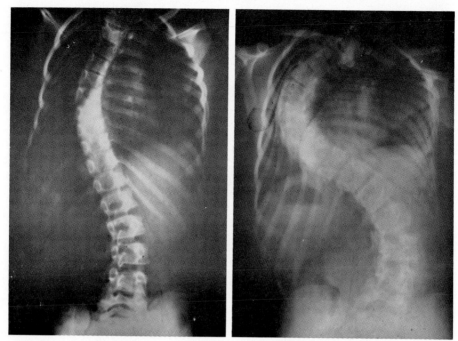

Figure 18.48. (*Left*) M.W., 8-year-old female with idiopathic scoliosis, 1948. Treatment consisted of the use of exercises and braces. Operative intervention was never suggested. (*Right*) X-ray of same patient taken in 1953; patient then aged 13. Correction and fusion resulted in very definite improvement, but certainly the ideal time for this procedure was missed. Serial x-ray observation at 3-month intervals would have graphically demonstrated the progression of angular deformity and indicated the need for surgical therapy.

enthusiastically pursued. At times it may be necessary, as in the infantile, to perform a limited fusion to aid in halting the progression of the spinal deformity. Secondary surgery may be necessary at a later date depending on the progression of the scoliosis.

The adolescent form is the most common type of scoliosis seen and will be discussed in greater detail (Fig. 18.50).

The neuromuscular and myopathic groups of patients deserve special consideration for they emphasize the importance of making the specific diagnosis associated with the clinically noted scoliosis. Appropriate treatment must be rendered for the primary disease and the management of the patient's scoliosis modified.[4]

Many advances have been made in the management of patients with congenital scoliosis, particularly those who have segmental variations and those who have scoliosis associated with a myelomeningocele. These pa-

tients are discussed in detail in another section of this chapter.

The remainder of the classification is directed to patients with specific etiologic classification who have the potential to develop scoliosis as a portion of their disease process.

It is extremely important in the management of the whole patient and, in particular, the existent scoliosis to recognize that these entities coexist. We must always remember that, in treating scoliosis, we are not just dealing with a roentgenograph filled with angular deformities, but rather with a patient who has the physical and roentgenographic findings of a structural scoliosis.

Idiopathic Scoliosis

In the past, a wide variety of etiologies were proposed for idiopathic scoliosis. Old wives' tales, such as carrying a heavy load on

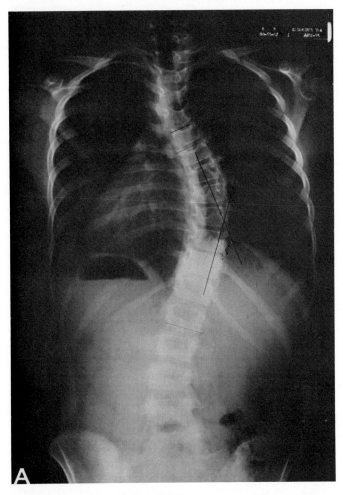

Figure 18.49.   (*A*) A.F. This patient was first seen at age 8 witn a typical juvenile idiopathic scoliosis. Treatment was recommended but refused by parents on the advice of the family physician. (*B*) When examined by us in 1966, the 38 degree curve had increased to 155 degrees. The patient did subsequently undergo surgical treatment, but the end result is certainly far from that desired. She has severe restrictive ventilatory defect and a vital capacity of 33%. Her scoliosis had been allowed to progress to the degree that she is a pulmonary cripple.

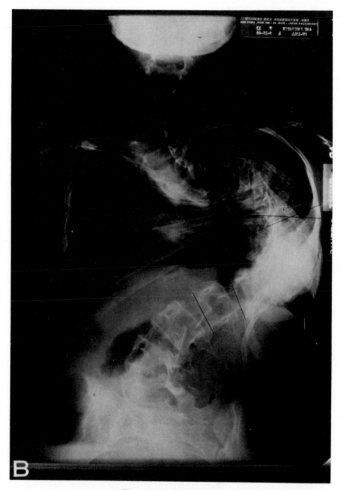

Figure 18.49 (B)

one side, the performance of asymmetrical exercise, the adoption of a pattern of a poor sitting or standing position, still persist. To associate these "facts" as cause and effect is to ignore the mechanics of the spine as related to scoliosis. It is mechanically impossible to demonstrate the forces of such suggested etiologies that could possibly produce a structural scoliosis with a three- or four-curve pattern.

Some have said that idiopathic scoliosis represents the unrecognized effect of anterior poliomyelitis. One can readily demonstrate mathematically that this is not true. Idiopathic scoliosis occurs predominantly in female patients, who account for approximately 85% of the cases. Recognizable postpoliomyelitis scoliosis occurs equally in male and female patients. Idiopathic scoliosis occurs within definite age limits, whereas postpoliomyelitis scoliosis might develop at almost any age. The spine in idiopathic scoliosis is almost always stable (Fig. 18.51). In a large percentage of the postpoliomyelitis scolioses, the spine is unstable. Postpoliomyelitis scoliosis often demonstrates marked telescoping and collapse in the erect position (Fig. 18.52). The characteristic curves of these two forms of scoliosis are different, and the prognosis and behavior of the curve in each instance are different. For example, postpoliomyelitis scoliosis may increase after growth is complete, or it may originate after growth is completed. Further and most significant, since the advent of the poliomyelitis vaccine, there has been no decrease in the incidence of idiopathic scoliosis. Idiopathic scoliosis, on the other hand, usually increases before the

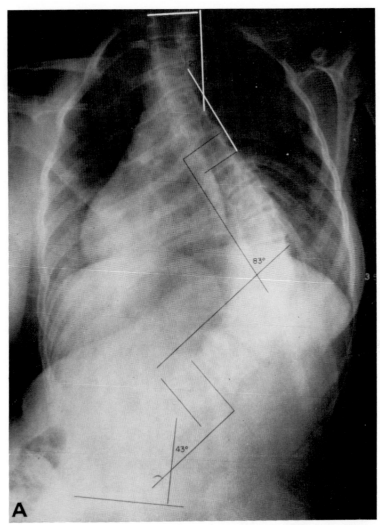

Figure 18.50. (A) S.T., age 14, with a typical idiopathic scoliosis. Major curve, D6 to L2, 83 degrees. Minor curves, D1 to D6, 29 degrees, and L2 to S1, 43 degrees. (B) Recumbent left bending film. Minor curve, D1 to D6, reduces to 16 degrees; L2 and S1 reduces to 10 degrees. This demonstrates considerable flexibility in the opposite curves and indicates that considerable reduction in the angular deformity of the major curve, D6 to L2, is permissible. (C) Postoperative film. Major curve, D6 to L2, 30 degrees. This degree of correction has been maintained.

completion of growth and only occasionally afterward. Urbaniak and Stelling[122] have shown that some of their patients, followed 2–20 years after iliac crest capping, demonstrated a mild increase in the degree of their curves. Certainly, though, the time for the greatest likelihood of an increase in the degree of angular deformity of a curve in idiopathic scoliosis is prior to skeletal maturity as evidenced by bone age, capping of the iliac

apophyses and, finally, closure of the vertebral ring apophyses. Comparative measurement of idiopathic scoliotic curves in the erect position and recumbent position seldom show a variation of more than 10–15 degrees, whereas postpoliomyelitis scoliotic curves may show considerably more variation than this.

The work of Wynne-Davies[123, 133] and that of MacEwen and Cowell[78] have demonstrated

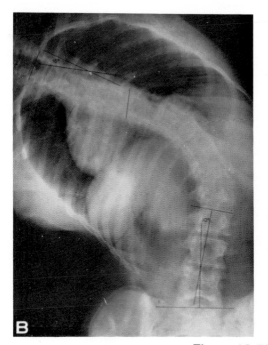
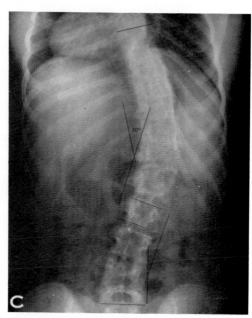

Figure 18.50 (*B* and *C*)

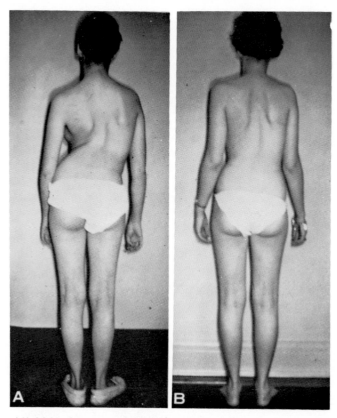

Figure 18.51. (*A*) M.K. Patient had a right dorsolumbar scoliosis with marked asymmetry of the flank creases and a list to the right of 4 cm. (*B*) Postoperatively, patient has

that there is more of a genetic factor in many of the families of patients with idiopathic scoliosis. We have all seen patients who have other family members with idiopathic scoliosis. Until these studies, the genetic pattern had not been well established. By examining and x-raying members of patients' families and collecting roentgenograms of persons unavailable for personal examination, MacEwen and Cowell[16, 78] were able to construct family trees of their patients and demonstrate the inheritance pattern. Admittedly, many of these angular deformities were small, but their curves did have structural characteristics. The pattern of inheritance they found was sex-linked and dominant, whereas Filho and Thompson[36] concluded that the pattern

was multifactoral (polygenetic). As a result, it is now our policy to inform the patients and their families that such potential does exist, that they should make a practice of checking the spines of their children on their birthdays and seek medical evaluation if there is any evidence of a developing scoliosis. We are equally positive in our recommendation that this factor alone should not influence the decision of the patient concerning future childbearing.

Still others have postulated that a nutritional deficiency is the responsible factor, but this has never been proven even by extensive biochemical studies. It is difficult to prove either a nutritional or endocrine variation. In a study of a large segment of patients with

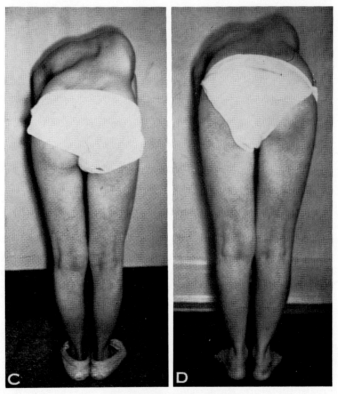

Figure 18.51 (*C* and *D*)

marked improvement in symmetry, but there is still some asymmetry. In most instances, surgical treatment results in improvement, not in elimination, of all the physical signs associated with scoliosis. (*C*) On forward flexion, the right dorsolumbar rib hump is evident preoperatively. (*D*) Postoperatively, it is improved but, of all the clinical stigmata of scoliosis, it is the angulation of the ribs that can be reduced the least. Even in patients in whom it is permissible and obtainable to reduce the angular deformity of the thoracic curve to 0 degrees, there will still be some residual deformity of the rib cage present both anteriorly and posteriorly.

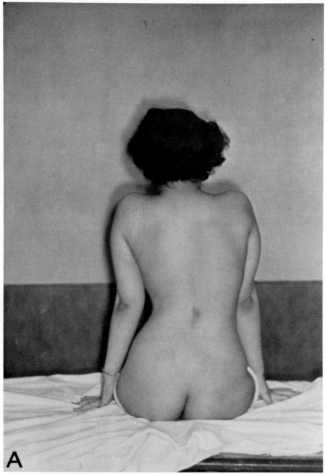

Figure 18.52. (*A*) M.W. Patient developed anterior poliomyelitis as an infant. She had involvement of her trunk and lower extremities. Her scoliosis developed within 2 years after onset of polio. Bracing became increasingly difficult. The patient eventually could sit only with support of her right hand because of the progressive scoliosis and the marked instability of her spine. (*B*) Patient is able to distract her unstable spine. Correction and fusion resulted in a stable, almost straight, spine and the patient became independent of bracing and able to perform most normal activities.

scoliosis at any one time, the vast majority show no increase in their angular deformity while they are under observation. Idiopathic scoliosis tends to increase at irregular and unpredictable intervals; therefore, the variations that might occur would be relatively infrequent and difficult to evaluate and check.

In idiopathic scoliosis, definitive curve patterns[61] can be identified and this is the only category in which such a classification is possible. The most common varieties are the single major or single structural curve with minor or compensatory curves above and below, and the double major or double structural in which there are two structural curves with two minor or compensatory curves, one above and one below. A third pattern is thoracolumbar structural curve, that usually extends from T10 or T11 to L3 or L4 with compensatory curves above and below. This usually has a convexity to the left. The single structural curve usually has its convexity to the right and extends from T5 or T6 to T11, T12, or L1 and the double major structural curve has its convexity to the right from T4

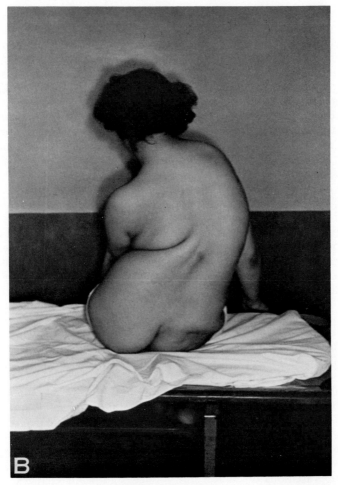

Figure 18.52 (B)

or T5 to T10 or T11 and to the left from T10 or T11 to L3 or L4. There is a fourth pattern of an upper dorsal curve that is the least common. It extends from T1 or T2 to T5 or T6. It is the most difficult of all curve patterns to manage with a nonoperative treatment program.

Much has been written concerning the transformation of a functional scoliosis into a structural one. In spite of all that has been said, no valid proof exists that such a true transition ever occurs. Even the earliest x-rays of true structural scoliosis usually show structural changes.

History

In evaluating the patient with scoliosis, we are interested in having a complete and ac-

curate history, not only of the scoliosis, but also of the general condition of the patient. Care must be taken to try to elicit a history of specific illnesses that have the potential to produce a structural scoliosis. It should be recorded that the family history does or does not reveal that other members of the family (siblings or maternal or paternal ancestors) have a scoliosis. As noted, recent studies in this area suggest that definite genetic patterns do exist.

Physical Findings

Again, the physical examination of the patient must not be limited to the scoliosis, but must be complete and general. If it is superficial or too narrow, the etiologic background of cases of known etiology is missed and, therefore, the proper management of the patient is not determined. We are particularly interested in trying to find evidence of neurologic deficit, muscular weakness, or significant skin lesions.

In a patient with scoliosis, the findings that are directly related to the scoliosis itself are asymmetrical prominence of the rib cage, an elevated shoulder, a prominent hip and asymmetry of the flank creases (Fig. 18.51). These findings are directly related to the lateral deviation of the spine and its associated rotation. We are also interested in such findings as café au lait spots, subcutaneous or pedunculated neurofibroma, and the various skin lesions associated with congenital malformations of the spine—for example, a hairy patch, a midline hemangioma, a skin dimple, a lipoma, or a myelomeningocele.[17, 23]

We have found it useful to grade the degree of rotation, as evidenced by clinical rib prominence, depending upon severity. Grade one is the mildest, grade four is the sharp razor back. While this method is empiric and fairly gross, it has been clinically useful. A number of attempts have been made to grade the degree of rib hump and the associated contralateral thoracic valley. The use of a spirit level, (and the recording in centimeters of the difference in height at the apex of the curve) appears to be the most accurate but, in a practical sense, has not resulted in significant follow-up variations of clinical importance. A list should be described as that distance to the right or left of the midgluteal crease that a plumbline reaches when dropped from the posterior spine of T1 or in patients with other than idiopathic scoliosis from the occiput down, i.e., a list of 1 cm to the right (Fig. 18.53 A).

X-ray Findings

The original x-ray studies should include anteroposterior views of the spine (standing, sitting, and recumbent) from the iliac crests up to and including the first thoracic vertebra. If there is a cervical component to the scoliosis, the cervical spine must also be included. These studies should be made on large films (preferably 14 × 36 inches but at least 14 × 17 inches) in order that the entire curve pattern, as it exists from the first thoracic vertebra to the sacrum, may be visualized (Charts 18.1–18.3). Segmental films do not permit accurate measurement of the curves. A lateral view of the spine must also be made as part of the original x-ray study. In patients with idiopathic scoliosis, we have been impressed with the higher incidence of spondylolisthesis than that seen in the population at risk. Several studies have documented this. The presence of spondylolisthesis certainly should modify one's approach to the surgical management of such a patient's scoliosis if it should be necessary. Follow-up films need include only anteroposterior standing and sitting x-rays of the spine. They should be made at 3- or 4-month intervals during the period of time when an increase in the angular deformity may be reasonably expected. The erect films of the standing and sitting positions serve as a mathematical countercheck against each other. By either method of measurement (Figs. 18.54 and 18.55), the variation between these two films usually is not more than 3–5 degrees. This countercheck excludes technician error. However, the variation may be greater if the patient has, for example, atrophy of a buttock and, therefore, a pelvic tilt in the sitting film. If an inequality of leg length is present, it will distort the spine in the standing films. Such deformities must be compensated for when the films are taken, for, depending on their severity, they produce significant changes in the degree of angular deformity and make comparative measurements imprecise.

All the curves must be measured and the measurement should be recorded each time for comparative study in the future. If a change in the degree of a measured curve exceeds 5 degrees in both the sitting and standing films, an increase in the angular deformity can be said to have occurred. Additional views, such as sitting tilt and lateral bending studies, are chiefly of value in the preoperative evaluation of the patient prior to correction and fusion. These studies are of particular value in establishing the flexibility of the major (structural) and minor (compensatory) curves. They are used to determine the amount of correction that is permissible as evidenced by the flexibility of the major curve or curves, thereby indicating how much correction might be obtained (Figs. 18.50 and 18.55). We are using forced bend lateral recumbent films (Fig. 18.56) to give us a better

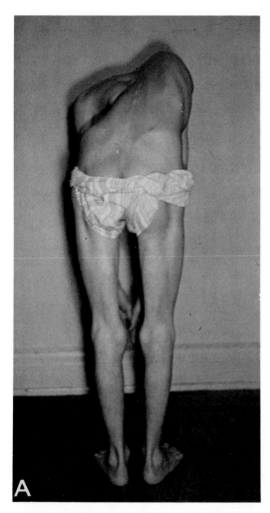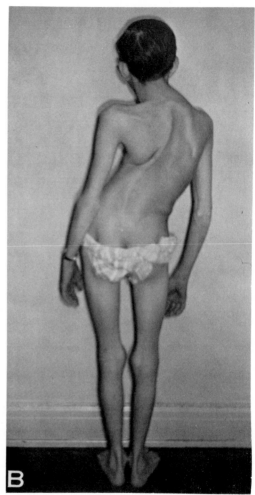

Figure 18.53.   R.E. This patient demonstrates severe but typical clinical findings of a structural scoliosis. (*B*) He has a major (structural) right cervical dorsal curve with a higher right shoulder and prominence of the right scapula. His left dorsolumbar curve is a minor (compensatory) curve as is his upper cervical curve. There is marked list to the right (6 cm). This list is a further automatic attempt to balance for the major, structural, curve. (*A*) On forward flexion the marked +4 razorback rib hump is seen on the convex side of the curve. On the left concave side of the thoracic curve, the deep thoracic valley is readily appreciated. The anterior chest mirrors these deformities. As the spine bends laterally, it also rotates bringing the ribs back on the convex side of a curve and forward on the concave side. As a juvenile, this patient had had empyema which was surgically treated. He was not followed for the development of scoliosis and, when recognized, it was ignored.

Chart 1
Scoliosis History

Name	Date	History of Number
Date of Birth	Age	Sex

Complaint: (High shoulder, prominent shoulder blade, high or prominent hip, prominent chest or breast, short leg, curvature, poor posture, awkward walk, pain in back, general fatigue, *etc.*)

Present History: Which deformity noted first
　　Age first noted　　　　　　　　　　　　by whom (patient, parents, doctor, teacher, nurse)
　　Age first treated　　　　　　　　　what treatment (corset, brace, frame exercises, traction)
　　Duration of treatment
　　Progress of deformity (stationary, increasing, decreasing, rapid, slow)

Family History: Give history of scoliosis or other deformity in each case (other side).
　　Maternal grandmother (descent . . . .) Paternal grandmother (descent . . . .)
　　　　″　grandfather (descent . . . .) 　 ″ 　grandfather (descent . . . .)

			standing height		sitting height	
Father	Age					
Mother	Age		″	″	″	″
Brothers	1	Age	″	″	″	″
(names)	2	″	″	″	″	″
	3	″	″	″	″	″
	4	″	″	″	″	″
Sisters	1	″	″	″	″	″
(names)	2	″	″	″	″	″
	3	″	″	″	″	″
	4	″	″	″	″	″

Past History: Birth difficult or normal. Evidence of trauma?
　　General health (robust, weak, normal weight, underweight, overweight, good color, pale, sickly, frequent illness.) Illness—(age and duration) scarlet fever , measles , mumps , chicken pox , whooping cough , polio , rickets , diphtheria , empyema , pneumonia , torticollis , Friedreich's ataxia , chorea , tonsillitis ; menses, age onset , (regular, irregular, scanty, profuse, duration)

Examination　　　　　　　　　　　　　　　　　　　　　Date
　　General posture (good, fair, poor). General development (good, fair, poor). Musculature (good, fair, poor). Nutrition (good, fair, poor). High shoulder (rt., left). Prominent scapula (rt., left). Prominent low ribs (rt., left). Exaggerated flank crease (rt., left). Prominent hip (rt., left). High hip (rt., left). List (rt., left). R.A. L.A. Rotation (no, mild, moderate, severe)
　　Standing height　　　　　　　　Sitting height　　　　　　　　　　　　Weight
　　Flexibility of spine (flexible, moderately fixed, fixed)
　　Curve　　　　　　　　　　　　　　　(Note muscle imbalance on other side of sheet)
　　Curve corrected on forward bending? (No, slight, moderate, complete)
　　Curve corrected on suspension? (No, slight, moderate, complete)

Diagnosis—Scoliosis　　{　A. Functional
　　(check which)　　{　B. Structural

I. Osteopathic　{　1. Congenital
　　　　　　　　　2. Thoracogenic
　　　　　　　　　3. Other osteopathic

II. Neuropathic.　{　1. Congenital
　　　　　　　　　2. Post polio
　　　　　　　　　3. Other neuropathic

III. Myopathic　{　1. Congenital
　　　　　　　　　2. Muscular dystrophy
　　　　　　　　　3. Other myopathic

IV. Idiopathic

Chart 2
Scoliosis Record

Name .... Doctor ....
Diagnosis .... History No. ....

Date					
Age					
Ht. Standing					
Ht. Sitting					
Weight					
L. A.					
R. A.					
List					
High Shoulder					
Low Hip					
Prominent Hip					
X-ray Date					
Born Age					
( ) Curve { Standing / Sitting / Supine					
Rotation (+, ++, etc.)					
Wedging (+, ++, etc.)					
( ) Curve { Standing / Sitting / Supine					
Rotation (+, ++, etc.)					
Wedging (+, ++, etc.)					
( ) Curve { Standing / Sitting / Supine					
Rotation (+, ++, etc.)					
Wedging (+, ++, etc.)					
( ) Curve { Standing / Sitting / Supine					
Rotation (+, ++, etc.)					
Wedging (+, ++, etc.)					

index of the correction that can be expected with the various methods of preoperative correction.

In addition to the degree of angular deformity of the curves, one also should record the amount of rotation and wedging. Both rotation and wedging may be graded from one plus to four plus. Rotation may be determined by the location of the apical posterior spinous process or by the outline of the vertebral pedicles. The former is easier to define, but the necessary landmark is destroyed when a spine fusion has been performed. Therefore, pedicle rotation, as described by Nash and Moe,[97] must be used if we are going to be able to compare preoperative and postoperative rotation as seen in the roentgenograph.

Many other things might be measured in the x-rays, but these fundamental findings have proven to be the most significant and valuable aids to an accurate follow up of the patient with scoliosis.

Adolescent Idiopathic Scoliosis

In our large scoliosis service where all degrees of scoliosis are seen and followed, the vast majority of the cases are idiopathic in nature. Idiopathic scoliosis is a self-limited disease characterized by the development of a structural scoliosis for which there is no known etiology. The probable genetic basis for it has already been referred to. Apparently the predisposition is inherited, but its expressivity is delayed. This, however, still does not explain why the scoliotic curve develops. The angular deformity does not progress at a constant rate but, rather, at unpredictable intervals. If an increase occurs, it almost always appears before age 15 in female patients and age 16 in male patients. Progression may or may not occur and, if it does, it may stop spontaneously with or without treatment. Growth is not the only factor associated with an increase in the angular deformity of an idiopathic scoliosis. Many patients show a marked increase in height without any significant change in the degree of angular deformity.

If the curves increase, they most often do so while growth is occurring, but not because of it (Fig. 18.49). These two, then, are concomitant occurrences and not cause and effect. Some patients show an increase in their curves after skeletal maturity and, therefore, these patients must be followed at least to age 21. After skeletal maturity, they may be checked at yearly intervals instead of every 3–4 months.

Chart 3
Scoliosis File

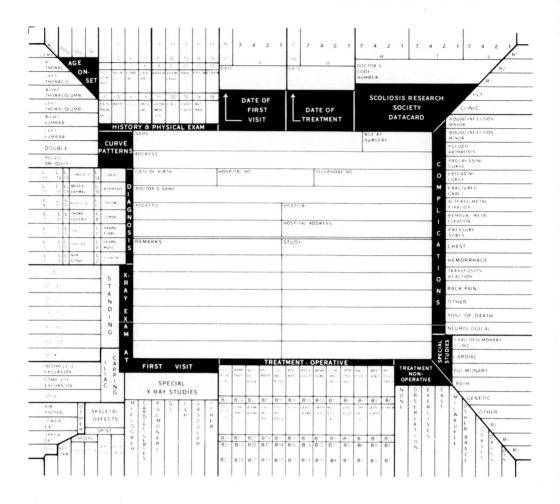

The observation by Risser[111] that, after the iliac crests are fully capped by their apophyses, idiopathic scoliosis does not usually increase, is of particular value in treating those patients whose spines mature before the age of 15 or 16. The crest may be considered to be fully capped when the mineralization of the apophysis has progressed from the lateral aspect medially to include the area of the posterosuperior iliac spine.[136] A better index of skeletal maturity is bone age and the maturity of the spine is best determined by the closure of the vertebral ring apophyses.

Approximately 85% of the cases of idiopathic scoliosis occur in female patients, many of whom have a very early or very late onset of sexual maturity as evidenced by the menarche.[68, 103] Many of the male patients who develop idiopathic scoliosis have a fairly feminine type of build, at least during their active growth period.

Nonoperative treatment of these patients is difficult to evaluate because of the lack of predictable progression of the angular deformity. Elsewhere, the use of the Milwaukee brace is discussed. Certainly, time has shown that exercises alone have no effect on the progression of the degree of the curves. Other forms of bracing have not tolerated the test of time. It is unfortunate that there are so few well documented series of the use of the Milwaukee brace and its associated exercise program.[30, 37, 91]

Operative treatment of a patient with idiopathic scoliosis must be based upon an accurate knowledge of the mechanics of the

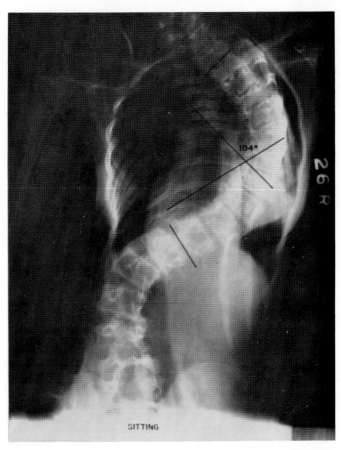

Figure 18.54. P.S. Neuropathic scoliosis with marked progression over a 4-year period. Pulmonary function studies, including blood gases, demonstrated less than 20% of the normal.

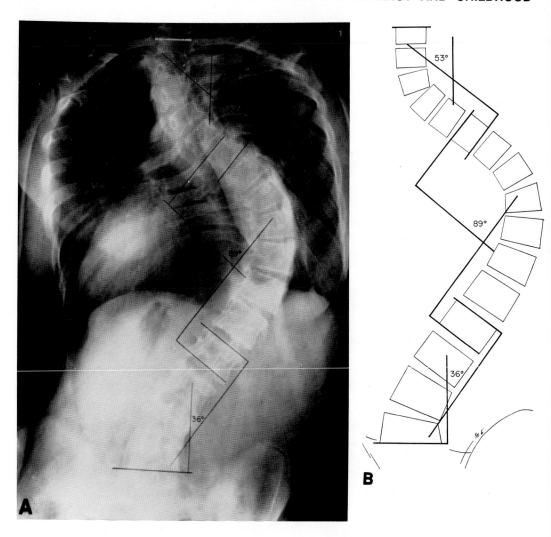

Figure 18.55. (A) Preoperative film of patient M.K., standing (See Figs. 18.51A and B). Major curve. D6 to L1, 89 degrees. Minor, D1 to D6, 53 degrees, and L1 to S1, 36 degrees. (B) Diagram of (A). (C) Preoperative lateral recumbent bending film. Minor curves, D1 to D6, 30 degrees, and L1 to S1, 1 degrees. (D) Diagram of (C). (E) Preoperative x-ray showing reduction in the major curve, D6 to L1, from 89 degrees to 34 degrees. Note the metal markers over the spinous processes of D6 and L1. The film is made through the Risser jacket. The opaque discs are the studs in the hinges. The central opaque disc is at the apex of the anterior hinge, the posterior hinge having been removed in excising the window for surgery. It is to be noted that even when the desired correction has been obtained, the apex of the hinges has just reached the concavity of the major curve from its original position eccentric to the convexity and at or about the apex of the major curve. (F) Diagram of (E). (G) Composite film showing the eventual angular pattern of the patient on completion of correction and fusion. The top and bottom portions, the minor curves, are taken from Figure 8.55B, bending film; superimposed between these is our preoperative correction film, Figure 8.55C. By this means we can determine that our patient is not overcorrected. More correction would have been permissible if it had been obtainable. Serial x-rays taken during correction showed that no further correction was obtainable. (H) Diagram of (G). (I) Postoperative films demonstrate maintenance of correction obtained. Note the neurologic clips which have been

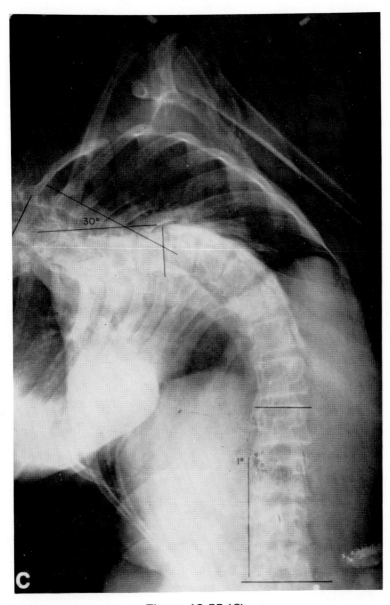

Figure 18.55 (*C*)
placed on the remaining tips of the spinous processes at the ends of the fusion area, D6 to L1. These readily identify the area fused in the follow-up x-ray studies. (*J*) Diagram of (*I*).

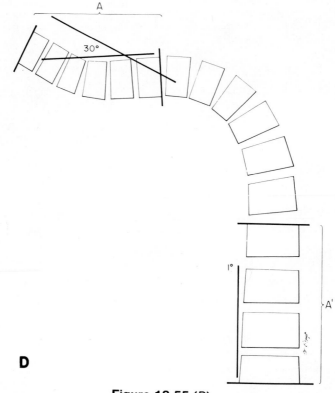

D

Figure 18.55 (*D*)

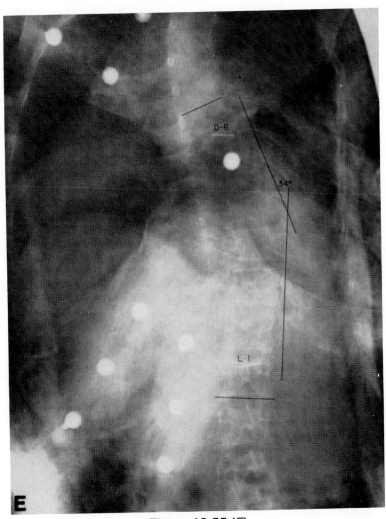

Figure 18.55 (*E*)

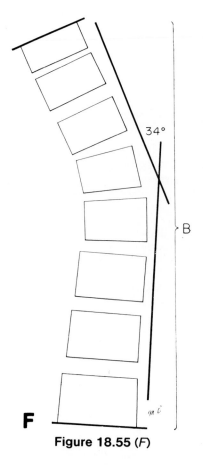

34°

B

F

Figure 18.55 (F)

longer be salvaged cosmetically and physiologically.

The preoperative evaluation of the patient must include a complete history, physical, and x-ray studies and certain baseline laboratory studies, not only for initial evaluation but, also, for the postoperative regulation of the patient who may in this period of time develop any disease. We routinely obtain a complete blood count with differential, urinalysis, sedimentation rate, serology for luetic infection, total protein and albumin-globulin (A/G) ratio, electrocardiogram, chest x-ray, and pulmonary function studies.[43, 45, 67, 72, 93, 106, 114, 115, 126–128] Many of these patients, particularly those with curves of at least 90 degrees, have significant pulmonary dysfunction. Up to 60 degrees, the pulmonary status is usually satisfactory in patients with stable spines. It is unfortunate but true that significant reduction in the degree of angular deformity by correction and fusion does not result in proportionate gains in pulmonary function. Therefore, patients must not be permitted to develop severe curves. Cor pulmonale secondary to scoliosis has not been seen in patients whose thoracic curve measures 60 degrees or less (Fig. 18.54). In addition, we also require a thorough dental check and, if significant difficulties are found, they are corrected before treatment is begun.

The amount of correction permissible may be determined by the use of standing and recumbent bending films (Fig. 18.55). The amount of correction to be expected is evaluated by forced lateral bend in recumbency (Fig. 18.56E).

In our hands, preoperative correction of the patient with idiopathic scoliosis has undergone significant modification. Essentially, we are using one of three different modalities: (1) Risser localizer cast (Fig. 18.57), (2) turnbuckle jacket (Fig. 18.46),[5, 70] (3) halo-femoral traction (Fig. 18.58),[102] halo-pelvic distraction (Fig. 18.59),[19, 20, 59, 99, 101, 134] or Cotrell traction. The choice of method depends upon the flexibility of the curve or curves undergoing treatment. For the more flexible curves, the localizer jacket has proven to be most satisfactory. If more correction is permissible than can be obtained by this method, then we resort to the turnbuckle jacket. For the still more rigid curves, we use halo-femoral traction, or at times halo-pelvic distraction. We have had a very limited experience with the

spine, both normal and abnormal. Surgical treatment is not indicated in a patient with a mild idiopathic scoliosis whose serial x-rays show that there has been no increase in the angular deformity.[15, 47, 64] It is indicated in those whose angular deformity, when first seen, is severe enough to warrant correction and in those in whom there has been a rapid and/or a significant increase. The procedure may be relatively contraindicated for patients in whom the amount of correction obtainable is not significant (20 degrees or less) or for those in whom no correction of the major curve is permissible, provided that the scoliosis is not progressive. It may also be contraindicated by the presence of other organic or psychologic conditions that make any surgical procedure unwise.

The ideal time for performing this procedure is between the ages of 12 and 16. However, as we must not fuse unnecessarily in the mild, nonprogressive cases, we must also not allow the young patients to become so progressively deformed that they can no

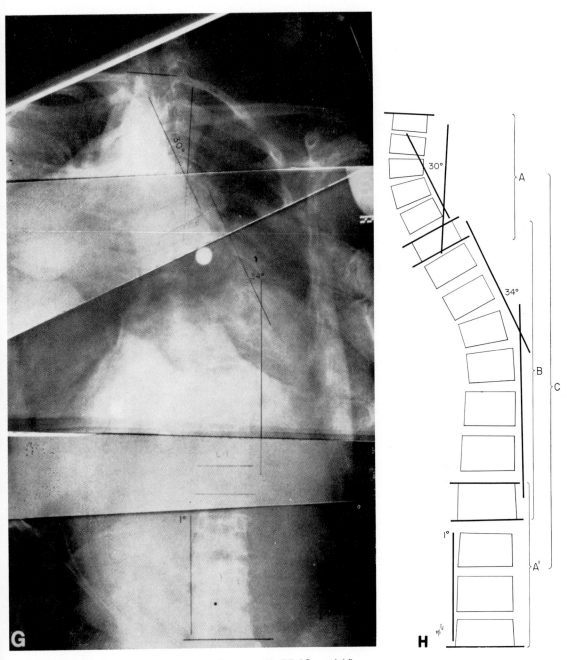

Figure 18.55 (*G* and *H*)

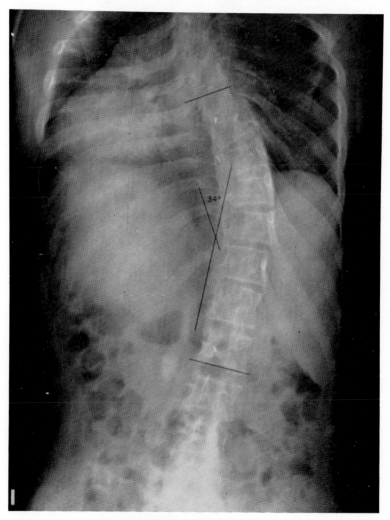

Figure 18.55 (*l*)

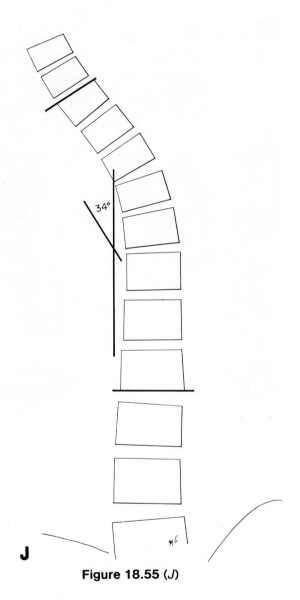

Figure 18.55 (J)

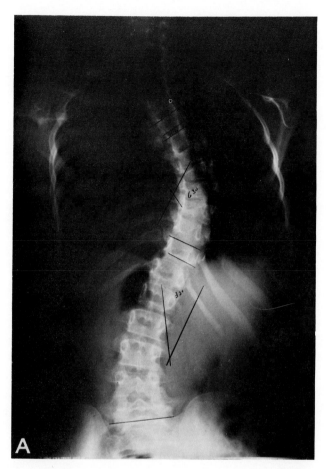

Figure 18.56. (*A*) B.E., age 11. Scoliosis first noted 1 year earlier. Received chiropractic treatment. Serial films demonstrated an increase in her major curve of adolescent idiopathic scoliosis. Her major, structural, curve extends from T4 to T11, 63 degrees standing with minor, compensatory, curves T1 to T4 above, 26 degrees, and below, T11 to sacrum, 32 degrees. She has +4 rotation of the apical vertebrae of the major curve as evidenced by the pedicles. (*B*) In recumbency, the major curve, T4 to T11, reduces to 54 degrees. (*C*) On lateral bend, recumbent, toward the concavity of the major curve, the minor compensatory curves reduce to 20 degrees, T1 to T4, and 8 degrees, T11 to the sacrum. (*D*) On lateral bend, recumbent, toward the convexity of the major curve, the major structural curve reduces to 40 degrees. This demonstrates very limited flexibility for the age of the patient and the degree of the curve present. (*E*) Forced lateral bend to the right demonstrates that reduction is possible of the major curve, T4 to T11, to 25 degrees. (*F*) After the posterior window has been removed for preoperative marking, the major curve now measures 34 degrees. The metal strips over two methylene blue intradermal marks injected into the skin overlie the posterior spinous processes of the end vertebrae of the selected fusion area. (*G* and *H*) After instrumentation, the curve now measures 25 degrees. As indicated in the text, most of the correction should be obtained preoperatively.

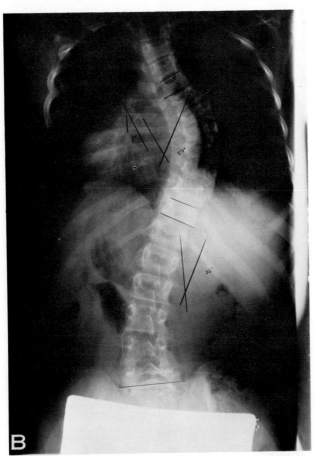

Figure 18.56 (*B*)

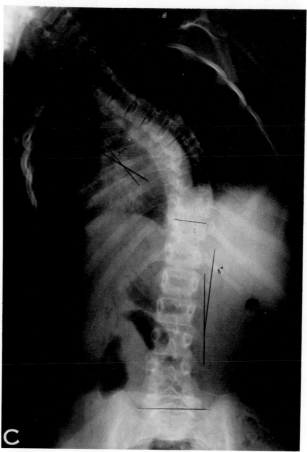

Figure 18.56 (*C*)

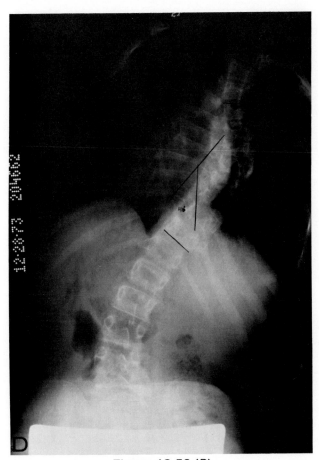

Figure 18.56 (*D*)

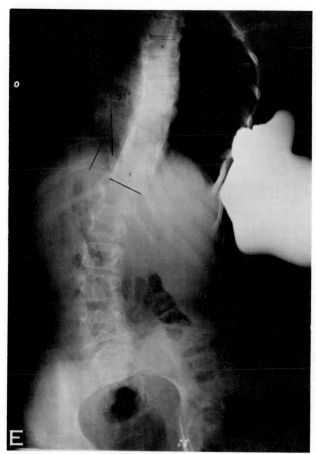

Figure 18.56 (*E*)

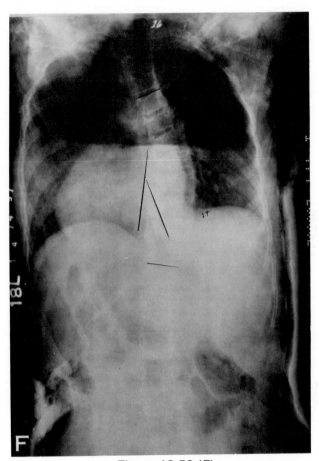

Figure 18.56 (*F*)

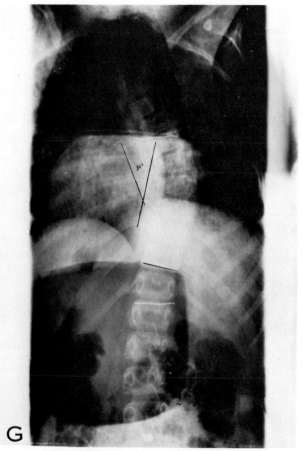

Figure 18.56 (*G*)

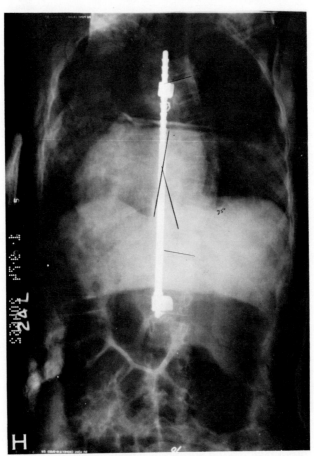

Figure 18.56 (*H*)

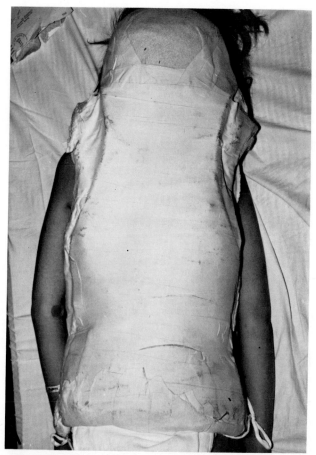

Figure 18.57.   (A) Risser localizer jacket extending well up over the posterior aspect of the head and down over the buttock. A posterior window will be cut out for preoperative level marking and through which the surgery will be performed. (B) Anterior view showing the molded chin piece, the throat, and abdominal windows. (C) Posterior window has been removed and the operative sites for both the fusion and the left posterior iliac crest donor site can be seen.

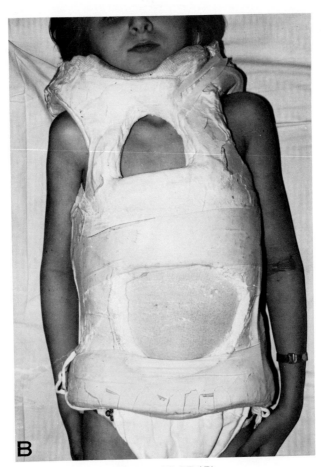

Figure 18.57 (*B*)

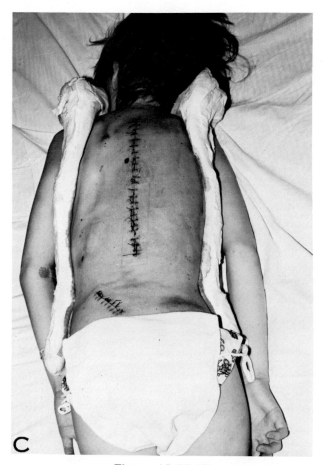

Figure 18.57 (*C*)

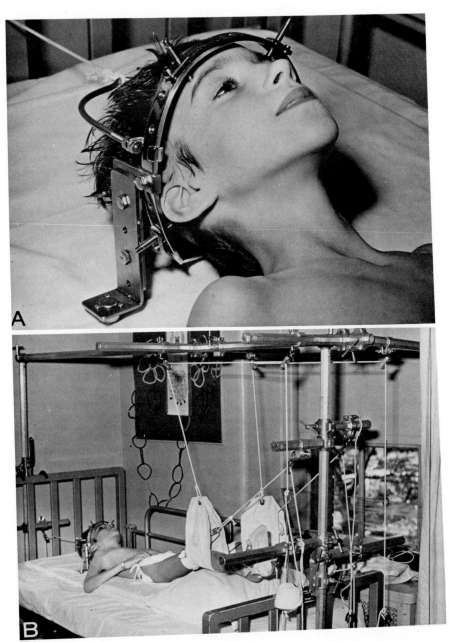

Figure 18.58. Halo-femoral traction (*A*) Halo. (*B*) Traction (*C*) Halo cast. This patient was treated in traction preoperatively. Postoperatively we could not use instrumentation. He was placed in a halo cast after primary wound healing.

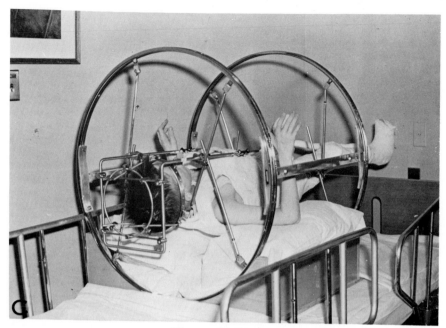

Figure 18.58 (C)

Cotrell method of traction and, therefore, are not in a position to express our own evaluation of its role.

The greater the forces used and the more rigid the curve undergoing correction, the more likely the patient is to develop complications such as pressure sores, neurologic deficit, etc. These patients demand close monitoring while undergoing preoperative correction.

Regardless of the preoperative method of correction used, we try to convert all patients into a localizer type of jacket immediately preoperatively (Fig. 18.57). Great care must be taken in transferring a patient from a turnbuckle jacket or halo-femoral traction so that significant correction is not lost.

The posterior aspect of the localizer cast is cut out exposing the entire length of the spine and both posterior iliac crests (Fig. 18.46D and 18.57).

The spine is marked at two levels, one at either end of the intended fusion area. We have found the methylene blue, metal marker technique, to be most satisfactory (Fig. 18.56F). Correct identification of the fusion levels is imperative (Fig. 18.60).

The selection of a fusion area in an idiopathic scoliosis must be done with extreme care if satisfactory results are to be obtained. Where a complete permissible correction has been obtained, the minimum fusion area in a stable idiopathic scoliosis is the extent of the major (structural) curve or curves. If it has not been possible to obtain the maximum amount of correction permissible, then the inclusion of some compensation by addition to the fusion area of an extra segment from the adjacent opposite curve or curves may be desirable. More recent work has shown in single major curves the extent of the fusion should be increased to include all those vertebrae that are rotated into the curve, that is, from the neutrally rotated vertebrae above (pedicle) to the neutrally rotated segment below the extent of the actual curve (Fig. 18.61). This has obviated apparent loss of correction caused by the angulation of adjacent vertebrae, particularly those inferior to the major curve. They can add to the length of the original curve and increases its angular deformity.

For some years now we have adopted Harrington spinal instrumentation combined with a spine fusion as our standard surgical technique for patients undergoing surgical treatment for idiopathic scoliosis. As a result, we have modified our spine fusion technique and now, in these instances, perform only a complete decortication of the posterior elements. If spinal instrumentation is not feasible, we still perform a modified Hibbs fusion

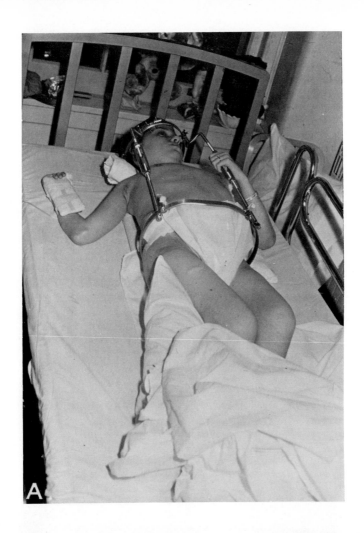

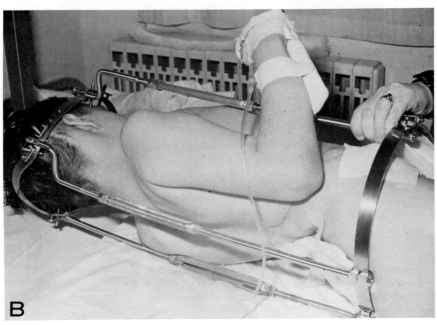

Figure 18.59. Halo-pelvic distraction: (*A*) anterior view. (*B*) lateral view.

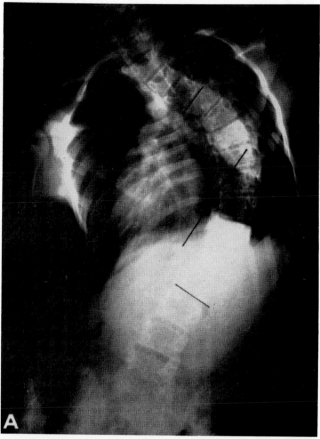

Figure 18.60.   (A) C.M. The original films demonstrate a major curve, D5 to L2. After correction and fusion, it was found that the fusion extended from D4 to L1. (B) C. M. Ten months postoperatively. Fusion area, D4 to L1, measures 23 degrees; L1 to L4 measures 7 degrees. (C) C.M. Thirty-one months postoperatively. Fusion area, D4 to L1, measured 32 degrees, and this measurement has been consistent since 12 months postoperatively. Note that there is recurrent angular deformity between L1 and L2; this deformity was originally part of the major curve and was omitted in error in the fusion area. The angular deformity between L1 and L4 is 44 degrees. (D) C.M. The patient was placed in a turnbuckle jacket and the angular deformity was reduced 7 degrees. Fusion was extended from L1 to L4. The patient has maintained this correction without loss.

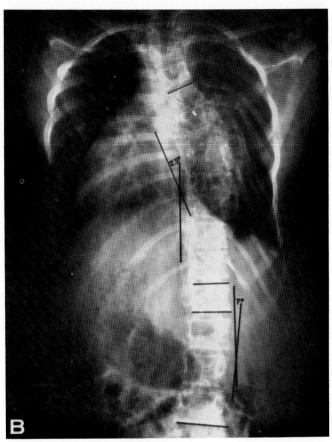

Figure 18.60 (*B*)

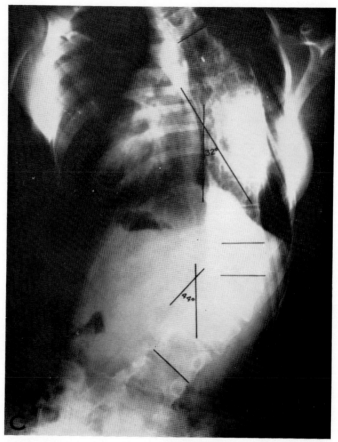

Figure 18.60 (*C*)

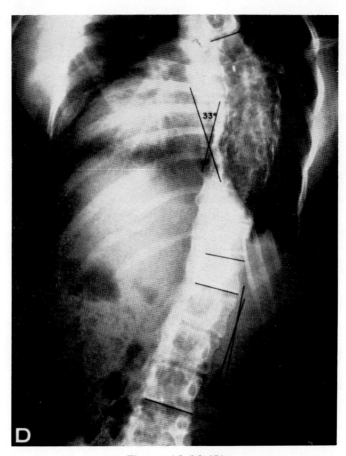

Figure 18.60 (*D*)

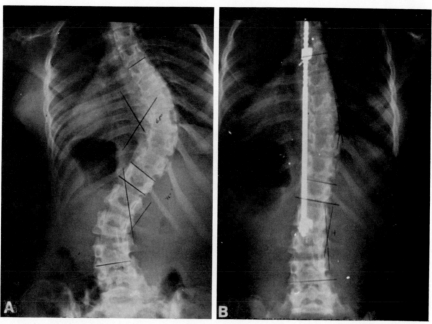

Figure 18.61.   K.R. Idiopathic scoliosis. (*A*) Major, structural, curve extends from T6 to T12. Pedicle rotation is not neutral until L1. Therefore, fusion is extended to L1 (*B*). This excellent correction has been maintained and there has been no adding to the major curve from below.

supplemented by autogenous posterior iliac crest bone (Fig. 18.62). In the thoracic area, the fusion bed extends from the tip of one transverse process across to the tip of its counterpart. In the lumbar area, we extend the fusion bed from facet to facet. We have found that, with the use of spinal instrumentation, the modified Hibbs type of fusion makes it technically more difficult to insert the distraction rod and its hooks. Further, since resorting to simple decortication over this same broad bed, our incidence of successful fusion in the presence of satisfactory instrumentation has not decreased but, rather, improved even though we permitted our patients to become ambulatory earlier.

We have discarded the use of the compression rods (Fig. 18.63) as a part of our standard procedure. In our hands it has not resulted in significantly increased correction or better maintenance of correction. As previously stated, we attempt to gain almost all the permissible correction preoperatively and, therefore, at the operating table we are attempting to gain only another 10–15 degrees. This limited goal of additional correction has a most important side benefit in that there is little opportunity for the operator to

produce a relatively sudden distraction with the potential for vascular embarrassment of the cord. We limit ourselves to that amount of force which can be applied to the distraction apparatus with one hand (approximately 40 inch-pounds).[94, 95] For similar reasons, we do not employ the outrigger to obtain correction.

The distraction hooks are placed into the facetal joint proximally on the concave side and beneath the superior laminal edge of the inferior lumbar vertebrae to be included in the fusion (Fig. 18.64). In a single major curve, the distal hook is placed on the concave side. In a double major curve, it is placed on the opposite side of the thoracic proximal hook, thus causing the rod to cross over to the opposite side.

Autogenous bone graft is obtained from the posterior iliac crest. Most patients have a sufficient volume of bone available from a single posterior crest.[41] Only occasionally is it necessary to supplement the graft volume with bone bank bone. We reserve the opposite crest for use, should a secondary procedure ever become necessary. In a few patients, particularly those with other forms of scoliosis because of the small posterior iliac crest, it may be necessary to rely entirely on bone bank bone. This is strictly second class bone as has been shown in our studies of consecutive patients whose spine fusions were explored routinely 6 months postoperatively (Table 18.4).[22, 24, 26, 82] Since the incidence of pseudoarthrosis was reduced so dramatically by the use of autogenous bone, we feel that routine exploration is not indicated in patients in whom autogenous graft can be used and particularly, in those in whom spinal instrumentation has been performed. We reserve exploration for those who show a significant amount of loss of correction (10 degrees or more).

With rare exception, all of our patients undergo a one-stage operative procedure. Blood loss is followed by weighing sponges and appropriate replacement is given with either whole blood or packed cells and plasma. The patient undergoes continuous monitoring with electrocardiogram, central venous pressure, and temperature and, in the more complicated or prolonged cases, blood gases are determined at intervals.

In spite of the use of spinal instrumentation, it is still the mature fusion that must be counted upon to maintain the corrected position against all the forces that have produced the curve. The necessity for a mature massive fusion is apparent.

Immediately postoperatively, the patient is maintained recumbent in the localizer jacket or the turnbuckle jacket, etc., until the sutures are removed on the tenth postoperative day. We routinely have a nasogastric tube in place

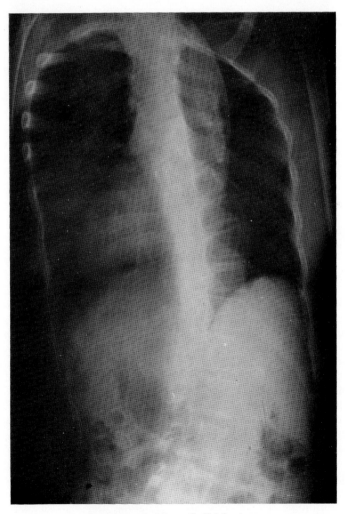

Figure 18.62. Solid fusion.

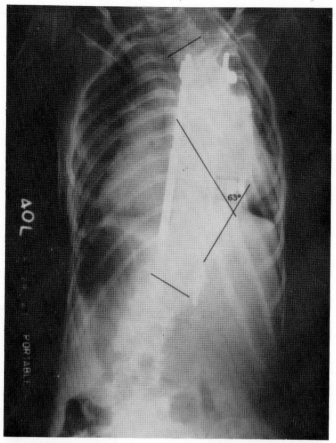

Figure 18.63. P.S. Spine instrumentation performed as described by Harrington. This patient has shown no significant loss of correction in 1 year.

and it is maintained until bowel sounds are present and the patient is able to tolerate liquids with the tube clamped off. By such a system, we have been able to avoid the "cast syndrome."[31, 52, 104] The hemoglobin and hematocrit are checked the day postoperative and 2–3 days later. Additional blood may be required in the early postoperative period, particularly if the amount of replacement blood and other maintainers of fluid volume has not been adequate. We do not use prophylactic antibiotic coverage in the routine idiopathic scoliosis patient. We emphasize pulmonary toilet and place all our patients on an "intermittent positive pressure breathing" program.

In the immediate postoperative period, it is imperative that the patient be carefully monitored[96] for the presence of, or the development of, neurologic deficit. We have not resorted to waking the patients during surgery to have them move their feet at the time instrumentation has been completed, as described by Hilal and Keim,[57] nor do we perform routine preoperative selective angiography. We do closely check the patient in the recovery room for neurologic deficit. The presence of acute anterior thigh pain is a prodromal symptom of impending neurologic deficit. If neurologic deficit is present or develops, it is an immediate indication for the removal of the rod and one should not try to reinsert it. Time is of the essence if recovery is to be expected. This has become abundantly clear in the reports of the morbidity committee of the Scoliosis Research Society.

Following suture removal and primary wound healing, a new localizer cast is applied and the patient is permitted to become ambulatory. If spinal instrumentation has not been used, the patient is not permitted to get

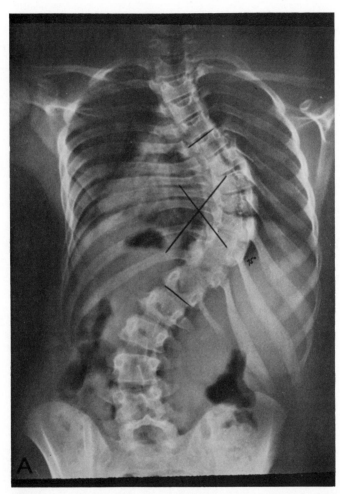

Figure 18.64. (*A*) K.S. Adolescent idiopathic scoliosis. Age 12 at time of surgery. Treated in a localizer cast preoperatively. (*B*) Discharged 11 days postoperative; ambulatory, wearing a newly applied localizer cast. This correction has been maintained.

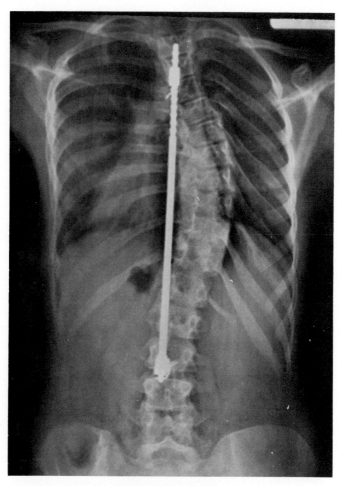

Figure 18.64 (*B*)

Table 18.4
Follow-up of Patients with Spinal Fusion

Graft	No. of Patients	Pseudoarthrosis No	%
A. Occurrence of pseudoarthrosis			
Homologous	54	18	33
Autogenous	81	8	9.9
B. Number of vertebrae in fusion area 4–8			
Homologous	54	20	37
Autogenous	63	2	3
C. Number of vertebrae in fusion area 9–14			
Homologous	26	9	35
Autogenous	37	8	22

up but, rather, remains recumbent. The vast majority of the patients are suitable for instrumentation and, therefore, are discharged to their homes ambulatory. They may return to school on a limited activity program (no gym, etc.). Six months postoperatively the cast is removed and x-rays are taken to determine the maintenance of correction and the progression of the fusion. The bony mass is best visualized in oblique projections of the fusion area. A body cast is then applied for another 4–5 months. If at 11 months follow-up roentgenographs are satisfactory, the patient is permitted to discard the body cast and gradually resume normal activities. We ask our patients not to engage in such sports as tumbling, the use of a trampoline, etc.

It is our experience that, with a solid mature fusion, there is no appreciable loss of correction. Since we have switched to using autogenous rather than homologous bone, the incidence of pseudoarthrosis has markedly decreased from about 30% to less than 10% in patients with idiopathic scoliosis. With spinal instrumentation, this has been further reduced to less than 3% in the patient with idiopathic scoliosis (Fig. 18.65) (Table 18.4).

Postpoliomyelitis Scoliosis

Patients with postpoliomyelitis scoliosis in the past accounted for approximately 10% of the cases of scoliosis seen. However, as we get further and further away from the pre-vaccine days, their numbers are rapidly diminishing; but there are still some cases being referred for their spinal problems.[9, 44, 62, 76, 100] Many of these people have unstable spines and, for them, correction and fusion may be indicated to obtain stability rather than for the amount of correction permissible.

All patients who have had anterior poliomyelitis must be watched for the development of scoliosis. Some of them do not develop a clinically evident scoliosis for as long as 10 years after the onset of the disease. One cannot predict which patients will develop scoliosis by the muscles involved. The muscles attached to the spine are numerous and the possible mathematical combinations in which they may be involved, as well as their effect upon the spine, cannot be comprehended. The use of bracing and casts in the postpoliomyelitis scoliosis may have definite value in providing stability for the trunk, but it must not be felt that they will stop the curve from progressing.

Patients with postpoliomyelitis requiring the use of respirators have been shown to develop and increase an angular deformity even though their activities are so completely confined and their recumbency so prolonged.

In selecting the area for fusion in these patients, at least the major (structural) curve and a segment or more below it must be included. At times it may be necessary to fuse a more extensive area in order to provide the necessary stability. In some patients it may be desirable to fuse to the sacrum. When the cervical region is severely involved (Fig. 18.66), it may be necessary to include the cervical spine and occiput in the fusion area. In these patients, it is usually desirable to use the halo technique. A preliminary tracheostomy may be desirable if they have severe respiratory involvement. The more severely involved the patients are, the more the spine telescopes and the more the patient needs stability. These patients must be stable sitters. Very early and extensive fusion in some patients has resulted in severe lordosis, but these patients were operated upon before spinal instrumentation was available. As in all cases of scoliosis, each patient must be individually evaluated, and therapy must be adapted to the evaluation.

It may be advisable to use halo-pelvic distraction for correction and immobilization for those patients with marked respiratory embarrassment who would not tolerate a plaster jacket. These patients may be operated upon

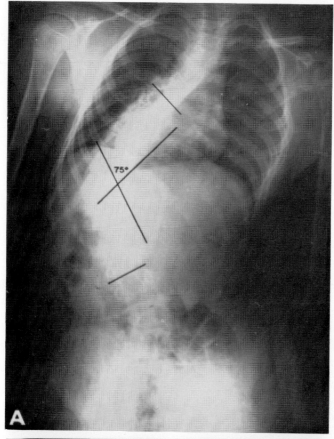

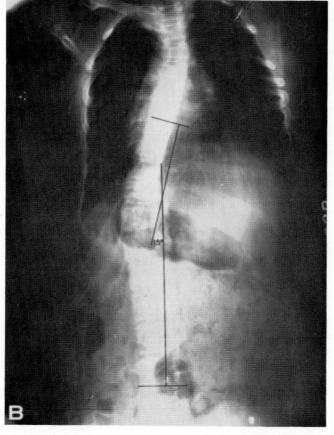

Figure 18.65. (*A*). K.W. Postpolio scoliosis with a major curve extending from D7 to L3 and measuring 75 degrees. This patient underwent correction and fusion. (*B*) K.W. One year postoperatively. Spine fusion, D7 to L4, measuring 15 degrees. (*C*). K.W. Sixteen months postoperatively. Loss of correction is 30 degrees. Patient has been ambulatory 6 months. Note loss of correction at apex. (*D*). K.W. Oblique films. *Arrows* point to pseudarthrosis. (*E*). K.W. Bending film to the concavity of the major curve, demonstrating that the opposite curves, D1 to D7, measuring 30 degrees, and L4 to the sacrum, measuring 7 degrees, would permit reduction of the major curve through pseudarthrosis. (*F*). K.W. Bending film toward the convexity of the major curve, D7 to L4, measuring 33 degrees as compared to 45 degrees in the standard film. This demonstrates obvious motion at the level of pseudarthrosis. (*G*). K.W. Postoperative film following Risser jacket correction and repair of pseudarthrosis, D11 to D12, measuring 22 degrees. Note the large mass of bony fusion at the level of repair. (*H*). K.W. Oblique film. Arrows pointing to the area of repair of pseudarthrosis. This patient has shown no further loss in more than 3 years.

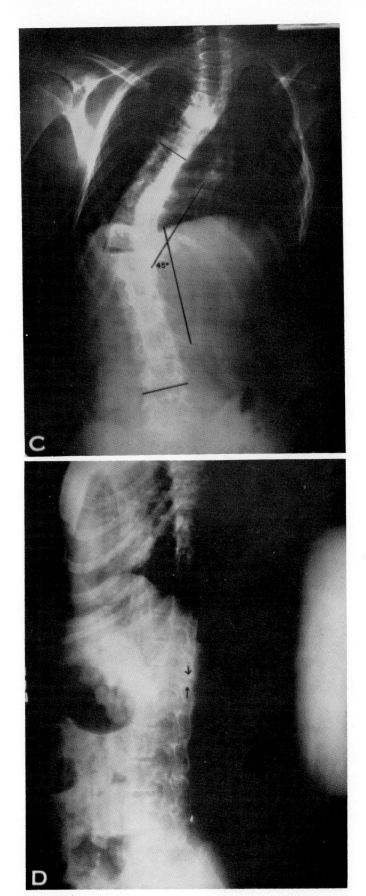

Figure 18.65 (*C* and *D*)

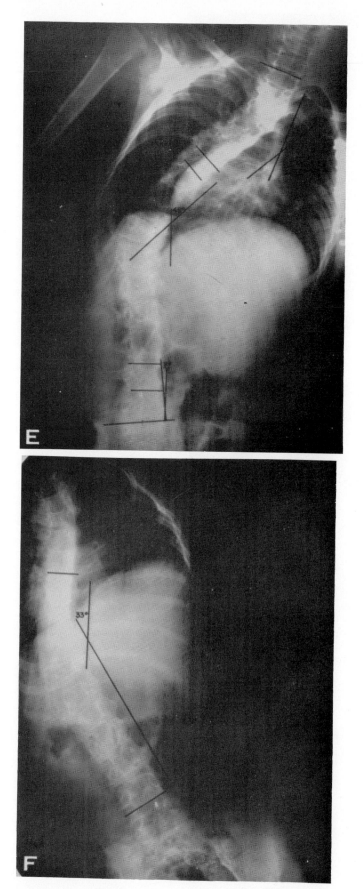

Figure 18.65 (*E* and *F*)

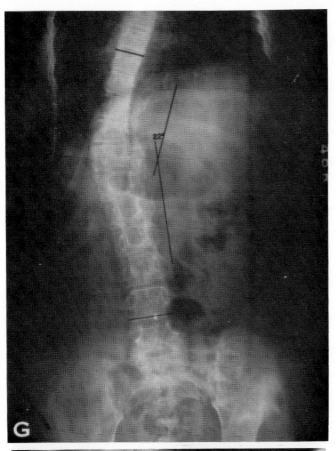

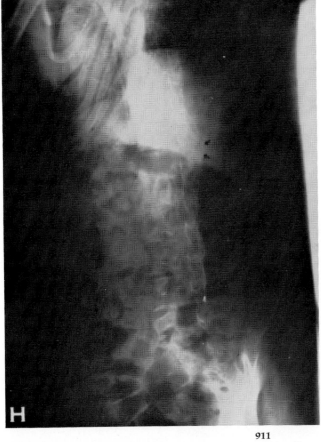

Figure 18.65 (*G* and *H*)

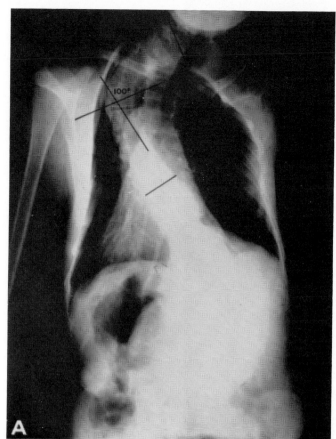

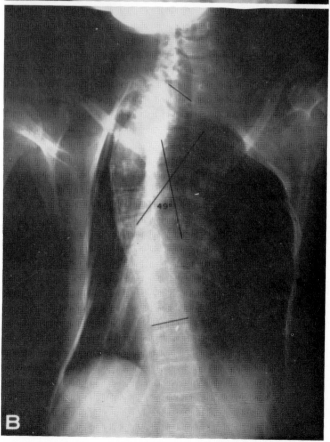

Figure 18.66. (*A*) Postpolio scoliosis with a cervical component to the major curve. (*B*) Postoperative film following correction and fusion. When the scoliosis involves the cervical region, tne serial films must include it.

while in the apparatus by temporarily removing one or two of the uprights during surgery. The avoidance of a prolonged period of immobilization in a plaster jacket may prevent further reduction of their already faulty pulmonary function.

For patients in whom it is necessary to fuse to the sacrum, we have found Harrington's spinal instrumentation in combination with the sacral bar to be of particular value because of the gross instability of their spines.

Congenital Scoliosis

In evaluating a congenital scoliosis, one cannot add up the segmental errors to determine the prognosis. It must be remembered that the x-rays show only the bony variations and not the associated soft-tissue changes. These patients must be closely observed, not only for a change in the scoliosis, but also for the development of neurologic deficits—motor, sensory, or sphincter changes (Fig. 18.67). Any of these suggests the possibility of such lesions as diastematomyelia, extradural lipomas, etc. Patients who have errors in segmentation usually have a trunk that is short in proportion to the extremeties. Most congenital scolioses are stable.[105, 118, 119] Elsewhere in this chapter the management of congenital scoliosis is discussed in detail. In general, procedures that shorten the spine and that can be performed in the lumbar area have

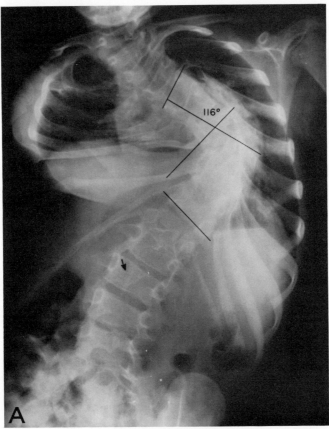

Figure 18.67. (A) C.W. Five-year-old female with congenital osteopathic scoliosis. Major curve, D5 to D11, 116 degrees. Serial x-rays have not shown any progression of the angular deformity, but repeated neurologic examination revealed development of diminished sensation of L5 and S1 and progressive loss of function in the right peroneals. On the original examination, and for a year thereafter, the neurologic examination of the extremity had been negative. (B) Myelogram demonstrating diastematomyelia, level of L1. Surgical correction resulted in return of sensation and no further progression of peroneal weakness.

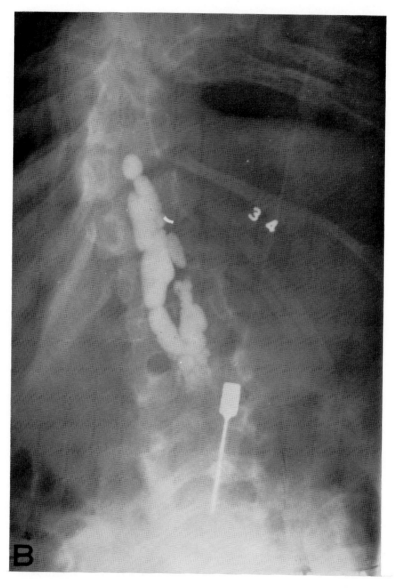

Figure 18.67 (*B*)

less chance of producing neurologic embarrassment.[58, 73, 84, 130–132] Other congenital anomalies should be sought in these patients, i.e., kidney.[80]

von Recklinghausen's Neurofibromatosis

The curve pattern in a patient who has a scoliosis associated with a neurofibromatosis is usually characteristic (Fig. 18.68). The curve presents a short, sharp angular pattern by x-ray (Fig. 18.69) and the structural changes are usually greater than those usually associated with the amount of angular deformity present.[113, 129] This is particularly evident in the milder curves. Many of these patients show the cutaneous manifestations of neurofibromatosis: café aulait spots, subcutaneous neurofibroma, or pedunculated

neurofibroma. Almost all of these patients require correction and fusion. It has been the experience of many that these curves usually progress and eventually produce the most severe deformity seen in the patient with scoliosis. Many believe that, once the diagnosis is made, correction and fusion should be performed. Their belief stems from an appreciation of the marked deformity that usually develops if correction and fusion are not done. The propensity for these patients to develop neurologic problems has been well defined by Cobb, and by Curtis.[18]

In the patient with neurofibromatosis and scoliosis, one must not consider performing a laminectomy for relief of the symptoms of spinal cord pressure secondary to neurofibroma before performing a spine fusion. It has been the experience of those who have performed such a procedure, prior to stabi-

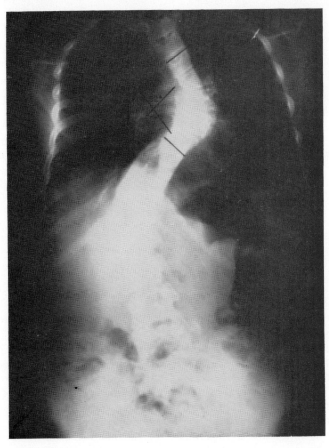

Figure 18.68. G.M. Neuropathic scoliosis, von Recklinghausen. This patient had all the characteristic skin manifestations of neurofibromatosis. Notice the short, sharp, angular major curve, D4 to D8, measuring 82 degrees. This curve pattern is typical of those seen in neuropathic scoliosis.

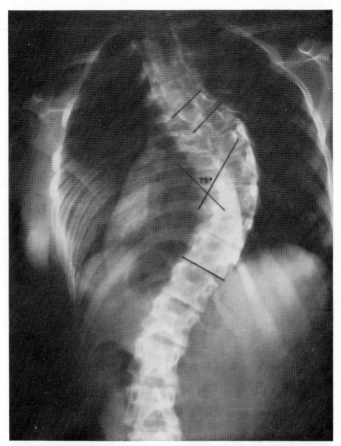

Figure 18.69. M.B. Neuropathic scoliosis, von Recklinghausen. This patient has all the characteristic skin manifestations. The fifth, sixth, seventh, and eighth ribs show "neurotrophic" effect. There is marked wedging of D7 out of proportion to the rest of the curve.

lization of the spine, that the results are often diastrous. The neurologic deficit may increase precipitously.

Postempyema and Post-thoracoplasty Scolioses

Postempyema and post-thoracoplasty scolioses[6, 7, 46, 71, 120] are becoming less of a problem because of the decreased incidence of empyema and thoracoplasty and the successful way in which the problems associated with them are currently handled. These scolioses should always be looked for, particularly in the skeletally immature. The patient who has had either empyema or a thoracoplasty should be followed by serial x-ray films of the spine if there is any suggestion of a developing scoliosis. Correction and fu-

sion are indicated when a significant curve develops or when definite progression is demonstrated. It is usually in childhood that a significant scoliosis develops from either of these causes.

Muscular Dystrophy

The patients with muscular dystrophy who develop scoliosis often develop an extreme amount of deformity. The recognition of the associated disease is extremely important. These patients must not be placed in recumbency during the period of time required for correction and fusion. To do so will cause the muscular atrophy to progress to the point where walking may no longer be possible. In selected patients, we have performed correction and fusion with spinal instrumentation in an effort to improve their sitting ability and prolong their useful life (Fig. 18.70). Again, the use of halo-pelvic distraction has proven to be valuable.

Postirradiation Scoliosis

This is a specific type of acquired scoliosis.[2, 3, 25, 69, 74] It is usually seen as a result of the irradiation therapy administered to infants in the course of treatment of either a Wilms' tumor or a neuroblastoma. A careful study of these patients reveals that no definite changes are seen in the irradiated segments until approximately 2 years after the therapy was administered. The changes that occur are attributable to the growth inhibition secondary to the irradiation. The vertebral bodies show irregular ossification and, in many instances, resemble lesions seen in osteochondrodystrophy. The scarred outline of the vertebral body may be visible and appear as an os within an os. This form of structural scoliosis may progress (Fig. 18.71). Since these patients have had their insult early in life, the

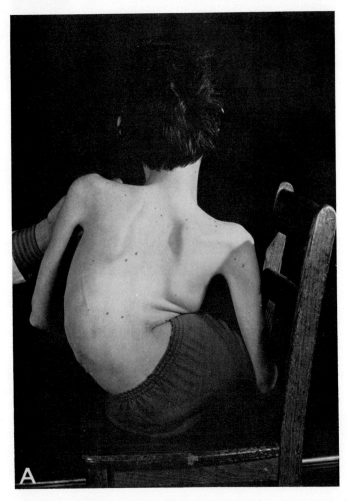

Figure 18.70. Muscular dystrophy. (*A*) This patient's muscular dystrophy is advanced. He is unable to sit alone without external support. (*B*) Simple manual suspension corrects most of his deformity. Patients of this category are, on occasion, considered for correction and fusion provided their life expectancy and general medical condition warrants. With such marked telescoping and limited extremity power, the desirability of stabilizing the spine is obvious. Since the advent of spinal instrumentation and halo-pelvic distraction, the possibilities for performing such surgery are improved.

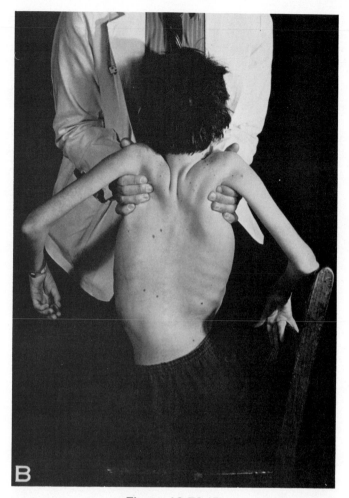

Figure 18.70 (*B*)

growth inhibition produced may be severe, and, therefore, the resulting deformity may be severe. In our series of 37 patients, all patients who have developed a postirradiation scoliosis have received more than 1,200 R tumor dose. All patients in whom the tumor or the surgery involved the spine were excluded from this study.

This type of scoliosis has the same characteristics as all other structural scolioses, i.e., wedging, rotation, and definitive curve pattern.

These patients should be subjected to the same careful clinical and roentgenographic follow-up. Correction and fusion should be performed on those who show continuing progression, or who have developed a significant angular deformity. In our series, only 2 patients have progressed to the degree that they required correction and fusion. Where the necessary surgery to remove the tumor included the excision of spinal elements or when the tumor itself invaded the structure of the spine of the patient, the degree of scoliosis that followed was almost without exception progressive and severe.

Summary

In summary, it would seem that intelligent management of a patient with scoliosis is dependent upon appreciation of etiology. The vast majority of patients do not require correction and fusion. When correction and fusion is indicated, it must be carefully

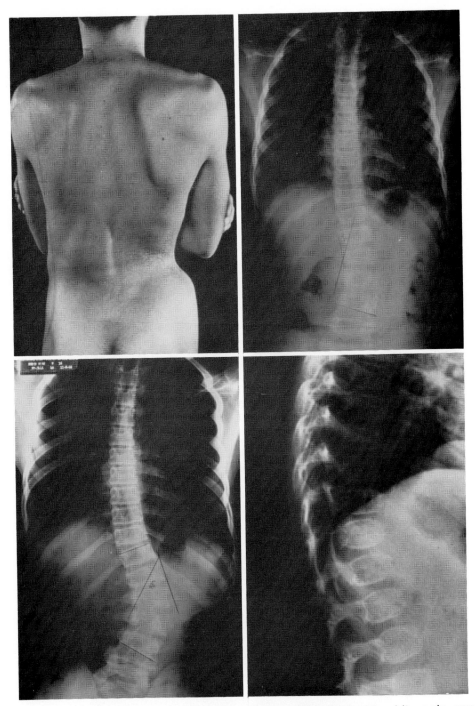

Figure 18.71. (*Top, left*) Postirradiation scoliosis, 1962. Patient is white male, age 12; Wilms' tumor excised at age 4. (*Top, right*) Progressive increase over next 2 years, but none since he became skeletally mature (*bottom, left*). Lateral roentgenogram demonstrates postirradiation change, os with os. This is "the scar of the insult of the irradiation" (*bottom, right*).

planned and carried out. If these criteria are met, successful correction and fusion can be obtained and the results are gratifying.

It is our considered opinion that in treating scoliosis surgically, the surgeon must have an extensive understanding of the mechanics of the spine. He should handle the problem frequently and he should have available an anesthesiologist who is familiar with scoliosis and who is capable of handling the endotracheal anesthesia required.

The surgeon must realize that the opportunity to obtain correction and fusion for the rest of the patient's life normally occurs only once during that lifetime. Salvage procedures for loss of correction or for inadequate fu-

sions are, at best, second rate. Time, therefore, is not of the essence, but adequate correction and a solid and mature fusion are.

Postlumboperitoneal Shunt Lordosis

For the past 10 years, we and others[23, 50] have become increasingly concerned about the effect upon the spine that lumboperitoneal shunting for communicating hydrocephalus can produce. Most often, the patient develops a fixed, progressive lordosis (Fig. 18.72). Less often, a significant degree of scoliosis develops.

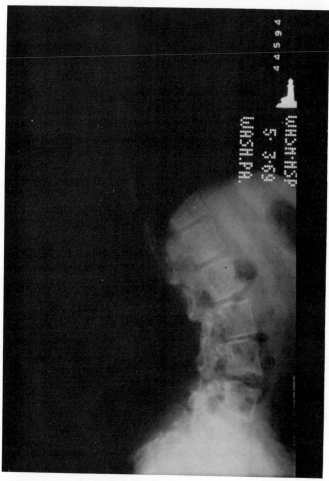

Figure 18.72. C.C. Lumboperitoneal shunt performed as an infant. His lordosis is fixed and progressive. Note the narrow disc space, L3-L4, level of the operative procedure posteriorly. Many of these patients show this particular change suggesting failure of the disc space to expand, similar to that seen when a fusion has been performed in early childhood.

Nonoperative treatment is ineffectual whether braces, traction, or exercises are employed.

We have found that in the patients with fixed lordosis, the posterior approach is ineffective. Therefore, our routine is to perform anterior wedge resection and place the patient in 90-90 skeletal traction. If the wedge does not close within 10 days to 2 weeks, we perform a second-stage procedure posteriorly. At that time, the facets opposite the level of the anterior wedge are resected and this permits desired correction (Fig. 18.73).

The scoliosis that occurs in these patients is also a very rigid type but does respond to turnbuckle jacket correction and fusion.

Removal of the shunt has no beneficial effect upon the spinal deformity or its progression. We feel that this type of shunting procedure should be avoided because of its destructive effect upon the spine. The unanswered question to date is how extensive a posterior spine fusion, if any, should be performed following the correction of lordosis. Based on our limited experience, it would appear that in the skeletally immature pa-

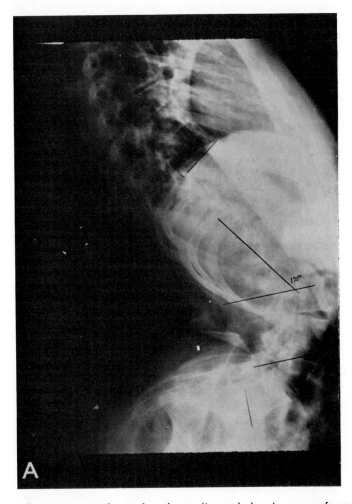

Figure 18.73. A.S., 14 years of age. Lumboperitoneal shunt was performed in infancy. Progressive lordosis was noted to have its onset at age 3 and obviously noticeable by age 8. (A) Preoperative roentgenogram demonstrating 125 degrees of fixed lordosis. (B) Following the first stage, anterior wedge resection L3-L4, the lordosis reduced only partially after 3 weeks in 90-90 traction. After second stage, the resection of the facets at L3-L4, the lordosis is corrected.

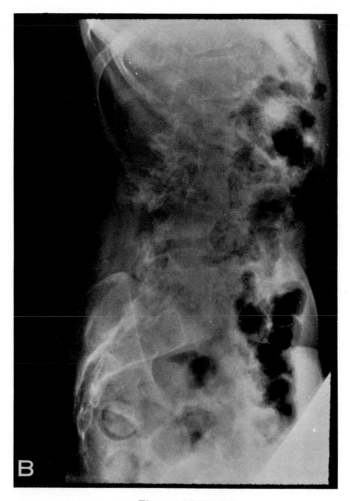

Figure 18.73 (B)

tient, a spine fusion and Harrington instrumentation should be added to the posterior procedure. We have had one patient whose deformity recurred at a higher level and required secondary surgery. She was skeletally immature. The older patients have not shown this.

References

1. Albee, F. H., and Kushner, A.: Albee spine fusion operation in treatment of scoliosis, *Surg. Gynecol. Obstet., 66:* 797, 1938.
2. Arkin, A. M., Pack H. F., Ransohoff, N. S., and Simon, N.: Radiation-induced scoliosis, *J. Bone Joint Surg., 32A:* 401, 1950.
3. Arkin, A. M., and Simon, N.: Radiation scoliosis; experimental study, *J. Bone Joint Surg., 31A:* 394, 1960.
4. Balmer, G. A., and MacEwen, G. D.: The incidence and treatment of scoliosis in cerebral palsy, *J. Bone Joint Surg., 52B:* 134, 1970.
5. Barr, J. S.: Turnbuckle brace, 3 point pressure brace for correction and treatment of ambulatory care of scoliosis, *J. Bone Joint Surg., 18:* 760, 1936.
6. Bisgard, J. D.: Thoracogenic scoliosis; influence of thoracic disease and thoracic operations, *Arch. Surg., 29:* 417, 1934.
7. Bjork, V. O.: Scoliosis and herniation after osteoplastic thoracoplasty, *J. Thorac. Cardiovasc. Surg., 38:* 81, 1959.
8. Blount, W. P., and Moe, J. H.: *The Milwaukee Brace:* Baltimore: Williams & Wilkins, 1973.
9. Bonnett, C., Perry, J., Brown, J. C., and Greenberg, B. J.: Halo-femoral distraction and posterior spine fusion for paralytic scoliosis, *J. Bone Joint Surg., 54A:* 202, 1972.
10. Cobb, J. R.: Treatment of scoliosis, *Conn. Med. J., 7:* 467, 1943.
11. Cobb, J. R.: Outline for study of scoliosis, *Instruct. Lect. Am. Acad. Orthop. Surg., 5:* 1948.
12. Cobb, J. R.: Technique, after-treatment and results

of spine fusion for scoliosis, *Instruct. Lect. Am. Acad. Orthop. Surg.,* 9: 65, 1952.

13. Cobb, J. R.: The problem of the primary curve, *J. Bone Joint Surg.,* 42A: 1413, 1960.

14. Cobb, J. R.: Scoliosis, quo vadis, *J. Bone Joint Surg.,* 40A: 507, 1968.

15. Collis, D. K., and Ponseti, I. V.: Long-term follow-up patients with idiopathic scoliosis not treated surgically, *J. Bone Joint Surg.,* 51A: 425, 1969.

16. Cowell, H. R., Hall, J. N., and MacEwen, G. D.: Genetic aspects of idiopathic scoliosis, *Clin Orthop.,* 86: 121, 1972.

17. Curtis, B. H.: Classification of myelomeningocele and congenital spinal defects, In *Symposium on Myelomeningocele,* pp. 3–10; St. Louis: C. V. Mosby, 1972.

18. Curtis, B. H., Fisher, R. L., Butterfield, W. L., and Saunders, F. P.: Neurofibromatosis with paraplegia; report of 8 cases, *J. Bone Joint Surg.,* 51A: 843, 1969.

19. Dewald, R. L., Mulcahey, T. M., and Schultz, A. B.: Force measurement studies with the halo-hoop apparatus in scoliosis, *Orthop. Rev.,* 2: 17, 1973.

20. Dewald, R. L., and Ray, R. D.: Skeletal traction for the treatment of severe scoliosis; The University of Illinois halo-hoop apparatus, *J. Bone Joint Surg.,* 52A: 233, 1970.

21. Donaldson, W. F.: Scoliosis associated with spina bifida and myelomeningocele, In *Post Graduate Course on the Management and Care of the Scoliosis Patient,* pp. 40–42; New York, 1969.

22. Donaldson, W.F.: The problem of pseudoarthrosis in scoliosis surgery, In *Post Graduate Course on the Management and Care of the Scoliosis Patient,* pp. 75–77; New York, 1969.

23. Donaldson, W. F.: Neural spinal dysraphism, In *Spinal Deformity in Neurological and Muscular Disorders;* St. Louis: C. V. Mosby.

24. Donaldson, W. F., and Wissinger, H. A.: The results of surgical exploration of spine fusion period for scoliosis, *West J. Surg.,* 72: 195, 1964.

25. Donaldson, W. F., and Wissinger, H. A.: Axial skeletal changes following tumor dose radiation therapy, *J. Bone Joint Surg.,* 47A: 1469, 1967.

26. Donaldson, W. F., Wissinger, H. A., and Stone, C. S.: Exploration of scoliosis spine fusions, *J. Bone Joint Surg.,* 51A: 205, 1969.

27. Dwyer, A. F.: Anterior instrumentation in scoliosis, *J. Bone Joint Surg.,* 52B: 782, 1970.

28. Dwyer, A. F.: Screw and cable correction of scoliosis, *J. Bone Joint Surg.,* 52B: 193, 1970.

29. Dwyer, A. F., Newton, M. C., and Sherwood, A. A.: An anterior approach to scoliosis; preliminary report, *Clin. Orthop.,* 62: 192, 1969.

30. Edmonson, A. S.: Evaluation of Milwaukee brace treatment in idiopathic scoliosis, *J. Bone Joint Surg.,* 51A: 202, 1969.

31. Evarts, C. M., Winter, R. B., and Hall H. E.: The spinal traction syndrome—arteriomesenteric-duodenal obstruction associated with correction of spinal curvature with report of 3 illustrative cases, *J. Bone Joint Surg.,* 53A: 198, 1971.

32. Ferguson, A. B.: Study and treatment of scoliosis, *South, Med. J.,* 23: 116, 1930.

33. Ferguson, A. B.: Roentgen diagnosis in extremities and spine, *Instruct. Lect. Am. Acad. Orthop. Surg.,* 2: 214, 1947.

34. Ferguson, A. B.: Roentgen interpretations and decisions in scoliosis, *Instruct. Lect. Am. Acad. Orthop. Surg.,* 7: 160, 1950.

35. Ferreira, J. H., and James, J. I. P.: Progressive and resolving infantile idiopathic scoliosis; differential diagnosis, *J. Bone Joint Surg.,* 54B: 648, 1972.

36. Filho, N. A., and Thompson, M. W.: Genetic studies in scoliosis, *J. Bone Joint Surg.,* 53A: 199, 1971.

37. Galante, J., Schultz, A., DeWald, R. L., and Ray, R. D.: Forces acting in the Milwaukee brace on patients undergoing treatment for idiopathic scoliosis, *J. Bone Joint Surg.,* 52A: 498, 1970.

38. George, K., and Reppstein, J.: A comparative study of the two popular methods of measuring scoliotic deformity of the spine, *J. Bone Joint Surg.,* 43A: 809, 1961.

39. Goldstein, L. A.: Results in the treatment of scoliosis with turnbuckle plaster cast correction and fusion, *J. Bone Joint Surg.,* 41A: 321, 1959.

40. Goldstein, L. A.: Surgical management of scoliosis, *J. Bone Joint Surg.,* 43: 167, 1966.

41. Goldstein, L. A.: Treatment of idiopathic scoliosis by Harrington instrumentation and fusion with fresh autogenous iliac-bone grafts, *J. Bone Joint Surg.,* 51A: 209, 1969.

42. Goldstein, L. A., and Evarts, C. M.: Follow up notes on articles previously published in the *Journal;* further experiences with the treatment of scoliosis by cast correction and spine fusion with fresh autogenous iliac-bone grafts, *J. Bone Joint Surg.,* 48: 962, 1966.

43. Graham, J. J., Schack, J. A., and Liggett, A. S.: Cardiopulmonary function in scoliosis; preoperative and postoperative study, *J. Bone Joint Surg.,* 52A: 399, 1970.

44. Gucker, T.: Experience with poliomyelitic scoliosis after fusion and correction, *J. Bone Joint Surg.,* 38A: 1281, 1956.

45. Gucker, T.: Changes in vital capacity in scoliosis; primary report on effects of treatment, *J. Bone Joint Surg.,* 44A: 469, 1962.

46. Gurd, F. B.: Scoliosis accompanying chronic infected open pneumothorax; its causation and correction, *Arch. Surg.,* 5: 366, 1922.

47. Hall, J. E.: The management of scoliosis, *J. Bone Joint Surg.,* 52A: 408, 1970.

48. Hall, J. E., Chan, D., Spira, I., and Roth, A.: Dwyer instrumentation and anterior spine fusion, Unpublished data.

49. Hall, J. E., and Gillespie, R.: Idiopathic scoliosis treated by Harrington instrumentation and spine fusion, *J. Bone Joint Surg.,* 53A: 198, 1971.

50. Hall, J. E., and King, J. D.: Hyperlordosis following lumbar peritoneal shunts for hydrocephalus, *J. Bone Joint Surg.,* 53A: 198, 1971.

51. Hall, J. E., and Spira, I. S.: Dwyer anterior instrumentation and interbody fusion of the spine in the management of scoliosis, *J. Bone Joint Surg.,* 54A: 201, 1972.

52. Hardy, J. H., Cooke, R. W., and Einbund, M.: Hyperalimentation in the treatment of "cast syndrome," *J. Bone Joint Surg.,* 54A: 200, 1972.

53. Harrington, P. R.: Treatment of scoliosis, *J. Bone Joint Surg.,* 44A: 591, 1962.

54. Harrington, P. R. First Progress Report: A Surgical Correction of Paralytic Scoliosis. Monograph.

55. Harrington, P. R.: Treatment of scoliosis; correction

and internal fixation by spine instrumentation, *J. Bone Joint Surg.*, 44A: 591, 1962.

56. Hibbs, R. A., Risser, J. D., and Ferguson, A. B.: Scoliosis treated by fusion operation, end-result study of 360 cases, *J. Bone Joint Surg.*, 13: 91, 1931.
57. Hilal, S. K., and Keim, H. A.: Selective spinal angiography in adolescent scoliosis, *Radiology*, 102: 340, 1972.
58. Hodgson, A. R.: Correction of fixed spinal curves, *J. Bone Joint Surg.*, 44A: 591, 1962.
59. Houtkin, S., and Levine, D. B.: The halo yoke; a simplified device for attachment of the halo to a body cast, *J. Bone Joint Surg.*, 54A: 881, 1972.
60. James, J.: Two curve patterns in idiopathic structural scoliosis, *J. Bone Joint Surg.*, 33B: 399, 1951.
61. James, J.: Idiopathic scoliosis, *J. Bone Joint Surg.* 36B: 36, 1954.
62. James, J.: Paralytic scoliosis, *J. Bone Joint Surg.*, 38B: 660, 1956.
63. James, J.: Symposium on the treatment of organic spinal deformities; the indications for correction and fusion, *Proc. R. Soc. Med.*, 51: 236, 1958.
64. James, J.: Infantile structural scoliosis, *J. Bone Joint Surg.*, 41: 719, 1959.
65. James, J.: Infantile idiopathic scoliosis, *Clin. Orthop.*, 21: 106, 1961.
66. James, J. I. P.: The etiology of scoliosis, *J. Bone Joint Surg.*, 52B: 410, 1970.
67. Johnson, B. E., and Westgate, H. D.: Methods of predicting vital capacity in patients with thoracic scoliosis, *J. Bone Joint Surg.*, 52A: 1433, 1970.
68. Kane, W. J., and Moe, J. H.: A scoliosis prevalence survey in Minnesota, *Clin. Orthop.*, 69: 216, 1970.
69. Katzman, H., Waugh, T., and Berdon, W.: Skeletal changes following irradiation of childhood tumors, *J. Bone Joint Surg.*, 51A: 825, 1969.
70. Kendrick, J.: Correction of scoliosis by use of modified turnbuckle jacket, *Cleve. Clin. Q.*, 4: 16, 1937.
71. Kergin, F. G., and Dewar, F. P.: Pleural decortication in prevention and treatment of thoracogenic scoliosis (resulting from fibrothorax), *Arch. Surg.*, 61: 705, 1950.
72. Lamarre, A., Hall, J. E., Weng, T. R., Aspin, N., and Levison, H.: Pulmonary function in scoliosis 1 year after surgical correction, *J. Bone Joint Surg.*, 53A: 195, 1971.
73. Leatherman, K. D.: Resection of vertebral bodies, *J. Bone Joint Surg.*, 51A: 206, 1969.
74. Leatherman, K. D.: Radiation deformities of the spine, *J. Bone Joint Surg.*, 52A: 405, 1970.
75. Levine, D. B., Wilson, R. L., and Doherty, J. H.: Operative management of idiopathic scoliosis; a critical analysis of 67 cases, *J. Bone Joint Surg.*, 52A: 408, 1970.
76. Lowman, C. L.: Relation of abdominal muscles to paralytic scoliosis, *J. Bone Joint Surg.*, 14: 763, 1932.
77. Loynes, R. D.: Scoliosis after thoracoplasty, *J. Bone Joint Surg.*, 54B: 484, 1972.
78. MacEwen, G. D., and Cowell, H. R.: Familial incidence of idiopathic scoliosis and its implications in patient treatment, *J. Bone Joint Surg.*, 52A: 405, 1970.
79. MacEwen, G. D., and Kirsch, P.: The structural response of the idiopathic curve to the Milwaukee brace, *J. Bone Joint Surg.*, 53A: 196, 1971.
80. MacEwen, G. D., Winter, R. B., and Hardy, J. H.: Evaluation of kidney anomalies in congenital scoliosis, *J. Bone Joint Surg.*, 54A: 1451, 1972.

81. Mankin, H. J., and Scheck, J.: Cardiopulmonary function in mild and moderate idiopathic scoliosis, *J. Bone Joint Surg.*, 46: 53, 1964.
82. Mathews, R. S., and Stelling, F. H.: Second look spinal exploration for scoliosis, *J. Bone Joint Surg.*, 52A: 409, 1970.
83. McCarroll, H. R.: Attempted treatment of scoliosis by unilateral vertebral epiphyseal arrest, *J. Bone Joint Surg.*, 43A: 965, 1960.
84. McKenzie, K. G., and Dewar, F. P.: Scoliosis with paraplegia, *J. Bone Joint Surg.*, 31: 162, 1919.
85. Moe, J. H.: The management of idiopathic scoliosis, *Clin. Orthop.*, 9: 169, 1957.
86. Moe, J. H.: Management of paralytic scoliosis, *South. Med. J.*, 50: 67, 1957.
87. Moe, J. H.: A critical analysis of methods of fusion for scoliosis on evaluation in 266 patients, *J. Bone Joint Surg.*, 40A: 529, 1958.
88. Moe, J. H.: Changing concepts of the scoliosis problem, *J. Bone Joint Surg.*, 43A: 471, 1961.
89. Moe, J. H.: Presidential address, *J. Bone Joint Surg.*, 54A: 1789, 1972.
90. Moe, J. H., and Gustilo, R. B.: Treatment of scoliosis; results of 196 patients treated by cast correction and fusion, *J. Bone Joint Surg.*, 46: 293, 1964.
91. Moe, J. H., and Kettleson, D. N.: Idiopathic scoliosis; analysis of curve patterns and the preliminary results of Milwaukee brace treatment in 169 patients, *J. Bone Joint Surg.*, 52A: 1509, 1970.
92. Nachemson, A.: A long-term follow-up study of nontreated scoliosis, *J. Bone Joint Surg.*, 51A: 203, 1969.
93. Nachemson, A., Bake, B., Bjure, J., Grimby, G., Kaslichy, J., and Lindh, M.: Clinical follow-up and regional lung function studies in patients with non-treated idiopathic scoliosis, *J. Bone Joint Surg.*, 52A: 401, 1970.
94. Nachemson, A., and Elfstrom, G.: A force-indicating distractor for the Harrington rod procedure, *J. Bone Joint Surg.*, 51A: 1660, 1969.
95. Nachemson, A., and Elfstrom, G.: Intravital wireless telemetry of axial forces in Harrington distraction rods, *J. Bone Joint Surg.*, 53A: 194, 1971.
96. Nash, C. L., Jr., Brodky, J. S., and Croft, T. J.: A model for electrical monitoring of spinal cord function in scoliosis patients undergoing correction, *J. Bone Joint Surg.*, 54A: 197, 1972.
97. Nash, C. L., Jr., and Moe, J. H.: A study of vertebral rotation, *J. Bone Joint Surg.*, 51A: 223, 1969.
98. Nastasi, A. J., LeVine, D. B., and Veliskakis, K. P.: Pain patterns associated with adolescent idiopathic scoliosis, *J. Bone Joint Surg.*, 54A: 199, 1972.
99. O'Brien, J. B.: Halo-pelvic traction in the correction of spinal deformities, *J. Bone Joint Surg.*, 52B: 801, 1970.
100. O'Brien, J. P., and Yau, A. C. M. C.: Anterior and posterior correction and fusion for paralytic scoliosis, *Clin. Orthop.*, 86: 151, 1972.
101. O'Brien, J. P., Yau, A. C. M. C., Smith, T. K., and Hodgson, A. R.: Halo-pelvic traction, *J. Bone Joint Surg.*, 53B: 217, 1971.
102. Perry, J., Bonnett, C., and Ulin, R.: Halo-femoral traction as a method of preoperative correction of paralytic scoliosis, *J. Bone Joint Surg.*, 51A: 402, 1970.
103. Ponseti, J., and Friedman, B.: Prognosis in idiopathic scoliosis, *J. Bone Joint Surg.*, 32A: 381, 1950.
104. Puranik, S. R., Keiser, R. P., and Gilbert, M. G.:

Arteriomesenteric duodenal compression in children, *Am. J. Surg., 124:* 334, 1972.

105. Raycroft, J. F., and Curtis, B. H.: Spinal curvature in myelomeningocele; natural history and etiology, In *Symposium on Myelomeningocele,* pp. 182–201; St. Louis: C. V. Mosby, 1972.

106. Riseborough, E. J., and Shannon, D.: The effects of scoliosis on pulmonary function as determined by studies with xenon-133, *J. Bone Joint Surg., 52A:* 400, 1970.

107. Risser, J. C.: Scoliosis treated by fusion, preliminary report on some observations in 348 cases, *Am. J. Surg., 4:* 496, 1928.

108. Risser, J. C.: Scoliosis; prognosis, *J. Bone Joint Surg., 18:* 607, 1936.

109. Risser, J. C.: Important practical facts in treatment of scoliosis, *Instruct. Lect. Am. Acad. Orthop. Surg., 5:* 1948.

110. Risser, J. C.: Scoliosis, *Instruct. Lect. Am. Acad. Orthop. Surg., 14:* 91, 1957.

111. Risser, J. C.: The iliac apophyses; an invaluable sign in the management of scoliosis, *Clin. Orthop., 11:* 111, 1958.

112. Risser, J. C., and Norquist, D. M.: A follow-up study of the treatment of scoliosis, *J. Bone Joint Surg., 40A:* 555, 1958.

113. Salerno, N. R., and Edeiken, J.: Vertebral scalloping in neurofibromatosis, *Radiology, 97:* 509, 1970.

114. Shannon, D. C., Riseborough, E. J., Laercio, M. V., and Kazemi, H.: The distribution of abnormal lung function in kyphoscoliosis, *J. Bone Joint Surg., 52A:* 131, 1970.

115. Silver, R. A., Nickel, V. L., Perry, J., and Bonnett, C.: The evaluation of pulmonary function in patients with scoliosis, *J. Bone Joint Surg., 52A:* 400, 1970.

116. Simmons, E. H., and Garside, H.: Biochemical and clinical study of anterior spinal instrumentation, *J. Bone Joint Surg., 52A:* 407, 1970.

117. Smith, A., Butte, F. L., and Ferguson, A. B.: Treatment of scoliosis by wedging jacket and spine fusion, *J. Bone Joint Surg., 20:* 825, 1938.

118. Sriram, K., and Bobechko, W. P.: Surgical management of spinal deformities in myelomeningocele, In *Proceedings, Scoliosis Research Society,* 1970.

119. Sriram, K., Bobechko, W. P., and Hall, J. E.: Surgical management of spinal deformities in spina bifida, *J. Bone Joint Surg., 54B:* 666, 1972.

120. Stauffer, E. S., and Mankin, H. J.: Scoliosis after thoracoplasty; a study of 30 patients, *J. Bone Joint Surg., 48:* 339, 1966.

121. Tambornino, J. M., Armbrust, E. N., and Moe, J.

H.: Harrington instrumentation in correction of scoliosis; a comparison with cast correction, *J. Bone Joint Surg., 46:* 313, 1964.

122. Urbaniak, J. R., and Stelling, F. H.: Progression of the scoliotic curve after completion of the excursion of the iliac epiphyses; a preliminary report, *J. Bone Joint Surg., 51A:* 205, 1969.

123. Vanderpool, D. W., James, J. I. P., and Wynne-Davis, R.: Scoliosis in the elderly, *J. Bone Joint Surg., 51A:* 446, 1969.

124. Van Lockum, W. H.: The surgical treatment of scoliosis, *Instruct. Lect. Am. Acad. Orthop. Surg., 5:* 1948.

125. Van Lockum, W. H.: Surgical scoliosis, *Surg. Clin. North Am.,* 1951.

126. Westgate, H. D., and Johnson, B. E.: Effects of scoliosis therapy on pulmonary function, *J. Bone Joint Surg., 52A:* 400, 1970.

127. Westgate, H. D., and Johnson, B. E.: Preoperative pulmonary evaluation and postoperative respiratory management of patients with severe thoracic scoliosis, *J. Bone Joint Surg., 53A:* 195, 1971.

128. Westgate, H. D., and Moe, J. H.: Pulmonary function in kyphoscoliosis before and after correction by the Harrington instrumentation method, *J. Bone Joint Surg., 51A:* 935, 1969.

129. Wilson, P. D., Jr., Veliskakis, K., and LeVine, D. B.: Neurofibromatosis and scoliosis; significance of the short, angular spinal curve, *J. Bone Joint Surg., 51A:* 203, 1969.

130. Winter, R. B., and Moe, J. H.: Scoliosis and the Marfan syndrome, *J. Bone Joint Surg., 51A:* 204, 1969.

131. Winter, R. B., Moe, J. H., and Eilus, V. R.: Congenital scoliosis; a study of 234 patients treated and untreated, *J. Bone Joint Surg., 50A:* 1, 1968.

132. Winter, R. B., Moe, J. H., and Leonard, A.: The anterior approach for deformities and diseases of the spine, *J. Bone Joint Surg., 52A:* 406, 1970.

133. Wynne-Davies, R.: *Heritable Disorders in Orthopaedic Practice,* pp. 166–171; London: Blackwell Scientific Publications, 1973.

134. Yau, A., O'Brien, J. P., Smith, T., and Hodgson, A. R.: The treatment of scoliosis in Hong Kong, *J. Bone Joint Surg., 53A:* 200, 1971.

135. Young, L. W., Oestreich, A. E., and Goldstein, L. A.: Roentgenology in scoliosis; contribution to evaluation and management, *Am. J. Roentgenol., 108:* 778, 1970.

136. Zaousses, A. L., and James, J. I.: The iliac apophyses and the evaluation of curves in scoliosis, *J. Bone Joint Surg., 40B:* 442, 1958.

Index

Acetabular angle, hip, 299
Acetabular index, 293
Acetabuloplasty hip dislocation, 330, 334
Acetabulum
  deformity of posterior rim, 56
  osteotomy, 328
    Legg-Perthes disease, 384
Achilles tendon, lengthening, cerebral palsy, 688
Achilles tendonitis, 239
Achondrogenesis, 439
Achondroplastic dwarfism, 126, 419
Adducted femurs, 508
  physical examination, 509
  treatment, 509
Adductor, lengthening, cerebral palsy, 686
Adolescent posture, treatment, 805
Affections
  diaphyseal, 140
  epiphyseal, 115
  metaphyseal, 124
Agenesis, 733
Akins procedure, bunions, 225
Amputation
  acquired, 28
  childhood, 27, 28
  congenital
    surgical conversion, 42
    upper extremity, 730
  exercise program, 29
  follow-up, 40
  forequarter, 33
  gait training, 38
  juvenile, 27
  limb prescription, 31, 33
  principles of care, 29
  prosthetic fitting, 31
  revision of, 46
  skin care, 30
  stump, 44, 45
    absent tibia, 406
    care, 29
    end bearing, 405
    os calcis, 44
    revision of, 46
  surgical principles of, 28
  treatment, 407
  use of heel, 45, 160
Amstutz osteotomy, coxa vara, 346
Anderson technique, lengthening, 101, 102
Aneurysmal bone cyst, 523
  pathology, 524
  roentgen appearance, 524
  treatment, 524
Ankle, epiphyseal center, 62
Annular grooves
  upper extremity, 730
  treatment, 732
Anterior tibialis   flat feet, 176
Anteversion
  hip, 298

in-toeing, 163
  osteotomy, 324
Antibiotics
  infections of bone and joint, 592
  septic arthritis treatment, 570
Arachnodactyly, 140
  system involvement, 144
Arteriovenous fistula, 396
Arthritis
  gonococcal, see Gonococcal arthritis
  monarticular, see Monarticular arthritis
  pauciarticular, see Pauciarticular arthritis
  preventive treatment, 467
  rheumatoid, see Rheumatoid arthritis
  septic, see Septic arthritis
Arthrocentesis, septic arthritis treatment, 570, 580
Arthrodeses
  hand, 757
  wrist, 752
Arthrogryposis, hip dislocation and, 323
Arthrogryposis multiplex congenita, 197
  clinical picture, 503
  etiology, 503
  pathology, 503
  roentgen picture, 503
  treatment, 504
Aseptic necrosis
  femoral head, 379
  hip, 360
  reduction and, 322
Astragalus
  flat-topped, 217
  osteotomy of, 219
Atmospheric pressure, joints, 23
Avascular necrosis, hip, 313

Back pain, children, 805
Baker's cysts, 260
Bands, congenital, 407
Benign cortical defect, 514
Bifid distal phalanx, 723
Bivalved cast routine, rheumatoid arthritis, 475
Bleck's classification, 175
Blind children, posture of, 162
Blocker's exostosis, 506
Blood supply
  hip, 57
  proximal femur, 56
Blount's Disease, 137
Bone
  calcified medullary defects, 435
  defective formation of, 419–442
  infections, 567–605
  shortening in spastic child, 689
Bone cyst
  aneurysmal, 523

simple, 522
  treatment, 523
Borden's osteotomy, coxa vara, 345
Bowlegs, apparent, 249
Brace, Milwaukee, 831, 850
Brachial palsy
  birth type, 795
  clinical picture, 801
  etiology, 799
  pathology, 801
  treatment, 802
Brachydactylism, 733
Bracing
  hip, 614
  knee, 614
  lower extremities, 614
  neck, 615
  trunk, 615
  upper extremities, 615
Bradford frame, hip dislocation, 325
Bunions, 222
Burns, hand, treatment, 789
Bursa, semimembranosus, 262

Caffey's disease
  pathology, 151
  treatment, 151
Calcaneonavicular bar, 187, 191
Calcaneovalgus feet, 167
Calve's disease
  clinical picture, 809
  treatment, 810
  x-ray picture, 809
Cartilage canals, 11
Cast syndrome, 824
Cavus feet
  Charcot-Marie-Tooth disease, 624
  clinical appearance, 229
  diagnosis, 231
  etiology, 229
  treatment, 232
C-E angle, hip, 298
Cerebral palsy
  assessment, 669
  care goals, 678
  classification, 666
  definition, 665
  flexor carpi ulnaris transfer, 701
  hand, 745
  intelligence rating in, 676
  neuromaturation, 674
  postural responses, 672
  prevalence, 666
  prognosis, 674
  surgical treatment, 681
  upper extremity in, 700
  wrist flexion deformity, 701
Cervical spine
  rotary subluxations, 564
    clinical picture, 565
    pathology, 565
    treatment, 565
  spina bifida, 549

Chamber's procedure, 175
Charcot-Marie-Tooth disease, 623
Chemotherapy
    hip tuberculosis, 582
    tuberculosis of hip, 582
Chiari osteotomy, hip dislocation,
    333
Childhood
    amputees, 27, 28
    back pain, 805
    blindness, 162
    disability, 1
    flat feet, 167
    heel pain, 236
    pseudoarthroses, 154
    rheumatoid arthritis, 470
    synovectomy, 475
    unequal growth, 81
Chondroblastoma
    pathology, 529
    roentgen appearance, 528
    treatment, 529
Chondrodysplasia, traumatic, 421,
    427
Chondrodystrophia
    calcificans congenita, 118
    fetalis, 419, 423
    multiplex congenita, 424
Chondrodystrophy
    involving spine, 807
    local, 419
    spinal, 807
    spine in, 425
Chondromyxoid fibroma
    pathology, 525
    roentgen appearance, 525
    treatment, 526
Cleft hand, 728
Cleidocranial dysostosis
    clinical picture, 408
    treatment, 408
Clubfoot
    anatomy, 63, 200
    clinical picture, 195
    congenital, 192
    etiology, 192
    external torsion, 216
    follow-up therapy, 206
    inversion, 210
    overcorrected, 212
    posteromedial release, 201
    recurrent, 206, 208
        factors in, 210
    resistant, 65, 197
    serial casting technique, 196
    tendon transplant, 208
    treatment, 196
    triple arthrodesis, 211
    wedging, 200
    x-ray picture, 192
Clubhand, 709
    splint, 713
Cobb's classification, structural
    scoliosis, 860
Codman's tumor, 117, 528
Coleman approach, vertical talus,
    182

Colonna procedure, hip disloca-
    tion, 332
Compression rods, scoliosis, 902
Congenital bands, 407
Congenital dislocation of radial
    head
    clinical picture, 412
    treatment, 412
Congenital kyphosis
    clinical picture, 808
    etiology, 807
    treatment, 809
Congenital orthopaedic conditions,
    395–417
Congenital posterior angulation of
    tibia, 408
Contracture
    hip adduction, 302
    knee flexion, 264
        leg lengthening, 104
Coxa plana
    arthritis development, 377
    metaphyseal involvement, 384
Coxa vara
    clinical picture, 343
    congenital, 340
    congenital short femur and, 401
    course of, 343
    Gaucher's Disease and, 444
    pathology, 343
    progression, 343
    retroversion in, 341
    roentgen findings, 342
    treatment, 344
        early, 344
        late, 344
Crutch gait, 628, 840
Curve measurement
    Cobb method, 856
    Ferguson method, 856
Cyst
    aneurysmal
        clinical picture, 134
        etiology, 134
        pathology, 135
        roentgen picture, 134
        treatment, 135
    bone, 129
        aneurysmal, 523
        clinical picture, 130
        etiology, 130
        pathology, 131
        roentgen findings, 131
        treatment, 131
    differential diagnosis, 134
    lining, 133
    solitary distribution of, 131
    solitary fracture in, 132

Deformity
    acquired, 560
    due to position in utero
        clinical picture, 560
        etiology, 560
        treatment, 560
Dennis-Browne splints, clubfoot,
    197

Dennison, infections of bone and
    joint, 593
Dermatomyositis
    clinical picture, 502
    etiology, 502
    pathology, 502
    treatment, 502
Derotational osteotomy, 166
Desmoplastic fibroma, 526
    pathology, 526
    roentgen appearance, 527
    treatment, 527
Diagnosis, x-ray, 66
Diaphyseal aclasia, 425
Diaphyseal affections, 140
    clinical picture, 144
    etiology, 141
    roentgen picture, 145
    treatment, 145
Diaphyseal dysplasia
    clinical picture, 147
    pathology, 147
    roentgen features, 147
    treatment, 147
Diastrophic dwarfism, 122, 123
    clinical picture, 124
    roentgen features, 124
    treatment, 124
Dilwyn-Evans procedure, clubfoot,
    212
Discoid growth plate, 8, 10, 15
Disc space
    infections
        course, 603
        laboratory findings, 601
        roentgen findings, 603
        treatment, 603
Dorsal spine, wedging of, 827
Dwarfism
    achondroplastic, 419
    diastrophic, 122–124
    polydystrophic, 447
Dwyer calcaneal osteotomy, Char-
    cot-Marie-Tooth   disease,
    626
Dwyer's instrumentation, spinal
    osteotomy, 833
Dysplasia
    diaphyseal, 146
    epiphysialis hemimelica, 115
    familial metaphyseal, 128, 129
    spondyloepiphyseal, 119
Dysplasia epiphysialis hemimelica,
    clinical picture, 115, 116
Dysplastic hip
    roentgen signs, 301
    treatment, 301
Dystrophy
    muscular, 497, 916
        enzymes in, 500
        progressive, 500

Ehlers-Danlos Syndrome
    clinical picture, 397
    treatment, 397
Elbow, development, 47
Ellis-van Crevald Syndrome, 122

treatment, 123
Enlargement of limbs, 396
Eosinophilic granuloma, 529
  clinical picture, 448
  differential diagnosis, 449
  pathology, 448
  roentgen findings, 448
  treatment, 450, 531
Epiphyseal affections, 115
Epiphyseal center
  ankle, 62
  foot, 62
Epiphyseal chondroblastoma
  clinical picture, 117
  Codman's tumor, 117
  pathology, 118
  roentgen picture, 118
  treatment, 118
Epiphyseal dysplasia, 393
Epiphyseal osteochondroma, 115,
  116, 432, 521
  pathology, 116
  treatment, 117
Epiphyseal plate, growth, 81
Epiphyseodesis, 91, 99
Epiphysiodesis, 96
  slipped epiphysis treatment, 350
Epiphysis
  capital femoral, slipped, 346
  circulation, 10–12
    disruption of, 14
  development, 4
  fracture, 87
    effect on growth, 86
  growth, 4, 28
  injury, 87
  osteochondroma, 521
  plate stapling, 99
  slipped capital femoral
    cartilage necrosis, 357
    clinical picture, 348
    etiology, 347
    pathology, 348
    roentgen diagnosis, 347, 348
    treatment, 348
  stipped
    prognosis, 119
    roentgen features, 118
Equinovarus feet, 208
Equinus of forefoot, 230
Ewing's sarcoma
  clinical picture, 541
  course, 543
  differential diagnosis, 543
  laboratory data, 542
  pathology, 542
  symptoms, 541
  treatment, 543
  x-ray examination, 542
Exercise
  progressive resistance, 616
  stretching, 616
Exostosis, 426
  Blocker's, 506

Fairbank's disease, 118

Familial metaphyseal dysplasia,
  128
Familial nuchal rigidity
  clinical picture, 559
  etiology, 559
  treatment, 559
Femoral head
  abduction cast, 375
  aseptic necrosis, 379
  blood supply, 369, 375
  containment of, 392
  excision of lateral aspect, 385
  stress within, 371
Femoral osteotomy
  exposure via medial approach,
    690
  hip dislocation, 338
Femur
  adducted, 508
  Aitken's classification, 402
  anteversion, 300
  growth percentages, 84
  head
    deformity in dislocation, 299
    improperly seated, 295
    lengthening techniques, 103
    medial metaphysis break, 138
    proximal femoral focal defi-
      ciency, 402
    shortening, 100
    two-headed, 294
Ferguson's sign, malignment of hip,
  296
Fibroma
  chondromyxoid, 525
  desmoplastic, 526
  nonosteogenic, 430, 514
  osteogenic, 511
Fibromatosis, congenital central-
  ized, 533
Fibrous dysplasia
  clinical picture, 478
  pathology, 482
  roentgen findings, 480
  treatment, 482
Fibula
  congenital absence of
    clinical picture, 403
    pathology, 404
    treatment, 404
  hypertrophy, 157
Finger, webbing, 718
Fixed foot, treatment, 218
Flat feet
  anterior tibialis effect, 176
  childhood, 167
  disabling, 174
  effect of Achilles tendon, 170
  exercises, 172
  heel cord action, 170
  hypermobile, 169
  neurogenic, 191
  posterior tibialis effect, 176
  spastic, 185
  surgery for, 175
Flexor carpi ulnaris transfer, cerebral palsy, 701

Foot
  congenital anomalies, 239
  disorders, 161–247
  epiphyseal center, 62
  examination, 161, 162
  ligament laxity, 171
  medial and lateral columns, 210
  proprioception, 162
  SACH prosthesis, 31
  subungual exostosis, 241
  support, 174
  unstable, reconstruction of, 617
  vascular disorders, 234
Forefoot varus, correction, 220
Foreign body knee, 263
Four point gait, 628
Fractures
  myelomeningocele patient, 651
  stress type, 437
Freiberg's Disease
  clinical picture, 236
  roentgen findings, 236
  treatment, 236
Functional training, 616

Gage and Winter, congenital hip
  dislocation, 311
Gait
  crutch, 628
  four point, 628
  three point, 628
  toeing in, 162
Galeazzi's sign, hip dislocation, 308
Gargoylism, 438
Gastrocnemius recession, cerebral
  palsy, 694
Gaucher's disease
  coxa vara due to, 444
  treatment, 444
Genu valgum
  developmental, 254
  lengthening, 271
  pronated feet, 251
  surgical correction, 272
  treatment, 251, 271
Giannestras procedure, flat feet,
  177–179
Giant cell tumor
  atypical, 528
  pathology, 532
  roentgen appearance, 531
  treatment, 532
Gigantism, local, 395
Gluteus medius, weakness of, 310
Gonococcal arthritis, 580
Graft
  bypass type, 159
  double onlay, 159
Green procedure, 754
  Sprengel's deformity, 552
Grice arthrodesis, 175
Grice procedure, subastragalar arthrodesis, 619
Growth
  anticipated discrepancy, 94

Growth—*continued*
  contribution
    femoral, 84
    tibial, 84
  curve, 82
  diagramming, 93
  discrepancy, 83
    surgical treatment, 98
  epiphyseal fracture effects, 86
  epiphyseal plate, 81
  epiphysis, 4, 28
  factors affecting, 2
  femoral, 83
  genetic, 82
  graph, 83, 91
  hip, 50, 86
  hormonal, 82
  longitudinal, 81, 82
  lower extremity, 50
  mechanical, 82
  orthopaedic conditions, 3
  percentages, 84
  prediction, 90
    errors, 91, 95
    straight line graph method, 92
  projection, 94
  rate
    age, 2
    male vs. female, 2
  scoliosis, 4
  sitting height vs. leg length, 3
  skeletal, 1
  spine, 86
  stimulation, 101
  surgery effects, 96
  tibial, 83
  unequal, 81
  vascular, 82
  vertebral column, 50
  x-ray measurement, 88
Growth plate
  development, 4, 7
  discoid, 8, 10, 15
  partial closure
    central bridge, 108
    peripheral bridge, 108
    treatment, 108
  proximal femur, 54
  spherical, 8, 10, 14
  variation in, 50
  vertebral, 9

Halo-femoral traction, 832
Hamstring
  lengthening, cerebral palsy, 687
  tightening, 826
Hand
  arthrodeses, 757
  burns, 788
  cerebral palsy, 745
  development, 47
  incomplete development, 733
    treatment, 735
  tendon transplantation, 757
Harness, toddler type, 32
Harris view, 187
Heel

end bearing amputation, 45
operative treatment, 237
pain, 236
stress fractures, 238
Heel cord, lengthening, 505
Hemangiomas, 396
Hemarthrosis, acute, 464
Hemihypertrophy, treatment, 395
Hemophilia
  clinical picture, 459
  diagnosis, 460
  etiology, 459
  history and incidence, 458
  joint hematoma in, 466
  knee flexion contractures, 459
  pathology, 460
  pseudotumor formation in, 460
  treatment, 461
Heyman-Herndon procedure, metatarsus varus, 219
Hilgenreiner line, 299
Hip
  abduction, 292
    roentgen sign in, 321
    weakness of, 308
  acetabular angle, 299
  anatomy, 286
  anteversion, 298
    etiology, 290
  apparent dislocation, 305
  avascular necrosis, 313
  birth fracture, 305
  blood supply, 57
  capsule, constriction of, 324
  C-E angle, 298
  centering, 304
  chemotherapy, 582
  closed reduction, 321
  congenital disease, 285
    breech presentation in, 285
    etiology, 289
    instance of, 285
    lax ligaments in, 285
    teratologic, 285
  degenerative arthritis, 288
  disarticulation, 32
  dislocation
    circulation in, 58
    differential diagnosis, 309
    due to spasticity, 684
    intrauterine, 286
    pathology, 304
    roentgen diagnosis, 286
    treatment age 2–4, 327
    treatment age 4 up, 328
  dysplastic, 301
  embryo development, 291
  flexion contracture, 584
  gluteal weakness, 620
  growth, 51
  joint, normal development, 290
  median adductor approach, 313
  neurogenic dislocation, 335, 338
    femoral osteotomy for, 338
    treatment, 338
  osteotomy of Southwick, 351
  osteotomy to produce varus, 621

pathology, 582
  newborn, 297
  primary anterior congenital dislocation, treatment of, 324
  progression of, 287
  prosthesis, 32
  pyogenic infection, 585
    clinical picture, 586
    roentgen picture, 586
    treatment, 586
  reduction
    aseptic necrosis following, 322
    criteria, 334
    evaluation of, 316
    obstacles, 310
  relation to spine, 299
  retroperitoneal abscess, 585
  roentgen picture, 582
  septic, reconstruction of, 589
  shelf of operation, 337
  subluxated, 302, 313
  synovitis, 357
    clinical features, 358
    differential diagnosis, 359
    etiology, 358
    roentgen findings, 358
    treatment, 360
    x-ray diagnosis, 359
  traction, 336
    internal rotation, 350
  treatment, 582
  tuberculosis
    chemotherapy, 582
    clinical picture, 581
    pathology, 582
    roentgen picture, 582
    treatment, 582
Histiocytosis
  clinical features, 443
  histologic features, 443
  roentgen features, 443
Hoke operation, flat feet, 177, 179
Hourglass constriction, iliopsoas, 60
Humerus, neonatal, 48
Humerus varus, 441
Hunter's syndrome, 446
Hurler's syndrome, 445, 808
  laboratory findings, 446
  roentgen findings, 446
Hypercalcemia, 454
Hyperostosis
  infantile cortical, 148
    clinical picture, 149
    mandible in, 150
    pathology, 151
    roentgen picture, 149
    treatment, 151
Hypertension, leg lengthening, 106
Hypertrophy
  congenital, 731
  fibula, 157

Iliofemoral approach, hip dislocation, 323, 329
Iliopsoas
  action of, 295

capsular defect, 293
hourglass constriction, 60
mechanics of, 291
Immobilization, effects of, 22
Infant, see Neonate
Innominate osteotomy, 108
principles, 331
Intelligence rating, cerebral palsy, 676
Intrauterine packing syndrome, illustration of, 252

Joints
atmospheric pressure effects, 23
infections, 567–605
stability, 22

Kidner operation, flat feet, 177, 178
Kite's method, clubfoot, 196
Klein procedure, slipped epiphysis, 352
Klippel-Feil syndrome
clinical picture, 549
etiology, 549
treatment, 549
Knee
aspiration, 266
congenital dislocation, 269
clinical picture, 269
treatment, 270
flexion, leg lengthening, 104
flexion contracture, 264
foreign body, 263
hemophilia and, 459
hyperextension, 270
deformity, 620
pain, 249
septic arthritis, 265
tuberculosis, 266
clinical picture, 267
etiology, 266
pathology, 266
roentgen findings, 267
treatment, 267
valgus, 250
varus, 249
weight bearing, 253
Köhler's disease
clinical picture, 234
etiology, 234
roentgen findings, 235
treatment, 235
Kyphectomy, 841, 842
Kyphoscoliosis
conservative treatment, 849
nonoperative treatment, 849
Kyphosis
adolescent
clinical picture, 823
etiology, 821
normal spine development in, 822
roentgen picture, 823
treatment, 823
anterior decompression in, 837
classification of, 834

clinical picture, 823
congenital, 834
anterior decompression in, 837
classification, 834
clinical picture, 808
diagnosis, 835
early fusion in, 836
etiology, 807
paraplegia in, 837
treatment, 809
diagnosis, 835
early fusion in, 836
lumbar, 660, 841
paraplegia in, 837
roentgen picture, 823
spine, normal development, 823
treatment, 823

Lapidus procedure, bunion, 227
Larson-Johansson disease, 280
Lasts
exercises, 172
shoe
straight, 172
Leg
length
discrepancy, 96
unequal, 84, 85, 93
lengthening, 96
first phase, 102
second phase, 104
Legg-Perthes disease
acetabular osteotomy
adults, 371
aseptic necrosis, 360
conservative treatment, 374
coxa plana, 360
early signs, 368
onset, 364
osteoarthritis, 377
osteotomy
proximal femur, 385
timing, 373
pathology, 366
prognosis, 365, 372
progression, 365
significance of, 360
synovitis of hip, 360
Lengthening gap, complications, 108
Ligaments
excess laxity, 143
foot, laxity, 171
hip dislocation and, 285
Limbs
congenital deficiencies, 27
enlargement, causes of, 396
prescription, 33
Lipochondrodystrophy, 438
Lordoscoliosis
developmental
conservative treatment, 849
treatment, 843
Lordosis, 627
lumbar, in myelodysplasia, 660
postlumboperitoneal shunt, 920
Lorenz osteotomy, hip dislocation,

337
Lower extremity, growth, 50
Ludloff, hip, 297
Lumbar kyphosis, 660
Lumbar lordosis, 660
Lymphangiosarcoma, 396
Lymphatic aberrations, 396

MacEwen's osteotomy, coxa vara, 345
Maffucci's syndrome, x-ray examination, 493
Malignant change in osteochondroma, 520
Mandible, infantile cortical hyperostosis, 150
Marfan's syndrome, 140
ocular manifestations, 144
Maroteaux-Lamy syndrome, 447
Master knot of Henry, 202
McFarland's bypass graft, 159
Mechan's approach, hip reduction, 318
Medial arch support, 174
Medial release, Bost, 207
Median adductor approach, congenital hip dislocation, 312
Megalodactylism, treatment, 730, 731
Melorheostosis, 430
Menelaus, indications for talectomy, 208
Meningocele, 635
Meniscus
clinical picture, 257
discoid, 256
etiology, 256
normal development of, 256
treatment, 257
Metacarpals, elongation, 142
Metaphysis
affections, 124
bone cyst, 522
chondrodysplasia, 424
Metaphysical circulation, 11
interruption of, 14
Metatarsus atavicus, 222
Metatarsus primus varus
clinical appearance, 222
roentgen appearance, 223
treatment, 223
Metatarsus varus, 213
clinical picture, 214
fixed foot, 218
treatment of, 214
Milroy's disease, 411
clinical picture, 412
treatment, 412
Milwaukee Brace, 831, 850
congenital scoliosis, 831
Mitchell procedure, metatarsus primus varus, 225
Mobile foot, 214
Monarticular arthritis, 472
clinical picture, 262
etiology, 262
laboratory findings, 263

Monarticular arthritis—*continued*
  treatment, 263
Moromeila
  fibular, 43
  tibial, 43
Morquio's syndrome, 124, 447, 808
  achondroplastic dwarfs, 126
  clinical picture, 126
  differential diagnosis, 127
  etiology, 126
  roentgen findings, 126
  treatment, 127
Morton's foot, 222
Moseley technique, lengthening, 102
Motor development, infant, 21
Mucin, 477
Mucopolysaccharidoses, 445
Multiple epiphyseal dysplasia congenita
  clinical picture, 393
  roentgen findings, 393
  treatment, 393
Muscle
  absence of, 559
  affections of, 497–509
  bleeding, 466
Muscular dystrophy, 916
Muscular torticollis, 561
Myelodysplasia
  clinical management, 657
  lumbar kyphosis, 660
  lumbar lordosis, 660
  scoliosis with lordosis, 660
  scoliosis with thoracic kyphosis, 660
  spinal deformities attributable to, 655
  surgical management, 658
Myelomeningocele, 635–663
  embryology, 636
  fractures in, 651
  lower lumbar level, 648
  orthopaedic management of, 640
  sacral level, 650
  spinal deformities due to, 646, 839
  thoracic level, 642
  treatment, 639
Myositis ossificans, 506
  clinical picture, 507
  pathology, 508
  treatment, 508

Nail-patella syndrome, 417
Navicular, excision, 183
Naviculectomy, 184, 185
Nélaton's line, hip dislocation, 309
Neonate
  humerus, 48
  vertebral growth, 9
Neuroblastoma, 544
  treatment, 545
Neurofibroma, 396
Neurofibromatosis
  clinical picture, 629
  nonunion in, 631

orbital defects in, 631
  overgrowth in, 631
  recognition, 630
  sarcoma in, 631
  scoliosis in, 631
  skeletal lesions of, 630
  von Recklinghausen's, 915
Neuromaturation, cerebral palsy, 674
Nonosteogenic fibroma, 430
  pathology, 515
  treatment, 515

Obturator neurectomy, cerebral palsy, 685
Ollier's disease, 426, 430
Opponens transfers, 759
Opposition, thumb, 758
Orthopaedic treatment, childhood disability, 1
Ortolani's sign, congenital hip dislocation, 306, 311
Osgood-Schlatter disease
  clinical picture, 258
  etiology, 258
  roentgen findings, 259
  treatment, 259
Ossification center, proximal tibia, 62
Osteoarthritis, Legg-Perthes disease, 377
Osteochondritis dissecans
  clinical picture, 253
  etiology, 253
  pathology, 252
  roentgen findings, 254
  treatment, 254
Osteochondroma
  clinical picture, 517
  distal femoral epiphysis
    surgery for, 283
    treatment, 281
  epiphyseal, 432, 521
  malignant change in, 520
  polarization of cartilage cap, 519
  produced experimentally, 516
  treatment, 521
Osteochondroses, 234
Osteogenesis imperfecta
  Bauze's classification of, 487
  clinical picture, 488
  collagen deficiency in, 488
  fracture healing, 489
  fragilitas ossium, 490
  mild, 487
  pathology, 489
  rodding, 490
  roentgen findings, 489
  severe, 488
  treatment, 489
Osteogenic sarcoma, 534
  classification, 536
  laboratory data, 536
  osteolytic, 540
  pathology, 536
  physical examination, 535
  sclerosing, 540

symptoms, 535
  treatment, 539
Osteoid osteoma
  clinical picture, 152
  etiology, 152
  pathology, 513
  roentgen examination, 152, 513
  treatment, 152, 513
Osteoma
  delayed, 156
  osteogenic, 511
  osteoid, 151
Osteomyelitis, 589
  antibiotics, 592
  clinical picture, 591
  etiology, 590
  pathology, 593
  roentgen picture, 594
  subperiosteal abscess, 598
  treatment, 597
  x-ray picture, 594
Osteo-onychodystrophy, 417
Osteopathia Condensus Disseminata, 139
Osteopathia striata, 491
Osteopetrosis, 483
Osteopoikilosis, 139
Osteotomy
  anteversion, 324
  derotational, 166
  lumbar spine, 848
  proximal femur, 385
  spinal, 832
  varus, 621
Overlapping fifth toes, 241

Pain, congenital indifference to, 632
Paralysis
  radial nerve, 632
  reconstruction, 617
Paraplegia
  congenital kyphosis, 837
  lordosis, 627
  pelvic obliquity, 627
  treatment, 627
Parathyroid hormone, action of, 452
Paraxial hemimelia (tibia), 405
Patella
  apprehension signs, 275
  dislocation, 272
    clinical picture, 274
    etiology, 273
    mechanism, 274
    roentgen findings, 275
    treatment, 275
  elevation, 278
  osteochondritis
    roentgen findings, 281
    treatment, 281
  tendon, swelling, 260
Pauciarticular arthritis, 472
Pectoralis major muscle, absence of, 559
Pelvic obliquity, 627

Pelvic tilt, 85
Peroneal atrophy
 clinical picture, 623
 Dwyer calcaneal osteotomy, 626
 inheritance of, 625
 neurophysiology, 625
 treatment, 625
Peroneal spastic flat foot, 185
 calcaneonavicular coalition, 187
 treatment, 187
Pes valgus, 165
PFFD, 41
Phalanx, developmental valgus, 420
Plantar-flexed talus, 167
Pleonosteosis
 clinical picture, 123
 treatment, 123
Poliomyelitis
 bracing, 614
 chronic, clinical description, 613
 clinical picture, 609
 convalescent stage, 610
  pathology, 610
  treatment, 610
 diagnosis, 608
 history, 607
 onset of, 608
 treatment, 609
Polydactylism, treatment, 726
Polydystrophic dwarfism, 447
Popliteal cysts
 clinical picture, 260
 roentgen findings, 260
 treatment, 261
Positional deformities
 lower extremities, 249
 tibia vara, 249
Posterior capsulotomy, cerebral
 palsy, 687
Posterior tibialis, flat feed, 176
Posteromedial release, clubfoot,
 201
Postirradiation scoliosis, 917
Postlumboperitoneal shunt lordosis, 920
Postpoliomyelitis scoliosis, 907
Post-thoracoplasty scolioses, 916
Postural responses, cerebral palsy,
 672
Posture
 adolescent, treatment, 805
 blind children, 162
 sitting, 165
 television, 165
Prehension, development by age,
 40
Programmed learning, x-ray, 66
Progressive resistance exercise, 616
Prosthesis
 above elbow, 35
 amputations, 31
 below elbow, 35
 harness, 32
 hip disarticulation, 32
 prescription, 31
 SACH foot, 31
 socket-suction type, 32

Syme's, 34
 timing of fitting, 42
Proximal femoral focal deficiency,
 42, 397
 Aitken's classification, 402
 classification, 398
 clinical picture, 398
 coxa vara and, 397
 treatment, 400
Proximal femur
 blood supply, 56
 growth plate, 54
Proximal tibia, ossification center,
 62
Pseudoachondroplasia, 119
Pseudoarthroses
 childhood, 154
 treatment, 155
Pseudohypertrophic muscular dystrophy
 clinical picture, 497
 etiology, 497
 pathology, 499
 serum enzymes in, 499
Pseudoparalysis, septic arthritis
 and, 568
Pyle's disease, 434
Pyogenic infection of hip, 585
 clinical picture, 586
 roentgen picture, 586
 treatment, 587

Quadriceps
 alignment, 274
 lengthening, 271
Quingel cast, 467

Rachischisis, 636
Radial meromelia, 709
Radial nerve, paralysis, 632
Radioulnar synostosis, treatment,
 410
Refractory rickets, 454
 vitamin D in, 452
Renal phosphate-losing rickets, 453
Renal phosphate-retaining rickets,
 453
Resistant rickets, 450
Reticulum cell sarcoma, 547
Retroperitoneal abscess, hip, 585
Retroversion, coxa vara, 341
Rheumatoid arthritis
 age and sex incidence, 471
 contractures due to, 474
 deformity corrections, 474
 juvenile, 470
 mode of onset, 471
 systemic manifestations, 471
 therapy, 476
 upper extremity, 764
  treatment, 765
 without metabolic involvement,
  471
  clinical picture, 472
  treatment, 474
Rickets

phosphate-losing, 453
phosphate-retaining, 453
refractory, vitamin D in, 452
vitamin D resistant, 450
Rocker-bottom foot, 209

SACH prosthesis, 31
Salter's osteotomy, hip dislocation,
 325
Sanfilippo's syndrome, 447
Sarcoma
 Ewing's, 541
 osteogenic, 534
 reticulum cell, 547
Scanogram, 88
Scheie's syndrome, 447
Schmorl's node, 438
Scoliosis
 Cobb method, 856
 compression rods in, 902
 congenital, 827, 842, 913
  Milwaukee Brace, 831
  natural history, 828
  surgical treatment, 831
  treatment plan, 829
 conservative treatment, 849
 curve measurement, 856
 diagnosis, 855
 Ferguson method, 856
 functional, 858
 growth increases, 5
 idiopathic, 862
  adolescent, 873
  history, 869
  physical findings, 869
  x-ray findings, 870
 lordosis, 660
 postirradiation, 917
 postpoliomyelitis, 907
 post-thoracoplasty, 916
 structural, 859
  Cobb's classification, 860
 thoracic kyphosis, 660
Scurvy, 456
 subperiosteal hemorrhage in, 457
Semimembranosus bursa, 262
Septic arthritis, 567
 clinical picture, 567
 diagnosis, analysis of synovial
  fluid, 569
 etiology, 567
 knee
  etiology, 265
  joint fluid findings, 265
  treatment, 265
 pathology, 568
 pseudoparalysis and, 568
 remission, 580
 treatment
  antibiotic therapy, 569, 570
  arthrocentesis, 570, 580
  x-ray appearance, 568
Septic hip, reconstruction, 589
Sesamiodoma, 427
Shenton's line, hip dislocation, 307
Shoe lasts, 172

Shoes
  high, 168
  toddler, 168
Shoulder, development, 47
Silver procedure, bunions, 224
Sitting posture, 165
Skeleton, growth, 1
Slipped capital femoral epiphysys, 346
Soft tissue, bleeding, 466
Southwick biplane osteotomy
  slipped epiphysis, 351
  postoperative treatment, 354
Spastic hip, dislocation, 684
Spasticity, bone shortening for, 689
Spherical growth plate, 8, 10, 15
Spina bifida, 635
  clinical picture, 549
  etiology, 549
  treatment, 549
Spinal dysraphism, 635
Spine, 805–925
  chondrodystrophy and, 425
  congenital deformities, 828
    embryology, 825
  curvature secondary to adduction contracture of hip, 300
  deformities
    cerebral palsy and, 693
    classification, 861
    myelodysplasia, 655
    myelomeningocele, 646
  development, 822
  dorsal, wedging effects, 827
  orthotic devices, cerebral palsy, 695
  osteotomy, 832
  primary curvature, 300
  relation to hip, 300
  strut grafting, 839
  tuberculosis, 814, 819
    clinical picture, 816
    etiology, 815
    fusion for, 820
    laboratory findings, 816
    paraplegia in, 819
    pathology, 815
    roentgen findings, 817
    treatment, 817
Split Russell traction, bone and joint infections, 591
Spondyloepiphyseal displasia
  clinical picture, 119
  roentgen picture, 119
  treatment, 120
Spondylolisthesis
  clinical picture, 810
  etiology, 810
  roentgen findings, 812
  treatment, 812, 813
Sprengel's deformity, 550
  clinical picture, 551
  etiology, 551
  Green procedure, 552
  treatment, 551
  Woodward's procedure, 553
Stapling procedure, epiphyseal

plate, 99
Steel wedge, flat feet, 174
Stenosis, thumb tendon, 716
Sternocleidomastoid muscle
  clinical picture, 563
  embryology, 561
  etiology, 562
  pathology, 563
  treatment, 564
Streeter's dysplasia, 732
Strut grafting, spinal, 839
Stump, 29
  os calcis, 44
  revision, 46
  skin care, 30
  using heel, 45
Subastragalar arthrodesis, Grice procedure, 619
Subluxated hip, treatment, 303
Subluxation, progression, 313
Subperiosteal abscess, osteomyelitis, 598
Subperiosteal hemorrhage, scurvy, 457
Supernumerary digits, 242
Surgery
  bone shortening, 100
  growth discrepancy, 98
  growth effects, 96
  lengthening procedures, 101
  timing of, 97
Syme's prosthesis, 34
Syndactylism, treatment, 718
Synostosis, excision of, 190
Synovectomy, rheumatoid arthritis, 475
Synovial fluid
  analysis, 569
  characteristics of, 23
Synovitis, chronic, preventive treatment, 467

Talectomy, 208, 209
Talipes Equinovarus, 192
Talocalcaneal bridge, 187
Tarsal anomalies, multiple, 242
Tarsal coalitions, treatment, 187
Telescoping V osteotomy, coxa vara, 346
Television posture, 165
Teloroentgenogram, 88
Tendon
  grafts, 783
  lacerations, hands and fingers, 779
  transplantation
    clubfoot, 208
    hand, 757
Tenodesis, finger function, 763
Teratologic dislocation, hip, 285
Three point gait, 628
Thumb
  absence of, 737
  flexion and adduction deformity, 715
  opposition, reconstruction of, 758

web, widening of, 744
Thumb-clutched hand, treatment, 715
Tibia
  absent
    amputation for, 406
    complete, 403
    treatment, 405
  anterior angulation, 158, 404
  anterior transplant, 208
  growth percentages, 84
  lengthening
    ankle stability in, 104
    hypertension, 106
    technique of, 104
  medial metaphysis break, 138
  posterior angulation of, treatment, 409
  posterior transplant, 202
  shortening, 100
  torsion, internal, in-toeing, 163, 164
  varus deformity
    Blount's disease, 137
    clinical picture, 136
    growth stress, 137
    positional, 249
    prognosis, 137
    rickets, 137
    roentgen findings, 136
    treatment, 137
Tibia tubercle, 258
Tissue, see specific type of tissue
Toe-in gait, 162
  treatment, 163
Torticollis, muscular, 561
Traction, split Russell, 591
Trigger thumb
  clinical picture, 716
  pathology, 716
  treatment, 716
Triphalangeal thumb, 745
Triple arthrodesis
  clubfoot, 211
  wedge resection, 235
Tumors
  benign, 511–534
  Codman, 528
  giant cell, atypical, 528
  malignant, 534–548
Turco procedure, clubfoot, 211
Two-headed femur, 294

Ulna, absence of, 416
Ulnar-deficient extremity, 416
Upper extremity, 709–804
  development, 47
  muscular defects, 711
  rheumatoid arthritis, 764
Uterine packing syndrome
  clinical findings, 249
  roentgen appearance, 249
  treatment, 250

Varus deformity, tibia, 136
Varus osteotomy, cerebral palsy,